PRINCIPLES OF DRUG ACTION
The Basis of Pharmacology

THIRD EDITION

Edited by

William B. Pratt, M.D.

Professor
Department of Pharmacology
University of Michigan Medical School
Ann Arbor, Michigan

Palmer Taylor, Ph.D.

Professor
Department of Pharmacology
University of California, San Diego,
School of Medicine
La Jolla, California

Churchill Livingstone
New York, Edinburgh, London, Melbourne, Tokyo

Library of Congress Cataloging-in-Publication Data

Principles of drug action : the basis of pharmacology. — 3rd ed. /
[edited by] William B. Pratt, Palmer Taylor.
    p.   cm.
    Rev. ed. of Principles of drug action / Avram Goldstein, Lewis
Aronow, Sumner M. Kalman, 2nd ed. [1973, c1974].
    Includes bibliographical references.
    ISBN 0-443-08676-1
    1. Pharmacology. 2. Drugs—Physiological effect. I. Pratt,
William B., date. II. Taylor, Palmer. III. Goldstein, Avram.
Principles of drug action.
    [DNLM: 1. Pharmacology. QV 38 P957]
RM300.P73 1990
615′.7—dc20
DNLM/DLC   90-1630
for Library of Congress   CIP

Third Edition © **Churchill Livingstone Inc.** **1990**
Second Edition © Churchill Livingstone Inc. 1974
First Edition © Harper & Row, Publishers, Inc. 1968

Distributed in the United Kingdom by Churchill Livingstone, Robert Stevenson
House, 1–3 Baxter's Place, Leith Walk, Edinburgh EH1 3AF, and by associated
companies, branches, and representatives throughout the world.

Accurate indications, adverse reactions, and dosage schedules for drugs are provided
in this book, but it is possible that they may change. The reader is urged to review
the package information data of the manufacturers of the medications mentioned.

The Publishers have made every effort to trace the copyright holders for borrowed
material. If they have inadvertently overlooked any, they will be pleased to make
the necessary arrangements at the first opportunity.

Acquisitions Editor: *Robert A. Hurley*
Copy Editor: *Elizabeth Bowman*
Production Designer: *Patricia McFadden*
Production Supervisor: *Christina Hippeli*

Printed in the United States of America

First published in 1990   7 6 5 4 3 2

PRINCIPLES OF
DRUG ACTION
The Basis of Pharmacology

THIRD EDITION

To Avram Goldstein,
who developed many of the principles
of drug action presented herein

Contributors

Alvito P. Alvares, Ph.D.
Professor, Department of Pharmacology, Uniformed Services University of the Health Sciences, F. Edward Hébert School of Medicine, Bethesda, Maryland

Brian M. Cox, Ph.D.
Professor, Department of Pharmacology, Uniformed Services University of the Health Sciences, F. Edward Hébert School of Medicine, Bethesda, Maryland

Paul A. Insel, M.D.
Professor, Departments of Pharmacology and Medicine, University of California, San Diego, School of Medicine, La Jolla, California

Eric F. Johnson, Ph.D.
Associate Member, Division of Biochemistry, Research Institute of Scripps Clinic, La Jolla, California

Daniel W. Nebert, M.S., M.D.
Chief, Laboratory of Developmental Pharmacology, National Institute of Child Health and Human Development, National Institutes of Health, Bethesda, Maryland

Richard R. Neubig, M.D., Ph.D.
Associate Professor, Departments of Pharmacology and Internal Medicine, University of Michigan Medical School, Ann Arbor, Michigan

William B. Pratt, M.D.
Professor, Department of Pharmacology, University of Michigan Medical School, Ann Arbor, Michigan

Raymond W. Ruddon, M.D., Ph.D.
Professor, Department of Pharmacology, University of Michigan Medical School, Ann Arbor, Michigan

Palmer Taylor, Ph.D.
Professor, Department of Pharmacology, University of California, San Diego, School of Medicine, La Jolla, California

Robert H. Tukey, Ph.D.
Assistant Professor, Departments of Pharmacology and Medicine, University of California, San Diego, School of Medicine, La Jolla, California

Wendell W. Weber, M.D., Ph.D.
Professor, Department of Pharmacology, University of Michigan Medical School, Ann Arbor, Michigan

Preface

In the 16 years since the publication of the second edition of *Principles of Drug Action*, there have been tremendous advances in understanding drug action. A textbook devoted to basic principles and major research directions within pharmacology is even more essential for the student of the pharmacologic sciences today. Often pharmacologic texts are organized around organ systems, the practice of clinical medicine, or classes of drugs; this approach makes it difficult to identify the chemical and biologic concepts that underlie pharmacology and are essential to understanding this science. We hope this book will serve to define pharmacology as a continually evolving discipline and emphasize its important place within the biomedical sciences.

In undertaking this revision, our aim was to present current concepts of pharmacology in an easily used textbook form. To achieve the goal of comprehensively presenting the basic principles without substantially increasing the length of the text, we deleted the chapters on drug toxicity, drug development, and drug evaluation. In their place, we added new chapters that further elucidate fundamental concepts in pharmacology. This edition begins with two new chapters dealing with chemical and physical bases of pharmacologic specificity and a review of the molecular basis of drug action for the various classes of receptors and other sites of drug action. This section is followed by a chapter on drug absorption, distribution, and elimination and one on the time course of drug action. These two chapters update the only substantial portion of the text that was retained from the previous edition. A chapter on the principles and pathways of drug metabolism is followed by another entirely new chapter reviewing recent advances in defining the structures of the drug-metabolizing enzymes and their regulation. These advances have been spurred on by the new techniques of molecular biology. Other chapters on pharmacogenetics, drug resistance, carcinogenesis, and drug tolerance and physical dependence also reflect the application of new technology to these areas of pharmacology. In all, we estimate that about 70 percent of the material in this edition is new; the remaining 30 percent covers basic concepts that are unlikely to change substantially as our knowledge of drug action expands.

The breadth of modern pharmacology does not allow one pharmacologist to be an expert in all areas of the discipline. To make this edition as authoritative and accurate as previous editions, contributing authors were selected to provide expertise in each subject. To achieve an integrated perspective of the previous editions, we made a concerted effort to edit the chapters to achieve a consistency in scientific content and style. Throughout the text, we have followed the first two editions in illustrating principles with specific examples that do not require any specialized knowledge of pharmacology on the part of the reader. The framework of pharmacology is presented in such a way that scientists in any branch of biology, chemistry, or medicine will find it readable and will be able to understand those factors that determine drug action.

We thank the original authors, Avram Goldstein, Lewis Aronow, and Sumner Kalman, for their support in publishing this third edition. We hope that their high standards of accuracy, scientific sophistication, and writing style have been maintained.

William B. Pratt, M.D.
Palmer Taylor, Ph.D.

Contents

1

Molecular Basis of Pharmacologic Selectivity

Palmer Taylor
Paul A. Insel

THE LIGAND-MACROMOLECULE COMPLEX

The common event in the initiation of pharmacologic responses is the formation of a complex between the ligand, or drug, molecule and its site of action. Since most pharmacologic responses are mediated through *receptors*, recognition of the more mobile drug molecules by the cellular receptor is the critical element determining the specificity of the response. Moreover, these same considerations extend to chemical neurotransmission and to responses to hormones and other mediators within the body. Thus, neurotransmitters, hormones, other extracellular signals, and many intracellular mediators initiate cellular responses by forming complexes with receptors. In an even broader perspective, complex formation is common to many fields of the biologic sciences, and it is only when we consider the subsequent fate of the complex that the individual fields diverge. For example, an enzymologist views complex formation (e.g., formation of the Michaelis complex between enzyme and substrate) as an event leading to a reaction product via a change in the covalent structure of the substrate, while an immunologist looks at the formation of an antigen-antibody complex as an event that initiates sequelae such as antigen ingestion by macrophages or disruption of a cell surface. In classical pharmacology, drug-macromolecule complex formation is linked typically to a contractile, hemodynamic, or secretory event; however, in recent years the capacity to identify intracellular mediators, to monitor complex formation on cell surfaces, and to detect voltage changes in individual cells has enabled investigators to examine events more proximal to complex formation than the physiologic response. An essential goal of pharmacologic research is to identify intermediate steps in the response and to obtain a quantitative understanding of the linkage between drug-receptor complex formation and the ultimate functional response of the cell or organ. Details of such coupling mechanisms will be developed in Chapter 2.

Intrinsic to complex formation is the ability of the macromolecule to recognize ligands of a particular structure, which imparts the necessary specificity for physiologic function as well as for pharmacologic intervention. From the time that drugs could be characterized structurally, modification of structure of the drug and structural correlations with pharmacologic activity (i.e., the study of structure-activity relationships[1-5]) have formed the basis for major research endeavors in synthetic organic chemistry conducted by the pharmaceutical industry and many academic institutions.

The specificity of pharmacologic responses does not reside in ligand recognition alone, since many molecules show a differential capacity for initiating a response upon binding or complex formation. This is the basis for distinguishing among *agonists* (agents that can elicit a maximal response), *partial agonists* (agents that elicit a response that at maximum is less than the maximal response to another agonist on the same receptor) and *antagonists* (agents that occupy the receptor but fail to elicit a response). This differential capacity to transduce responses is attributed either to conformational changes in the receptor or to different states of association of the receptor with active complexes of coupling proteins.

With the above considerations of ligand recognition and signal transduction, we have defined the features that distinguish receptors from other macromolecules in biologic systems. Thus, a formal definition of *receptors* should encompass both their unique recognition properties and their primary function to transduce the binding of ligands into a cellular response.

Definition and Classification of Receptors

A strict definition of receptors connotes that the macromolecule has been designed by nature to confer a response or transduce a signal to a naturally occurring ligand. Thus, a receptor for neurotransmitter or hormone should be distinguished from serum albumin although both types of molecules can influence drug action. As will become evident in subsequent chapters, serum albumin can transport drugs in the circulation to various organs, and it can also sequester drugs, preventing them from gaining access to their site of action. Albumin might then be considered an *acceptor* site for the drug rather than a true receptor.

Pharmacologic Classification of Receptors

Receptors are commonly classified by the mediator to which they respond and hence by their chemical specificity. The mediator may be a hormone, neurotransmitter, drug, growth factor, paracrine, or an intracellular messenger. The name given to a receptor is usually derived from this classification (e.g., cholinergic receptor, insulin receptor). In some cases the endogenous compound to which the receptor responds is not known, and it is therefore classified according to an exogenous agent to which it responds. This has occurred in the case of opiate (morphine) receptors, which are now known to respond to a range of naturally occurring opioid peptides (endorphins, enkephalins, and dynorphins). Thus, this basis for classification requires modifications as additional knowledge is acquired.

The classification based solely on the endogenous agent eliciting response was found long ago to be inadequate to explain the effects of various agonists and antagonists on animals and tissues. In 1914 Sir Henry Dale proposed that acetylcholine exerts two distinct actions, termed *nicotinic* and *muscarinic*, because of the resemblance of acetylcholine's responses to those the plant alkaloids nicotine and muscarine. This necessity for *sub-*

classification of receptors upon which neurotransmitters or hormones act has been found to be the rule rather than the exception. Indeed, both the nicotinic and muscarinic cholinergic receptors have been further subclassified according to their responses to agonists and antagonists, and this has proved useful in designing cholinergic drugs of improved selectivity. Another early example of receptor subclassification is that of division of adrenergic receptors into α and β subtypes, as proposed by Ahlquist in 1948 on the basis of quantitative measurements of potency for a series of natural and synthetic agonists. In general it is most useful to have both selective agonists and antagonists to study the receptor subclasses. Pharmacologic classifications of receptors are critical to structure-activity considerations.

Biochemical or Biophysical Classification of Receptors

Another useful classification of receptors is based on the cellular *responses* elicited. This depends on the tremendous advances in molecular pharmacology since the late 1950s, which have permitted an understanding of receptors and the responses they produce at a biochemical and biophysical level. Many different types of responses can be studied for a single receptor, ranging from biochemical responses, such as changes in cyclic AMP concentrations or glucose production, to electrical or mechanical responses, such as membrane depolarization and muscle contraction. The understanding of receptor mechanisms at a molecular level requires a knowledge of the initial stimulus that the receptor produces in the cell or tissue.

Molecular or Structural Classification of Receptors

Such a classification is inherent to the primary amino acid sequence of the receptor, which may now be deduced from the sequence of the gene encoding the protein. Ultimately, one would hope for a convergence in the classification of receptors such that a receptor of known sequence could be expressed in a cell previously deficient in that or related receptors but possessing the necessary cellular machinery to confer a response. The ensuing cellular, biochemical, or biophysical responses and the chemical specificity of the receptor to a sufficient number of discriminating ligands could then be correlated with structure. Hence, each receptor could be defined on the basis of these three parameters for classification.

Other Classifications of Receptors

Receptors may also be classified by their anatomic location. Often nature's design has been convenient for this taxonomy since different tissues will express a predominant receptor subtype. Smooth (involuntary) muscle typically contracts in response to acetylcholine, and this is mediated by muscarinic receptors, while skeletal muscle in the voluntary motor system contracts in response to acetylcholine by activation of nicotinic receptors. Neurotransmission in the efferent or outward direction in the autonomic nervous system proceeds through a ganglion containing a synapse. Chemical neurotransmission occurs between preganglionic and postganglionic fibers. The primary transmitter is acetylcholine, and the initial electrical event (depolarization) is elicited through nicotinic receptors. These nicotinic receptors differ in chemical specificity and primary structure from the nicotinic receptors in skeletal muscle. Because of this they have been termed N_1 and N_2 or N_N and N_M (for neuronal and muscle, respectively). Efferent neurotransmission in the voluntary motor nervous system, in contrast to the autonomic nervous system, involves no ganglion.

Receptors also might be classified as *extracellular* or *intracellular*. Since polar molecules such as biogenic amines, amino acids, peptides, and proteins cannot rapidly transverse membranes, receptors for such molecules reside on cell surfaces. A major task for cells is the transduction of signals across cell membranes. Typically, extracellular receptors contain only a portion of their structure on the extracellular surface and contain domain(s) integral to the membrane or the cytoplasmic surface. This facilitates signaling across the cell membrane either through opening of an ion channel or through a change in conformation. Intracellular receptors are typically found for substances that are sufficiently nonpolar to cross the membrane (e.g., steroids) or that are generated within the cell itself.

The General Problem of Structure-Activity Relationships

Our considerations of the structure and conformation of drug molecules will attempt to bridge the disciplines of medicinal chemistry and pharmacology. Many of our considerations will require a background knowledge of bonding forces and protein structure, which will not be covered in this chapter. The reader might be referred to one of several texts on protein structure for this information.

Even though manipulation of the structure of the ligand (drug, hormone, or neurotransmitter) has usually proved inadequate for describing the precise mechanism of specificity of drug action, the ligand is usually the only component of the complex that is readily accessible to structural modification. This is beginning to change with the application of recombinant DNA technology to pharmacologic systems, whereby site-specific mutagenesis and the development of chimeric receptor constructs permit defined modifications of receptor structure (cf. Ch. 2). Nevertheless, a comprehensive understanding of pharmacologic selectivity and responses cannot be dissociated from a knowledge of the fundamentals of molecular structure.

Structure-activity relationships might be viewed from four distinct perspectives of study, which depend largely on how well we know the structure of the target site for drug action.

1. *An unidentified target molecule or site*: Studies in this arena must be largely correlative, and the best example is the action of general anesthetics. As developed in this chapter and in Chapter 2, correlations of the chemical structure of a ligand or a physical parameter inherent to it with biologic activity enable one to exclude potential sites of drug action but do not usually allow one to define a unique site. This arises because distinct subcellular loci (e.g., a phospholipid bilayer, a hydrophobic pocket on a protein, and an interface between a membrane lipid and a membrane-associated protein) may have similar physical properties.

2. *A target site that has been identified but whose primary structure (amino acid sequence) is unknown*: Sites of drug action falling in this category include the majority of drug-receptor systems. Studies of structure-activity relationships can be used to infer certain characteristics of the recognition site on the macromolecule. Information about the number of binding sites, the nature of binding forces, steric and size limitations of the recognition site, and requirements for activation can be deduced for these systems. Newer computational and graphic methods aided by computers enable one to estimate binding energies for congeneric series of compounds and to predict conformations of the bound state of the ligand-macromolecule complexes. The rapid advances in recombinant DNA technology should limit the number

of receptors studied at this level since primary structures of various receptors are being rapidly elucidated.

3. *A target site whose primary but not tertiary structure is known*: If the primary structure is known, some information on tertiary structure and location of binding sites can be inferred from sequence homology with proteins of known three-dimensional structure, from site-specific labeling of the recognition site, or from characteristic structural features of particular domains of the molecule. Such considerations further delimit the variables and increase the knowledge base from which structure-activity studies can be pursued. For example, homologous sequences between the guanine nucleotide-binding, or G proteins, involved in signal transduction and the oncogene *ras* and between the G protein-coupled receptors and bacteriorhodopsin provide critical reference points for structural predictions, since crystal structures have been solved for *ras* and bacteriorhodopsin (cf. Ch. 2).

4. *A target site of known tertiary structure*: Only in this case is structural information available at the atomic level. Few examples that relate to the specificity of pharmacologic agents exist to date, but such information greatly increases the power of computational and graphic methods for detailing structure-activity relationships and predicting activities of untested structures. To date, most of our knowledge of structures of macromolecules comes from x-ray crystallography[6]. Although nuclear magnetic resonance (NMR) has the potential for achieving comparable structural resolution[7], at present this technology is restricted to proteins of smaller mass ($\leq$ 10^4 daltons). In Chapter 2 we examine the structure of complexes of selective chemotherapeutic agents with various dihydrofolate reductases. Such three-dimensional structures provide a detailed frame of reference for examining defined protein mutants with different inhibitor selectivity and also for designing inhibitors with enhanced selectivity of action.

Distinguishing Receptor Types and Subtypes Using Structure-Activity Relationships

The delineation of nicotinic and muscarinic subtypes of acetylcholine receptors actually preceded the structural characterization of the two alkaloids (nicotine and muscarine). However, a knowledge of the structure of these alkaloids and many congeners allows one to infer distinctive features of the respective receptors.

Nicotinic agonists have common structural features, shown at the top of Figure 1-1. In addition to a cationic center, there is a group, whose van der Waals radius is 5.9 Å distant, that can act as an acceptor for a hydrogen bond. In acetylcholine and some of its congeners this is the carbonyl oxygen, but in nicotine it is the pyridine nitrogen. In the muscarinic series (Fig. 1-1 bottom) the hydrogen bond acceptor is an oxygen atom located 4.4 Å from the center of positive charge. This is the ester oxygen in acetylcholine and the ring oxygen in muscarine. In addition, a methyl group corresponding to the acetyl methyl in acetylcholine or the ring methyl in muscarine strongly reinforces the interaction. These intersite distances suggest that acetylcholine binds to the nicotinic and muscarinic receptors in rather different conformations, and studies with conformationally rigid analogs of acetylcholine that are agonists further support this contention.

The disparate structures of the prototypical cholinergic antagonists *d*-tubocurarine and atropine for the nicotinic and muscarinic subtypes of receptors, respectively, are indicative of even greater diversity in the recognition sites of the respective receptors. It is now

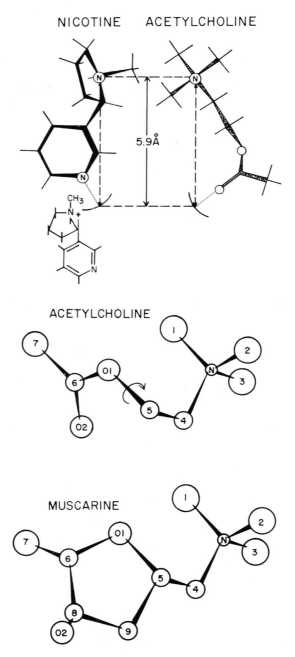

Fig. 1-1. Relationship of the molecular structures of nicotine and muscarine to that of acetylcholine. (Top) 1-Nicotine and corresponding conformation of acetylcholine, with 5.9 Å distance between cationic N and hydrogen bond acceptor group. (Bottom) L(+)-Muscarine and the corresponding conformation of acetylcholine, with 4.4 Å distance between cationic N and H-bond acceptor group 01. Group 7 is CH_3. (From Beers and Reich[8] and Chothia and Pauling[9], with permission.)

known that these receptors have evolved from very different gene families. Their protein sequences and the relationship of the binding site to the membrane surface show a wide divergence. Hence, it is not surprising that both agonist and antagonist specificities for these two receptor types are quite distinct.

A good example of a congeneric series of acetylcholine antagonists is the polymethylenebismethonium family, whose members selectively block the nicotinic class of acetylcholine receptors. The prototypical structure is:

$$H_3C - \overset{\overset{\displaystyle CH_3}{|}}{\underset{\underset{\displaystyle CH_3}{|}}{N}}\overset{+}{} - (CH_2)_n - \overset{\overset{\displaystyle CH_3}{|}}{\underset{\underset{\displaystyle CH_3}{|}}{N}}\overset{+}{} - CH_3$$

Polymethylenebismethonium

These molecules, containing two cationic groups separated by a simple aliphatic chain, can be bisected by two axes of symmetry. The only molecular variable to be considered here is n, the number of carbon atoms in the polymethylene chain, or in other words, the distance between the two positively charged nitrogen atoms.

Two distinct biologic effects of importance are produced by compounds in this series: ganglionic blockade and neuromuscular blockade, which, as considered previously, results from block of nicotinic acetylcholine receptors. We shall examine structure-activity data for both kinds of action in the cat.[10,11] It is instructive to describe representative preparations since many analyses of structure versus activity still derive from intact tissue preparations. A classic pharmacologic assay system for ganglionic blockade employs the nictitating membrane of the eye. This structure is composed largely of smooth muscle at the effector site, innervated by postganglionic sympathetic nerve fibers originating in the superior cervical ganglion (Fig. 1-2). The ganglion cells whose axons carry impulses from the nerve cell body out to the nictitating membrane receive impulses from preganglionic sympathetic nerve fibers, which emerge in the ventral roots of the spinal cord. These preganglionic fibers are cholinergic (i.e., they liberate acetylcholine), and the ganglion cells upon which they impinge are called *cholinoceptive* or *cholinergic* (i.e., they contain acetylcholine receptors). In the assay system the nictitating membrane is attached to a lever or strain gauge for recording its contractions. A continuous train of electrical stimuli is applied to the preganglionic fibers, and the nictitating membrane responds with a sustained contraction. If synaptic transmission from the preganglionic terminals to the ganglion cells is blocked during stimulation, then no impulses will arrive at the nictitating membrane, which will therefore relax. If this happens, a simple way to confirm that the blockade is at the ganglion rather than at a more peripheral site is to stimulate the postganglionic fiber electrically and elicit a normal response of the nictitating membrane. In the assay a drug to be tested is injected intravenously at appropriate dosage to produce a certain degree of blockade (Fig. 1-3). The relative potencies of various drugs may then be expressed in terms of the ratios of the respective doses that produce the same degree of blockade.

An assay system for skeletal neuromuscular blockade employs any convenient muscle (e.g., tibialis anterior) and the appropriate motor nerve (e.g., sciatic). Motor nerves are cholinergic, and skeletal muscle contains specialized cholinoceptive structures (endplates) where the nerve fibers terminate (Fig. 1-2). In the assay the motor nerve is stim-

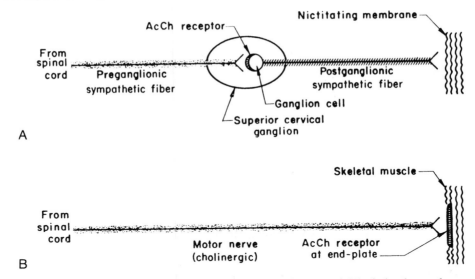

A

B

Fig. 1-2. Innervation of (**A**) the nictitating membrane and (**B**) skeletal muscle.

ulated at regular intervals by single stimuli large enough to elicit maximal contractions from the muscle. These muscle contractions are recorded. A drug-induced blockade of transmission between nerve ending and muscle end-plate manifests itself as a decline in amplitude and ultimate disappearance of the muscle twitches (Fig. 1-4). During such neuromuscular blockade direct electrical stimulation of the muscle fibers will confirm that their intrinsic capacity for contraction is unimpaired (arrow 2 in Fig. 1-4). The procedure for determining relative drug potencies is like that described for the cat nictitating membrane preparation.

Eight different compounds were tested in both assay systems, with the results shown in Figure 1-5. Two distinct optima were found, one at $n = 5$ to 6 (hexamethonium) for ganglionic blockade, another at $n = 10$ (decamethonium) for neuromuscular blockade. It is apparent, therefore, that even though the ganglionic and muscle end-plate nicotinic receptors are both stimulated by local release of acetylcholine from nerve endings, these receptors cannot be identical.

As has been done in the past, data in Figure 1-5 might be used to infer a structure of the ligand binding site. However, the mechanism of action of these polymethylene bismethonium compounds is more complex. First, decamethonium acting on the muscle receptor can stimulate the receptor weakly, but its occupation of the receptor prevents

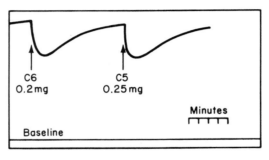

Fig. 1-3. Typical effects of ganglionic blocking agents on the nictitating membrane of the cat. Sustained contraction of nictitating membrane excited by stimulation of cervical preganglionic sympathetic nerve; hexamethonium (C6) and pentamethonium (C5) given intravenously at arrows. (From Paton and Zaimis,[10] with permission.)

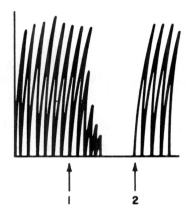

Fig. 1-4. Typical effect of a neuromuscular blocking agent on cat nerve-muscle preparation in situ. Tension recording from tibialis muscle stimulated by nerve shock every 10 seconds: at arrow 1, decamethonium (0.1 mg) injected intravenously; at arrow 2, muscle was stimulated directly. (From Paton and Zaimis,[10] with permission.)

binding of the full agonist acetylcholine. Decamethonium also has a secondary action whereby at higher concentrations it blocks the functional channel in the receptor (cf. Ch. 2). This second action occurs at a distinct site on the receptor, and as it renders the receptor nonfunctional, it is noncompetitive with acetylcholine.[12] The complex action of decamethonium was only delineated with techniques suitable for measuring events occurring at single receptor channels (cf Ch. 2). When the same technology is applied to ganglionic receptors, hexamethonium is found not to be competitive with acetylcholine, as in the primary action of decamethonium on the muscle receptor; rather, it blocks the channel in a noncompetitive fashion.[13] Hence, when taken further, these considerations illustrate that a single assay on intact tissues may not be sufficient for structure-activity analyses if details about receptor recognition sites are to be inferred from such studies.

The qualitative and quantitative properties of receptors in the same tissue of various species may also be compared. The length of the polymethylene chain was varied, and the resulting compounds were tested for neuromuscular blockade in the cat, rabbit, mouse, and rat.[10] Regardless of species, the C_{10} compound was the most potent, which implies that the muscle end-plate receptors in all four animal species have anionic sites at the same separation. The potencies differed, however, over a nearly 1,000-fold range. Recent

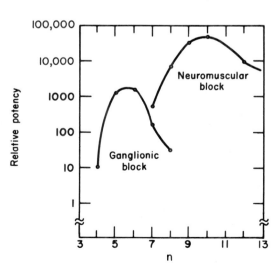

Fig. 1-5. Structure-activity data for ganglionic and neuromuscular block by polymethylenebis-methonium compounds. The number of -CH_2- groups between cationic groups is n: relative potency has a logarithmic scale. (From Paton and Zaimis[10] with permission.)

studies on the molecular structures of these receptors enable us to begin to understand the structural basis of these similarities and differences. Although the ganglionic and neuromuscular receptors are oligomers (both are probably pentamers) of subunits of homologous but not identical sequences, the sequences of the subunits differ. Moreover, the amino acid sequences of the individual subunits in the different animal species are also distinct (cf. Ch. 2).

Correlation of Physical Parameters with Biologic Activity

The correlation of physical parameters of a ligand with its potency in eliciting a response has been a long-standing approach toward understanding the mechanism of drug action and predicting pharmacologic activity on the basis of structure. The second objective has, by far, been the more successful. For example, in their early attempts to predict anesthetic potency on the basis of the partitioning of the anesthetic between olive oil and water, Overton[14] and Meyer demonstrated that the concentration of anesthetic actually found in the olive oil phase was relatively constant when aqueous phase concentrations required to produce general anesthesia were compared. Thus, anesthetic potency could be directly correlated with the oil/water partition coefficient of the anesthetic. This basic approach has been refined through the use of solvents of defined composition and known solubility parameters as well as by consideration of other physical parameters such as molecular volume and thermodynamic activity coefficients (cf. Ch. 2); yet the simple experiments of Overton and Meyer have provided a conceptual framework for understanding the mode of action of one class of drugs.

Substituent Constants

The overall correlative approach of Overton and Meyer has been extended to examine substituent group modification in relation to biologic activity.[15,16] In this approach the potencies of a series of congeneric compounds are correlated with a chemical or physical property. For example, modification of a substituent may change a physical parameter, such as the partition coefficient between immiscible phases, and may alter the electronic structure of the compound itself. In the simplest case, one may find that a physical constant is logarithmically related to biologic activity. As developed later in this chapter, the logarithmic relationship has its origin in the relationship between equilibrium dissociation constants and the free energy of complex formation. Since activity or potency is inversely related to the concentration [C] producing the defined action, then

$$\log 1/[C] = ax + b \qquad \text{(equation 1)}$$

where a and b are constants derived by correlation and x is a substituent constant relating the physical properties of a series of compounds to a standard (usually the unsubstituted compound). Typical substituent constants are:

1. The hydrophobicity constant[15] π_x

$$\pi_x = \log P_x - \log P_H \qquad \text{(equation 2)}$$

   P_x and P_H are the octanol-water or other two-phase solvent partition coefficients for the compound in question (x) and the unsubstituted compound (H), respectively. An increase in π reflects increased hydrophobicity.
2. The Hammett constant[16] σ_x

$$\sigma_x = \log K_x - \log K_H \qquad \text{(equation 3)}$$

This substituent constant was originally defined by the effect of meta, para, and sometimes ortho substituents on the dissociation constant of benzoic acid (K_H). It provides a quantitative expression of the electron-donating and electron-withdrawing properties of the substituents. Both inductive and resonance effects mediated through the aromatic ring will influence the Hammett value.

3. The Taft steric constant E_{sx}

$$E_{sx} = \log K_{XCOOCH_3} - \log K_{CH_3COOCH_3} \qquad \text{(equation 4)}$$

This parameter relates the hydrolysis rate of methyl acetate to those of the substituted carboxymethyl esters. Both steric and inductive effects will influence the Taft constant.

Shown in the quadrants of Figure 1-6 are the hydrophobicity and Hammett constants for a series of substituents substituted para on an aromatic ring.[3] The overall procedure involves the correlation of the individual constants and biologic activity. Correlations need not be restricted to the above substituent constants. Molar volumes, molecular orbital parameters, and polarizability coefficients have also been used in such regression anal-

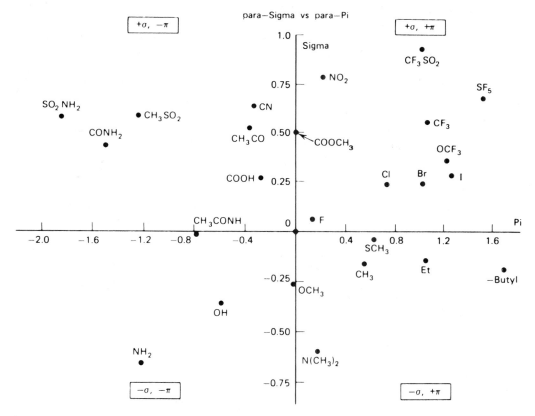

Fig. 1-6. Two-dimensional plot of sigma (σ) Hammett substituent constants versus pi (π) hydrophobicity constants for para substitution on an aromatic ring. The equations for the individual parameters are described in the text. (Reproduced by permission from Wolff[3].)

yses. In other cases combinations of parameters have been employed in the analysis. For example,

$$\log 1/[C] = a\pi + b\sigma + cE_{sx} + d \qquad \text{(equation 5)}$$

where a, b, c, and d are the coefficients determined by curve fitting and the variables are as defined above. If only the data in Figure 1-6 were employed, the best fit of a and b would be determined for the set of hydrophobicity (π) and Hammett (σ) values. Finally, in cases such that increases in the parameter increase activity over a limited range of values, after which activity decreases, higher-order terms may be used to refine the correlations. For example

$$\log 1/[C] = -a\pi^2 + b\pi + c \qquad \text{(equation 6)}$$

If $a < b$, increases in hydrophobicity or lipophilicity will increase activity up to a certain point, after which activity will decrease. For equations 1-1, 1-5, and 1-6, regression analyses are usually made to optimize the fit and determine the coefficients. This correlative approach, which was developed in large part by Hansch and Leo,[15] is often called *quantitative structure-activity relationships* (QSAR). A recent application has been to expand these considerations to three dimensions. The energy contours developed around the surface of the molecule allow visualization of portions of the ligand structure where electrostatic or steric features are dominant.[17,18]

QSAR analyses have a useful predictive value in ranking the order of potencies of a series of close congeners, but they fall short of providing an understanding of actual mechanisms of drug action. Several reasons for this limitation are apparent. First, the physical parameter is usually measured in a homogeneous solvent, and the loci of drug action, such as the active sites of enzymes or the recognition sites of receptors, are not isotropic and usually do not show such spatial uniformity. Second, stabilization of ligand-macromolecule complexes is likely to be a consequence of multipoint attachments, which include distinct orientation factors in the stabilization. Third, both the ligand and receptor may change in conformation as part of the binding process. In fact, the change in conformation of the macromolecular receptor may be the critical parameter for eliciting biologic activity.

Use of QSAR methods considered above to calculate binding affinity is also inadequate for estimating the role of changes in solvation arising upon ligand complex formation. Moreover, the calculations largely relate to binding enthalpies of anticipated stabilization energies for bond formation (i.e., van der Waals forces, hydrogen bonds, electrostatic forces) and are limited in estimating the entropy changes associated with complexation. However, entropic differences in binding between members within a congeneric series of compounds may be relatively small, or in other circumstances they may be roughly proportional to the enthalpy differences. In such cases the energetics of complexation as calculated from the interactions predicted on the basis of ligand structure may correlate closely with experimental values.

Molecular Orbital Theory

By using quantum mechanics to predict the configuration of small molecules, it has proved possible to describe the electronic features of drug molecules and predict the overall conformation of flexible molecules. Summation of all the attractive and repulsive forces between bonds in each potential conformation permits calculation of the minimum energy, corresponding to the preferred conformation.[19–21] Over the years several approaches to the description of molecular orbitals have been employed to give a global estimation of conformation and molecular structure. Molecular orbital calculations have proven valuable for molecules of simpler structure, but the number of uncertainties and permutations increases greatly as the number of flexible bonds increases. As molecular size increases, more approximations must be introduced, or calculations become unwiedly and computer costs exorbitant. Thus, ligand-receptor systems and even more complex ligand structures place severe constraints on computational capacities. Moreover, molecular orbital calculations are often based on considering molecular structure in vacuo, and solution forces may have a dominant effect in determining conformational preferences for flexible molecules.

Computational and Computer Graphic Approaches to Structure Activity Relationships

The computational power of the newer computers allows use of more sophisticated methods to examine molecular complexes.[22–25] Developments in the computation of preferred structures of ligands in solution and in molecular graphics confer an additional dimension on structure-activity considerations. Three-dimensional structures, energy differences between conformations, and binding energies can now be estimated for ligands of increasing complexity. Statistical mechanics evaluates the respective energies of an ensemble of complexes of different conformation, molecular dynamics simulates internal motions of the complex to predict entropy contributions and equilibrium or thermodynamic cycle perturbation techniques modify one point in the structure and examine the change in energy associated with this perturbation. These techniques, like the less intensive approaches, are most valuable when three-dimensional structural information on the complex is available. Without such information one can only assume that the receptor surface is complementary to the ligand and that the complex possesses a nondeforming surface with fixed recognition points positioned in three-dimensional space. Thus, one presents a candidate receptor site with appropriately positioned functional groups and asks whether a series of ligands with known binding energies provides a best fit to the model. Changing the functional groups, their positions in three-dimensional space, and hence the overall atomic pattern of functional groups may result in an improved or a worse fit. Operationally the number of variables is large, and the problem becomes far more manageable as structural information provides reference points.

Optical Enantiomers and Stereoselectivity

One of the limitations in correlating physical parameters with biologic activity is that selectivity of optical enantiomers for receptors would not be predicted by simple correlative techniques. True *enantiomers*, for which chirality is detected as optical asymmetry at a single atom, show no differences in physiochemical properties in the absence of a dissymmetric surface, and thus parameters that predict hydrophobicity or electronic arrangements do not differ between optical isomers. If more than a single center of asymmetry is present in the molecule (a *diastereomer*), then physical properties will differ. This is the basis for derivatization of enantiomers to form diastereomers for optical isomer separation.

Geometric isomers, such as cis-trans configurations around a double bond, chair-boat configurations of ring systems, and epimers of rigid ring system (Fig. 1-7) all lead to

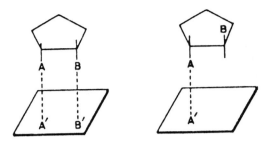

Fig. 1-7. Geometric isomerism. The rectangle represents a receptor surface. (From Beckett,[26] with permission.)

molecules that differ physicochemically and will have distinct properties in the absence of a dissymmetric surface.

Differences in biologic activity that exist between enantiomers have been known for several decades[26-31] and often approach three to four orders of magnitude; differences of such magnitude encroach upon the limits of optical purity. It may therefore be appropriate to consider such compounds as being *stereospecific* rather than simply *stereoselective*. Differences in activity between enantiomers have provided a long-standing argument in support of the existence of receptors. More recently, assessment of enantiomeric potencies has been an important criterion for determining whether the association of agonists and antagonists in vitro reflects binding to a biologic receptor. Because binding of an agonist to the receptor reflects the initial step in drug action and because occupation by competitive antagonists should directly reflect the ability of the antagonist to block the functional response, the resultant functional activity should reflect the ratios of affinities of enantiomeric pairs. Moreover, an appropriate control is presented by enamtiomeric pairs because the chemical properties of each of the enantiomers in the absence of a dissymmetric surface should be identical.

The fundamental principles of enantiomeric selectivity were delineated long before investigators contemplated the isolation of receptors. Easson and Stedman[27] in 1933 suggested that if selectivity of enantiomeric pairs could be seen in a biologic system, then a three-point attachment must occur between the enantiomer and a dissymmetric surface. The concept becomes apparent in considering Figure 1-8. Compounds 1 and 2 are optical

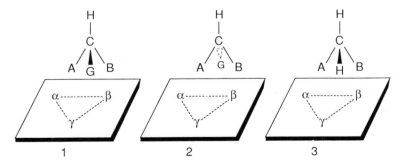

Fig. 1-8. Hypothetical model of two enantiomers (1 and 2) containing a chiral carbon C and a non-optically active congener (3) interacting with a receptor surface. Upon association with the receptor surface, one enantiomer is capable of making a three-point contact with corresponding loci on the receptor (i.e., A-α, B-β, and G-γ), while the other enantiomer and the optically inactive compound contact only two of the loci.

enantiomers with four distinct groups, A, B, G, H, tetrahedrally disposed around the carbon atom, C. Compound 3 does not have enantiomeric pairs. With compound 1 the A-α, B-β, and G-γ interactions can all be achieved, but with compound 2 only two at most of the interactions are possible on the surface (i.e., A-α and B-β). Compound 3 is not optically active because of the identity of two substituents; it also cannot achieve a distinctive three-point interaction.

The active enantiomer has a configuration and chirality complementary to the surface of the binding site. The planar and rigid surface for the receptor depicted in the above examples is an obvious oversimplification. Moreover, as we learn more about protein structure, it has become increasingly evident that conformational changes accompany the binding process. In this circumstance the three-point attachment required for the fit and hence the stereoselectivity may be thought of as being induced selectively by one of the enantiomers in the ligand binding process.

Biologic chirality should be distinguished from optical rotation [dextrorotatory $d(+)$ or levorotatory $l(-)$] or the *R, S* classification of the Cahn-Prelog-Ingold convention.[32] The d,l designation relates to rotation of polarized light, which depends on electronic properties around the chiral atom, while the R,S classification depends on mass assignments around the chiral atom. Usually, but not always, biologic activities of homologous structures correlate with the direction of light rotation or a particular R or S notation (i.e., all the $d(+)$ enantiomers in a series of congeners are more active than the $l(-)$ enantiomers if one compound in the series shows this preference).

Three examples of the Easson-Stedman principle are illustrated below. In the case of norepinephrine directly interacting with α-receptors (Fig.1-9), the R($-$) or *l*-enantiomer is more potent than the desoxy compound dopamine,[31] which in turn is more potent than the S($+$) or *d*-enantiomer. This suggests that the hydroxyl group when oriented in one direction enhances activity, while in the opposite orientation it may reduce activity. By contrast, an examination of stereoselectivity for the indirect actions of these three agents (e.g., their uptake into the nerve ending) shows little enantiomeric preference. Thus, discrete sites with which norepinephrine interacts (e.g., the α-receptor at the postsynaptic effector site and the transport carrier for presynaptic uptake of the neurotransmitter) are likely to differ in enantiomeric preference. Similarly, many β-adrenergic antagonists exhibit local anesthetic action in addition to selective blockade at β-adrenergic receptors, yet within a series of agents the enantiomeric preference for competitive antagonism at the β-adrenergic receptor is high while it is virtually nonexistent for local anesthetic activity.[31]

Marked stereoselectivity is seen in both the cyclic and noncyclic opiates. For the methadone enantiomers, the R compound is analogous to compound 1 in Figure 1-8, while the S isomer is analogous to compound 2. The enhanced potency of compound 1 on the opioid receptor is realized by virtue of the interaction of the three groups around the asymmetric carbon (Fig. 1-10). Loss of one of these interactions is seen in both the *S* enantiomer and the corresponding *nor* compound (6-desmethylmethadone). Presumably, orientation of the methyl group in one direction enhances either the affinity or the efficacy (i.e., the ability to confer a response) of this agonist on the opiate receptor, and its absence decreases either or both parameters. Additionally, orientation of the methyl group in the opposite direction further decreases the interaction or response. Ostensibly this arises because of a steric factor that precludes close apposition of the three contact points.[29] As will be considered later in this chapter, steric factors dictate a particular spatial configuration for methadone, and free rotation around many of the bonds in this structure is not possible.

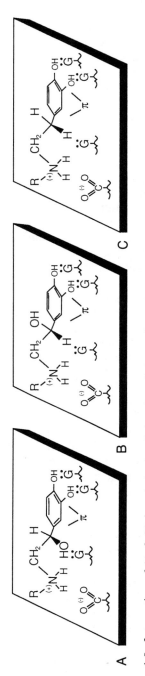

Fig. 1-9. Interaction of (**A & B**) *l*- and *d*-epinephrine, *l*- and *d*-norepinephrine and (**C**) dopamine with an α-adrenergic receptor. For epinephrine R=CH₃, while for norepinephrine and dopamine, R=H. G denotes a hydrogen bond acceptor and π represents π orbital bonding.

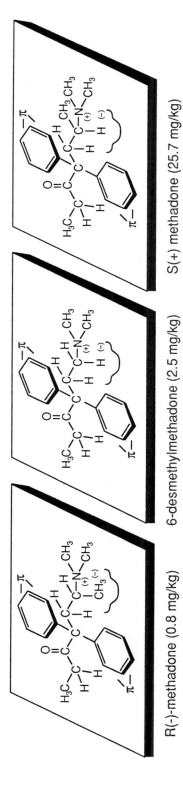

R(-)-methadone (0.8 mg/kg)   6-desmethylmethadone (2.5 mg/kg)   S(+) methadone (25.7 mg/kg)

Fig. 1-10. Interaction of R(−)-methadone, S(+)-methadone, and 6-desmethylmethadone with the mu (μ) opioid receptor. The numbers designate equivalent doses for analgesia when given systemically.

The third example of stereoselectivity shows a marked reduction of stimulation of the muscarinic acetylcholine receptor with one enantiomer of methacholine (β-methylcholine). This behavior can be compared with that of the corresponding enantiomers for related antagonists (Fig. 1-11). pD_2 and pA_2 are the negative logarithms of the concentration yielding half-maximal response for agonists and half-maximal occupation of the receptor for antagonists. A greater pD_2 or pA_2 increases the potency of the agonist or antagonist, respectively. Here we observe that R(−)-methacholine and acetylcholine have virtually identical potencies; this suggests that the trimethylammoniomethyl and the acetoxy groups, which protrude from the optically active carbon, are able to bind in a similar fashion for the two compounds. Presumably the methyl group in the active enantiomer neither enhances nor hinders interaction with the receptor surface, but should it be oriented in the opposite direction, a reduction in capacity to stimulate the receptor is evident. This could well arise from steric factors on the surface of the receptor, which when the methyl group is oriented in one direction, precludes optimal interaction between A and α and B and β in Figure 1-8. In this situation the potencies of compounds 1 and 3 are equal and much higher than that of compound 2.

It is also instructive to compare the enantiomeric preference for agonists and antagonists on a single receptor. Interestingly, the 300-fold preference for R(−)-methacholine is lost when similar substitutions are made on the choline moiety of the benzilylcholine antagonist[33,34] (Fig. 1-11). Benzilylcholine is a competitive antagonist, and we presume that its binding site overlaps that of acetylcholine. Close apposition of the choline portion of the molecule to the receptor surface is presumably required either for the smaller agonist to bind or to elicit a response upon binding. In the case of the antagonist, the fit in the binding site at this end of the molecule may be less critical. Hence, stabilization of the complex occurs primarily for the antagonist through the acyl end (the benzilyl group) of the molecule. Two additional elements of structure-activity relationships buttress these arguments. First, substitution of cyclohexyl group for one of the phenyl groups (Fig. 1-11) yields two enantiomers with a chiral carbon at the substituted glycolic acid moiety. While this results in little overall loss of activity, there is a partial return of enantiomeric preference (to about 25-fold). Accordingly, fit in the acyl region of the molecule is a determinant in antagonist binding affinity.[34]

The substitution of carbon for the quaternary nitrogen in the choline moiety is an isosteric substitution (i.e., the methyl groups remain tetrahedrally disposed around the carbon atom in the 3,3′-dimethyl-l-butanol moiety, as was the case around the nitrogen atom in choline). This substitution renders the agonist virtually inactive (it undergoes a greater than 3,000-fold loss of activity) while only a seven fold loss of activity is seen with uncharged antagonist.[34] Thus, the above structure-activity relationships systematically demonstrate the importance of the hydrophobic acyl portion of the ester in stabilizing the antagonist-receptor complex, whereas the cation in the choline moiety of the ester and its close apposition to the receptor surface appear critical for receptor activation. What cannot be distinguished in these measurements is whether losses of agonist activity are a consequence of diminished binding or of an inability of the bound agonist to activate the receptor.

In addition, stereoselectivity in drug action is not limited to pharmacodynamic action but may be a consequence of the pharmacokinetics of drug disposition or drug metabolism. Both the drug-metabolizing enzymes and specialized transport systems can show stereoselectivity.[35] These points will be developed further in subsequent chapters.

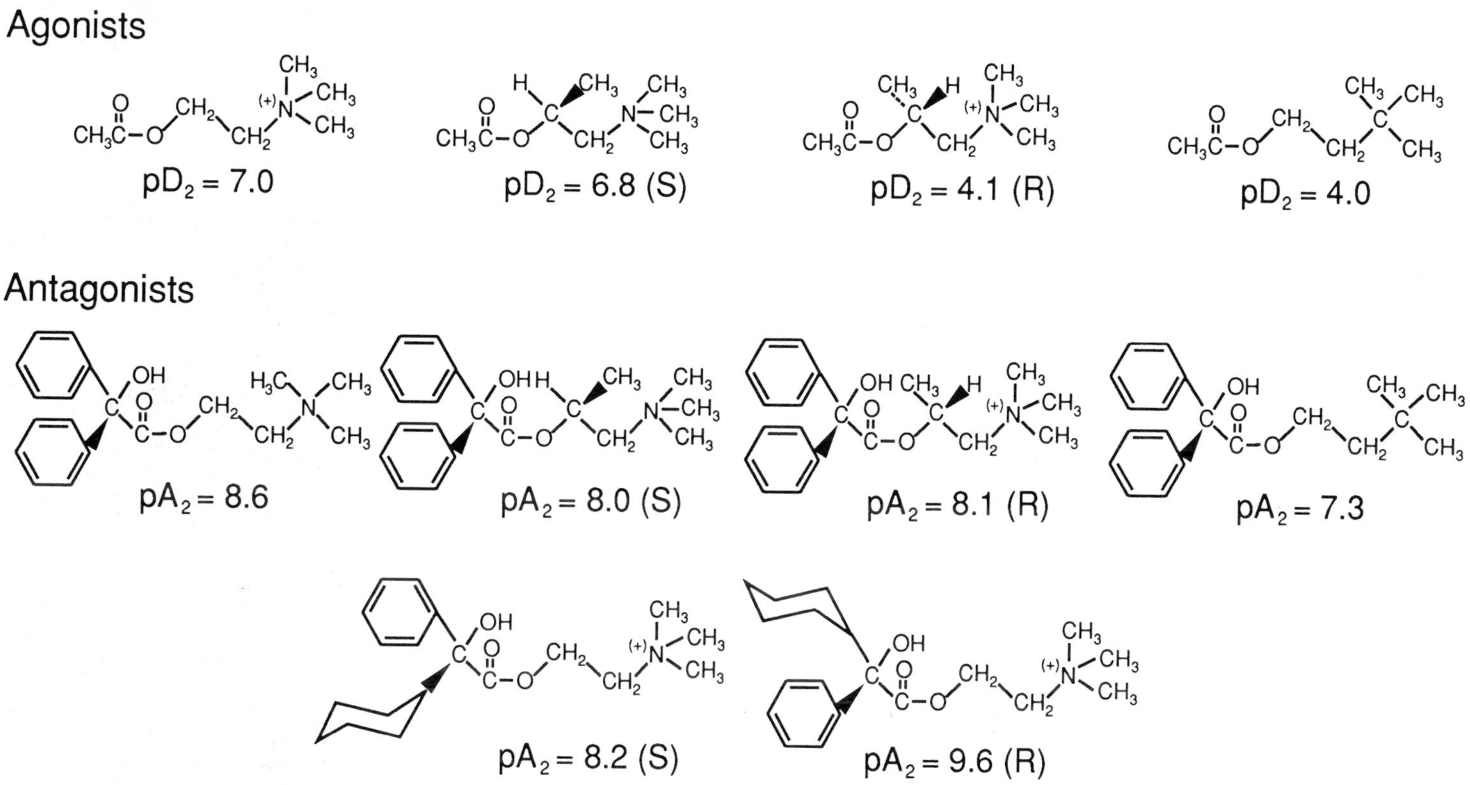

Fig. 1-11. Values pD$_2$ for acetylcholine, R(−)-β-methacholine, S(+)-β-methacholine, and 2,2'-dimethylbutyl acetate when tested as agonists on the muscarinic acetylcholine receptor and pA$_2$ values for benzilylcholine, R-phenylcyclohexylglycolylcholine, and S-phenylcyclohexylglycolylcholine when tested as antagonists on the muscarinic receptor (pD$_2$ and pA$_2$ are the negative logarithms of the concentrations yielding half-maximal responses to the agonists and giving half-maximal occupation by the antagonists, respectively).

Conformation of Flexible Ligands

Ligands that exhibit free rotation around bonds present additional considerations in arriving at the active conformation of flexible drugs with the receptor. This behavior is best illustrated with a simple structure such as acetylcholine:

$$CH_3\overset{\overset{O}{\parallel}}{C} - O \overset{\tau_1}{\rightthreetimes} CH_2 \overset{\tau_2}{\rightthreetimes} CH_2 \overset{\tau_3}{\rightthreetimes} N \overset{CH_3}{\underset{CH_3}{\diagup}} {}^{(+)}$$

where τ_1, τ_2, and τ_3 can be considered as torsion angles and designate the degree of twist around these bonds of free rotation. If we view acetylcholine in the plane of the paper from the left side (from the arrow in the above representation), projections (typically called *Newman* projections) around τ_2 would appear as in Figure 1-12A.

The projections consider only the bond τ_2 between the two methylene groups; τ_1 becomes somewhat less important because the ester oxygen lacks eclipsing hydrogens and the acetoxy group itself tends to be planar. Because of the identity of the methyl groups

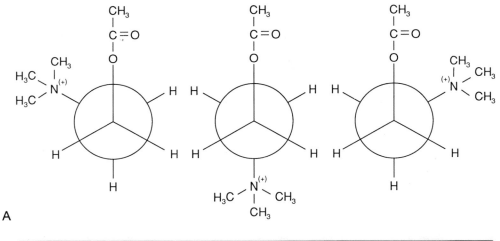

A

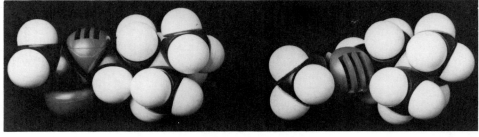

B

Fig. 1-12. **(A)** Newman projections of acetylcholine achieved by rotation around the bond joining the two methylene carbons (see text for details). **(B)** Corey, Pauling, Koltun (CPK) space-filling models for the trans (left) and gauche (right) conformation of acetylcholine.

around the quarternary nitrogens, symmetry minimizes the role of conformation at the τ_3 bond. Thus, the critical torsion angle in acetylcholine conformation is at τ_2. The three Newman projections differ by 120-degree angle rotations around τ_2, since the three torsion angles will maximize the distance between the three groups and as a first approximation correspond to the three lowest-energy forms. Rotation to positions at which the functional groups are eclipsing will result in a higher-energy conformation. The two forms in which the bulkiest groups (acetoxy and trimethylammonio) are separated by 60 degrees (or 60 and 300 degrees if rotation is considered in the same direction) are denoted as the *gauche* forms, and symmetry considerations dictate that their energy states be identical. The form with the 180-degree separation is the *trans* form. These gauche and trans forms differ substantially in configuration, as is evident in space-filling models (Fig. 1-12B). Thus, it becomes important to ask which of the forms is preferred in aqueous solution and which may be the preferred conformation on the receptor.

Three approaches are available for examining the conformation of compounds in aqueous solution. The first entails calculations on the basis of molecular orbital theory, and we have alluded to the limitations of this approach to calculating preferred conformation. Nevertheless, useful predictions of conformation have been achieved with small molecules such as acetylcholine and its congeners.

The second approach involves x-ray analysis of crystal structure. Although this approach has proved invaluable for larger protein macromolecules, in which *intra*molecular forces dominate in determining the folding pattern of the peptide chain, in small molecules *inter*molecular forces are significant, so that the conformations preferred in the crystal often differ from those in solution. For example, the various salts of the bis-quaternary cation decamethonium crystallize with discrete but different distances between the cationic nitrogens. This depends on the size of the counteranion with which it crystallizes.

The third technique, nuclear magnetic resonance (NMR), actually measures conformation in solution. The most used NMR technique for studying conformation to date has been proton magnetic resonance, since the resonances of the protons will be coupled to neighboring proton resonances, all of which contain a net spin. Thus, in the case of acetylcholine the two methylene groups will show coupling constants characteristic of whether they are proximal to two other methylene protons or to one methylene proton and another substituent group. Such determinations have shown that the gauche forms (i.e., those with a 60-degree torsion angle between the quaternary and acetoxy groups) of acetylcholine predominate in solution.[36] It is likely that coulombic attractive forces between the carbonyl oxygen, which possesses a partial negative charge in the dipole, and the positive charge of the quaternary nitrogen stabilize this conformation of the molecule.

Two-dimensional nuclear magnetic resonance analyses and *nuclear Overhauser* enhancement[37,38] allow for more detailed interpretation of solution conformation. The nuclear Overhauser effect is a change in signal intensity resulting from cross relaxation when a resonance signal of an adjacent nucleus is perturbed. Its value in elucidating conformation arises from the signal being dependent on the inverse sixth power of the distance between the observed and perturbed nuclei. By using a precise sequence for pulsing neighboring nuclei in specified directions, the integrated areas of the off-diagonal elements in the resonance signal are correlated with dipolar interactions between pairs of protons. The technique makes it possible to specify interproton distances of relatively complex molecules, and from these considerations a series of bond angles for many compounds can often be uniquely determined. Plate 1-1 shows the bond angles determined by the nuclear Overhauser method for acetylcholine when free in solution and when bound to the acetylcholine receptor. The solution conformation agrees with that determined by nonpulse coupling-constant methods. As considered below, the conformations of the free and bound acetylcholine species differ substantially, particularly when viewed in terms of exposure of hydrophobic surfaces.

Accordingly, it becomes important to estimate the difference in conformational energy from the differences in populations of the trans and gauche forms in solution. If, as indicated by the NMR studies, gauche forms predominate over trans by 10:1 in solution, then the free energy difference between the two forms can be described by

$$\Delta G = RT \ln p \qquad \text{(equation 7)}$$

where p is the population ratio of the two forms as determined by the physical measurement, R is the gas constant, and T is the absolute temperature. At 37°C the free energy difference between the gauche and trans forms is 1.4 kcal. Thus, if we plot the free energy as a function of bond angle, we see a profile like that shown in Figure 1-13.

The importance of these considerations can now be related to two principles involved in association of the ligand with the receptor surface. First, should the receptor prefer the gauche form of acetylcholine, virtually no loss of energy from a change in acetylcholine conformation would occur upon binding. If the trans form is preferred by the receptor, nearly 1.4 kcal will be lost and must be compensated for in the energy of interaction of

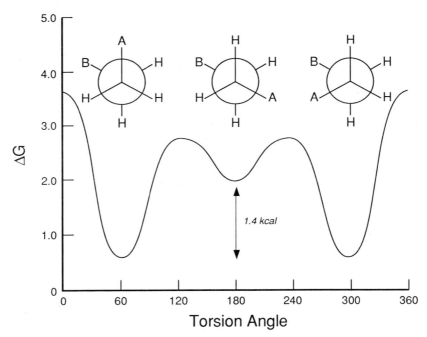

Fig. 1-13. Relationship between the torsion angle between the two methylene carbons in A-CH$_2$-CH$_2$-B and conformational free energy ΔG. A torsion angle of 0 degrees reflects the eclipsing of the two groups of largest volume. The energy differences show that the two gauche forms are each in a 10-fold excess over the trans form. The heights of the transition barriers at 0, 120, and 240 degrees are arbitrary.

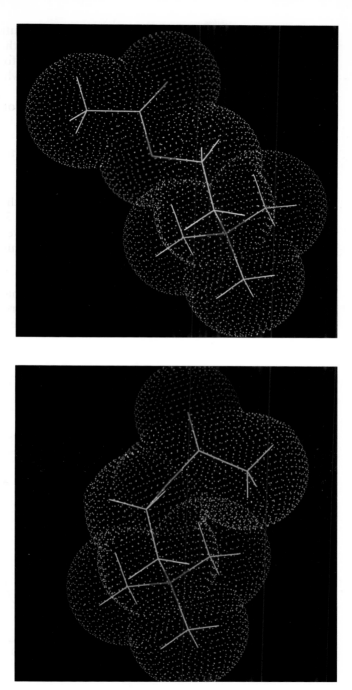

Plate 1-1. Preferred conformations of acetylcholine in solution (top) and bound to the nicotinic receptor (bottom) with two-dimensional NMR used to assign bond angles. The dark blue colors designate the quaternary nitrogen, and the light blue colors designate the hydrophobic methyl and methylene groups. The carboxyl and ester oxygens are shown in red. The dotted surfaces represent the van der Waals surface of the molecule. (Reproduced from Behling et al.,[38] with permission.)

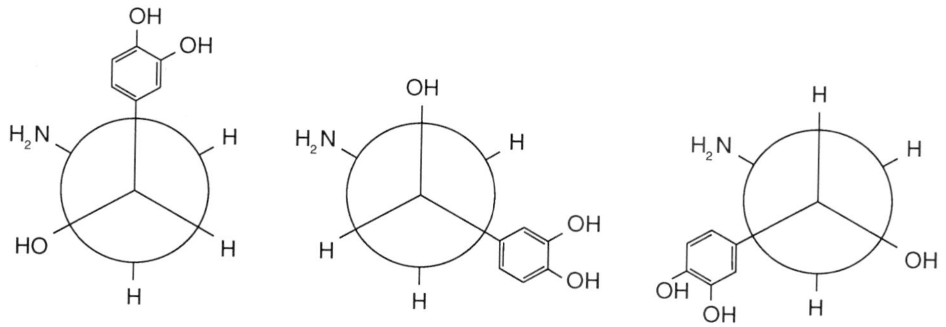

Fig. 1-14. Newman projection illustrating two distinct gauche and one trans species for norepinephrine upon bond rotation around the two aliphatic carbon atoms.

the complex. Changes in other bond angles in the conformation of bound ligand (e.g., τ_1 in Fig. 1-12) that differ from the lowest-energy conformation of the free ligand will also contribute to a loss of binding energy. Second, the compound upon binding may traverse an activation barrier for bond rotation when the residues are eclipsed. These barriers are reflected in the maxima resulting from bond rotation in Figure 1-13. Should these barriers be high, a rate-determining factor in the kinetics of interaction between ligand and receptor would come into play.

Accordingly, if we return to Plate 1-1, it can be estimated that the bound conformation of acetylcholine itself would be in a considerably higher energy state than the acetylcholine when free in solution, and this energy can be thought of as being compensated for by the energy of the complex. Moreover, to achieve the determined bound conformation, bond rotation requires transcending activation energy barriers. If these are substantial, the probability of transcending these barriers per unit time diminishes, and reaction kinetics could be limited by these bond rotation rates. Since acetylcholine activates its receptor at rates close to those of a diffusion-controlled reaction, at first inspection a bound conformation of acetylcholine that is remarkably different from the solution conformation would be unexpected. However, the times required for completing the pulse sequence to measure NMR relaxation by the nuclear Overhauser method are long, and almost certainly the receptor would reside in its high-affinity, desensitized conformation by the end of the sequence. Whereas binding to the activable receptor is rapid, the transition to the desensitized receptor state is slow and hence perfectly compatible with transcending high energy barriers (cf. Ch. 2).

As ligand structures become more complex, the factors influencing preferred conformation become much more complex. For example, with *l*-norepinephrine (Fig. 1-14) the torsion angle determined by the α and β carbons will yield two distinct gauche species, each possessing a different conformational energy. This results because the asymmetric center on the β carbon dictates that the proximal groups in the two gauche conformations are nonidentical.

Conformationally Rigid Compounds

Opioid Analgesics

A significant proportion of ligands or drug molecules do not exhibit free bond rotation and thus would have a unique conformation in solution that will be maintained upon binding; morphine would be an example[40,41] (Fig. 1-15). Early methods of measuring

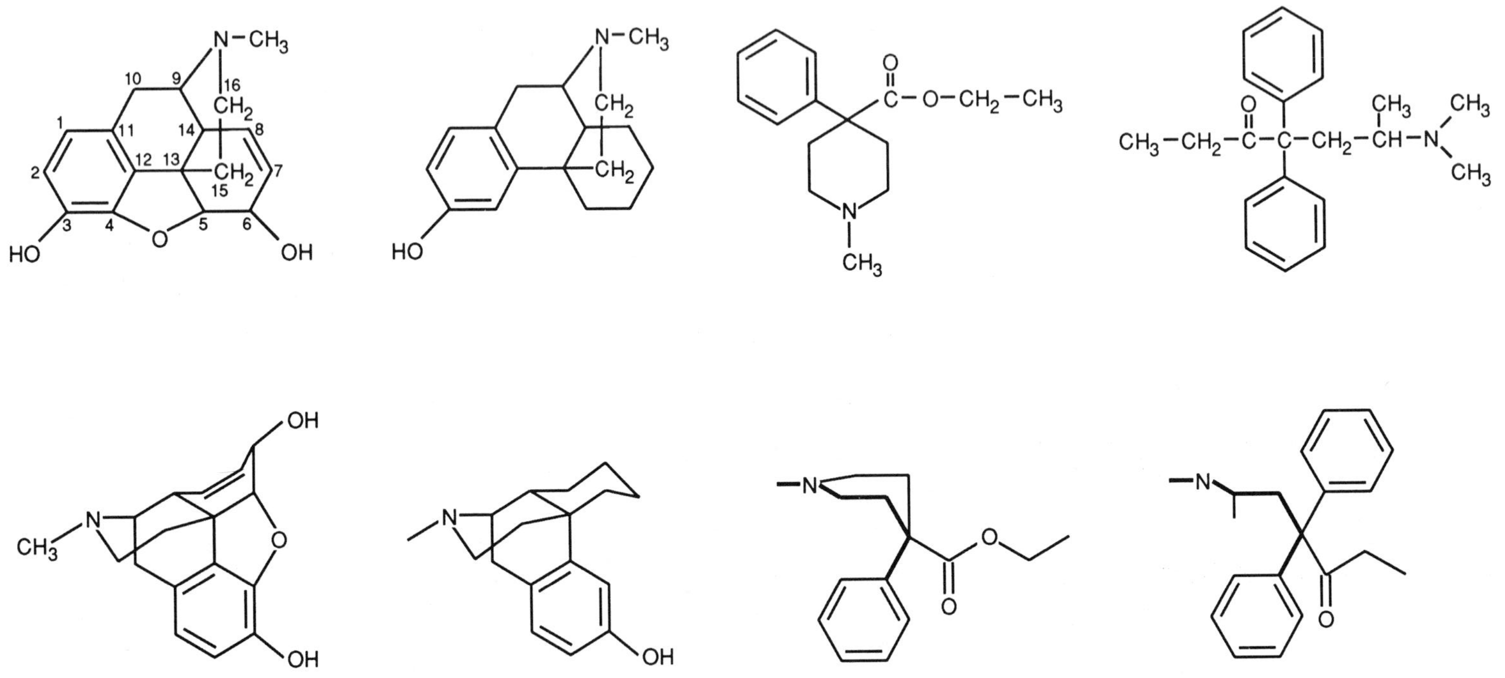

A Morphine (phenanthrene alkaloid) | B Levorphanol (morphinan) | C Meperidine (phenylpiperidine) | D Methadone (phenylheptylamine)

Fig. 1-15. Structure of morphine and related opioid analgesics. (**A**) Planar structure and stereochemical representation of D(−)-morphine, showing the relationship between the phenolic (carbons 1, 2, 3, 4, 11, 12) and piperidine (carbons 9, 14, 13, 15, 16) ring systems. Planar and stereochemical structures of (**B**) levorphanol, (**C**) meperidine, and (**D**) methadone. (*Figure continues.*)

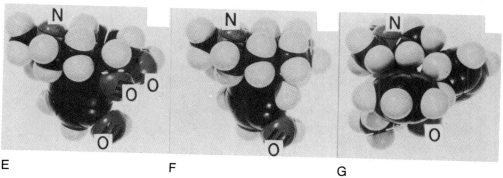

Fig. 1-15. (*Continued*). Space-filling (CPK) structures of (**E**) morphine, (**F**) levorphanol, and (**G**) methadone.

analgesia from morphine involved a rather simple but crude assay. Constant heating is applied to a rat's tail so that in about 10 seconds a tail "flick" is observed. After injection of an analgesic agent into a rat, the tail flick is delayed or even abolished. Since this is a dose-related phenomenon, potencies of various compounds may be compared. Analgesia involves multiple sites of action in the spinal cord and higher central nervous system centers, and several distinct types of opioid receptors are involved. The most important in supraspinal analgesia is the mu (μ) receptor, in which morphine is the prototypic agonist. The analogs that we will compare with morphine also have their primary action on the μ receptor.

Although there are several positions in the morphine molecule for stereoisomerism, the carbon at position 13 gives rise to active D(−) and inactive L(+) enantiomers. The stereochemistry of the biologically active D(−) morphine is shown below the conventional representation in Figure 1-15A. Since the multiple ring system imparts rigidity to the compound and precludes ring inversion, the corresponding enantiomers will have very different three-dimensional dispositions of their atoms. Levorphanol (Fig. 1-15B) shows a similar stereospecificity and slightly greater potency when compared with morphine, yet its structure is greatly simplified in that it lacks the aliphatic hydroxyl group at C-6, the ether oxygen between C-4 and C-5 and the unsaturation at C-7–C-8. Photographs of the space-filling models for morphine (Fig. 1-15E), levorphanol (Fig. 1-15F), and methadone (Fig. 1-15G) show similar surfaces on the left-hand side of the molecule and a similar distance between the bridged nitrogen and the phenolic hydroxyl moieties.

The analogs meperidine (Fig. 1-15C) and methadone (Fig. 1-15D) appear to be very different from morphine in terms of their planar structures. Methadone, for example, appears as a single aliphatic chain bearing a keto group, two benzene rings, and a dimethylamine group. It might be assumed that methadone, lacking a bridged ring system, could assume multiple conformations through bond rotation. However, the stereochemical configurations yield distinct and fixed conformations for the molecule. This becomes even more evident upon construction of a space-filling model, which shows that the sheer bulk of the aromatic and aliphatic groups would severely restrict bond rotation (Fig. 1-15G). In fact, the size of these groups governs the positions of the two polar groups nitrogen and oxygen. Hence, methadone adopts a rather similar conformation to morphine when examined in terms of the positions of the bridged nitrogen and the phenolic hydroxyl groups.

A characteristic T shape is apparent in the sterochemical and space-filling models for morphine. The nitrogen atom is positioned in a flat hydrophobic surface containing nine carbon atoms, those of the piperidine ring (C-9, C-13, C-14, C-15, C-16) and those of the partially unsaturated ring (C-13, C-5, C-6, C-7, C-8, C-14). The other two rings protrude in a perpendicular plane, with the phenolic hydroxyl group at C-3 positioned at a maximum distance from the nitrogen. The oxygen bonding perhaps to an amino group in the receptor, should also contribute to stabilizing the ligand-receptor complex. The alcoholic hydroxyl at C-6, the C-7–C-8 unsaturation, and the oxygen bridge are not critical, as evidenced in levorphanol and several benzomorphans to be considered later.

It is evident from the molecular model that the two essential groups (nitrogen and phenolic hydroxyl) could not both interact on a flat receptor site. It is surmised, therefore, that the receptor must have the shape of an irregular pouch, into which the opioid molecule can fit, making the essential contacts on different walls of the pouch. A large part of the hydrophobic regions comprising the cross-piece and stem of the T would ideally come into close contact with hydrophobic areas on the receptor surface to provide binding through van der Waals forces. This view is supported by the pharmacologic inertness of the L(+) enantiomers throughout the opioid series; that they have neither agonistic nor antagonistic activity suggests that they are excluded from the μ receptor site by their geometry.

With methadone, a pseudopiperidine ring is formed, and the benzene rings themselves are not free to rotate about C-4 of the aliphatic chain (as might have been expected on the basis of the flat structural representation) but are restricted to a conformation like that of the corresponding rings in the phenanthrene nucleus of morphine. Again, of the two optical isomers only D(−)-methadone, which fits the postulated receptor, is analgesic. Meperidine (Fig. 1-15C), a seemingly simple phenylpiperidine carboxylic acid ester, has no center of asymmetry, but one of its possible conformations corresponds to the D(−) compounds in the opioid series.

As discussed in connection with stereospecificity, certain minor modifications of the D(−)-methadone molecule emphasize further the principle of "goodness of fit" in drug-receptor interactions. If the $-CH_3$ attached to the carbon atom adjacent to the nitrogen atom is removed, analgesic potency decreases but the compound is still an effective analgesic. If, instead, a second $-CH_3$ is attached to the same carbon atom, the analgesic effect is destroyed. Evidently, the groove on the receptor surface will accept

$$-CH_2-CH- \atop | \atop CH_3$$

somewhat better than $-CH_2CH_2-$, as would be expected from the fact that the additional methyl group is free to orient outward from the groove. The difficulty with the structure

$$-CH_2-\overset{\displaystyle CH_3}{\underset{\displaystyle CH_3}{\overset{|}{\underset{|}{C}}}}-$$

is presumably that the groove cannot accommodate the additional width at all or that one methyl group will necessary project downward; in either case the entire molecule will be prevented from achieving the necessary perfect fit to the receptor surface. In short, the similarity of activities of methadone and morphine on brain μ receptors can be better understood when the space-filling models of these two ligands are compared.

Substitution of allyl ($-CH_2CH=CH_2$) or cyclopropylmethyl moieties or to a lesser extent other groups for methyl on the bridged nitrogen atom of morphine and its analogs produces a remarkable change (Fig. 1-16). Such compounds behave as specific competitive antagonists of analgesia (and other effects) produced by any of the opioid agonists. It is assumed, therefore, that they interact with the same site on the receptor. When morphine itself is changed in this way, the resulting compound, nalorphine (Fig. 1-16), displays a curious mixture of agonistic and antagonistic actions; it produces some analgesia but also is capable of blocking morphine-induced analgesia, depending upon the dose ratio of the two compounds. The associated dysphoria of nalorphine (disorientation, sedation, and hallucinations) may be related to interactions with other opioid receptor subtypes and the sigma receptor discussed in Chapter 10. Pure antagonists also exist; the most widely used (and the antidote of choice for opiate overdose) is naloxone, N-allyloxydihydromorphi-none (Fig.1-16). Many investigators now classify receptors as being opioid on the basis of antagonism of agonist binding and the pharmacologic response by naloxone. Naloxone is also of structural interest because a contribution to the complete abolition of agonistic properties (as compared with nalorphine) must also be attributed to the hydroxyl group at C-14. This substitution places a hydroxyl moiety directly adjacent to the nitrogen atom, sterically blocking any interaction with the receptor at this position. In many of the receptor systems considered in the next chapter, considerable latitude exists in the structural requirements for competitive antagonists. On the other hand, full agonist activity is achieved only within narrow boundaries of structural modification. A contrast is found in the case of opiates; few antagonists devoid of agonist activity have been synthesized. A similar situation has been encountered with other peptide receptors, for which few examples exist in which peptide modifications have yielded selective antagonists.

Nicotinic Receptor Antagonists

A structural comparison of the two isomers of the competitive neuromuscular blocking agent *d*-tubocurarine and its analog *O, O'*, *N*-trimethyltubocurarine (metocurine) illustrates another property of rigid molecules. Metocurine is two to three times as potent as *d*-tubocurarine. Both *d*- and *l*-trimethyltubocurarine have their two quaternary nitrogen atoms separated by 10.5 A. If the spatial disposition of quaternary ammonium groups were the sole criterion for activity, then *d* and *l* isomers would be equivalent in their potencies for neuromuscular blockade[42]; yet we find that the two isomers differ in potency by at least two orders of magnitude. An examination of the structures reveals that only the *d* isomer contains a separation of hydrophobic and hydrophilic residues on the respective surfaces (Fig. 1-17). With *d*-trimethyltubocurarine, hydrophobic residues may be found on the concave surface, shown in Figure 1-17C and D, while the hydrophilic residues (oxygens) shown in Figure 1-17A and B are localized entirely on the convex surface. This is not the case for *l*-trimethyl tubocurarine, in which the hydrophilic oxygens are found on both sides of the molecule. In general, the enantiomers of structurally rigid compounds reveal marked differences in the geometric positions of critical moieties in

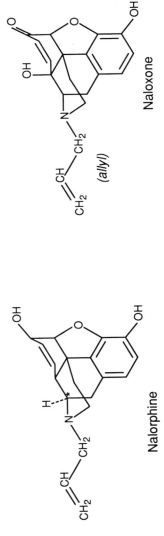

Nalorphine

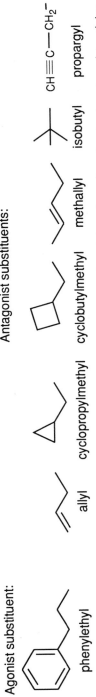

Naloxone

Agonist substituent:

phenylethyl

Antagonist substituents:

allyl   cyclopropylmethyl   cyclobutylmethyl   methallyl   isobutyl   propargyl

Fig. 1-16. Structures of moieties attached to the bridged nitrogen in the piperidine ring of the opiates that give rise to antagonist activity. The most selective moieties for antagonism are the allyl and cyclopropylmethyl groups; the phenylethyl group yields potent agonist activity. The structures of nalorphine and naloxone are shown.

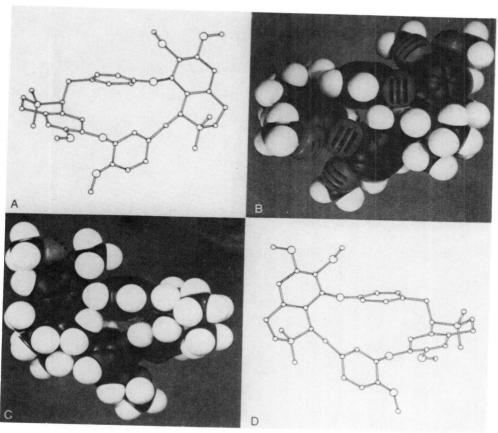

Fig. 1-17. TEP computer-drawn (ball-and-stick) and space-filling (CPK) models of the O,O′,N-trimethyl-*d*-tubocurarine molecule. (**A & B**) The convex surface is hydrophilic (note abundance of oxygen) while (**C & D**) the concave surface is almost entirely hydrophobic. In Figs. A and D the larger spheres are oxygen, the intermediate size nitrogen, and the smallest carbon. (From Sobell et al,[42] with permission.)

the structure, so that simple considerations regarding a three-point attachment presented earlier for the flexible compounds are no longer sufficient in the analysis of binding loci.

Ligands of Partial Conformational Flexibility

Peptides represent an intermediate case in flexibility-rigidity considerations, small peptides often having multiple degrees of freedom. Other peptides, particularly the larger ones, may adopt a secondary structure in solution, such as an α-helix, a β-pleated sheet, and various specialized turns; the energy of interaction with the receptor may govern whether a preferred conformation in solution is altered upon binding. Other peptides such as oxytocin have their degrees of freedom constrained by disulfide bonds, which limit conformational options.

An example might be considered to illustrate this point. It is known that the enkephalin pentapeptides and opiate alkaloids interact with several of the subtypes of opioid recep-

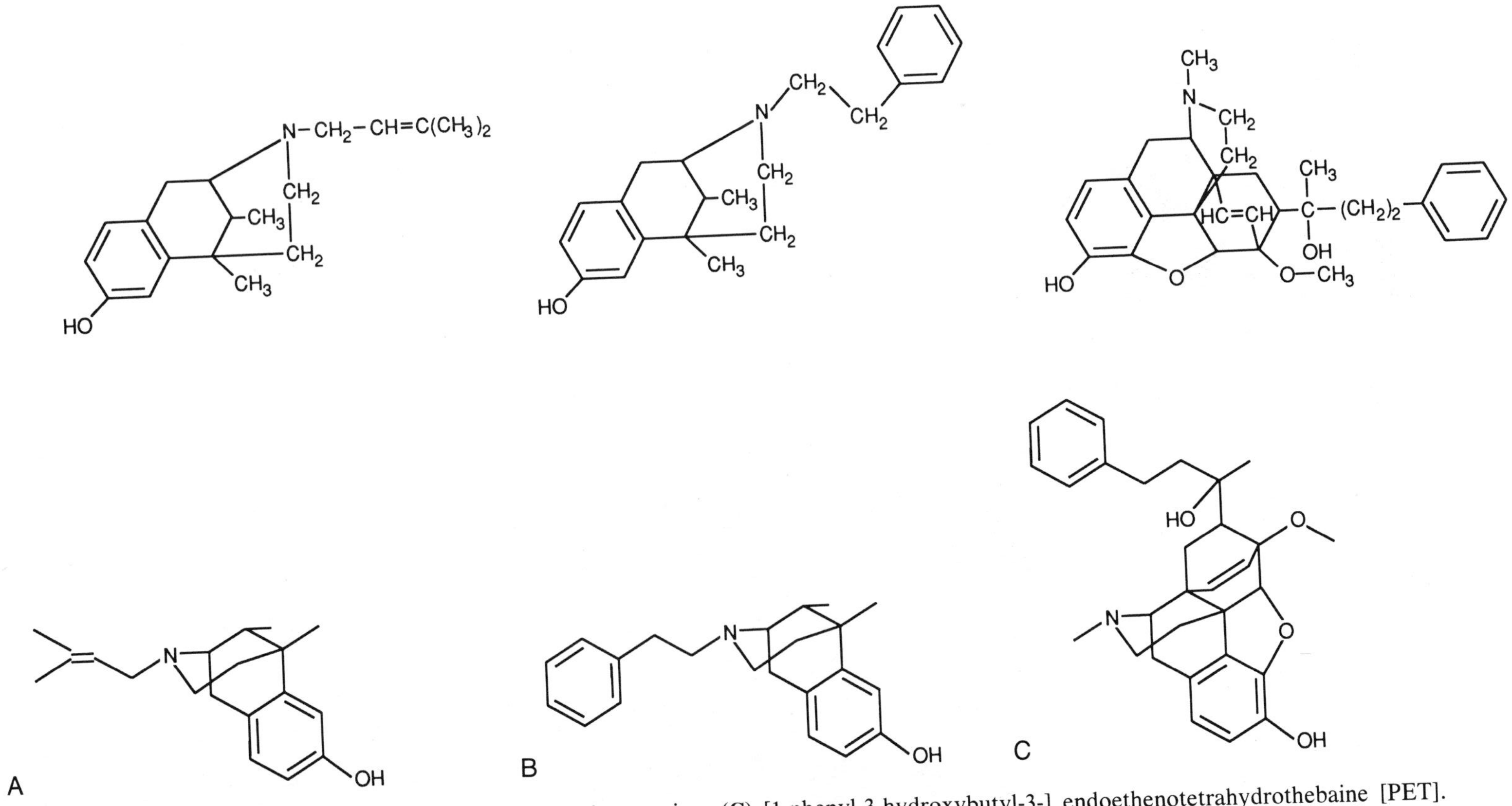

Fig. 1-18. Structures of (**A**) pentazocine, (**B**) phenazocine, (**C**) [1-phenyl-3-hydroxybutyl-3-] endoethenotetrahydrothebaine [PET]. (*Figure continues.*)

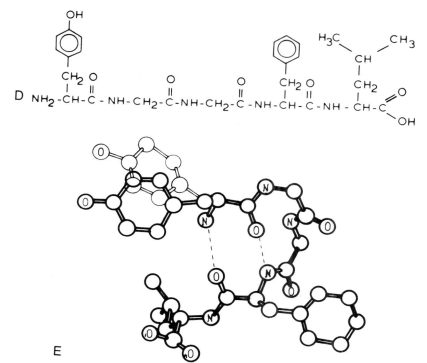

Fig. 1-18. (*Continued*). (**D**) & (**E**) Structure and conformation of [leu]-enkephalin determined from the crystal structure showing β bend and antiparallel hydrogen bonding. The light lines represent a second orientation of the N-terminal tyrosine residue. (Fig. E from Smith and Griffin,[43] with permission.)

tors, yet the planar structures of the enkephalin pentapeptides and opiate alkaloids are very different (Fig. 1-18). We know that all the determinants of the morphine structure are not required for binding, and an extensive structure-activity analysis reveals that levorphanol, meperidine, methadone (Fig. 1-15), and the benzomorphans (pentazocine) (Fig. 1-18A), which lack the nonaromatic ring system, elicit strong opioid agonist activity. Yet these structures maintain a T-like conformation, with approximately equivalent distances between the nitrogen atom and a dipole at the base of the T. On the other hand, the more potent thebaine opiates contain an additional ring system (Fig. 1-18C). This class of ligands is more potent than morphine by two to three orders of magnitude.

For the flexible peptide to bind to the same complement of opioid receptors as the plant alkaloids, we might also expect them to adopt similar conformations. Various investigations of opioid peptide structure by NMR or crystallography indicate a folded conformation resembling that of the alkaloids. For example, the crystal structure of leu-enkephalin (Fig. 1-18D) shows a β bend in the Tyr-Gly-Gly-Phe sequence, which is probably stabilized by hydrogen bonds between the amino nitrogen of Tyr and the carbonyl oxygen of Phe and between the amino nitrogen of Phe and the carbonyl oxygen of Tyr.[43] This conformation would superimpose the aromatic hydroxyl groups in ring A of morphine on the Tyr hydroxyl in enkephalin, the amino nitrogen of tyrosine in enkephalin on the tertiary nitrogen of morphine, the C-7–C-8 face of morphine on the Leu or Met side chain in

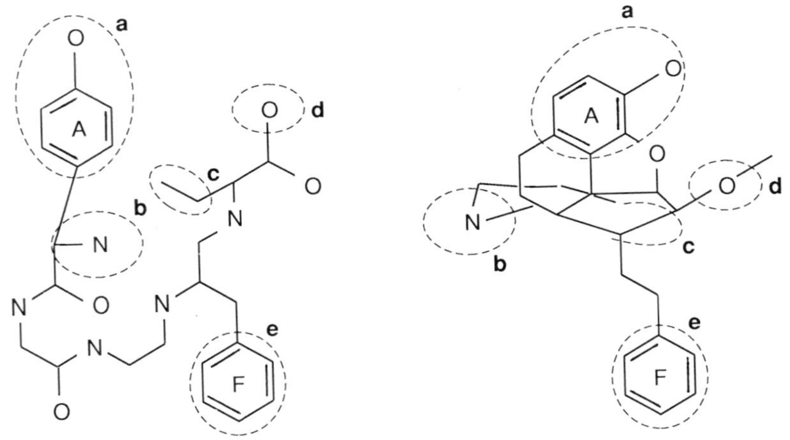

Fig. 1-19. Stick drawings of [leu]enkephalin and [1-phenyl-3-hydroxybutyl-3-]endoethenotetrahy-drothebaine [PET], with analogous regions shown by letter. (**a**) The phenyl ring of tyrosine and the aromatic portion of the opiate phenanthrene ring. (**b**) The N-terminal amino group of enkephalin and the bridged nitrogen of the opiate. (**c**) The hydrophobic side chain of the C-terminal amino acid of enkephalin (Leu or Met) and the aliphatic alcohol ring of the opiate. (**d**) The C-terminal carboxy group of enkephalin and the aliphatic OH group of the opiate. (**e**) The aromatic region encompassed by the phenylalanine ring of the enkephalins and the aromatic ring in phenazocine or in PET. A and F denote the two aromatic ring systems. (Adapted from Smith and Griffin,[43] with permission.)

enkephalin and the carboxy terminus of enkephalin on the polar group at the O-6 position of morphine (Fig. 1-19). The phenyl ring in the thebaine series would correspond with the Phe in enkephalin; this additional energy of interaction for thebaine series would arise from the aromatic residue. Alternatively, the aromatic residue attached to the bridged nitrogen in phenazocine (Fig. 1-18B), which is also a potent agonist, could correspond to the Phe position.

It still remains uncertain how far such inferential considerations of conformation can be carried. For example, none of the peptides possesses the selectivity of morphine for the μ receptor subtype, and specific peptides show greater selectivity at κ (dynorphin), δ (leu-enkephalin), and ε (endorphin) receptors than do the alkaloids. Moreover, slightly different peptide conformations have been deduced from solution analyses of conformation so that there is no consensus on the fine details of a preferred conformation for the enkephalins.[44]

Nonpeptidic Analogues of Peptides

The major limitations for peptides as therapeutic agents stem from their susceptibility to proteases and their inability to be absorbed orally and cross the blood-brain barrier. If the peptide or a particular region of the peptide could be mimicked in conformation by a nonpeptide analogue, such limitations might be circumvented. Several examples of peptide mimics have been described.

Cholecystokinin Antagonists

Cholecystokinin (CCK) is a octapeptide found in the gastrointestinal tract and brain (Fig. 1-20). Cholecystokinin stimulates distinct receptors in the gut and brain which have been designated CCK receptors. Removal of the sulfate on the tyrosine of CCK gives

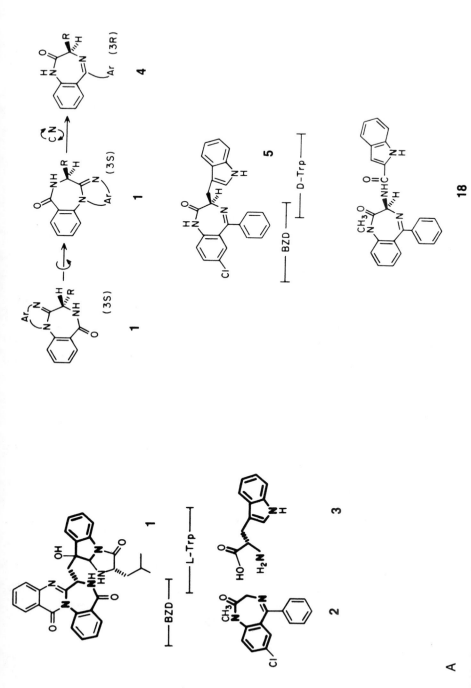

Fig. 1-20. Structures of cholecystokinin antagonists and cholecystokinin. (A) Asperlicin (compound 1) is a naturally occurring antagonist; the benzodiazepine and hydroxyindoline moieties are darkened in the structure. By rotation around the connecting bond and inversion of the carbonyl and nitrogen bonds, asperlicin can be compared with a conjugate between chlordiazepoxide (compound 2) and tryptophan (compound 3). Compound 5 shows potency as a cholecystokinin antagonist comparable with that of asperlicin (compound 1). Addition of the linking amide bond yields compound 18 and a large increase in potency as an antagonist (cf. Table 1-1). The numbering corresponds to that of the compounds in the original synthetic series. (*Figure continues.*)

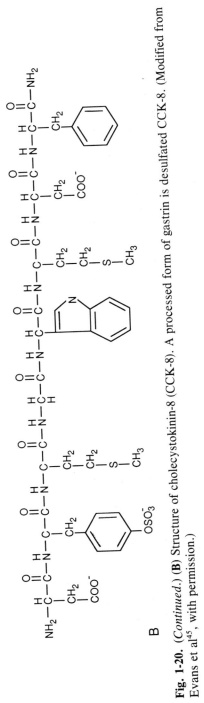

Fig. 1-20. (*Continued.*) (**B**) Structure of cholecystokinin-8 (CCK-8). A processed form of gastrin is desulfated CCK-8. (Modified from Evans et al[45], with permission.)

rise to an active form of gastrin, which has a distinct spectrum of activity in the gastrointestinal tract. Gastrin and CCK exert their actions through distinct receptors. A predominant activity of gastrin is the promotion of gastric acid secretion. In the gut CCK influences pancreatic secretion, gallbladder contraction, and gut motility. The role of CCK and several of its peptide precursors in brain is less clear, but they may serve as neurotransmitters or neuromodulators. They appear to be released together with some of the better characterized central nervous system neurotransmitters.

Asperlicin, a naturally occurring nonpeptide analogue of cholecystokinin isolated from fermentation, has been shown to be a moderately potent antagonist and selective for peripheral (i.e., gastrointestinal tract) cholecystokinin receptors (Fig. 1-20 and Table 1-1). Asperlicin (compound 1) contains a benzodiazepine moiety, and the 3-hydroxylindoline may be an analog of the critical tryptophan residue in cholecystokinin. Synthesis of a fusion product between *D*-tryptophan (compound 3) and chlordiazepoxide (compound 2), a benzodiazepine, yielded a cholecystokinin antagonist (compound 5) of simplified structure and equal potency equal to that of asperlicin.[45,46] The relationship between this structure and asperlicin can be seen by rotation of the benzodiazepine moiety 180 degrees around its connecting bond and inversion of the carbonyl and nitrogen groups. The addition of an amide bond between the indole and benzodiazepine rings greatly enhances activity (compound 18). Stereospecificity is also maintained at the 3' position.

Several orally effective CCK antagonists of this prototype structure with sustained activity have been synthesized, and the compounds appear selective towards gastrointestinal CCK receptors (CCK-A) in relation to brain CCK receptors (CCK-B), gastrin receptors, or receptor sites for antianxiety action (Table 1-1). 3-Acylamino and 3-amino substituents on the benzodiazepine ring diminish antianxiety activity but enhance CCK antagonist potency. The stereochemical preferences of the benzodiazepine and CCK receptors also differ. Certain 3-benzoylamino substitutions diminish the potency for the CCK-A receptors but enhance the potency for CCK-B and gastrin receptors (Table 1-1). Other studies have revealed a similar ligand specificity for gastrin and CCK-B receptors. Thus, a relatively rigid and nonpeptide analog that mimics a portion of CCK structure serves as an effective CCK-A antagonist and shows substantial receptor subtype specificity. Modification of this structure has also yielded antagonists specific for the CCK-B and gastrin receptors. These findings reveal that substitution of the benzodiazepine moiety can markedly change the receptor specificity of this nucleus. In a more general sense, the rigid benzodiazepine moiety, with its inherent amide bond, may mimic certain conformations of a peptide backbone. In the cases of chlordiazepoxide, diazepam, and other antianxiety agents, the benzodiazepines with their rigid ring structures may mimic the active conformation of an endogenous antianxiety peptide.

Angiotensin-Converting Enzyme Inhibitors

The development of an orally active inhibitor of angiotensin-converting enzyme had its genesis in the early 1970s, when it was recognized that a nonapeptide from the venom of the pit viper *Bothrops jararaea* was an inhibitor of this enzyme.[47] Angiotensin-converting enzyme is a peptidyldipeptide carboxyhydrolase of approximately 150 kDa apparent mass. One of its natural substrates is angiotensin I, in which a C-terminal dipeptide is cleaved to form the octapeptide angiotensin II (Fig. 1-21). Angiotensin II has numerous actions, including vasoconstriction, enhancement of evoked release of norepinephrine, and promotion of release of aldosterone from the adrenal cortex. The angiotensins are derived

Table 1-1. Activity of Benzodiazepine Analogs for Cholecystokinin (CCK), Gastrin, and Benzodiazepine (BDZ) Receptors

Compound	X	R_1	R_2	3-Stereo[a]	CCK-A (IC_{50})[b]	CCK-B (IC_{50})[c]	BDZ (IC_{50})[d]	Gastrin (IC_{50})[e]
Chlordiazepoxide	Cl	CH_3		—	>100	—	0.007	—
Asperlicin (Fig. 1-20)				S	1.4	—	—	>100
5 (Fig. 1-20)	Cl	H	CH_2–indolyl	R	3.4	—	>100	—
6 (Fig. 1-20)	Cl	H	CH_2–indolyl	S	32	—	5.6	—
18 (Fig 1-20) (L-364, 718)	H	CH_3	NHC(O)–indolyl	S	0.0008[f]	0.245	>100	0.30
19 (Fig. 1-20)	H	CH_3	NHC(O)–indolyl	R	0.065	—	>100	—
L-365, 260	H	CH_3	NHC(O)NH–(tolyl)	S	0.003	0.151	—	0.130
L-365, 260	H	CH_3	NHCNH–(tolyl)	R	0.280	0.002	—	0.0011

[a] The preferred orientation of the 3′-substituent of the more active compounds is spatially the same; the change in preferred stereochemistry from R to S between the alkyl (5 and 6) and acylindolyl (18 and 19) is due to convention in assigning the stereochemical designator.

[b] Half-maximal inhibition of binding of ^{125}I-CCK-33 to pancreatic CCK receptors in μMs. The IC_{50} for compound 18 yields a K_i of 0.1 nM, compared with the K_d for CCK-8 of 0.11 μM.

[c] IC_{50} in μM for displacement of ^{125}I-CCK-8 from guinea pig cerebral cortex.

[d] IC_{50} in μM for displacement of [^{3}H]-diazepine from benzodiazepine receptors (values for 18 and 19) are displacement of [^{3}H]-flunitrazepine from guinea pig brain benzodiazepine receptors.

[e] IC_{50} in μM for displacement of ^{125}I-gastrin from guinea pig gastric glands.

[f] Compound 18 shows greater than 10^3 selectivity for pancreatic CCK receptors when compared with brain CCK receptors or gastrin receptors.

(Data from Evans et al.[45] Chang and Lott,[46] and Bock et al.[109])

SUBSTRATES

K_M

$^{+}$Asp–Arg–Val–Tyr–Ile–His–Pro–Phe$\backslash$His–Leu^{-} 30–80 µM
Angiotensin I

$^{+}$Arg–Pro–Pro–Gly–Phe–Ser–Pro$\backslash$Phe–Arg^{-} 0.9 µM
Bradykinin

INHIBITORS

K_I

<Glu–Lys–Trp–Ala–Pro^{-} 0.09 µM
BPP$_{5a}$

<Glu–Trp–Pro–Arg–Pro–Gln–Ile–Pro–Pro^{-} 0.84 µM
Teprotide

A

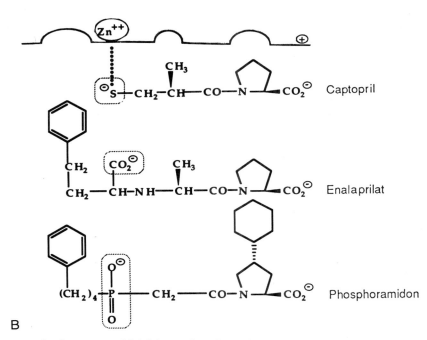

B

Fig. 1-21. (**A**) Sequences of substrates and inhibitors of angiotensin-converting enzyme. The numbers on the right show the approximate K_m for hydrolysis at the designated peptide bond or the K_1 for inhibition of proteolysis. (**B**) Proposed attachment sites for various inhibitors of converting enzyme. The three inhibitors shown from top to bottom are captopril, enalaprilat, and phosphoramidon. (Figure B from Wyvral and Patchett,[48] with permission.)

from a larger peptide, angiotensinogen, a substrate for renin. The renin-angiotensin-aldosterone system plays a critical role in the regulation of blood pressure in humans. Angiotensin-converting enzyme also catalyzes the cleavage of bradykinin, a potent vasodilator, to inactive peptides. Inhibitors of angiotensin-converting enzyme have antihypertensive actions, primarily by preventing the formation of angiotensin II and secondarily by enhancing the stability of bradykinin. This was initially shown in clinical studies with the *B. jararaea* peptide. A pentapeptide, BPP$_{5a}$ was shown to be more active in vitro but less stable in vivo.

These observations led Ondetti[47] to examine a series of even smaller peptides and peptide analogs. The tripeptides Trp-Ala-Pro and Phe-Ala-Pro showed maximum activity among the peptides. The mercaptoalkanoyl amino acids, of which captopril[47] (2(*S*)-methyl-3-mercaptopropanoyl-(*S*)-proline) is a member, and the carboxyalkyl dipeptides, represented by enalapril and enalaprilat (N^α-[(*S*)-1-carboxy-3 phenylpropyl]-L-alanyl-L-proline)[48] evolved from modifications of the tripeptide structure. The rationale behind the structure-activity studies emerged from two considerations of the catalytic mechanisms of angiotensin-converting enzyme: (1) the enzyme is similar in catalytic mechanism and probably in active site structure to the zinc-containing metalloproteases carboxypeptidase and thermolysin, for both of which crystal structures have been determined; and (2) the reaction product or collected products of catalysis are inhibitors of the enzyme catalyzing their formation. The following seem essential for substrate interaction: (1) the carboxyl group on the C-terminal proline; (2) the amide carboxyl between the amino acids; (3) hydrophobic interactions on the proline and the α-methyl group on the adjoining amino acid; and (4) a sulfhydryl, carboxylic, or phosphinic acid moiety for interaction with the coordinated Zn^{2+} in the enzyme. Many of the inhibitors such as captopril contain only a single amide linkage with the proline. As such they are absorbed from the gastrointestinal tract and are relatively stable in vivo. With other compounds such as enalapril, systemic absorption after oral administration is enhanced by esterification of the carboxyl groups. Thus, the active species is administered as the inactive ester enalapril, which is hydrolyzed after absorption to form the active inhibitor enalaprilat. Both captopril and enalapril have been widely used in the treatment of hypertension and congestive heart failure. The success with nonpeptidic or partially peptidic substances in inhibiting angiotensin synthesis and bradykinin degradation suggests that receptor antagonists that are nonpeptidic in nature and cross biologic membranes might be developed for peptide receptors. Initial progress has been made with a series of antagonists acting on angiotensin receptors.[49]

Opiates

Based on the structure-activity analyses in the previous section, the opiate alkaloids might also be considered as another example in which a nonpeptidic substance possessing the capacity to cross membranes mimics the conformation of a naturally occurring peptide. Although the various opiates have different rates of absorption from the gastrointestinal tract and penetration into the central nervous system, they exhibit far more rapid rates of transmembrane permeation than do the opioid peptides (cf. Chs. 3 and 10). Moreover, the slower rates of metabolism of the alkaloids or their synthetic analogs (cf. Ch. 5) obviate the other limitation in the peptides.

Conformation of Bound Ligand

Physicochemical Measurements of Conformation

The conformation of the ligand when bound to a receptor can generally only be inferred from indirect studies; nevertheless it is an important determinant in predicting specificity in drug action. As noted above, the additional energy of the conformational change of the ligand must be considered if receptor binding prefers a ligand conformation not favored in solution. Second, conformational flexibility of the ligand may be a critical determinant in enabling the entire drug-receptor complex to adopt the conformation associated with activation by agonists. Obviously, structurally rigid compounds whose conformation is fixed by ring systems or by steric hindrance can only bind the same conformation that exists in solution. In fact, this situation will also hold for partially flexible compounds whenever the energy required for a change in conformation would approach or be greater than that gained in the binding interaction.

To examine the conformation of the bound ligand one must again turn to techniques suited to atomic level resolution, but the problem becomes even more formidable since it is necessary to obtain high concentrations of the ligand-macromolecule complex. In only a few selected cases has it been possible to ascertain the conformation of the drug when bound to its site of action. X-ray crystallography and two-dimensional NMR studies have yielded detailed information on the torsion angles between ring systems when trimethoprim and other analogs bind to dihydrofolate reductase. This information has been employed for the design of new dihydrofolate reductase inhibitors (see Ch. 2).

NMR has also been employed to examine the binding affinity, dissociation rate and conformation of bound acetylcholine.[38,39] If the rate of ligand dissociation exceeds the rate of relaxation of the bound nuclei when excited in a magnetic field, then a composite signal reflecting the free and bound ligand is obtained. This is usually advantageous for detection of binding, since the resonance signal of the bound species is not obscured by its efficient relaxation. Consideration of the reaction $L + R \rightleftharpoons LR$, where L is the ligand and R the receptor, yields the following equation for relaxation of nuclei in a ligand that is associating with and dissociating from a receptor.

$$\frac{1}{T_{1,\text{obs}}} = \frac{1}{T_{1,\text{free}}} + \frac{F}{T_{1,\text{bound}} + \tau} \qquad \text{(equation 8)}$$

where $T_{1,\text{obs}}$ is the observed spin-lattice relaxation time for a particular nucleus; $T_{1,\text{bound}}$ and $T_{1,\text{free}}$ are the respective relaxation times for the particular nucleus when the ligand is free in solution or bound to the macromolecule; τ is the reciprocal of the dissociation rate constant; and F is the fraction of total ligand that is bound. $T_{1,\text{obs}}$ provides a time constant for the major means by which nuclei, when in a magnetic field, relax after radio-frequency excitation in circumstances where τ, the time constant for exchange, is smaller than $T_{1,\text{bound}}$. These parameters are governed by the mobility of neighboring molecules and the nuclei of interest. $T_{1,\text{bound}}$ and $T_{1,\text{free}}$ will differ usually by several orders of magnitude.

The equilibrium dissociation constant and rate constants for association and dissociation can be determined from NMR relaxation. Since $T_{1,\text{bound}}$ is usually much less than $T_{1,\text{free}}$ as F becomes a significant fraction ($10^{-4} \rightarrow 0.1$), the observed relaxation depends on the second term. If $\tau > T_{1,\text{bound}}$, exchange will determine $T_{1,\text{obs}}$, whereas if $T_{1,\text{bound}} > \tau$, then $T_{1,\text{bound}}$ will affect the signal even at small values of F. Accordingly, even at low fractional occupation $T_{1,\text{obs}}$ will be affected by $T_{1,\text{bound}}$.

The above techniques require large quantities of macromolecule for detection of the signal and selective ligand binding because the ligand is often in stoichoimetric excess of the macromolecule. To date, these constraints have limited NMR studies on most receptors and the conformation of bound acetylcholine on its receptor is the prototype example (Plate 1-1). However, expression systems designed for producing high yields of recombinant DNA gene products should make several other receptor systems accessible to this approach.

Rigid Analogs of Acetylcholine

Rigid analogs of agonists have been employed to gain insight into the bound conformation of flexible agonists such as acetylcholine, catecholamines, peptides, and the excitatory and inhibitory amino acids.[29,30] Since our knowledge of structure-activity relationships is perhaps greatest in the case of acetylcholine, we might use this example for illustrative purposes. Figure 1-22 shows several analogs of acetylcholine, all of which have had their activity on muscarinic acetylcholine receptors determined.[29] In each case the positions of the acetoxy or quaternary groups in the two isomers can be compared with the distances between these groups in the gauche or trans conformations of acetylcholine. Either the bicyclic ring systems or steric hindrance between bulky groups preclude facile interconversion between the conformations. The tropane, decalin, bicyclooctane, and cyclopropane analogs shown in Figure 1-22 will not show ring inversion, and the α,β dimethylcholine analog will require an energetically unfavorable eclipsing of methyl groups to achieve one of the two conformations. The series also illustrates the principal limitation of the approach, namely that in all the compounds steric bulk is added to the parent acetylcholine structure. Perturbation of the acetylcholine structure is minimal in the cyclopropane derivative, and even here one does not have a precise steric representation of acetylcholine. Nevertheless, these studies show that rigid analogs that mimic the trans conformation of acetylcholine (Fig. 1-12) are most active on the muscarinic receptor. A change in conformation from the gauche form preferred in solution appears to be associated with muscarinic receptor binding. Hence, the dipole of the carbonyl group and the positive charge are positioned farther apart than in the preferred conformation of acetylcholine in solution.

A similar conformation for the ligand in the bound state may not necessarily exist for the nicotinic acetylcholine receptor. In fact, distinct specifications of cholinergic agonists as being primarily nicotinic or muscarinic have been attributed to the appendages existing on one side or the other of the basic structural skeleton[8,9] (Fig. 1-1). Finally, structures of certain potent rigid analogues of acetylcholine such as anatoxin (Fig. 1-23) point to a conformation resembling a gauche conformation when bound to the nicotinic receptor. The conformation of anatoxin shown in Fig. 1-23B reflects its most stable conformation.[50] These considerations are intuitively satisfying since changes in ligand conformation require both energy and time. Conformational changes with large activation barriers should be precluded for rapidly binding, activating, and dissociating ligands such as acetylcholine acting on nicotinic receptors. Hence, it might be anticipated that as a first approximation the conformation of a bound flexible ligand would resemble the conformation of the more potent rigid analogs.

The bound acetylcholine conformation predicted from the rigid analog study of the

→

Fig. 1-22. Rigid analogs of acetylcholine. The various analogs of acetylcholine have been synthesized and their activities tested on the muscarinic receptor. The bicyclic ring systems and the cyclopropyl ring system do not show ring inversion and in each case give rise to two distinct orientations for the acetoxy and trimethylammonium moieties, with distances between the carbonyl oxygen and the center of the positive charge that approximate either the gauche or trans conformation of acetylcholine. The most active isomers are: dimethylacetoxytropane, equatorial; trimethylaminoacetoxydecalin, trans diaxial; acetyl-α,β-dimethylcholine, erythro; acetoxytrimethylaminobicyclooctane, trans; acetoxytrimethylaminocyclopropane, trans.

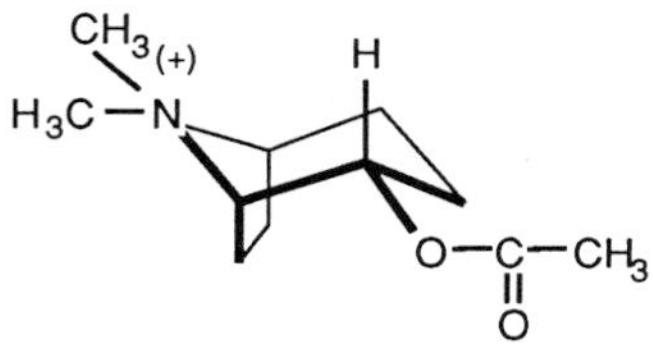

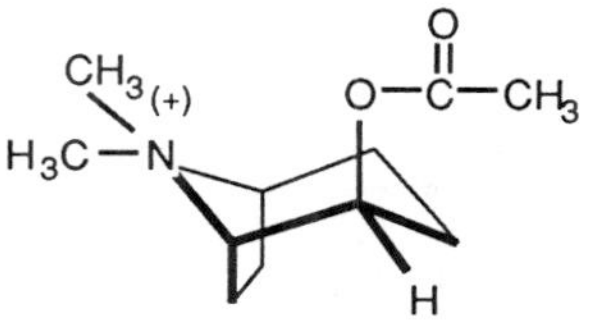

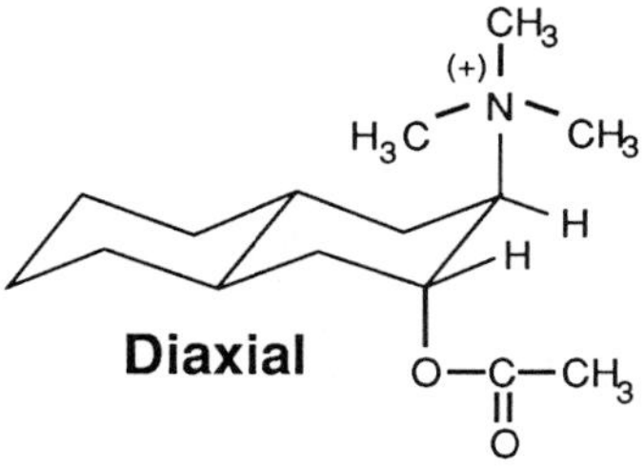

Diaxial

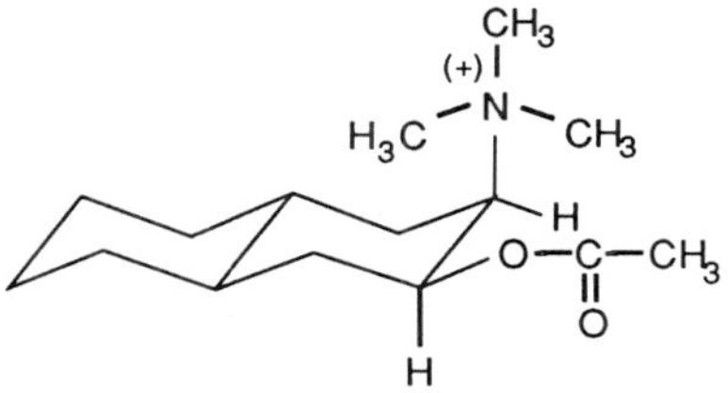

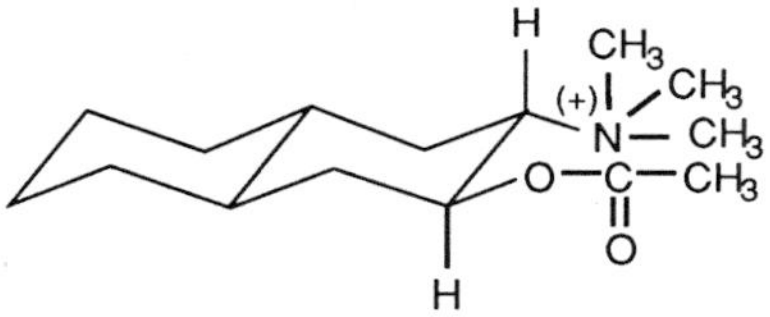

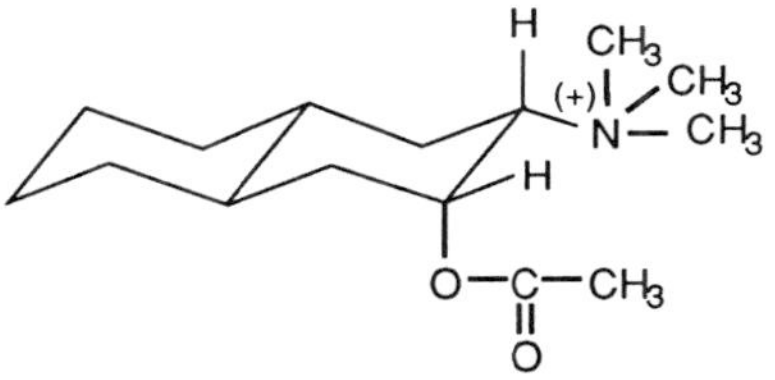

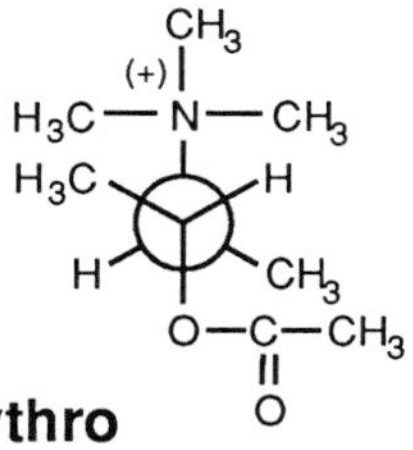

erythro

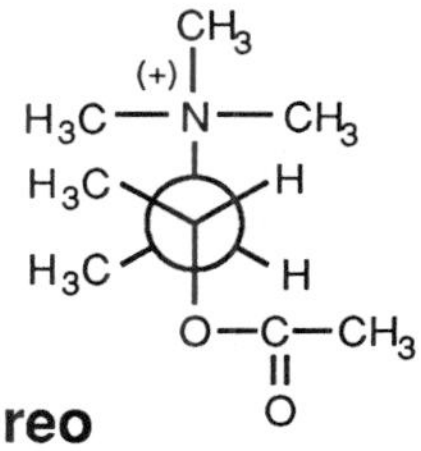

threo

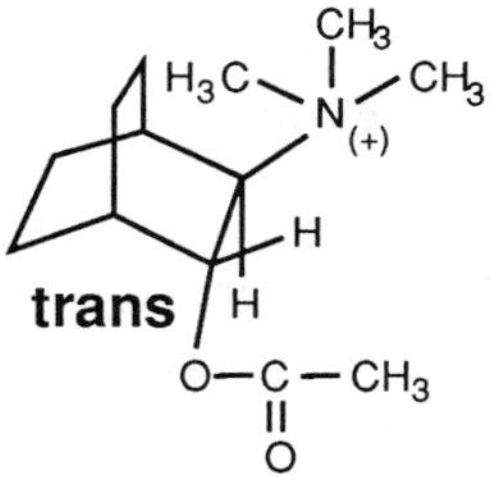

trans

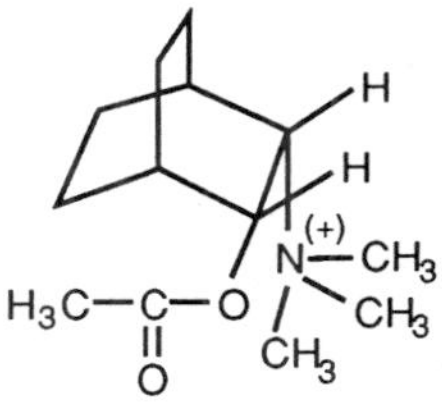

cis

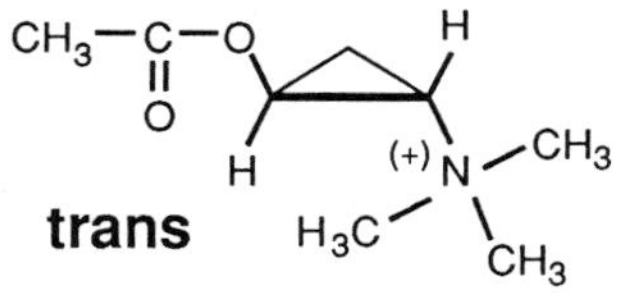

trans

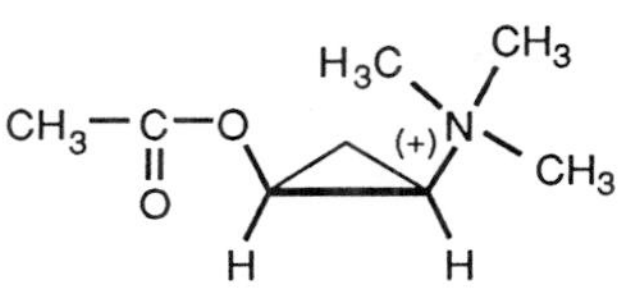

cis

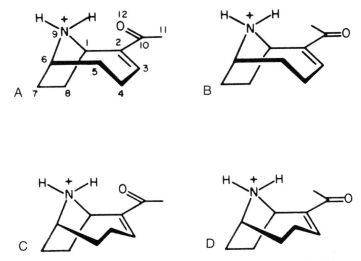

Fig. 1-23. Potential conformations of anatoxin, a potent agonist on nicotinic receptors. The abundant conformation ascertained by NMR, x-ray crystallography, and molecular orbital calculations is that shown in Fig. B. (From Koskinen and Rapoport,[50] with permission.)

anatoxins differs substantially from that determined by two-dimensional NMR (Plate 1-1). However, as previously discussed, the NMR study required long periods for agonist equilibration, and the NMR spectra should reflect a conformation of a ligand-receptor complex in a desensitized rather than an activated receptor state.[38] Accordingly, the bound conformation of a ligand may depend on the receptor state.

Rigid Analogs of Gamma-Aminobutyric Acid

γ-Aminobutyric acid (GABA), an inhibitory amino acid transmitter, is another widely studied example in which rigid analogs enable one to analyze the stereospecificity and complementarity of functional groups necessary for pharmacologic activity. The three methylene groups in GABA allow for multiple degrees of torsional movement around the bonds, which will place the opposite charges in this zwitterion in very different positions. GABA is known to act on two distinct receptor subtypes, GABA-A and GABA-B, each of which has a distinct coupling mechanism for eliciting a cellular response (see Ch. 2). In addition, GABA is actively transported into neurons and glia to terminate its action after being released from neurons by nerve stimulation. Its chemical conversion to succinic semialdehyde takes place within neurons and surrounding glial cells. This transamination reaction resulting in GABA catabolism is catalyzed by GABA transaminase. The two receptor subtypes, the transport processes, and the degradative enzyme each exhibit distinct chemical specificities, and these may be exploited by the rigid analog approach.[30]

Shown in Figure 1-24 are measures of agonist activity, determined by iontophoresis, and ligand occupation of GABA-A receptors for several rigid analogs of GABA. Because of the absence of potent rigid analogs and antagonists at the GABA-B receptor, less can be said about the active conformation of GABA at the GABA-B receptor. Nevertheless, GABA-A and GABA-B receptors exhibit opposite stereochemical requirements. Since several potent GABA-A agonists are completely inactive at GABA-B receptors and since baclofen does not stimulate GABA-A receptors, the active conformations of GABA at the two receptor subtypes should prove to be very different.

Rigid Analogs and Intersite Distances

Rigid analogs fix the relative positions of functional groups. In the case of the GABA analogs, the intersite distances between the hydrated cationic amino and anionic carboxyl groups are defined. For the acetylcholine analogs, distances may be calculated between the nonhydrated quaternary ammonium groups and the dipole on the carbonyl or the ester oxygen. Imperfect as the rigid analog approach is, it is likely to be some time before crystallographic or NMR investigations provide the resolution to examine structures of bound ligands on a variety of receptors. A second problem with the NMR techniques will be the development of a rapid method to entrap the receptor in its active conformation.

QUANTITATION OF RECEPTOR OCCUPATION AND RESPONSE

The Law of Mass Action

Interpretation of the relationship between ligand (drug) concentration and observed response depends upon the molecular model used to describe the overall reaction scheme. One can fit models by a variety of methods for graphical presentation. The simple bimolecular association and unimolecular dissociation scheme involves the association of two combining molecules and the dissociation of a single species:

$$[L] + [R] \underset{k_{-1}}{\overset{k_1}{\rightleftharpoons}} [LR] \qquad \text{(equation 9)}$$

where [L] is the ligand concentration, [R] is the receptor concentration, and [LR] is the concentration of the ligand-receptor complex. This reaction forms the starting point for analysis of receptor occupation.

In this reaction scheme, based on the law of mass action, unbound ligand reversibly binds to unbound receptor at a rate dependent on the concentration of the two reactants, and the resulting ligand-receptor complex breaks down at a rate proportional to the concentration of complex. Thus, drug-receptor complexes are formed by a bimolecular association reaction, the rate of which is described by:

$$\text{Rate of association} = k_1[L][R] \qquad \text{(equation 10)}$$

where k_1 is the association rate constant and is expressed in reciprocal units of the product of concentration and time. Breakdown (dissociation) of ligand-receptor complexes is unimolecular and its rate can be described by

$$\text{Rate of dissociation} = k_{-1}[LR] \qquad \text{(equation 11)}$$

where k_{-1} is the dissociation rate constant, expressed in reciprocal units of time.

At equilibrium (which is more appropriately termed *apparent equilibrium* or *steady*

Inhibition of Receptor Binding

Compound	Structure	GABA-A Agonism	GABA-A IC$_{50}$ (µM)	GABA-B IC$_{50}$ (µM)
GABA	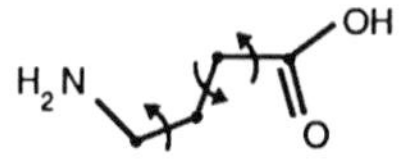	– – –	0.03	0.03
(S)-DHM	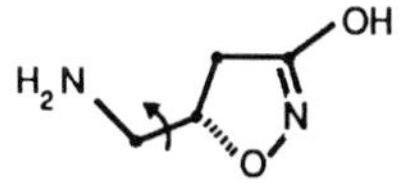	– – –	0.004	13
(R)-DHM	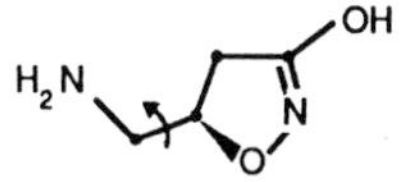	– –	0.3	5
Muscimol	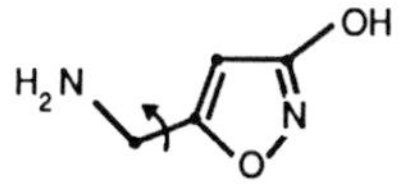	– – –	0.006	2.4
Thiomuscimol	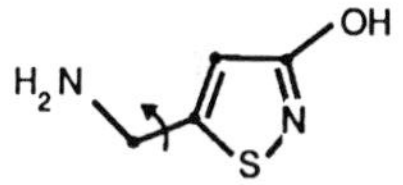	– – –	0.02	N.T.
THIP	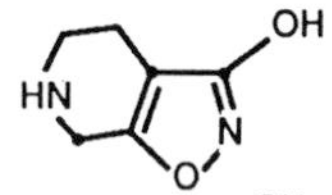	– – – (-)	0.1	>100
Homo-β-proline	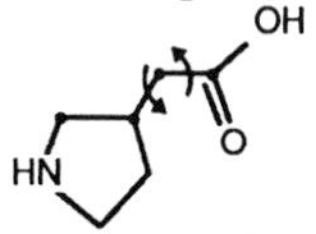	– – –	0.3	25
Isonipecotic acid	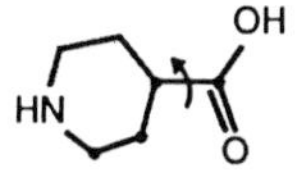	– – –	0.3	>100
Isoguvacine	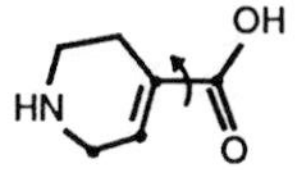	– – –	0.04	>100

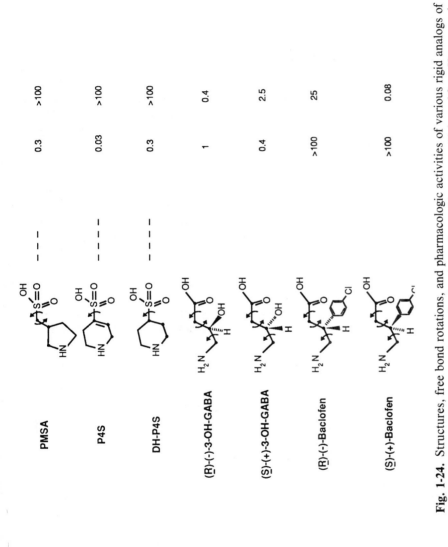

Fig. 1-24. Structures, free bond rotations, and pharmacologic activities of various rigid analogs of gamma-aminobutyric acid. Freely rotating bonds are denoted by arrows. (Adapted from Krogsgaard-Larsen[30], with permission.)

45

state, since unequivocal evidence of achievement of equilibrium is often not possible in pharmacologic systems), the rate of association equals the rate of dissociation:

$$k_1[L][R] = k_{-1}[LR] \qquad \text{(equation 12)}$$

which can be rearranged to

$$\frac{k_{-1}}{k_1} = \frac{[L][R]}{[LR]} = K_D \qquad \text{(equation 13)}$$

Hence the dissociation constant determined at equilibrium can be defined both by a ratio of rate constants for dissociation and association and by the ratio of the concentration of free species to that of the associated species or the complex. It is convenient and usually conventional to describe the equilibrium constant as a dissociation constant K_D rather than as its reciprocal, an association constant. Hence, in the simple bimolecular association–unimolecular dissociation system K_D will be defined in units used to express concentration, typically molarity (M). A low dissociation constant designates high affinity.

It is important to emphasize that several assumptions are made when the above scheme is used:

1. The binding reaction is totally reversible, so that association depends only on the interaction of L and R and dissociation only on the breakdown of LR.
2. The two reactants exist as either free or bound species, and measured concentrations of these species do not include degradation products or other forms unavailable for the reaction such as "nonspecific" binding or "acceptor" sites for L (i.e., sites other than R to which L can bind and at which its free concentration is effectively diminished). In the subsequent discussion it is generally assumed that correction has been made for these sites.
3. All receptor sites are considered to have equivalent affinity for L and to be independent, so that occupancy of some receptor sites does not alter the binding of unoccupied sites (cooperative interactions). These considerations will be developed further later in this chapter.

Although these assumptions are implicit in the use of the above equations, rigorous tests to validate them often have not been adequately performed in published studies of ligand-receptor interactions.

Assessment of Receptor Occupation

We can assay the binding component of ligand-receptor interactions by a variety of techniques, most commonly the use of labeled drugs binding to receptors in intact cells or in subcellular fractions. One widely used approach involves the incubation of a receptor-containing tissue with radioactively tagged drug (radioligand) molecules and subsequent separation and quantitation of bound and unbound radioactive material. The development of radioligand binding methods for a vast number of drug receptors was a major achievement in molecular pharmacology during the middle to late 1970s. Such methods have yielded a large amount of new information regarding biochemical and biophysical properties of receptors and in addition have provided assays required for purification of receptor molecules. A monograph by Limbird provides an excellent description of methods and planning for radioligand binding studies.[51]

Fluorescence, NMR, and other spectroscopic and spectrometric techniques provide alternative means to examine ligand-receptor interactions. These techniques use nondisruptive detection methods (i.e., the free and bound species need not be separated) and allow for continuous monitoring of the kinetics of interaction from a single reaction sample. Further, as alluded to previously, spectroscopy or spectrometry can yield valuable information regarding the bound state of the molecule. However, few molecules have physicochemical characteristics suitable for such detection. One system that has begun to prove amenable to use of cytofluorimetric methods to assess ligand-receptor interactions on multiple intact cells is the f-Met-Leu-Phe receptor, a receptor for chemotactic peptides of human polymorphonuclear leukocytes.[52]

Plotting Methods

Graphical representation provides an important tool for analysis of drug-receptor interactions. Results obtained from kinetic and equilibrium binding studies are the two principal types of experimental data available from such analyses.

Kinetic Analyses

Kinetic analysis involves estimating the rate of formation or breakdown of [LR]. Thus,

$$\frac{d[\text{LR}]}{dt} = k_1[\text{L}][\text{R}] - k_{-1}[\text{LR}] \qquad \text{(equation 14)}$$

so that at equilibrium, $d[\text{LR}]/dt = 0$, and $k_1[\text{L}][\text{R}] = k_{-1}[\text{LR}]$, as described above. Determination of k_1 usually involves assay of the rate of formation of LR by use of labeled L under conditions such that [R] is known and [L] >> [R]. These so-called pseudo-first-order conditions simplify estimates of k_1 by keeping [L] essentially constant during the formation of LR, while [R] decreases as LR is formed. Under these conditions

$$\ln\frac{[\text{LR}]_{\text{eq}}}{([\text{LR}]_{\text{eq}} - [\text{LR}]_t)} = (k_1 [\text{L}] + k_{-1})t \qquad \text{(equation 15)}$$

As shown in Figure 1-25, plotting LR as a function of time yields an asymptotic relationship for the formation of LR as equilibrium is approached ([LR]$_{\text{eq}}$), and when data are plotted logarithmically (inset, Fig. 1-25), this approach to equilibrium is described by a straight line whose slope is $(k_1[\text{L}] + k_{-1})$ and whose intercept is zero. The value of k_1 can be determined from this expression either by using independent estimates of k_{-1} (as described below) or by estimating the rate of formation of LR at several different concentrations of L and then calculating k_1 and k_{-1} from the slope and intercept of a plot of the formation rate of LR versus [L].

The rate constant for receptor-ligand dissociation k_{-1} is determined experimentally by blocking further formation of LR after a certain amount has been formed (conventionally estimated as the amount at steady state) by infinite (greater than 100-fold) dilution or by addition of a large excess of unlabeled competing ligand if LR is radiolabelled. Thus, equation 1-14 reduces to

$$\frac{d[\text{LR}]}{dt} = -k_{-1}[\text{LR}] \qquad \text{(equation 16)}$$

As shown in Figure 1-26, the exponential rate of decay of LR and k_{-1} can be estimated from the slope of the logarithmic plot of this decay.

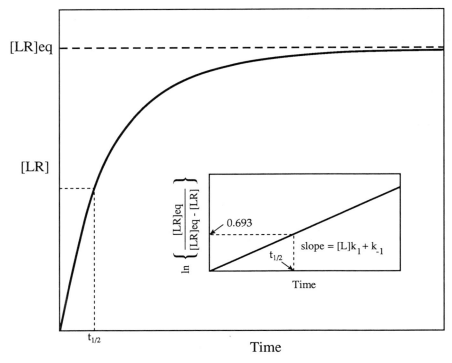

Fig. 1-25. Rate of association of a ligand and receptor to form a ligand-receptor complex. Tissue receptors (R) are incubated with radioligand (L), and bound complex (LR) is determined at various times. Under the conditions such that $[L] \gg [R]$ (i.e., pseudo-first-order conditions), the logarithm of the fractional approach to equilibrium ($[LR]_{eq}$) is linear, as shown in the inset, with slope = $k_1[L] + k_{-1}$.

Equilibrium Binding Analysis

As indicated above, $k_{-1}/k_1 = K_D$, and thus kinetic studies can permit estimation of K_D as an overall measure of the binding reaction. Equilibrium binding studies provide an alternative means for determining K_D as well as an experimental approach to the further characterization of the properties of receptor binding sites. Incubation of a fixed concentration of receptor with varying concentrations of radiolabeled ligand under equilibrium binding conditions is the typical protocol used to determine K_D. Several graphical means are commonly utilized to analyze such data, including linear, semilogarithmic, Scatchard, double reciprocal, and Hill plots (Figs. 1-27 to 1-31), although an approach that is increasingly used involves computer-assisted fitting of data to various possible models.[53]

The linear plot is the most direct means of graphing experimental data. As shown in Figure 1-27, data from binding studies require values for both total binding and nonspecific binding. Nonspecific binding is the "noise" attributable to usually lower affinity interaction of drug with sites other than the specific receptor site of interest. Nonspecific binding is usually determined in the presence of a high concentration of unlabeled drug or preferably of another chemically distinct receptor-specific compound and is typically nonsaturable and a linear function of drug concentration. Subtraction of values for the nonspecific binding from those for total binding yields the *specific binding*, which appears to reach a plateau or saturation value. The plateau of this line, which is the maximum

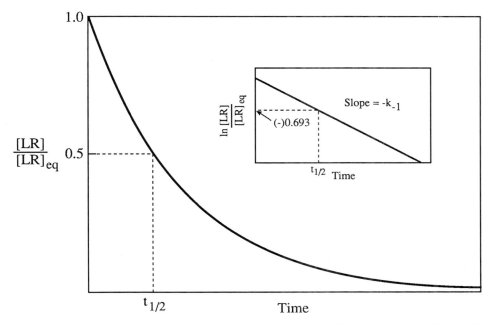

Fig. 1-26. Rate of dissociation of ligand-receptor (LR) complex. Tissue receptors (R) are first incubated with ligand (L). At zero time, association of R and L is blocked, and dissociation of [LR] is measured at various times. This dissociation event is a first-order process and therefore is linear on a natural logarithm of 2 semi-logarithmic plot (inset). The half-life of LR is ln $2/k_1$ or $0.693/k_1$.

amount of drug bound, $[LR]_{max}$ or B_{max}, is approached asymptotically and thus is difficult to measure from a linear plot. K_D, which can be determined as the free ligand concentration [L] at which [LR] is 50 percent of $[LR]_{max}$, is also difficult to define with accuracy and precision from the linear plot.

Plotting logarithmically transformed values of [L] versus [LR] (Fig. 1-28A) yields a sigmoidal curve for LR formation when the law of mass action applies to a single class of binding sites. The advantage of the semilogarithmic plot in which the logarithmic scale is on the abscissa is that one can visualize binding processes when the concentrations of various ligands differ from each other by several orders of magnitude. As with the linear plot, however, one must usually extrapolate to determine $[LR]_{max}$ value at the upper plateau of the curve. Nevertheless, the semilogarithmic plot is a very useful method and the most widely employed means to analyze data from pharmacologic studies in which a response (rather than "bound ligand") is measured and then plotted as a function of agonist concentration. In these log dose versus response curves one commonly plots response as a percentage or fraction of the maximal response (Fig. 1-28B).

A commonly employed graphical transformation that can be used to convert the curves of the linear or semilogarithmic plots of binding data into straight lines is the Scatchard method. The Scatchard plot was originally derived for the binding of ligands to a class of independent sites, which all possess an identical K_D for the ligand.[54,55] At a particular unbound ligand concentration $[L]_{free}$:

$$K_D = \frac{\left(\dfrac{LR_{max}}{R_{total}} - \dfrac{LR}{R_{total}}\right)[L]_{free}}{\dfrac{LR}{R_{total}}} \qquad \text{(equation 17)}$$

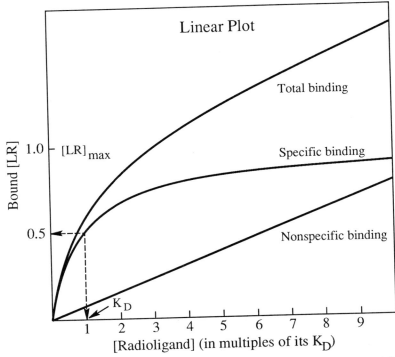

Fig. 1-27. Linear plot of saturation binding isotherm for ligand-receptor binding. Tissue receptors (R) are incubated with various concentrations of radioligand (L), and bound radioligand (LR) is determined after equilibrium is achieved. The reaction is measured in the absence (total binding) and presence (nonspecific binding) of a compound known to occupy the receptor sites. Subtracting values for nonspecific binding from total binding yields specific binding. At $[L] = K_D$, the receptors are half-saturated relative to LR_{max}.

where LR_{max}/R_{total} is the maximal attainable amount of ligand bound per unit receptor protein, LR/R_{total} is the amount of ligand bound per unit receptor at the molar concentration of free ligand $[L]_{free}$, and $[R]$ is the molar concentration of receptor. Thus (LR/R_{total}) $[R]$ is the molar concentration of bound ligand and $(LR_{max} - LR/R_{total})$ $[R]$ is the molar concentration of unoccupied sites. Rearrangement of this equation yields

$$\frac{LR}{R_{total}} \cdot K_D = \frac{LR_{max}}{R_{total}} \cdot [L]_{free} - \frac{LR}{R_{total}} [L]_{free}$$

or

$$\frac{\dfrac{LR}{R_{total}}}{[L]_{free}} = \frac{\dfrac{LR_{max}}{R_{total}}}{K_D} - \frac{\dfrac{LR}{R_{total}}}{K_D} \qquad \text{(equation 18)}$$

then

$$\frac{[LR]}{[L]_{free}} = \frac{[LR]_{max}}{K_D} - \frac{[LR]}{K_D}$$

An alternative derivation of the Scatchard plot is to consider $\bar{Y}$ as the fractional saturation of R with L so that

$$\bar{Y} = \frac{[LR]}{[R]_{total}} = \frac{[LR]}{[LR]_{max}} \qquad \text{(equation 19)}$$

Log-Linear Plot

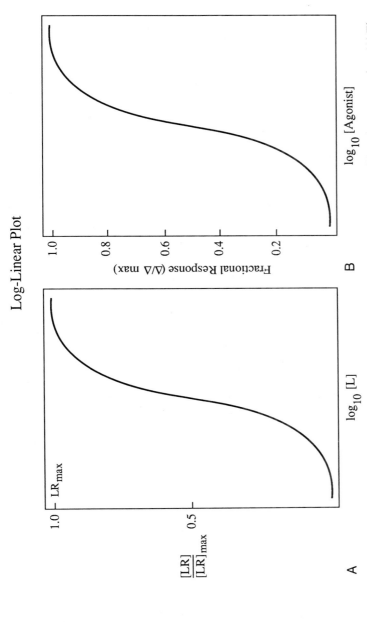

Fig. 1-28. Semilogarithmic plot of ligand-receptor binding and of drug response as a function of ligand concentration. (**A**) Tissue receptors (R) are incubated with various concentrations of radioligand L, as described in Fig. 1-27. (**B**) Drug response is plotted as a function of agonist concentration. In both panels, drug (ligand or agonist) concentration is expressed in logarithmic units.

where $[R]_{total}$ = total concentration of receptors. In this formulation $[LR] = \overline{Y} \cdot [R]_{total}$ and $(1 - \overline{Y})$ is the fraction of unoccupied receptors such that $[R] = (1 - \overline{Y}) \cdot [R]_{total}$. Thus, the rate of association $= k_1[L][R] = k_1[L](1 - \overline{Y})[R]_{total}$ and the rate of dissociation $= k_{-1}[LR] = k_{-1}(\overline{Y})[R]_{total}$.

At equilibrium, when the rate of association equals the rate of dissociation

$$k_1[L](1 - \overline{Y})[R]_{total} = k_{-1}\overline{Y}[R]_{total} \qquad \text{(equation 20)}$$

which can be rearranged to

$$\overline{Y} = \frac{k_1[L]}{k_{-1} + k_1[L]} \qquad \text{(equation 21)}$$

and in turn to

$$\overline{Y} = \frac{[L]}{\dfrac{k_{-1}}{k_1} + [L]} = \frac{[L]}{K_D + [L]} \qquad \text{(equation 22)}$$

or

$$[LR] = \frac{[L][R]_{total}}{K_D + [L]} \qquad \text{(equation 23)}$$

This formulation, which is that for a rectangular hyperbola, explains the asymptotic nature of $[LR]_{max}$ when data are plotted as in Figure 1-27. Equation 1-23 can also be rearranged so that $[LR]_{max} = [R]_{total}$ and

$$\frac{[LR]}{[L]} = \frac{[LR]_{max} - [LR]}{K_D} = \frac{[LR]_{max}}{K_D} - \frac{[LR]}{K_D} \qquad \text{(equation 24)}$$

which is identical to equation 1-18. This equation can be plotted in the form of a line with $[LR]/[L]$ (bound/free) ligand or drug as a function of $[LR]$, the bound ligand or drug. As shown in Figure 1-29, the line derived from the data obtained when a given ligand L, interacts with a single class of receptors that possess a single affinity for the ligand is a straight line with a slope of $-1/K_D$. The intercept on the abscissa is $[LR]_{max}$, and the intercept on the ordinate is $[LR]_{max}/K_D$. Although the Scatchard plot used in drug-receptor binding studies is not identical to that which Scatchard originally derived,[54] it provides a useful means to determine values for both K_D and $[LR]_{max}$. As will be discussed subsequently, curvilinear Scatchard plots are sometimes obtained in studies with receptors, and there are a variety of explanations for this result.

Another linear transformation of receptor binding data is the double reciprocal plot. Equation 1-23 is quite similar to the Michaelis-Menten equation, which characterizes the interaction of enzyme (E) and substrate (S) to form an enzyme-substrate complex (ES) and in turn a product (P):

$$E + S \underset{k_{-1}}{\overset{k_1}{\rightleftharpoons}} ES \overset{k_2}{\longrightarrow} E + P \qquad \text{(equation 25)}$$

Enzyme velocity (v) as a fraction of maximal velocity (v_{max}) can be expressed by

$$\frac{v}{v_{max}} = \frac{[S]}{K_m + [S]} \quad \text{with } K_m = \frac{k_{-1} + k_2}{k_1} \qquad \text{(equation 26)}$$

K_m and K_D have the same units, and when $k_2 < k_{-1}$, K_m will equal K_D, the dissociation

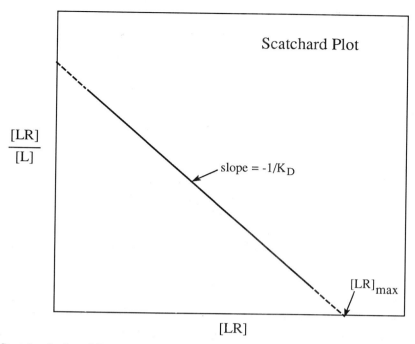

Fig. 1-29. Scatchard plot of ligand-receptor binding. Data derived from an experiment like that in Figure 1-27 have been plotted as bound/free or [R]/[L] versus bound or [LR]. The intercept on the abscissa is $[LR]_{max}$ and the slope is $-1/K_D$. The dotted parts of the line represent extrapolations for which experimental data have not been obtained.

constant of a substrate. However, from a mechanistic perspective the two constants are designed to quantitate quite different processes—the concentration of substrate at which its enzymatic transformation to a product is one-half the maximal rate versus the equilibrium dissociation constant for a ligand receptor complex. Even so, just as plotting the reciprocal values of v as a function the reciprocal value of [S] (Lineweaver-Burke plots) is a widely used method to ascertain K_m (the intercept on the abscissa, $-1/K_m$) and v_{max} (the intercept on the ordinate), the double reciprocal method can be used to determine K_D and $[LR]_{max}$, as shown in Figure 1-30. Reciprocal plots are not generally used with pharmacologic data, primarily because these studies are often conducted over wide concentration ranges, where reciprocals are subject to broad error ranges, especially at lower ligand concentrations.[55] The wide concentration ranges commonly employed in pharmacologic studies also preclude plotting reciprocal values on the same coordinates.

The semilogarithmic and the Scatchard plots have an additional advantage in that the bounds of error are not enlarged excessively at small or large values on the abscissa. With both plots the errors are smallest near 50 percent occupation or response but do increase somewhat at small or large values; however, the large bias in error seen in the reciprocal plot when [L] is small and 1/[L] is large is not evident. Several studies have analyzed the relative errors inherent in data plotting by logarithmic, reciprocal, and Scatchard plots.[55–57]

The Hill plot is another linear transformation of data obtained in studies assessing receptor binding or drug responses. This method of data analysis was originally developed

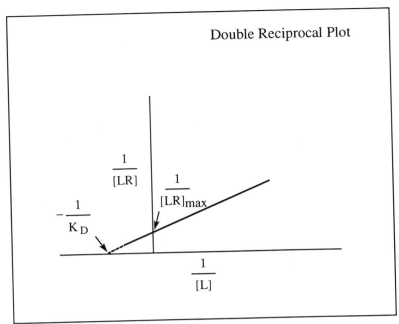

Fig. 1-30. Double reciprocal plot of ligand-receptor binding. Data derived from an experiment like that in Figure 1-27 have been plotted in double reciprocal format; the intercept on the abscissa is $(-1/K_D)$ and that on the ordinate ($1/[LR]$). The dotted portions of the line represent extrapolated values for which experimental data have not been obtained.

by A. V. Hill in attempting to define the cooperative binding of oxygen to hemoglobin.[51,58] The Hill formulation, now used as an empiric means of analyzing data, is

$$[LR] = \frac{[L]^n \cdot [LR]_{max}}{K_D{}^n + [L]^n} \qquad \text{(equation 27)}$$

This equation is analogous to equation 1-23 except that $[L]$ and K_D now have the exponent n. This exponent can be any positive value. Formal considerations now show that n cannot exceed the number of binding sites but may be less than an integral number. Equation 1-27 is a general equation that describes settings in which binding sites can interact ("cooperate") with another. General mechanisms of cooperativity will be considered in a subsequent section. Thus, the value for n, more commonly designated n_H, the Hill coefficient, is a measure of this cooperativity. The Hill equation can be rearranged to

$$\frac{[LR]}{([LR]_{max} - [LR])} = \frac{[L]^n}{K_D{}^n} \qquad \text{(equation 28)}$$

and taking the common logarithm of both sides

$$\log \left[\frac{[LR]}{([LR]_{max} - [LR])} \right] = n \log [L] - n \log K_D \qquad \text{(equation 29)}$$

Therefore a plot of $\log [[LR]/([LR]_{max} - [LR])]$ as a function of $\log [L]$ yields a line whose slope is n_H (also called the Hill slope) and whose intercept on the ordinate is $-n \log K_D$ (Fig. 1-31). When a ligand binds to a single class of noninteracting ("noncoopera-

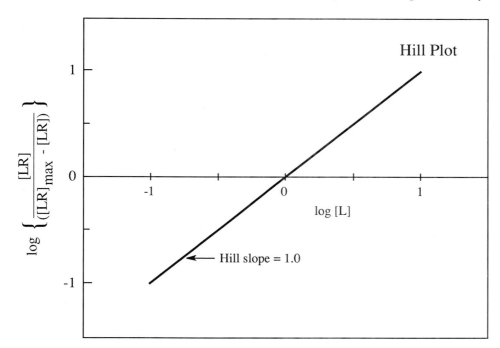

'ig. 1-31. Hill plot of ligand-receptor binding. Data derived from an experiment like that in Figure -25 have been plotted in the Hill format, a type of log-logit plot. Values for the ligand L are plotted 1 logarithmic units such that the intercept on the abscissa equals K_D, because when [LR] = 0.5 LR]$_{max}$, the value of the ordinate is 0. The slope of the line in the Hill slope is 1.0, indicating no cooperativity in the binding of L to R.

ive'') receptors, this binding is described by the law of mass action, n_H = 1.0. When n_H > 1.0, this indicates positive cooperativity, whereby occupancy of one binding site by a gand enhances the likelihood that other coupled sites on the same oligomeric molecule vill preferentially bind the same ligand or a related ligand. When n_H < 1.0, several ex-lanations are possible, including negative cooperativity (where a linkage between sites xists and occupation of one site decreases the likelihood that other sites on the same ligomeric molecule will bind the ligand) and multiple classes of noninteracting or non-nterconvertible binding sites. If n_H > 1 or n_H < 1, one observes curvilinear Scatchard lots. In settings with n_H > 1.0, Scatchard plots are convex upward, while in settings vith n_H < 1.0, Scatchard plots are concave upward.

An important operational feature of the Hill plot relates to the concentration range of .R that can be meaningfully evaluated by this graphical method. At both low (≤ 20 ercent) and high (≥ 80 percent) fractional occupation of R, there is considerable error 1 accurately estimating the value of log [LR]/([LR]$_{max}$ − [LR]) because either the nu-merator or denominator is a small value, and the logarithmic relationship amplifies the rror. In addition, at low fractional occupation all the sites are effectively unoccupied, nd binding of multiple ligand molecules to the oligomer is a low probability event, whereas t high fractional occupation, very large concentration changes are required to achieve aturation. Thus, accurate estimates of n_H cannot be made with observations at the two extremes of fractional occupation of R by L. In fact, slopes of Hill plots tend to converge on 1.0 when fractional occupation either is very low or approaches saturation.

An additional feature to note is that $n_H = 1.0$ when the concentration range corresponding to 10 to 90 percent occupancy is slightly less than two orders of magnitude (81-fold to be exact). When a greater concentration range is needed, n_H is < 1.0, and if a smaller concentration range is needed, n_H is > 1.0.

Competitive Binding

Other types of data can be readily generated in equilibrium binding studies of receptors. The most important of these studies are competitive binding experiments that ascertain the specificity of the interaction between a radioligand and its binding site(s) by examining the ability of various drugs, hormones, or neurotransmitters to compete with a radiolabeled or other reference probe for the binding sites. Typically, these experiments are performed by incubating a constant concentration of radioligand with numerous concentrations of an unlabeled compound under equilibrium binding conditions and then determining the amount of labeled probe specifically bound. Results of such experiments are usually plotted in terms of specific binding expressed as a percent of control value (i.e., in the absence of competitor) on the ordinate against the logarithm of the concentration of competitor (Fig. 1-32). Several key features can be noted for the data obtained in competitive binding experiments, namely, the potency, extent, and concentration range of a ligand or series of ligands in competing with the labeled probe.

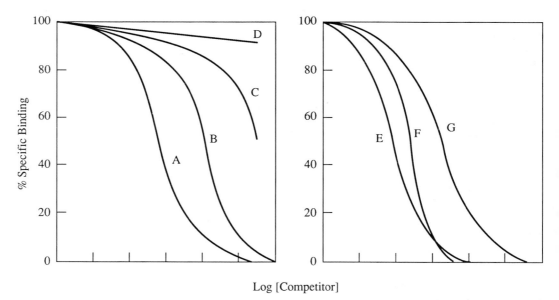

Log [Competitor]

Fig. 1-32. Competitive binding experiments assessing ligand-receptor interaction. A radioligand has been incubated with tissue receptors in the absence and presence of varying concentrations of several compounds (A through G), which compete for the radioligand binding sites. In the left panel, the rank order of potency in competing for sites is A > B > C ≫ D. In the right panel, Drug E competes in a manner compatible with interaction at a single class of sites, while drug F shows a steeper curve and competes over a narrower concentration and drug G shows a shallower curve and competes over a larger range of concentration.

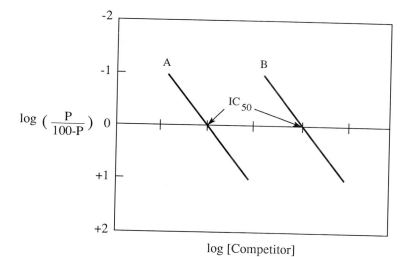

Fig. 1-33. Logit-log plot (pseudo-Hill plot) of competitive binding curves. The specifically bound percentage P for competing drugs A and B is used to calculate log (P/[100 − P]), which is plotted against the logarithm of the concentration of A and B. The intercept on the abscissa is IC_{50}. The slope of the curve is sometimes termed the *pseudo-Hill slope* or *slope factor*.

Potency refers to the concentration of the compound that is effective in competing for labeled sites. Most commonly, one defines the IC_{50} (i.e., the concentration that inhibits specific binding by 50 percent). In a given experiment one might rank a series of candidate competing ligands (as shown in Fig. 1-32) in their order of potency. A commonly used approach involves testing drugs of known selectivity or rank order of potency in eliciting response at a particular class of receptors in order to "prove" that a labeled radioligand is recognizing that class of receptor.

Values for IC_{50} are ascertained by visual inspection (a rather inaccurate technique), by logit-log analyses, sometimes termed pseudo-Hill plots (Fig. 1-33), or by computer-assisted nonlinear regression (the most objective and statistically valid method).[53] The equation of the pseudo-Hill plot is

$$\log \frac{P}{(100 - P)} = n \log[I] + n \log IC_{50} \qquad \text{(equation 30)}$$

where P is the percent competition of specific binding in presence of [I], a given concentration of inhibitor. The slope of the plot of log P/(100 − P) versus − log[I] yields n, which relates K_D to IC_{50} by the relationship $K_{D(apparent)} = (IC_{50})^n$. This expression should be distinguished from the Hill equation (equation 27), in which occupation of a receptor by one compound is examined.

The equilibrium dissociation constant of a competitive inhibitor, generally termed K_I, is a more quantitative property of the ability of a drug to compete for binding site than is the IC_{50}. An experimentally determined IC_{50} depends on K_I, K_D, and the concentrations of labeled and unlabeled ligand used in a given competition experiment. In competitive binding studies obeying the law of mass action, two simultaneous sets of equilibria occur, one for the labeled ligand, $[L] + [R] \rightleftarrows [LR]$ where $K_D = [L][R]/[LR]$ (equation 19), and one for the competitor, $[I] + [R] \rightleftarrows [IR]$. Thus one can define

$$K_I = \frac{[I][R]}{[IR]}$$ (equation 31)

and $$[R]_{total} = B_{max} = [LR] + [IR] + [R]$$

One can combine this equation from the law of conservation of mass with equations 1-23 and 1-31 and after rearrangement obtain

$$[LR] = \frac{[R]_{total} [L]}{K_D (1 + [I]/K_I) + [L]}$$ (equation 32)

This equation shows that values of [LR] that are obtained in competitive binding studies depend on K_D, K_I, [L], and [I]. When no inhibitor is present, equation 32 reduces to equation 1-23. When $[I] = IC_{50}$, [LR] in the presence of I is equal to 0.5 of the [LR] observed in absence of [I], then

$$[LR] = \frac{0.5[L][R_{total}]}{[L] + K_D} = \frac{[L][R_{total}]}{K_D (1 + IC_{50}/K_I) + [L]}$$ (equation 33)

Equation 1-32 can be simplified and solved for K_I:

$$K_I = \frac{IC_{50} \cdot K_D}{[L] + K_D} = \frac{IC_{50}}{1 + [L]/K_D}$$ (equation 34)

This formulation[59,60] is useful for defining values for K_I, although several assumptions are involved. These include: (1) both I and labeled L interact with a single population of R; (2) these interactions are assayed at equilibrium for binding of R with L at all concentrations of I; (3) simple competitive relationships apply; and (4) $[R] \ll K_D$ and K_I. Other calculations are necessary to obtain K_I when these assumptions are not valid.

The extent of competition represents the ability of a competing ligand to compete either fully or only partially for sites identified by a labeled ligand. If the competitor can compete to only a limited extent even at higher concentrations (e.g., compound D in Fig. 1-32), such a compound cannot be considered to bind to the same site as the radioligand.

The *concentration range* over which competition occurs can provide further useful insights into the nature of drug receptors. The 10 to 90 percent range of competition by an unlabeled ligand for sites identified by a labeled probe occurs over an 81-fold concentration range if the interactions represent simple bimolecular reactions (pseudo-Hill slope equal to 1.0). Competitive binding curves that require a larger concentration range for the 10 to 90 percent competition are described by pseudo-Hill slopes of less than 1.0. These competition curves, which are sometimes termed "shallow," are most commonly observed in the setting of multiple classes of binding sites. Multiple classes of binding sites are typically identified in two situations: (1) when a competing ligand selectively recognizes more than one *receptor subtype*, each of which is recognized as identical by the radioligand; and (2) when a competitor can distinguish between *different states of the receptor* that differ in affinity for competitor yet are recognized as identical by the labeled ligand. Experimental data in many different drug-receptor systems have validated the usefulness of competitive binding curves with shallow pseudo-Hill slopes to identify receptor subtypes and/or discrete states of receptors. Different states are most commonly observed in the studies that examine competition by unlabeled agonists for binding sites identified by using labeled antagonists. In such settings receptor states may correspond to different molecular species or conformations of receptors. For example, for receptors linked to guanosine triphosphate (GTP)-binding proteins (G proteins) high-affinity and low-affinity states have been proposed to represent the receptor–G protein complex and the free receptor species, respectively (see Ch. 2).

Quantitation of Agonist Responses

Drug-receptor interactions have been described thus far in terms of assessment of receptor occupation by use of labeled drug molecules. Although examination of receptor binding is very important for molecular characterization of drug receptors, the key feature that distinguishes a true receptor from a binding site is the ability of a receptor to produce an alteration in function of a target cell. Assessment of functional responses is still the principal means by which various classes of drug receptors have been defined. In addition, quantitative evaluation of such responses forms the basis for describing how receptors regulate target cell function.

A.J. Clark[61] described the first equations that relate occupation of receptors by an agonist to response promoted by that agonist. Clark's proposal, the theory of occupancy, provides the simplest, and in some cases an accurate, means of defining the relationship between occupation and response. The key feature of this formulation is that response is proportional to the number of occupied receptors (i.e., a linear relationship exists between binding and response):

$$L + R \rightleftarrows LR \xrightarrow{k_e} \text{response} \qquad \text{(equation 35)}$$

Thus, if k_e is known, for any given [LR] one can predict the extent of response. From the previous discussion of the law of mass action and receptor occupation, it was shown (equation 23) that

$$[LR] = \frac{[L][R]_{total}}{K_D + [L]} = \frac{[L][LR]_{max}}{K_D + [L]} \qquad \text{(equation 36)}$$

Thus, Clark's equation predicts that maximal response Δ_{max} will occur at $[LR]_{max}$ and that at any fraction of $[LR]_{max}$, response Δ will be a fraction of maximal response (i.e., $\Delta/\Delta_{max} = [LR]/[LR]_{max} = [L]/(K_D + [L])$). From this relationship it can be shown that half-maximal response will occur when $[L] = K_D$. Because of the hypothesized proportionality between occupancy and response, one can use the same graphical means to relate [L] to *response* that are used to relate equilibrium *binding* and the kinetics of formation of LR from L and R. Figure 1-28B shows the classical log dose-response curve, although other graphical representations are sometimes used. One of these is the probit plot, which is mathematically similar to the Hill plot and which converts the sigmoidal patterns of log-dose response curves into straight lines, thereby allowing more precise estimates of EC_{50}, the concentration of a drug that elicits a half-maximal response (Fig. 1-34). The slope of the probit plot (akin to a Hill slope) relating [L] to response will be 1.0 for systems that are described by Clark's equation.

The rank order of potency of a series of drugs in eliciting a particular response is a key criterion conventionally used to define different classes of drug receptors. The relative potency of such compounds is usually reported as a comparison of EC_{50} values (note that EC_{50} value for compound A is between one and two orders of magnitude lower than that

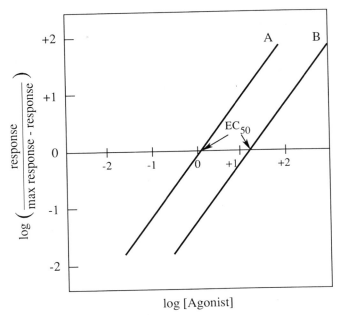

Fig. 1-34. Logit-log (probit) plot to assess agonist response. Responses to agonists A and B as related to maximal response have been used to calculate log (response/[max response-response]), which is plotted against the logarithms of the concentrations of A and B. The intercept on the abscissa is EC_{50}. Note the similarity to the Hill plot shown in Fig. 1-31 and to the plot of competitive interaction shown in Fig. 1-33.

of compound B in Figure 1-34). This method of analysis requires that the agonists that are being compared elicit the same maximal response. If very high concentrations of L are unable to elicit maximal response, rank ordering EC_{50} values will not necessarily reflect receptor occupation. As discussed in the next section, receptor reserves also preclude correlating EC_{50} values with receptor occupation.

Quantitation of Pharmacologic Antagonism

The use of antagonists to block responses elicited by agonists has been one of the principal approaches of classical pharmacology. Such blockade must generally fulfill certain criteria if it is to be useful in examining properties of a single type or subtype of drug receptors where a simple binding relationship exists:

1. Blockade must be selective for the family of agonists acting on this receptor type.
2. Blockade of responses in different tissues by a series of antagonists (if available) should show an identical rank order of potency for individual members of the series. Ideally, a single receptor system in different tissues should show identical values for the K_I of each antagonist (see below).
3. Blockade should be sufficiently rapid so as to allow precise quantitative measurements.

4. In the case of competitive antagonists, blockade of response should be reversible.
5. If a particular competitive antagonist is studied, one should obtain an identical value for its K_I in antagonizing different agonists that act at the same receptor.
6. Values for the dissociation constants (K_I) derived from studies assessing tissue response should be identical to antagonist dissociation constants obtained in studies of binding to a particular type of receptor.

Pharmacologic antagonism can be described by several different criteria: pharmacologic end point, reversibility of the interaction, mutual interaction at the same site, and linkages between binding sites. These criteria may be used to distinguish the following types of antagonism: functional, irreversible, competitive, noncompetitive, and mixed.

Functional Antagonism

Functional antagonism is defined as antagonism of tissue response that is unrelated to blockade at drug receptors but instead represents blockade of tissue response at a site distal to receptors. This precludes its precise quantitation or delineation of its site of action. Functional antagonists may or may not affect second messenger production. *Nonspecific antagonism* which might depress all cellular excitability by affecting the energy charge, physicochemical state of the membrane, or capacity to generate second messengers, is one type of functional antagonism. General anesthetics, which may act to perturb overall membrane structure and function (see below), would be an example of such functional antagonism. Agonists producing opposing actions through different receptors would be another example. Thus, agonists that promote relaxation of smooth muscle are functional antagonists of agonists that promote smooth muscle contraction.

Competitive Antagonism

Competitive antagonists are ligands that compete with agonists, usually for a common binding site in a receptor. The following scheme describes the response to an agonist L in the presence of antagonist I where k_e is a proportionality constant or function relating fractional occupancy and response:

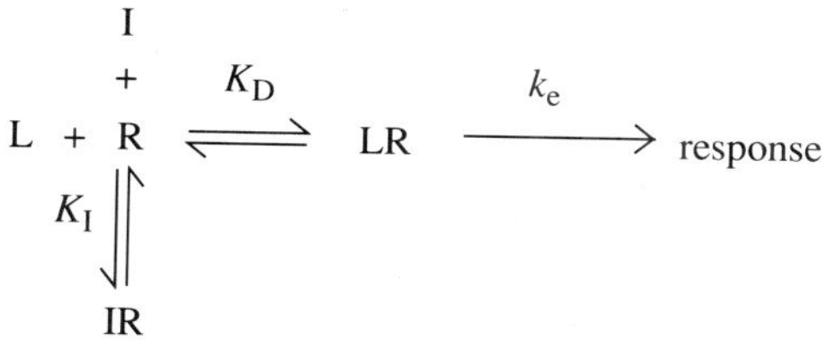

$$
\begin{array}{ccccc}
 & \text{I} & & & \\
 & + & K_D & & k_e \\
\text{L} + \text{R} & \rightleftharpoons & \text{LR} & \xrightarrow{} & \text{response} \\
K_I \Big\updownarrow & & & & \\
 & \text{IR} & & &
\end{array}
$$

Then

$$
\frac{\Delta}{\Delta_{max}} = k_e \left(\frac{[LR]}{[R]_{total}} \right) = k_e \left(\frac{[LR]}{[R] + [LR] + [IR]} \right)
$$

$$
= k_e \left(\frac{[L][R]/K_D}{[R] + [L][R]/K_D + [I][R]/K_I} \right)
$$

$$
= k_e \left(\frac{[L]/K_D}{1 + [L]/K_D + [I]/K_I} \right) \qquad \text{(equation 46)}
$$

$$
= k_e \left(\frac{[L]}{[L] + K_D (1 + [I]/K_I)} \right)
$$

This equation is analogous to equation 1-32, and it can be seen that the extent of competitive antagonism depends on both the agonist and antagonist concentrations and their dissociation constants.

In the presence of the competitive inhibitor I, fractional occupation $[LR]/[LR]_{max}$ decreases as a consequence of an increase in the *apparent* equilibrium dissociation constant of the agonist L from a value of K_D in the absence of inhibitor to a value of $K_D (1 + [I]/K_I)$ in the presence of I. The increase in apparent dissociation constant by the factor $(1 + I/K_I)$ yields an equation with the same incremental concentration dependence on [L]; only the constant has changed. Hence, rightward and parallel shifts in agonist dose–response curves as a function of increasing [I] are observed without a decrease in maximal response (Fig. 1-35 left panel). Since the competitive antagonist acts simply by excluding agonist from binding, it should not change the relationship between agonist occupation and response elicited. Accordingly, at equal fractional occupancies, equal responses should be observed. When Δ/Δ_{max} in the absence of competitor equals Δ'/Δ_{max} in the presence of competitors [I], then

$$\frac{[L]}{[L] + K_D} = \frac{[L']}{[L'] + K_D (1 + [I]/K_I)} \qquad \text{(equation 47)}$$

Here [L] and [L'] are the respective concentrations of L required to generate equivalent responses Δ/Δ_{max} and Δ'/Δ_{max} in the absence and presence of [I]. By rearrangement, this equation becomes

$$\frac{[L']}{[L]} - 1 = \frac{[I]}{K_I} \qquad \text{(equation 48)}$$

In this formulation K_I can be determined regardless of the value of K_D for the agonist.

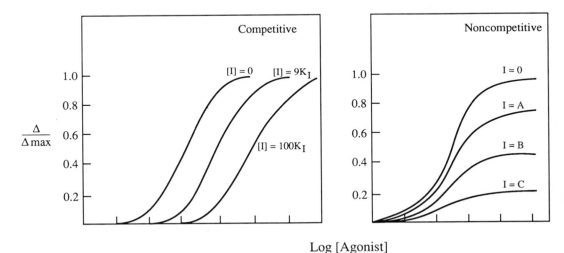

Log [Agonist]

Fig. 1-35. Analysis of antagonism by semilogarithmic plots. The left panel shows the pattern for competitive antagonism of a response to an agonist produced by increasing concentration of competitive inhibitor I. A parallel rightward shift in the response curve without a change in maximal response occurs. The extent of rightward shift is a consequence of the ratio of [I] to K_I, the equilibrium dissociation constant of the inhibitor. The right panel shows the pattern expected for noncompetitive antagonism, in which the maximal response decreases, without a change in the concentration producing half maximal-response, as the inhibitor concentration increases, A < B < C.

The term *dose ratio* is applied to the expression [L′]/[L] (commonly referred to as D'/D, where D refers to agonist concentrations). Dose ratios depend only on the concentration of antagonist I and its dissociation constant K_I. A caveat to the use of this equation is that the dose ratio for an antagonist is independent of the agonist provided that the agonist is acting on a single receptor type. Schild[62] was the pharmacologist who pointed out the usefulness of analyzing data from studies with antagonists by determining dose ratios. The basic procedure can be regarded as a *null procedure*, in which equivalent responses are analyzed in the presence and absence of antagonist. Schild defined the pA_x as the negative logarithm of an antagonist concentration that yielded a dose ratio of x. Thus, taking the logarithm of both sides of equation 48 yields

$$\log \left(\frac{[L']}{[L]} - 1 \right) = \log [I] - \log K_i \qquad \text{(equation 49)}$$

$$\text{or} \quad \log (x - 1) = - \log K_I - pA_x \qquad \text{(equation 50)}$$

When the dose ratio $x = 2$, $pA_2 = - \log K_I$, since $\log 1 = 0$. The concentration of antagonist that yields a dose ratio of 2 (i.e., causes twofold shift to the right in agonist dose-response curve) is equal to K_I.

As shown in Figure 1-36 (left) the Schild plot is a graph of values for log (dose ratio -1) as a function of log [I]. The intercept on the abscissa is $- \log K_I$ or pA_2, and the slope is -1. Alternatively, equation 50 can be plotted in a form, sometimes termed the Schild regression, in which the intercept on the abscissa is K_I and the anticipated slope is 1 for competitive antagonist (Fig. 1-36 right). These linear transformations of data from studies of functional response tested in the presence of various concentration of antagonist readily permit determination of K_I or pA_2. A number of technical or tissue-specific problems[63] (e.g., inadequate equilibration times, uptake or degradation of antagonist, or interaction of antagonist with uptake or degradation sites or with sites that release endogenous agonist) can contribute to the generation of nonlinear Schild plots, plots with

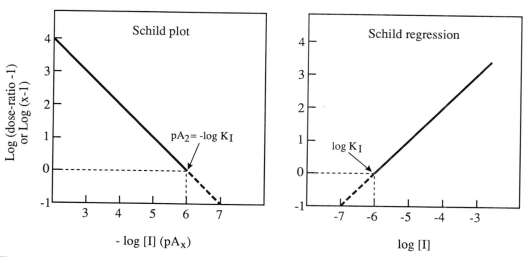

Fig. 1-36. Schild plot to assess competitive antagonism. Data for competitive antagonism by an inhibitor I can be analyzed by the Schild plot (left panel) in which the logarithm of the dose ratio, also called x as defined in the text, minus 1 is plotted as a function of the negative logarithm of [I], also known as pA_x. The intercept pA_x of the extrapolated subsample value on the abscissa at a dose ratio of 2, is equal to $- \log K_I$. On the right panel, response data are plotted as a function of log [I], and the Schild regression yields K_I as the intercept on the abscissa.

slopes other than 1.0, or difficulties in equating pA_2 with K_I. Nevertheless, this approach is a standard and reliable means of estimating antagonist dissociation constants or potencies from experiments in which agonist responses are blocked.

There are alternative means to analyze competitive antagonism, although these are not generally used in pharmacologic studies. One of these is the double reciprocal (Lineweaver-Burke) method, which can be used to show a change in K_D (derived from the intercept on the abscissa) without a change in maximal response (from the intercept on the ordinate). See Figure 1-37.

Noncompetitive Antagonism

A nonconpetitive antagonist produces quantitative changes in the agonist dose-response curves that involve parameters different from those affected by competitive antagonists. Thus maximal response is decreased, but the EC_{50} of the agonist is not changed (Fig. 1-35, right). One model for such antagonism is as follows:

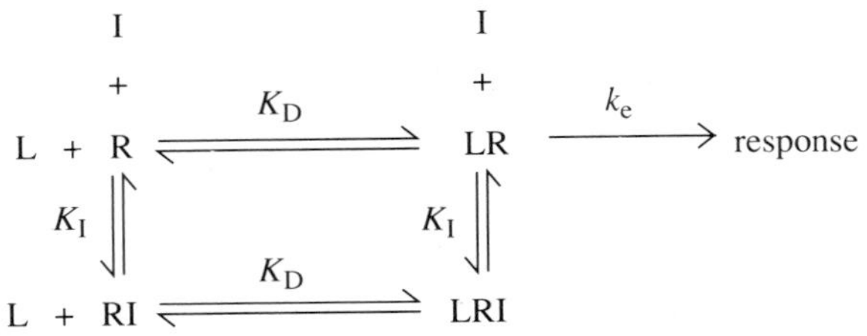

$$
\begin{array}{ccccc}
I & & & I & \\
+ & & & + & \\
L + R & \underset{K_D}{\overset{K_D}{\rightleftharpoons}} & LR & \xrightarrow{k_e} & \text{response} \\
K_I \updownarrow & & K_I \updownarrow & & \\
L + RI & \underset{K_D}{\overset{K_D}{\rightleftharpoons}} & LRI & &
\end{array}
$$

The antagonist does not alter the concentration of bound agonist ([LR] + [LRI]), but the LRI complex is nonfunctional. The response to agonist, which is proportional to [LR], is decreased. The relationship for noncompetitive antagonism may be derived as follows:

If

$$\frac{\Delta}{\Delta_{max}} = k_e \left(\frac{[LR]}{[R]_{total}} \right)$$

then

$$\frac{\Delta}{\Delta_{max}} = k_e \left(\frac{[LR]}{[R] + [LR] + [IR] + [ILR]} \right)$$

$$= k_e \left(\frac{\dfrac{[L][R]}{K_D}}{[R] + \dfrac{[L][R]}{K_D} + \dfrac{[I][R]}{K_I} + \dfrac{[I][L][R]}{K_I K_R}} \right)$$

$$= k_e \left(\frac{\dfrac{[L]}{K_D}}{1 + \dfrac{[L]}{K_D} + \dfrac{[I]}{K_I} + \dfrac{[I][L]}{K_I K_D}} \right) \qquad \text{(equation 51)}$$

$$= k_e \left(\frac{[L]}{K_D + [L] + K_D \dfrac{[I]}{K_I} + \dfrac{[L][I]}{K_I}} \right)$$

$$= k_e \left(\frac{[L]}{([L] + K_D) \left(1 + \dfrac{[I]}{K_I} \right)} \right)$$

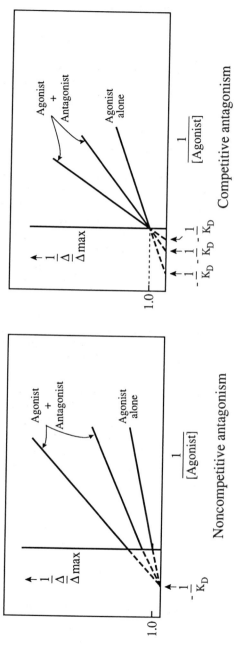

Fig. 1-37. Analysis of antagonism by double reciprocal plots. Noncompetitive antagonism: The lower line represents data obtained with agonist alone, and the upper lines are data for agonist in the presence of two different concentrations of antagonist. Δ_{max} is changed by each antagonist concentration, but K_D remains apparently the same. Competitive antagonism: Δ_{max} is unchanged in the presence of antagonist, but each antagonist concentration yields an apparently different value of K_D.

As shown in equation 1-51, the response is decreased by a factor whose magnitude is increased by [I] and by low values of K_I (i.e., high affinity of the antagonist). For noncompetitive antagonists $K_I = IC_{50}$, the concentration of antagonist that inhibits the response 50 percent.

Graphical analysis can be used to discriminate between competitive and noncompetitive antagonism. Both the semilogarithmic plot (Fig. 1-35, right) and the double reciprocal plot (Fig. 1-37, left) indicate a decrease in maximal response without a change in K_D. Noncompetitive antagonism occurs most commonly by an inhibitor binding a site other than the agonist binding site and acting allosterically to modulate coupling of binding with the response.

Irreversible and Pseudoirreversible Antagonism

Some types of antagonists produce irreversible antagonism of agonist-mediated responses (i.e., antagonism that persists after repeated washing of a target tissue to remove antagonist free in solution). This is most commonly observed when an antagonist produces a covalent modification in a receptor. Such antagonists have been identified for many different types of receptor systems (e.g., phenoxybenzamine for α_1-adrenergic receptors, propylbenzilylcholine mustard for muscarinic acetylcholine receptors). Irreversible antagonism will yield curves identical to those for noncompetitive antagonism if the response is proportional to the number of receptors occupied by agonist. As we will see in subsequent sections, if the receptor number exceeds that necessary for a full response, irreversible antagonism will shift the dose-response curve to higher concentrations (rightward shift) without depressing the maximal response.

Competitive antagonists are also able to produce irreversible (more appropriately termed pseudoirreversible) antagonism if they are tightly bound to the receptor and do not dissociate within the time frame of measurement of the agonist response. The data may give the appearance of noncompetitive antagonism. Alternatively, antagonists can be sequestered in a tissue and thus be difficult to remove by washing, thereby producing higher local concentrations ("unstirred layers") of antagonist. Tissue-localized compartments in which drugs act have been termed the *biophase*, a concept that reflects the nonuniformity of tissue compartments into and out of which drugs can diffuse or be taken up; drugs are thought to be readily accessible to receptors and therefore functionally active in only certain of these compartments. Thus far, rigorous identification of such biophases has not been possible.

Noncompetitive, irreversible, and pseudoirreversible antagonism share the common properties of not regaining the original response by addition of higher agonist concentrations. This behavior is sometimes referred to as *nonsurmountable antagonism*.

Mixed Antagonism

Mixed antagonism is observed for antagonists that can have multiple types of interaction with receptor systems. In some cases an antagonist may initially block receptors in a competitive manner, but with increasing time of incubation blockade can become irreversible and give the appearance of being noncompetitive. An example is the β-haloalkylamine phenoxybenzamine, which initially blocks α-adrenergic receptors competitively but subsequently alkylates and thereby blocks these receptors.[64,65]

Another reaction scheme that can produce mixed antagonism is the following:

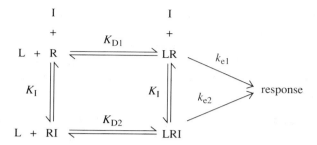

whereby an inhibitor I can react with receptors in either agonist-bound LR or free R forms, the agonist L can react with either inhibitor-bound RI or free R, and both LR and LRI are able to produce a response. Depending on the values for K_{D1}, K_{D2}, k_{e1}, and k_{e2}, a variety of different responses might be produced. For example, if $K_{D2} > K_{D1}$ and $k_{e2} < k_{e1}$, mixed antagonism will occur such that the agonist EC_{50} value will be increased and the response to maximally effective concentration of agonist will be decreased.

Still another scheme for mixed antagonism is actually a hybrid of competitive and noncompetitive antagonism. In noncompetitive antagonism, K_I is identical for I binding to R and LR, and K_D is identical for L binding to R and IR. For competitive antagonism, L will only bind to R and not to IR, and I will also bind to R but not to LR. Hence K_D and K_I are dissociation constants for only the LR and IR species, respectively, and do not describe ligand association to form a ternary complex. Mixed antagonism can result from a situation intermediate between competitive and noncompetitive antagonism where in the scheme

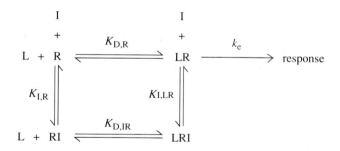

$K_{D,R} < K_{D,LR}$ and $K_{I,R} < K_{I,LR}$. This relationship of dissociation constants will also apply to mixed antagonism in which a depression of the maximum response and a shift of the half-maximal responses to higher agonist concentrations will be seen.

Partial Agonists

Partial agonists were defined in the beginning of this chapter, and a quantitative formulation of the behavior of a partial agonist is detailed in the receptor theory section. Partial agonists may elicit distinct molecular events; for example, a partial agonist may induce a conformation in the receptor that is intermediate between the conformations induced by agonists and antagonists. Alternatively, the partial agonist may only partially shift the equilibrium in receptor states between active and inactive states (two or more conformational states). Finally, the ligand could bind to two discrete sites on the receptor, of which one elicits activation of the receptor and the other serves to diminish the response. For example, binding to the agonist site may open the channel, while binding to the channel itself partly occludes it (multiple sites of ligand binding for activation and inhibition).

KINETICS AND ENERGETICS OF LIGAND-MACROMOLECULE COMPLEX FORMATION

As mentioned in the previous section, the fraction of ligand bound to the receptor, its rate of binding (association), and the rate of dissociation are important to analyzing drug-receptor interactions. Both the fraction bound at equilibrium and the binding rates depend on free energy considerations for the system. Accordingly, it becomes important to understand the relationship between free energy and the equilibrium dissociation constants and rate constants.

Equilibrium Thermodynamics

Several concepts that arise from fundamental physicochemical principles can be generalized for ligand-macromolecule complexes. Given the reaction

$$\text{L} + \text{R} \underset{k_{-1}}{\overset{k_1}{\rightleftharpoons}} \text{LR} \qquad \text{(equation 9)}$$

as before, we can define the equilibrium dissociation constant in terms of

$$K_{\text{D}} = \frac{[\text{L}][\text{R}]}{[\text{LR}]} = \frac{k_{-1}}{k_1} \qquad \text{(equation 13)}$$

Equilibrium constants are governed by the energetics of the interaction (i.e., the differences in free energy between the conditions in which all reactants are free and in which the binding sites are fully occupied). Hence, equilibrium constants can be related to the free energy of reaction ΔG (the change in free energy of the system produced by the reaction) by

$$K_{\text{D}} = e^{-\Delta G/RT} \qquad \text{(equation 52)}$$

or
$$\ln K_{\text{D}} = -\Delta G/RT \qquad \text{(equation 53)}$$

where ΔG is the free energy of reaction, R is the gas constant 1.98 cal/degree·mole, and T is the absolute temperature. Thus, for every 10-fold change in K_{D} at 37°C (310K), ΔG amounts to 1.4 kcal/mole. The system of interacting species always seeks a minimal free energy. Hence the lower the ΔG value on a free energy profile (i.e., the larger the negative value), the greater the stabilization energy of the complex and the higher the fractional population of complex versus free species.

Free energy may be defined in terms of temperature-dependent and temperature-independent terms as follows:

$$\Delta G = \Delta H - T\Delta S \qquad \text{(equation 54)}$$

The enthalpy of interaction ΔH primarily reflects the energetics of bond making and

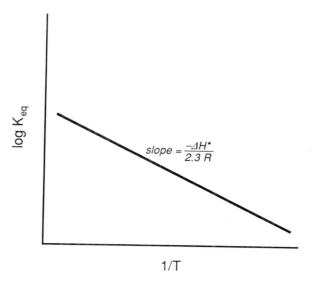

Fig. 1-38. Van't Hoff plot used to determine the enthalpy and entropy of a reaction at equilibrium. T is in degrees, Kelvin. Since the slope shown yields a positive enthalpy (ΔH), this reaction is driven by a positive entropy value (ΔS). Reactions driven by a negative enthalpy would have a positive slope. Since equation 54 may be rearranged to log $K_{eq} = \dfrac{-\Delta H}{2.3\ RT} + \dfrac{\Delta S}{2.3\ R}$, the intercept on the ordinate is $\Delta S/2.3\ R$.

breaking, whereas the entropy change ΔS reflects the change in degree of order of all molecular structures, including solvent, accompanying the reaction. Stabilization of a complex through a hydrogen bond, for example, will yield a negative ΔH and hence a favorable energy of interaction. Likewise, complex formation may be favored by increasing the disorder or randomness of the system (a positive ΔS). Thus, providing more degrees of freedom for the solvent H_2O leads to a positive increase in entropy and a favorable, or more negative, free energy of reaction. This might be envisioned in the situation where water molecules assist the reaction by forcing two hydrophobic surfaces together, thus maximizing the number of potential hydrogen bonds that the H_2O molecules form and increasing the degree of freedom of the H_2O molecules.

Several drug-receptor interactions have been analyzed to ascertain thermodynamic parameters.[66,67] The procedures involve plotting the logarithm of the dissociation constant against reciprocal temperature (equation 1-53). A simplified relation is shown in Figure 1-38. ΔH can be ascertained from the slope of the plot and ΔS from the intercept on the abscissa. Thermodynamic parameters have been analyzed for agonist and antagonist binding to receptors, but it should be recognized that ΔH and ΔS reflect the global changes of all interactions in such systems. Contributions to binding energy are not only due to interactions between the ligand and its binding site but in addition conformational changes in the receptor, changes in associated solvent, changes in membrane state, and association or dissociation of linking proteins all can contribute to the thermodynamic parameters. Hence, contributions of the thermodynamic parameters to particular processes or steps can only be inferred from differences between values for individual ligands. Determination of specific molecular forces involved is usually not possible from an analysis of the thermodynamics in such complex systems.

Free Energy of Activation and the Reaction Kinetics Profile

Kinetic constants can be related to energetic parameters in a manner analogous to that used to relate equilibrium dissociation constants to the free energy of the reaction. Hence, absolute rate theory predicts for the association and dissociation rate constants.[66]

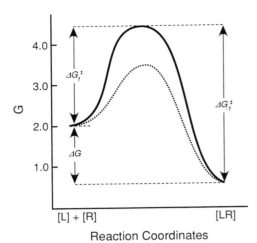

Reaction Coordinates

Fig. 1-39. Relationship between the free energy of complex formation ΔG and the free energies of activation for the association $\Delta G_1\ddagger$ and the dissociation $\Delta G_{-1}\ddagger$ for a slowly (solid line) and for a rapidly (dashed line) associating and dissociating complex. The two complexes have equivalent free energies of equilibrium binding.

$$k_1 = \frac{RT}{nh} e^{-\Delta G_1^{\ddagger}/RT} \qquad \text{(equation 55)}$$

and

$$k_{-1} = \frac{RT}{nh} e^{-\Delta G_{-1}^{\ddagger}/RT} \qquad \text{(equation 56)}$$

where n is Avagadro's number, h is Planck's constant, R is the gas constant, T is the absolute temperature, and $\Delta G^{\ddagger}_1$ and $\Delta G^{\ddagger}_{-1}$ are free energies of activation for the association and dissociation steps. The expression RT/nh is directly proportional to the rate constant and depends on temperature and the three constants defined above. From

$$K_D = \frac{k_{-1}}{k_1}$$

and from the exponential relationships between kinetic and equilibrium constants and free energies of activation and equilibrium, respectively

$$\Delta G = \Delta G^{\ddagger}_{-1} - \Delta G^{\ddagger}_1 \qquad \text{(equation 57)}$$

The relationship between the free energy of activation for association and dissociation and the overall free energy of the reaction can be plotted along hypothetical reaction coordinates as shown in Figure 1-39.

In the two reaction profiles shown by the solid and dashed lines the ΔG values are equivalent; thus both reactions have identical equilibrium dissociation constants K_D. Also, as shown in Figure 1-39, LR at equilibrium will be the predominant species, since it has a lower free energy than dissociated L and R. If ΔG were -1.4 kcal/mole at 37°, LR would be favored over the dissociated species L and R by a factor of 10 at the concentration of reactants employed.

The two profiles, however, reveal very different free energies of activation, which may be viewed as the activation barriers that must be transcended in the association and dissociation processes. The greater the activation energy, the slower the reactions of both association and dissociation. It also can be seen that the same ratio k_{-1}/k_1, despite differences in absolute values of numerator and denominator, will yield the same difference between $\Delta G^{\ddagger}_{-1}$ and $\Delta G^{\ddagger}_1$. Accordingly, at equilibrium the same ratio of reactants to product would exist, and the two reactions would only differ by the time required to achieve equilibrium following a perturbation of the equilibrium condition or admixture of the reactants.

Since

$$\Delta G_1^\ddagger = \Delta H_1^\ddagger - T\Delta S_1^\ddagger \qquad \text{(equation 58)}$$

upon separation of the free energy of activation into its temperature-dependent and temperature-independent components, the rate constant may be related to the enthalpy and entropy of activation as follows:

$$k_1 = \frac{RT}{nh} e^{-\Delta H_1^\ddagger/RT} e^{\Delta S_1^\ddagger/R} \qquad \text{(equation 59)}$$

Since the Arrhenius activation energy, E_a, is defined as

$$\frac{d\ln k_1}{dT} = \frac{E_a}{RT^2} \qquad \text{(equation 60)}$$

one finds that the enthalpy from absolute rate theory can be related to the free energy of activation by the relationship

$$\Delta H_1^\ddagger = E_a - RT \qquad \text{(equation 61)}$$

The energy maximum for each reaction profile reflects the transition state for complex formation. Although we cannot establish a physical picture for a ligand and macromolecule at this point in the reaction coordinate for ligand-receptor complex formation, some general principles can be developed for the association and dissociation steps.

Kinetics of Association of the Complex

In our simple scheme, association is a bimolecular process. If each collision between ligand and macromolecule were productive and resulted in formation of a complex, the association process would be controlled by diffusional translocation of the ligand in the medium. Hence, the activation energy would be that for moving a solute through water. Typically, diffusion-controlled reactions in aqueous solvents have enthalpies of activation between 2.0 and 2.5 Kcal/mole, yielding relatively low temperature coefficients for association. Associations occurring at rates slower than the diffusion rate reflect additional energy requirements in complex formation. These requirements could arise from several sources. Should the site on the receptor binding the ligand be located within a cleft, diffusion will be limited by geometric limitations on the angle of access or on the tortuosity of the diffusional pathway. The ligand may have certain orientational constraints such that only collisions with a certain orientation are productive. Similarly as we have observed, a population of ligand conformations may exist, collisions with only particular conformations being productive. Analogous arguments can be advanced for conformational states of the macromolecule.

Kinetics of Dissociation of the Complex

Dissociation shown in the mass action scheme of equation 1-9 is a simple unimolecular process and can be viewed as the probability that the ligand molecule with a given kinetic energy will leave the energy well on the macromolecular surface on which it resides. Those molecules acquiring sufficient energy will transcend the barrier and dissociate into the medium. The higher the barrier, the less likely will be the molecule to acquire sufficient thermal energy to ascend the barrier and hence the slower the rate of dissociation. Usually the dissociated ligand is thought to enter the bulk solvent phase rather than a separate compartment where reassociation is more probable.

Theoretical constructs have also been developed for collision-limited reaction rates and for diffusion-limited dissociation of ligands from restricted compartments; however, the number of biologic systems where restricted or buffered diffusion may exist and that are accessible to rapid detection methods is limited.[69,70]

The Reaction Pathway

The pathway of complex formation also influences the energetics of formation and dissociation of the complex. For example, additional energy is required when the receptor species able to accept the ligand is not the abundant species in absence of a ligand or when the ligand induces a change in conformation of the macromolecule upon complex formation. The scheme in equation 62 shows the receptor in two states. If we assume that the R form or state of the receptor is in greater abundance than R' in the absence of ligand and that LR' is a more stable complex than LR, the reaction will proceed as a two-step process, and at high ligand concentrations the overall rate may be limited by either of the isomerization steps $R \rightleftarrows R'$ and $LR \rightleftarrows LR'$. It may then be possible to detect both binding and isomerization steps in the reaction.

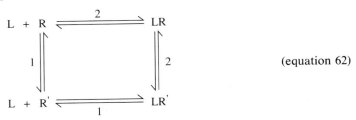

(equation 62)

Does the ligand select the receptor in a conformation R' acceptable for forming the stable complex LR' (pathway 1) or does the ligand combine with the R state of the receptor to form LR and then isomerize to form the more stable complex LR' (pathway 2)? Such questions have an important bearing on the nature of the transition states but can only be approached by methods that can detect short-lived transients in the reaction pathway.

Diffusion-Controlled Complex Formation

Theoretical considerations of diffusion-controlled reactions have allowed investigators to estimate the limitation of diffusion on reactions, which may be developed as follows.[71,72] If we assume that a ligand of radius r_L will combine with a receptor site of radius r_R (Fig. 1-40), then

$$k_1 = \frac{4\pi r_R D_L n}{1,000}$$

(equation 63)

where k_1 is the bimolecular rate constant for association in units of $M^{-1} sec^{-1}$, n is Avagadro's number, and D_L is the diffusion coefficient of the ligand. D_L can be defined by the Stokes-Einstein equation

$$D_L = \frac{kT}{6\pi r_L \eta}$$

(equation 64)

where k is the Boltzmann constant, T the absolute temperature, and η the solvent viscosity. Substitution for D_L yields

$$k_1 = \frac{2RT}{3,000} \cdot \frac{r_L}{r_R}$$

(equation 65)

Should r_R and r_L be of comparable value as reflected in Figure 1-40, then

$$k_1 \simeq 2.5 \times 10^9 M^{-1} sec^{-1}$$

(equation 66)

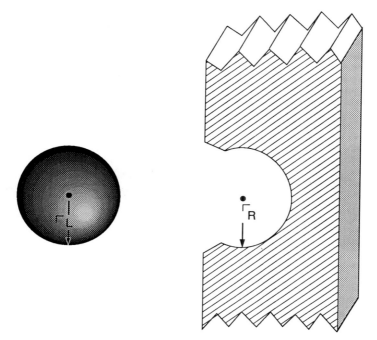

Fig. 1-40. Model for a diffusion-controlled reaction in which a spherical ligand of radius r_L combines with a receptor site of radius r_R. See text for details.

These theoretical estimates of the rates of diffusion-controlled reactions have been borne out in estimates of carbon dioxide association with carbonic anhydrase and of oxygen with hemoglobin. Few detailed kinetic studies of agonist interactions with receptors have been reported, but voltage-jump relaxation, single channel recordings, and stopped-flow measurements of association of acetylcholine with the nicotinic receptor have yielded values near 10^8 $M^{-1}sec^{-1}$ for the bimolecular association constants, about one order of magnitude below the theoretical diffusion-limited rate (cf. Ch. 2). This is to be expected because of the nonspherical nature of the ligand and a presumed limited sector of access to the binding site. Rates of association approaching the diffusion limitation are also evident for amino acid agonists at their respective receptors.

By contrast, the elapid (snake venom) α-toxins, which are peptide antagonists at the nicotinic receptor, show rates of association of ~10^5 $M^{-1}sec^{-1}$ (four orders of magnitude below that predicted for a diffusion-limited reaction). The large activation barrier for association indicates that substantial changes in conformation occur in the α-toxin, the receptor, or both upon association. The α-toxins also exhibit extremely high affinities (i.e., low dissociation constants). To accommodate these values dissociation rates must also be extremely slow with half-lives ($t\frac{1}{2}$) of several hours to days, and in fact it is the low rates of dissociation that have made the α-toxins, which may be radiolabeled, useful for identifying the receptor in vitro and in situ.

Competitive antagonists at other types of receptors also exhibit rates of association well below those predicted for diffusion and those found for agonists on the same receptor. For example, the benzilylquinuclidines (antagonists at muscarinic acetylcholine receptors) and prazosin (an antagonist at α_1-adrenergic receptors) have equilibrium dissociation con-

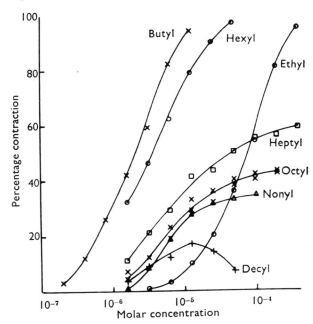

Fig. 1-41. Dose-response relationships generated for a series of C_2 through C_{10} alkyltrimethylammonium ions on guinea pig ileum. The ethyl through hexyl congeners produce maximal responses while the heptyl through decyl agents produce smaller than maximal responses and are termed *partial agonists.* (From Stephenson,[81] with permission.)

stants near 1.0×10^{-10} M. Their association rate constants are in the vicinity of 10^6 to 10^7 M^{-1} sec^{-1}. Given these values, dissociation rate constants would be predicted to be 10^{-3} to 10^{-4} sec^{-1}. These findings have been verified in both isolated preparations and intact cells. Rate constants of this magnitude will give a $t\frac{1}{2}$ for dissociation of several minutes. A knowledge of these values is important to the design and interpretation of pharmacologic experiments. For example, if prazosin has a dissociation rate constant of 4×10^{-4} sec^{-1} ($t\frac{1}{2} \simeq 30$ minutes), and after equilibration with prazosin responses to agonists are measured in a much shorter time frame (say 1 minute), prazosin antagonism will appear irreversible instead of reversible since its dissociation rate is far slower than the agonist response rate. Also, in equilibrium binding experiments, the dissociation rate constant is the important determinant in dictating equilibration times. In a bimolecular association–unimolecular dissociation reaction, the rate constant for equilibration equals k_1 [L] + k_{-1}, and under conditions such that [L] is less than K_D, the rate constant for equilibration equals k_{-1}. Hence the *minimal* rate of equilibration is determined by k_{-1}. At a time equal to $1/k_{-1}$, the fractional approach to equilibrium will be 0.63 of that achieved at complete equilibration.

RECEPTOR THEORY

The first reference to the principles of mass action and antagonism of responses in relation to drug action came from Langley's 1878 studies,[73] in which he examined the antagonism of pilocarpine by atropine in salivary glands and heart. In 1904 Langley[74] defined *receptive substances* as the sites of action of these agents and many other alkaloids he had studied in the interim. While studying antagonism by nicotine and curare, Langley also suggested that the receptive substances could exist on the muscle surface and that the transmission of an impulse from nerve to muscle involves neural secretion of a chemical substance rather than mediation via an electrical discharge. These concepts were also germinal to the concepts of chemical neurotransmission put forward by Langley and his student Eliott.

During this period Ehrlich[75,76] was studying the chemical specificity of tissue-selective dyes, the antimicrobial activity of arsenicals, and the process of immunity development by formation of antitoxins. On the basis of different apparent degrees of reversibility of the reactions, he initially envisioned that antitoxins and drugs may act differently. Nevertheless, he contended that specificity resided in the rule; *Corpora non agunt nisi fixata* "agents cannot act without binding." His later contributions drew closer parallels between the toxin receptors and chemoreceptors. Ehrlich and Langley recognized each other's contributions to the development of receptor theory. Interesting accounts of the development of receptor theory and chemical neurotransmission concepts may be found in several recent texts.[77,78]

As mentioned earlier, *occupation theory*, as originally proposed by Ehrlich and developed quantitatively by Clark,[79] simply regarded fractional occupation of receptors as proportional to the biologic response. Thus, occupation theory permitted prediction of responses from the ligand concentration and an apparent dissociation constant but provided no means of distinguishing between agonists, partial agonists, and antagonists.

Receptor Reserve and Spare Receptors

Clark, Ariens, and other investigators[79,80] recognized the limitations of directly equating fractional occupation and biologic response, but significant quantitative modifications of occupation theory did not develop until Stephenson[81] in the mid-1950s analyzed a series of dose-response relationships that were difficult to rationalize on the basis of occupation theory. He applied to the muscarinic receptor in guinea pig ileum a series of alkyltrimethylammonium ligands of the following general structure:

$$CH_3-(CH_2)_n-\overset{\overset{\displaystyle CH_3}{|}}{\underset{\underset{\displaystyle CH_3}{|}}{N_{(+)}}}-CH_3 \qquad \text{where} \qquad n = 1 \text{ to } 9$$

His experimental data revealed three findings that led him to conclude that receptor occupancy alone could not account for agonist potency. First, within a congeneric series of alkyltrimethylammonium ions, full agonist activity was seen with increasing potency from $n = 1$ (ethyltrimethylammonium) to $n = 5$ (hexyltrimethylammonium). Then, although the threshold dose remained low, compounds of increasing chain length showed a diminishing maximal activity. It appeared that there was a conversion from the behavior of full agonists to that of partial agonists and then to that of a nearly complete antagonist. As chain length increased, threshold responses nevertheless occurred in a progressively lower concentration range (Fig. 1-41). The data for $n = 6$ to $n = 9$ could be interpreted in terms of an increased affinity of the alkytrimethylammonium ligands concomitant with a diminished capacity to confer a response as chain length increased.

For those agents not eliciting a full response (heptyl through decyl) it was possible to determine their dissociation constants by a procedure analogous to the dose ratio methods

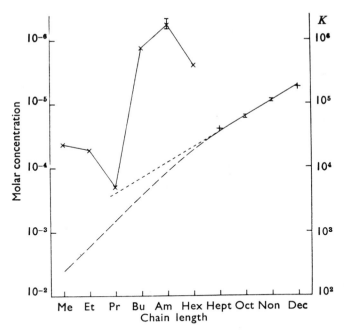

Fig. 1-42. A comparison of the calculated association constant K (equivalent to $1/K_D$) (right ordinate) for partial agonists with the molar concentrations giving half-maximal responses (left ordinate). The association constants for the partial agonists could be ascertained from their capacity to block the response of a full agonist. It was reasoned that one might observe a smooth progression of dissociation constants for a series of congeneric compounds. Since the concentrations for achieving 50% of a maximal response are lower than the dissociation constants predicted by extrapolation, lower occupancies might be required to achieve these responses. (From Stephenson,[81] with permission.)

described previously. The determined dissociation constants for the partial agonists directly reflect receptor occupation since a null procedure is employed to obtain equiactive concentrations of a full agonist in producing an additional incremental response in the presence and absence of a partial agonist. Hence, the Schild method can be applied to assess occupation of partial agonists by their capacity to shift the responses of the test agonist to higher concentrations. This approach cannot be applied to determination of dissociation constant of full agonists since the test agonist has no capacity for an additional response.

If we assume that 50 percent occupancy by full agonists also yields a 50 percent response, then the concentration yielding a 50 percent response might be expected to fall upon the extrapolated line of the logarithm of concentration versus chain length (Fig. 1-42). The observation that concentrations lower than those predicted by the extrapolation are necessary to elicit a response for the full agonists with shorter alkyl chains suggests that fractional occupancies of receptors by full agonists might be smaller than their fractional responses.

Second, Stephenson observed that if butyltrimethylammonium (a full agonist) and octyltrimethylammonium (a partial agonist) were added together at concentrations giving near maximal responses when each is added alone, the response of the combination of agents was closer to that for octyltrimethylammonium than to that for butyltrimethylam-monium.

Third, following addition of atropine a far longer time was necessary for washing out an effective concentration of antagonist when stimulation by octyltrimethylammonium was compared with stimulation by butyltrimethylammonium. Accordingly, recovery of the response after washout of atropine appeared to be more rapid when the test agonist was a full agonist.

From these findings Stephenson reasoned that the potency of agonists could be deter-mined by two properties, their affinity and their capacity to confer a response. The latter property he defined as *efficacy*. Both affinity and efficacy can be dependent on the ligand as well as on the receptor subtype.

Since the maximal response elicited by agonist was increased as chain length was short-ened, the enhanced capacity to confer a response at a fixed fractional occupation may continue to increase even after chain length is sufficiently short to obtain a full response. If so, a situation could exist where occupation of less than 100 percent of the receptors gives a full response. This consideration would be consistent with the trends in structure-activity relationships seen in Figures 1-41 and 1-42.

The results of Stephenson's second experiment can be rationalized in the following manner. If different fractional occupations of two agonists will give the same response, simultaneous addition of two agonists will yield primarily the response of the ligand with the greater occupation. Accordingly, the agonist with the greater fractional occupation (i.e., the partial agonist when compared with a full agonist) will dominate the composite response, as Stephenson observed with the combination of octyl- and butyltrimethylam-monium.

Finally, upon washing the preparation in the third experiment, atropine should vacate its occupied sites at a rate independent of the agonist, but, when near maximal concen-trations of agonist are employed, the agonist requiring occupation of the smaller fraction of receptors to achieve an equivalent response will demonstrate the more rapid apparent rate of response recovery.

Stephenson developed the following equation to explain his observations:

$$\frac{\Delta}{\Delta_{max}} = f(S) = f\left[\epsilon\left(\frac{[LR]}{[R_t]}\right)\right] = f\left[\epsilon\left(\frac{[L]}{K_D + [L]}\right)\right] \qquad \text{(equation 67)}$$

Here the fractional response is a function of a stimulus S, which, in turn, is related to the product of the fractional receptor occupation $[LR]/[R_t]$ and the efficacy ϵ. Fractional occupation can then be related to the ligand concentration and the dissociation constant K_D by our previous considerations. Efficacy is a ligand-dependent quantity, which con-notes the efficiency of transducing ligand occupation into the stimulus S. Importantly, the function that relates the stimulus to the fractional response is not linear but approaches a maximum value asymptotically (Fig. 1-43); thus, as long as the product of efficacy and occupation is sufficiently large, a maximal response can be achieved regardless of the magnitudes of the individual values. Fractional occupation extends between values of zero and unity, but in theory the range of efficacy values can be much larger. Should efficacy be of sufficient magnitude, it is no longer necessary to have a high fractional occupation to elicit a maximal or near maximal response. Stephenson defined an agonist with an efficacy of 1.0 as one in which full occupation will yield a 50 percent response.

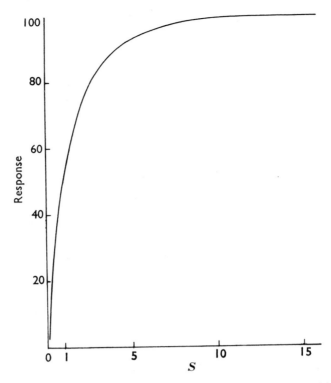

Fig. 1-43. Functional relationship between the stimulus and response proposed by Stephenson. The stimulus is the product of efficacy and fractional occupation, and a full response is denoted by 100. (From Stephenson,[81] with permission.)

In a series of hypothetical curves he showed how a change in efficacy will affect the position of the dose-response curve and hence the apparent potency of an agonist (Fig. 1-44). From these suggestions he predicted that the alkyltrimethylammonium compounds of shorter chain length would have sufficiently large efficacies that full occupation was not necessary to achieve a maximal response.

By using partial agonists to block the response of full agonists, Stephenson was able to rank the affinities or dissociation constants of partial agonists. By substitution into equation 1-67 the relative efficacies of the partial agonists could also be determined. Stephenson's analysis did not extend to quantitating affinity and efficacy of full agonists. Nevertheless, his formulation of efficacy could account for the differential capacities of agonists and antagonists to transduce occupation into a response. Importantly, his theoretical considerations predicted *receptor reserves* or *spare receptors* for the muscarinic receptors in guinea pig ileum.

Subsequent studies by Stephenson and his colleagues measuring tissue responses to rapid- and slow-acting agonists and antagonists have yielded kinetic profiles that are entirely consistent with the view that distinct fractional occupations for two agonists can elicit equivalent responses.[82,83] Analysis as presented in these references of the basis for the onset and offset of the intensity of response provides a worthwhile exercise in understanding the original formulations of the spare receptor concept.

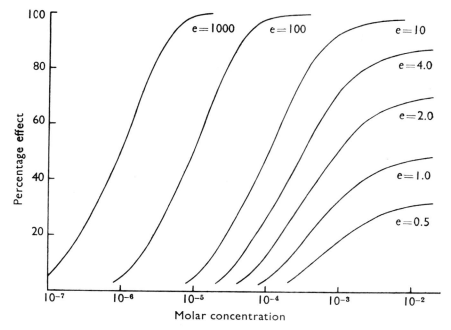

Fig. 1-44. Hypothetical dose-response curves generated by a series of agonists with differing efficacies and a dissociation constant of 10^{-3}M. An efficacy of 1.0 is defined for an agonist giving a 50 percent response at saturating concentrations. (From Stephenson,[81] with permission.)

Quantitation of Receptor Reserves

In subsequent studies Furchgott[84] extended the Stephenson concept of efficacy to quantitate efficacies and dissociation constants (K_D's) for full agonists. His approach permitted assessment of whether the relative potencies of agonists are reflected in their affinity or efficacy. To accomplish this, he reasoned that fractional inactivation of the receptor by an irreversibly acting compound would affect the dose-response relationship in a manner dictated by the receptor reserve. Hence, by diminishing the number of receptors, the shape of the dose-response curve that would be generated could predict the extent of receptor reserve.

Consider a simplified model of a cellular system composed of 10 identical receptors, in which a partial agonist A and three full agonists B, C, and D stimulate the 10 receptors (Fig. 1-45). The partial agonist can occupy all 10 receptors, yet not elicit a maximum response. Agonist B requires occupation of all 10 receptors to achieve a full response. Agonist C requires occupation of five receptors, and agonist D requires occupation of a single receptor for a full response. From a simple dose-response analysis it is only possible to determine fractional occupation for the partial agonist A by the dose ratio procedure outlined by Stephenson. Without a means for measuring receptor occupation, the products of efficacy and occupation for B, C, and D are not separable into their components on the basis of their responses.

Upon irreversible inactivation of the receptors, it becomes possible to determine fractional occupation and to rank the efficacies for the three agonists. If 50 percent of the receptors are inactivated, the maximal response of the partial agonist A and full agonist B will be reduced by 50 percent, since only one-half of the receptors necessary to achieve

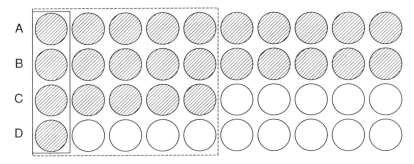

Fig. 1-45. Hypothetical model for a receptor system in which the occupation-response relationship is dependent on the agonist, partial agonist, and antagonist.

the original response are now present on the cell. For agonist C sufficient receptors to achieve a full response are still present, but now 100 percent occupation of the remaining receptors is necessary to accomplish this. On the basis of statistical mechanical considerations, a higher concentration of agonist will be required to occupy 100 percent than 50 percent of a field of receptors despite the requirement for an identical number of occupied receptors to achieve the same response. Thus, the dose-response curve will shift to the right. Similar behavior will occur with agonist D, yet a more substantial receptor reserve exists. Upon inhibition of 90 percent of the receptors, the maximal responses to agonists B and C will be approximately 10 and 20 percent of the original response, respectively. Agonist D will still elicit a nearly full response despite a rightward shift of the curve. Thus, following irreversible inactivation, the extent of a rightward shift of the dose-response curve without a depression of the maximum response will reflect the receptor reserve, and a ranking of efficacy can be achieved. Drawing the dose-response curves for agonists B and D (Fig. 1-46) reveals the dissociation constants and degree of receptor reserve for each. For agonist B no receptor reserve is present, as adduced from the absence of a rightward shift. The dissociation constant can be ascertained from the value on the abscissa, at which the response is 50 percent of maximal. In the case of C and D, the dissociation constant would be reflected in an extrapolated value achieved by convergence of the concentrations yielding 50 percent of the maximal responses with successive irreversible blockade of the receptors.

Dibenamine, an alkylating agent, was used by Furchgott to inactivate muscarinic receptors from the stomach fundus muscle, and dose-response curves were generated following alkylation of increasing fractions of the receptor population. Furchgott used the term *intrinsic efficacy*, which is equal to efficacy as defined by Stephenson divided by the total receptor number.[84]

Prior to alkylation

$$\frac{\Delta}{\Delta_{max}} = f\left[\epsilon\left(\frac{[LR]}{[R_t]}\right)\right] = f\left[\epsilon\left(\frac{[L]}{K_D + [L]}\right)\right] \qquad \text{(equation 68)}$$

Following inactivation, q is the fraction of receptors remaining and $[L^*]$ the ligand concentration

$$\frac{\Delta^*}{\Delta_{max}} = f\left[\epsilon q\left(\frac{[L^*]}{K_D + [L^*]}\right)\right] \qquad \text{(equation 69)}$$

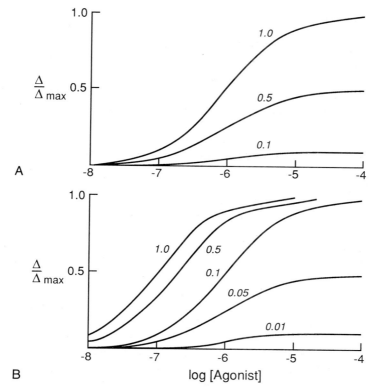

Fig. 1-46. Dose-response relationships for two receptor systems; **(A)** agonist B in Fig. 1-45; occupation of 100 percent of the receptors is necessary to achieve a full response, **(B)** agonist D in Fig. 1-45; occupation of 10 percent of the receptors will yield a full response. In both cases the dissociation constant is 10^{-6} M. (It should be noted that in the actual experimentation the transition from a rightward shift of the curve to depression of a maximum response may not be as abrupt as shown). The numbers above each curve show the fraction of receptors remaining after irreversible inhibition.

If we then equate responses prior to and after alkylation,

$$f\left[\epsilon\left(\frac{[L]}{K_D + [L]}\right)\right] = f\left[\epsilon q\left(\frac{[L^*]}{K_D + [L^*]}\right)\right] \qquad \text{(equation 70)}$$

Since we assume that alkylation will not affect either the coupling function between stimulus and response or the efficacy term

$$\frac{[L]}{K_D + [L]} = q\left(\frac{[L^*]}{K_D + [L^*]}\right) \qquad \text{(equation 71)}$$

Rearranging yields

$$\frac{1}{[L]} = \frac{1 - q}{q K_D} + \frac{1}{q[L^*]} \qquad \text{(equation 72)}$$

Thus a plot of $1/[L^*]$ on the abscissa versus $1/[L]$ on the ordinate will yield a slope of $1/q$ and intercept on the ordinate of $(1 - q)/q K_D$.

Hence q and K_D can be determined directly. Moreover, efficacies may be ranked for a series of agonists. Fig. 1-47 shows data obtained for the stomach fundus muscle and the analysis of efficacy and affinity. Shown in Table 1-2 are the values for several cholinergic agonists. Two means of validation reveal self-consistency in the approach. First, the relative efficacies and dissociation constants of the ligands examined agree with the predictions of Stephenson for relative efficacy and affinity. Second, since the efficacy of pilocarpine differs substantially from that of acetylcholine, it is to be expected that a reduction of receptor number to small fractions of those originally present could reduce pilocarpine's responses while still maintaining a full response to acetylcholine. Thus, after alkylation of a sufficient number of receptors to virtually eliminate the pilocarpine response, it should be possible to employ pilocarpine as a reversible antagonist of acetylcholine. The K_D for pilocarpine determined by the dose ratio method discussed previously for reversible antagonists agrees closely with that obtained by analysis of dose-response curves prior to and following receptor alkylation. Furchgott also conducted studies with α-adrenergic receptors and found that efficacy among full agonists varied far less than in the case of cholinergic agonists.[85]

Several caveats in the interpretation of these data were noted in the original studies and should be borne in mind. First, the irreversible agent used to diminish receptor number should only affect the number of sites but not affect the dissociation constant or the efficacy of the remaining sites. This is self-evident in the equations, since upon equating responses (equation 1-70), the functional relationship between stimulus and response, the efficacy terms, and the dissociation constants are identical and therefore should not be affected by the alkylating agent. Second, the population of responding receptors being rendered inactive should be homogeneous. Radioligand binding techniques now permit analysis of receptor numbers upon covalent inactivation, and receptor number can be compared with the pharmacologic response. In general, muscarinic cholinergic receptors in smooth muscle show substantial receptor reserves.[84,85] By contrast, there is little evidence for substantial receptor reserves in α-adrenergic receptors.[86,87]

Spare Receptors in Subcellar Systems

Simplified models for analysis of spare receptors can be developed from the analysis of the function of receptors in subcellular organelles or isolated reconstituted systems. They also illustrate two other principles important to the quantitation of receptor occupation and response. First, occupation and response should be measured over the same time interval, and second, keeping this measurement interval short (and approximating initial rate conditions) avoids complications of nonlinearity of response. Receptors can rapidly change conformational states in response to agonist occupation, and changes in state are often reflected in the ligand dissociation constant, the ratio of active to inactive species of the receptor, and the coupling to the effector molecule. Hence, one strives to achieve a constant response during the interval of agonist exposure although this is not always feasible. For example, this might be accomplished by demonstrating linearity of agonist-elicited mediator generation or ion permeability during the interval of agonist occupation.

In an elegant demonstration of an apparent receptor reserve, Neubig and Cohen[88] have shown that shifts of dose-response curves quantitatively similar to those obtained by Furchgott could be achieved by inactivating nicotinic receptors with α-bungarotoxin in sealed membrane vesicles and then generating dose-response curves to carbamylcholine. The vesicles are small, and the large surface area to volume ratio ensures that rapid

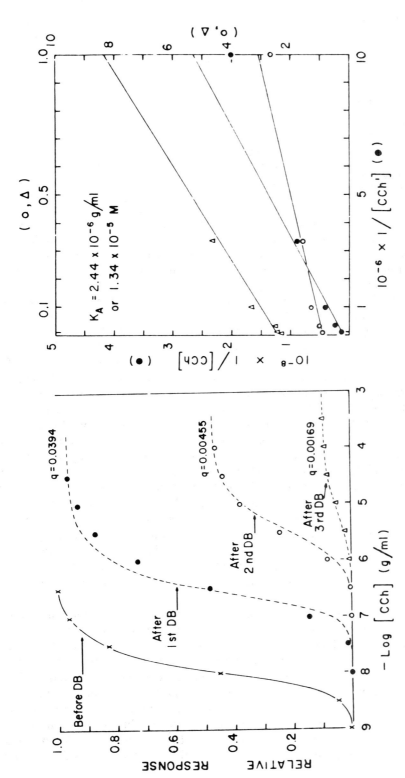

Fig. 1-47. Determination of the dissociation constant K_A for carbamylcholine (CCh) prior to and after each of three successive exposures to dibenamine (DB), and irreversible antagonist. Contractile responses on stomach fundus muscle are measured on the ordinate of the left panel and q represents the fraction of receptors remaining. In the right panel, the reciprocal concentrations of agonist, given equivalent responses in the presence and absence of alkylating agent, are plotted according to equation 1-72, and the dissociation constant (designated K_A) is calculated. (From Furchgott and Bursztyn,[84] with permission.)

Table 1-2. Analyses of the Potency of Various Agonists on the
Muscarinic Receptors in Stomach Fundus Muscle

Agonist	Dissociation Constant[a] (M)	Relative Efficacy[b]
Acetylcholine	2.0×10^{-6}	1.0
Carbamylcholine	1.6×10^{-5}	1.0
Pilocarpine	6.9×10^{-6}	0.054
Methacholine	2.4×10^{-6}	0.73

[a] Determined from analysis of equation 1-72.
[b] Efficacy determined from concentrations producing equivalent responses in the presence and absence of alkylating agents.
(Data from Furchgott and Bursztyn.[84])

equilibration of $^{22}Na^+$ occurs upon opening of the ion channel associated with the nicotinic receptor. Measurements using time intervals of several seconds allow for complete equilibration of the $^{22}Na^+$ inside and outside the vesicle even when a small fraction of receptors are activated. Therefore, an accumulation of $^{22}Na^+$ is half-maximal when a small fraction of receptors are occupied by agonists (Fig. 1-48).

α-Bungarotoxin binds to the receptors in an essentially irreversible manner, which effectively reduces receptor number. If the flux interval is 20 seconds, the concentration of carbamylcholine associated with a half-maximal response is 13 μM. Occupancy of 47 percent of the receptors by α-bungarotoxin increased the EC_{50} by a factor of 5 with only a small decrease in the maximal response. With 73 percent of the sites blocked, the EC_{50} was shifted further with the maximal response decreased by 40 percent. In contrast, phenyltrimethylammonium, a partial agonist, shows largely a decrease in the maximal response with little shift in the EC_{50} upon bungarotoxin inactivation of similar fractions of receptors. Analysis of the responses by the method of Furchgott and Bursztyn[84] described previously yields a dissociation constant for carbamylcholine of 150 μM. The analysis of spare receptors is complicated by the requirement for agonist occupation of two sites for activation[88] (see also Ch. 2). Hence, random block of 50 percent of the sites yields 25 percent of the original response. Nevertheless, the analysis clearly reveals the spare receptor behavior. By examining efflux by rapid flow methods, in which rate constants of Na^+ efflux can be ascertained at short time intervals, an EC_{50} of 600 μM is found for carbamylcholine, a value converging on the point determined by analysis of the responses following bungarotoxin inactivation. The rapid kinetic analysis more clearly reveals the partial agonist nature of phenyltrimethylammonium, since its EC_{50} changes little from the 20-second values, and the maximal flux it elicits is 2 percent of that achieved with carbamylcholine.

β-Adrenergic receptor coupling to guanosine triphosphate (GTP) binding proteins, which in turn activate adenylyl cyclase, provides another simplified example of apparent spare receptors. Ross and colleagues used a lipid vesicle to which a purified β-adrenergic receptor and G protein (G_s) were added; the stoichiometry of the two proteins could then be defined.[89] A comparison of the concentration dependence of agonist-elicited GTP binding with the concentration dependence of receptor occupation by agonist (isoproterenol) reveals the response (GTPγS binding) curve occurs at concentrations two orders of magnitude lower than the binding curve (Fig. 1-49). This indicates that occupation of a small fraction of receptors yields a maximal response. Nevertheless, determination of the stoichiometry of G proteins and β-adrenergic receptors in the reconstituted system, in which

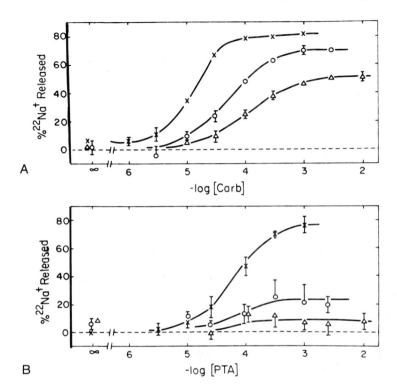

Fig. 1-48. Carbamylcholine (Carb)- and phenyltrimethylammonium (PTA)-stimulated Na$^+$ efflux from nicotinic receptor-containing membrane vesicles. Responses are measured 20 seconds after addition of agonist. The family of curves in **A** reflects responses when none (x), 47 percent ($\bigcirc$), and 73 percent ($\triangle$) and in **B** when none (x), 49 percent ($\bigcirc$), and 81 percent ($\triangle$) of the sites are blocked by α-bungarotoxin, a slowly dissociating inhibitor. (From Neubig and Cohen,[88] with permission.)

the numbers of molecules can be quantitated, reveals that the G protein is in large stoichiometric excess. Hence, the apparent *receptor reserve* can not be accounted for by a low ratio of G protein to receptor. Despite being in stoichiometric deficiency, the receptor has the capacity to activate multiple G proteins, and the amplification occurs because the receptor association and dissociation rates allow for activation of multiple G protein molecules in the time frame of the measurement. GTP hydrolysis or GTPγS dissociation is relatively slow, which in effect produces a cumulative activation, presumably through sequential association events. Hence, a single receptor has the capacity and a sufficient time interval to activate multiple G protein molecules. The apparent dissociation constant for functional antagonism determined for the β-adrenergic antagonist, propranolol was virtually identical to the dissociation constant measured for propranolol binding, as would be expected if a single population of receptor sites were involved.

In the two examples described using purified systems, the stoichiometry of the participating molecules can be ascertained, and a response linked to receptor occupation can be monitored. By measuring responses in short time intervals (i.e., the initial rates of Na$^+$ flux in the case of the nicotinic receptor and the initial rate of enhanced GTP binding

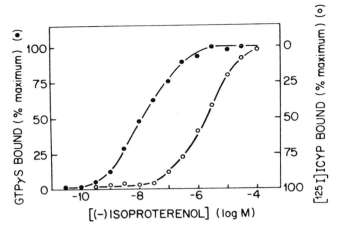

Fig. 1-49. A comparative assay of the concentration dependence of isoproterenol binding to reconstituted receptors and stimulation of GTPγS binding was made over a 2-minute interval. Isoproterenol binding was measured by competition with an antagonist at a concentration equal to its K_D. The calculated K_D for isoproterenol is 870 nM. The total GTPγS bound was 66 fmoles in the presence of isoproterenol and 18 fmoles in its absence. Total agonist sites were 1.1 fmoles. (From Asano et al,[89] with permission.)

for the β-adrenergic receptor), a convergence of the concentration dependence for receptor occupation and the respective functional responses would be anticipated.

Spare Receptors, Intracellular Mediators, and Cellular Responses

The quantitation of stoichiometry of receptors and G proteins in intact cellular systems requires separate assays of numbers of G protein and effector molecules by approaches such as antibody titrations. Applications of these techniques show that cells typically possess a large excess of G proteins over a single receptor. Receptors in intact cells may also exhibit high catalytic activity by interacting with and activating multiple G proteins within a given time frame.[90]

One has also observed with G protein-coupled receptors that the degree of receptor reserve may also depend on the intracellular response[91] or mediator[92] being analyzed. The studies of Brown and Goldstein show that inhibition of adenylyl cyclase by stimulation of muscarinic acetylcholinic receptors in chick heart cells shows a considerably larger receptor reserve than does the production of inositol phosphates by receptor-elicited hydrolysis of phosphoinositides.[92] Although this phenomenon could be a consequence of distinct muscarinic receptor subtypes, it seems more likely that it reflects the capacity of two distinct G proteins to interact with the receptor. Each G protein possesses a distinct coupling efficiency. The receptor reserve can be analyzed by use of a specific alkylating agent, propylbenzilylcholine mustard, for the muscarinic receptor (Fig. 1-50). A smaller number of receptors are needed to achieve maximal activation of adenylyl cyclase. The data also show a convergence of dissociation constants when receptor reserve is analyzed, which is to be expected if the agonist is acting through a single receptor. Experiments that now enable investigators to clone individual muscarinic receptors and G proteins and express them in cells devoid of these molecules should enable a more detailed analysis of receptor–G protein coupling efficiency.[93,94]

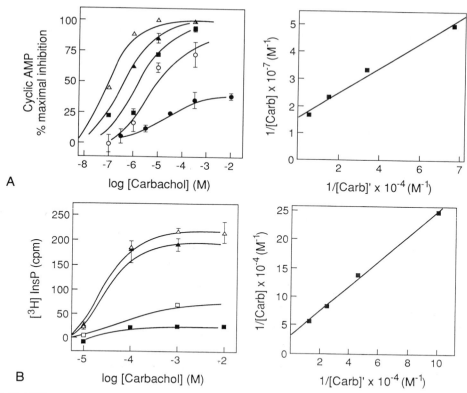

Fig. 1-50. Effect of propylbenzilylcholine mustard (PrBCM) on concentration-response curves for **(A)** inhibition of cyclic AMP (cAMP) formation and **(B)** stimulation of inositol phosphate formation. Cells were untreated ($\triangle$—$\triangle$) or treated with PrBCM at 0.5 nM (▲), 5 nM (□), 10 nM (■), 0.5 μM (○), or 1 μM (●), washed, and then challenged with a single dose of isoproterenol and carbachol at various concentrations to assess inhibition of cAMP formation and with carbachol to assess inositol phosphate formation. In separate experiments, PrBCM inhibited antagonist binding to 50 percent of the receptors at 0.1 μM, and the alkylating agent was found not to affect basal and isoproterenol-stimulated cAMP production or basal inositol phosphate production. The panels on the right show reciprocal plots of equiactive doses of carbachol in control cells and cells treated with 1 μM PrBCM. The straight lines fitted by linear regression analysis show values of $K_D = 27$ μM and $q = 2 \cdot 2 \times 10^{-3}$ for PrBCM in A and $K_D = 39$ μM and $q = 0.45$ for 10 nM PrBCM in B.

It becomes far more difficult to assign a basis for receptor reserves in complex cellular systems. Spare receptors require that another process in addition to receptor occupation should determine the saturation function for the response. Inherent in cell signaling are amplified systems. For example, the steps in a metabolic cascade (e.g., β-receptor-elicited glycogenolysis) show amplification, and each succeeding metabolic step involves the turnover of greater quantities of substrate[95] and is usually catalyzed by greater quantities of enzyme. The spread of a depolarization event across the muscle surface from the small focus of a motor end-plate on skeletal muscle (see Fig. 1-2) is a second example of amplification. Saturation of one step, making it rate-limiting, will result in a spare capacity or a reserve in the macromolecules participating in the upstream steps. This yields a situation in which lower agonist concentrations are required for the functional response than for ligand binding to the receptor.

Strickland and Loeb[96] developed an empirical equation to describe the process of a hormone-generated intracellular mediator interacting with an intracellular receptor to elicit a response:

$$K_{total} = \left(\frac{K}{K + aR_t}\right) K_d \qquad \text{(equation 73)}$$

where R_t is the total number of hormone receptor sites, K_d the ligand dissociation constant, K is the dissociation constant for the binding of intracellular mediator to its intracellular receptor, and a is a constant relating the abundance of intracellular mediator to R_t. Since $K_{total} \leq K_d$, the concentration-response curve for function will lie to the left of the receptor occupancy curve.

Despite the development of formulas permitting calculation of efficacy, the definition of efficacy in terms of mechanistic events or chemical equilibria is not intrinsic to the above spare receptor theories. Hence, spare receptor theory provides equations consistent with the experimental observations but falls short of describing affinity and efficacy in terms of chemical equilibria.

An early attempt to conceptualize efficacy in terms of rate constants resulted in Paton's *rate theory of drug action*,[97] which proposes that efficacy is related to the number of drug-receptor association events. Hence, ligands showing rapid rates of association and dissociation with the receptor would be agonists whereas those exhibiting slow rates of association and dissociation would be antagonists. Crossing the transition state barrier depicted in Figure 1-39 would be sufficient for a unit of activation. Accordingly, efficacy could be related to a transient activation state achieved in association or dissociation of the ligand while the dissociation constant or affinity would govern occupation at a particular ligand concentration. While this rate theory for drug action does not seem realistic in terms of fundamental physicochemical principles of ligand binding to a macromolecule and the conformational changes that might ensue, the theory is largely notable as an attempt to define occupation and efficacy as distinct physical events.

Ligand Binding to Multisubunit Proteins

Several examples of receptors or enzymes important to drug action exist in which the protein is oligomeric and contains more than a single site critical for drug action (see Ch. 2). This molecular arrangement allowing for coupled binding sites in theory not only changes the range of concentrations over which drug action is seen (i.e., the steepness of the dose-response relationship) but also may result in nonlinearity in the receptor occupation-response relationship.

In 1925 Adair[98] developed a more formal statistical relationship for ligand binding to a multisubunit protein, which expanded on the empirical proposal of Hill to explain the cooperative behavior of oxygen binding to hemoglobin. Although requiring far more constants for the fit of the relationship, such equations can be used to model cooperative binding in terms of individual microscopic dissociation constants.

We may represent the equation below in terms of the fractional occupation of a tetrameric receptor:

$$4L + R \underset{k_{-1}}{\overset{k_1}{\rightleftharpoons}} 3L + LR \underset{k_{-2}}{\overset{k_2}{\rightleftharpoons}} 2L + L_2R \underset{k_{-3}}{\overset{k_3}{\rightleftharpoons}} L + L_3R \underset{k_{-4}}{\overset{k_4}{\rightleftharpoons}} L_4R$$

If the sites behave in an identical fashion and we define K_{di} as the intrinsic microscopic dissociation constant and K_1, K_2, K_3, and K_4 as dissociation constants corrected for the fractional occupation of sites, then

$$K_{di} = \frac{k_{-1}}{k_1} = \frac{k_{-2}}{k_2} = \frac{k_{-3}}{k_3} = \frac{k_{-4}}{k_4} \qquad \text{(equation 74)}$$

and

$$K_1 = \frac{k_{-1}}{4k_1} \quad K_2 = \frac{2k_{-1}}{3k_1} \quad K_3 = \frac{3k_{-1}}{2k_1} \quad K_4 = \frac{4k_{-1}}{k_1} \qquad \text{(equation 75)}$$

then

$$K_{di} = 4K_1 = \frac{3}{2}K_2 = \frac{2}{3}K_3 = \frac{1}{4}K_4 \qquad \text{(equation 76)}$$

If we then consider fractional site occupation

$$\overline{Y}_s = \frac{\text{moles of ligand bound}}{\text{moles of sites}} \qquad \text{(equation 77)}$$

$$= \frac{[LR] + 2[L_2R] + 3[L_3R] + 4[L_4R]}{4([R] + [LR] + [L_2R] + [L_3R] + [L_4R])}$$

If we also consider sites of bound ligand per mole of macromolecule

$$\overline{Y} = \frac{[LR] + 2[L_2R] + 3[L_3R] + 4[L_4R]}{[R] + [LR] + [L_2R] + [L_3R] + [L_4R]} \qquad \text{(equation 78)}$$

At saturation L₄R should be the only species and

$$\overline{Y}_s = 1 \qquad \overline{Y} = 4$$

Substitution of the appropriate dissociation constants yields

$$\overline{Y}_s = \frac{\dfrac{[L]}{K_1} + \dfrac{2[L]^2}{K_1K_2} + \dfrac{3[L]^3}{K_1K_2K_3} + \dfrac{4[L]^4}{K_1K_2K_3K_4}}{4\left(1 + \dfrac{[L]}{K_1} + \dfrac{[L]^2}{K_1K_2} + \dfrac{[L]^3}{K_1K_2K_3} + \dfrac{[L]^4}{K_1K_2K_3K_4}\right)} \qquad \text{(equation 79)}$$

Since

$$K_1 = \frac{K_{di}}{4}$$

$$K_1K_2 = \frac{K_{di}}{4} \cdot \frac{2}{3}K_{di} = \frac{1}{6}K_{di}^2$$

$$K_1K_2K_3 = \frac{K_{di}}{4} \cdot \frac{2}{3}K_{di} \cdot \frac{3}{2}K_{di} = \frac{1}{4}K_{di}^3 \qquad \text{(equation 80)}$$

$$K_1K_2K_3K_4 = \frac{K_{di}}{4} \cdot \frac{2}{3}K_{di} \cdot \frac{3}{2}K_{di} \cdot 4K_{di} = K_{di}^4$$

$$\overline{Y}_s = \frac{\dfrac{4[L]}{K_{di}} + \dfrac{12[L]^2}{K_{di}^2} + \dfrac{12[L]^3}{K_{di}^3} + \dfrac{4[L]^4}{K_{di}^4}}{4\left(1 + \dfrac{4[L]}{K_{di}} + \dfrac{6[L^2]}{K_{di}^2} + \dfrac{4[L^3]}{K_{di}^3} + \dfrac{[L]^4}{K_{di}^4}\right)}$$

By factoring $4/K_{di}$ from the numerator and then factoring the resultant polynominals, we obtain:

$$\overline{Y}_s = \frac{\frac{[L]}{K_{di}}\left(1 + \frac{[L]}{K_{di}}\right)^3}{\left(1 + \frac{[L]}{K_{di}}\right)^4} = \frac{\frac{[L]}{K_{di}}}{1 + \frac{[L]}{K_{di}}} \qquad \text{(equation 81)}$$

This equation is identical to equation 22 for a single class of binding sites. Hence, if there are no interactions between sites and the sites are identical, the statistical relationship between binding constants allows one to describe binding in terms of a single constant K_{di}. The individual constants for the microscopic processes can be related to K_{di} by the statistical constraints considered above. In the case of cooperativity, the individual constants can be modified to reflect changes in dissociation constant associated with ligand occupation of neighboring sites. Hence, the Adair equations can be readily adjusted to reflect cooperative relationships.

Equation 1-81 should be distinguished from the situation in which the sites exist on different macromolecules, each containing a single site. Here

$$\overline{Y} = \frac{n_1\frac{[L]}{K_{d1}}}{1 + \frac{[L]}{K_{d1}}} + \frac{n_2\frac{[L]}{K_{d2}}}{1 + \frac{[L]}{K_{d2}}} + \frac{n_3\frac{[L]}{k_{d3}}}{1 + \frac{[L]}{K_{d3}}} + \frac{n_4\frac{[L]}{K_{d4}}}{1 + \frac{[L]}{K_{d4}}} \qquad \text{(equation 82)}$$

where n_1, n_2, n_3, and n_4 are the fractional populations of total sites on each macromolecule and $n_1 + n_2 + n_3 + n_4$ equals the total number of sites divided by the total number of macromolecules. When $K_{d1} = K_{d2} = K_{d3} = K_{d4}$, multiple site binding can be fit to either equation 81 or equation 82, since the two equations yield a formal identity.

Both the existence of multiple sites with different dissociation constants and cooperativity in binding at a single class of sites can be described by the above equations, and it becomes necessary to develop more sophisticated approaches to distinguish mechanisms.

Multiple Sites of Ligand Binding

If we consider the situation in which we have two sites on a macromolecule and both are behaving independently, then $n_1 + n_2 = \overline{Y} = 2$. If K_{d1} is $10^{-3} K_{d2}$, $\overline{Y}_s$ may be described by curve A shown in Figure 1-51. The two binding sites are clearly separated by the inflection on the curve occurring at $\overline{Y}_s = 0.5$. In addition, the two dissociation constants can be estimated from the concentrations at which $\overline{Y}_s = 0.25$ and $\overline{Y}_s = 0.75$. There are also the points of maximum slope. The two aspects of the curve could also be easily distinguished on a Hill plot Fig. 1-51A with slopes near 1.0 when $0.1\ K_{d1} < [D] < 10.0\ K_{d1}$ and $0.1\ K_{d2} < [D] < 10.0\ K_{d2}$.

By contrast, when $K_{d1} = 0.1\ K_{d2}$, Y_s shows far less change in curvature, and it becomes far more difficult to distinguish the inflection point (curve C in Fig. 1-51). The data may be fitted to K_{d1} and K_{d2}, but additional information is required to distinguish a two-site mechanism from alternative schemes of negative cooperativity or binding to a more complex array of multiple sites with distinct but quantitatively similar dissociation constants. These considerations have several implications for drug-receptor interactions. First, when a heterogeneity of binding sites exists, it will prove difficult to assign dissociation constants and fractional populations of sites as the dissociation constants converge. Distinction of receptor subtypes is also best done with ligands whose dissociation constants differ by large values. As clearly revealed for the opiate receptors,[99] the problem is compounded as the number of receptor subtypes increases. Second, heterogeneity or impurities in the

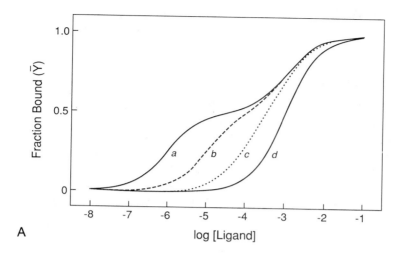

A

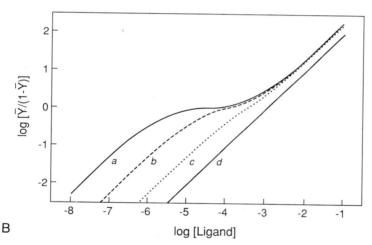

B

Fig. 1-51. **(A)** Semilogarithmic and **(B)** Hill plot of profiles for ligand binding to two receptor sites of equal population, where the differences in dissociation constants differ by 10^3, 10^2, 10^1, and 10^0. Binding in each case is described by the following equation:

$$Y_s = 0.5 \frac{[L]}{[L] + K_1} + 0.5 \frac{[L]}{[L] + K_2}$$

where $K_1 = 10^{-6}$ M and $K_2 = 10^{-3}$ M in curve a, $K_1 = 10^{-5}$ M and $K_2 = 10^{-3}$ M in curve b, $K_1 = 10^{-4}$ M and $K_2 = 10^{-3}$ M in curve c, and $K_1 = 10^{-3}$ M and $K_2 = 10^{-3}$ M in curve d. Note that in curves a through d the Hill coefficients approach a value of 1.0 at the extreme values and that a distinct inflection or plateau in the curves can only be discerned when K_1 and K_2 differ by large values.

binding ligand itself (either chemical or isomeric impurities) will yield Hill coefficients less than 1.0. Very often such heterogeneity has been incorrectly equated with negative cooperativity or site multiplicity.

Cooperative Interactions

We may define *cooperative binding* as that which occurs in a oligomer when binding of the ligand to the first site enhances or diminishes binding to the neighboring sites. Hence, in equations 1-80 and 1-81, although K_{di} for all sites are initially identical (i.e., there is an equal probability of L landing on each square in the tetramer on page 88), occupation of one or more of the sites can change the K_{di} for the remaining vacant sites by an allosteric mechanism. Hence the previous statistical considerations will not alone determine the dissociation constants for binding to remaining sites. In general, for *positive cooperativity*

$$4K_1 > \frac{3}{2} K_2 > \frac{2}{3} K_3 > K_4$$

This ordering of inequalities in dissociation constants is to be expected, since in positive cooperativity the binding of one ligand at a neighboring site will enhance the binding of the second ligand and so on until occupation is complete. For negative cooperativity, in general we see ligand binding at neighboring sites decreasing the probability of binding on that oligomer, so that

$$4K_1 < \frac{3}{2} K_2 < \frac{2}{3} K_3 < K_4$$

Hence, a true linkage relationship, in which each dissociation constant is coupled to the extent of occupation, is intrinsic to cooperativity. This is so because the binding energy contains a component that is affecting the conformation of a neighboring site. Hence, in positive cooperativity the binding of the first ligand on a vacant oligomer may have a higher dissociation constant (lower affinity), owing to its need to induce a conformational change in a neighboring subunit, but as ligand occupation proceeds, binding is facilitated by the conformational change being effected by prior binding of ligands at neighboring sites. In negative cooperativity the induced conformational change associated with the binding of the first ligand makes it even more difficult for the remaining sites on the oligomer to be filled.

The overall mechanisms for cooperativity have been proposed, and a schematic illustration is shown in Figure 1-52. The *Monod-Wyman-Changeux*[100,101] model considers the oligomeric protein to exist in multiple (usually two) states, the driving force being the maintenance of symmetry or conformational identity between the subunits. The *induced-fit model*[102,103] proposes that the ligand induces a change in conformation of the binding subunit, and it is the ease of conformational change that contributes to cooperativity.

Coupled Equilibria between Receptor Occupation and Response

Receptor activation typically involves associations of the binding subunit with other proteins or a change in conformation within the receptor itself. Such events are usually described by coupled equilibria, which in themselves will produce a disparity between

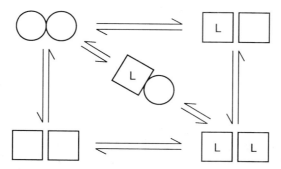

Fig. 1-52. Schematic comparisons of cooperative behavior of a dimeric receptor for a model involving symmetry-driven state transition and for an induced-fit model. The outer square depicts the symmetry-driven model, where in the absence of ligand the conformation represented by the circles is preferred. Ligand binding is preferred by the square conformation, and the requirement to maintain symmetry drives both subunits to the same conformation. Accordingly, ligand binding to the neighboring subunit is facilitated. The induced-fit model is represented along the diagonal. Ligand binding to one of the subunits induces the conformational change. Binding to the second subunit in the pair facilitates the conformational change, thus contributing to the positive cooperativity.

the dependences of occupation and function on ligand concentration. To illustrate this point, consider the equilibrium

$$L + R \underset{}{\overset{K_1}{\rightleftharpoons}} LR \underset{}{\overset{K_2}{\rightleftharpoons}} LR^*$$

where LR is the inactive and LR* the active (i.e., open channel or effector-coupled) state of the receptor, K_1 is a typical dissociation constant ($K_1 = [L][R]/[LR]$), and $K_2 = [LR^*]/[LR]$. Fractional occupation is defined by the ratio of the ligand-bound to the total receptor species. Then

$$\frac{[LR] + [LR^*]}{[LR] + [R] + [LR^*]} = \frac{\dfrac{[L][R]}{K_1} + K_2 \cdot \dfrac{[L][R]}{K_1}}{\dfrac{[L][R]}{K_1} + [R] + K_2 \cdot \dfrac{[L][R]}{K_1}} = \frac{[L](1 + K_2)}{K_1 + [L](1 + K_2)} \quad \text{(equation 83)}$$

By contrast, fractional activation is defined by

$$\frac{[LR^*]}{[LR] + [R] + [LR^*]} = \frac{\dfrac{K_2[L][R]}{K_1}}{[L][R]/K_1 + [R] + K_2[L][R]/K_1} = \frac{[L]K_2}{K_1 + [L](1 + K_2)} \quad \text{(equation 84)}$$

Hence, only when K_2 is large do we observe equality between the occupation and response and in a relatively simple scheme we have shown that occupation and activation have distinct concentration dependencies.

Binding and State Functions of Receptors

The concepts that (1) proteins exist in multiple conformational states with discrete functions and (2) ligand binding could control the conformational states provide a basis for developing reaction schemes in which at equilibrium the fraction of occupied receptor species will *not* be identical to the fraction of active species. As mentioned above, multiple states of a protein that are controlled by ligand binding are also used to explain cooperativity in ligand binding.

Monod et al.[100] originally proposed that multisubunit oligomeric proteins existed in more than a single state and that ligands that bind to the protein show a preference for a particular state. Ligand association can then alter the fraction of the protein in a particular state. This theory also was based on the concept that in a multisubunit protein maintenance of symmetry between subunits is the predominant driving force. Thus, in either the presence or absence of ligand, the individual subunits within an oligomer will try to maintain an identity of conformational state. The energy of interaction at subunit interfaces could be the driving force to achieve conformational identity among the subunits or symmetry at their interfaces. Such a model gives rise to a concerted mechanism for ligand binding and alterations in functional state of the protein.[100,101] In this case the multiple states of the protein exist before the binding of ligand, and we do not detect populations of oligomeric molecules with subunits in different states (Fig. 1-52).

The alternative to Monod et al.'s model would be an induced-fit model in which ligands can alter the state of the protein by inducing a change in conformation of the individual subunits.[102,103] In this model the conformational states do not exist before the binding of ligand, and symmetry among the subunits or their interfaces is not maintained. The associating ligand induces a conformational change in the binding subunit, and this either facilitates or hinders binding to the neighboring subunit, (positive or negative cooperativity, respectively).

Both models can account for positive cooperativity in ligand binding, but only the induced-fit model will explain negative cooperativity. In the induced-fit model a linkage relationship must also be demonstrated whereby the binding of ligand to the first site on an oligomer enhances or diminishes the affinity for binding to the second site. A Hill coefficient less than unity does not establish negative cooperativity, and in fact virtually all circumstances in which low Hill coefficients have been found can be described by (1) heterogeneity in the receptor population, (2) nonequivalence of sites on an oligomeric receptor, or (3) impurity of the radioligand. Positive cooperativity requires a multisubunit protein, but Hill coefficients cannot distinguish between a symmetry-controlled and an induced-fit model.[104]

The value of a multiple-state receptor system is that it also allows for description of the relationship between fractional occupation and fractional response when they are not identical. The initial applications of state functions and binding functions to receptor systems were made independently by Karlin[105] and Thron.[106] Other operational models of receptor function involving coupled equilibria have also been developed.[107,108]

Receptor Existing in Two States

The simplest scheme for a receptor existing in multiple states that differ in their capacities to bind and activate ligand is shown below:

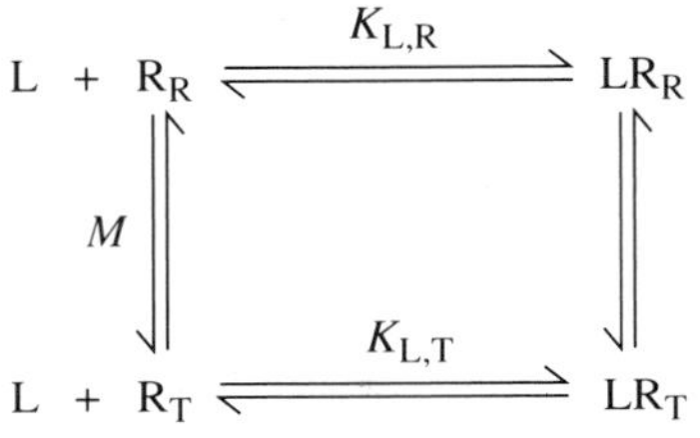

$$
\begin{array}{ccc}
L + R_R & \xrightleftharpoons{K_{L,R}} & LR_R \\
M \Updownarrow & & \Updownarrow \\
L + R_T & \xrightleftharpoons[\phantom{K_{L,T}}]{K_{L,T}} & LR_T
\end{array}
$$

$K_{L,R}$ and $K_{L,T}$ are the two "microscopic" dissociation constants for ligand (L) binding to the R and T states, and M is an equilibrium constant defining the ratio R_T/R_R. If we define R as the active and T as the inactive state, we might anticipate that $M > 1$. The ratio of LR_R to LR_T is defined by $K_{L,T}M/K_{L,R}$, which is consistent with the microscopic reversibility of the above cyclic scheme for equilibration. A binding function $\overline{Y}$ for the above scheme can be defined as follows:

$$\overline{Y} = \frac{[LR_T] + [LR_R]}{[LR_T] + [LR_R] + [R_R] + [R_T]} \qquad \text{(equation 85)}$$

By substitution of the appropriate equilibrium constants

$$\overline{Y} = \frac{[L]}{[L] + \dfrac{1 + M}{\dfrac{1}{K_{L,R}} + \dfrac{M}{K_{L,T}}}} \qquad \text{(equation 86)}$$

Accordingly, a "macroscopic" equilibrium constant K_{app} can be defined as

$$K_{app} = \frac{1 + M}{\dfrac{1}{K_{L,R}} + \dfrac{M}{K_{L,T}}} \qquad \text{(equation 87)}$$

Similarly, if we define all R states of the receptor as active, then the state function for activation R is:

$$\overline{R} = \frac{[LR_R] + [R_R]}{[LR_R] + [R_R] + [LR_T] + [R_T]} \qquad \text{(equation 88)}$$

Substitution of the appropriate equilibrium constants yields

$$\overline{R} = \frac{1}{1 + M\left(\dfrac{1 + \dfrac{[L]}{K_{L,T}}}{1 + \dfrac{[L]}{K_{L,R}}}\right)} \qquad \text{(equation 89)}$$

Thus, we can see that although the binding and state functions depend on the same parameters, they are not identical. Accordingly, fractional occupancy $\overline{Y}$ will no longer equal fractional response $\overline{R}$, and we have a means for accounting for distinct ligand-dependent occupation and efficacy terms. The equilibrium constant to which occupation is related is given by equation 87. Efficacy can be approximated by the relationship

$$\epsilon = \frac{K_{L,T}}{K_{L,R}} - 1 \qquad \text{(equation 90)}$$

In this simple scheme the ratio of microscopic dissociation constants will dictate the efficacy of the agonist. Assuming $K_{L,T} = K_{L,R}$, then $\epsilon = 0$. An efficacy of zero defines an antagonist, since equal dissociation constants dictate that ligand association does not change the state function or the ratio of R to T species. We find that $K_{L,R} \leq K_{L,T}$ for agonists, and we can see how adjustment of these parameters will shift the ratio of R to

T species. A scheme of this nature could also yield a ligand with negative efficacy, but this would be indistinguishable from a zero efficacy in the absence of competition with an agonist.

Other relationships between state and occupation functions can be derived for more complex equilibria, but the basic principle of nonidentity of the occupation and state function will hold. A more satisfying scheme for certain receptor systems might only consider the liganded receptor species (i.e., LR) as active. In this situation the state function for activation would differ from equation 89, but the binding function would remain as in equation 86.

Binding of Multiple Ligands

In the scheme of a dimeric receptor where two ligands bind

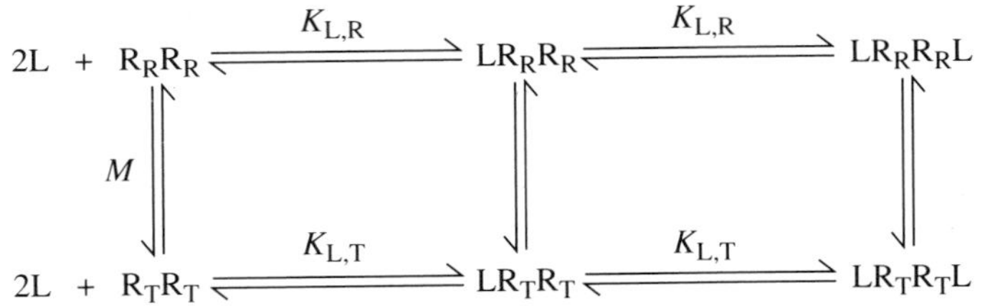

$$2L + R_R R_R \xrightleftharpoons{\quad K_{L,R} \quad} LR_R R_R \xrightleftharpoons{\quad K_{L,R} \quad} LR_R R_R L$$

$$\Big\updownarrow M \qquad\qquad\qquad \updownarrow \qquad\qquad\qquad \updownarrow$$

$$2L + R_T R_T \xrightleftharpoons{\quad K_{L,T} \quad} LR_T R_T \xrightleftharpoons{\quad K_{L,T} \quad} LR_T R_T L$$

For the binding function the following equation can be derived:

$$\bar{Y} = \frac{\dfrac{[L]}{K_{L,R}}\left(1 + \dfrac{[L]}{K_{L,R}}\right) + M\,\dfrac{[L]}{K_{L,T}}\left(1 + \dfrac{[L]}{K_{L,T}}\right)}{\left(1 + \dfrac{[L]}{K_{L,R}}\right)^2 + M\left(1 + \dfrac{[L]}{K_{L,T}}\right)^2} \qquad \text{(equation 91)}$$

where $M = R_T R_T / R_R R_R$ and $K_{L,T}$ and $K_{L,R}$ define the microscopic dissociation constants for the two sites.

For the state function

$$\bar{R} = \frac{1}{1 + M\left(\dfrac{1 + \dfrac{[L]}{K_{L,T}}}{1 + \dfrac{[L]}{K_{L,R}}}\right)^2} \qquad \text{(equation 92)}$$

From an examination of equation 1-92 it is evident that the exponential relationship for the portion of the equation in the parentheses means that the state function can be markedly influenced by the presence of multiple binding sites. Hence, the dissociation constants and the ligand concentrations are influenced by the exponential function, while M is not affected. We also observe from a comparison of equations 91 and 92 that the state and binding functions will have a different dependence on [L]. Hence, the apparent Hill coefficients for occupation and response can differ. Moreover, the Hill coefficient n_H will depend on n, $K_{L,R}/K_{L,T}$, and M. Also, $n_H \leq n$; by varying the constants in equation 91 one may analyze the extent to which n_H and n differ depending on how the various equilibria are positioned.[106] The above equations not only describe the binding and state functions but also define the extent of homotropic cooperativity seen in these systems.

Heterotropic Ligands

The definition of a *heterotropic ligand* is based on a lack of identity between its site of binding and that of the primary ligand. Hence, if the heterotropic ligand H and the primary ligand L (usually the agonist) bind to different sites, the potential exists for an interaction. Often the site to which the heterotropic ligand binds is termed an *allosteric* site, that is, a site physically removed from the site of reference. These terms have been used interchangeably in the literature.

A generalized scheme for heterotropic ligand binding is shown below:

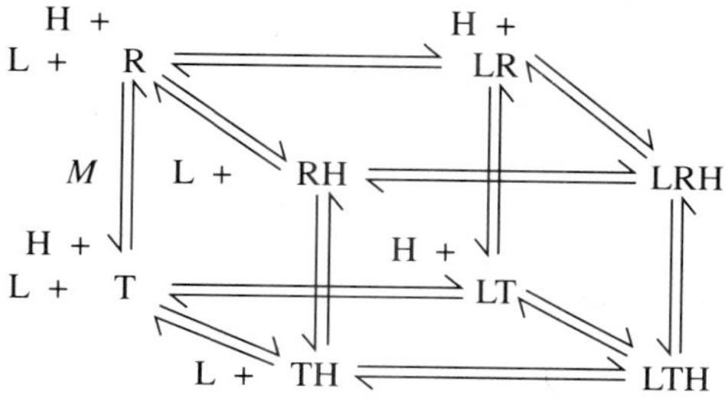

$$
\begin{array}{c}
\text{H +}\\
\text{L +}\quad \text{R} \rightleftharpoons \text{LR}
\end{array}
\qquad
\begin{array}{c}
\text{H +}\\
\text{LR}
\end{array}
$$

(equation 93)

where $K_{H,R} = \dfrac{[R][H]}{[RH]}$ $\qquad$ $K_{H,T} = \dfrac{[T][H]}{[TH]}$

From this equation

$$
M' = M \left(\frac{1 + \dfrac{[H]}{K_{H,T}}}{1 + \dfrac{[H]}{K_{H,R}}} \right)
$$

(equation 94)

Hence, we can see that H as a heterotropic ligand can affect the state and binding functions of the primary ligand L by altering the equation of state in the absence of L. Accordingly, allosteric activation would increase the fraction in the R state while allosteric inhibition would increase the fraction of receptor in the T state. Allosteric activators require $K_{H,R} < K_{H,T}$ while allosteric inhibitors require $K_{H,T} < K_{H,R}$. Both activators and inhibitors define a new value M' in the equation of state in the absence of L; as seen in equation 94, M' depends on [H], $K_{H,R}$, and $K_{H,T}$. Allosteric ligands effectively add another dimension to our cyclic, two-state scheme. Four species now exist to which the primary ligand can bind.

The importance of these equations of receptor state is that they permit description of binding and functional responses to agonist, antagonist, heterotropic activator, and heterotropic inhibitor in terms of chemical equilibria and conformational states of receptors. A formidable challenge awaits those attempting to detect receptor states and distinguish mechanistic pathways by physicochemical approaches. This cannot be accomplished without information on receptor structure, and appropriately this subject will be a central topic in Chapter 2.

REFERENCES

1. Martin YC: Quantitative Drug Designs. Marcel Dekker, New York, 1978
2. Nogrady T: Medicinal Chemistry: A Biochemical Approach. Oxford University Press, New York, 1985
3. Wolff ME (ed): The Bases of Medicinal Chemistry. 4th Ed. Wiley Interscience, New York 1980.
4. Dean PM: Molecular Foundations of Drug-Receptor Interaction. Cambridge University Press, Cambridge, England, 1987
5. Topliss JG (ed): Quantitative Structure-Activity Relationships. Academic Press, Orlando, FL, 1983
6. Kraut J, Matthews DA: Dihydrofolate reductase p.l. In Jurnak F, and McPherson A (eds): Biological Macromolecules and Assemblies. Vol. 3. John Wiley & Sons, 1987
7. Birdsall B, Feeney J, Pascual, C et al: A ^{1}H NMR study of the interactions and conformations of rationally designed trimethoprim analogues in complexes with *Lactobacillus casei* dihydrofolate reductase. J Med Chem 27:1672, 1984
8. Beers WH and Reich E: Structure and activity of acetylcholine. Nature 228:917, 1970
9. Chothia C, Pauling P: Conformations of acetylcholine. Nature 219:1156, 1968
10. Paton WDM, Zaimis EJ: The pharmacological actions of polymethylene bis trimethylammonium salts. J Pharmacol 4:381, 1949
11. Paton WDM, Zaimis EJ: The methonium compounds, Pharmacol Rev 4:219, 1952
12. Adams PR, Sakmann B: Decamethonium both blocks and opens endplate channels. Proc Natl Acad Sci USA 75:2994, 1978
13. Gurney AM, Rang HP: The channel-blocking action of methonium compounds on rat submandibular ganglion cells. Br J Pharmacol 82:623, 1984
14. Overton E: Studien über die Narkose Zugleich ein Beitrag zu allgemeinen Pharmakologie. G. Fischer, Jena, 1901
15. Hansch C, Leo A: Sustituent Constants for Correlation Analysis in Chemistry and Biology. Wiley Interscience, New York, 1979
16. Hammett LP: Physical Organic Chemistry. 2nd Ed. McGraw-Hill, New York, 1970
17. Marshall, G.R: Computer-aided drug design. Annu Rev. Pharmacol, Toxicol 27:193, 1987
18. Cramer RD, Bunce JD: p. 3. In Hadzi D, Jerman-Blazic B (eds): QSAR in Drug Design and Toxicology. Elsevier, Amsterdam, 1987
19. Weinstein H, Green JP (eds): Quantum chemistry in biomedical sciences. Ann NY Acad Sci 367, 1981
20. Beveridge DL, Jorgensen WL: Computer simulation of chemical and biomolecular systems. Ann NY Acad Sci 482:1, 1986
21. Bergman E, Pullman B (eds): Molecular and Quantum Pharmacology. Reidel, Dordrecht, Netherlands, 1974
22. Goodford PJ: Drug design by method of receptor fit. J Med Chem 27:557, 1984
23. Kollman PA: Theory of complex molecular interactions: Computer graphics, distance geometry, molecular mechanics and quantum mechanics. Accounts Chem Res 18:105, 1985
24. McCammon JA: Computer-aided molecular design. Science 238:486, 1987
25. Bash P, Singh UC, Brown FK, et al: Calculation of the relative change in binding free energy of a protein-inhibitor complex. Science 235:574, 1987
26. Beckett AH: Stereochemical factors in biological activity. Fortschr Arzneimittelforsch 1:455, 1959
27. Easson LH and Stedman E: Studies on the relationship between chemical constitution and physiological action. Biochem J 27:1257, 1933
28. Ariens EJ: Stereochemistry in the analysis of drug action. Parts I, II, and III. Res Rev 6:461, 1986; 7:367, 1987; 8:309, 1988
29. Portoghese PS: Relationships between stereostructure and pharmacological activities. Annu Rev Pharmacol Toxicol 10:51, 1970

30. Krogsgaard-Larsen P: GABA synaptic mechanisms: Stereochemical and conformational requirements. Medicinal Res Rev 8:27, 1988
31. Patil P, Miller D, Trendelenburg U: Molecular geometry and adrenergic drug activity, Pharmacol Rev 26:323, 1975
32. Cahn RS, Ingold CK, Prelog V: The specification of asymmetric configuration in organic chemistry. Experientia 12:81, 1956
33. Ariëns EJ, Simons M: Cholinergic and anticholinergic drugs. Do they act on common receptors? Ann NY Acad Sci 144:892, 1967
34. Burgen ASV: The role of ionic interaction at the muscarinic receptor. Br J Pharmacol 25:4, 1965
35. Drayer DE: Pharmacodynamic and pharmacokinetic differences between drug enantiomers in humans. Clin Pharmacol Ther 40:125, 1986
36. Partington J, Feeney J, Burgen ASV: The conformation of acetylcholine and related compounds in aqueous solution as studies by nuclear magnetic resonance spectroscopy. Mol Pharmacol 8:269, 1972
37. Shulman RG (ed): Magnetic Resonance Studies in Biology. Academic Press, Orlando FL, 1979
38. Behling RW, Yamane T, Navon G, Jelinski LW: Conformation of acetylcholine bound to the nicotinic acetylcholine receptor. Proc Natl Acad Sci USA 85:6721, 1988
39. Behling RW, Yamane T, Navon G, et al: Measuring relative acetylcholine receptor binding by proton nuclear magnetic resonance relaxation experiments. Biophys J 53:947, 1987
40. Bentley KW, Cardwell HME: The absolute stereochemistry of the morphine, benzylisoquinoline, aporphine, and tetrahydroberberine alkaloids. J Chem Soc 1955:352
41. MacKay M, Hodgkin DC: A crystallographic examination of the structure of morphine. J Chem Soc 1955:3261
42. Sobell HM, Sokure TD, Tovale SS, et al: Stereochemistry of a curare alkaloid. O', O'N-trimethyl-*d*-tubocurarine. Proc Natl Acad Sci USA 69:2212, 1972
43. Smith GD, Griffin JF: Conformation of [Leu^5] enkephalin from X-ray at diffraction: Features important for recognition at opiate receptors. Science 199:1214, 1979
44. Schiller PW, DiMaio J: Opiate receptor subclasses differ in their conformational requirements. Nature 297:74, 1982
45. Evans BE, Bock MG, Rittle KE, et al: Design of potent, orally effective, nonpeptidal antagonists of the peptide hormone cholecystokinin. Proc Natl Acad Sci USA 83:4918, 1986
46. Chang RSL, Lotti VJ: Biochemical and pharmacological characterization of an extremely potent and selective non-peptide cholecystokinin antagonist. Proc Natl Acad Sci USA 83:4923, 1986
47. Ondetti MA: Structural relationships of angiotensin converting enzyme inhibitors to pharmacologic activity. Circulation 77:I-74, 1988
48. Wyvral MJ, Patchett AA: Recent developments in the design of angiotensin-converting enzyme inhibitors. Med Res Rev 5:483, 1985
49. Wong PC, Price WA, Chiu AT, et al: Non-peptide angiotensin II receptor antagonists. IV. EXP 6155 and EXP 6803. Hypertension 13: 489, 1989
50. Koskinen AMP, Rapoport H: Synthetic and conformational studies on anatoxin-a: A potent acetylcholine agonist. J Med Chem 28:1301, 1985
51. Limbird LE: Cell Surface Receptors: A Short Course on Theory and Methods. Martinus Nijhoff, Boston, 1986, 196 pp.
52. Sklar LA: Ligand-receptor dynamics and signal amplification in the neutrophil. Adv Immunol 39:95, 1986
53. Munson PJ: LIGAND: A computerized analysis of ligand binding data. Methods Enzymol 92:543, 1983
54. Scatchard G: The attractions of proteins for small molecules and ions. Ann NY Acad Sci 51:660, 1949
55. Klotz IM: Numbers of receptor sites from Scatchard plots. Facts and fantasies. Science 217:1247, 1982

56. Deranleau DA: Theory of measurements of weak molecular complexes. J Am Chem Soc 91:4044, 1969
57. Dahlquist FW: The meaning of Scatchard and Hill plots. Methods Enzymol 48:270, 1978
58. Hill AV: The combinations of haemoglobin with oxygen and with carbon monoxide. Biochem J 7:471, 1913
59. Cheng Y, Prusoff WH: Relationship between the inhibition constant (K_I) and the concentration of an inhibitor that causes a 50% inhibition (I_{50}) of an enzymatic reaction. Biochem Pharmacol 22:3099, 1973
60. Chou TC: Relationship between inhibition constants and fractional inhibition in enzyme-catalyzed reactions with different numbers of reactants, different reaction mechanisms, and different types and mechanisms of inhibition. Mol Pharmacol 10:235, 1974
61. Clark AJ: General Pharmacology. Springer Verlag, Berlin, 1937
62. Schild HO: pA, a new scale for measurement of drug antagonism. Br J Pharmacol 2:189, 1947
63. Kenakin T: The classification of drugs and drug-receptors. Pharmacol Rev 36:165, 1984
64. Kenakin TP: Pharmacologic Analysis of Drug-Receptor Interaction. Raven Press, New York, 1987, 335 pp.
65. Nickerson M, Goodman LS: Pharmacological properties of a new adrenergic blocking agent: N,N-dibenzyl-β-chloro-ethylamine (dibenamine). J Pharmacol Exp Ther 89:167, 1947
66. Hitzemann R: Thermodynamic aspects of drug-receptor interactions. Trends Pharmacol Sci 9:408, 1988
67. Weiland GA, Minneman KP, Molinoff PB: Fundamental differences between the molecular interactions between agonists and antagonists with the β-adrenergic receptor. Nature 281:114, 1979
68. Eyring H: The activated complex and the absolute rate of chemical reactions. Chem Rev 17:65, 1935
69. Abbott AJ, Nelsestuen GL: The collisional limit: An important consideration for membrane associated enzymes and receptors. FASEB J 2:2858, 1988
70. Armstrong DL, Lester HA: The kinetics of d-tubocurarine action and restricted diffusion in the synaptic cleft. J Physiol (Lond) 294:365, 1979
71. Burgen ASV: The drug-receptor complex. J Pharm Pharmacol 18:137, 1966
72. Alberty RA, Hammes GG: Application of the theory of diffusion-controlled reactions to enzyme kinetics. J Phys Chem 62:154, 1958
73. Langley JN: On the physiology of the salivary secretion. Part II. J Physiol 1:339, 1878
74. Langley JN: On the contraction of muscle, chiefly in relation to the presence of "receptor" substances. Part IV. J Physiol 33:374, 1904
75. Ehrlich P: Experimental researches on specific therapy (1907 and 1914) pp. 106, 505. In Himmelweit F (ed.): The Collected Papers of Paul Ehrlich Vol. 3. 1960
76. Ehrlich P: Ueber den jetzigen Stand der Chemotherapie. Ber dtsch chem Ges 42:17, 1909
77. Parascandola J: The development of receptor theory. In Parnheim MJ, Bruinvels J (eds): Discoveries in Pharmacology. Elsevier, Amsterdam 1987
78. Von Euler US: Historical perspective: Growth and impact of the concept of chemical neurotransmission. p. 3. In Stjärne L., Hedquist P, Largercrantz O, Wennmalm A (eds). Chemical Neurotransmission: 75 Years. Academic Press, London, 1981
79. Clark AJ, Raventos J: The antagonism of acetylcholine and quaternary ammonium salts. Q J Exp Physiol 26:375, 1937
80. Ariens EJ: Affinity and intrinsic activity in the theory of cooperative inhibition. Arch Int Pharmacol Biochim 99:32, 1954
81. Stephenson RP: A modification of receptor theory. Br J Pharmacol 11:379, 1956
82. Stephenson RP, Ginsborg BL: Potentiation by an antagonist. Nature 222:770, 1969
83. Ginsborg BL, Stephenson RP: On the simultaneous action of two competitive antagonists. Br J Pharmacol 51:287, 1974

84. Furchgott RF, Bursztyn P: Comparison of dissociation constants and relative efficiencies of selective agonists acting on parasympathetic receptors. Ann NY Acad Sci 139:882, 1967
85. Besse JC, Furchgott RF: Dissociation constants and relative efficacies of agonists acting on *alpha* adrenergic receptors in rabbit aorta. J Pharmacol 197:66, 1976
86. Minneman KP: α_1-Adrenergic receptor subtypes, inositol phosphate and sources of cell Ca^{2+}. Pharmacol Rev 40:87, 1988
87. Amitai G, Brown RD, Taylor P: The relationship between alpha$_1$-adrebnergic receptor activation and the mobilization of intracellular Ca^{2+}. J Biol Chem 259:7554, 1986
88. Neubig RR, Cohen JB: Permeability control by cholinergic receptors in *Torpedo* postsynaptic membranes: Agonist dose response relations measured at second and millisecond times. Biochemistry 19:2770, 1980
89. Asano T, Pedersen S, Scott CW, Ross, EW: Reconstitution of catecholamine-stimulated binding of guanosine 5'-0-(3-thiotriphosphate) to the stimulatory GTP-binding protein of adenylate cyclase. Biochemistry 23:5460, 1984
90. Ransnäs LA, Insel PA: Subunit dissociation is the mechanism for hormonal activation of the G_S-protein in native membranes. J Biol Chem 263:17239, 1988
91. Burgen ASV, Spero L: The action of acetylcholine and other drugs on the efflux of potassium and rubidium from smooth muscle of guinea pig intestine. Br J Pharmacol 34:99, 1968
92. Brown JH, Goldstein D: Differences in muscarinic receptor reserve for inhibition of adenylate cyclase and stimulation of phosphoinositide hydrolysis in chick heart cells. Mol Pharmacol 30:566, 1986
93. Ashkenazi A, Winslow JW, Peralta EG, et al: An M2 muscarinic receptor subtype coupled to both adenylyl cyclase and phosphoinositide turnover. Science 238:672, 1987
94. Ashkenazi A, Peralta EG, Winslow JW, et al: Functionally distinct G proteins selectively couple different receptors to phosphatidylinositol hydrolysis in the same cell. Cell 56:487, 1989
95. Goldberg ND: Cyclic nucleotides and cell function p. 185. In Weissmann G, Glaiborne R (eds): Cell Membranes: Biochemistry, Cell Biology and Pathology. Hospital Practice Publishing, New York, 1975
96. Strickland S, Loeb JN: Obligatory separation of hormone binding and biological response curves in systems dependent on secondary mediators of hormone action. Proc Natl Acad Sci USA 78:1366, 1981
97. Paton WDM: A theory of drug action based on the rate of drug-receptor combination. Proc R Soc Lond [Biol] 154:21, 1961
98. Adair GS: The hemoglobin system, VI. The oxygen dissociation curve of hemoglobin. J Biol Chem 63:529, 1925
99. James IF, Goldstein A: Site directed alkylation of multiple opioid receptors. Mol Pharmacol 25:337, 1984
100. Monod J, Wyman J, Changeux, JP: On the nature of allosteric transitions: A plausible model. J Mol Biol 12:88, 1965
101. Changeux J-P, Podleski TP: On the excitability and cooperativity of the electroplax membrane. Proc Natl Acad Sci USA 59:944, 1968
102. Koshland DE, Nemethy G, Filmer D: Comparison of experimental binding data and theoretical models of proteins containing subunits. Biochemistry 5:565, 1966
103. Cornish-Bowden A, Koshland DE: Diagnostic uses of the Hill (Logit and Nernst) plots. J Mol Biol 95:201, 1975
104. Janin J: The nature of allosteric proteins. p. 77. In Butter JAV, Nobel D (eds): Progress of Biophysics and Molecular Biology. Pergamon Press, New York, 1973
105. Karlin A: On the application of a ''plausible model'' of allosteric proteins to the receptor of acetylcholine. J Theor Biol 16:306, 1967
106. Thron CD: On the analysis of pharmacological experiments in terms of an allosteric receptor model. Mol Pharmacol 9:1, 1973

107. Colquhoun D: The relation between classical and cooperative models for drug action. In Rang HP (ed): Drug Receptors. University Park Press, Baltimore, 1978
108. Black JW, Leff P: Operational models of pharmacological agonism. Proc R Soc Lond [Biol] 220:141, 1983
109. Bock MG, DiPardo RM, Evans BE, et al: Gastrin and brain cholecystokinin receptor ligands L-365,260. J Med Chem 32:16, 1989

2

Molecular Basis of Drug Action

Palmer Taylor
Paul A. Insel

RECEPTOR SPECIFICITY AND SIGNAL TRANSDUCTION

The biochemical and molecular characterization of drug, hormone, and other cell surface receptors has proceeded rapidly since the late 1970s, and from this work several general principles of signal transduction via receptors have emerged. Although a diverse group of neurotransmitters, neuromodulators, hormones, and autacoids exert their actions through receptors, nature has evolved only a limited number of basic routines for mediating receptor activation. Discrete extracellular or intracellular receptors that recognize endogenous chemical messengers now number in the several hundreds, with an unknown but large number yet to be characterized. By contrast, the totally unique signal generation mechanisms are likely to number about 10 (Table 2-1). Thus, one can envision a far greater multiplicity of receptors than of the pathways through which the ultimate response is conferred.

By far the greatest specificity arises from the recognition capacity of the individual receptor. Nevertheless, a second order of selectivity arises through polymorphism of coupling proteins, intracellular enzymes, and the branching of signal pathways that amplify or mediate the cellular response.

The general problem of signal transduction relates to eliciting a specific cellular response with an extracellular chemical messenger. The vast majority of these messengers are polar and cannot rapidly enter the cell. Typically, small numbers of receptors are present on the cell surface, and thus amplification represents a critical element in the overall process. As we will see, signal generation relies heavily on inherent changes in conformation of the receptor molecule. These conformational changes are not well understood in molecular terms and yet are often associated with changes in ion permeability or linked to activation of intracellular enzymatic processes. By consideration of the well studied examples, models for related receptors can be deduced. No attempt will be made in this chapter to be comprehensive in covering all receptor types. Rather, receptors representative of particular mechanisms will be highlighted.

Table 2-1. Cellular Receptors and Their Signaling Mechanisms

Receptors	Mode of Action
Plasma Membrane Active	
Cation channels	Na^+, K^{+a}, Ca^{2+a}
Anion channels	Cl^-
Adenylyl cyclase	Stimulation[a], inhibition[a]
Phospholipase C	Stimulation[a], inhibition[a]
Tyrosine kinase	Stimulation
Other candidates	Guanylyl cyclase stimulation, phospholipase A_2 stimulation[a], Na^+/H^+ exchange stimulation[a]
Intracellular	
Transcriptional regulation	Direct binding to promoter or enhancer regions of the gene in 5′ regions or selected introns or by association and regulation of other DNA binding proteins that bind to these regions
Translational regulation	Affects RNA secondary structure and its stability or translation efficiency

[a] Involve regulation by guanine nucleotide–binding proteins.

CHANNEL-CONTAINING RECEPTORS

Several cell-surface molecules possess the capacity to recognize and form complexes with extracellular mediators and, as a result of complex formation, open a channel that selectively allows ions to move down their concentration gradients. The channel and the recognition capacity for the ligand can be intrinsic to the same macromolecule, and the association of subunits or proteins with distinct functions subsequent to ligand binding is not necessary for activation. Other channels are activated by a change in transmembrane potential, and their activity may be modulated by associated receptors that bind ligands or directly by the ligands themselves. In general, there are structural and functional parallels between potential-sensitive (voltage-gated) and chemosensitive (ligand-gated) channels.

Nicotinic Acetylcholine Receptors

The best-characterized receptor system—and in fact one of the most widely studied membrane proteins—is the nicotinic acetylcholine receptor. The fortuitous circumstances of having available a source of receptors in high density and abundance and highly selective markers for this receptor enabled investigators to purify the nicotinic receptor about a decade before purification of other receptor types was possible. Electric organs of the *Torpedo* species are heavily endowed with nicotinic receptors; these electric organs consist of stacks of electrocytes, which emerge from a similar embryonic origin as skeletal muscle. Upon differentiation, the electrogenic bud in the electrocyte proliferates while the contractile elements actually atrophy. Thus, the excitable membrane surface encompasses most of the ventral surface of the electrocyte, instead of being localized to focal junctional areas as in skeletal muscle. The electrical impulse in *Torpedo* relies solely on a postsynaptic excitatory potential resulting from the depolarization of the postsynaptic membrane. The depolarization arises directly from opening of receptor channels, whereas in skeletal muscle and in the freshwater electric eel (*Electrophorus electricus*) depolarization activates a voltage-sensitive Na^+ channel, which in turn causes the depolarization to spread across the surface of the muscle cell or the eel electrocyte. Thus, the absence of a second type of channel in the *Torpedo* electrocyte to amplify the initial depolarization helps explain the requirement for a higher density of nicotinic acetylcholine receptors in this tissue. Receptor densities in *Torpedo* electric organs approach 100 pmol/mg of protein, which may be compared with densities of 0.1 pmol/mg of protein in skeletal muscle. The latter values are typical of many other receptor types.

An ideal marker for a receptor should display specificity or at least marked selectivity for the receptor type in question. In addition, a high affinity and slow rate of dissociation for the monitoring ligand can also prove advantageous in the isolation of receptors. Studies of Chang and Lee in the 1960s established that several snake α-toxins irreversibly inactivated receptor function in intact skeletal muscle,[1] and this finding was applied initially by Changeux and colleagues in 1970 for the identification and subsequent isolation of the nicotinic acetylcholine receptor from the more abundant source of *Torpedo* electric organs.[2] α-Bungarotoxin, a 7,800-dalton peptide from snake venom, was radiolabeled. By virtue of its high affinity and slow rate of dissociation, the labeled toxin served as a marker of the receptor during solubilization and purification.

The purification of this receptor facilitated a detailed examination of its overall structure over the next decade.[3-5] Antibodies were raised to the purified protein, and sufficient amino acid sequence of the receptor itself became available to enable the cloning of the genes encoding the individual subunits of the receptor.[6] Predictions of functional domains and membrane-spanning regions were made from the amino acid sequences deduced from cDNA sequences. Owing to the high density of nicotinic acetylcholine receptors in the postsynaptic membranes of *Torpedo*, sufficient order of the protein is achieved in isolated membrane fragments that image reconstruction could be attempted from electron microscopy and, in initial studies, from x-ray diffraction.[7-9] The high density of receptors has also facilitated investigation of its structure by optical and magnetic resonance spectroscopy. Finally, laborious studies involving the labeling of functional sites, determination of subunit structure, and ascertaining ligand specificity and stoichiometry have contributed and continue to contribute importantly to the interpretations of nicotinic receptor structure.[3-7]

Acetylcholine Receptor Structure

From these approaches we now know that the nicotinic acetylcholine receptor in muscle consists of four distinct subunits of partially homologous amino acid sequence (30 to 40 percent identity of amino acid residues) arranged around a pseudoaxis of symmetry. One of the subunits, designated α, is expressed in two copies, while the other three (β, γ, and δ) are present as single copies (Fig. 2-1). Thus, the receptor is a pentamer of molecular mass near 280 kDa. Structural studies show the subunits to be arranged around a central cavity with the largest portion of the protein exposed towards the extracellular surface. The central cavity is believed to be the ion channel, which in the resting state is impermeable to ions but upon activation opens to a diameter of about 6.5Å. The open channel is selective for cations, but among the cations permeation of the channel appears limited primarily by the 6.5Å diameter. The α subunits form the site for binding of agonists and competitive antagonists and the primary surface with which the larger snake α-toxin molecules associate. A site for ligand binding exists on each of the α subunits. Electrophysiologic and ligand-binding measurements, together with analysis of the functional states

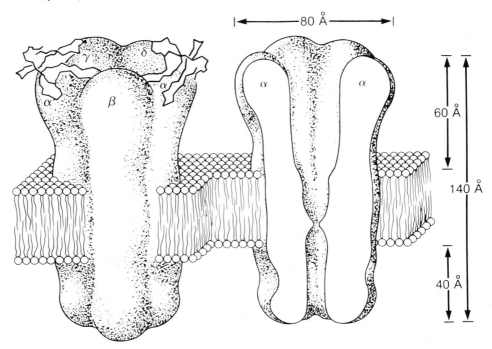

Fig. 2-1. Structure of the acetylcholine receptor from image reconstruction analyses employing electron microscopy on isolated membrane tubes enriched in receptor. The receptor is a pentamer of four distinct subunits ($\alpha_2\beta\gamma\delta$); this illustration shows one proposed subunit arrangement. The internal channel surrounded by the five subunits appears funnel-shaped, with the primary constriction near the membrane surface. Most of the membrane protein projects from the membrane on the outer or extracellular surface. A nonintegral membrane peptide, often termed *43k*, is associated with the cytoplasmic surface of the receptor. Although it is not essential to the function of the receptor and can be dissociated by mild alkaline treatment of the receptor, this peptide appears to play a role in immobilization and aggregation of receptors in junctional regions. This peptide may contribute to much of the cytoplasmic density seen in the proposed structure. Two α-toxin molecules bind per receptor oligomer, presumably one on each α subunit. The stoichiometry of agonists such as acetylcholine and antagonists such as *d*-tubocurarine is equivalent to that of the α toxins: two bound ligands per oligomer. The outlined structures at the outer perimeters of the top of the α subunits represent the peptide chains of bound cobra α toxin. (Adapted from Brisson and Unwin,[9] with permission.)

of the receptor, indicate positive cooperativity in the association of agonists; Hill coefficients greater than unity have been described for agonist-elicited channel opening, agonist binding, and agonist-induced desensitization of the receptor.[3-5]

The sequences of the individual subunits are shown in Figure 2-2. Sequence identity among the subunits appears greatest in the hydrophobic regions, which indicates that the subunits have evolved from a common primordial gene. Various models for the disposition of the peptide chains have been proposed on the basis of hydropathy (Fig. 2-3) and reactivity of various residues to modifying agents and antibodies. Five candidate membrane-spanning regions (domains) have been proposed. Four of these are hydrophobic (M_1 to M_4), while one (M_A) can be constructed as an amphipathic α helix containing negative charges aligned to one surface of the helix (Fig. 2-4). All these regions appear after residue

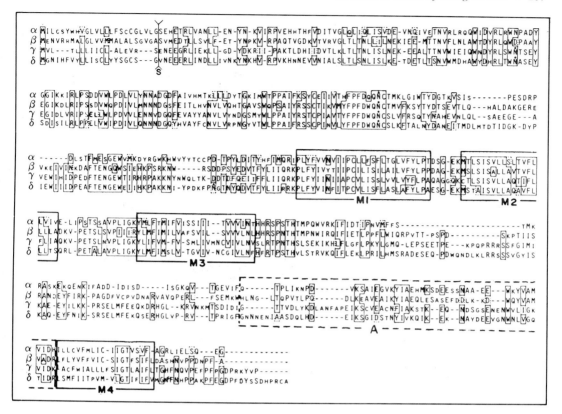

Fig. 2-2. Sequence homology between the four subunits (α, β, γ, δ) of the *Torpedo californica* acetylcholine receptor. Amino acid positions identical in at least three of the four subunits are enclosed in solid boxes. Cases in which the fourth residue is replaced with a residue of equivalent hydrophilic/hydrophobic character are denoted by a dotted line. The four hydrophobic α-helical domains and one amphipathic α helix, which are candidates for spanning the membrane, are denoted by M_1 to M_4, and M_A, respectively. The arrow denoted by S represents the cleavage point of the signal peptide. (The single-letter code is used: A = alanine, C = cysteine, D = aspartate, E = glutamate, F = phenylalanine, G = glycine, H = histidine, I = isoleucine, K = lysine, L = leucine, M = methionine, N = asparagine, P = proline, Q = glutamine, R = arginine, S = serine, T = threonine, V = valine, W = tryptophan, Y = tyrosine.) (From Changeux et al.,[3] with permission.)

210, with the N-terminal portion of the molecule on the extracellular surface. The homology between the α, β, γ, and δ subunits strongly suggests that the same folding pattern is found in all subunits (Fig. 2-4). The validity of such models should continue to be tested by rigorous structural studies. There is substantial evidence that at least the four hydrophobic regions contributed by each subunit traverse the membrane, but it has not been rigorously established that the amphipathic helix or other domains also span the membrane.[7] Analysis of primary structure allows for predictions on overall structure, but further details on structure of the receptor are likely to emerge from analysis of disulfide linkages, reactivity of particular residues, and higher-resolution structural methods.

In the α subunit, Asp 141 is glycosylated and hence is on the outside surface. After reduction of the receptor by dithiothreitol to convert disulfide bonds to free thiols, bro-

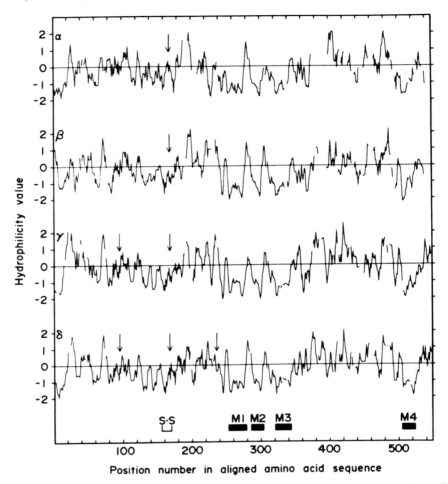

Fig. 2-3. Hydropathy profiles of the four subunits of the acetylcholine receptor from *Torpedo*. Membrane-spanning regions are shown by the shading. Values above zero denote hydrophilicity and values below zero hydrophobicity.[3,6] The arrows denote glycosylation sites. The numbering system includes the leader peptide so that 24 amino acids must be subtracted to obtain the positions in the processed peptides for α and β, 17 for γ, and 21 for δ. (From Numa et al.,[6] with permission.)

moacetylcholine and 4-(*N*-maleimido)benzyltrimethylammonium (MBTA)[4] react with cysteine 192 or 193. Since the adjacent cysteines at residues 192 and 193 are unique to the α subunit, this region is believed to play a role in agonist binding. Cysteine 192 and 193 appear disulfide-linked with each other as are cysteines 128 and 142. The latter linkage results in an extracellular disulfide loop in the receptor. Additional labeling studies and higher-resolution structural analysis should more precisely define chain folding in this region, but it appears that about the first 200 residues are largely, if not totally, in the extracellular domain. When the subunits from the muscle and the subtypes of neuronal receptor from the rat are compared, similar structural motifs involving the disulfide loops, glycosylation sites, and membrane-spanning domains are evident (Fig. 2-5). Residues in the β (serine 254) and δ chain (serine 262) have been labeled with the noncompetitive inhibitors chlorpromazine and tetraphenylphosphonium. The labeled residues are part of the regions that span the membrane (M2), and conformational changes in this region could be critical to channel opening. The cobra α-toxins and α-bungarotoxin have a leaflike structure[10] (Fig. 2-6) and bind to an extended surface area, which is mainly encompassed by the two α subunits (Fig. 2-1). Fluorescence energy transfer measurements and electron microscopic imaging indicate that the α-toxin and agonist binding sites are closer to the outer perimeter of the receptor than to the pseudoaxis of symmetry running down the center of the molecule.

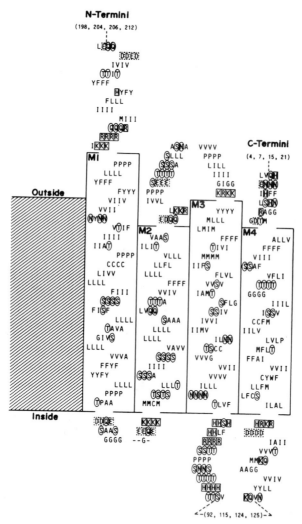

Fig. 2-4. Proposed membrane-spanning regions for the four subunits (α, β, γ, δ) of the *Torpedo* acetylcholine receptor. The numbers indicate the residues not shown in the sequence. Cationic residues are shown in solid rectangles, anionic residues in broken rectangles, and neutral polar residues in ovals. In this representation M_A, the amphipathic helix, does not span the membrane, leaving the N- and C-terminal peptides on the same side of the membrane. (From Numa et al.,[6] with permission.)

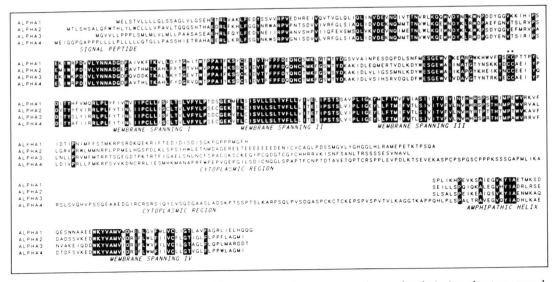

Fig. 2-5. Alignment of the amino acid sequences of mouse muscle α subunit (α_1) and rat neuronal α_2, α_3, and α_4 subunits. The two cysteines (corresponding to 192 and 193 in *Torpedo*) are marked by the double asterisks. Darkened areas show residue identities. (From Wada et al.,[22] with permission.)

Functional States of the Acetylcholine Receptor

The cooperative events associated with ligand binding and activation of the receptor have been studied by analysis of opening and closing events of individual channels using high-resistance patch electrodes.[11] These electrodes form tight seals on the membrane surface over a diameter of 1 to 2 μm and have the capacity to record conductance changes of individual channels within the lumen of the electrode. The patch of membrane with the electrode may be excised, inverted, or studied on the intact cell. The individual opening events for acetylcholine elicited responses achieve a conductance of 25 picosiemens (10^{-12} ohms^{-1}) across the membrane and have an opening duration that is exponentially distributed around a value of about 1 msec. The durations of channel-opening events are dependent on the particular agonist, while the conductance of the open channel state appears to be independent of the agonist provided the agonist itself does not block the channel. Analyses of the frequencies of opening events have permitted estimation of the kinetic constants for channel opening and ligand binding. Overall, activation events can be described by the following scheme:

$$2L + R \underset{k_{-1}}{\overset{2k_1}{\rightleftharpoons}} L + LR \underset{2k_{-1}}{\overset{k_1}{\rightleftharpoons}} L_2R \underset{k_{-2}}{\overset{k_2}{\rightleftharpoons}} L_2R^* \qquad (1)$$

(Closed)   (Closed)   (Closed)   (Open)

Two ligands L associate with the receptor R prior to the isomerization step to form the open-channel state L_2R^*. For acetylcholine $k_1 = 1 - 2 \times 10^8$ M^{-1}sec^{-1}, a value about one order of magnitude below that for a diffusion-limited process on a fully exposed target site (cf. Ch. 1). The constants k_2 and k_{-2} yield rates of isomerization consistent with opening events in the millisecond time frame. Since k_2 and k_{-2} are greater than k_{-1}, several opening and closing events with the fully liganded receptor are likely to occur prior to dissociation of the first ligand. Binding of the first and second ligands appears not to be identical even allowing for the statistical differences arising from occupation of the two sites. Such a conclusion is not inconsistent with receptor structure, since the subunits adjacent to the α subunits cannot be identical in the pentamer. Moreover, evidence has been obtained that processing of the respective glycosylation sites (Asp 141) in two α subunits may not be equivalent even though the two α-subunits are transcribed by a common gene.

Desensitization of Nicotinic Receptors

It has been well known since the 1950s that continued exposure of nicotinic receptors to agonist leads to a diminution of the response even though the concentration of agonist available to the receptor is not changed. The loss of response from prior agonist exposure is called *desensitization*. Katz and Thesleff[12] examined the kinetics of the desensitization process with microelectrodes and found that the rate of desensitization was dependent on agonist concentration (up to a limiting concentration), while the recovery rate was slow and independent of both the specific agonist and the agonist concentration used to achieve desensitization. Moreover, the recovery rate was intermediate between the rates of desensitization onset at low and high agonist concentrations. From these kinetic considerations, a cyclic scheme for the process was proposed according to which the receptor existed in two states, R and R', prior to exposure to the ligand:

$$
\begin{array}{ccc}
\text{L} + \text{R} & \overset{K_R}{\rightleftharpoons} & \text{LR} \\
\text{M} \updownarrow & & \updownarrow \\
\text{L} + \text{R}' & \underset{K_{R'}}{\rightleftharpoons} & \text{LR}'
\end{array}
\tag{2}
$$

where $M = [\text{R}']/[\text{R}]$, R denotes the resting or activatible state, and R' is the desensitized state. In this scheme M is less than unity and the dissociation constant K_R' is less than K_R. Accordingly, in the absence of L the receptor exists primarily as R or in an activatible state. Addition of ligand will eventually result in an increased fraction of R' species because K_R'/K_R is less than unity. Since the equilibria represented horizontally are fast and the vertical ones are slow, upon dilution of such a system the ligand rapidly dissociates and the slower R' → R transition should dictate the rate of recovery from desensitization. The driving force for desensitization is simply the higher affinity of receptor in the R' state, and no external energy is required. In this basic scheme the existence of an activatible R and a desensitized R' state precede the binding of ligand. The hypothesis by Katz and Thesleff[12] in 1957 of two receptor states controlled by ligand occupation in fact antedated the proposal of allosteric theories of protein conformation (cf. Ch. 1). Both the cyclic model for receptor desensitization and the concerted model for cooperativity of multisubunit proteins[13] are based on the existence of the protein in multiple states and on their population distribution being influenced by the associating ligand.

The presence of multiple states of the receptor and the slow transitions to states possessing higher affinity for agonists have been confirmed by direct binding experiments. As expected, agonists exhibit a greater tendency for promoting the conversion to the high-affinity state than do antagonists.

Since the early 1980s it has been possible to examine desensitization by single-channel kinetics, rapid flow methods with isolated membrane vesicles containing receptor, and

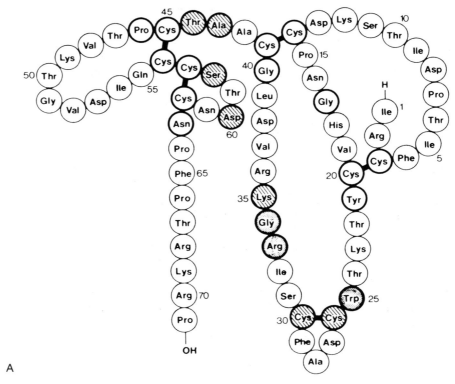

Fig. 2-6. Structure of the cobra α toxins (*Naja naja siamensis*). These toxins and related toxins—α-bungarotoxins from *Bungaris multicintis*—bind essentially irreversibly to the nicotinic acetylcholine receptor. The α toxins are extensively linked by internal disulfide bonds, which confer a rigid structure. Stabilization energy of the toxin complex with the receptor arises from a multipoint attachment between α toxin and the receptor, although it is felt that the loop encompassing the cysteines between 14 and 41 may be the most important. (**A**) Amino acid sequence showing disulfide attachments. (*Figure Continues*).

electrophysiologic procedures that allow rapid concentration changes of agonist.[14] The overall process appears more complex; a rapid and a slow desensitization step (of about 100 msec and about several seconds duration, respectively) can be detected. Even with this additional complexity, it appears that multiple states of the receptor provide the best means of modeling the kinetics of desensitization. Phosphorylation of the receptor at particular residues on a cytoplasmic loop of the molecule influences the kinetics of desensitization, but this is not obligatory for desensitization. Phosphorylation of neuronal nicotinic receptors may also provide a means for controlling the fraction of active and inactive receptors.

   In the functioning neuromuscular junction, a question arises as to whether desensitization would be detectable when quantal release and rapid destruction of acetylcholine prevail. Under conditions in which miniature end-plate currents from acetylcholine are prolonged by acetylcholinesterase inhibition, desensitization can be observed following repetitive nerve stimulation.[15] Receptor states resembling the desensitized state are also evident when the intact neuromuscular junction is treated with agonists or partial agonists,

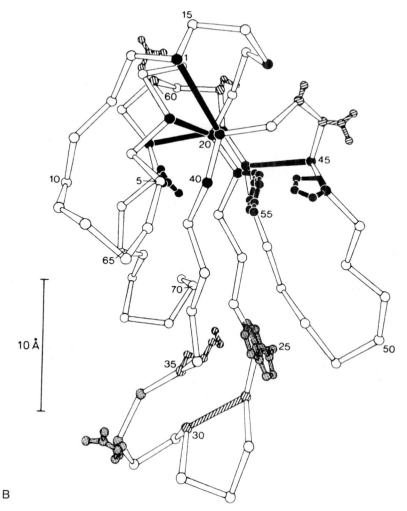

Fig. 2-6. (*Continued*). (**B**) Structure of cobra α-toxins from x-ray crystallographic analysis. Positions of certain side chains and the disulfide bonds are shown. (From Walkinshaw et al.,[10] with permission.)

such as decamethonium, that are not susceptible to acetylcholinesterase-catalyzed hydrolysis.

Scheme for Nicotinic Receptor Activation and Desensitization

To achieve receptor desensitization and activation by a single ligand, multiple conformational states of the protein must be proposed. As before, the binding steps are represented in the horizontal equilibria and are rapid, while the vertical steps reflect the slow unimolecular isomerizations involved in desensitization. A rapid isomerization of channel opening must be added to the scheme. To accommodate the additional complexities of the observed fast and slow steps of desensitization, additional states would also have to be considered.

A simplified scheme in which only one desensitized and one open-channel state of the receptor exist could be represented as follows (Eq. 3 and Fig. 2-7).

$$2L + R \rightleftharpoons LR \rightleftharpoons L_2R \rightleftharpoons L_2R^*$$
$$M \updownarrow \qquad \updownarrow \qquad \updownarrow \qquad \qquad (3)$$
$$2L + R' \rightleftharpoons LR' \rightleftharpoons L_2R'$$

Electrophysiologic studies have enabled investigators to assign most of the kinetic constants involving the individual steps, even though activation and desensitization are the only parameters measured. This results from the fact that measurements can be made over a range of concentrations. Statistical analyses can be applied to the bursts of opening events in the presence of high and low concentrations of agonist. Measurements obtained from fast kinetic (stopped-flow) studies, in which ligand occupation and ligand-elicited permeability changes (ion fluxes) in membrane vesicles enriched in receptors are measured, yield kinetics in accord with those observed in the electrophysiologic analyses.[14]

Requirements for Activation and Antagonism of Nicotinic Receptors

It has long been known that reversible neuromuscular blocking agents typified by *d*-tubocurarine can block receptor function competitively under appropriate conditions (see Fig. 2-8). Accordingly, parallel rightward shifts of the agonist dose–response curves with no depression of the maximum response can be achieved with *d*-tubocurarine inhibition in intact muscle preparations. Although it cannot be stated with certainty that the binding of agonists and antagonists occurs at overlapping sites, their binding is mutually exclusive. The same mutually exclusive binding occurs with the α-toxins and agonists, although in this case the slow rate of toxin dissociation precludes equilibration of agonist and α-toxin. Hence, one cannot demonstrate competitive behavior between α-toxins and agonists over normal time intervals for equilibration. Nevertheless, it can be shown that the α-toxins

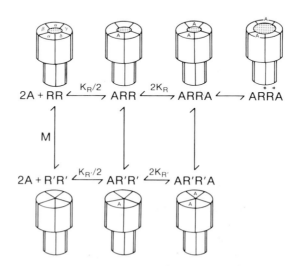

Fig. 2-7. Representation of the dominant states of the acetylcholine receptor during ligand binding, activation, and desensitization. The ligand is represented by A for acetylcholine.

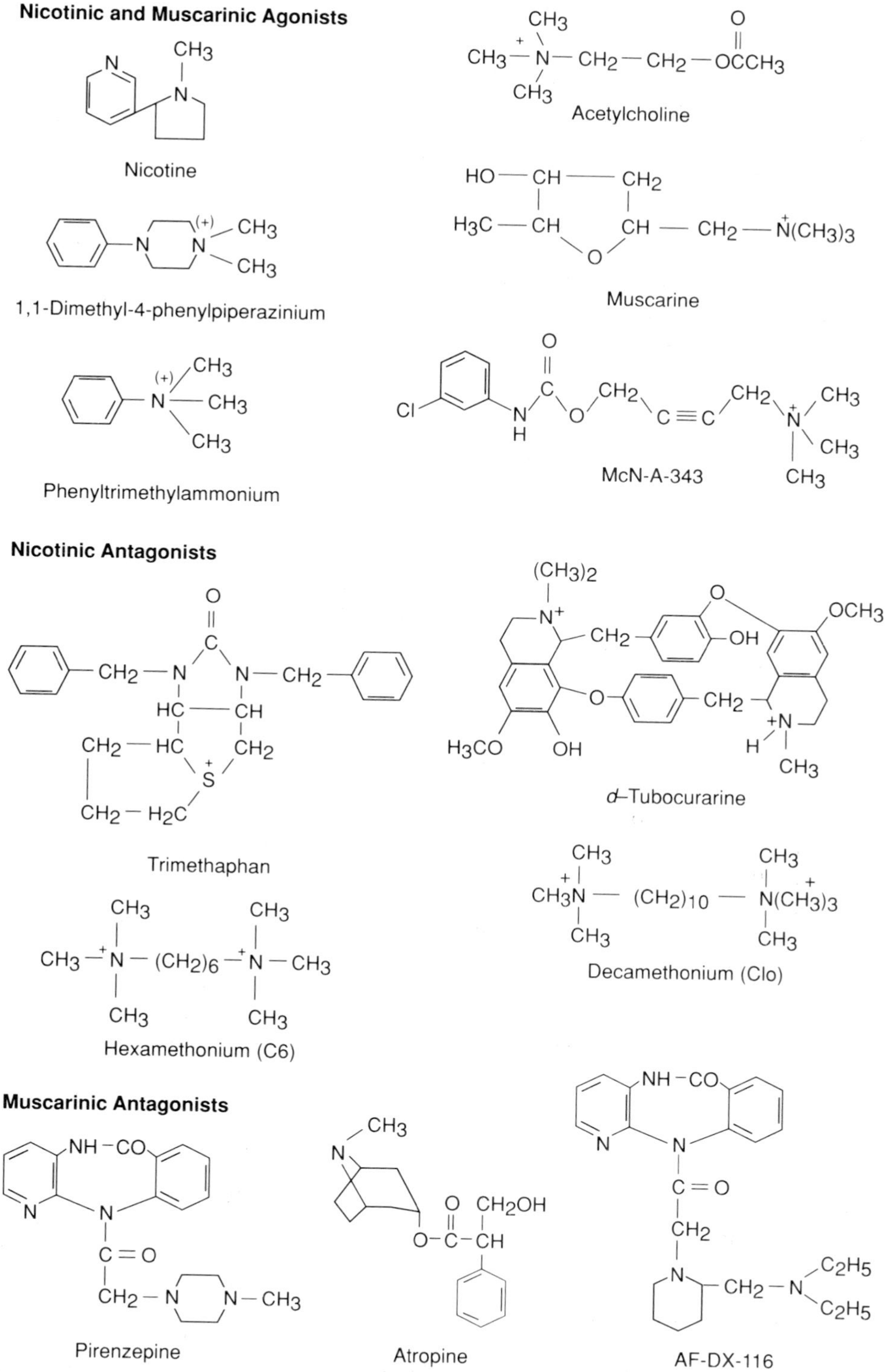

Nicotinic and Muscarinic Agonists

Nicotine

Acetylcholine

1,1-Dimethyl-4-phenylpiperazinium

Muscarine

Phenyltrimethylammonium

McN-A-343

Nicotinic Antagonists

Trimethaphan

d–Tubocurarine

Hexamethonium (C6)

Decamethonium (Clo)

Muscarinic Antagonists

Pirenzepine

Atropine

AF-DX-116

Fig. 2-8. Structures of some nicotinic and muscarinic agonists and antagonists.

inhibit occupation of the receptor by agonists and that agonists competitively inhibit the initial rate of α-toxin binding.

Since occupation of more than one site by agonist is required to achieve the cooperative activation profiles obtained for nicotinic receptors, it might be asked whether occupation of a single site on each receptor oligomer by an antagonist is sufficient to block receptor function. When the fractional occlusion of binding sites is examined with an α-toxin whose slow rate of dissociation allows it to be treated as an irreversible ligand, the populations of binding species would be defined by a binomial distribution (Fig. 2-9). If the two sites show no distinction for the association of α-toxin, then the fraction of sites binding α-toxin, y, would be defined by the following equation:

$$y = \frac{n_{1A}/2 + n_{1B}/2 + n_2}{\Sigma n} \tag{4}$$

The fraction of sites that remain vacant and should be available for agonist binding will be:

$$m = \frac{n_0 + n_{1A}/2 + n_{1B}/2}{\Sigma n} = 1 - y \tag{5}$$

The fraction of unoccupied receptor species is described by $n_0/\Sigma n$ or $(1 - y)^2$, the fraction of receptor species occupied by α-toxin at both sites is defined by y^2, and the fraction of hybrid species containing one of the two sites occupied is defined by $2y(1 - y)$. Analysis of the loss of functional response with fractional occupation by α-toxin is shown in Figure 2-10, and the data are best fitted by the parabola described by $(1 - y)^2$. Thus it appears that only the doubly unoccupied receptor species is able to respond upon addition of agonist and that the hybrid species containing an agonist and α-toxin on the receptor are nonfunctional. Should this condition hold, a corollary would be that fractional occupation by α-toxin should not change the shape (i.e., the concentration dependence and Hill coefficient) of the agonist dose–response curve. This is to be expected, since it is only the doubly unoccupied species that will lead to a response upon addition of agonist. On the other hand, analysis of occupation of the residual sites not blocked by α-toxin should reveal a change in concentration dependence if occupation is cooperative. Occupation of the vacant site in the hybrid species should have a linkage relationship with the neighboring site different from that of the sites on the doubly unoccupied species. The above observations on agonist occupation and the functional response following fractional occupation by α toxin have been borne out for nicotinic receptors in intact cells and isolated vesicles.[16–18]

Antagonism by Reversible Ligands

The binding of reversible antagonists is not equivalent at the two sites on the individual α subunits,[19,20] and binding can be described by a two-site model in which the sites are present in equal populations.[20] For a series of antagonists we would expect the fractional population of the two sites to be constant, but the binding constants for each site would be dependent on the ligand and would not necessarily be equivalent. This, in fact, has been shown for the nicotinic receptor for several competitive antagonists (Fig. 2-11). The block of the functional response can also be examined and correlated with occupancy of the sites. As in the case of antagonism by the α-toxins, a hybrid receptor containing an agonist and a reversible antagonist on the respective sites is nonfunctional. These considerations may further distinguish between models in which the nonequivalence in binding

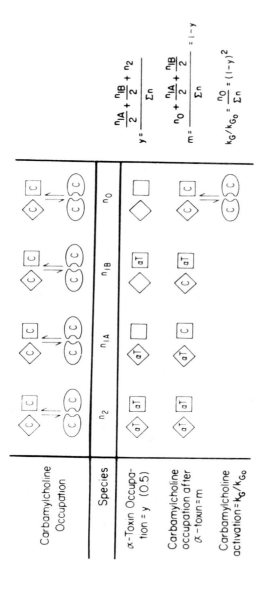

Fig. 2-9. Description of occupied species of the acetylcholine receptors, showing the relationship between prior α-toxin (αT) occupation and agonist (i.e., carbamylcholine (C)) occupation and activation of the acetylcholine receptor. The receptor is depicted as a dimer of nonequivalent binding sites. α-Toxin association does not distinguish between sites. (From Taylor et al.,[5] with permission.)

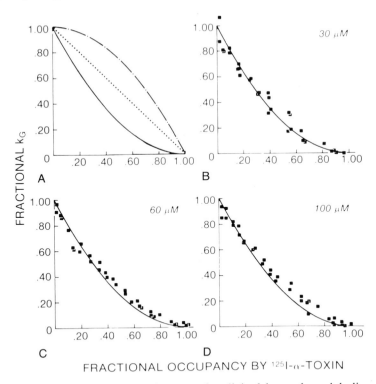

Fig. 2-10. Reduction of the permeability increase k_G elicited by carbamylcholine resulting from progressive occupancy of receptors by ^{125}I-labeled α-toxin. **(A)** Theoretical relationships for the fractional permeability response versus fractional occupancy of receptors by the irreversible binding of α-toxin generated from models 1 to 3 (——·——· , Model 1; ····· , model 2; ——— , model 3). *Model 1*: Functional receptor contains two binding sites, and full activation results when one or two binding sites are occupied under saturating agonist concentrations. Occupation of both sites by toxin is required to block function. Therefore, $k_G = k_{Go}(1 - y^2)$, where k_G is the observed response, k_{Go} the observed response in the absence of fractional α-toxin occupation, and y fractional occupation by α-toxin. *Model 2*: Functional receptor contains two binding sites, and activation results when one or two binding sites are occupied under saturating agonist concentrations. Occupation of each site by α-toxin reduces the response capacity of the receptor molecule by one-half; therefore $k_G = k_{Go} (1 - y)$. *Model 3*: Functional receptor contains two binding sites, and activation requires occupation of both binding sites by agonist. Occupation of either site by α-toxin will completely block function. Therefore $k_G = k_{Go} (1 - y)^2$ **(B–D)** Experimentally determined fractional k_G following progressive degrees of occupancy by ^{125}I-labeled α-toxin. Permeability increases, determined from the rates of sodium influx elicited by 30 (Fig. B), 60 (Fig. C), and 100 μM (Fig. D) carbamylcholine. In each panel the solid line corresponds to the function $k_G = k_{Go} (1 - y)^2$ resulting from model 3. (Adapted from Taylor et al.[5] and Sine et al.,[16] with permission.)

affinity at the two sites is confined to a single receptor molecule as opposed to a model with two discrete populations of receptor molecules in which the binding affinities are identical on each molecule.[20] If we define overall fractional occupation by y

$$y = 0.5 (X_A) + 0.5 (X_B) \tag{6}$$
$$= 0.5 [[L]/([L] + K_A)] + 0.5 [[L]/([L] + K_B)]$$

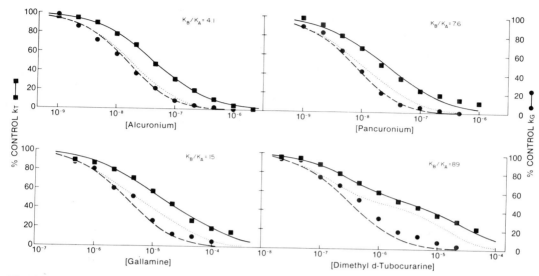

Fig. 2-11. Relationship between antagonist binding and functional antagonism of the nicotinic receptor. Assume the two sites are present in equal populations and the data are fitted to two dissociation constants in the ratios of dissociation constants indicated. The fit is shown by the solid line. Occupation is measured from the inhibition of the initial rates of α-toxin binding k_T, and the solid squares show the data points. The dashed and dotted lines reflect the predicted functional antagonism of agonist-elicited ion permeability, k_G, using the same ratio of dissociation constants if the nonequivalent sites exist on a single receptor population (dashed line) or exist on two distinct receptor populations in which the sites are identically paired (dotted line). The solid circles are experimental measurements of the block of the functional response.

where X_A and X_B reflect the fractional occupation of the A and B sites by reversible antagonist with dissociation constants K_A and K_B, respectively.

Thus, if the respective populations of A and B sites are nearly equal, binding experiments alone will not distinguish a model involving a single receptor species with nonequivalent sites from one involving two populations of receptors with equivalent sites. However, measurement of the functional response adds an additional dimension to the analysis.

In the case in which a single receptor molecule with nonequivalent sites exists, the fractional response (Δ/Δ_0) can be described by:

$$(\Delta/\Delta_0) = (1 - X_A)(1 - X_B)$$
$$= [K_A/([L] + K_A)][K_B/([L] + K_B)] \tag{7}$$

The other limiting case, in which the two sites exist on different receptor molecules but each receptor contains identical sites, is described by:

$$(\Delta/\Delta_0) = 0.5(1 - X_A)^2 + 0.5(1 - X_B)^2$$
$$= 0.5\left(\frac{K_A}{[L] + K_A}\right)^2 + 0.5\left(\frac{K_B}{[L] + K_B}\right)^2 \tag{8}$$

The data in Figure 2-11 are best described by a limiting model in which the nonequivalence of sites is confined to a single receptor molecule (Eq. 7).

With the multiple sites on each receptor molecule, fractional occupation of antagonist sites would not be equivalent to fractional antagonism of the permeability response. In the extreme case in which one site is of much higher affinity (i.e., K_A is smaller than K_B), then K_{ant}, the dissociation constant for functional antagonism, will equal K_A. Alternatively, when K_A equals K_B, then K_{ant} will equal $K_A/(1 + \sqrt{2})$ (i.e., $K_A/2.4$). These equations allow for the enhanced statistical probability of functional antagonism when occupation of either site by antagonist leads to a nonfunctional receptor. Antagonism of receptor function where occupation of two or more sites is required for activation would be an exception to the rule that the calculated dissociation constant from the pharmacologic experiment is equal to the dissociation constant of the antagonist calculated from binding studies (cf. Ch. 1).

Subtypes of Nicotinic Receptors

Early pharmacologic comparisons showed that nicotinic receptors in ganglia of the autonomic nervous system possessed a different pharmacologic specificity than did those found in the neuromuscular junction. Hexamethonium is the most potent in the series of bisquaternary ammonium ligands in blocking at ganglia, while decamethonium is the most potent in producing depolarization blockade at the neuromuscular junction. Hexamethonium blocks depolarization in the neuromuscular nicotinic receptor, but treatment of this receptor with a reducing agent such as dithiothreitol causes hexamethonium to become a partial agonist. These early findings from classical assays of receptor function also pointed to minor structural modifications of the receptor protein, such as disulfide bond reduction, affecting the specificity and functional responses of interacting ligands.

Several other reversible antagonists and a few agonists show partial, but not complete, selectivity for the ganglionic and neuromuscular subtypes of nicotinic receptors. A more striking difference in specificity is seen with α-bungarotoxin and cobra α-toxin (elapid α-toxins). These peptides have dissociation constants not greater than $10^{-10}M$ for the neuromuscular receptor and are virtually inactive in ganglia or other nicotinic receptors derived from the embryonic neural crest. The peptidic α-conotoxins from marine snails are also only active on the muscle receptor while the κ-toxins (also called neuronal bungarotoxin), which are peptides from snake venom, are active on ganglionic and central nervous system nicotinic receptors. The lophotoxins, diterpenoid toxins from coral, block nicotinic receptors from neurons and muscle.

Nevertheless, the absence of an enriched source of nicotinic receptors from ganglia or brain has meant that progress in the direct isolation of these nicotinic receptor subtypes lagged behind that for receptors in the neuromuscular junction. However, the cDNAs isolated from the neuromuscular receptor appear to have provided the necessary key to obtaining detailed structural information on neuronal nicotinic receptors. Since considerable sequence homology exists between nicotinic receptor subtypes, cross-hybridization using muscle or electrocyte cDNA clones in neuronal libraries has yielded several candidate cDNAs encoding subunits for nicotinic receptors from the central nervous system and tissues of neural crest origin.[21,22] That these cDNAs encode functional subunits of a nicotinic receptor can be demonstrated by injection of their transcripts into oocytes and detection of changes in permeability elicited by acetylcholine. The evidence to date indicates that the neuronal nicotinic receptors consist of only α and β subunits in some combination that gives rise to a tetramer or, more probably, a pentamer. Localization of mRNA that hybridizes with the cDNA clones to particular regional areas in the central nervous system documents their central origin and distinct regional distributions. A more

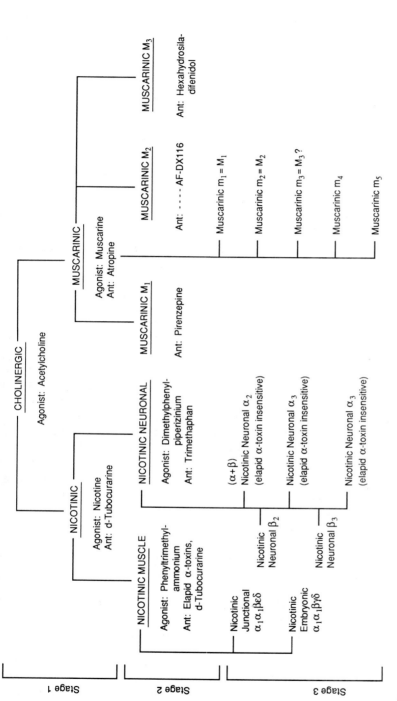

Fig. 2-12. Evolution of acetylcholine receptor classification. Parallel to identification of a presumed neurotransmitter, responses were subtyped in the 1910s and 1920s on the basis of crude alkaloids from *Amanita muscaria* and *Nicotiana tabacum* (stage 1). Additional discrimination was possible by rank ordering of potencies with alkaloids whose structures were determined and with synthetic compounds (stage 2). A third stage has emerged from the molecular cloning of the receptors; expression in cells, and an analysis of their pharmacologic properties. In the case of the nicotinic receptor, two distinct types in muscle have been identified; they differ in expression of one of the subunits γ and ϵ. In neurons (brain and ganglia), three types of receptors based on different α subunits have been identified: α_1 is the muscle subunit, whereas α_2, α_3, and α_4 are distinct neuronal subunits. Activity results from coinjection with a neuronal subunit β_2 or β_3, giving rise to a pentamer composed of α and β subunits. Studies involving the purification of brain nicotinic receptors have yielded α and β subunits. Molecular cloning of muscarinic receptors has yielded five receptor subtypes, m_1, m_2, m_3, m_4, and m_5. Subtype m_1 was cloned from brain and corresponds functionally to the M_1 subtype pharmacologically; m_2 was cloned from heart and corresponds to M_2; and the pharmacologic specificity of m_3 resembled that of the glandular receptor, termed M_3 by some groups. The pharmacology and anatomical locations of m_4 and m_5 have not been fully resolved. The nomenclature of the cloned receptors corresponds to that of Bonner et al.[164]

difficult task will be the assignment of particular cDNAs to receptor subtypes that are actually isolated from these brain regions.

Acetylcholine (Cholinergic) Receptor Classification

Although information on the structures and ligand specificity of central nervous system nicotinic receptors is incomplete, it is instructive to examine acetylcholine receptor subtypes in order to see how classical receptor classifications deduced from ligand specificity (i.e., pharmacologic classification) can now be extended by a knowledge of receptor coupling mechanisms, protein sequence, and subunit composition. This approach enables one to subtype receptors at the molecular level. In Figure 2-12 we see that the initial classification of nicotinic receptors and muscarinic receptors and subsequently the designation of their subtypes were based on pharmacologic specificity of agonists and antagonists in different tissues. The first stage of classification occurred prior to the availability of chemically synthesized analogs of natural agonists or antagonists; hence, classification relied on the use of plant alkaloid extracts. The terms *nicotinic* and *muscarinic* were based on eliciting activity with rather crude extracts containing nicotine and muscarine before the structures of the alkaloids were known. The availability of chemically synthesized antagonists revealed enhanced selectivity and enabled further discrimination between receptor subtypes. Hence, the second stage of receptor classification was at least partially reliant on the skills and persistence of the organic chemist. It is also fortunate that in the peripheral nervous system the subtypes of acetylcholine receptors have largely segregated themselves to particular tissues or anatomic regions.

Different genes encode the α subunits of the neuronal and neuromuscular nicotinic receptors, and the neuronal receptors appear to lack γ and δ subunits. Molecular cloning studies in brain have revealed at least three different neuronal α subunits and two β subunits (Figs. 2-5 and 2-12). Expression of functional receptor from cDNA clones is achieved by in vitro transcription of the cDNAs and injection of the transcribed mRNAs from the various subunits into oocytes[22] or by direct transfection of the cDNAs into somatic cell lines.[23] Electrophysiologic measurements from the cell surface reveal that the cDNAs yield functional gene products and the encoded α subunits have different specificities for the snake α- and κ-toxins.[21,22] In addition to their discrete regional locations and cell type distribution in brain and other tissues, different nicotinic receptor subtypes may appear at a particular stage in development. For example, small differences in antagonist affinity and channel-opening kinetics have been detected between junctional and extrajunctional (embryonic) nicotinic receptors in skeletal muscle. This difference appears to arise from the γ subunit being expressed in embryonic muscle and being replaced by an ε subunit in adult tissue, where the receptor is primarily localized in the junctional endplate. Although junctional and extrajunctional receptors in muscle have slightly different voltage sensitivities and affinities for *d*-tubocurarine, it would have been difficult to make a case for a discrete subtype of muscle nicotinic receptor on the basis of the pharmacologic data alone.

These examples reveal the third stage of the evolution of receptor classification, in which functional differences can be measured as primary responses (i.e., opening and closing of single receptor channels) in a defined cell system to which the gene or mRNA can be added to achieve expression of the pharmacologic response. In turn, the functional response can be related to an absolute parameter, namely, the primary structure of the receptor, which is deduced from the sequence of the encoding gene. If the α and β subunits were to associate in various permutations, the number of subtypes of receptor oligomers would be bewildering.

Muscarinic acetylcholine receptors couple to guanine nucleotide-binding (G) proteins and only share with nicotinic receptors the property of acetylcholine recognition. Hence, there is no reason to expect that these receptor proteins are at all related beyond the point that both recognize acetylcholine. The recent cloning of muscarinic receptor cDNAs reveals no sequence homology with nicotinic receptors; their structures will be considered in a subsequent section. Here again, knowledge of primary structures has rapidly expanded the number of distinct receptor subtypes.

Voltage-Sensitive Channels

A family of channels is known to mediate the conductance of Na^+, Ca^{2+}, and K^+ in response to a change in membrane potential.[24,25] Hence these channels have been termed *potential-sensitive* or *voltage-gated* to distinguish them from *chemosensitive* or *ligand-gated* channels. The voltage-gated channels propagate action potentials in electrically excitable cells and are involved in the regulation of membrane potential and intracellular Ca^{2+} transients in most cells. These channels are highly selective for a particular cation, yet have comparatively large single-channel conductances. They are characterized by a marked voltage dependence for activation, which is much greater than that exhibited by ligand-gated channels.

Examination of the voltage-gated channels has revealed several common structural and functional features with the ligand-gated channels. Electrophysiologic measurements show that the channel-opening kinetics for the nicotinic receptors considered in the previous sections are voltage-sensitive. Thus, voltage can modify both the duration of individual opening events and the probability of opening in the presence of agonist. Similarly, although voltage-sensitive channels function in the absence of endogenous ligands and are documented to be triggered by a change in transmembrane potential, several naturally occurring activators and inhibitors of the voltage-sensitive channels have been identified. It is of clear evolutionary advantage for smaller organisms to produce such toxins, for they can activate excessively or block voltage-sensitive channels in a predator or an incompatible neighbor. Moreover, these toxins have proved invaluable in both the isolation and characterization of Na^+ and Ca^{2+} channels. From the listings in Table 2-2 and 2-3, it is also evident that the evolutionary processes at work in the development of these toxins have capitalized on more than one region of the protein to achieve either activation or blockade of channel function.[24,25] In general, voltage-sensitive channels exhibit high ion selectivities, voltage sensitivities, and single-channel conductances.

Sodium Channels

The voltage-sensitive sodium channel plays the critical role in initiation of the action potential, and since the pioneering studies of Hodgkin and Huxley on the giant squid axon, it has been widely studied electrophysiologically. Activation of the channel results from abrupt changes in membrane potential, and channel opening allows for the inward movement of Na^+ from extracellular space. The permeability to Na^+ rapidly rises and then slowly declines even when the potential is maintained.

Inward movement of Ca^{2+} through calcium channels contributes to the plateau phase of the action potential. The action potential is terminated by activation of voltage-sensitive

Table 2-2. Classification of Chemical Effectors of the Voltage-Sensitive Sodium Channel

Structure	Representative Agents	Physiologic Activity	Presumed Molecular[a] Site of Action
Caged hydroxylic antagonists	Tetrodotoxin Saxitoxin	Block ion permeability	Interior of channel or channel mouth; site 1
Lipid-soluble activators	Veratridine Batrachotoxin Acotine Grayanotoxin	Persistent activation	Allosteric site 2
Peptides: group A	African α-scorpion toxin Sea anemone toxin	Slow the inactivation step	Allosteric site 3
Peptides: group B	American β-scorpion toxin	Enhance activation	Allosteric site 4
Dinoflagellate toxins	*Ptychodiscus brevis* toxins	Induce repetitive activity	Allosteric site 5

[a] The allosteric sites differ from the locus of ion permeation; their exact locations are unknown.

Table 2-3. Plasma Membrane Calcium Channels

	Voltage-Sensitive Channels			Receptor-Operated Channels
	T Channels	*N Channels*	*L Channels*	
Voltage sensitivity Activation Inactivation	(+) to −70 mV −100 to −60 mV	(+) to −20 mV >−100 to −40 mV	(+) to −10 mV −60 to −10 mV	Modulated by agonists
Single-channel conductance	8–9 pS	13 pS	25 pS	
Cd^{2+} sensitivity (IC$_{50}$)	100 μM	10 μM	10 μM	
ω-Conotoxin sensitivity	+/−	(+)	(+)	(−)
Dihydropyridine modulation	No	No	Yes	Yes/no
Single-channel kinetics	Late opening, brief burst	Long burst, inactivates	Persistent activation	
Location[a]	Endocrine, cardiac, smooth muscle, glia, sensory neurons, CNS neurons	Sensory, autonomic, and CNS neurons	Virtually all cell types where T and N channels are found	Many excitable cells

[a] Skeletal muscle cells are excluded from the classification.

potassium channels, which repolarize the cell through outward movement of K^+. Sodium channels exhibit transitions from a resting (closed) to a conducting (open) and an inactivated (again closed) state. The slow decline has been attributed to the inactivation rate. Some pharmacologic agents and agents that modify protein structure selectively eliminate the inactivation mechanism. Sodium channels have also been examined by single-channel methods,[26] and details on the kinetics of the activation and inactivation processes have become known. In particular, the inactivation process is rapid, and slow activation of a fraction of the channels accounts for the slow decline in the Na^+ permeability when observed on a large population of channels.

As shown in Table 2-2, several toxins block sodium channel function, whereas others cause activation in the absence of a change in membrane potential. The structures of some of these substances are shown in Figure 2-13.

Subunit Structure

The voltage-sensitive sodium channel has been purified to homogeneity by employing several of these toxins, either as affinity ligands or as a means to monitor functional or binding parameters of the purified fractions. The solubilized and isolated channel is approximately 300 kDa in mass and consists of as many as three subunits (α, β_1, β_2)[25] (Fig. 2-14). Each of the subunits has been purified. Interest focuses on the α (260-kDa) subunit, since the smaller β subunits have not been detected in the solubilized sodium channel from *Electrophorus*. Messenger RNA encoding the α subunit in brain when injected into frog oocytes is sufficient to form functional channels of the brain type.[27,28]

At least one peptide of the β type (39 kDa) has been identified in mammalian muscle. Mammalian brain sodium channels, when solubilized and purified, appear as a heterotrimer and contain two β-peptides of 33 and 36 kDa. Molecular cloning and expression of the mRNA from the cloned cDNAs reveal additional polymorphisms of structure of the α subunit in brain sodium channels.[28,29] Three distinct central nervous system cDNAs encoding sodium channel α-subunits have been isolated, two of which appear to be expressed only in brain and not in the peripheral nervous system.

The α subunit is heavily glycosylated. It contains four repeating domains, composed of about 250 residues each, in which clear similarities in sequence can be demonstrated. Between six and eight segments in each of these domains are believed to span the membrane. The four domains, and hence 24 to 32 membrane-spanning segments, encircle the central ion channel (Fig. 2-15). Accordingly, the channel structure resembles a bracelet in which a pseudosymmetric array of homologous but not identical domains surrounds the hydrated pore. Four of the putative membrane-spanning segments in each domain are hydrophobic and should form intramembranous α-helices, while two show less hydrophobicity and are candidates for forming the inner lining of the channel. One of these segments (S_4) contains cycles of alternatively spaced positively charged residues with an intervening dipeptide of hydrophobic residues (Fig. 2-16). This region may function as a sensor for voltage-dependent gating. Voltage-dependent gating currents that initiate the activation process involve the outward movement of four to six positive charges from within the channel structure to its surface.[30] Various voltage gating models involving the sliding or torsional movement of a positively charged helix structure have been proposed[25] (Fig. 2-17). Regions containing potential *N*-linked glycosylation sites should exist on the extracellular surface, whereas another region between domains 1 and 2 contains potential phosphorylation sites and can be expected to be disposed on the cytoplasmic surface of the membrane. A site for scorpion α-toxin binding has been found between membrane-spanning segments 6 and 7 in domain 1.

Several of the functional properties of the sodium channel have been demonstrated following reconstitution of the solubilized and purified protein in phospholipid vesicles. Among these have been binding of saxitoxin, tetrodotoxin, and scorpion α-toxin, block

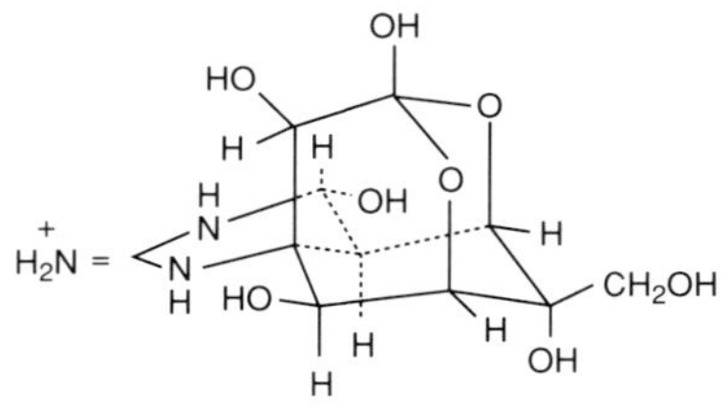

Tetrodotoxin

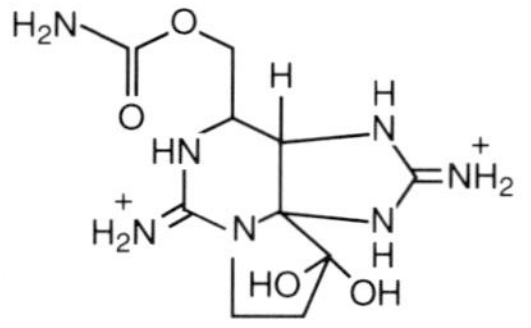

Saxitoxin

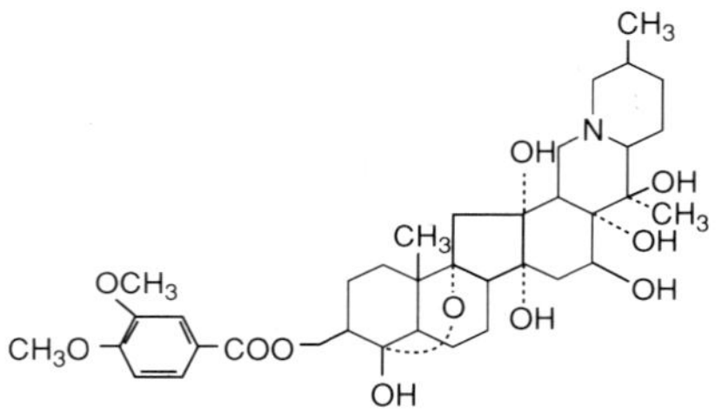

Veratridine

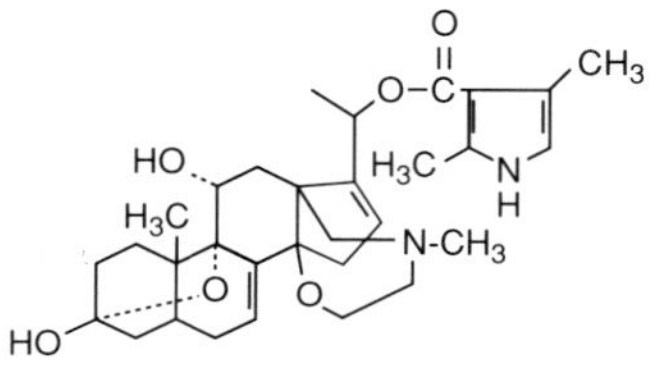

Batrachotoxin

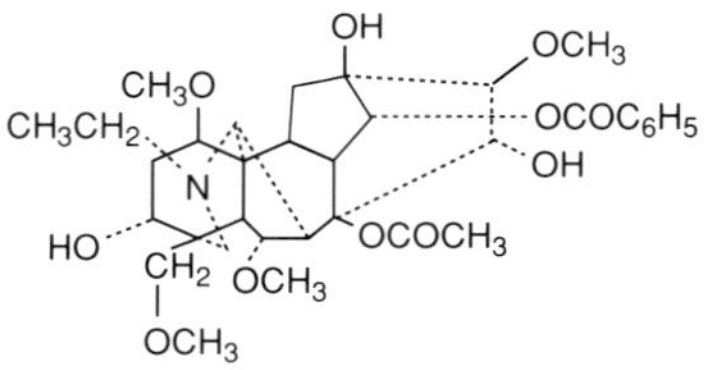

Aconitine

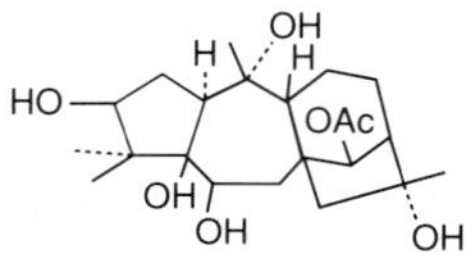

Grayanotoxin I

```
      Ile*              5                      10                      15                      20
Gly-Val-Pro-Cys-Leu-Cys-Asp-Ser-Asp-Gly-Pro-Ser-Val-Arg-Gly-Asn-Thr-Leu-Ser-Gly-
                     25                      30                      35                      40
Ile-Ile-Trp-Leu-Ala-Gly-Cys-Pro-Ser-Gly-Trp-His-Asn-Cys-Lys-Lys-His-Gly-Pro-Thr-Ile-Gly-
           45
Trp-Cys-Cys-Lys-Gln-
```

Sea anemone toxin (ATX II)

Fig. 2-13. Ligand structures that affect sodium channels.

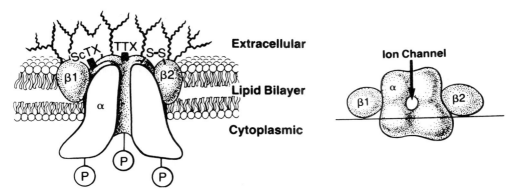

Fig. 2-14. Subunit arrangement and structure of the mammalian sodium channel. The model is shown in cross section, cut perpendicular to the plane of the membrane (*left*) and parallel to the plane of the membrane (*right*). The probable distribution of the three subunits (α, β_1, β_2) of the mammalian channel in brain is represented along with glycosylation sites, neurotoxin-binding sites, the disulfide bond between subunits, and sites of phosphorylation (left). The four homologous domains of the α subunit are shown forming a central transmembrane pore when viewed from the top of the membrane surface (right). (From Catterall,[25] with permission.)

of voltage-sensitive activation by these toxins, and batrachotoxin- and veratridine-stimulated Na^+ flux.[25] In the case of the brain Na^+ channel, the α subunit and only one of the two β subunits are necessary for reconstitution of function.[25,31]

The β subunits have yet to be cloned, so detailed structural information on these subunits is lacking. They appear to be glycosylated and hence exist on the outside surface of the membrane. The precise function of the β subunits remains unclear. They may represent unique specializations found in particular tissues and play a role in modulation of the permeability response. Alternatively, they may be involved in the assembly and extracellular transport of the newly biosynthesized channel to the cell surface.

Analysis of the sodium channel and the nicotinic acetylcholine receptor reveals several common structural features. Both oligomeric proteins are of similar mass (250 to 300 kDa), are glycosylated and contain amino acid residues located on the cytoplasmic surface that can be phosphorylated. The two channel proteins contain at least 20 hydrophobic segments of about 22 to 25 amino acids, which span the membrane as α-helices. Four repeating domains flanked by intervening sequences in a single subunit subserve the structural role of encircling the voltage-sensitive sodium channel. This gives rise to a structure of covalently linked homologous domains. In the case of the nicotinic acetylcholine receptor, the similar repeating domains are found in homologous but distinct subunits, which noncovalently associate in a precise order within the membrane to encircle a channel. The divergences in structure of the two proteins presumably are necessary to achieve their distinctive ligand-binding and ion-gating properties.

It should be recognized that the current models of the channel structures are based largely on assignments of hydropathy of the peptide chains and that the application of physical techniques to test rigorously details of these models is only in its infancy. Thus, analysis of secondary structure, reactivity of sequence-specific antibodies toward a particular membrane surface, site-specific covalent labeling, high-resolution crystallographic studies, two-dimensional nuclear magnetic resonance measurements, and electron microscopic analyses of structure will be necessary to provide a more refined description of the structure of channel-linked proteins.

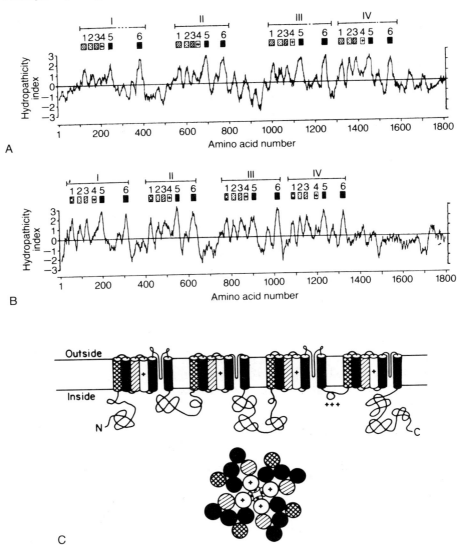

Fig. 2-15. **(A)** Plot of hydrophobicity versus amino acid sequence number for the *Electrophorus* sodium channel. Hydrophobicity is reflected in an increased positive value. The four homologous domains (I, II, III, IV) and six of the helical segments within each domain (S1, S2, S3, S4, S5, S6) are noted. **(B)** Similar analysis for the calcium channel (dihydropyridine-binding receptor). **(C)** Linear display of the proposed transmembrane topology of the sodium channel viewed in the plane of the membrane and from the top of the membrane. The six segments (S_1 through S_6) in each of the four repeating domains (labeled I, II, III, and IV above) are indicated by cylinders. Segments 1, 3, 5, 6 are the most hydrophobic. Segment 4 contains four to eight positive charges in each of the domains and may play a role in gating of ions or stabilization of the negatively charged segments. Segment S_2 contains glutamic acid and lysine residues in each segment and may form the inner wall of the channel. Shown below is a cross-sectional view of the sodium channel, in which the ion channel is the central pore and is surrounded by four units of homology. The shading denotes similar membrane-spanning segments. (Figs. A and B from Noda et al.,[27] with permission.)

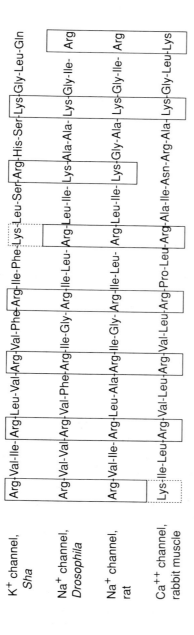

K$^+$ channel, *Sha*
Arg-Val-Ile-Arg-Leu-Val-Arg-Val-Phe-Arg-Ile-Phe-Lys-Leu-Ser-Arg-His-Ser-Lys-Gly-Leu-Gln

Na$^+$ channel, *Drosophila*
Arg-Val-Val-Arg-Val-Phe-Arg-Ile-Gly-Arg-Ile-Leu-Arg-Leu-Ile-Lys-Ala-Ala-Lys-Gly-Ile- Arg

Na$^+$ channel, rat
Arg-Val-Ile-Arg-Leu-Ala-Arg-Ile-Gly-Arg-Ile-Leu- Arg-Leu-Ile-Lys-Gly-Ala- Lys-Gly-Ile- Arg

Ca^{++} channel, rabbit muscle
Lys-Ile-Leu-Arg-Val-Leu-Arg-Val-Leu-Arg-Pro-Leu-Arg-Ala-Ile-Asn-Arg-Ala-Lys-Gly-Leu-Lys

The K$^+$ channel is from the Shaker locus in Drosophila; Na$^+$ channels have been sequenced from Drosophila, *Electrophorous* electric organs, and rat brain.

Fig. 2-16. Sequences of the putative voltage gating (S4) segment of voltage-sensitive sodium, calcium and potassium channels. The potassium channel is from the *Shaker* locus in *Drosophila*; sodium channels have been sequenced from *Drosophila*, *Electrophorus* electric organs, and rat brain; calcium channel from skeletal muscle.

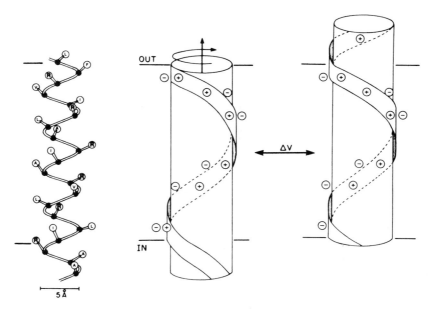

Fig. 2-17. Proposal for the voltage-dependent torsional movement of the charged α-helices (segment S4) that gives rise to gating currents. The helices are found in each of the domains; they span the membrane containing positively charged amino acids with an intervening hydrophobic dipeptide. The torsional movement causes the charge displacement discussed in the text. (From Catterall,[25] with permission.)

Calcium Channels

Calcium has long been known to play a diverse and critical role as a mediator of cell function, both as a transmembrane charge carrier and as an intracellular second messenger. Although the cell possesses substantial stores of calcium, intracellular free calcium ($[Ca^{2+}]_i$) is maintained in the submicromolar range by sequestration into organelles such as the endoplasmic reticulum and sarcoplasmic reticulum. Ultimately, the low $[Ca^{2+}]_i$ must be maintained by pumps or exchange systems, which act to transport Ca^{2+} from the cytoplasm to the outside of the cell. Transient increases in $[Ca^{2+}]_i$ provide a critical link in cellular activation processes such as excitation-contraction and excitation-secretion coupling. Prolonged increases in $[Ca^{2+}]_i$, which can be localized or dispersed throughout the cell, play roles in mitogenesis, cell division, cell differentiation, and perhaps oncogenesis.

Since Ca^{2+} gradients larger than 4 orders of magnitude exist across the cell membrane and between subcellular organelles and the cytoplasm, a potential mechanism for rapid activation is present. Transient increases of $[Ca^{2+}]_i$ occur by two mechanisms, both presumably involving channels. The first is release from intracellular storage sites, most importantly those in the endoplasmic reticulum. This release apparently involves channels that can be activated by inositol 1,4,5-trisphosphate and other putative intracellular mediators. The mechanism of generation of the inositol phosphate will be considered in a subsequent section. The second involves channels in the plasma membrane that allow extracellular Ca^{2+} present at millimolar concentrations to pass down a concentration gradient into the cell.

Plasma membrane Ca^{2+} channels may be subdivided into two types. The first are receptor-operated channels, in which Ca^{2+} influx is directly coupled to occupation of a receptor. *N*-methyl-D-aspartate receptors appear to act in this manner,[32] and several other ligands are known to activate Ca^{2+} channels. Apart from having the receptor site and channel located on the same oligomeric protein, receptor-operated Ca^{2+} channels also function by direct linkages through G proteins and by production of intracellular mediators that activate the channel. The second type of plasma membrane Ca^{2+} channel is the voltage-sensitive calcium channel, in which rapid depolarization of the cell membrane leads to opening of the channel and entry of calcium. Less is known about the receptor-operated channels than about the voltage-sensitive channels, which are becoming well characterized.

The voltage-sensitive Ca^{2+} channels have been subclassified primarily through electrophysiologic and ligand-binding studies. Ligands that activate and block Ca^{2+} channels are shown in Figure 2-18. The Ca^{2+} channels in smooth muscle, exocrine glands, and skeletal muscle seem to be dihydropyridine-sensitive, while voltage-sensitive channels in brain appear to be largely dihydropyridine-insensitive. The dihydropyridines, in fact, have proved useful not only for the subclassification but also for the molecular characterization of the channels. Dihydropyridines that act as agonists and antagonists have been identified.

Other compounds bearing no structural similarity to the dihydropyridines can act as Ca^{2+} channel antagonists but usually are of lower selectivity for the L-type channel (Table 2-3). All dihydropyridine-sensitive channels may not be identical, and differences in antagonist-binding and channel-opening properties have been detected; for example, certain smooth muscle cells show exquisite sensitivity to the dihydropyridines. Subtypes of dihydropyridine-sensitive and dihydropyridine-insensitive channels have been implicated on the basis of channel activation and gating behavior. It is entirely possible that the dihydropyridine-sensitive channel found in the central nervous system is identical to one of the subtypes in peripheral tissue, but these considerations await the determination of their primary structures.

Multiple channels have been extensively characterized by electrophysiologic means in the dorsal root ganglion, and three distinct types—T, N, and L—have been detected with incremental increases in depolarizing voltages. They also can be distinguished on the basis of sensitivity to the dihydropyridines, cadmium, and a 27–amino acid peptide, ω-Conotoxin, which comes from the marine snail *Conus geographica*[32-35] (Table 2-3). Calcium channels also exhibit distinct activation, inactivation, and conductance properties. It is

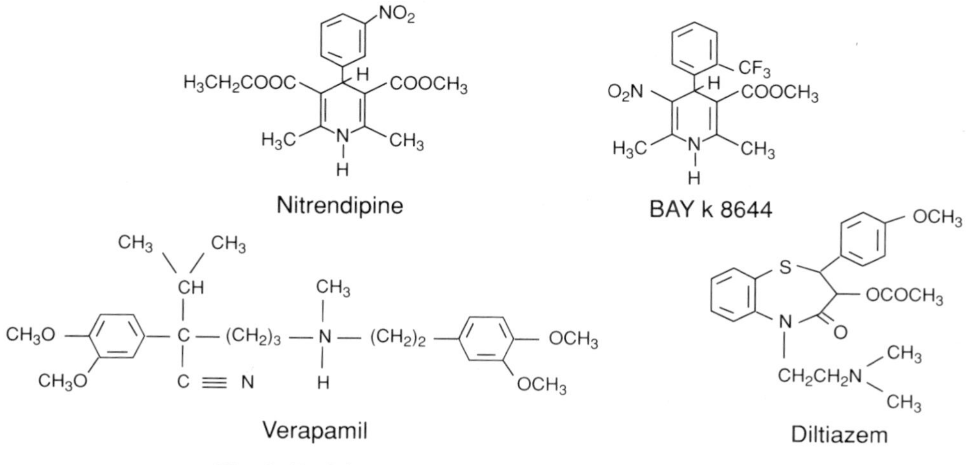

Fig. 2-18. Ligand structures that affect calcium channels.

quite possible that the three types of channels carry distinct functions in the neuron. For example, it has been proposed that the N channel may be preferentially localized near neurotransmitter release sites.[32] The other channels may play roles in cellular bursting activity, late post-tetanic potentiation, or increasing intracellular Ca^{2+} for activation processes involved in intermediary metabolism.

In skeletal muscle two types of calcium channels have been identified in the transverse (T) tubule system, although the precise function played by the calcium channels is not resolved. Muscle shows both fast (I_{fast}) and slow (I_{slow}) Ca^{2+} currents; the slow currents are caused by L-type channels and are blocked by the dihydropyridines, but it has proved difficult to correlate muscle Ca^{2+} channels with the properties described in Table 2-3. Some investigators have proposed that the T-tubule calcium channels produce a local Ca^{2+} current, which triggers Ca^{2+} release from the sarcoplasmic reticulum. Alternatively, these channels may act as a voltage sensor in the T tubule to trigger the Ca^{2+} release. In addition to triggering or gating Ca^{2+} release for excitation-contraction coupling, either as a voltage sensor or by producing a local Ca^{2+} current, T-tubule calcium channels may act to slowly replenish Ca^{2+} in the cell following release. This secondary role of replenishing these sites is effected through the slow dihydropyridine-sensitive channel. Another type of Ca^{2+} channel in skeletal muscle that may be coupled to the above channels is the ryanodine receptor.[36] The plant alkaloid ryanodine binds to a Ca^{2+} release channel, which likely forms the feetlike structures in the muscle triad that connect the sarcoplasmic reticulum and the tubular foldings of the plasma membrane (T-tubules). It appears involved in intermembrane signal transduction in excitation-contraction coupling.

Owing to its abundance in T tubules, the dihydropyridine-sensitive Ca^{2+} channel has been purified, its binding function has been reconstituted, and the gene encoding its major subunit (α_1) has been isolated and sequenced by recombinant DNA techniques.[37] The isolated T-tubule Ca^{2+} channel appears to consist of five subunits (α_1, α_2, β, γ, and δ), although the precise stoichiometry and obligate function of all the subunits remain to be established.[37,38] The α_1 subunit contains the dihydropyridine binding site, binding sites for phenylalkylamines, and the phosphorylation sites. Its molecular weight is 212 kDa, somewhat larger than would have been predicted from estimates by biochemical techniques such as polyacrylamide gel electrophoresis in the presence of sodium dodecyl sulfate. Four units, or domains, of internal homology have been identified, and each of these units is also homologous with the corresponding regions of the voltage-sensitive Na^+ channel[37] (Fig. 2-19). As in the case of the Na^+ channel, each internal repeat has five hydrophobic segments (S_1, S_2, S_3, S_5, and S_6) and one positively charged segment (S_4). The S_4 segment contains the positive charges disposed in such a manner that it also may serve as a voltage sensor for gating. Like the Na^+ channel, the α_1 subunit of the Ca^{2+} channel is devoid of a leader sequence which suggests that the amino terminal sequence lies on the cytoplasmic side of the membrane. Overall, this subunit shows 29 percent sequence identity with the α subunit of the Na^+ channel.

The α_2 subunit is a heavily glycosylated 143 kDa subunit; it is disulfide linked to the δ subunit, also a 27 kDa glycosylated peptide. The β subunit is 54 kDa. Like α, it is sensitive to phosphorylation, but β shows low hydrophobicity and is not glycosylated. The γ subunit is glycosylated and is hydrophobic. The combination of α, β, and γ will mediate conductance in reconstituted systems, so the functional roles of α_2 and δ remain to be established.[38,39] As is the case for the β subunits in the Na^+ channel, the subunits other than α_1 may be important as modulators of function or for the assembly and export of an active α_1 subunit to the membrane.

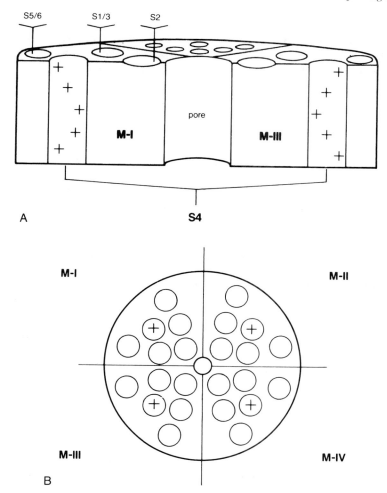

Fig. 2-19. Schematic structure of the Ca^{2+} channel. **(A)** Cross section normal to the plane of membrane; **(B)** cross section in the plane of membrane. Membrane-spanning domains are deduced from hydropathy plots (see Fig. 2-17B). The fourfold symmetry is shown from the top. M-I and M-III denote two of the domains from the plane of the membrane. (From Alsobrook and Stevens,[165] with permission.)

Potassium Channels

An extensive variety of potassium channels have been identified by electrophysiologic means, and their conductances are regulated by membrane potential, receptor ligands, intracellular Ca^{2+}, ATP, and probably several other cellular mediators. Various K^+ currents exhibit characteristic voltage activation patterns and sensitivities to 4-aminopyridine or to naturally occurring peptide toxins such as dendrotoxin from snake venom or apamin from bee venom. In general, these channels repolarize or hyperpolarize excitable membranes. As such, they control cellular excitability by regulating duration of the action potential, frequency of nerve activity, and efficiency of synaptic transmission.

A family of potassium channels has been cloned from the *Shaker* locus of *Drosophila*.[40] In *Drosophila* structurally related but functionally distinct potassium channels are expressed by alternate mRNA processing of a 65-kilobase gene. The potassium channel appears to be composed of a 70-kDa subunit containing six identifiable membrane-spanning regions. As was observed in the sodium and calcium channels, a 22-residue hydrophobic stretch containing positive residues alternating with largely hydrophobic dipeptides was also identified (Fig. 2-16). The retention of this motif throughout the voltage-gated channels but not the ligand-gated channels is further evidence for the role of this sequence as a voltage sensor. The various cDNAs encoding the potassium channels use identical exons in this internal core region, and the alternative exon usage encodes for variation in the N-terminal and C-terminal ends of the molecule. When expressed in oocytes, each cDNA species yields different conductance properties. The lower molecular weight of the potassium channel suggests that the functioning unit is an oligomer of the 70-kDa subunit giving rise to a molecular weight similar to that of the α subunit of the sodium channel. However, the participation of ancillary subunits yielding a heteroligomeric structure, as seen with the calcium and some of the sodium channels, cannot be ruled out.

Channel-Containing Receptors Activated by Amino Acids

The action of the excitatory amino acids (aspartate and glutamate) and inhibitory amino acids (γ-aminobutyric acid and glycine) are mediated through ion channels. Despite some estimates that up to 60 percent of the central neurotransmission is mediated by amino acids, our knowledge of the molecular details of these systems is surprisingly sparse. This is due in part to the fact that the amino acid transmitters, except γ-aminobutyric acid, have other biologic functions in addition to neurotransmission. Moreover, we have lacked sufficiently selective agonists—and in some cases have also lacked high-affinity, selective antagonists—to fully characterize subtypes of amino acid receptors.

Isolation and characterization of the excitatory amino acid receptors also have been limited by the low potency and the limited selectivity of agonists and antagonists. However, more selective antagonists are available for the inhibitory amino acid receptors. Accordingly, purification and molecular cloning studies are at a far more advanced stage for the inhibitory receptors. As was the case with the neuronal nicotinic acetylcholine receptors, the expected homology between all the amino acid receptor-linked channels may well offer a means to determine receptor structures for the excitatory amino acids by the screening of libraries at low stringency with cDNAs that encode subunits of the inhibitory amino acid receptors.

Excitatory Amino Acid Receptors

The natural excitatory amino acids acting as transmitters are glutamate and aspartate, and because of a higher affinity for the receptor subtypes, glutamate is the predominant excitatory transmitter in mammals. Since the natural agonists and virtually all the more selective agonist congeners carry two negative charges at physiologic pH values, the term *diacidic amino acid* appropriately characterizes this neurotransmitter-receptor system. Diacidic amino acids are the neurotransmitters functioning in afferent excitatory transmission and in many excitatory central pathways. Thus, the system is found in the dorsal horn of the spinal cord and in cortex, midbrain, and cerebellum. Curiously, arthropods use aspartate as an efferent motor transmitter for excitation and several of its properties (i.e., receptor-linked rapid sodium conductance, congregation of receptor, and formation of active zones in apposition to the nerve ending) are similar to those observed for the nicotininc acetylcholine receptor. Attempts have been made to subclassify the diacidic acid receptor systems primarily on the basis of limited selectivity of agonists.[41,42] Two distinct terminologies have evolved for the three receptor subtypes: AA_1 (*N*-methyl-D-aspartate), AA_2 (quisqualate), and AA_3 (kainate) (Tables 2-4 and 2-5). All these receptors rely on primarily Na^+ conductance, but the AA_1 subtype shows slower responses and a marked voltage sensitivity. Long-term potentiation can be seen upon repetitive stimulation of this receptor system, and the enhanced activity associated with the potentiation may be a result of the reduction of membrane potential. AA_2 and AA_3 show essentially identical physiology and are distinguished largely on the basis of agonist selectivity (Table 2-5). As these systems become further characterized, expansion to additional subtypes or coalition of the existing subtypes is still possible.

The AA_1 [*N*-methyl-D-aspartate(NMDA)] receptor has received the greatest attention since its unusual conductance properties, giving rise to short- and long-term potentiation, suggest that it may be involved in plasticity, information processing, and memory. The NMDA receptor gives more prolonged conductance changes in Na^+ and Ca^{2+}. Its activation by glutamate only occurs when depolarization via the kainate and quisqualate receptor relieves a Mg^{2+}-dependent block. Na^+ and Ca^{2+} move through the NMDA channel, leading to a more prolonged depolarization and intracellular biochemical events. Excessive stimulation of the amino acid receptors may result from cerebral ischemia and gives rise to necrosis of neurons, perhaps through elevated intracellular Ca^{2+}. This has raised the possibility of using antagonists of these receptors, such as MK801, in the prophylaxis and treatment of stroke.[42] Several well recognized pharmacologic agents modulate the function of the AA_1 receptor. Included within this group are the phencyclidines (PCP), glycine, and certain synthetic opioids such as SKF 10,008 and ketocyclazine.[41] Analysis of the specificity of opioid ligands on excitatory amino acid junction suggests that sigma (σ_1) sites, which were originally designated as opioid receptors, actually are found on the AA_1 (NMDA) receptor channel. Occupation of these sites modulates NMDA function, and the functional response can be blocked allosterically by MK-801. This site is termed the σ_1 or PCP_1 site. A second sigma site, termed σ_2 or PCP_2, has been identified; it is not affected by MK-801 but is blocked by haloperidol. The absence of sensitivity of either σ_1 or σ_2 receptors to naloxone has led investigators not to classify them among the opioid receptors.[42]

Inhibitory Amino Acid Receptors

The major inhibitory transmitters are glycine and γ-aminobutyric acid (GABA), and recent progress in the characterization of these neurotransmitter-receptor systems has been substantial (Fig. 2-20, Table 2-6). The inhibitory transmitters function by opening an anion (Cl^-) channel. Since the Cl^- concentration gradient usually is directed inward, opening of the channel initiates an inward flow of Cl^- and a resultant hyperpolarization.[43] These receptor channels stabilize the potential of the cell during activation of excitatory channels, or by hyperpolarization they decrease the spontaneous depolarization and firing of cells.

Glycine is the major inhibitory transmitter in the spinal cord and brain stem. In the spinal cord glycine is found in interneurons, where it plays a role in conjunction with Renshaw cells to dampen excitability and coordinate motor responses. Strychnine is a competitive antagonist of glycine and possesses the selectivity and high affinity required for characterization of glycine receptors. The excruciating pain associated with strychnine poisoning is attributable to blockage of the inhibitory influences of interneurons on excitability of the motor neurons innervating the muscles of posture. Strychnine-binding

Table 2-4. Structures of Some Amino Acid Agonists and Antagonists

Receptor Type	Agonist	Antagonist	Allosteric
Non-selective	L-Glutamate	cis-2,3 - PDA	
NMDA	NMDA	D-AP5 CPP	MK-801 Phencyclidine (PCP)
Quisqualate	Quisqualate	GAMS	
Kainate	Kainate	GAMS	

PDA, piperidine dicarboxylate; NMDA, *N*-methylᴅ-aspartate; CPP, 3-(2-carboxypiperazam-4-yl)-propyl-1. phosphonate, GAMS, 6-ᴅ-glutamylaminomethylsulphonate.

Table 2-5. Classification of Diacidic Amino Acid Receptors

Receptor Subtype	AA_1 (N-*methyl*-D-aspartate)	AA_2 (Quisqualate)	AA_3 (Kainate)
Location in mammals	Spinal dorsal roots; subcortical brain areas	Spinal dorsal roots; subcortical brain areas	Spinal dorsal roots; subcortical brain areas
Physiology	Slower signal transduction (long-term potentiation) of polysynaptic pathways	Monosynaptic rapid response	Monosynaptic rapid response
Receptor-linked channel	Mg^{2+}-voltage sensitive Na^+ channel Ca^{2+} channel	Fast Na^+ channel excitatory postsynaptic potential	Fast Na^+ channel excitatory postsynaptic potential
In situ transmitter	Glutamate (aspartate)	Glutamate (aspartate)	Glutamate (aspartate)
Selective agonist	N-methyl-D-aspartate	Quisqualate	Kainate
Selective antagonists	MK-801 DAP$_5$, DAP$_7$	Glutamylamino-methylsulfonate	Glutamylamino-methylsulfonate

sites and glycine-induced hyperpolarization appear localized primarily to the thoracolumbar region of the spinal cord. Glycine and its analogs compete for strychnine binding with an effectiveness that parallels their activities in situ as agonists. All the actions of glycine may not be coupled directly to Cl^- channels. As noted above, glycine is also a heterotropic inhibitor of the NMDA receptor, and this finding has prompted a reevaluation of glycine action.

The glycine receptor has been purified with the aid of strychnine as a ligand for affinity chromatography. Purification has yielded an oligomer of 48-, 58-, and 93-kDa subunits. The 93-kDa subunit may be entirely cytoplasmic and thus neither has a direct ligand-binding function nor is involved in the intrinsic channel structure. The basic functional unit of the receptor may arise from association of the two smaller subunits in a pentameric arrangement.[44] Strychnine, in fact, has been shown to bind to the 48-kDa subunit, and the 48-kDa and 58-kDa subunits are homologous in sequence. A cDNA encoding the 48-kDa subunit has been cloned from spinal cord,[45] and the deduced amino acid sequence shows limited homology with the subunits of the GABA and the nicotinic acetylcholine receptors. Particularly striking are four hydrophobic and candidate membrane-spanning regions that are found in the same position in the linear sequence as these regions in the nicotinic receptor.[45] As will be discussed in a subsequent section, comparison of structural properties of anion and cation receptor-linked channels further delimits the potential permutations for spanning the membrane and for the peptide chain folding of those subunits that contribute to channel formation.

γ-Aminobutyric Acid Receptors

γ-Aminobutyric acid is the other major, well characterized inhibitory amino acid transmitter. It is a prevalent transmitter in the mammalian central nervous system, being localized in the spinal neurons, cortex, midbrain, and cerebellum. Its localization in the midbrain indicates that it may have a major inhibitory function in the central coordination of excitability, motor, and autonomic function. Although GABA is not a major transmitter in the peripheral nervous system of mammals, an inhibitory motor component involving GABA is present in arthropods, and hyperpolarization results in inhibitory motor responses.

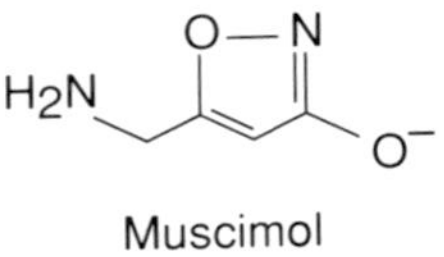

Muscimol

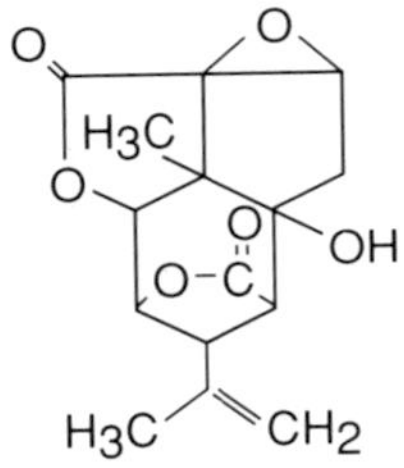

Picrotoxinin

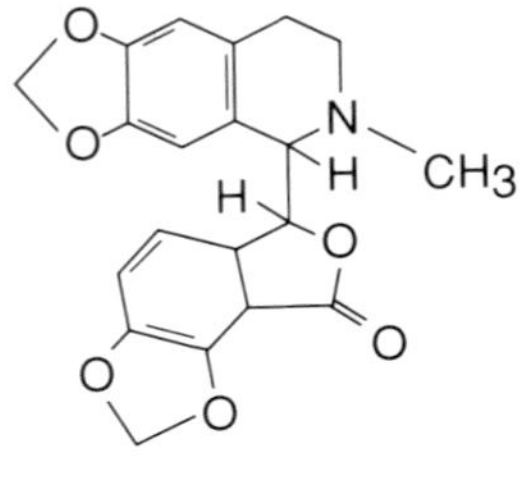

Bicuculline

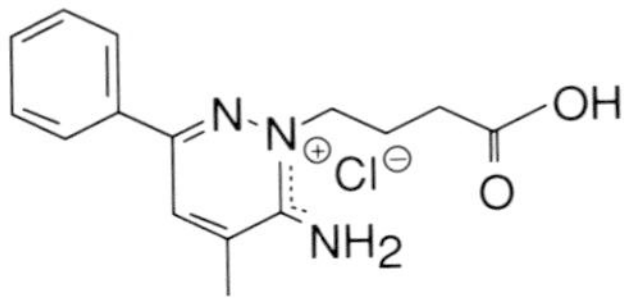

SR 95103

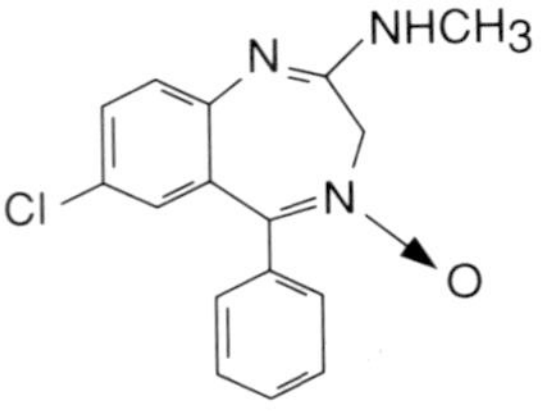

Chlordiazepoxide

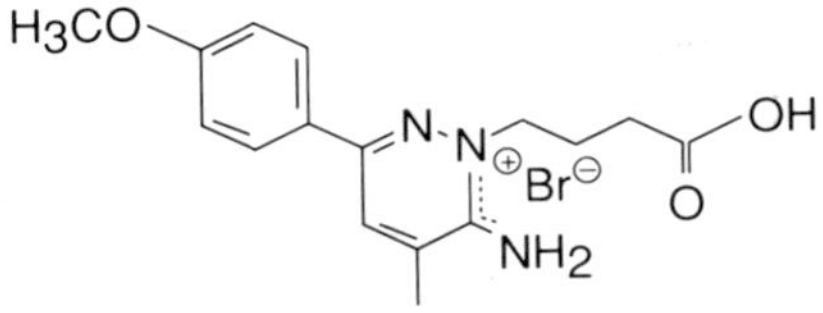

SR 95531

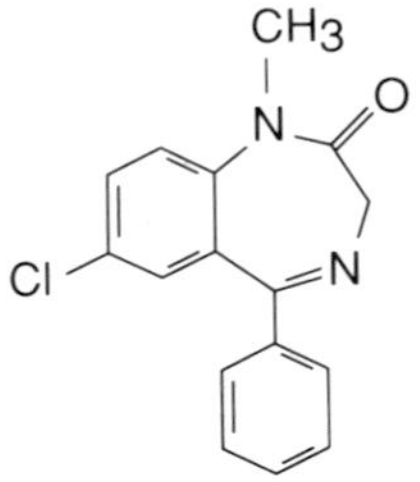

Diazepam

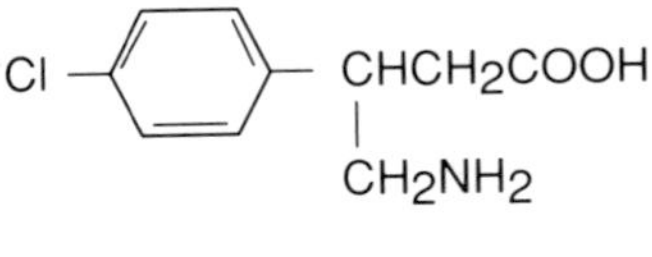

Baclofen

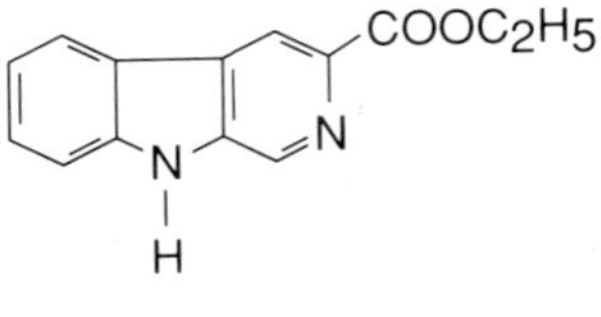

β–Carboline

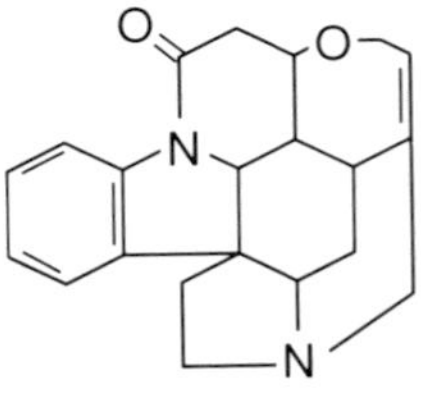

Strychnine

Fig. 2-20. Agonists and antagonists of γ-aminobutyric acid and glycine receptors.

Table 2-6. Major Inhibitory Amino Acid Transmitter Receptor Systems

Receptor Type	Glycine	GABA$_A$	GABA$_B$
Location in mammals	Central nervous system: brain stem, spinal cord (particularly thoracolumbar region)	Central nervous system: midbrain-cerebellum	Central nervous system
Receptor-linked channel	Cl$^-$ (Intrinsic)	Cl$^-$ (Intrinsic)	Ca^{2+}, K$^+$ (through G proteins)
Agonists	Glycine (β-alanine)	γ-Aminobutyric acid, muscimol, δ-aminovaleric acid	γ-Aminobutyric acid, baclofen
Allosteric activators	—	Benzodiozepines Barbiturates Alphaxolone	—
Allosteric inhibitors	THIP Avermectin B$_{la}$	β-Carbolines	—
Antagonists	Strychnine	Bicuculline Pyridazinyl-GABA analogs: SR 95531 and SR 42641	—
Channel blockers		(Picrotoxin)	—

Two types of GABA receptors, GABA$_A$ and GABA$_B$, have been distinguished on the basis of distinct differences in agonist selectivity, antagonist selectivity, modulation by drugs of the benzodiazepine class, and coupling mechanisms (Table 2-6).[46,47] GABA$_A$ receptors contain an intrinsic Cl$^-$ channel while GABA$_B$ receptors appear to be linked to Ca^{2+} and K$^+$ channels via guanine nucleotide-binding proteins. These latter actions of the GABA$_B$ receptor may be mediated through production of arachidonic acid.

Dose-response relationships for GABA and other agonists on GABA$_A$ receptors show Hill coefficients greater than unity.[46,47] Thus, as in the case of the nicotinic acetylcholine receptor, binding of more than a single agonist molecule is required for channel opening. Relatively large open-channel conductances of near 30 picosiemens (pS) are observed. Channel opening results in bursts lasting about 30 msec and containing two or three interruptions. Desensitization occurs in a similar fashion to that described for acetylcholine receptor.[46] Several ligands appear to affect GABA$_A$ receptors in a noncompetitive fashion, although details on precise mechanisms are lacking. Two important classes of pharmacologic agents, the barbiturates and the benzodiazepines, appear to be heterotropic activators of GABA receptors. They enhance the binding and activity of agonists by binding to a site distinct from the agonist and antagonist recognition site in the receptor. The benzodiazepines appear to enhance GABA binding and functional activity. In this sense the benzodiazepines behave as *allosteric* or *heterotropic activators* of the receptor, where their binding is coupled to GABA binding. This action of potentiating the effect of an inhibitory transmitter may be responsible for the antianxiety (anxiolytic) actions of these drugs. The β-carbolines also bind to the benzodiazepine site and in so doing diminish the response of agonist. Although the term *inverse agonist* has been used for these agents, it may be more appropriate to consider them to be *allosteric* or *heterotropic inhibitors*. The barbiturates may also act allosterically. Their effect on binding affinity is less evident, and they increase the duration of channel opening when agonist binds.

A potential mechanism by which heterotropic activators and inhibitors act may be represented as

$$
\begin{array}{ccccc}
& \text{H} & & \text{H} & & \text{H} \\
& + & & + & & + \\
2\,\text{GABA} + \text{R} & \underset{}{\overset{K_G}{\rightleftharpoons}} & \text{GABA}_2\cdot\text{R} & \underset{}{\overset{K^*_G}{\rightleftharpoons}} & \text{GABA}_2\cdot\text{R}^* \\
K_H \updownarrow & & \updownarrow & & \updownarrow \\
2\,\text{GABA} + \text{RH} & \underset{}{\overset{K_{G,H}}{\rightleftharpoons}} & \text{GABA}_2\cdot\text{RH} & \underset{}{\overset{K^*_{G,H}}{\rightleftharpoons}} & \text{GABA}_2\cdot\text{RH}^*
\end{array}
\qquad (9)
$$

where K_G, $K_{G,H}$, and K_H are the dissociation constants for GABA binding to the unmodified receptor, for GABA binding to the heterotropic ligand–GABA receptor complex, and for the heterotropic ligand binding [H] to the receptor, respectively. K^*_G and $K^*_{G,H}$ are isomerization constants (i.e., $K^*_G = \text{GABA}_2\cdot\text{R}^*/\text{GABA}_2\text{R}$) for receptor activation. Heterotropic activators such as the benzodiazepines produce activation since $K_{G,H}$ is smaller than K_G, which will enhance GABA binding; $K^*_{G,H}$ would not necessarily be altered. The β-carbolines would diminish $K^*_{G,H}$, relative to K^*_G, which should reduce GABA-induced receptor activation. Barbiturates could act by increasing $K^*_{G,H}$ through occupation of a separate allosteric site.

This mechanism is analogous to the allosteric theories of drug action discussed in Chapter 1. A heterotropic activator binds to a site distinct from the agonist. In so doing it enhances the affinity of the agonist for the receptor ($K_{G,H} < K_G$) and/or increases the fraction of receptors in the activated state ($K^*_{G,H} > K^*_G$). A heterotropic inhibitor would also bind to a site distinct from the agonist (but in this case $K_{G,H} > K_G$ and $K^*_{G,H} < K^*_G$).

Two endogenous peptides that affect GABA receptors have been identified, and some investigators have considered these entities also to be allosteric, heterotropic ligands.[48,49] One is GABA-modulin, a peptide of 16.5 kDa, which inhibits GABA binding and GABA enhancement of benzodiazepine binding; it may do this by noncompetitively reducing the number of GABA binding sites. The other peptide is a diazepam binding inhibitor of 11 kDa, which blocks benzodiazepine binding but upon occupation of its site acts in an opposite fashion to the benzodiazepine. Hence, its functional activity appears to resemble that of the β-carbolines, which promote rather than diminish anxiety. The physiologic role of either of these peptides has not been assessed, and it remains to be shown whether they are found in brain in concentrations sufficient to be active *in vivo*. Nonpeptidic benzodiazepine mimetics have also been reported to exist in brain and may originate from plant sources. The limited data available suggest that endogenous substances may regulate these channels and that certain drugs may stimulate or antagonize function by acting at these regulatory sites for endogenous substances.

GABA receptors have been solubilized, purified, and characterized. They appear to exist as pentamers of three distinct subunits in the arrangement $\alpha_m\beta_n\gamma$,[50] but other associated subunits may contribute to the full range of GABA receptor function. Although mRNA encoding β subunits is sufficient when injected into oocytes to produce a GABA-activated Cl^- channel, it appears that γ subunits are necessary to confer benzodiazepine regulation. The overall molecular weight of the receptor molecule is comparable with the oligomeric channels we have considered previously. The β subunit appears to have the recognition capacity for GABA and related agonists. The α, β, and γ subunits have all been cloned and sequenced; they show about 35 percent residue identity. Moreover, the amino acid sequences are similar to those of the mammalian nicotinic receptor (15 to 19 percent residue identity), the glycine receptor (34 to 39 percent residue identity), and the

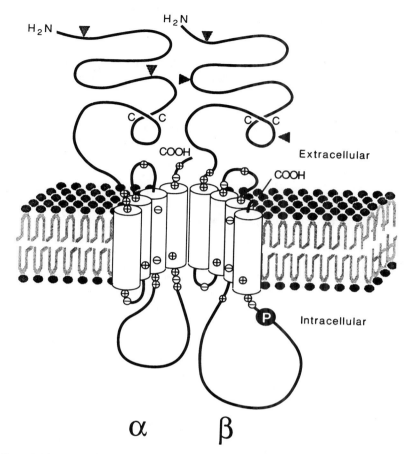

Fig. 2-21. Proposed topography of the γ-aminobutyric acid receptor (GABA$_A$) in the membrane. The four membrane-spanning helices in α and β subunits are shown as cylinders. The loop formed by disulfide-bonded cysteines 139 and 153 is denoted by the proximal Cs. Charged residues near the membrane surface are circled. Sites of phosphorylation and glycosylation are denoted by P and triangles, respectively. Presumably, two copies or more of the α and β subunits form the tetramer or pentamer, so that only some of the membrane-spanning helices form the inner wall of the central channel. (From Schofeld et al.,[50] with permission.)

nicotinic receptor anion channel in *Drosophila*. The α and β subunits have molecular weights of 48.8 and 51.4 kDa, respectively. Again, the similar motif of an N-terminal extracellular domain and four discrete membrane-spanning regions starting just beyond residue 210 is evident. Thus, clear evidence has emerged that these ligand-gated channels are part of a superfamily of proteins. A proposed structure for the GABA receptor based on hydropathy of residues is shown in Figs. 2-21 and 2-22.

Common Structural Features of Ligand-Gated Channels

Based on their primary structure, several common features of ligand-gated cation and anion channels have been identified:

1. Although the evidence is far from conclusive, the region between amino acids 180 and

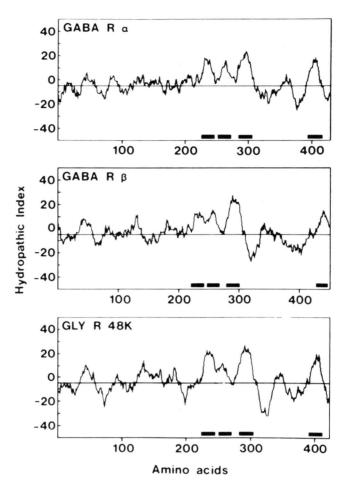

Fig. 2-22. Hydropathy profiles of the α and β subunits of the GABA receptor and the 48-kDa subunit of the glycine receptor. The four candidate membrane-spanning regions are denoted by the bars. (Adapted from Grenninghol et al.[45] and Schofeld et al.,[50] with permission.)

200 is a likely recognition site for agonists and antagonists. Covalent antagonists, maleimidobenzyl trimethylammonium and lophotoxin, react with cysteine 192 or 193 and with tyrosine 190, respectively, in the nicotinic receptor. Blotting of peptides derived from the receptor with α-toxin also implicates this region as the surface of α-toxin binding. In the case of the glycine receptor, strychnine labels an extracellular region, and partial proteolytic digestion indicates that this site is not in the first 100 residues. Moreover, the nicotinic receptor from mammals and *Drosophila*, the glycine receptor, and the GABA receptor all show a conserved intrasubunit disulfide loop between amino acids 100 and 200. If the nicotinic receptor is used as a frame of reference, the loop extends between Cys 128 and 145, forms a hairpin around a conserved region at position 134, and contains several conserved residues (Fig. 2-23). This loop extends between Cys 139 and 153 in the anion channel receptors.
2. The four hydrophobic regions that are candidates to span the membrane are present

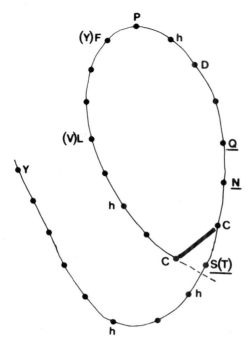

Fig. 2-23. Proposed disulfide loop region common to the ligand recognition site in the nicotinic and GABA$_A$ receptors (cysteines 139 and 153 in the GABA$_A$ receptor and cysteines 128 and 142 in the acetylcholine receptor). Positions that are identical or have a conserved substitution are shown as capital letters, and hydrophobic residues are marked by h. The hairpin is formed around the invariant proline. A similar loop is found in the glycine receptor. (From Schofield et al.,[50] with permission.)

in all cases. Each has a similar position in the linear sequence (see Figs. 2-3 and 2-22), which suggests that the polypeptide chains follow the same route in traversing the membrane. Thus, corresponding positions of the individual residues within the linear sequence would be on the same side of the membrane. Also, the positions of phosphorylation (cytoplasmic surface) or glycosylation (extracellular) sites would be maintained. Interestingly, an amphipathic helix is not found in the anion channels but is found only in the nicotinic receptor family. This would argue against this region playing an essential functional role in channel structure. Otherwise, we might have expected an amphipathic helix carrying a positive charge in anion channels. Without a conserved amphipathic helix in the ion channel receptors, one is limited to four membrane-spanning regions per subunit and the possibility that the N-terminal and C-terminal regions of the peptide are on the same side of the membrane.

3. Ion selectivity appears to be a consequence of amino acid residues of charge opposite to that of the permeant ion that exist at the channel entry point rather than within the channel itself. A comparison of the anion and cation channel receptors indicates differences in charged residues in regions proximal to (within eight residues of) the hydrophobic membrane-spanning regions rather than within them.

4. Membrane-spanning regions M-1 and M-2 possess some unusual properties, which appear to be conserved. M-1 contains a proline, which is a candidate region for a conformational change to allow channels to open transiently. M-2 contains an abun-

dance of noncharged polar side chains. Perhaps the four to seven serine and threonine hydroxyl groups found in the M-2 regions are essential for the rapid changes in hydrogen bonding needed for channel opening or replacement of the water of hydration as the ion traverses the channel pore.[51]

RECEPTORS LINKED TO GUANINE NUCLEOTIDE BINDING PROTEINS

Historically, much work in pharmacology has emphasized efforts directed at understanding responses of target tissues to stimulation by the autonomic (sympathetic and parasympathetic) nervous system. Autonomic control of visceral tissues (cardiovascular, gastrointestinal, genitourinary, etc.) is mediated by postganglionic neurons, which release norepinephrine at sympathetic fibers and acetylcholine at parasympathetic fibers. In addition, norepinephrine and epinephrine circulate in the blood, partially as a consequence of autonomic activation of chromaffin cells located in the adrenal medulla. These circulating catecholamines, along with neuronally released norepinephrine and acetylcholine, combine with receptor sites on postsynaptic cell membranes and thereby elicit responses.

A large number of pharmacologic studies have been conducted in which selective agonists and antagonists have been used to define the adrenergic and cholinergic receptors that mediate responses to catecholamines and acetylcholine (Fig 2-24). Use of these selective agents has permitted the description of schemes for classifying subtypes of cholinergic (Fig. 2-12) and adrenergic (Table 2-7) receptors. Such evidence distinguishes three types of muscarinic receptors (M_1, M_2, and M_3), two types of α_1-adrenergic (α_{1A}, α_{1B}), two types of α_2-adrenergic (α_{2A}, α_{2B}) and two or possibly three types of β-adrenergic (β_1, β_2 and β_3) receptors.

In addition to postsynaptic receptors on target cell membranes, receptors for acetylcholine and catecholamines are found on certain presynaptic neurons as well. Thus, for example, presynaptic α_2-adrenergic receptors on sympathetic neurons feed back and inhibit release of norepinephrine; conversely, presynaptic β_2-adrenergic receptors enhance norepinephrine release. Muscarinic acetylcholine receptors also modulate release of neurotransmitters in certain tissues.

At a cellular level, regulation of functions such as smooth and cardiac muscle function, glandular secretion, and release of neurotransmitters appears to involve the complex interplay of several biochemical mechanisms. These include changes in membrane potential, ion concentrations, and enzyme activities. A common theme that has emerged for all subtypes of adrenergic and muscarinic acetylcholine receptors is their linkage to one or more guanine nucleotide binding proteins in the plasma membrane. As such, receptors for autonomic nervous system transmitters have provided important paradigms for other classes of receptors linked to such proteins.

Receptors Coupled to Adenylyl Cyclase

The discovery by Sutherland and Rall in 1957 of adenosine 3′,5′-cyclic monophosphate (cyclic AMP) as an intracellular second messenger for certain hormones and neurotransmitters active at membrane receptors was a landmark observation in modern pharmacology.[52] Prior to this discovery, ideas about the molecular basis of drug action were dominated by the view that drug responses (and receptors) were only amenable to study in intact tissues. The evidence that agonists could trigger production of a second messenger that was responsible for mediating tissue responses revolutionized thinking as well as

Table 2-7. Adrenergic Receptor Classification

	α₁ *Receptors*	α₂ *Receptors*	β₁ *Receptors*	β₂ *Receptors*
Distribution	Many sympathetic nervous system effector cells	Sympathetic postganglionic neuronal cells (some effector cells, platelets, adipocytes, CNS)	Certain sympathetic nervous system effector cells (heart, adipocytes, some smooth muscle, CNS)	Many effector cells (glands, smooth muscle, leukocytes, CNS); sympathetic postganglionic neuronal cells
Responses	Smooth muscle contraction; glandular secretion; neuronal regulation	Feedback inhibition of norepinephrine release; smooth muscle contraction; stimulation of secretion and aggregation of platelets; antilipolysis; inhibition of secretion (insulin, renin)	Stimulate rate and force of cardiac cell contraction; lipolysis; stimulate renin secretion; smooth muscle relaxation	Smooth muscle relaxation; glandular secretion; stimulation of norepinephrine release from sympathetic nerves
Linkage to G protein	? G_p	G_i ? G_o	G_s	G_s
Mechanisms of action	Phospholipase C activation; other (?) (Ca^{2+} mobilization, phospholipase A_2; activation of other ion channels)	Adenylyl cyclase inhibition; activation of K^+ channel conductance; other (?) (stimulate Na^+/H^+ exchange, Ca^{2+} channels)	Stimulation of adenylyl cyclase; ?other (stimulate Ca^{2+} channel conductance)	Stimulation of adenylyl cyclase; other (?) (regulate Mg^{2+} flux)
Selective agonist	Phenylephrine	Clonidine	Dobutamine	Terbutaline
Selective antagonist	Prazosin	Yohimbine	Betaxolol	ICI 118.551
Molecular size	~80-kDa glycoprotein	~62-kDa glycoprotein	~60-kDa glycoprotein	~60-kDa glycoprotein

experimental approaches. The subsequent description by Sutherland and his colleagues of adenylyl cyclase (also formerly called adenylate cyclase) and phosphodiesterase as the enzymes involved in cyclic AMP formation and degradation, respectively, provided the starting point for the dissection of the biochemical mechanisms that regulate cyclic AMP concentrations. With the discovery of cyclic AMP–dependent protein kinase as the intracellular receptor and mediator of cyclic AMP action via phosphorylation of tissue proteins,[53,54] one could formulate a general scheme whereby a large number of drugs and hormones modulate tissue responses (Fig. 2-25).

Agonists that increase tissue concentrations of cyclic AMP generally accomplish this by the receptor-mediated activation of adenylyl cyclase (which converts ATP to cyclic AMP) (Table 2-8). Certain classes of drugs (e.g., methylxanthines) are able to increase these concentrations by inhibition of the degradative enzyme cyclic AMP phosphodiesterase. Combined treatment of a target cell with an agonist whose receptor stimulates adenylyl cyclase and with a phosphodiesterase inhibitor will typically increase cyclic AMP concentration severalfold over its level in the absence of inhibitor.

In addition to agonists whose receptors increase adenylyl cyclase activity, a large number of agonists interact with receptors that decrease the activity of this enzyme (Table 2-

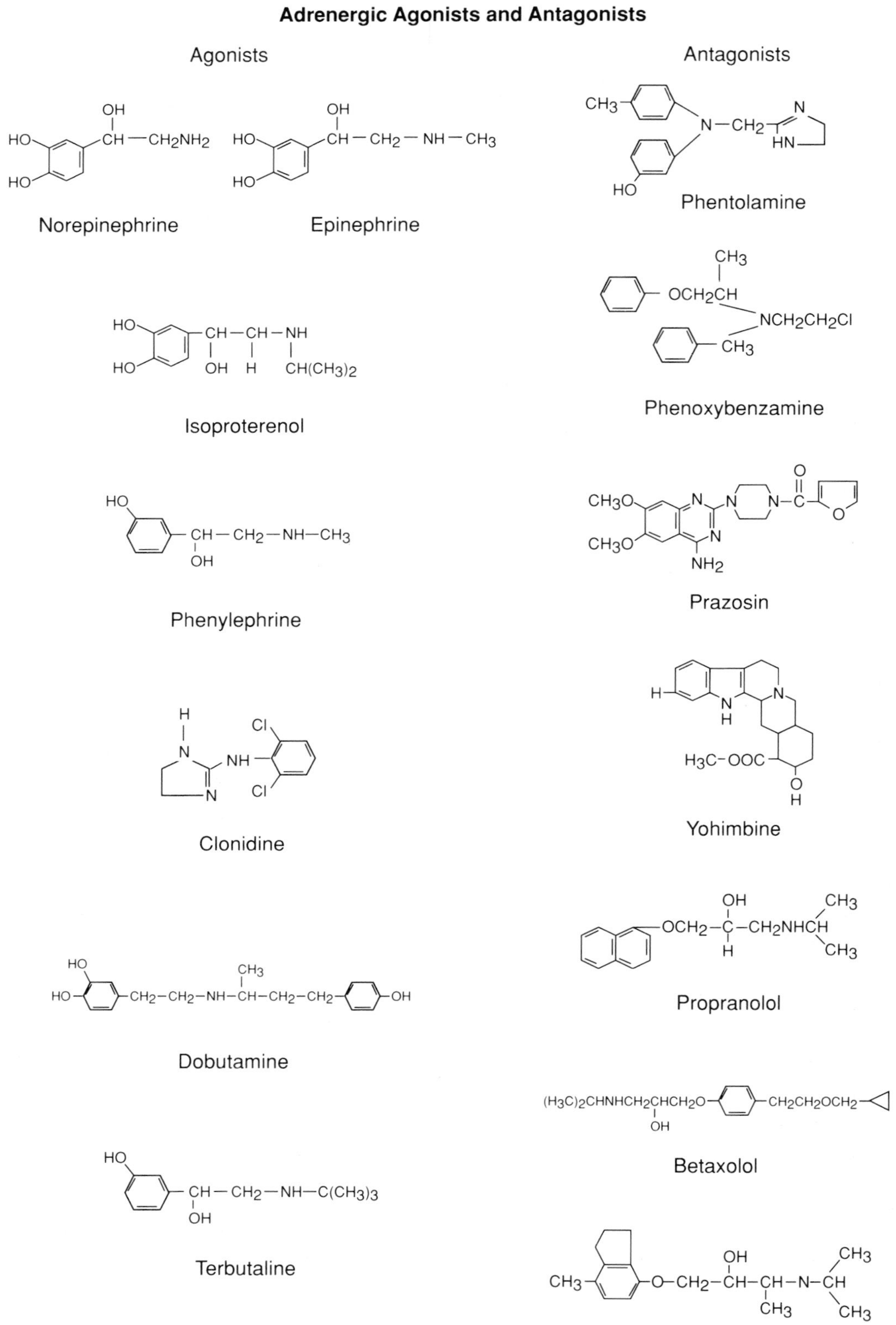

Adrenergic Agonists and Antagonists

Agonists

Norepinephrine

Epinephrine

Isoproterenol

Phenylephrine

Clonidine

Dobutamine

Terbutaline

Antagonists

Phentolamine

Phenoxybenzamine

Prazosin

Yohimbine

Propranolol

Betaxolol

Fig. 2-24. Structure of ligands that distinguish adrenergic receptor subtypes.

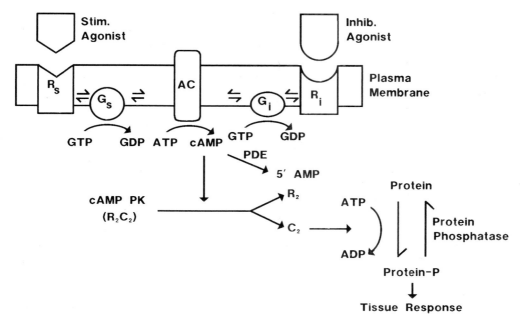

Fig. 2-25. Scheme for regulation of cellular response by neurotransmitters and hormones that regulate cellular cyclic 3′,5′-adenosine monophosphate (cAMP) concentrations. The scheme indicates that agonists interact with plasma membrane receptors that can either stimulate (R_s) or inhibit (R_i) the catalyst of adenylyl cyclase activity (AC) via specific guanine nucleotide-binding proteins (G_s, G_i). Activation of AC leads to formation of cyclic AMP, which can be degraded by phosphodiesterase (PDE) or can activate cyclic AMP-dependent protein kinase activity (cAMP PK). The activation of this kinase involves dissociation of the inactive holoenzyme into its regulatory (R) and catalytic (C) subunits and promotes the phosphorylation of specific proteins, thereby altering their function. One or more protein phosphatases reverses the action of the kinase and the functional activity of the proteins.

Table 2-8. Agonists and Receptor Systems That Regulate Adenylyl Cyclase Activity

Increase Activity	*Decrease Activity*
β_1 and β_2-adrenergic	α_2-adrenergic
H_2-histamine	A_1-adenosine
A_2-adenosine	D_2-dopamine
S_1-serotonin (5-HT$_{1A}$)	S_1-serotonin (5-HT$_{1A}$)
D_1-dopamine	Muscarinic acetylcholine
Certain prostaglandins (E_1, E_2, I_2)	Opiates and enkephalins
Many peptides and proteins (e.g., glucagon, corticotropin, TSH[a], FSH[a], vasopressin V_2, parathyroid hormone, calcitonin, etc.)	Certain prostaglandins (e.g., E_1, in fat cells)
	Certain peptides and proteins (e.g., somatostatin, neuropeptide Y, atriopeptin)

[a] FSH = follicle-stimulating hormone; TSH = thyroid-stimulating hormone.

8). Even so, there is as yet limited evidence that inhibition of adenylyl cyclase activity can fully account for the physiologic actions of agonists at those receptors; other mechanisms, such as linkage to K^+ channels and to Na^+/H^+ exchange, have also been proposed as possibly involved in inhibitory responses.[55] In some cases, "inhibitory" agonists decrease responses elicited by cyclic AMP analogs, thus strongly suggesting the involvement of mechanisms other than inhibition of adenylyl cyclase activity. Nevertheless, assessment of the mechanism for receptor-mediated inhibition of adenylyl cyclase has been important for understanding the regulation of this enzyme.

A key advance in the understanding of the regulation of adenylyl cyclase activity by drugs and hormones was the discovery by Rodbell and co-workers that the nucleotide guanosine triphosphate (GTP) was required for the activation of this enzyme.[56] Those workers demonstrated that enzyme activity in hepatic membrane preparations was unresponsive to the hormone glucagon unless GTP was included in the enzyme assay. This important observation, which has subsequently been confirmed for virtually every receptor-stimulated adenylyl cyclase system that has been carefully examined, pointed to a key role for guanine nucleotides, and GTP in particular, as a cofactor for the activation of this enzyme. Receptor-mediated inhibition of adenylyl cyclase activity was also shown to require addition of guanine nucleotides.[57] The requirement for guanine nucleotides is somewhat different for stimulation of adenylyl cyclase activity, which typically requires less than 0.3 μmolar concentrations of GTP, than for inhibition, which generally requires at least micromolar concentrations of GTP.

The important role of guanine nucleotides in control of adenylyl cyclase activity was extended by the evidence that GTP analogs (Fig. 2-26) that were not susceptible to hydrolysis at the γ phosphate linkage—such as guanosine 5'-β,γ-imidotriphosphate (Gpp NH p), and guanosine 5'-(γ-thio)triphosphate (GTPγS)—were able to promote sustained activation of the enzyme independently of drug or hormonal agonists.[58] Subsequently, it was found that agonists that regulated adenylyl cyclase activity were able to promote hydrolysis of GTP via GTPase.[59] These findings, together with the observation that added guanine nucleotides regulate the binding of agonists (but not antagonists) to receptors linked to the stimulation or inhibition of adenylyl cyclase, led to the notion that one or more guanine nucleotide-binding proteins (termed G or N proteins) are responsible for the transduction of signals or "coupling" of receptors to the catalyst of adenylyl cyclase.

Guanine Nucleotide–Binding Proteins

Knowledge regarding G proteins has evolved rapidly within the past several years. This progress has resulted from the application of many approaches including: (1) study of mutant cells that lack G proteins and enable one to reconstitute their activity; (2) purification of G proteins and reconstitution of purified proteins with other components; (3) identification of probes to label such proteins covalently; and (4) molecular cloning of the proteins and determination of their primary structures.[60–63] The combined use of these approaches has definitively shown that at least two different classes of G proteins are involved in the regulation of adenylyl cyclase activity (Table 2-9). One of these has been termed G_s because it is responsible for stimulation of adenylyl cyclase activity, and the other has been termed G_i because it mediates inhibition of adenylyl cyclase activity.

As summarized in Table 2-9, both these proteins are heterotrimers of the subunit composition αβγ. The α subunits of the various G proteins are structurally homologous but distinct in terms of functional properties, amino acid sequence, and molecular mass; thus

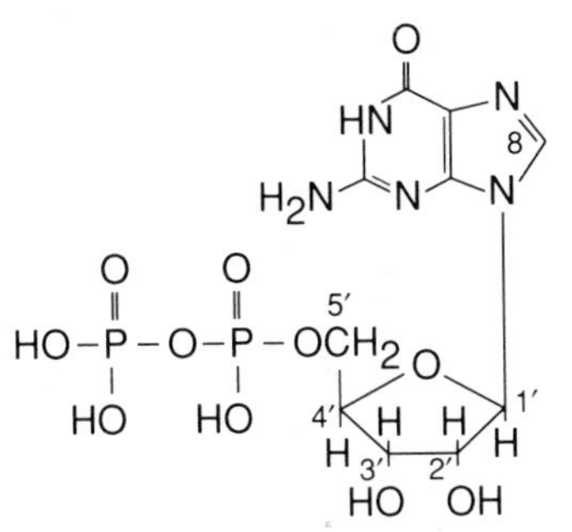

GDP

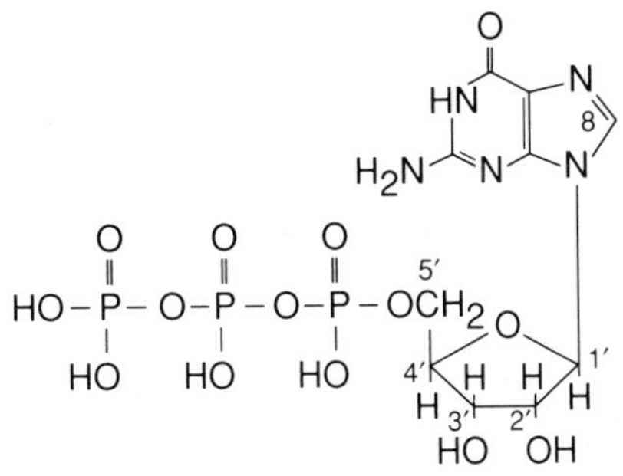

GTP

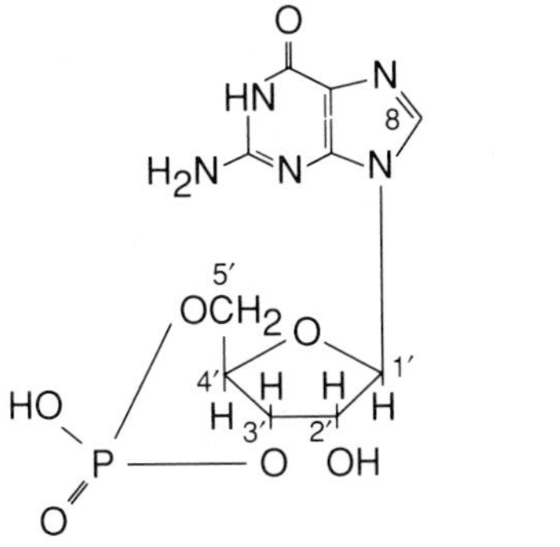

Guanosine 3′, 5′ - cyclic phosphate

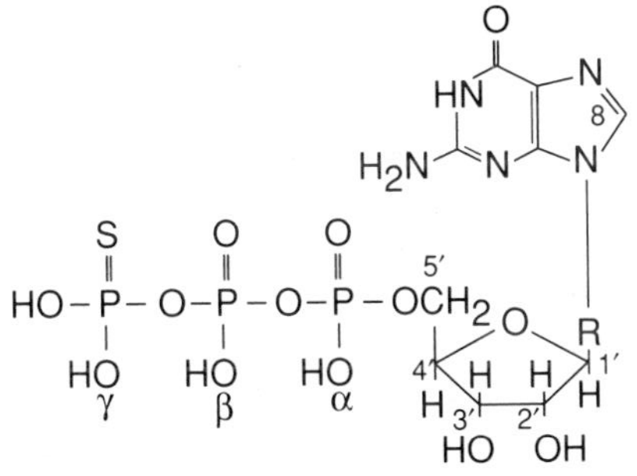

GTPγS

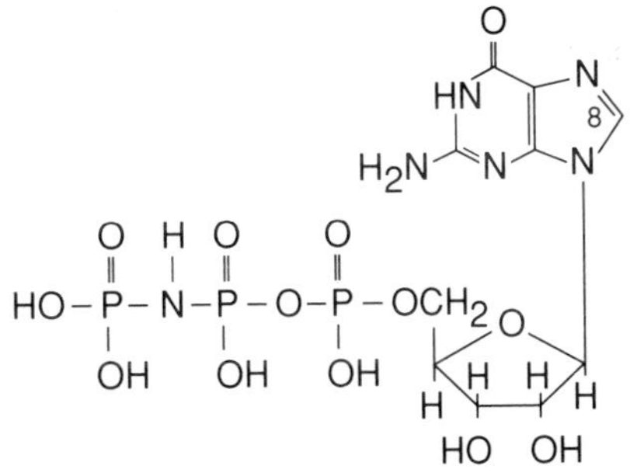

Gpp(NH)p

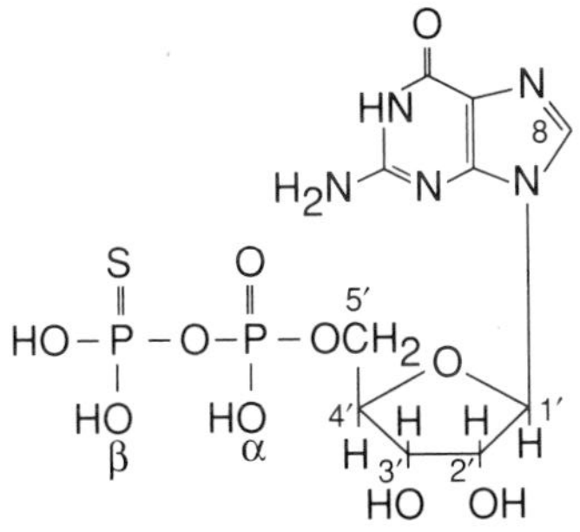

GDPβS

Fig. 2-26. Structure of guanosine phosphate derivatives. The molecular structures of guanosine triphosphate (GTP), guanosine diphosphate (GDP), guanosine cyclic 3′,5′-monophosphate (cyclic GMP), guanosine 5′-(βγ-imidotriphosphate) or 5′-guanylylimidodiphosphate (GppNHp), guanosine 5′-O-3-thiotriphosphate (GTPγS), and guanosine 5′-O- (2-thiodiphosphate) (GDPβS) are shown.

Table 2-9. Properties of G_s and G_i Proteins

	G_s	G_i
Effect	↑ Adenylyl cyclase (AC) activity, Ca^{2+} channel conductance; other (?) including Mg transport, Ca-Mg ATPase	↓ Adenylyl cyclase (AC) activity, K^+ channel conductance; other (?) including phospholipases A_2 and C, Na^+/H^+ exchange, Ca^{2+} channel
Activators	Hormones/neurotransmitters GTP (< 0.3 μM) Nonhydrolyzable guanine nucleotides (GN) AlF_4^-	Hormones/neurotransmitters GTP (> 1 μM) Nonhydrolyzable GN AlF_4^-
Cation dependence	Monovalent: None Divalent: Mg^{2+}	Monovalent: Na^+ may stimulate Divalent: Mg^{2+} ($K_a < 1$ μM)
GTPase activity	Present	Present
Toxin effect	Cholera toxin ADP ribosylates ↑ GTP (but not nonhydrolyzable GN) effect to increase AC activity; no effect on receptor binding	Pertussis toxin ADP ribosylates, ↓ GTP effect to decrease AC activity; blocks GTP effect on receptor binding, does not usually block nonhydrolyzable GN inhibition of AC
Stoichiometry	Receptor $<G_s$	Receptor $\ll G_i$, ($G_i \gg G_s$)
Structure	Heterotrimeric (α, β, γ) α = 42–52 (binds GN, Mg^{2+} (?), receptor; stimulates catalysis by AC; cholera toxin substrate) β = 35–36 kDa (deactivates α) γ = 5–10 kDa: (unknown function: (?) anchors G_s in membrane	Heterotrimeric, (α, β, γ) α = 40–41 kDa (binds GN, Mg^{2+}, receptor; inhibits (?) catalysis by AC; pertussis toxin substrate) myristoylated at NH_2 terminus β = 35–36 kDa (identical to β of G_s) γ = 5–10 kDa (unknown function: (?) anchors G_i in membrane)
Molecular mechanism	Dissociation of heterotrimer by GN/Mg^{2+}, AlF_4^-, hormone Hormone promotes GTP/GDP exchange and decreases K_a for Mg^{2+} Termination by GTPase	Dissociation of heterotrimer by GN/Mg^{2+}, AlF_4, hormone Hormone promotes GTP/GDP exchange $\beta\gamma$ associates with α_s to form inactive $\alpha_s\beta\gamma$ heterotrimer; $\beta\gamma$ direct inhibition of C (?); GN-bound α_i can inhibit C (?); termination by GTPase (?)

α_s is 42 to 55 kDa and exists in at least two different forms, while α_i is 40 to 41 kDa and also has multiple forms. The α subunits contain the GTP-binding and GTP-hydrolytic domains of these proteins. The bacterial toxins of *Vibrio cholerae* and *Bordatella pertussis* are able to catalyze the adenosine diphosphate (ADP) ribosylation and thereby to covalently modify α_s and α_i, respectively, according to the following reaction scheme:

$$\alpha_S + NAD + V.\ cholerae\ \text{toxin} \rightleftharpoons \alpha_S\ ADPR + \text{nicotinamide} + H^+$$
$$\alpha_i + NAD + B.\ pertussis\ \text{toxin} \rightleftharpoons \alpha_i\ ADPR + \text{nicotinamide} + H^+$$

(10)

Use of labeled NAD for these reactions allows the direct identification of α_s and α_i by autoradiography following polyacrylamide gel electrophoresis in the presence of sodium dodecyl sulfate. ADP ribosylation of α_s by *V. cholerae* toxin or of α_i by *B. pertussis* toxin blocks the GTPase activity of the subunits and alters the activity of adenylyl cyclase. With *V. Cholerae* toxin treatment, cellular cyclic AMP rises as a consequence of irreversible activation of adenylyl cyclase activity. *B. pertussis* toxin treatment blocks the ability of G_i to mediate the action of receptors linked to G_i and thereby also increases cellular cyclic AMP. At least one other G protein (termed G_o for "other" G protein) can be identified by use of labeled NAD and *B. pertussis* toxin as a 39- or 40-kDa α subunit,[64,65] and G proteins linked to second messengers other than adenylyl cyclase are sensitive to *B. pertussis* toxin.[66,67] These observations complicate interpretation of experiments in which *B. pertussis* toxin, which is also known as islet-activating protein (IAP), is used to block receptor-mediated responses. The β subunits of G_s, G_i, and G_o appear to be identical 35- to 36-kDa proteins.[60,63] Few details are known regarding the 5- to 10-kDa γ subunits, but it has been proposed that these subunits are tightly bound to the β subunits and may be responsible for anchoring the G proteins to the cytoplasmic surface of the plasma membrane.

The availability of antibodies to G proteins and the application of molecular cloning techniques has revealed that the G proteins of the adenylyl cyclase system are part of a larger family of GTP binding proteins, many of which appear to be involved in signal transduction across plasma membranes.[60-63] Examples include:

1. Transducin, a G protein of the retinal photoreceptor (rod) cells, which is activated by light, regulates a guanosine 3',5'-monophosphate (cyclic GMP) phosphodiesterase activity. Transducin also is a heterotrimer of $\alpha\beta\gamma$ structure. The α subunit of transducin, α_t, has a 39-kDa molecular mass and its amino acid sequence is homologous to that of α_s and α_i (Fig. 2-27). Moreover, α_t (T_1 in Fig. 2-27) can partially substitute for the other α subunits to reconstitute adenylyl cyclase activity in vitro, and it can be labeled by both *V. cholerae* and *B. pertussis* toxins. The β subunit of transducin appears to be similar or identical to that of G_s, G_i, and G_o. A transducin specific for retinal cones has also been identified (T_2 in Fig. 2-27).
2. G_o, which was briefly described above, is a membrane protein found in high abundance in the central nervous system (approximately 1 percent of membrane protein) and in other tissues as well. Its function in vivo is poorly understood. In reconstitution studies α_o, the purified α subunit from G_o, is able to regulate GTP-dependent binding of certain agonists to receptors and can substitute for α_i[68]; other data suggest that this protein is linked to the regulation of Ca^{2+} channels.[69]
3. G_p is a protein whose existence has been inferred from data showing that certain receptors regulate phospholipase C activity in membranes in a GTP-dependent manner and that such activity can also be regulated by guanine nucleotides independently of receptor agonists.[70,71]
4. G_z is a protein that has been cloned and sequenced, although its physiologic role and mechanism of action are controversial.[72]

The prospect that other G proteins will be identified seems quite likely, as does the likelihood that GTP-binding proteins involved in signal transduction will be part of a larger family of GTP-binding proteins, such as those that regulate microtubule assembly and protein synthesis in eukaryotes and prokaryotes.[62,74] Moreover, individual G proteins appear to be multifunctional in terms of their ability to link to more than one effector system.[63,72,73]

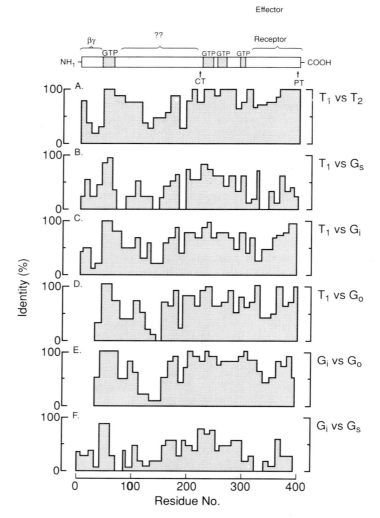

Fig. 2-27. Comparison of the amino acid sequences of the α subunits of G proteins T_1 (transducin of retinal rods), T_2 (transducin of retinal cones), G_s, G_i, and G_o. The percent sequence identity has been averaged over sequential blocks of 10 residues and is plotted versus residue number for various pairs of α subunits. The abscissa refers to residue number in α_s, which is larger than the others—hence gaps in the plots. At the top are illustrated the regions in the α chain that may correspond to protein domains that interact with receptors and effectors, bind GTP, and are ADP-ribosylated by cholera toxin (CT) and pertussis toxin (PT). (Adapted from Stryer and Bourne,[61] with permission.)

Binding of agonists to many classes of membrane receptors is sensitive to addition of guanine nucleotides (Fig. 2-28). In the absence of added nucleotide, unlabeled agonists compete for radiolabeled antagonist sites over a wide concentration range, and the competitive binding curves yield a pseudo-Hill coefficient less than unity. Addition of GTP or other guanine nucleotide typically produces two principal changes in this competitive binding curve: the overall potency of the agonist in competing for binding is decreased,

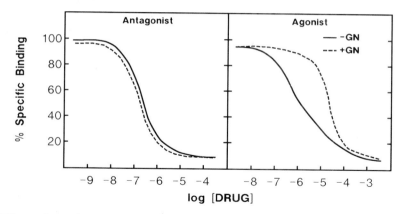

Fig. 2-28. Effect of guanine nucleotides on interaction of agonist and antagonist with G-protein-linked receptor. This schematic figure demonstrates the typical curves observed with varying concentrations of an antagonist (left) and agonist (right) competing with an antagonist radioligand for specific binding sites in experiments conducted in the absence (solid line) or presence (broken line) of a guanine nucleotide such as GTP, Gpp (NH)p, or GTPγS.

and the pseudo-Hill coefficient approaches 1.0. Computer modeling of these data has indicated that the results can be described by two classes of binding sites (one with high affinity and the other with low affinity for agonists in the absence of guanine nucleotides), which are converted to a single lower-affinity class of sites in the presence of guanine nucleotides. The results have suggested that in the absence of guanine nucleotides a ternary complex is formed between agonist, receptor, and G protein.[60,75]

In some cases (e.g., the β-adrenergic receptor of frog erythrocytes), the ability of various agonists to form or "stabilize" this complex correlates closely with the efficacy of the agonist.[76] Thus, full agonists promote formation of a higher percentage of high-affinity complexes than do partial agonists, and antagonists fail to form such complexes. Moreover, efficacy, as introduced in Chapter 1, also seems to correlate with the ratio of K_D values for the high- and low-affinity states of β-adrenergic receptors that bind agonists. Such results provide one molecular interpretation for the concept of drug efficacy, although the applicability of this model to a large number of receptor systems has not yet been rigorously tested. Studies with purified receptors and purified G proteins indicate that high- and low-affinity states of binding sites that bind agonists can be reconstituted in phospholipid vesicles, indicating that this transition can be documented in a simpler system.[77,78] Rigorous investigations of G protein coupling in relation to agonist efficacy are likely to require reconstituted systems to which components of defined stoichiometry can be added.

As indicated above, a large number of membrane receptors exhibit guanine nucleotide-sensitive binding of agonists. Thus, when agonists are used to identify receptors by radioligand binding, only a fraction of the total population of binding sites may be detected—those that bind the agonist with high affinity (dissociation constants typically less than 30 nM). Because addition of guanine nucleotides decreases the receptor affinity for the agonist, it is difficult or perhaps impossible to detect binding of a labeled agonist in the presence of the guanine nucleotide. This is particularly true when one tries to identify receptors in intact cells, in which the cellular GTP concentrations would be expected to convert most of the receptors to the low-affinity form.

The guanine nucleotide sensitivity of agonists in binding to receptors has sometimes been interpreted as evidence that a particular receptor is "linked to adenylyl cyclase." The discovery of G proteins that are not involved in regulating adenylyl cyclase activity indicates that it would be more accurate to interpret this sensitivity as evidence that the receptor likely interacts with a G protein, but not necessarily with G_s or G_i. Future studies are likely to be designed to identify the specific G proteins with which particular receptors interact.

Structure of G Protein-Linked Receptors

The application of molecular cloning techniques has facilitated the elucidation of the amino acid sequences for the G protein-linked receptors.[51,79–81] The receptors that have been cloned—including α_1, α_{2A}, α_{2B}, β_1, β_2, and β_3-adrenergic receptors, angiotensin receptor (*mas* oncogene), the neurokinin receptors, serotonin 1a and 1c receptors, and five types of muscarinic acetylcholine receptors—show sequence homology with each other and also with the opsin family of retinal proteins involved in photoreception, with mating factor receptors in yeast, and with a cell surface cyclic AMP receptor in slime molds. Analysis of hydropathy profiles of the deduced amino acid sequence has suggested that all these proteins possess seven membrane-spanning domains (Fig. 2-29). In addition, certain asparagine residues have been identified as likely sites of glycosylation and hence positioned on the extracellular surface. Intracellular residues have been identified that contain amino acids capable of being phosphorylated by cyclic AMP-dependent protein kinase or other protein kinases. All the classes of receptors linked to G proteins show substantial regions of sequence identity, in particular within the membrane-spanning re-

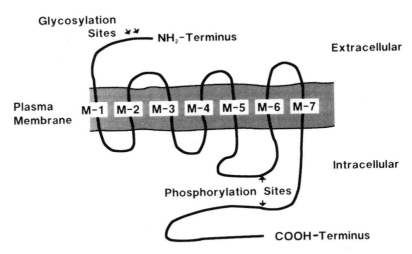

Fig. 2-29. Schematic representation of the membrane organization of plasma membrane receptors (such as adrenergic receptors, muscarinic acetylcholine receptors, substance K receptors, or opsins; see text) that are linked to G proteins. An extracellular amino terminal region with sites of glycosylation on asparagine residues is followed by seven membrane-spanning domains (M1 to M7) interspersed with three intracellular and three extracellular loops and then an intracellular carboxy terminus. The consensus sequences expected at sites for phosphorylation are found in the third intracellular loop and carboxy terminal regions.

gions. Thus, these receptors all appear to be members of a family of proteins that have evolved from a common ancestral gene. It is of interest that the receptor genes (with the possible exception of α_1-adrenergic receptors[82]), unlike those of the opsins, appear to possess no introns and thus may have evolved later in the evolutionary scale. It is to be expected that other G-linked receptors will have similarities in structure and functional domains to the receptors that have already been cloned and sequenced.

With the purification of the key components of adenylyl cyclase system receptors, G proteins, and catalyst (termed C) and the reconstitution of purified components in phospholipid vesicles, it has been possible to develop tentative molecular models that describe how receptors and G proteins regulate adenylyl cyclase activity.[60,63] Purification of the β-adrenergic receptor to homogeneity and its reconstitution with G proteins has indicated that a single receptor protein could possess both the recognition function for agonists and antagonists and the ability to interact with and regulate a G protein.[77,78] It is worth noting that the retention of recognition and effector coupling within a single protein subunit for G protein-linked receptors is in contrast to the behavior of channel-linked receptors, which possess multiple subunits.

Results obtained with chimeric receptors constructed by using molecular genetic techniques and expressed in *Xenopus laevis* oocytes have indicated that the specificity of coupling of the β_2-adrenergic receptors to G_s appears to be determined by a region extending from the amino terminus of the fifth hydrophobic domain to the carboxy terminus of the sixth hydrophobic domain, whereas key regions involved in defining specificity of antagonist binding to α_2- and β_2-adrenergic receptors are within the seventh membrane-spanning domain.[80] Further efforts directed at the use of mutational analysis and construction of receptor chimeras should prove useful in defining the precise structural domains and specific amino acids of receptors that are responsible for agonist binding, G protein interaction, and other functions of the G-linked receptors.

Molecular Mechanism for Stimulation and Inhibition of Adenylyl Cyclase

The use of a purified receptor, purified G_s, and purified adenylyl cyclase (the catalyst C) has indicated that these three components are necessary and sufficient to mediate a receptor-stimulated activation of adenylyl cyclase.[83] The detailed mechanism of activation is not precisely understood, in part because limited studies have been undertaken with only these three purified components. Most studies have involved the reconstitution of purified G_s proteins into membranes of cells that lack G_s but retain receptors and C (e.g., the cyc⁻ mutant of murine S49 lymphoma cells). Reconstitution of the adenylyl cyclase system in the cyc⁻ cells has indicated that the α_s subunit of G_s is responsible for the activation of C and that the activation process requires that $\alpha_s\beta\gamma$, the inactive holoenzyme form of G_s (Fig. 2-30), be dissociated to yield α_s.[60-63,72] GTP and certain GTP analogs are able to promote this activation, but GDP and the GDP analog, GDP β-thiosulfide, are unable to activate G_s. Thus, it is believed that the deactivation of the G_s protein results from the hydrolysis of GTP to form GDP. Another cofactor that seems to play a key role in the activation reaction is Mg^{2+}, which may be required for a conformational change in the α_s protein.[60]

Receptors are thought to stimulate adenylyl cyclase via G_s by facilitating an exchange of GTP for bound GDP, which is believed to occupy the α_s protein in its ground state (Fig. 2-30). Receptors may also enhance conformational changes required for the α_s protein to be activated. Receptor-promoted binding of GTP to the α_s protein has two effects: with

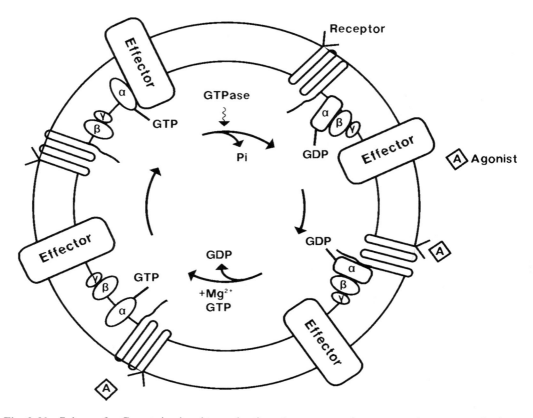

Fig. 2-30. Scheme for G protein signal transduction. A seven-membrane-spanning receptor is shown as it becomes occupied by agonist (A) and forms a ternary complex with the G protein ($\alpha\beta\gamma$) to which GTP is bound. The exchange of GTP for GDP in the presence of Mg^{2+} leads to the activation of the G protein, dissociation of α_{GTP} from $\beta\gamma$, and dissociation of the receptor from the G protein. Agonist also dissociates from the receptor in its low-affinity form. The α_{GTP} is able to activate the effector molecule, although conceivably $\beta\gamma$ may also regulate effectors. The intrinsic GTPase activity of the α subunit hydrolyzes GTP to GDP, releasing inorganic phosphate (P_i), and α_{GDP} reassociates with $\beta\gamma$ to end the activation cycle. (Adapted from Neer and Clapham,[63] with permission.)

GTP binding to α_s, the receptor dissociates from α_s, enabling α_s to activate C; and the activation of C is terminated by the hydrolysis of GTP to GDP, allowing the G_s to return to its ground state.

The mechanism for inhibition of adenylyl cyclase activity by the G_i protein is controversial.[60,62,63,84,85] This inhibition is thought to require dissociation of the heterotrimer $\alpha_i\beta\gamma$. The close similarity of the $\beta\gamma$ subunits between G_s and G_i provides at least two possible mechanisms for inhibition of the catalyst: direct inhibition by α_i or indirect inhibition involving formation of the inactive heterotrimer $\alpha_s\beta\gamma$ through promotion of reassociation of the $\beta\gamma$ subunits with α subunits. Much of the available data suggest that the latter mechanism is the principal, although perhaps not the exclusive, means by which adenylyl cyclase activity is inhibited. The substantial molar excess of G_i compared with G_s in cells in which the two proteins have been quantitated is consistent with the idea that G_i may mediate inhibition of adenylyl cyclase activity by providing $\beta\gamma$ subunit. As with the stimulatory pathway, GTP hydrolysis appears to terminate G protein-mediated inhibition of adenylyl cyclase. Receptors that mediate inhibition of adenylyl cyclase are thought to enhance exchange of GTP from GDP bound to an inactive α_i protein, although other mechanisms may also be involved. ADP ribosylation of α_i by *B. pertussis* toxin blocks the ability of receptors to promote inhibition of adenylyl cyclase activity. In addition, *B. pertussis* toxin treatment blocks the GTPase activity of α_i, as well as the ability of guanine nucleotides to alter the binding of agonists to "inhibitory receptors." By contrast, *V. cholerae* toxin blocks the GTPase activity of α_s, thereby converting α_s to a more persistently active state, but unlike the situation with *B. pertussis* toxin, *V. cholerae* toxin does not perturb the ability of agonists to bind to "stimulatory receptors."

Studies with purified and reconstituted components of the adenylyl cyclase system have yielded additional insights regarding the regulation of adenylyl cyclase activity. Thus, it has been possible to define the site of action of a variety of regulators of activity. These include: AlF_4^-, which is commonly used as an activator of adenylyl cyclase and which appears to interact with α_s, perhaps by enhancing the ability of GDP-bound α_s to activate the enzyme[86] (under appropriate conditions AlF_4^- can also be shown to activate α_i); and the diterpene forskolin, which stimulates adenylyl cyclase activity via a primary interaction with C (although interaction of G_s is required for full responses to forskolin).[87]

The cloning of adenylyl cyclase has revealed an unexpected structure of two alternating hydrophilic and hydrophobic domains; each hydrophobic domain contains 6 transmembrane spans.[88] Although there is no direct sequence homology, its topographical structure resembles that of membrane channels and transporters. The closest resemblance is to the P glycoprotein, a multidrug resistance gene product that binds ATP and exports small molecules from cells (see Ch. 9). A domain with homology to the guanylyl cyclase has also been identified. Adenylyl cyclases may have, in addition to catalyzing the formation of cyclic AMP, a transporter function.

Receptors Linked to Phosphoinositide Hydrolysis and Ca^{2+} Mobilization via G Proteins

A large number of drug and hormone receptors have been shown to utilize a second major pathway for transmembrane signaling.[89] These membrane receptors activate hydrolysis of a specific class of membrane phospholipids, the phosphoinositides[89,90] (Table 2-10).

In 1953 Hokin and Hokin first reported that acetylcholine stimulated the incorporation of ^{32}P into phospholipids in the pancreas.[91] Subsequent work showed that a variety of agonists could regulate incorporation of labeled phosphate into phospholipids, in particular phosphatidylinositol. Two key features emerged from these studies: (1) agonists that pro-

Table 2-10. Agonists and Receptor Systems That Increase Membrane Phosphoinositide Hydrolysis and Intracellular Calcium

α_1-Adrenergic
H_1-Histamine
S_1-Serotonin
Muscarinic acetylcholine (e.g., m_1 and m_3)
Certain peptides and proteins (e.g., vasopressin V_1, bradykinin, bombesin, angiotensin, F-Met-Leu-Phe, thyrotropin-releasing hormone, platelet-derived growth factor)

moted incorporation of label into phosphatidylinositol also were generally able to increase free intracellular calcium concentrations in cells; and (2) agonist-promoted labeling of membrane phosphatidylinositol appeared to represent one limb of a cyclic pathway whereby this class of membrane phospholipids was first hydrolyzed and then resynthesized. Michell integrated some of these ideas in the mid-1970s and proposed that phosphoinositide turnover was likely to be a general mechanism for agonists that raise intracellular free calcium.[92] For several years thereafter this intriguing hypothesis had not been readily amenable to study. Several problems contributed to this. One was the difficulty in producing agonist-mediated changes in phospholipid metabolism in broken cell preparations on which detailed mechanistic studies might be conducted. Instead, most experiments on phosphoinositide metabolism were performed with intact cells or tissue slices. A second problem was the lability of certain substrates and products and the difficulty in establishing whether changes in cytosolic calcium were the cause or effect of changes in phosphatidylinositol.

A substantial increase in understanding of receptor-mediated alteration in phosphoinositide metabolism has subsequently been achieved as the result of several key observations:

1. The demonstration that certain polyphosphatidylinositols, in particular phosphatidylinositol 4,5-bisphosphate (PIP$_2$), which occurs in very low abundance, is the critical substrate for the formation of inositol 1,4,5-trisphosphate (IP$_3$), a second messenger capable of liberating calcium from intracellular stores[89-91]
2. The recognition that hormone-stimulated activation of phospholipases, in particular phospholipase C, is likely to be responsible for liberation of the IP$_3$ from PIP$_2$ (Fig. 2-30) and that this enzyme can be studied in broken cell preparations[70,90,93]
3. The observation that diacylglycerol, the other product of phospholipase C-mediated hydrolysis of phosphoinositides, is also able to function as a second messenger, because it can activate a calcium/phospholipid-dependent protein kinase, protein kinase C.[89,90,94,98]

A concept that can unify studies of transmembrane signaling via regulation of adenylyl cyclase activity with studies of receptor-mediated phosphoinositide hydrolysis is that receptors that activate either of those two effector systems are linked to G proteins[61-63,66, 67,70,90,93] Several observations lead to this conclusion. Guanine nucleotides modulate binding of agonists to receptors that mediate phosphoinositide breakdown. They may be necessary cofactors in receptor-mediated activation of phospholipase C in membrane preparations, and in some cases *B. pertussis* toxin blocks phosphoinositide hydrolysis under conditions in which cyclic AMP concentrations are not substantially altered. Thus, for some receptor systems a *B. pertussis* toxin-sensitive G protein may be responsible for phosphoinositide hydrolysis.[54,55,58] In other receptor systems phosphoinositide hydrolysis is not sensitive to treatment with *B. pertussis* toxin even though binding to receptors is altered by added guanine nucleotides. Hence G$_p$, which is a G protein not sensitive to pertussis toxin, may be involved. Details of how G$_p$ activates phospholipase(s) are poorly understood, although requirements for the activation of phospholipase C in membrane preparations include added Mg^{2+} and guanine nucleotide.

Few mechanistic details are known regarding the phospholipase (phosphodiesterase, phosphoinositidase) that mediates the receptor-activated breakdown of membrane phosphoinositides. As noted above, breakdown of membrane phosphatidylinositol 4,5-bisphosphate to inositol 1,4,5-trisphosphate and *sn*-1,2-diacylclycerol appears to be a key step in the generation of second messengers for these types of receptors. Phosphatidy-linositol 4,5-bisphosphate is a minor (5 percent) component of membrane phosphatidy-linositols and is formed by stepwise phosphorylation of phosphatidylinositol, initially to phosphatidylinositol 4-phosphate and then to phosphatidylinositol 4,5-biphosphate. Different lipid kinases appear to be responsible for these sequential phosphorylations.

Inositol 1,4,5-trisphosphate, the water-soluble product formed by the action of phospholipase on phosphatidylinositol 4,5-bisphosphate, is susceptible to a variety of fates. One of these is hydrolysis by a specific phosphatase to inositol 1,4-bisphosphate, which in turn is hydrolyzed by an inositol bisphosphatase to inositol 1-phosphate. Inositol 1-phosphate is hydrolyzed by an inositol 1-phosphatase to free inositol. Inositol can then be utilized to regenerate phosphatidylinositol when combined with cytosine diphosphate diacylglycerol, thus defining the cyclic nature of the formation and breakdown of membrane phosphoinositides (Fig. 2-31).

Inositol 1-phosphatase is prominently inhibited by Li^+, an observation of experimental and perhaps also of therapeutic importance.[96] Li^+ blocks the formation of free inositol and thus the continuous cycling of the pathway. Addition of lithium thus provides a means to examine the hydrolysis of phosphatidylinositols, so that resynthesis from inositol phosphate products is minimized. Conceivably this action of lithium contributes to its usefulness as an agent for the therapy of manic-depressive disorders, since cells in the brain may require the generation of free inositol by inositol 1-phosphatase for the continuous cycling of the phosphoinositide/inositol phosphate pathway.

Inositol 1,4,5-trisphosphate can also be converted to a form with four phosphate groups, inositol 1,3,4,5-tetrakisphosphate, which in turn can be hydrolyzed to form inositol 1,3,4-trisphosphate.[97] Some evidence suggests that inositol 1,3,4,5-tetrakisphosphate may enhance calcium entry into cells.[98] When cells are treated with agonists, inositol 1,3,4-trisphosphate appears to accumulate more slowly than does inositol 1,4,5-trisphosphate, and it appears to be far less active than inositol 1,4,5-trisphosphate in mobilizing calcium from intracellular sites.

A third fate for inositol 1,4,5-trisphosphate is to bind to specific receptors that have been detected at nonmitochondrial, presumably endoplasmic reticulum, sites.[90.99] Molecular details are scanty regarding the nature of these membrane receptors, but data from several cell types indicate that inositol 1,4,5-trisphosphate can promote calcium efflux from a nonmitochondrial site into the cytosol as a consequence of this receptor interaction. These receptors sites preferentially interact with inositol 1,4,5-trisphosphate rather than with other trisphosphates, bisphosphates, or monophosphate. Kinetic studies in some systems have suggested that the rate of formation of inositol 1,4,5-trisphosphate and its rate of interaction with these putative receptors can account for the rapid increase in cytosolic calcium produced by agonists that act via cell surface receptors linked to phosphoinositide hydrolysis; in other systems it may be insufficient.

The other product of phospholipase C action on membrane phosphoinositides, *sn*-1,2-diacylglycerol, is thought to play other important roles in receptor-mediated signal transduction.[89,91,94,95] Nishizuka and co-workers were the first to demonstrate that a unique protein kinase was activated by calcium and utilized phospholipids (of which acidic phospholipids, such as phosphatidylserine, appear most active) as a cofactor.[94,95] It was later discovered that this calcium/phospholipid-dependent protein kinase, termed protein kinase C, is present in many tissues and that its activity is enhanced by *sn*-1,2-diacylglycerols. The diacylglycerols act in a stereospecific manner to increase the affinity of the enzyme

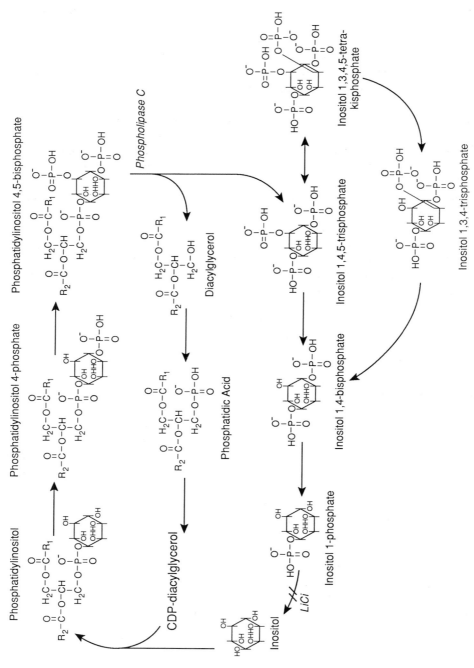

Fig. 2-31. The phosphoinositide cycle. Several forms of phosphatidylinositols are shown, with their hydrolysis by phospholipase C to diacylglycerol and respective inositol phosphates. Diacylglycerol can be converted via diacylglycerol kinase to phosphatidic acid, which in turn can be joined to inositol (derived from hydrolysis of inositol phosphates) via cytosine diphosphate diacylglycerol to form phosphatidylinositol.

for calcium. The enzyme appears to have a stoichiometry of 1 mole protein kinase C:1 mole diacylglycerol:1 mole Ca^{2+}:4 moles phosphatidylserine. Multiple forms of protein kinase C have been identified.[100-102]

Protein kinase C has been shown to be the cellular receptor for a class of tumor-promoting phorbol esters, which include 12-O-tetradecanoyl phorbol 13-acetate (TPA), also known as phorbol myristylacetate (PMA).[94] The phorbol esters show some similarities in conformation to the diacylglycerols but are not susceptible to the relatively rapid metabolism of those compounds. Thus, phorbol esters produce a prominent and long-lived activation of protein kinase C, perhaps by modifying the phospholipid microenvironment of the enzyme and also by increasing its affinity for calcium.

Diacylglycerols can be cleaved by monoacylglycerol or diacylglycerol lipases.[90,91] Activation of these enzymes yields a free fatty acid, typically arachidonic acid, because it is one of the unsaturated fatty acids preferentially found in the sn-2 position of membrane phospholipids (Fig. 2-32). Arachidonic acid is the rate-limiting precursor in the formation of fatty acid derivatives that act via membrane receptors to modulate function of a wide variety of cell types. These fatty acids derivatives appear to function primarily as "local hormones" that regulate cells in a given tissue in an autocrine (i.e., on the same cell) or paracrine (i.e., on a nearby cell) fashion.

As shown in Fig. 2-32, the fatty acid derivatives formed from arachidonic acid are generated by the action of a variety of enzymes. Cyclooxygenase yields intermediates that generate prostaglandins (e.g., PGD_2, PGE_2, PGI_2) and thromboxanes (e.g., TXA_2). Several lipoxygenases yield various intermediates that are converted to leukotrienes (e.g., LTA_4, LTC_4, LTD_4, LTE_4) and lipoxins (e.g., lipoxin A and B). Thus, hydrolysis of diacylglycerol to yield arachidonic acid represents a means by which prostaglandins, thromboxanes, leukotrienes, and lipoxins can be formed. In addition, another phospholipase, phospholipase A_2, can release arachidonic acid from membrane phospholipids or from phosphatidic acid formed by phosphorylation of diacylglycerol by diacylglycerol kinase. Drug and hormone receptors may be able to stimulate phospholipase A_2 and perhaps also phospholipase D, an enzyme that yields phosphatidic acid and the polar head group of this phospholipid[103-105] (Fig. 2-33). Phosphatidic acid serves as a substrate for cytosine triphosphate in the synthesis of phosphatidylinositols and perhaps also as a weak calcium ionophore in some cell types.[106]

The ability of diacylglycerol to act as an intracellular second messenger in the activation of protein kinase C appears to be the most important consequence of formation of this product from membrane phosphoinositides. Receptor-mediated generation of diacylglycerol may also occur from membrane phospholipids other than phosphoinositides.[107-109] Activation of protein kinase C by diacylglycerol has been implicated in a large number of cellular processes, including glandular secretion, activation of blood platelets and neutrophils, and regulation of gene expression, cell growth, cell differentiation, and metabolism.[80,84,85] It seems likely that in some of these cases the activation of protein kinase C occurs in concert with the increase in cytosolic Ca^{2+} produced by inositol 1,4,5-trisphosphate.[94] Calcium is able to activate not only protein kinase C but also calcium-calmodulin–regulated protein kinases.[110,111] Together with protein kinase C, these kinases modulate the phosphorylation of a variety of proteins that are involved in regulation of cellular function, including ion channels, receptors, and G proteins. Thus, calcium-dependent protein kinases regulate cellular responses directly but also can indirectly modulate (via "cross-talk") receptor systems not themselves linked to protein kinase C or to phosphoinositide hydrolysis.

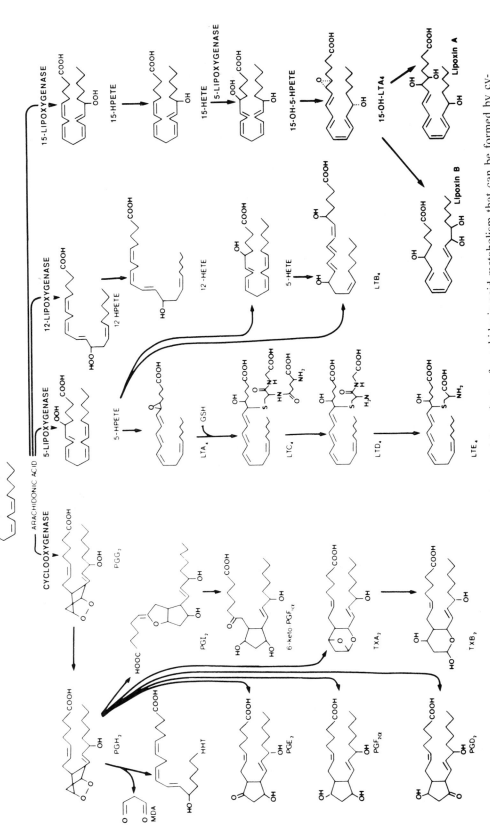

Fig. 2-32. Arachidonic acid metabolism. The multiple potential products of arachidonic acid metabolism that can be formed by cyclooxygenase and 5-, 12-, and 15-lipooxygenase action are shown.

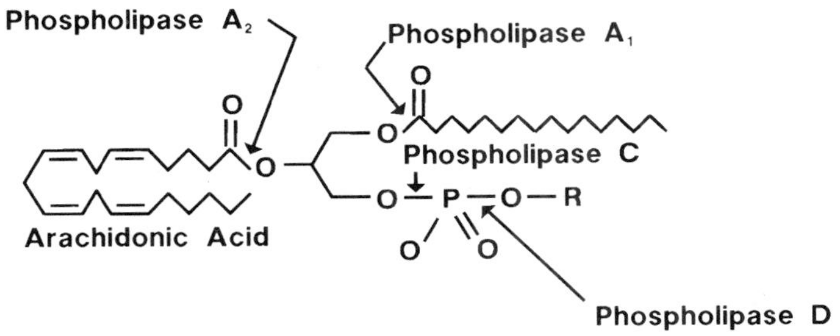

Fig. 2-33. Sites of action of various phospholipases. R = inositol(s), choline, ethanolamine, serine.

Protein kinase C is a cytosolic or peripheral membrane enzyme whose weak association with membrane components appears to be enhanced by phorbol esters or by diacylglycerols.[111,112] Thus receptors that lead to activation of protein kinase C will be expected to promote a "translocation" of the enzyme from cytosolic to plasma membrane fractions. This translocation is synergistically enhanced by increases in intracellular calcium.[112]

The general features described for receptors that act via phosphoinositide hydrolysis summarize considerable data in this area. A large number of unanswered questions or conflicting observations remain. A partial list includes: the nature of the several G proteins involved in these responses; the difficulty in showing or, in some cell types, the inability to show receptor-mediated increases in inositol 1,4,5-trisphosphate levels even though calcium mobilization occurs; the possible role of the slower, more sustained formation of inositol 1,3,4-trisphosphate and of inositol phosphates other than inositol-1,4,5-trisphosphate; the ability of certain types of receptors to activate phospholipase A_2 and perhaps phospholipase D, apparently independently of phospholipase C; evidence that diacylglycerol may be derived from phospholipids other than phosphoinositides; the demonstration that inositol phosphates and phosphatidylinositols with more than three phosphate groups may be formed in some cell types; the precise role of the inositol phosphates in cellular activation; the multiplicity of forms of protein kinase C that have been identified; and the several forms of calcium-dependent protein kinases that exist in agonist-responsive cells. It is evident that phospholipid hydrolysis, which yields a large complement of candidate mediators, is well suited to contribute to cell-specific responses. Future efforts are likely to be directed at refining the general scheme.

Ion Channels Coupled through G Proteins

Electrophysiologic studies have provided clear evidence that certain receptors may couple to ion channels through associated G proteins. The best studied example is muscarinic receptor activation of K^+ channels,[63,73] although G-protein-regulated K^+ channels may exemplify a far more generalized signaling mechanism.[113] In addition, G-protein-mediated regulation of Ca^{2+} channels has also been demonstrated.[63,69,72,73]

The fortunate circumstances of the selective inhibition of a G protein by pertussis toxin and the sensitivity of these proteins to GTP for coupling provided the essential tools by which the G protein coupling mechanism could be demonstrated. For example, in single-channel studies using isolated membrane patches, it was shown that muscarinic activation of K^+ channels required GTP on the cytoplasmic surface and could be inhibited by pertussis toxin.[63,73] The K^+ channel would not be expected to be an integral component of the receptor; rather, it would exist as linked, and perhaps fully dissociable, subunits in the membrane. As described above, the nature of the G protein that couples to K^+ and Ca^{2+} channels and the mechanism(s) for G protein action have not been precisely identified.

Peptide Receptors

A wide variety of peptide receptors have been characterized with respect to ligand specificity and coupling mechanisms. Since the peptides selective for individual receptors are usually derived from larger precursor peptides and the intermediates in processing usually are active, considerable potential exists for a wide diversity in agonist structure. Accordingly, for the peptides an unusually strong pressure may exist for the formation of multiple receptor subtypes. This may be the reason why we find at least four subtypes of opioid receptors. The opioid receptors are discussed in further detail in Chapter 10. Structural properties of peptides as receptor ligands are discussed in Chapter 1.

There is as yet no clear classification of the peptide receptors as large superfamilies. Since coupling mechanisms unique to peptide receptors are not evident, the different peptide receptors may have evolved independently. It might be most appropriate to organize the receptors in relation to the peptide families, as has been done in Table 2-11 for representative peptides, some of which react selectively with distinct receptor subtypes. It is also worth noting that in general it has been difficult to develop receptor subtype-selective peptide antagonists for most classes of peptides. This problem has contributed to difficulty in defining relationships between various peptide receptors and in precisely characterizing various types of peptide receptors.

The mechanisms of mediation of responses by peptide receptors are multiple. The receptor for substance K or neurokinin A (a member of the neurokinin family) has been

Table 2-11. Representative Peptide Families in which Receptor Subtypes Have Been Identified or Appear to Exist

Peptide Class	Agonists	Receptors
Opioids	Enkephalins, dynorphins, endorphins	μ, κ, δ, ϵ
Neurokinins	Substance P, neurokinin A, neurokinin B	NK_1, NK_2, NK_3
Neurohypophyseal hormones	Vasopressin, oxytocin	V_1, V_2, OT
Neurotensin	Neurotensin	NT_1, NT_2
Angiotensin	Angiotensin II	AII, *mas* gene product
Bombesin	Bombesin	BB_1, BB_2
Cholecystokinin	Cholecystokinin octapeptide	CCK-A, CCK-B
Kinins	Bradykinin, Lys-bradykinin, Met-Lys-bradykinin	B_1, B_2, B_3
Atriopeptins	Atriopeptin	Atriopeptin, C-Atriopeptin
Hypothalamic-derived releasing factors	LHRH, GnRH, CRF, TRH	LHRH, GnRH, CRF, TRH

Several other peptides have been shown to have actions that may be mediated through distinct receptors. These include the pituitary-derived trophic hormones, endothelin, neuropeptide Y, glucagon, and parathormone.

cloned by expression cloning, and it appears to be a G-protein-linked receptor.[113] Many other peptide receptors will almost certainly prove to be members of the G protein-linked receptor family in that the peptides increase or decrease adenylyl cyclase activity, activate K^+ channels, or stimulate phosphoinositide hydrolysis. It is possible that as further information regarding the structure of peptide receptors becomes available, new evolutionary and "family" relationships will be revealed and, in turn, reclassification of peptide receptors will be required. The mechanism of transduction of signals for some larger peptides such as insulin appear not to be linked to G proteins and will be considered in the subsequent section of this chapter. In addition, certain peptides have been demonstrated to modulate receptor function and hence may act as heterotropic activators or inhibitors of function of other types of receptors. For example, substance P enhances nicotinic receptor desensitization, but it remains to be seen whether this modulation occurs physiologically in the central nervous system.

MEMBRANE RECEPTORS WHOSE MECHANISM INVOLVES TYROSINE KINASE ACTIVITY

Another major class of membrane receptors appears to activate cellular events by a different pathway—phosphorylation of tyrosine residues in receptors themselves. We present only an abbreviated discussion of these types of receptors as they have been recently reviewed elsewhere.[115–118] Several hormonal agonists (e.g., insulin, insulin-like growth factor, epidermal growth factor, and platelet-derived growth factor) appear to use this mechanism of action. Regulation of other known second messenger systems, such as changes in cyclic AMP or Ca^{2+} concentrations, ion channel conductance, or phosphoinositide hydrolysis, have not been consistently shown for these types of receptors, although evidence has accrued implicating either those second messenger systems or other novel intracellular mediators (e.g., intracellular release of inositol phosphate–glycan after insulin stimulation) in some cell types.[115–119]

That this class of receptors undergoes autophosphorylation on tyrosine residues has been demonstrated for receptors from many tissues.[115–118,120] Phosphorylation of tyrosine is a less common mode of protein phosphorylation compared with the roughly 100-fold higher level of phosphorylation of serine and threonine residues in cellular proteins.[120] The demonstration that several of these types of receptors undergo autophosphorylation and can promote phosphorylation of other proteins appears to define a unique mechanism for cellular regulation. Exactly how phosphorylation of tyrosine occurs and how this phosphorylation leads to changes in intracellular events have not yet been fully defined, but in vitro studies indicate that autophosphorylation of receptors can prominently increase the ability of the receptors to catalyze phosphorylation of exogenous proteins without substantially altering ligand binding to the receptor. It appears likely, although not definitively proven, that autophosphorylation activates receptor kinase activity by conformational changes in the receptor protein.

Structural data obtained from molecular cloning indicate that tyrosine kinase-linked membrane receptors are quite different in several respects from the receptors that are linked to G proteins.[116,118] As depicted schematically in Figure 2-34, the tyrosine kinase receptors span the membrane bilayer only once, in contrast to the seven times that G-linked receptors span the bilayer. In addition, the tyrosine kinase receptors have two functional domains: an extracellular ligand binding domain, which is enriched in cysteine residues, and a cytoplasmic domain, which possesses the tyrosine kinase activity as well

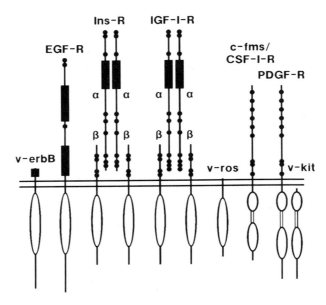

Fig. 2-34. Schematic model of structure of receptors that possess tyrosine kinase activity. Cysteine-rich domains of the receptors are shown as solid boxes, other cysteine residues in extracellular domains as filled circles. Tyrosine kinase domains are shown as ovals, with insertions in *c fms/* CSF1-1R and PDGF-R as parallel lines. Receptors include: EGF-R, human epidermal growth factor receptor; CSF-1-1R, colony-stimulating factor-1 receptor; PDGF-R, platelet-derived growth factor receptor; INS-R, human insulin receptor; and IGF-1-R, insulin-like growth factor-1. Similarity in the organization and structure of these receptors and several retroviral gene products—v-erbB, v-ros, v-kit—are shown. (Adapted from Yarden and Ullrich[118] and Ullrich et al.,[166] with permission.)

as the sites of autophosphorylation. The tyrosine kinase domains appear to be similar among these receptors, but while certain of the receptors possess a single polypeptide chain (e.g., epidermal growth factor, EGF, receptors), others contain two dissimilar chains (α,β) linked as a dimer (e.g., insulin and insulin-like growth factor I). For the latter type of receptors the β chains possess the tyrosine kinase activity.

Receptors produced by site-specific mutagenesis have helped to define domains of receptors involved in certain aspects of functional activity.[116,117,121–124] Thus, deletions in the terminal 112 amino acids of the β chain of the insulin receptor, which are in the cytoplasmic domain, produce receptors that lack tyrosine kinase activity and the ability to promote insulin-mediated glucose uptake. Mutant receptors that lack tyrosine kinase activity can still bind insulin but fail to show several metabolic responses to the hormone. Deletion of the cytoplasmic domain of EGF receptors leads to receptors that are secreted from the cell. Moreover, production of chimeric receptors that possess extracellular binding domains of the insulin receptor but transmembrane and cytoplasmic domains of the EGF receptor respond to insulin with enhanced tyrosine kinase activity, thus indicating the likely similarity in molecular mechanisms of the functional response for these types of receptors.

A common feature of this class of receptors is their ability to produce both rapid and delayed effects on target cells. Metabolic responses are sometimes observed within a few minutes, whereas other effects, such as regulation of DNA synthesis, often occur after a lag of many hours. A universally observed feature is that exposure of target cells to agonists that stimulate tyrosine kinase-linked receptors promotes a prominent feedback regulation of receptors in the target cells. Thus, agonists elicit a rapid internalization (endocytosis) of receptors, which commonly leads to loss of receptors from the cell (down regulation) as well as to recycling of some receptors back to the cell surface. The precise roles of the autophosphorylation of tyrosine in this cellular "processing" of receptors and of the intracellular movement of receptors in the mediation of cellular responses are not yet clearly defined. Studies with mutagenized insulin receptors indicate that protein tyrosine kinase activity of the receptors may be essential for ligand-mediated endocytosis and down regulation.[124]

RECEPTORS LINKED TO GUANYLYL CYCLASE

Guanosine 3'5'-cyclic monophosphate (cyclic GMP) is a purine nucleotide, which is synthesized by the enzyme guanylyl (guanylate) cyclase and which, like cyclic AMP, is metabolized by one or more phosphodiesterases. Although it has been proposed that cyclic GMP and cyclic AMP exhibit opposing actions in various systems, this hypothesis has not achieved general acceptance. Instead, considerable data indicate that cyclic GMP can regulate a variety of responses, including vasodilatation, intestinal secretion, and retinal phototransduction, apparently independently of an antagonism of cyclic AMP responses.[125]

Certain types of receptors appear to be linked to the stimulation of guanylyl cyclase.[125] These include: receptors for at least one peptide hormone, atrial natriuretic factor (atriopeptin); receptors involved in fertilization in some species; a heat-stable enterotoxin of *E. coli*; and "receptors" that mediate response of cells to agents such as the organic and inorganic nitrate vasodilators (e.g., nitroprusside and the so-called endothelium-derived relaxant factor, which is thought to be responsible for the ability of endothelium to promote vasodilatation and perhaps bronchodilatation and has been tentatively identified as nitric oxide[126]). Other classes of receptors may indirectly or secondarily promote formation of cyclic GMP as a consequence of increases in cytosolic calcium or generation of fatty acids and other lipid breakdown products by cyclooxygenase or lipoxygenase.

Unlike adenylyl cyclase, a plasma membrane-associated enzyme whose activity is regulated by G proteins, guanylyl cyclase is found both in membranes and in cytosol. Activation of guanylyl cyclase is thought to occur in part by an oxidative mechanism. The precise manner by which various agents regulate the enzyme is not well understood.

Cloning and sequencing of membrane forms of guanylyl cyclase has revealed glycoproteins with a deduced molecular mass based on amino acid content of 130–160 kDa.[127] Upon expression of the cloned receptor, cells respond to atriopeptins (peptides secreted from cardiac atria) by dramatically increasing cyclic GMP. Thus, the membrane-associated guanylyl cyclase is an atriopeptin receptor. Hydropathic analysis suggests a single membrane-spanning domain, which divides the protein into an extracellular amino terminal and intracellular carboxy-terminal domains. Guanylyl cyclase is thus an example of a membrane receptor where binding of a peptide to an extracellular site transmits a signal by a presumed conformational change to a catalytic site on the intracellular face of the protein where it enhances the conversion of GTP to cyclic GMP.

INTRACELLULAR RECEPTORS FOR DRUGS AND HORMONES

Additional classes of drug and hormone receptors are found in intracellular locations. Those include receptors for steroids (glucocorticoids, mineralocorticoids, sex steroids, vitamin D), for thyroid hormone, and for inducers of drug metabolism, such as tetrachlorodibenzodioxan (TCDD) and barbiturates (see Ch. 5). A brief review of the molecular mechanism of steroid hormone action is considered here; the description of other intracellular receptors will be considered in subsequent chapters of this book. The steroid hormone receptor provides a useful prototype for receptors that alter cellular function by virtue of their capacity to regulate gene expression.[128]

Receptors for steroid hormones were one of the first classes of drug receptors whose existence was inferred from the use of labeled analogs.[129] Animals injected with such analogs preferentially concentrated labeled material in target cells specific for particular classes of steroids (e.g., localization of labeled estrogen in responsive tissues such as ovary and uterus). In subsequent studies the binding of radiolabeled derivatives to intact target cells or subcellular fractions prepared from such cells was utilized to identify receptors (typically about 60,000 per cell) that had appropriate affinity ($K_D < 10^{-9}$ M) for physiologic hormones.

A general model has evolved from these types of studies[128,130] (Fig. 2-35). Unoccupied steroid receptors ar found in the cytoplasm for some classes of receptors (e.g., the glucocorticoids) but in the nucleus for certain other classes (e.g., sex steroids, vitamin D). Because of their hydrophobic nature, steroid molecules can readily enter cells by crossing the plasma membrane by diffusion through the lipid bilayer. With the exception of receptors for certain sex steroids, steroid receptors in general appear to be composed of a single hormone-binding polypeptide. Binding of steroid to the receptor produces a "transformation," presumably an allosteric conformational change in the receptor molecule, which cannot occur when steroid and receptor are at 0° to 4°C but which proceeds rapidly at temperatures above 20°C.

Inactive receptors appear to exist as heteromeric complexes with sedimentation values of 8 to 9 S and molecular masses of about 300 kDa. The heteromeric 9S complexes consist of a single molecule of the steroid binding protein in association with other components, one of which is the 90-kDa heat shock protein (hsp90).[131] "Transformed" receptors possess a less negative charge (pI values 5.5 to 7.0), have lower sedimentation values (typically 3 to 4 S) and lower apparent molecular mass (60 to 120 kDa). Thus, transformation appears to involve dissociation of the receptor-hsp90 complex to yield a monomeric receptor with DNA binding activity.

The transformation of the steroid receptor associated with agonist binding is required for the steroid-receptor complex to bind to sites in chromosomal DNA in the nucleus, probably at specific DNA sequences. The binding of the steroid to the receptors enhances the affinity of the steroid-receptor complex for these sequences, and this interaction then leads to an alteration in the level of transcription of steroid-responsive genes (a small subset of the cellular genome). Altered rates of transcription of these genes change the rates of synthesis and in some cases the stability or processing of the steroid-responsive proteins.[132]

A definitive understanding of how the steroid-receptor complex alters gene expression is not yet available, although some information has now emerged.[128,131] For several types of these receptors, discrete genomic regions that are typically found 5′ (upstream) of transcriptional start sites have been identified as regulatory sequences that are able to modulate transcription independently of their orientation. These regulatory sequences have been termed *hormone response elements* (HREs), sometimes denoted by the specific hormone (e.g., glucocorticoid response elements, GREs). They are considered *cis*-acting (i.e., acting on the same genome) regulatory sequences, called *enhancers*, which can confer hormonal regulation upon promoters and which are necessary for efficient tran-

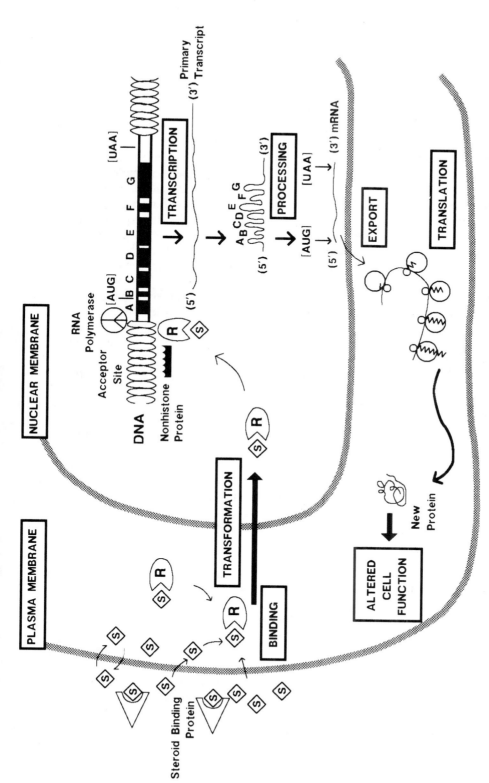

Fig. 2-35. Schematic model for steroid hormone action. Circulating steroid is free or bound to one or more plasma-binding proteins. Free steroid can diffuse across the membrane and bind to cytoplasmic (or, in some cases, to nuclear) receptor (R). Transformation of the steroid-bound receptor facilitates entry into the nucleus and interaction with chromosomes at or near 5' flanking DNA of regulated genes on acceptor sites. Gene activation occurs, leading to the synthesis of primary transcript, which is spliced and processed, and mature mRNA is then transported to the cytoplasm. Translation of the mRNA or ribosomes produces the new protein, which can then alter cell function.

scription of certain genes. The steroid receptor complex is thus viewed as a *trans*-acting factor, which is recognized by the HRE to mediate transcriptional control. The precise roles of other nuclear proteins that may be involved in the interaction of steroid receptor complexes with regulatory sequences in the genome are not yet well defined. Moreover, although their positions within the genome can be precisely mapped by footprinting or deletion analysis, molecular details are scanty with respect to exactly how hormone response elements facilitate alterations in rates of transcription.

The cloning and sequencing of the genes encoding steroid hormone receptors (including those for estrogen, androgen, progesterone, glucocorticoid, mineralocortoid, and vitamin D receptors) have revealed several intriguing features of these proteins (Fig. 2-36) (see Evans[133] and references therein). The C terminal half of the receptor proteins, as well as the v-*erb A* oncogenes with which the receptors are homologous, all contain highly homologous regions rich in cysteine, lysine, and arginine. Interspecies differences in this region of the receptor for particular classes and among different classes appear to be relatively small. Such results suggest that all the steroid receptors may have arisen from a family of genes derived from a common ancestry. This homologous cysteine-rich region is the DNA-binding domain, and it is required for receptor-mediated enhancement of transcription. Other functional domains of the receptors have been demonstrated, including the presence of the steroid-binding domain and nuclear localization signals in the carboxy-terminal protein of the molecules and an immunogenic region located in the amino-terminal half of the protein. The N-terminal region of the receptor, which is also N-terminal to the DNA binding domain, is the region with the greatest variability in length and sequence among the various classes of steroid receptors. The amino acid sequences of hormone-binding domains of glucocorticoid, estrogen, and progesterone receptors show only about 20 to 30 percent identity, but within the steroid-binding domain there lies a short, highly conserved region which is rich in hydrophobic amino acids. This is called the C_2 domain (second conserved domain) in order to distinguish it from the C_1 domain, which determines DNA binding.

The thyroid hormone receptor is also a member of this receptor superfamily in that its structure possesses a DNA-binding domain like that of the steroid hormone receptor and a carboxy-terminal region distantly related to the steroid-binding domain.[133] In addition, other members of this superfamily of receptors have been tentatively identified by molecular cloning techniques, including a receptor for the vitamin A-related metabolite retinoic acid. Further structural and functional mapping of steroid hormone receptors and other members of this superfamily should be forthcoming when expression of the mutagenized and chimeric forms of the receptor are examined.

One intriguing and unexpected observation that has already emerged from application of such mutational analysis to the study of the glucocorticoid receptor is that the loss of the hormone-binding region of the receptor yields a constitutively active molecule in terms of DNA binding and transcriptional enhancement. Thus, the steroid hormone acts to relieve an ongoing inhibition of DNA binding and transcriptional activation produced by the hormone-binding region of the receptor. The steroid-binding domain contains the binding site for hsp90, and it has been proposed that the free energy of steroid binding is transduced into a conformational change in the C_2 domain that results in the dissociation of hsp90 and resulting derepression of the DNA binding function.[134] The steroid-binding domain has been called a "regulatory cassette" because it contains the features required for both repression of receptor function and hormone-mediated derepression and because it can be moved to various positions in the molecule and still render the receptor hormone-responsive.

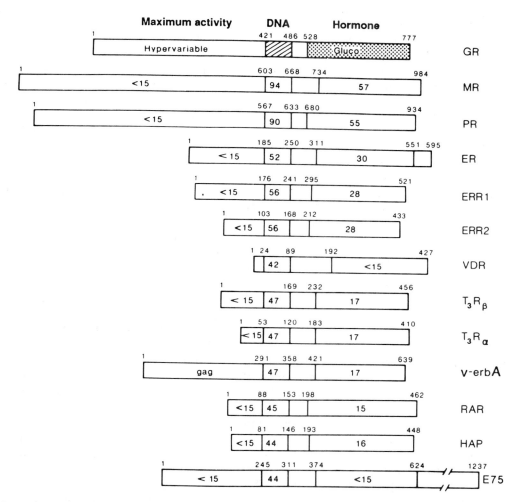

Fig. 2-36. Schematic diagram of structure of steroid and thyroid hormone receptor family members. Amino acid sequences have been aligned on the basis of region of maximum amino acid similarity with the percentage identity shown within the boxes for each region in relation to the human glucocorticoid receptor (GR). Domains shown are the domain of amino-terminal end that is required for "maximum activity," a 66- to 68-amino acid DNA-binding core (DNA) and the binding domain for hormones with DNA sequences of about 50 amino acids (Hormone). Amino acid position is indicated by numbers at the top of each structure for human mineralocorticoid receptor (MR), progesterone receptor (PR), estrogen receptor (ER), estrogen receptor-related 1 or 2 (ERR$_1$, ERR$_2$), vitamin D receptor (VDR), thyroid hormone receptors (T$_3$R$_\alpha$, T$_3$R$_\beta$), and retinoic acid receptors (RAR). The structure of retroviral oncogene product v-*erbA* is also shown. (Adapted from Evans,[133] with permission.)

RECEPTOR DESENSITIZATION, REGULATION, AND TURNOVER

An important concept that has emerged with the development of techniques to assess receptors as discrete molecular entities is the recognition that receptors are not stable entities but instead are subject to the dynamics of cellular metabolism.[135,136] A variety of physiologic states and pharmacologic interventions have been shown to regulate receptor number and affinity. The application of radioligand binding and other methods has provided new insights into the molecular mechanisms involved in regulation of receptor expression.

Studies conducted many decades ago had indicated that functional responses to some classes of agonists are very transient. The loss in response has been most commonly termed *tachyphylaxis* (implying a very rapid loss in response), *refractoriness*, or *desensitization*. The last term is the one most widely used now, especially with isolated systems. The phenomenon of desensitization subsumes a variety of molecular events, which differ for different classes of receptors. In examining these, it is useful to consider both the *kinetics* and the *specificity* of desensitization. Thus, some types of receptors (e.g., nicotinic acetylcholine receptors) desensitize very rapidly, the fast step occurring within 1 second, whereas other types of receptors, such as many of those coupled to G proteins or tyrosine kinase-linked receptors, desensitize over many seconds to minutes or even hours. The differing kinetics suggest that distinct molecular mechanisms are responsible, and this is indeed the case. Moreover, many types of cells demonstrate more than one phase of desensitization, often showing both a rapid and a more slowly developing loss in response to agonist.[137,138] Again, different molecular mechanisms appear to be involved.

With respect to specificity of response, in some systems agonists promote a desensitization that has been termed *homologous* because it only involves the specific class of receptors that the agonist occupies. In other systems a *heterologous* desensitization can be demonstrated in which response is diminished, not only to the agonist with which a target cell has been treated but to other classes of agonists as well. Heterologous desensitization often develops more slowly than does homologous desensitization. Since many different receptors can utilize a common pathway for cellular activation—for example, a G_s-mediated stimulation of adenylyl cyclase, leading to increased cellular levels of cyclic AMP and thus to stimulation of cyclic AMP-dependent protein kinase activity—heterologous desensitization typically results from a change in one or more components that are common to multiple types of agonists. Thus, alterations in the G_s or G_i component of adenylyl cyclase and enhanced cyclic AMP phosphodiesterase activity may be associated with heterologous desensitization of receptors that act by enhancing cellular cyclic AMP concentrations.

The precise mechanisms responsible for such alterations are poorly understood. Covalent modification, in particular, phosphorylation of components involved in producing agonist responses (receptors, G proteins, etc.) have been proposed for certain cell types,[139] while in other settings the actual amounts of the components are changed by agonist treatment. For example, cyclic AMP phosphodiesterase can be induced in some cell types in response to elevations in cellular cyclic AMP. This induction of phosphodiesterase serves to increase the rate of degradation of cellular cyclic AMP, thereby yielding a negative feedback mechanism for maintaining homeostasis of cyclic AMP concentrations. Different target cells appear to utilize more than one molecular mechanism for heterologous desensitization. As discussed in more detail in Chapter 10, tolerance to opiates (and perhaps to other types of drugs) may involve changes in components distal to receptors such that chronic stimulation by agonists that inhibit adenylyl cyclase activity can elicit compensatory, slowly developing increases in adenylyl cyclase activity.

Homologous desensitization is a more specific form of desensitization, whose specificity for a given class of agonists implies changes in receptors or components selectively linked to a particular class of receptor. The first well studied example of homologous desensitization was that of agonist-mediated desensitization of nicotinic acetylcholine receptors.[12] Thus, the ion channel integral to these receptors opens in response to a cholinergic agonist. As discussed earlier, this opening is rapidly followed by a closure of the ion channel within a time frame of 0.1 to 10 seconds. No input of cellular energy or components, other than agonist occupation, is required for the receptor to convert to the desensitized state; the driving force is the higher agonist affinity of this state. Withdrawal of the agonist leads to a spontaneous reversal from the desensitized state.

For receptors linked to G proteins, homologous desensitization appears to involve a quite different series of events.[137-139] Most current knowledge has derived from studies of a limited number of receptor systems linked to the G_s protein. Whether these events will be applicable to all, or even most, G-linked receptors is unknown. The kinetics of desensitization are much slower for these types of receptors than for nicotinic acetylcholine receptors. At least two discrete kinetic phases of loss of responsiveness can be discerned: a phase that transpires over many seconds to several minutes, in which receptors appear to become "uncoupled" from the G_s protein; and a later phase that requires many minutes to several hours and involves a decrease in receptor number (receptor down regulation). The early, uncoupling phase has been associated with a decrease in receptor affinity for agonist, with a decreased ability of receptor to stimulate adenylyl cyclase, and in some cell types with a physical sequestration of receptors from G_s. Sequestered receptors are relatively inaccessible to hydrophilic agonists and antagonists and in some cases can be identified in cellular compartments that appear to be distinct from the plasma membrane. An event that precedes this sequestration appears to involve a cyclic AMP–independent phosphorylation of receptors, perhaps via a distinct type of receptor kinase that phosphorylates agonist-occupied receptors after translocation of the kinase from the cytosol to the cytoplasmic surface of the plasma membrane.[139]

The later down regulation phase of G_s-linked receptor desensitization and the type of desensitization commonly observed in tyrosine kinase-linked receptors are likely to involve a series of events that may depend upon covalent modification (perhaps phosphorylation) and ultimately upon an endocytosis of receptors from the plasma membrane to locations inside cells. As such, this movement of receptors probably represents one phase of the receptor "life cycle" that has been described for a wide variety of membrane receptors[135,136,140,141] (Fig. 2-37). Prolonged exposure to agonist may serve to alter one or more portions of the life cycle.

Receptor Turnover

The life cycle of receptor turnover is characterized by the following series of events upon transcription of the receptor gene. Messenger RNA coding for receptors is translated, and the nascent peptide adopts a tertiary structure and may assemble with other subunits in the endoplasmic reticulum. In addition, the initial phase of receptor glycosylation occurs co-translationally. Some processing events, such as removal of leader sequences or C-terminal processing, occur directly following translation. Subsequent processing of receptors, in particular modification of carbohydrate moieties, occurs as the receptors pass

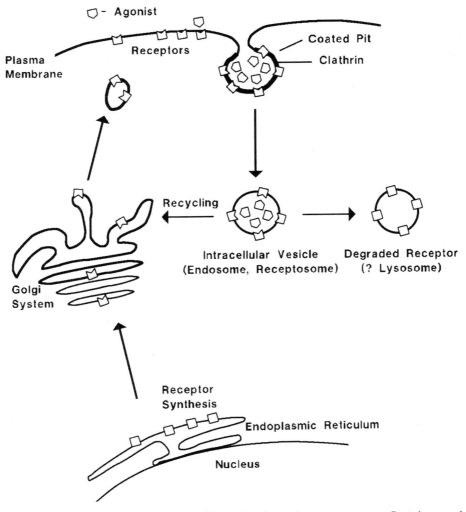

Fig. 2-37. A diagrammatic scheme for the life cycle of membrane receptors. Certain morphologic components of the scheme are shown but are not drawn to scale. See text for explanation.

through the Golgi system. Ultimately, Golgi vesicles containing receptors fuse with the plasma membrane, thereby inserting the receptor into the mobile lipid domain of the cell surface. Depending on their type, the receptors may be distributed randomly and diffusely in the surface membranes, they may cluster in receptor-rich microaggregates (perhaps closely allied with certain cytoskeletal structures), or they may congregate in specialized regions of the membrane known as *coated pits*. The coated pit regions, of which there are typically 500 to 1,000 per cell (occupying about 3 percent of the cell surface), are so named because of their fuzzy, indented appearance in electron microscopic studies; the fuzzy coat consists of a unique protein, clathrin.

Treatment of target cells with agonist promotes a movement of receptors in the plane of the membrane, an event which for many (or perhaps most) types of receptors leads to a concentration of the receptors in coated pit regions. These coated pit regions appear to be the principal sites from which agonist-occupied receptors are internalized into cells, a process known as *receptor-mediated endocytosis* (as distinguished from less selective mechanisms such as pinocytosis and phagocytosis). Internalized coated pit regions appear intracellularly as coated and later as uncoated vesicles, which are about 0.5 μm in diameter and are known as endosomes or receptosomes. These intracellular vesicles appear to be subject to one or more fates, which include fusion with other similar vesicles; possibly recycling of some of the vesicle contents (including receptors) to the plasma membrane after fusion with the Golgi system (in particular, elements of what has been termed trans-Golgi or transreticular Golgi[132]), in which the agonist and receptors may be sorted; and transfer (perhaps via the trans-Golgi) to intracellular sites for storage or degradation. In some cases ligands and receptors appear to become dissociated in intracellular endosomes by a process that may be secondary to a decrease in vesicular pH (about 5.5), thereby facilitating potentially different fates for the agonist and the receptor. Intracellular degradation of receptors is thought to occur predominantly in lysosomes, which have a low pH (about 4.5) and possess a variety of acid hydrolases and proteases.

Thus, agonist-mediated down regulation of receptors is hypothesized to result from a delivery of surface receptors via coated pits and intracellular vesicles to lysosomes. It should be noted that this hypothesis derives from data obtained in studies conducted primarily for "nutrient" and "transport" receptors (such as those for low-density lipoproteins, transferrin, and asialoglycoproteins) and to some extent for receptors for polypeptide hormone and growth factors (e.g., insulin, epidermal growth factor).[135,136,140] Relatively limited information is currently available on whether most types of pharmacologic (such as G-protein-linked) receptors undergo a similar fate when a target cell is exposed to agonist.

Current information on the turnover of pharmacologic receptors has been derived by a variety of techniques.[141] These include: (1) use of protein synthesis inhibitors to block receptor formation and to assess receptor degradation; (2) growth of target cells in media containing heavy isotope-labeled (^{15}N, ^{13}C, ^{2}H) amino acids instead of the natural abundance (^{14}N, ^{12}C, ^{1}H) amino acids, followed by density gradient separation of "light" and "heavy" receptors after target cell membranes are solubilized; and (3) blockade of receptors with irreversible antagonist, followed by assessment of the kinetics of reappearance of receptor binding to control levels. In addition, various perturbants have been added as potential probes of different cellular membranes that may be involved in receptor formation or turnover. All these methods have certain limitations, some practical and some theoretical, for the study of receptor metabolism. Most importantly, all the methods require the ability to detect binding to receptors, a function that may not necessarily be conserved during the various phases, especially during the intracellular events in the receptor life cycle. Further insights into receptor regulation will almost certainly require use of appropriate probes to tag receptors in order to study their disposition in intact cells. Advances in fluorescent detection and electron microscopy should help to further resolve receptor location and distribution in situ. Antireceptor antibodies may prove particularly valuable for these types of studies.

Agonist-mediated regulation of receptor number and affinity is but one of a number of treatments that can regulate expression of target cell receptors. Table 2-12 lists other physiologic states and pharmacologic interventions that can influence receptor expression in a homologous manner. *Homologous* regulation refers to regulation by agonists and antagonists that can occupy a particular class of receptor, in analogy with homologous desensitization described above. In addition, *heterologous* regulation by treatments other

Table 2-12. Pharmacologic Manipulations That Change Expression of Receptors in a Homologous Manner

Change	Observed
Agonist treatment	Desensitization/down regulation
Inhibition of degradation or uptake of cognate neurotransmitter or hormone	Desensitization/down regulation
Antagonist treatment	Supersensitivity/up regulation
Inhibition of synthesis/release of cognate neurotransmitter or hormone	Supersensitivity/up regulation

than with the cognate agonist or antagonist can produce a wide variety of changes in receptor expression, including up and down regulation, sensitization (supersensitivity), and desensitization. Steady-state changes in receptor number imply that one or more phases of the receptor life cycle (Fig. 2-37) have been altered, although which of these phases is altered in most settings of homologous and heterologous regulation of receptors has not been determined. This major gap in understanding seems likely to be filled as suitable reagents and experimental systems become available.

DRUG ACTION ON CELLS NOT MEDIATED THROUGH RECEPTORS

For pharmacologic agents to be effective clinically, they must be able to alter the function of a target site, cell, tissue or invading organism without modifying other cells or tissues. Selectivity in drug action can arise from several mechanisms of a *pharmacokinetic* or *pharmacodynamic* nature. As considered in Chapter 3, the pharmacokinetic properties may allow the drug to be concentrated within or excluded from particular tissues. We have already considered in this chapter and in Chapter 1 the pharmacodynamic features that contribute to the selectivity of drugs acting on receptors. Selectivity arises either from the ligand recognition properties or from cell- or tissue-specific transduction mechanisms. However, several important families of drugs do not act on receptors; hence their selectivity must arise from other factors.

Drug Action Mediated through Enzymes

Many therapeutically useful drugs have been shown to be inhibitors of particular enzymes. As such, these agents have shown a wide variation in their modes of inhibition, which include competitive blockade at a substrate or cofactor binding site, noncompetitive inhibition of activity, and irreversible inhibition in which the number of active enzyme molecules is actually diminished.

A common mode of action of antimicrobial agents and antineoplastic agents is inhibition of enzymes critical to function of the cell. Such agents are considered to be *antimetabolites*, and to be effective they must exert a degree of *selective toxicity* toward the invading organism in relation to the host.[142] This may be achieved either by a unique metabolic pathway existing in one species or by species differences in enzyme selectivity for a common metabolic pathway.

Selective Toxicity Achieved through Inhibition of a Unique Metabolic Pathway

Sulfonamides are effective antibacterials because the invading organism acquires folates by synthesis from pteridine, *p*-aminobenzoic acid, and glutamic acid (Fig. 2-38), whereas

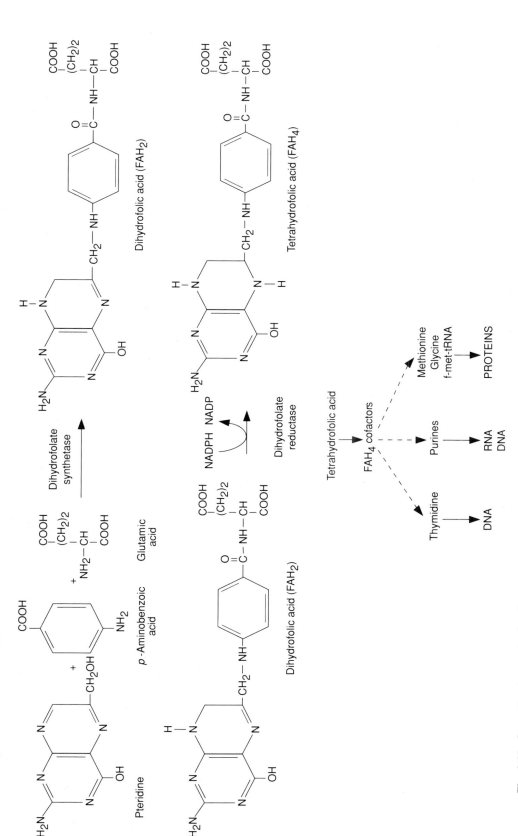

Fig. 2-38. Steps for the synthesis of tetrahydrofolic acid. The tetrahydrofolate cofactors are involved in one-carbon transfers required for the synthesis of protein and nucleic acid precursors.

folates are actively transported into mammalian host cell and synthesis is not required. Sulfonamides inhibit dihydrofolate synthesis by inhibiting the incorporation of *p*-amino-benzoic acid. Selective action on the pathogenic organism versus the host arises from the fact that the dihydrofolate synthesis pathway is obligatory only for the invading organism.

The sulfonamides are structural analogs of *p*-aminobenzoic acid and inhibit the condensation of *p*-aminobenzoic acid with the glutamylpteridine. Figure 2-39 compares the structure of *p*-aminobenzoic acid with the sulfonamide. It is not surprising, on the basis of structure, that the sulfonamides can combine with folate synthetase condensing enzyme, thereby competitively inhibiting the normal conjugation of *p*-aminobenzoic acid into folic acid.[143,144]

In the series of antibacterial sulfonamides biologic potency is modified by substituents which do not themselves seem to partake in binding to the enzyme but rather influence the ionic character of another group on the molecule. The simplest member of the sulfonamide series is sulfanilamide, in which both hydrogen atoms on the amide nitrogen are unsubstituted. The other sulfonamides carry substituents; a few out of the hundreds that have been synthesized and tested are shown in Table 2-13. Just as a free *p*-amino group is essential for substrate activity in *p*-aminobenzoate (PAB), so in a sulfonamide drug a free *p*-amino group is essential for antibacterial action. In contrast, there are almost no limitations to the possible substituents on the sulfonamido nitrogen compatible with antibacterial efficacy.

What then is the role of substituents? A plausible explanation is suggested by the relationship between the $-SO_2-$ group in the sulfonamides and the $-CO_2-$ group of PAB. The latter is completely ionized at neutral pH, and there is independent evidence that a negative charge here promotes combination with the enzyme. Thus it may be inferred that sulfonamides should become more potent with increasing electron density in the $-SO_2-$ region, and this property should be influenced by electron-withdrawing substituents on the amide nitrogen. Any tendency to draw electrons away from the N–H bond will be reflected in an increased ease of proton dissociation, which can be measured by the pK_a' value of each compound. That various R substituents are capable of altering pK_a' profoundly is seen in Table 2-13. Sulfanilamide itself is a very weak acid (i.e., its

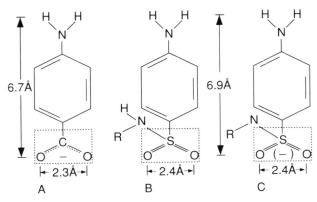

Fig. 2-39. *p*-Aminobenzoate (PAB) and sulfonamide structures. **(A)** PAB ionized form. **(B)** Sulfonamide, nonionized form. **(C)** Sulfonamide, ionized form. Although the negative charge that can result from loss of a proton is shown associated with the sulfonamide N atom, delocalization of the charge occurs. (From Bell and Robin,[145] with permission.)

Table 2-13. Some Sulfonamides with Different Acid Strengths

Compound	−R	pK'_a
Sulfanilamide	−H	10.43
Sulfapyridine	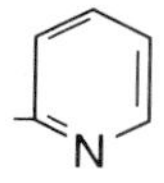 (pyridine ring attached at N)	8.43
Sulfathiazole	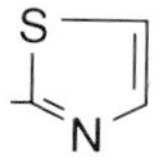 (thiazole ring)	7.12
Sulfadiazine	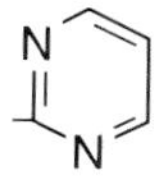 (pyrimidine ring)	6.48
Sulfacetamide	$-\overset{\overset{\text{O}}{\|\|}}{\text{C}}-CH_3$	5.38

(Data from Bell and Robin.[145])

proton is tightly bound); but electrophilic substituents in the other compounds increase the acid strength to varying degrees.

To explore the relationship between pK$'_a$ and antibacterial potency, the minimum molar concentration of each sulfonamide required to inhibit growth of *E. coli* cultures at pH 7.0 was estimated, and the pK$'_a$ was also determined for each compound. The observations are presented in Figure 2-40. The graph shows reciprocals of bacteriostatic concentrations as indices of potency (since lower effective concentration means greater potency), and in order to span several orders of magnitude in potency a logarithmic scale is used. Beginning at the extreme right with the weakest acids and moving toward the left, antibacterial potency is seen to increase as acid strength increases. Since the tests were performed at pH 7, this portion of the curve shows that an increasing degree of ionization favors antibacterial activity. Thus, under the experimental conditions a compound with a pK$'_a$ of 11 would be practically nonionized, whereas one with a pK$'_a$ of 6 would be 91 percent ionized.

The findings thus far are consistent with the conclusion that the anionic form of a sulfonamide is the active form. One would predict, however, that all compounds with pK$'_a$ less than 6 should be maximally active, since they would be nearly completely ionized at pH 7. A special explanation is therefore required to account for the decreasing potency of the more acidic sulfonamides. One such explanation focuses more closely upon the charge distribution in the sulfone group itself. As the substituent R is made more electrophilic so that the amide proton dissociates (as described above), the sulfone group shares in the electronegative character of the resulting anionic amide. Beyond a certain point, however, when complete ionization has already been attained, a still more strongly electrophilic substituent will begin to draw electrons away from the sulfone group. The altered charge distribution, with diminished electron density in the $-SO_2-$ region, will cause a diminution in antibacterial potency.

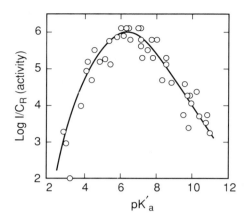

Fig. 2-40. Relation of antibacterial potency to acid strength in the sulfonamide series. The logarithm of the reciprocal of the bacteriostatic concentrations is the measure of potency. Each point represents a different sulfonamide. One discrepant point has been eliminated for justifiable reasons. All the testing was done at pH 7. (From Bell and Robin,[145] with perimission.)

Selective Toxicity through Species Differences in Enzyme Selectivity

The pathogenic microbe and host may use the same enzymatic pathway yet the specificity of inhibitors for the enzyme in the two species can be widely divergent. The antimalarial activity of pyrimethamine and the antimalarial and antibacterial activities of trimethoprim are due to these agents being effective inhibitors of dihydrofolate reductase in the respective microbes but not in the host. Dihydrofolate reductase catalyzes the reduction of dihydrofolate to tetrahydrofolate (Fig. 2-38). Tetrahydrofolate and other reduced analogs of folic acid are involved as cofactors in one-carbon transfer reactions, which are essential for the biosynthesis of purines and thymidylate and the interconversion of glycine and serine. Table 2-14 presents the K_I values measured for the inhibitors on dihydrofolate reductase.[146,147] Pyrimethamine shows selective inhibition towards the dihydrofolate reductase from the *Plasmodium* sp., while trimethoprim is effective in both plasmodium and the bacterium. In contrast, methotrexate, a closer structural analog to the substrate and product (see Fig. 2-41), inhibits all forms of the enzyme, with dissociation constants in the neighborhood of 10^{-11} to 10^{-12} M.

Since the crystal structures of several dihydrofolate reductases have been analyzed at high resolution and altered forms of the enzyme prepared by site-specific mutagenesis have been expressed,[148-150] it becomes possible to examine drug specificity in this system

Table 2-14. Inhibition of Purified Dihydrofolate Reductases by Pyrimethamine and Trimethroprim

	Concentration Required for 50% Inhibition (nM)		
Inhibitor	*Mammalian (Human Liver)*	*Bacteria (E. coli)*	*Protozoa (P. berghei)*
Pyrimethamine	1,800	2,500	0.5
Trimethoprim	300,000	5	70

(Data from Burchall and Hitchings[146] and Ferone et al.[147])

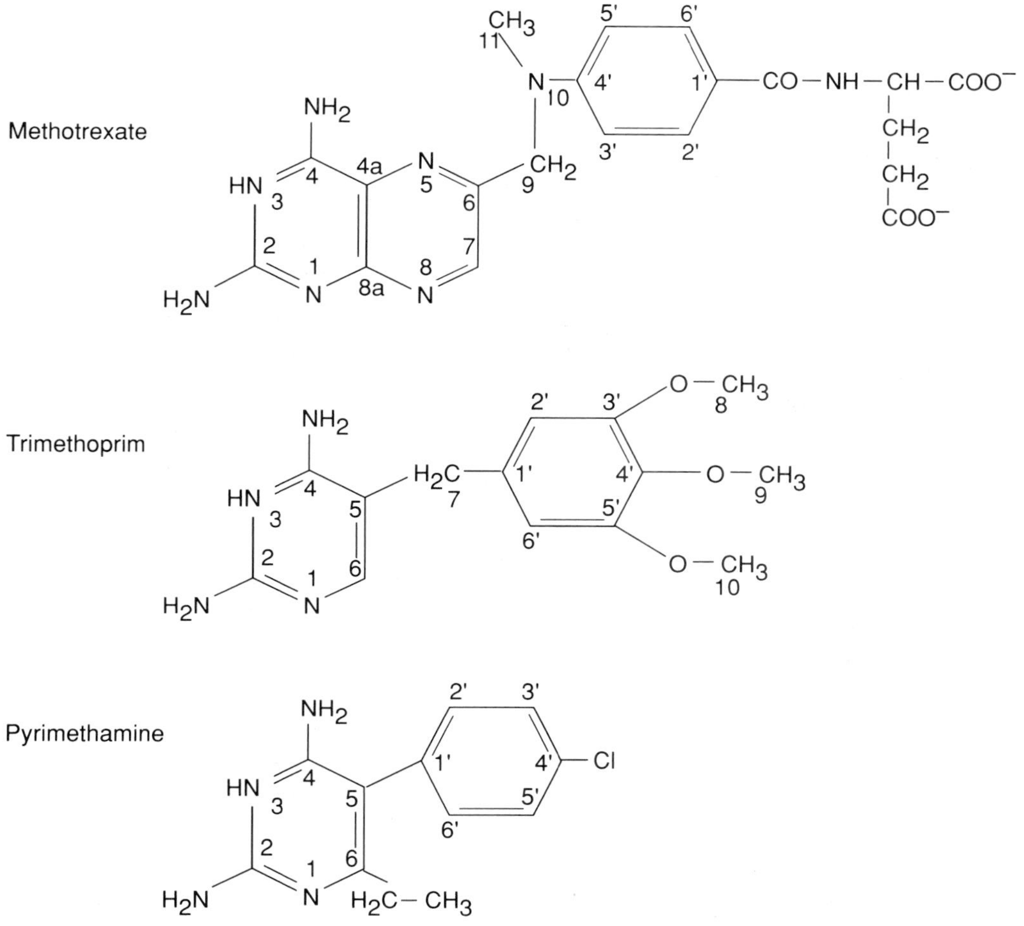

Fig. 2-41. Structures of pyrimethamine, trimethoprim, and methotrexate.

in terms of substitution of individual amino acid residues in the protein. As represented in the stereopair view in Fig. 2-42, trimethoprim binds at the active site of *E. coli* dihydrofolate reductase with its pyrimidine ring within a deep cleft, where it is stabilized by van der Waals forces, hydrogen bonding, and ionic (coulombic) interactions with the protein. The trimethoxybenzyl group extends toward the mouth of the binding cavity, making van der Waals contact with two α-helices in the protein.

A comparison of the crystal structures of methotrexate, trimethoprim, and other inhibitor complexes with dihydrofolate reductase from *E. coli* (invading microbe) and chicken (host) shows that small differences in the dimensions of the active-site cleft give rise to the marked differences in inhibitor specificity. Several features of the active center clefts of folate reductase from the various microbe and host species can be resolved at atomic level. First, an intricate system of hydrogen bonding gives rise to the positioning of the 2,4-diaminopyrimidine ring and the enhanced affinity of the diamino-substituted congener (i.e., methotrexate) when compared with folate itself. The positions of the py-

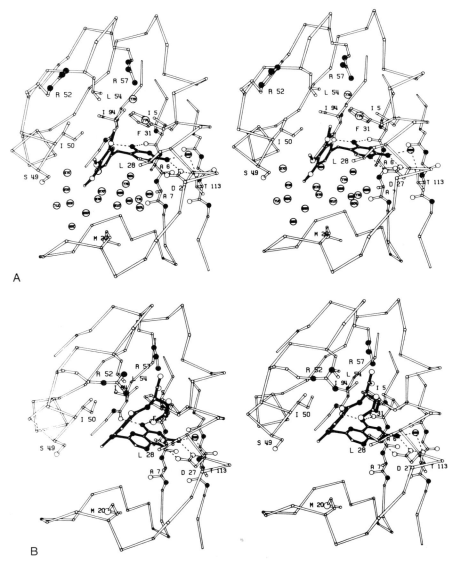

Fig. 2-42. **(A)** Stereopair depiction of the binding of trimethoprim to *E. coli* dihydrofolate reductase. Trimethoprim is indicated by solid bonds and protein by open bonds. Carbon atoms are represented by small open circles, oxygen by larger open circles, and nitrogen by blackened circles. Large numbered circles represent fixed solvent (water). Van der Waals forces from I-5, A-6, A-7, L-28, F-31, and I-94 form the pocket for the pyrimidine ring, while L-28, F-31, S-49, I-50, and L-54 contribute van der Waals interactions for the trimethoxybenzyl ring. Hydrogen bond formation is critical for the stabilization of the pyrimidine ring. These are formed between (1) the carboxylate of D-27 and the N_1 and 2 amino group; (2) the carbonyl of I-5 and the 4-amino group; (3) the carbonyl of I-94 and the 4-amino group; and (4) perhaps T-113 through H_2O to the 2-amino group of the pyrimidine ring. The area below the binding site contains a substantial number of H_2O molecules. Many of these are displaced by the nicotinamide ring when the inhibitor-NADPH-enzyme ternary complex is formed, but cofactor binding does not change the position of the inhibitor. The cofactor is known to enhance cooperatively the binding of methotrexate. (*Figure Continues*).

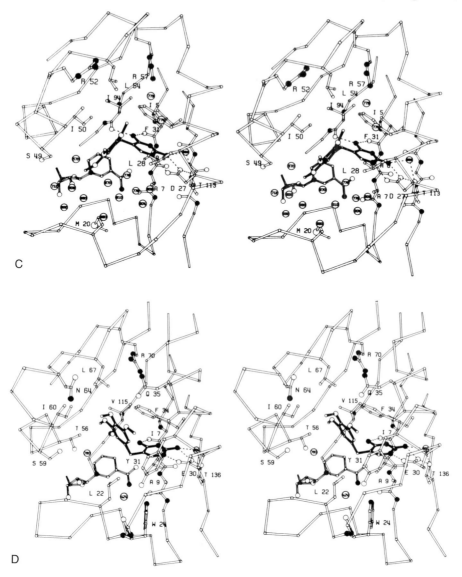

Fig. 2-42 (*Continued*). The hydrogen-bonded salt bridge between D-27 and the N_1 nitrogen increases the pk_a of trimethoprim from 7.5 to 10, indicating that N_1 is protonated and D-27 is deprotonated in the complex. Definition of the single-letter amino acid codes is found in Fig. 2-2. See structures of the individual ligands for the assignments of substituent groups. (**B**) Binding of methotrexate to the *E. coli* enzyme. (**C**) Binding of trimethoprim and NADPH in a ternary complex with *E. coli* dihydrofolate reductase. The relevant portion of the NADPH molecule is shown by the striped bonds. (**D**) Binding of trimethoprim and NADPH to chicken dihydrofolate reductase. Note in comparison with Figs. A and C that the pyrimidine ring is inserted more deeply into the cleft and that the bond angles for the ring system are different. This affects: (1) hydrogen bonding between V-115 and the 4-amino substituent of the pyrimidine ring; (2) different interactions with the trimethoxybenzyl group; and (3) a different torsion angle for the ring system and a specific conformational change for tyrosine (Y-31). (From Matthews et al.,[150] with permission.)

rimidine ring in methotrexate and trimethoprim are virtually the same in the *E. coli* enzyme (Fig. 2-42A andB). Second, the different dimensions of the cleft appear to force distinct orientations for the ring system of trimethoprim in both the chicken and the bacterial enzyme. In the chicken enzyme the torsion angles of the C5–C7 and C7–C1 bonds are −85 and 102 degrees, respectively, while in the *E. coli* enzyme these angles are 177 and 76 degrees, respectively (Fig. 2-42C). The pyrimidine ring is forced deeper into the cleft of the chicken enzyme, and the different torsion angles forces distinct positions for tyrosine (Y) 31. Third, the opposite sides of the cleft appear larger in the chicken enzyme, and this may give rise to the loss of a hydrogen bond between the 4-amino group in the pyrimidine ring of trimethoprim and the carbonyl group of valine (V) 115 in the enzyme. Finally, mutagenesis of aspartate (D) 27 with the loss of activity shows the critical role played by this appropriately positioned diacidic amino acid in catalysis and in methotrexate binding.

Incorporation of Drug into a Macromolecule

A "counterfeit incorporation" mechanism, wherein a drug replaces a normal metabolite in the synthesis of an important cellular constituent, certainly requires the activity of enzymes. The effect of the drug, however, is not attributable directly to interaction with an enzyme. Rather, the drug participates as a substrate; the reaction product rather than the drug produces the characteristic biologic response.

A case of counterfeit incorporation that has been studied intensively is that of the thymine analogs 5-bromouracil (BU), and 5-iodouracil (IU).

Thymine   5-Bromouracil

The van der Waals radii of Br, I, and –CH$_3$ are very nearly the same (Table 2-15), so that BU and IU resemble thymine quite closely. They enter all the preliminary reactions that ordinarily lead to the synthesis of thymidine triphosphate; bromodeoxyuridine triphosphate then enters the DNA polymerase reaction, pairing opposite adenine. Depending upon the ratio of BU to thymine in the cellular environment, DNA can be synthesized in which up to 40 percent of the thymine is replaced by BU, without significant short-term adverse effect. Under these conditions, cell populations grow and divide normally; it is obvious, therefore, that practically all the incorporated BU molecules function as though they were thymine, both at replication and at transcription. Because of the increased density of BU (compared with thymine), BU-substituted DNA has proved useful in experiments requiring density labeling of one DNA strand. Despite its generally normal function, BU-containing DNA shows an increased mutation rate, presumably because of a heightened probability that BU will pair anomalously with guanine instead of with adenine. Other abnormalities resulting from the presence of BU and other base analogs in DNA are increased sensitivity to x-rays, increased frequency of chromosome breakage, and mitotic abnormalities in mammalian cells. These effects are discussed at greater length in Chapter 11.

Table 2-15. Atomic Radii (van der Waals) of Halogens and Related Groups

Atom or Group	Radius (Å)
H	1.20
F	1.35
Cl	1.80
Br	1.95
CH₃	2.00
I	2.15

5-Fluorouracil (FU) presents an interesting contrast.[151,152] This compound is not incorporated into DNA at all but acts readily as a counterfeit of uracil, consistent with the small van der Waals radius of the fluorine atom.

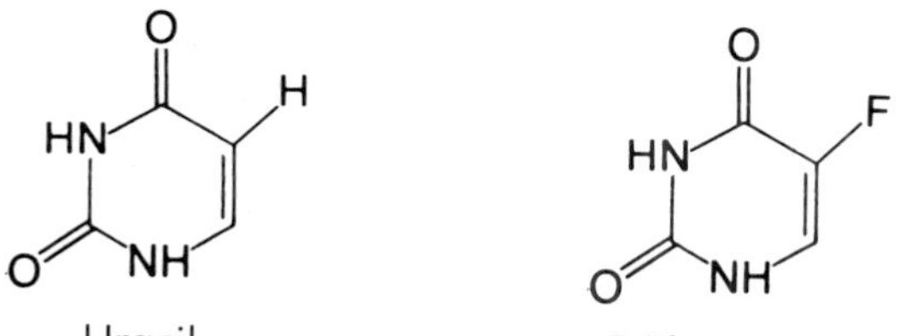

Uracil   5-Fluorouracil

There are two primary effects of FU. It is handled metabolically like uracil, forming a riboside and riboside phosphates. The monophosphate strongly inhibits the enzyme thymidine synthetase (which normally converts deoxyuridine monophosphate to thymidine monophosphate), thereby blocking the de novo synthesis of thymine. At the same time, FU is converted to the nucleoside triphosphate and then incorporated into messenger RNA in place of uracil. "Miscoding" may result through misreading of codons containing FU during the assembly of polypeptide chains, so that incorrect amino acids are inserted. Phenotypically altered proteins are thus formed, which may be nonfunctional, partly functional, or even fully functional, depending upon the particular protein and the nature and position of each amino acid substitution.

Inhibitors of Enzyme Activity in Specialized Cells

Several agents that influence the function of the central autonomic and motor nervous systems affect the synthesis or degradation of neurotransmitters. These drugs alter concentrations of neurotransmitter and thus influence the metabolism of a critical mediator in specialized cells. Hence, selectivity of drug action is manifest because such enzyme inhibitors work in specialized locations and thereby dramatically affect neurotransmission. Examples include (1) α-methyl-*p*-tyrosine, an inhibitor of tyrosine hydroxylase, the enzyme catalyzing the rate-limiting step in catecholamine biosynthesis; and (2) monoamine oxidase inhibitors, which block the degradation of various monoamines. Figure 2-43 shows the pathway for synthesis and degradation of the catecholamines. Substrate specificity and other features of the reaction steps are considered in Chapter 5. From this scheme α-methyl-*p*-tyrosine can be expected to lower the concentration of catecholamines in the

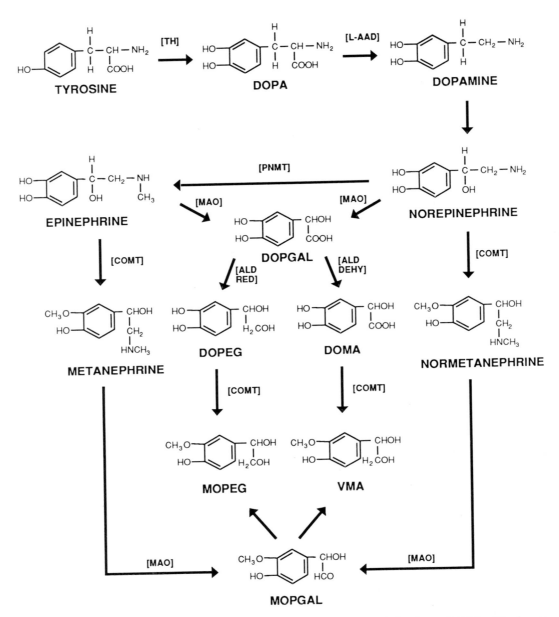

Fig. 2-43. Pathways of biosynthesis and degradation of the catecholamines. DOPA, dihydroxy-phenylalanine; DOPGAL, 3,4-dihydroxyphenylglycolaldehyde; DOPEG, 3,4-dihydroxyphenyl-ethyleneglycol; DOMA, 3,4-dihydroxymandelic acid; MOPEG, 3-methoxy-4-hydroxyphenylethy-lene glycol; VMA, 3-methoxy-4-hydroxymandelic acid; MOPGAL, 3-methoxy-4-hydroxyphenyl-glycolaldehyde; ALD RED, aldehyde reductase; ALD DEHYD, aldehyde dehydrogenase; COMT, catecholamine-*O*-methyltransferase; MAO, monoamine oxidase; TH, tryosine hydroxy-lase; L-AAD, l-amino acid decarboxylase; PNMT phenylethylamine N-methyltransferase.

adrenergic nerve ending by inhibiting the initial step in biosynthesis. Since oxidation of the primary amine is one of the mechanisms of degradation of catecholamines and the mechanism of degradation of serotonin, monoamine oxidase inhibitors will increase tissue concentrations of catecholamines and serotonin (5-hydroxytryptamine). An inhibitor of aromatic amino acid decarboxylase might also be expected to decrease catecholamine biosynthesis. However, these inhibitors are far less selective in their actions, in part because several decarboxylases are inhibited and this step is not rate-limiting in catecholamine biosynthesis. The influence of the inhibition of each mediator will depend on the extent of inhibition required before the individual step becomes rate-limiting.

A more general consideration of drug action in excitable cells is the inhibition of Na^+,K^+-sensitive ATPase by the digitalis family of cardiac glycosides. By strict definition this enzyme would not be considered a receptor, since its function in situ is to maintain ion gradients and cellular water balance rather than to recognize and transduce signals of known mediators. These considerations could change if endogenous compounds with intrinsic cardiac glycoside activity and regulatory function were isolated and characterized. Na^+,K^+-sensitive ATPases exist in virtually all cells, but the consequences of their inhibition at lower concentrations of the digitalis glycosides are most prominent in cardiac tissue. Digitalis glycosides bind specifically to an extracellular site on the Na^+,K^+ ATPase. Inhibition of activity results in an impairment of the active transport process for exit of intracellular Na^+ and entry of extracellular K^+. Intracellular Na^+ thereby rises, while intracellular K^+ may decrease slightly. In cardiac muscle intracellular Ca^{2+} is influenced by Na^+ concentrations in that an Na^+/Ca^{2+} transport system is driven by the concentrations of these ions. When intracellular Na^+ is increased, intracellular Ca^{2+}/extracellular Na^+ exchange is diminished, and intracellular Ca^{2+} will rise. It is likely that under these circumstances more Ca^{2+} is accumulated in the sarcoplasmic reticulum and is therefore available for release with each action potential. Thus, an incremental increase in activation of the cardiac contractile apparatus is achieved by inhibiting an enzyme that regulates ion homeostasis. This action may be augmented by the influence of intracellular Ca^{2+} altering the slow inward current of Ca^{2+}. Since the slow inward current is carried by Ca^{2+}, greater quantities of this ion may be carried during the plateau of the action potential.[153,154]

Stoichiometric and Irreversible Inhibition

Several agents are known to inhibit enzymes irreversibly or pseudoirreversibly and the precise mechanism of inhibition gives rise to subtle differences in the inhibition profiles and the duration of inhibition. For example, methotrexate possesses an extremely high affinity ($K_D = 10^{-10}$ to 10^{-12} M) for dihydrofolate reductase and thymidylate synthetase. Because these dissociation constants are actually far lower than the concentration of enzyme in tissue, inhibition is largely *stoichiometric* with the enzyme sites. Substantial inhibition is achieved with a total body load of drug equal to the number of enzyme sites. Accordingly, amplification of the number of enzyme molecules as a mechanism for acquiring drug resistance can dramatically increase the requirements for the drug. The implications of such changes are considered in Chapter 9. Despite the high affinities of these inhibitors, the enzyme-inhibitor linkage is not covalent but rather only slowly reversible.

Many inhibitors of acetylcholinesterase react covalently with the enzyme to form an acyl enzyme that deacylates more slowly than the acetyl enzyme formed with the natural substrate acetylcholine[155,156] (Fig. 2-44). The acetyl enzyme forms rapidly by attack of

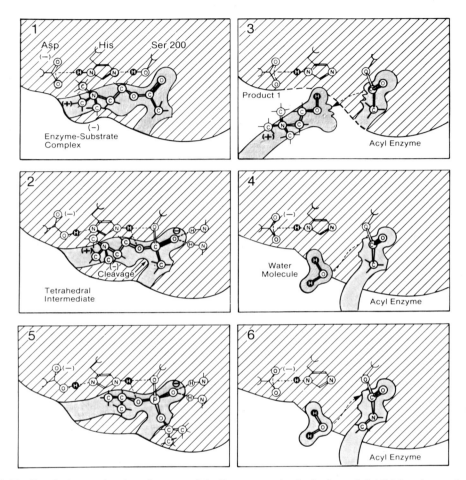

Fig. 2-44. Catalytic mechanism for acetylcholinesterase hydrolysis and inhibition by carbamoyl esters and alkylphosphorates. *Panels 1, 2, 3, and 4* show the progressive steps in acetylcholine ester hydrolysis. *Panels 5 and 6* depict the conjugates formed with hemisubstrate inhibitors. Substrate encounter with the active center (*Panel 1*) is, in part, governed by hydrophobic and coulombic interactions between the quaternary group and anionic subsite within the active center. Substrate ester hydrolysis proceeds through formation of a tetrahedral transition state, in which the active site serine is rendered nucleophilic by a charge-relay system involving a histidine and presumably a negatively charged proton sink. Attack by the nucleophilic serine is facilitated by stabilization of the carbonyl group through hydrogen bonding (*Panel 2*). The acetyl enzyme is formed with the liberation of choline (*Panel 3*). In the case of acetyl enzyme hydrolysis ensues rapidly, ($t_{1/2} = 60$ μsec), forming the free enzyme (*Panel 4*). *Panels 5 and 6* depict the modifications of active center of the enzyme that occur upon reaction with a carbamoylating agent such as physostigmine or a phosphorylating agent such as diisopropyl phosphorofluoridate.

the active site serine on the substrate. Transfer of the acyl group to the enzyme occurs through a tetrahedral intermediate. The acetyl enzyme is rapidly hydrolyzed, with a half-time of 10 μsec. These rapid acylation and deacylation steps give rise to a turnover rate of 10^5 substrate molecules per enzyme molecule per second. Cholinesterase inhibitors such as physostigmine and neostigmine form methylaminocarbamoyl and dimethylaminocarbamoyl enzymes which have half-times for deacylation of several minutes. Thus, by providing the enzyme with an *alternative substrate*, catalysis of acetylcholine is precluded during the catalytic cycle for the carbamoylating agent. The kinetic constants for the respective acylation steps for the acetoxy and carbamoxy ester substrates do not greatly differ; hence the longer residence time of the carbamoyl enzyme conjugate is the important factor in favoring inhibition.

The alkyl phosphates, such as diisopropyl phosphorofluoridate or echothiophate, have an alkylphosphoryl group as the acyl moiety. Alkylphosphoryl and alkylphosphonyl compounds with good leaving groups such as fluorine or thiocholine react rapidly with the enzyme (Fig. 2-44). These compounds have tetrahedral geometry around the phosphorus atom and hence resemble the transition state in hydrolysis of the acetyl substrate. This acyl species has a half-life of several hours to days. For practical purposes the alkyl phosphates are hemisubstrates, in which only the acylation step occurs at an appreciable rate. In this case inhibition is both covalent and irreversible.

Several other enzymes are inhibited by covalent attachment of the inhibitor, giving rise to irreversibility. The hydrazines (phenelzine, isocarboxazid metabolites) and the acetylenic agents (pargyline) are oxidized to reactive intermediates by monoamine oxidase. These intermediates attack the associated flavin cofactor on the enzyme. Such agents have been termed *suicide substrates*[157,158] since their activation requires catalysis by the very enzyme that they inactivate. Hence the inactivation process is mechanism-based. There are now many examples of such substrates, activation of which by the enzyme results in covalent modification of the enzyme or of an associated cofactor. Often this occurs by conjugation or association of the enzyme and substrate followed by a neighboring group attack. Several of the targets of suicide substrates have therapeutic significance. These include the penicillinases and alanine racemases in antibacterial design; GABA transaminase inhibitors for antiepileptic agents; lipoxygenase and cyclooxygenase inhibitors to control leukotriene and prostaglandin biosynthesis, respectively; aromatase inhibitors to block formation of estrogenic hormones; ornithine decarboxylase inhibitors as antiparasitic agents; and dopamine β-hydroxylase inhibitors to control catecholamine biosynthesis. A myriad of other suicide substrates serve as antimetabolites and are potential antineoplastic agents. The effectiveness of these inhibitors depends not only on their relative dissociation constants or K_m values compared with those of the endogenous substrate but also on kinetic competition between turnover of the suicide substrate and the inactivation event. The structures of some monoamine oxidase inhibitors are shown in Figure 2-45.

Perturbation of Structure of Excitable Cells

Several arguments can be marshalled to suggest that general anesthetics block cellular excitability not by an action on specific receptors but instead as generalized perturbants of membrane structure. Many of these considerations also apply to local anesthetics. First, there are great variations in molecular structure among the anesthetics, extending from nitrogen, nitrous oxide, the noble gases (such as xenon) to certain steroids, halogenated

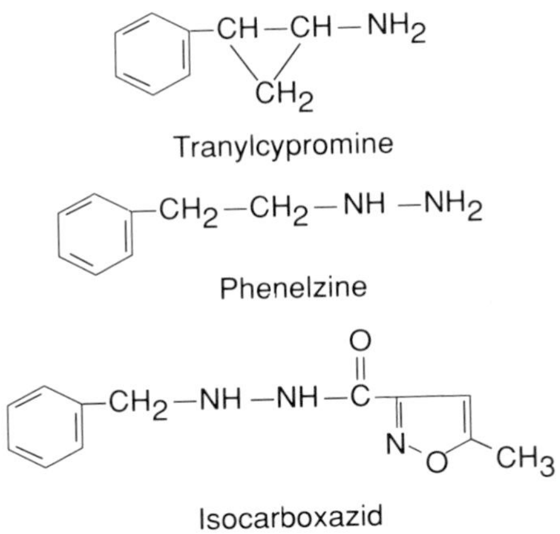

Fig. 2-45. Structures of some monoamine oxidase inhibitors.

hydrocarbons, alcohols, alkanes, and ethers. Second, anesthetics show virtually no stereoselectivity when enantiomeric pairs are compared. Third, quantitative correlations of anesthetic potencies with physical parameters of the anesthetics themselves show simple relationships between the various anesthetics; these correlations are well maintained within the phylogenetic tree. Hence the rank ordering of anesthetic potencies in producing a loss of cellular excitability in *Paramecium* will be comparable to production of consciousness loss in humans.[159,160]

At the turn of the century Overton and Meyer assessed the potency of various general anesthetics and related these potencies to lipid solubility.[161] Their studies suggested that anesthetic potency could be directly correlated with lipid/water partitioning, and that when the concentration of anesthetic, irrespective of its structure, reached 0.03 to 0.08 molal in the membrane, anesthesia ensued (Fig. 2-46). Minor refinements of the Overton-Meyer correlations have been made over the years by considering thermodynamic activities (rather than concentrations) of the anesthetic, molar volumes of the anesthetic (Fig. 2-46), and solubility parameters of the lipid (solvent) phase. Moreover, alternative theories that relate anesthetic activity to clathrate formation within the cell have also been entertained. These clathrates form inclusion crystals in the cell cytoplasm or on the cell membrane, thereby increasing electrical impedance. Both lipid solubility and clathrate formation by these compounds depend on the polarizability of the electron cloud of the anesthetic molecule. If the same molecular forces are responsible for the two physical phenomena, equally good correlations of anesthetic potency with lipid/water partition coefficients and with hydrate dissociation pressure of the clathrate can be achieved. Thus correlations of anesthetic potency with physical parameters have not provided an unequivocal means of distinguishing the basic mechanism or site of action of anesthetics.

Fortunately, our knowledge of membrane structure and of the mode of membrane protein association with lipids has also increased in recent years. Should membrane proteins that control excitability and membrane lipids be involved, a theory of anesthetic action must incorporate the basic tenets of structure and function of membranes and membrane-associated proteins likely to influence cellular excitability. Also, since it has long been known that hyperbaric pressure will reverse anesthesia in a graded manner, theories of anesthesia should accommodate this observation.

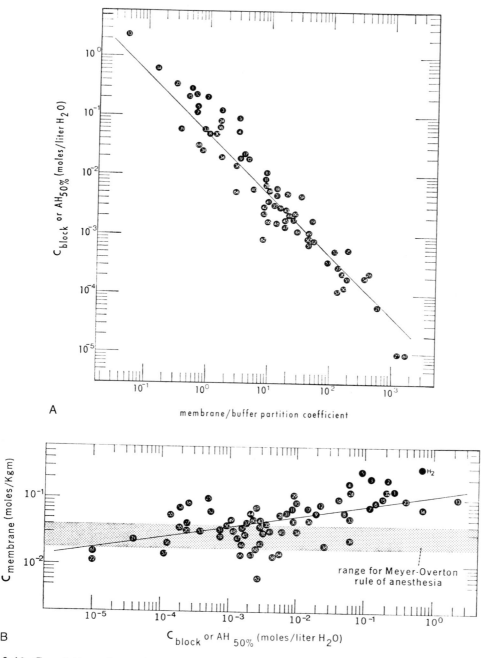

Fig. 2-46. Correlation of experimental data with Overton-Meyer theory of anesthesia. **(A)** shows the inverse correlation between the concentration required for block of nerve conduction with the membrane/buffer partition coefficient. **(B)** shows the membrane concentrations of anesthetic for equivalent activity plotted against the external concentration. Over a 250,000-fold variation in external concentration, the concentration within the membrane varies by a factor of approximately 50. (*Figure Continues*).

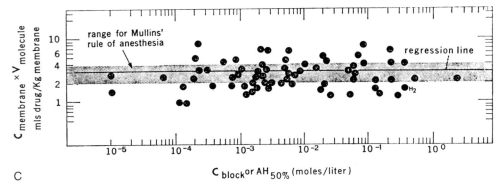

C

Fig. 2-46 (*Continued*). (C) shows that this value can be delimited further by correcting for the partial molar volume of the anesthetic, as originally suggested by Mullins. In this case a 250,000-fold variation in external concentration gives approximately a 10-fold variation in the product of membrane concentration and molecular volume. (From Seeman,[160] with permission. Reference 160 gives the codes for the individual agents.)

The critical volume hypothesis developed in recent years by Miller and colleagues[162,163] extends the basic concepts of Overton and Meyer and has provided the most consistent framework for a model of anesthesia. The hypothesis is compatible with pressure reversal of anesthesia, the rank ordering of anesthetic potencies, and physical measurements of membrane expansion in response to anesthetic administration. The basic equation contains expansion ($\overline{V}_2X_2P/V_\mathrm{m}$) and compression ($\beta P$) terms, and expresses the fractional expansion E as

$$E = \frac{\overline{V}_2X_2P}{V_\mathrm{m}} - \beta P \tag{12}$$

where $\overline{V}_2$ and X_2 are the partial molar volume and mole fraction of the anesthetic partitioned in the lipid phase, V_m is the molar volume of the membrane phase, P is the pressure of anesthetic, and β is a coefficient of isothermal compressibility. When $\overline{V}_2X_2P/V_\mathrm{m}$ exceeds βP by a critical value, anesthesia results. The threshold for expansion E would then yield the critical volume. Physical pressure without increasing the partial pressure of the anesthetic gas would increase only the second term in the equation and hence be compatible with pressure reversal of anesthesia. Helium and neon at all partial pressures do not produce anesthesia, and this is predicted by the low polarizability of the comparatively small electron clouds of these elements. Hence van der Waals forces are minimal for these gases, and little partitioning into the hydrophobic phase would occur even at higher partial pressures of the gas. At all partial pressures the compression term is never greatly exceeded by the expansion term for helium and neon; thus the critical volume is never reached. In contrast, nitrogen gas (N_2), with a larger electron cloud, becomes an anesthetic at a pressure of 34 atm. Accordingly, studies with subjects at hyperbaric pressure or studies on pressure reversal of anesthesia cannot employ nitrogen as the inert gas.

Physical measurements of membrane expansion, magnetic resonance-derived order parameters for anesthetics imbedded in membranes and for membrane lipids themselves, and other assessments of fluidity of the membrane following anesthetic perturbation have buttressed the arguments that membrane expansion is associated with anesthesia.[160] Such studies document that membrane expansion is greater than the volume that would be accounted for by the partial molar volume of the anesthetic itself. Hence, an increased disorder of the membrane phase ensues upon insertion of the anesthetic molecule into the membrane. However, such concepts fall short of delineating the actual site of anesthetic action or, for that matter, of distinguishing between mechanisms of local and general anesthesia. To extend anesthetic mechanisms to this level, one must consider the membrane proteins involved in cellular excitability that are susceptible to anesthetic action. Moreover, such proteins should in some way be linked to the maintenance of consciousness or the block of sensory responses.

Substantial evidence exists that amine-containing local anesthetics act on the cytoplasmic surface of the voltage-sensitive sodium channel to block nerve conduction.[159] This site has been demonstrated most convincingly in the squid giant axon, in which the inner and exterior surface of the membrane can be independently perfused and block of conduction can be measured. Whether the anesthetic binds within a hydrophobic crevice in the channel or serves to displace annular (boundary) lipids essential for channel function has not been ascertained. Presumably, the site(s) differ from the five sites specified in Table 2-2 as affecting the voltage-sensitive sodium channel. Electrophysiologic experiments show that an activated channel conformation is more susceptible to inhibition. Hence, a use dependence for local anesthetic block of nerve conduction can be demonstrated. The potent local anesthetics usually are tertiary amines, which tend to be protonated at physiologic pH values. These compounds would only slowly transfer across a membrane bilayer and would not partition deep within the bilayer. By contrast, general anesthetics are far more hydrophobic and they can accordingly cross the bilayer more rapidly and partition more deeply into it.

Most workers believe that in the case of general anesthesia the loss of consciousness results from a deficit in neurotransmission, not nerve conduction as is the case for local anesthetics. The site of general anesthetic action is not at all obvious. Polysynaptic pathways appear more sensitive to general anesthetics than are monosynaptic pathways or pathways of nerve conduction. Although there is no compelling evidence ruling out an impairment of neurotransmitter release in anesthesia, anesthetics may noncompetitively inhibit membrane-associated protein(s) involved in excitatory function, possibly by affecting the membrane environment in which such proteins reside. Alternatively, anesthesia might be mediated by activation of an inhibitory neurotransmitter receptor. Such an action would be analogous to that seen with benzodiazepines and barbiturates on γ-aminobutyric acid receptors. However, it is difficult to envision how discrete regulatory sites could accommodate the binding of the wide array of general anesthetic agents. Accordingly, we are again forced to consider that a general perturbation of a hydrophobic environment may activate an inhibitory receptor or inhibit an excitatory receptor system within excitable membranes.

The general perturbations of cellular or membrane structure constitute a realistic mechanism of anesthetic action even though identification of specific loci of the anesthetic action on excitable membranes remains a vexing problem.

REFERENCES

1. Chang CC, Lee CY: Isolation of neurotoxins from the venom of *Bungarus multicinctus* and their modes of neuromuscular blocking action. Arch Int Pharmacodyn Ther 144:241, 1969
2. Changeux J-P, Kasai M, Lee CY: Use of a snake venom toxin and characterize the cholinergic receptor protein. Proc Natl Acad Sci USA 67:1241, 1970

3. Changeux JP, Devilers-Thierry A, Chemouilli P: Acetylcholine receptor: An allosteroic protein. Science 225:1335, 1984

4. Karlin A: Molecular properties of nicotine acetylcholine receptors. p. 191. In Poste G, Nicholson GL, Cotman CW (eds): The Cell Surface and Neuronal Function. Elsevier, Amsterdam, 1982

5. Taylor P, Brown RD, Johnson DA: The linkage between occupation and response of the nicotinic acetylcholine receptor. p. 407. In Kleinzeller A, Martin BR (eds): Current Topics of Membranes and Transport. Vol. 18. Academic Press, Orlando, FL, 1983

6. Numa S, Noda M, Takahashi H, et al: Molecular structure of the acetylcholine receptor. Cold Spring Harbor Symp Quant Biol 48:57, 1983

7. Maelicke A (ed): Nicotinic Acetylcholine Receptor: Structure and Function. pp. 359–387. NATO ASI Series, vol. H3, Springer-Verlag, Berlin, 1986

8. McCarthy MP, Earnest JP, Young EF, et al: The molecular neurobiology of the acetylcholine receptor. Annu Rev Neurosci 9:383, 1986

9. Brisson A, Unwin PNT: Quaternary studies of the acetylcholine receptor. Nature 315:414, 1986

10. Walkinshaw MD, Saenger W, Maelicke A: Three dimensional structure of the "long" neurotoxin from cobra venom. Proc Natl Acad Sci (USA) 77:2400, 1980

11. Neher E, Sakmann B: Single channel currents recorded from membrane of denervated fragment fibers. Nature 260:799, 1976

12. Katz B, Thesleff S: A study of "desensitization" produced by acetylcholine at the motor end plate. J Physiol (Lond) 138:63, 1957

13. Monod J, Wyman J, Changeux J-P: On the nature of allosteric transmissions, a plausible model. J Mol Biol 12:86, 1965

14. Hess G, Cash DJ, Aoshima H: Acetylcholine receptor-controlled ion translocation: Chemical kinetic investigations of mechanism. Annu Rev Biophys Bioeng 12:443, 1983

15. Magleby KL, Pallotta BS: A study of desensitization of acetylcholine receptors using nerve released transmitter in the frog. J Physiol (Lond) 316:225, 1981

16. Sine S, Taylor P: The relationship between agonist occupation and the permeability response of the cholinergic receptor revealed by bound cobra α-toxin. J Biol Chem 255:10144, 1980

17. Neubig R, Cohen JB: Permeability control by cholinergic receptors in *Torpedo* postsynaptic membranes: Agonist dose-response relations measured at second and millisecond times. Biochemistry 19:2770, 1980

18. Anholt R, Fredkin PR, Deernick T, et al: Incorporation of acetylcholine receptors into liposomes. J Biol Chem 257:7122, 1982

19. Neubig RR, Cohen JB: Equilibrium binding of [³H]tubocurarine and [³H]-acetylcholine by *Torpedo* postsynaptic membranes: Agonist dose-response measured at second and millisecond times. Biochemistry 19:2770, 1979

20. Sine SM, Taylor P: Relationship between reversible antagonist occupancy and the functional capacity of the acetylcholine receptor. J Biol Chem 256:6692, 1981

21. Boulter J, Evans K, Goldman D, et al: Isolation of a cDNA clone coding for a possible neural nicotinic acetylcholine receptor subunit. Nature 319:368, 1986

22. Wada K, Ballivet M, Boulter J, et al: Functional expression of a new pharmacological subtype of brain nicotinic acetylcholine receptor. Science 740:330, 1988

23. Claudio T, Greece WM, Mortman DS, et al: Genetic reconstitution of functional and acetylcholine receptor channels in mouse fibroblasts. Science 238:1688, 1987

24. Hille B: Ion channels of excitable membranes. Sinauer Associates, Sunderland, MA, 1984

25. Catterall WA: Structure and function of voltage sensitive ion channels. Science 242:50, 1988

26. Aldrich RW, Corey DP, Stevens CF: A reinterpretation of mammalian sodium channel gating based on single channel recording. Nature 506:436, 1987

27. Noda M, Ikeda T, Suzuki H, et al: Expression of functional sodium channels from cloned cDNA. Nature 322:826, 1986

28. Noda M, Iheda T, Kayano T, et al: Existence of distinct sodium channel messenger RNA's in rat brain. Nature 320:188, 1986
29. Noda M, Shimizu S, Tanabe T, et al: Primary structure of *Electrophorus electricus* sodium channel deduced from cDNA sequence. Nature 312:188, 1984
30. Armstrong CM: Sodium channels and gating currents. Physiol Rev 61:644, 1951
31. Messner DJ, Feller DJ, Scheuer T, Catterall WA: Functional properties of rat brain sodium channels lacking the β_1 or β_2 subunit. J Biol Chem 261:14882, 1986
32. Miller RJ: Multiple calcium channels and neuronal function. Science 235:46, 1987
33. Triggle DJ, Janis RA: Calcium channel ligands. Annu Rev Pharmacol Toxicol 27:347, 1987
34. Trimmer JS, Agnew WS: Molecular diversity of voltage sensitive Na^+ channels. Ann Rev Physiol 51:401, 1989
35. Tsien RW, Lipscombe D, Madison DV, et al: Neuronal calcium channels and their selective modulation. Trends Neurosci 11:431, 1988
36. Fill M, Coronado R: Ryanodine receptor channel of sarcoplasmic reticulum. Trends Neurosci 11:453, 1988
37. Tanabe T, Takeshima M, Mikawi A, et al: Primary structure of the receptor for calcium channel blockers from skeletal muscle. Nature 328:313, 1987
38. Takahashi M, Seagar MJ, Jones JF, et al: Subunit structure of dihydropyridine-sensitive calcium channels from skeletal muscle. Proc Natl Acad Sci USA 84:5478, 1987
39. Campbell K, Leung AT, Sharp AH: The biochemistry and molecular biology of the dihydropyridine sensitive calcium channel. Trends Neurosci 11:425, 1988
40. Papazian DM, Schwartz TL, Tempel BL, et al: Cloning of genomic and complementary DNA from Shaker, a putative potassium channel gene from *Drosophila*. Science 237:749, 1987
41. Fagg CE, Foster AG, Canong AH: Excitatory amino acid synaptic mechanisms and neurological function. Trends Pharmacol Sci 7:357, 1986
42. Cotman CW, Iversen LL (eds): Excitatory amino acids. Trends Neurosci 10:263, 1987
43. Curtis DR, Johnston GAR: Amino acid transmitters in the mammalian central nervous system. Ergeb Physiol 69:97, 1974
44. Langosch D, Thomas L, Betz H: Conserved quaternary structure of ligand gated ion channels: The postsynaptic glycine receptor is a pentamer. Proc Natl Acad Sci 85:7394, 1988
45. Grenninghol G, Rienitz A, Schmitt B, et al: The strychnine-binding subunit of the glycine receptor shows homology with nicotinic acetylcholine receptors. Nature 328:215, 1987
46. Bomann J: Electrophysiology of $GABA_A$ and $GABA_B$ receptor subtypes. Trends Neurosci 11:112, 1985
47. Olsen RW, Venter JC (eds): Bendodiazepine/GABA Receptors and Chloride Channels: Structural and Functional Properties. Alan R. Liss, New York, 1986
48. Alho H, Costa E, Ferrero P, et al: Diazepam-binding inhibitor: A neuropeptide located in selected neuronal populations of rat brain. Science 229:179, 1985
49. Guidotti A, Forchetti CM, Corda MG, et al: Isolation, characterization and purification to homogeneity of an endogenous polypeptide with agonistic action on benzodiazepine receptors. Proc Natl Acad Sci USA 80:3531, 1983
50. Schofeld PR, Darlison MG, Fujita N, et al: Sequence and functional expression of the $GABA_A$ receptor shows a ligand-gated receptor superfamily. Nature 328:221, 1987
51. Lear JD, Wasserman ZR, DeGrado WF: Synthetic amphiphilic peptide models for protein ion channels. Science 240:1177, 1988
52. Sutherland EW: Studies on the mechanism of hormone action. Science 177:401, 1972
53. Walsh DA, Perkins JP, Krebs EG: An adenosine 3'5'-monophosphate-dependent protein kinase from rabbit skeletal muscle. J Biol Chem 243:3763, 1968
54. Kuo JF, Greengard P: Cyclic nucleotide-dependent protein kinase. IV. Widespread occurrence of adenosine 3'5'-monophosphate-dependent protein kinase in various tissues and phyla of the animal kingdom. Proc Natl Acad Sci USA 64:1349, 1969

55. Limbird LE: Receptors linked to inhibition of adenylate cyclase: Additional signalling mechanisms. FASEB J 2:2686, 1988

56. Rodbell M, Birnbaumer L, Pohl SL, Krans HMJ: The glucagon-sensitive adenylate cyclase system in membranes of rat liver. V. An obligatory rate of guanyl nucleotides in glucagon action. J Biol Chem 246:1877, 1971

57. Cooper DMF: Bimodal regulation of adenylate cyclase. FEBS Lett 138:157, 1982

58. Schramm M, Rodbell M: A persistent active state of the adenylate cyclase system produced by the combined actions of isoproterenol and guanyl imidodiphosphate in frog erythrocyte membranes. J Biol Chem 250:2232, 1975

59. Cassel D, Selinger Z: Catecholamine stimulated GTPase activity in turkey erythrocyte membranes. Biochim Biophys Acta 452:538, 1976

60. Gilman AG: G proteins: Transducers of receptor-generated signals. Annu Rev Biochem 56:615, 1987

61. Stryer L, Bourne HR: G proteins: A family of signal transducers. Annu Rev Cell Biol 2:391, 1986

62. Spiegel AM: Signal transduction by guanine nucleotide binding proteins. Mol Cell Endocrinol 49:1, 1987

63. Neer EJ, Clapham DE: Roles of G protein subunits in transmembrane signalling. Nature 333:129, 1988

64. Sternweis PC, Robishaw JD: Isolation of two proteins with high affinity for guanine nucleotides from membranes of bovine brain. J Biol Chem 259:13806, 1984

65. Neer EJ, Lok JM, Wolf LG: Purification and properties of the inhibitory guanine nucleotide regulatory unit of brain adenylate cyclase. J Biol Chem 259:3586, 1984

66. Snyderman R, Smith CD, Vergnese M: Model for leukocyte regulations by chemoattractant receptor: Roles of a guanine nucleotide regulatory protein and polyphosphoinositide metabolism. J Leukocyte Biol 40:785, 1986

67. Bokoch GM, Gilman AG: Inhibition of receptor-mediated release of arachidonic acid by pertussis toxin. Cell 39:301, 1984

68. Cerione RA, Regan JW, Nakata H, et al: Functional reconstitution of the α_2-adrenergic receptor with guanine nucleotide regulatory proteins in phospholipid vesicles. J Biol Chem 261:3901, 1986

69. Hescheler J, Rosenthal W, Trautwein W, Schultz G: The GTP-binding protein, G_o, regulates neuronal calcium channels. Nature 325:445, 1987

70. Cockcroft S: Polyphosphoinositide phosphodiesterase: Regulation by a novel guanine nucleotide binding protein, G_p. Trends Biochem Sci 12:75, 1987

71. Fain JM, Wallace MA, Wojcikiewicz RJH: Evidence for involvement of guanine-nucleotide binding regulatory proteins in the activation of phospholipase by hormones. FASEB J 2:2569, 1988

72. Freissmuth M, Casey PJ, Gilman AG: G proteins control diverse pathways of transmembrane signalling. FASEB J 3:2125, 1989

73. Brown AM, Birnbaumer L: Direct G protein gating of ion channels. Am J Physiol 254:H401, 1988

74. Allende JF: GTP-mediated macromolecular interactions: The common features of different systems. FASEB J 2:2356, 1988

75. Lefkowitz RJ, Stadel JM, Carson MG: Adenylate cyclase-coupled beta-adrenergic receptors: Structure and mechanisms of activation and desensitization. Annu Rev Biochem 52:159, 1983

76. Kent RS, DeLean A, Lefkowitz RJ: A quantitative analysis of beta-adrenergic receptor interactions. Resolution of high and low affinity states of the receptor by computer modeling of ligand binding data. Mol Pharmacol 17:14, 1980

77. Kurose H, Katada T, Haga T, et al: Functional interaction of purified muscarinic receptors with purified inhibitory guanine nucleotide regulating proteins reconstituted in phospholipid vesicles. J Biol Chem 261:6423, 1986

78. Cerione RA, Strulovici B, Benovic JL, et al: Pure β-adrenergic receptors: The single poly peptide contains catecholamine responsiveness to adenylate cyclase. Nature 306:562, 1983
79. Dohlman HG, Caron MG, Lefkowitz RJ: A family of receptors coupled to guanine nucleotide regulatory proteins. Biochemistry 26:2657, 1987
80. Kobilka BK, Kobilka TS, Daniel K, et al: Chimeric α_2-β_2-adrenergic receptors: Delineation of domains involved in effector coupling and ligand binding specificity. Science 240:1310, 1988
81. Peralta EG, Winslow JW, Ashkenazi A, et al: Structural basis of muscarinic acetylcholine receptor subtype diversity. Trends Pharmacol Sci (suppl):6, 1988
82. Cotecchia S, Schwinn DA, Randall RR, et al: Molecular cloning and expression of the cDNA for the hamster α_1-adrenergic receptor. Proc Natl Acad Sci 85:7159, 1988
83. May DC, Ross EM, Gilman AG, Smigel MD: Reconstitution of catecholamine-stimulated adenylate cyclase actively using three purified proteins. J Biol Chem 260:15829, 1985
84. Katada T, Dinuma M, Ui M: Mechanisms for inhibition of the catalytic activity of adenylate cyclase by the guanine nucleotide binding proteins serving as the substrate of islet-activating protein, pertussis toxin. J Biol Chem 261:5215, 1986
85. Cerione RA, Storiszewski C, Gierschik P, et al: Mechanism of guanine nucleotide regulating protein-mediated inhibition of adenylate cyclase. J Biol Chem 261:9514, 1986
86. Bigay J, Deterre P, Pfister C, Chabre M: Fluoride complexes of aluminium or beryllium act on G proteins as reversibly bound analogues of the γ phosphate of GTP. EMBO J 6:2907, 1987
87. Seamon K, Daly JW: Forskolin: Its biological and chemical properties. Cyclic Nucleotide Protein Phosphorylation Res 19:1, 150, 1986
88. Krupinski J, Coussen F, Bakalyar HA et al: Adenylyl cyclase amino acid sequence: possible channel or transporter-like structure. Science 244:1558, 1989
89. Putney JW (ed): Phosphoinositides and Receptor Mechanisms. Alan R. Liss, New York, 1986
90. Berridge MJ: Inositol trisphosphate and diacylglycerol: Two interacting second messengers. Annu Rev Biochem 56:159, 1987
91. Hokin LE: Receptors and phosphoinositide-generated second messengers. Annu Rev Biochem 54:205, 1985
92. Michell RH: Inositol phospholipids and cell surface receptor function. Biochim Biophys Acta 415:81, 1975
93. Litosch I, Wallis C, Fain J: 5-Hydroxytryptamine stimulates inositol phosphate production in a cell free system from blowfly salivary glands. J Biol Chem 260:5464, 1985
94. Nishizuka Y: The role of protein kinase C in cell surface signal transduction and turnover promotion. Nature 308:693, 1984
95. Nishizuka Y: Turnover of inositol phospholipids and signal transduction. Science 224:1365, 1984
96. Berridge MJ, Downes CP, Hanley MR: Lithium amplifies agonist-dependent phosphatidylinositol responses in brain and salivary glands. Biochem J 206:587, 1982
97. Batty IR, Nahorski SK, Irvine RF: Rapid formation of inositol 1,3,4,5-tetrakisphosphate following muscarinic receptor stimulation of rat cerebral cortical slices. Biochem J 232:211, 1985
98. Irvine RF, Moor RM: Micro-injection of inositol 1,3,4,5-tetrakisphosphate activates sea urchin eggs by a mechanism dependent on external Ca^{++}. Biochem J 240:917, 1986
99. Streb H, Irvine RF, Berridge MJ, Schulz I: Release of Ca^{++} from a nonmitochondrial intracellular store in pancreatic acinar cells by inositol 1,4,5-trisphosphate. Nature 306:67, 1983
100. Ganong BR, Loomis CR, Hannun YA, Bell RM: Specificity and mechanism of protein kinase C activation by *sn*-1,2 diacylglycerols. Proc Nat Acad Sci USA 83:1184, 1986
101. Coussens L, Parker PJ, Rhee L, et al: Multiple distinct forms of bovine and human protein kinase C suggest diversity in cellular signalling pathways. Science 233:859, 1986
102. Nishizuka Y: The molecular heterogeneity of protein kinase C and its implications for cellular regulation. Nature 334:661, 1988
103. Burch RM, Luini A, Axelrod J: Phospholipase A_2 and phospholipase C are activated by distinct

GTP-binding proteins in response to α_1-adrenergic stimulation in FRTL-5 thyroid cells. Proc Natl Acad Sci USA 83:7201, 1986

104. Slivka SR, Insel PA: α_1-Adrenergic receptor-mediated phosphoinositide hydrolysis and prostaglandin E_2 formation in Madin Darby canine kidney cells. Possible parallel activation of phospholipase C and phospholipase A_2. J Biol Chem 262:4200, 1987

105. Exton JH: Mechanisms of action of calcium mobilizing agonists: Variations on a young theme. FASEB J 2:2670, 1988

106. Putney JW: Recent hypotheses regarding the phosphatidylinositol effect. Life Sci 29:1183, 1981

107. Besterman JM, Duronio V, Cuatrecasas P: Rapid formation of diacylglycerol from phosphatidylcholine: A pathway for generation of a second messenger. Proc Natl Acad Sci USA 83:6785, 1986

108. Irving HR, Exton JH: Phosphatidylcholine breakdown in rat liver plasma membranes. Roles of guanine nucleotides and P_2 purinergic agonists. J Biol Chem 262:3440, 1987

109. Slivka SR, Meier KE, Insel PA: Alpha$_1$-adrenergic receptors promote phosphatidylcholine hydrolysis in MDCK-D$_1$ cells: A mechanism for rapid activation of protein kinase C. J Biol Chem 263:12242, 1988

110. Nairn AC, Hemmings HC, Greengard P: Protein kinases in the brain. Annu Rev Biochem 54:931, 1985

111. Edelman AM, Blumenthal DK, Krebs EG: Protein serine/threonine kinases. Annu Rev Biochem 56:567, 1987

112. Wolf M, LeVine H, May WS, et al: A model for intracellular translation of protein kinase C involving synergism between Ca^{2+} and phorbol esters. Nature 317:546, 1985

113. North RA, Williams JT, Suprenant A, Christie MJ: μ and δ receptors belong to a family of receptors that are coupled to potassium channels. Proc Natl Acad Sci USA 84:5487, 1987

114. Masu Y, Nakayama K, Tamaki H, et al: cDNA cloning of bovine substance-K receptor through oocyte expression system. Nature 329:836, 1987

115. Carpenter G: Receptors for epidermal growth factor and other polypeptide mitogens. Annu Rev Biochem 56:881, 1987

116. Goldfine ID: The insulin receptor: Molecular biology and transmembrane signalling. Endocr Rev 8:235, 1987

117. Rosen OM: After insulin binds. Science 237:1452, 1987

118. Yarden Y, Ullrich A: Growth factor receptor tyrosine kinases. Annu Rev Biochem 57:443, 1988

119. Low MG, Saltiel AR: Structural and functional roles of glycosyl phosphatidylinositol in membranes. Science 239:268, 1988

120. Hunter T, Cooper JA: Protein-tyrosine kinases. Annu Rev Biochem 54:892, 1985

121. Ellis L, Clauser E, Morgan DO, et al: Replacement of insulin receptor tyrosine residues 1162 and 1163 compromises insulin-stimulated kinase activity and uptake of 2-deoxyglucose. Cell 45:721, 1986

122. Chou CK, Dull TJ, Russell DS, et al: Insulin receptors mutated at the ATP-binding site lack protein tyrosine kinase activity and fail to mediate postreceptor effects of insulin. J Biol Chem 262:1842, 1987

123. Riedel H, Dull TJ, Schessinger J, Ullrich A: A chimeric receptor allows insulin to stimulate tyrosine kinase activity of epidermala growth factor receptor. Nature 324:68, 1986

124. Russell DS, Gherzi R, Johnson EL, et al: The protein-tyrosine kinase activity of the insulin receptor is necessary for insulin-mediated receptor down-regulation. J Biol Chem 262:11833, 1987

125. Waldman SA, Murad F: Cyclic GMP synthesis and function. Pharmacol Rev 39:163, 1987

126. Palmer RM, Ferrige AG, Moncada S: Nitric oxide release accounts for the biological activity of endothelium-derived relaxing factor. Nature 327:524, 1987

127. Garbers DL: Guanylate cyclase, a cell-surface receptor. J Biol Chem 264:9103, 1989

128. Ringold GM: Steroid hormone regulation of gene expression. Annu Rev Pharmacol Toxicol 25:529, 1985

129. Jensen EV, DeSombre ER: Mechanism of action of female sex hormones. Annu Rev Biochem 41:203, 1972

130. Gustafson JA, Carlstedt-Duke J, Pellinger L, et al: Biochemistry, molecular biology and physiology of the glucocorticoid receptor. Endocr Rev 8:185, 1987

131. Pratt WB: Transformation of glucocorticoid and progesterone receptors to the DNA-binding state. J Cellular Biochem 35:51, 1987

132. Firestone G, Payvar F, Yamamoto KR: Glucocorticoid regulation of protein processing and compartmentation. Nature 300:221, 1982

133. Evans RM: The steroid and thyroid hormone receptor superfamily. Science 240:889, 1988

134. Pratt WB, Jolly DJ, Pratt DV, et al: A region in the steroid binding domain determines formation of the non-DNA-binding, 9S glucocorticoid receptor complex. J Biol Chem 263:267, 1988

135. Pastan I, Willingham MC: Endocytosis. Plenum, New York, 1985

136. Goldstein JL, Brown MS, Anderson RGW, et al: Receptor-mediated endocytosis. Annu Rev Cell Biol 1:1, 1985

137. Sibley DR, Lefkowitz RJ: Molecular mechanisms of receptor desensitization using the beta-adrenergic receptor-coupled adenylate cyclase as a model. Nature 317:124, 1985

138. Harden TK: Agonist-induced desensitization of the β-adrenergic receptor-linked adenylate cyclase. Pharmacol Rev 35:5, 1983

139. Sibley DR, Benovic JL, Caron MG, Lefkowitz RJ: Regulation of transmembrane signalling by receptor phosphorylation. Cell 48:913, 1987

140. Bergernon JJM, Cruz J, Khan MN, Posner BI: Uptake of insulin and other ligands into receptor-rich endocytic compartments of target cells. The endoxomal apparatus. Annu Rev Physiol 147:383, 1985

141. Mahan LC, McKernan RM, Insel PA: Metabolism of alpha- and beta-adrenergic receptors in vitro and in vivo. Annu Rev Pharmacol Toxicol 27:215, 1987

142. Albert A: Selective Toxicity: The Physiochemical Basis of Theory. 7th Ed. Chapman & Hall, New York, 1985

143. Woods DD: The biochemical mode of action of sulfonamide drugs. J Gen Microbiol 29:687, 1962

144. Woods DD: The biosynthesis of folic acid. II. Inhibition by sulfonamides. J Biol Chem 237:536, 1962

145. Bell PK, Robin RO Jr: Studies in chemotherapy. VII. A theory of the relation of structure to activity of sulfanilamide type compounds. J Am Chem Soc 64:2905, 1942

146. Burchall JJ, Hitchings GH: Inhibitor binding analysis of dihydrofolate reductase from various species. Mol Pharmacol 1:126, 1969

147. Ferone R, Burchall JJ, Hitchings GH: *Plasmodium berghei* dihydrofolate reductase: Isolation, properties and inhibition by antifolates. Mol Pharmacol 5:49, 1969

148. Howell EE, Meyer RJ, Warren MS, et al: Active site mutations in dihydrofolate reductase. p. 251. In Protein Engineering. Alan R. Liss, New York, 1987

149. Kraut J, Matthews DA: Dihydrofolate reductase. p. 1. In Jurnak F, McPherson A (eds): Biological Macromolecules and Assemblies. Vol. 3. Wiley & Sons, New York, 1987

150. Matthews DA, Bolin JT, Burridge JM, et al: Refined crystal structures of *Escherichia coli* and chicken liver dihydrofolate reductase containing bound trimethoprim. J Biol Chem 260:381, 1985

151. Brockman RW, Anderson EP: In Hochster RM, Quastel JH (eds): Pyrimidine Analogs in Metabolic Inhibitors. Vol. 1. Academic Press, Orlando, FL, 1963

152. Heidelberger C, Danenberg PV, Moran RC: Fluorinated pyrimidines and their nucleosides. Adv Enzymol 54:57, 1983

153. Blinks JR, Wier WG, Morgan JP, Hess P: Regulation of intracellular (Ca^{2+}) by cardiotonic

drugs. p. 205. In Hoshida H, Hagiwara Y, Ebashi S (eds): Advances in Pharmacology and Therapeutics II. Vo. 3. Cardio-Renal and Cell Pharmacology. Pergamon Press, Oxford, 1982

154. Hoffman BF: The pharmacology of cardiac glycosides. p. 387. In Rosen NR, Hoffman BF (eds): Cardiac Therapy. Martinus Nijhoff, Amsterdam, 1983
155. Quinn DM: Acetylcholinesterase enzyme structure, reaction dynamics and virtual transition states. Chem Rev 87:955, 1987
156. Rosenberry TL: Acetylcholinesterase. Adv Enzymol 43:103, 1975
157. Walsh CT: Suicide substrates, mechanism based inactivators: Recent developments. Annu Rev Biochem 53:493, 1984
158. Singer TP, Von Kroff DW, Murphy DL (eds): Monoamine oxidase: Structure, function and altered functions. Academic Press, Orlando, FL, 1979
159. Miller K, Roth SH (eds): Molecular and Cellular Mechanisms of Anesthetics. Progress in Anesthesiology. Vol. 3. Plenum, New York, 1986
160. Seeman P: The membrane actions of anesthetics and tranquilizers. Pharmacol Rev 24:583, 1972
161. Overton E: Studien über die Narkose zugleich ein Beitrag zur allgemeinen Pharmakologie. G. Fischer, Jena, 1901
162. Miller KW, Paton WDM, Smith RA, Smith EB: The pressure reversal of general anesthesia and the critical volume hypothermia. Mol Pharmacol 9:131, 1973
163. Miller KW: The nature of the site of general anesthesia. Int Rev Neurobiol 27:61, 1985
164. Bonner TI, Buckley NJ, Young AC, Brann MR: Identification of a family of muscarinic acetylcholinic receptor genes. Science 237:527, 1981
165. Alsobrook JP II, Stevens CF: Cloning the calcium neurochannel. Trends in Neuroscience 11:1, 1988
166. Ullrich A, Gray A, Tam AW, et al: Insulin-like growth factor I receptor primary structure: comparison with insulin receptor suggests structural determinants that define functional specificity. EMBO J 5:2503, 1986

3

The Entry, Distribution, and Elimination of Drugs

William B. Pratt

We now turn our attention to the factors that determine the access of a drug to its site of action.[1-6] Regardless of the site of entry, drugs are distributed throughout the body in the water phase of the blood plasma. In order to act, therefore (unless it acts directly at the site of administration) a drug must first enter the blood. It will then reach the tissues of each organ at a rate determined by the blood flow through that organ and by the rapidity of passage of the drug molecules across the vascular endothelium through intervening interstitial fluid, and into the cells of that particular organ.

Within the blood plasma some of the drug molecules may be bound to proteins and thus may not be freely diffusible out of the plasma. As a general rule the amount of any drug in the tissues in which it acts is but a very small part of the total drug in the body. Most of the drug remains in the various fluid compartments in solution or is localized by adsorptive or partition processes in subcellular particles, at macromolecular surfaces, or in fat depots. Even within the target cells themselves, cellular fractionation studies and radioautography usually reveal that most drug molecules are associated with structures having nothing to do with the specific drug effect.

Finally, even if no cell components other than the specific receptors were capable of binding drug molecules, we should nevertheless expect to find only a small fraction of the drug associated with these receptors. The reason is that approximately 80 percent of the cell mass is water and only a very small fraction of the cell dry weight is likely to be represented by the specific receptors. Moreover, the receptors are macromolecules of high molecular weight, each bearing only one or a few specific drug-binding sites. Thus, even at complete receptor occupancy and even with fairly high drug-receptor affinity, provided that the drug interacts reversibly, most of the drug molecules will be in the ambient water phase in equilibrium with those bound to the receptor. This general view of drug distribution is represented schematically in Figure 3-1.

A drug enters the circulation by being injected there directly (intravascular route) or by absorption from depots in which it has been placed. The commonest such depot is the

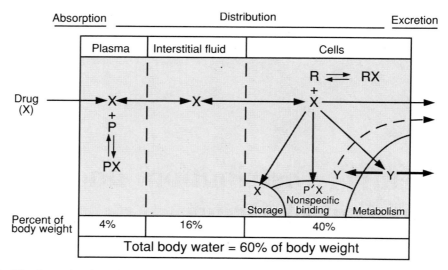

Fig. 3-1. The fate of a drug in the body. Broken lines represent membranes. Numbers at bottom are percentages of body weight represented by each fluid compartment in the adult man. X is free drug; PX, drug-protein complex in plasma; P'X, complex of drug with nonspecific binding sites in tissues; Y, a metabolic product of X; and RX, drug-receptor complex.

gastrointestinal tract, the drug having been taken orally or, rarely, administered by rectum. The other common routes of administration are subcutaneous and intramuscular. Several less usual routes are also employed, for example, through the skin (transdermal) and by inhalation. Drugs are sometimes injected for their local effects, minimizing entry into the general circulation. Examples include the injection of a local anesthetic agent subcutaneously and into spaces adjacent the spinal column or infusion of the drug into the arterial blood supply entering a target organ.[7]

A drug leaves the circulation by distribution into tissues, where it may be metabolized or excreted. Some drugs are metabolized in the plasma by various esterases. The rate of each of these processes that contribute to initiation or termination of drug action is determined by the chemical and physical properties of the drug and its interaction with the specialized tissues responsible for the pharmacologic effects or elimination processes. The kidney plays a major role in drug excretion. However, other excretory routes may be of prime importance for one or another drug. An example is excretion into the gastrointestinal tract by way of the bile. Volatile agents may be eliminated via the lungs. The liver is of chief importance in drug metabolism, but drugs are also biotransformed in other tissues. Often, metabolic alteration of structure, converting a lipid-soluble drug into a more water-soluble one, is a prerequisite to renal excretion. Accumulation at any site must obviously occur at the expense of other sites. Thus, lipid-soluble drugs may be localized in the large depots of neutral fat that comprise a significant fraction of the body weight. It is not unusual, long after administration of such a drug, to find practically all the drug molecules in the body stored in this way, exiting very slowly from the fat depot.

It follows from this brief review that the time course of drug action, determined by the effective concentration of drug at receptor sites, depends in a complex way upon the relatives rates of all the processes cited. In this chapter we shall first examine the various routes by which drugs may be administered and the important characteristics of each route. Then the factors influencing the distribution of drugs into the tissues will be considered, with special attention to the passage of drugs into the central nervous system and across the placenta into the fetus. Finally, routes of drug elimination will be analyzed. In Chapter 4 we shall consider the combined effects of absorption, distribution, and elimination upon the time course of drug action. The principles and pathways of drug metabolism will be deferred to Chapters 5 and 6.

DRUG ENTRY: ROUTES OF ADMINISTRATION

The possible routes of drug entry into the body may be divided into two classes—*enteral* and *parenteral*. In enteral administration the drug is placed directly in the gastrointestinal tract by placing it under the tongue (sublingual), by swallowing it (oral, PO, per os), or by rectal administration. In parenteral administration the gastrointestinal tract is bypassed. There are many parenteral routes. The commonest are subcutaneous (SC), intramuscular (IM), and intravascular, but drugs may also be injected intradermally or applied to the skin, for local effect or to be absorbed transcutaneously; they may be introduced intranasally, or they may be inhaled for direct action on the bronchial tree or to be absorbed into blood at the alveoli; they may be injected into or near the spinal column (epidural, intrathecal); they may be introduced intravaginally or directly into other body cavities (e.g., by intraperitoneal, intrapleural, or intra-articular injection or intracystically into the urinary bladder); and they may be injected directly into pathologic cavities, such as abscesses and tumor cavities. We shall discuss the principal routes of administration, their peculiar advantages and disadvantages, and the various determinants of the rate of onset and the duration of drug action.

Intravascular Administration

The common method of introducing a drug directly into the bloodstream is to inject it intravenously, usually into the antecubital or subclavian vein, or into a superficial vein of the hand or scalp. The obvious advantage of this route is that the drug is placed in the circulation with minimum delay, a matter of importance when speed is essential. Another advantage is control. The injection can be made slowly, and it can be stopped instantaneously if untoward effects should develop. The drug can be introduced slowly over a long time by means of an infusion pump, and thus the rate of drug administration can be held constant for indefinite periods. Sometimes it is important that the drug concentration in plasma be held within fairly narrow limits or that it not fall below some desired minimum or rise above a safe maximum concentration; in such instances the establishment and maintenance of a plasma plateau concentration by means of continuous infusion (Ch. 4) renders the intravenous route attractive. However, this is not the only route of administration capable of effecting a plasma plateau (e.g., sustained release enteral dosage forms and transdermal drug delivery may yield quite constant plasma drug concentrations).

Intravenous infusion may be the safest way to administer a drug that has a narrow margin of safety between therapeutic and toxic blood levels. This is especially true of drugs that are rapidly excreted or metabolized; excessive concentrations can be reduced rapidly by merely stopping the infusion or reducing its rate. An important practical example is the use of lidocaine to prevent dangerous ventricular arrhythmias and fibrillation in the wake of coronary occlusions.[8] The effective antiarrhythmic plasma concentration in most patients is in the range 1.5 to 5 μg/ml. If this is not achieved or is not maintained, the patient is exposed to the risk of potentially fatal arrhythmia; if it is exceeded, serious

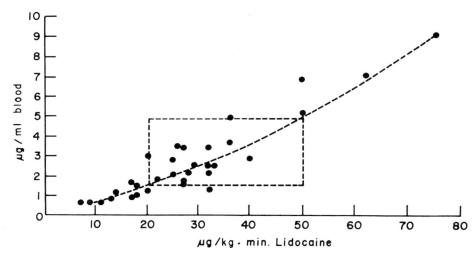

Fig. 3-2. Relation between rate of infusion and blood level of lidocaine. Data for 21 patients are given. Blood levels were measured after 2 hours of constant infusion. Area within rectangle is considered to be the appropriate therapeutic range. (From Gianelly et al.,[8] with permission.)

toxicity, including convulsive seizures, may be produced. Therefore, a carefully regulated constant rate of intravenous infusion is the method of choice. As shown in Figure 3-2, there is a nearly linear relationship between infusion rate and blood level of lidocaine, but the variability between patients is considerable, indicating the desirability of individualizing the infusion rate. The principles underlying establishment of steady-state plasma levels by constant intravenous infusion are considered in Chapter 4.

The intravenous route is also suited for substances that cannot be absorbed well from tissue depots or the gastrointestinal tract or that would be destroyed before appreciable entry into the general circulation could occur (e.g., blood products, such as plasma and cryoprecipitate that are too large to pass across absorptive barriers, or drugs that undergo extensive biotransformation during passage in intestinal venous blood through the liver on the way to the general circulation). Finally, drugs that would be intolerably painful in the subcutaneous or muscle tissues by virtue or their irritant properties may often be injected slowly into a vein without any difficulty; an example is nitrogen mustard, which is used in cancer chemotherapy.

The intravenous route has drawbacks. Once injected into a vein a drug cannot be recalled, whereas a stomach pump, emetic, or binding substance such as activated charcoal can prevent further drug entry from the gastrointestinal tract, while various procedures can delay absorption from a subcutaneous depot. Too rapid an injection rate may create a bolus of drug in the circulation, which can evoke catastrophic effects in the cardiovascular, respiratory, and central nervous systems. Blood pressure may fall to dangerous levels, cardiac arrhythmias or arrest may ensue, respiration may become shallow and irregular, or convulsions may occur.

Some of these effects may be seen even with simple salt solutions or other pharmacologically inert substances if these are injected rapidly enough. The effects are probably precipitated when a bolus of concentrated solute suddenly reaches the highly perfused tissues such as the myocardium and the chemoreceptors located in the aortic arch, carotid sinus, brain, or myocardium. The high drug concentration to which these tissues may be exposed can be appreciated from the following rough calculation. Suppose a total dose of 100 mg of a drug is to be injected intravenously in order to achieve a target therapeutic concentration throughout the body water at eventual equilibrium. In a 70-kg man with about 42 L of body water, this eventual concentration (if partitioning and elimination processes are ignored) will be 2.4 mg/L. Now suppose the injection is made into a vein over a period of 1 second. The blood returning to the heart in 1 second is one-sixtieth of the cardiac output (6 L/min), or about 0.1 L. Since all the injected drug will pass through the lungs, reach the heart, and be expelled into the aorta, we shall have a drug concentration of approximately 1,000 mg/L for a period of 1 second in these tissues. This is a 420-fold higher concentration than the therapeutic level that will be reached eventually at equilibrium. Even if we assume that the concentration is tolerable when the total amount of drug is dissolved in the whole volume of circulating plasma (about 3 L), the bolus would contain a transient 14-fold excess over this concentration after a 1-second injection.

Safety, therefore, demands that all intravenous injections be performed slowly, preferably over a period not much less than that required for a complete circulation of the blood (i.e., 1 to 2 minutes). In some cases, injection must be even slower. The therapeutic dose of theophylline, for example, must be given over 20 to 30 minutes to avoid gastrointestinal and central nervous system toxic effects. Quite apart from the need to avoid high transient drug concentrations, one wishes to be able, if necessary, to discontinue the administration if anything untoward happens; and many seconds may be required for adverse reactions to develop. The circulation time, for example, between the antecubital vein and the brain is roughly 10 to 15 seconds. If sudden loss of consciousness or convulsions were to occur 15 seconds after the start of drug injection, the difference between having emptied the syringe and having it still three-quarters full could be very significant for the patient's welfare. The same argument applies to the consequences of accidentally injecting a wrong solution, whether of a wrong drug or the right drug at a wrong concentration.

Embolism is another possible complication of the intravenous route. Particulate matter may be introduced if a drug intended for intravenous use precipitates for some reason or if a particulate suspension intended for intramuscular or subcutaneous use is inadvertently injected into a vein. Hemolysis or agglutination of erythrocytes may be caused by injection of hypotonic or hypertonic solutions or by more specific mechanisms. Some drugs damage the vascular wall and lead to phlebitis and local venous thrombosis, especially after prolonged infusions.

Infection by bacterial contaminants was commonplace until the development of aseptic technique, and the infectious hepatitis virus was sometimes spread from person to person by syringes and needles until disposable sets came into use. Self-administration of drugs, particularly by addicts, remains a cause of infections, such as hepatitis, acquired immune deficiency syndrome (AIDS), and endocarditis, because asepsis is usually ignored. Intravenous injection of drugs was long complicated by the development of fever due to pyrogens in water, especially when large volumes were infused. The pyrogenic substances (bacterial lipopolysaccharides) are heat-stable but can be removed by special procedures; thus, solutions for injection are now prepared in pyrogen-free water. Finally, excessive amounts of fluid (e.g., salt solutions given intravenously) may lead to or aggravate congestive heart failure, especially when renal or myocardial function is already impaired.

The intra-arterial route is used principally for the injection of diagnostic substances such as the radiopaque dyes used for radiologic imaging of critical arterial beds, as in coronary or cerebrovascular angiography. Specialized techniques in cancer chemotherapy call for regional infusions of drugs by an arterial route. This mode of administration may be advantageous when the drug has a high affinity for the target tissues, since regional arterial infusion maximizes binding of the drug to target cells while minimizing competition from other clearance mechanisms.[8]

Intramuscular Administration

Drugs injected into skeletal muscle (usually in the deltoid or gluteal regions) are generally absorbed rapidly. Blood flow through the muscles at rest is about 0.02 to 0.07 ml/min per gram of tissue, and this flow rate may increase many times during exercise as additional vascular channels open. Quite large amounts of solution can be introduced intramuscularly, and there is usually less pain and local irritation than is encountered by the subcutaneous route. Ordinary aqueous solutions of drugs are usually absorbed from an intramuscular site within 10 to 30 minutes, but faster or slower absorption is possible, depending upon the vascularity of the site, the ionization and lipid solubility of the drug, the volume of the injection, and the osmolality of the solution. Small molecules are absorbed directly into the capillaries from an intramuscular site, whereas larger molecules (e.g., proteins) gain access to the circulation by way of the lymphatic channels. Radiolabeled compounds of low molecular weight (maximum 585) but differing physical properties were found to be absorbed from rat muscle at virtually the same rate, about 16 percent per mintue.[9] This implies that the absorption process is usually limited by the blood flow. Drugs that are insoluble at tissue pH or that are in an oily vehicle form a depot in the muscle tissue, from which absorption proceeds very slowly.

At times, intramuscular administration may be disadvantageous, as in the case of diazepam, which enters the general circulation more consistently and predictably when administered orally than when injected into muscle. Because frequently repeated injections are inconvenient to patients and physicians alike, much ingenuity has been expended in developing *depot preparations* of various drugs for intramuscular use.[10] For example, the procaine salt of penicillin is injected as a microcrystalline suspension, which dissolves and enters the bloodstream over a period of 12 to 24 hours.

Subcutaneous Administration

Absorption of drugs from the subcutaneous tissues is influenced by the same factors that determine the rate of absorption from intramuscular sites.[11] Blood flow is said to be poorer than in muscle and the absorptive surface area may be less, so that the absorption rate is usually considered to be slower. Actually, there seems to be no simple way to measure blood flow in a subcutaneous area. Some drugs, at least, are known to be absorbed as rapidly from subcutaneous tissues as from muscle. It should be stressed that the subcutaneous route may give rise to considerable variability in drug entry. For example, both rapid-acting and intermediate-acting insulins have been shown to be absorbed at different rates after subcutaneous injection in the thigh or the arm of the same individual, leading to significant differences in postprandial blood glucose levels.[12]

If a patient has poor peripheral perfusion, drugs may not be absorbed rapidly enough from sites of subcutaneous or intramuscular injection to achieve effective plasma concentrations. This is particularly a problem when administering antibiotics to patients who are in shock, and these patients should receive intravenous therapy.[13]

Certain drugs produce severe pain when injected subcutaneously; local necrosis and sterile abscesses may also occur. Some agents have to be administered intravenously because no solution concentrated enough to be useful can be given subcutaneously or intramuscularly.

The rate of absorption from a subcutaneous depot may be retarded by immobilization of the limb, local cooling to cause vasoconstriction, and application of a tourniquet proximal to the injection site to block the superficial venous drainage and lymphatic flow. These techniques, customarily applied to slow down venom absorption in snake bites, are also of value in the emergency treatment of adverse drug reactions after subcutaneous or intramuscular administration. Epinephrine, in minute amounts, may be incorporated with a subcutaneous injection in order to constrict the local vasculature and thereby retard absorption. This is of special value when the injected drug is meant to act locally at the injection site rather than systemically. The best example is the inclusion of epinephrine in preparations of local anesthetic agents to prolong their action on sensory nerve fibers passing through the subcutaneous tissues. Drugs may affect the rate of their own absorption if they alter the blood supply or capillary permeability locally. Methacholine, for example, causes vascular dilation as part of its cholinergic action; consequently it enters the bloodstream so rapidly from a subcutaneous site that it causes systemic effects as early as 1.5 min after injection.

An effective way of achieving slow absorption for a long time is to incorporate a drug into a compressed pellet that can be implanted under the skin. The drug must be relatively insoluble, and the pellet must resist disintegration or rapid dissolution by the subcutaneous fluid environment. These conditions have been achieved with certain steroid hormones.[10,14] Cylindrical pellets of testosterone about 5 mm in diameter, 5 mm thick, and weighing 100 mg were implanted subcutaneously into human subjects. Upon removal at different intervals for individual subjects, the pellets were weighed carefully, and the weight loss was thus determined. Figure 3-3 shows that the absorption rate was nearly

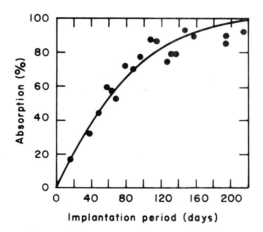

Fig. 3-3. Rate of absorption of testosterone pellets in human subjects. Pellets weighed 100 mg and were cylindrical (diameter 5 mm, thickness 5 mm). Implantation sites were subcutaneous. Each point represents a pellet in a single subject. Pellets were weighed initially and again after removal. The curve is a theoretical one calculated from an arbitrary rate constant of absorption on the assumption that absorption rate is proportional to surface area throughout the dissolution process. (From Bishop and Folley[14] with permission.)

constant at about 1 percent per day for 2 months and then diminished gradually, with absorption essentially complete at 5 to 6 months. For spherical pellets the ratio of surface area to volume increases with decreasing diameter. Thus, when drugs are prepared as spheres of known diameter, the rate of absorption can be predicted; the larger the spheres, the slower the rate of absorption of a given amount of drug.[10] This principle has been used in the design of long-acting insulin preparations; the so-called Lente insulins are small zinc insulin crystals of uniform size (about 30 μm) to provide a reproducible rate of absorption. However, as degradation of insulin may occur at the subcutaneous injection site, prolongation of absorption may not always be an advantage.

The ideal shape of a subcutaneous pellet for achieving a constant rate of absorption would be a flat disk. Absorption should occur almost exclusively from the two opposite surfaces, since the area of the edge is negligible by comparison. Moreover, the exposed area for absorption would hardly change at all as the disk becomes thinner, so that the absorption rate would be nearly constant until practically all the drug is absorbed. Studies in rats and mice have verified the correctness of these predictions. A useful experimental technique for establishing morphine tolerance and dependence in various small laboratory animals employs subcutaneously implanted pellets of morphine. The drug is released into the body at a constant rate for several days, producing a steady-state level, much as would be attained by a constant intravenous infusion.

Absorption of Drugs Through the Skin

The skin efficiently retards the diffusion and evaporation of water except at the sweat glands. The epidermis, although only about 0.2 mm thick, is largely responsible. The outer, horny layer (stratum corneum) consists of a sheet of keratinized lamellae of anucleate, thin flat cells, densely packed but associated with surface and intercellular lipids, which constitutes a barrier to the penetration of water-soluble substances. Thus, the intact epidermis behaves qualitatively as do cellular membranes in general.[15] Drugs penetrate at rates determined largely by their lipid/water partition coefficients, water-soluble ions and polar molecules (except for the very smallest) being virtually excluded.[16] Even substances that are very lipid-soluble penetrate solwly in comparison with their rates of penetration of other, thinner, cell membranes. The underlying dermis, which consists of loosely arranged connective tissue and is vascularized, is freely permeable to water-soluble compounds. The properties of the principle layers of skin are summarized in Table 3-1.

Two problems have to be considered in relation to percutaneous absorption of drugs: the use of this route for therapy and the absorption of toxic substances through the skin. The therapeutic application of drugs presents no special problem of penetration if the action is to be upon the exposed surface (as in treatment of wounds or burns) or within the superficial layers of the epidermis. Drugs may be incorporated into vehicles (creams, ointments) that adhere to the skin and permit local diffusion, or baths containing the drug may be employed. As would be expected from their lipid solubility, retinoids and steroids such as the anti-inflammatory glucocorticoids and the sex hormones diffuse readily into the skin after topical application. They are retained in the skin for long periods, and they are also metabolized there. However, if the drug is water-soluble and if the pathologic condition is in the deeper layers of the epidermis or in the dermis, systemic administration may be necessary. Antibacterial and antifungal agents, for example, are often more ef-

Table 3-1 Stratified Organization of the Skin

Layers	Epidermis	Dermis	Subcutaneous Fat
Function	Barrier	Connective tissue support	Thermal insulation, cushion
Embryonic origin	Ectoderm	Mesoderm	Mesoderm
Thickness (mm)	0.2	3–5	Variable
pH	4.2–6.5	7.2–7.3	—
H₂O content (%)	10–25	Up to 70	Low
Cellular activity	Actively dividing cells	Mostly noncellular	Closely packed cells
Cellular contents	Keratinocytes → keratin Melanocytes → melanin	Fibrocytes → collagen Fibroblasts, histiocytes, mast cells	Adipocytes → lipids
Vasculature	None	Blood vessels, lymphatics, sweat glands	Blood vessels

(From Katz and Poulsen,[16] with permission.)

fective in skin infections when given by mouth or by injection than when applied to the skin surface.

Much investigation has been directed toward developing pharmacologically inert organic solvents that might facilitate drug penetration through the skin. Dimethyl sulfoxide CH_3SOCH_3 (DMSO) is an example.[17] This liquid is miscible with water and with many organic solvents and is capable of increasing the penetration of ionized drugs into the deeper layers of skin. Unfortunately, these effects are accompanied by (or even in part attributable to) local tissue damage, and some generalized toxicity has also been observed in animal experiments. A variety of other chemicals have been shown to enhance skin permeability of drugs, including N_1N_1-dimethylacetamide, N_1N_1-dimethylformamide, certain pyrrolidones, azocycloalkan-2-ones, and tetrahydrofurfuryl alcohol.[18]

Toxic effects are often produced by the accidental absorption through the skin of highly lipid-soluble substances used for various industrial purposes. General experience leads people to suppose that the skin is a reliable protection against the environment, so little thought is given to the possibility of poisoning by this route. Carbon tetrachloride, other organic solvents, and tetraethyllead penetrate the body in this way and can cause serious toxic effects. Organic phosphate insecticides (DFP, parathion, malathion) have caused deaths in agricultural workers as a result of percutaneous absorption. Hexachlorophene, an antiseptic agent effective against gram-positive microorganisms, was once used in human neonates to cleanse the skin. However, its use was curtailed when it was associated with a devastating myelinopathy in preterm, low birthweight infants. This neurotoxicity was traced to excessive absorption of the antiseptic through the intact skin.[19]

Electrical gradients have been used to drive drugs into the skin in the method known as *iontophoresis*. An ionized drug in solution is placed in an absorbent material on the skin in contact with an electrode. By applying a galvanic current to this electrode and to another place elsewhere on the body surface, the drug ions are made to migrate through the epidermis. Studies with iodine 131 have shown that this method is quite efficient, at least for introducing very small amounts of drugs into the skin and general circulation. The reproducibility, however, between subjects and even between different skin areas in the same subject leaves much to be desired. The method has been investigated in attempts to induce transcutaneous delivery of anti-inflammatory drugs and insulin,[20] but its general utility is obviously rather limited.

The concept of controlled transdermal drug delivery has been demonstrated and commercialized with a skin patch system in which scopolamine is delivered to the skin surface at a preprogrammed rate.[21] Control of delivery rate may be achieved by interposing a microporous membrane between a drug reservoir and the skin surface or by formulating the drug in high concentration in a polymer matrix. Transdermal drug delivery systems of this nature have been developed to administer nitroglycerin, clonidine, and estradiol.[10,22] In theory, controlled transdermal drug delivery may mimic a constant intravenous infusion if the drug diffuses transdermally at a sufficient rate to maintain effective plasma drug concentrations. In practice, regional dermal permeation differences and variability between patients in dermal permeation and systemic pharmacokinetics, as well as drug tolerance (e.g., nitroglycerin) or intolerance must be overcome in order to achieve widespread acceptance of this class of transdermal delivery systems. Transdermal scopolamine patches were originally developed for astronauts, but they have become quite popular with travelers prone to motion sickness.[23]

Inhalation of Drugs

Drugs may be inhaled as gases and enter the circulation by diffusing across the alveolar membranes. This is the mode of administration of the volatile anesthetics. These drugs all have relatively high lipid/water partition coefficients, and inasmuch as their atomic or molecular radii are quite small and the alveolar membrane is quite permeable, they all equilibrate practically instantaneously with blood in the alveolar capillaries. The interesting differences among these agents in the kinetics of their equilibration in whole body water and in the rates of onset and decline of their anesthetic effects depend primarily upon their aqueous solubilities (blood/air partition coefficients). This will be discussed fully in Chapter 4.

Drugs may also be inhaled as *aerosols*,[24,25] and many toxic substances enter the body in this way. Aerosols are liquid or solid particles so small that they remain suspended in air for a long time instead of sedimenting rapidly under the force of gravity. Table 3-2 gives sedimentation rate as a function of particle diameter, computed from Stokes' law for the viscous drag on a moving sphere.

Stokes' law states:

$$f = 6\pi nrv$$

where f is force in dynes, n is viscosity of air at 20°C and atmospheric pressure and is equal to 1.9×10^{-4} g sec^{-1} cm^{-1}, r is radius of the sphere in centimeters, and v is constant velocity of movement when force f is balanced by the viscous drag.

Table 3-2 Rate of Gravitational Sedimentation in Quiet Air as a Function of Particle Size

Particle Diameter, μm	*a*Sedimentation Rate, cm sec^{-1}
100	28.7
50	7.17
25	1.79
10	0.287
5	0.072
1	0.0029

a Sedimentation rates are computed from Stokes' law as described in the text

For a sphere moving under the force of gravity, $f = \text{mass} \times g$, where $g = 980$ cm sec^{-2}; and assuming unity density,

$$f = \frac{4}{3}\pi r^3 g$$

When the viscous drag opposes the force of gravity so that the rate of fall is constant,

$$6\pi n r v = \frac{4}{3}\pi r^3 g$$

$$v = \frac{D^2 g}{18n}$$

$$v = 2.87 \times 10^5 D^2$$

where D is the diameter of the sphere in centimeters.

Particles below about 10 μm in diameter are of interest for the present discussion. Examples are bacteria and viruses, smoke, industrial fumes, dust laden with fission products from nuclear explosions, pollens, plant spores, insecticide dusts or sprays, and inhalant sprays used in the therapy of pulmonary disease.[26]

Impaction is the term used to describe the deposition of aerosol particles in the respiratory tract. The degree of impaction is determined by the rates of sedimentation, diffusion, and inertial precipitation. In considering the rate of movement of substances within the respiratory tract, diffusion may be ignored, except for very small particles. Inertial precipitation arises from the tendency of a particle moving in a stream of air to continue in its original direction when the air current changes direction, and thus to impact upon some tissue. This occurs, for example, at bronchial branch points.

The extent of impaction in different parts of the respiratory tract may be computed for particles of various sizes, and such computations have been confirmed by some experimental data.[26,27] In the nasal passages large particles (>10 μm) are almost completely removed; about half of the particles 5 μm in diameter and about one-fifth of the particles 2 μm in diameter are removed. Below 1 μm, nasal impaction is negligible. Table 3-3 gives theoretical results for particle sizes between 0.2 and 20 μm, at two extreme values of the

Table 3-3 Percent Retention of Inhaled Aerosol Particles in Various Regions of the Respiratory Tract

	Percent Retention									
	450 cm³ Tidal Air					1,500 cm³ Tidal Air				
	20	6	2	0.6	0.2	20	6	2	0.6	0.2
Mouth	15	0	0	0	0	18	1	0	0	0
Pharynx	8	0	0	0	0	10	1	0	0	0
Trachea	10	1	0	0	0	19	3	0	0	0
Pulmonary bronchi	12	2	0	0	0	20	5	1	0	0
Secondary bronchi	19	4	1	0	0	21	12	2	0	0
Tertiary bronchi	17	9	2	0	0	9	20	5	0	0
Quarternary bronchi	6	7	2	1	1	1	10	3	1	1
Terminal bronchioles	6	19	6	4	6	1	9	3	2	4
Respiratory bronchioles	0	11	5	3	4	0	3	2	2	4
Alveolar ducts	0	25	25	8	11	0	13	26	10	13
Alveolar sacs	0	5	0	0	0	0	18	17	6	7
Totals	93	83	41	16	22	99	95	59	21	29

[a] The figures in the columns are percent retention; the column headings are particle sizes in μm. A 4-second respiratory cycle is assumed.
(From Hatch and Gross,[28] with permission.)

tidal air. The following conclusions may be drawn: (1) The larger the particle, the greater its tendency to impact and be retained in the upper respiratory tract. (2) At high tidal volumes and the same respiratory rate the air stream velocity is greater, and thus particles of all sizes tend to be driven deeper into the pulmonary tree before impacting. (3) As particles become smaller, their retention is primarily limited to the most peripheral parts of the pulmonary tree, beyond the terminal bronchioles, but the total retention is substantially less than for larger particles. (4) When particles become extremely small (0.2 μm), the total retention begins to increase again, probably because diffusion becomes a significant factor in the translocation of particles from the lumen to the walls of the bronchioles and alveoli.

A mucous blanket, propelled cephalad by ciliary movements, covers the upper respiratory tract down to the terminal bronchioles, and impacted aerosol particles are cleared by this mechanism. Particles that deposit in the alveolar sacs must first be transported up to the mucous layer, presumably in a fluid film covering the epithelium. Particles in the alveoli are also ingested by phagocytic cells. The efficiency of clearance of solid particles from the lungs is remarkable. For example, not more than a minute fraction of all the mineral dust inhaled during a lifetime is retained in the lungs. However, a small decrease in the clearance capacity of the lungs could cause a marked increase in the amount of retained particulate matter; this may be a factor leading to the development of pneumoconiosis in miners exposed to silica dusts.

Particle size strongly influences the rate at which material is absorbed through the alveolar epithelium, probably because of the greatly increased surface area for solubilization as particle diameter becomes smaller. For example, particles of uranium dioxide larger than 3 μm had no toxic effect whatsoever when introduced into the trachea in rats, but the same relatively insoluble material was absorbed into the circulation and caused kidney damage when smaller particles were employed.

Exposure to lead in aerosol form presents a potentially serious occupational and environmental hazard, largely because of the widespread use of organic lead compounds (e.g., tetraethyllead) in gasoline. Lead is released from motor vehicles largely as lead halides, which are converted in the atmosphere to carbonates and oxides. The median diameter of airborne lead particulates is 0.1 to 0.2 μm, small enough to be absorbed with good efficiency (25 to 50 percent) from the respiratory tract.[29,30] Rural areas typically have atmospheric lead concentrations as low as 0.5 μg m^{-3}, whereas in urban centers such as Los Angeles the concentrations were found to be 5 to 16 μg m^{-3} and even higher during busy traffic hours. Figure 3-4 gives the observed relationship between average exposures to atmospheric lead and the mean blood level. The data are from various subjects living and working in different environments—farmers, city dwellers, traffic policemen, and so on. Also included are data from volunteers exposed to atmospheres of known lead content. Blood levels of about 100 ng ml^{-1} (at extreme left of figure) reflect the enteral absorption of about 10 percent of the average 300 μg dietary intake.[31] It is clear that lead aerosols, derived almost entirely from leaded fuels, can contribute significantly to the body burden of this heavy metal. An atmospheric concentration of 10 μg m^{-3}, yielding about 320 ng ml^{-1} in blood, has been considered to be a "safe" exposure level,[32] but the long-term toxic effects of chronic exposure to low concentrations have not been sufficiently studied. Recent studies indicate that levels well below 250 ng ml^{-1} currently defined as the highest acceptable level for young children, may in fact adversely affect the fetus.[33]

Drugs in aerosol form can elicit very rapid responses when inhaled. Histamine or pil-

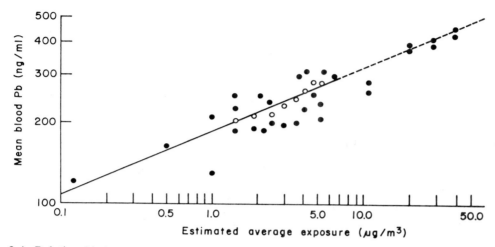

Fig. 3-4. Relationship between respiratory exposure to lead and the mean blood level. Open circles are epidemiologic data, solid circles are data from experimental subjects. (From Goldsmith and Hexter,[29] with permission.)

ocarpine administered in this way to dogs or guinea pigs can cause bronchiolar constriction and fatal asphyxia within 1 minute. An aerosol containing atropine can reverse within a minute the bronchospasm caused by a carbachol aerosol.

Particles larger than 6 μm in diameter probably do not reach the alveolar sacs, as shown in Table 3-3. Although aerosol particles in the range of 1 to 5 μm are most efficiently deposited in the lower respiratory tract,[27] aerosol generators used in therapy produce particles that are 0.5 to 35 μm in diameter.[34] Only 13 percent of particles produced by a metered-dose inhaler are in the 1 to 5 μm range.[35] Nebulizers produce an even smaller percentage of particles in this size range.[36] A technique that promotes deposition of particles is for subjects to hold their breath after inhalation to maximize the effective time for particle diffusion. Another technique is to add hygroscopic substances to the aerosol; the droplets then become larger as they traverse the moist respiratory tract, and the rate of impaction due to sedimentation is increased.

With aerosols of small particle size the amount of drug reaching the alveoli may be large, and since the rate of absorption into the bloodstream is much more rapid at the alveolar sacs than elsewhere in the pulmonary tree, the systemic absorption of the drug may be appreciable. Hence, care must be exercised in giving drugs such as the sympathomimetic bronchodilators by aerosol to avoid side effects on the cardiovascular system. Isoproterenol, for example, in a 0.5 percent aerosol, is an effective bronchodilator, but a 1 per cent aerosol is apt to cause undesirable cardioaccelerator and hypotensive actions after only a few inhalations.

Drug delivery by aerosol is becoming increasingly widespread, particularly in the treatment of bronchial asthma, for which a number of bronchodilating aerosols based on β₂ sympathomimetic amines or atropine-like peripheral anticholinergics as active principles are in use.[36] Between 1961 and 1966 there was a marked increase in prescriptions and sales of pressurized isoproterenol aerosols in England and Wales, which was paralleled by an increase in asthma mortality, particularly in the 10- to 14-year age group.[37] Following a general alert regarding overuse and misuse of pressurized aerosol canisters, asthma mortality quickly declined to its former level. After considerable debate and controversy, the most widely accepted conclusion was that, in general, patients died from the disease rather than from its treatment. When excessive use of bronchodilators does occasionally coincide with asthma death, it is felt that this indicates inadequate treatment with other drugs, such as corticosteroids, and that excessive aerosol use is not itself the cause of death.[36] However, the debate on aerosol-associated mortality in asthmatics in the 1960s still continues. With the development of selective β_2 sympathomimetics as well as better controlled delivery devices, the problem has diminished.

Drugs may be delivered by inhalation, not only as aerosols but as fine powders. One example is the mast-cell modifier cromolyn sodium, which is effective in the prevention of allergic asthma and is not absorbed from the gastrointestinal tract. Although most of an inhaled dose is eventually swallowed, the small portion reaching the alveoli is rapidly absorbed, producing blood concentrations detectable over 4 hours. Finally, mention should be made of the intranasal route of administration, which is occasionally utilized for systemic delivery of drugs such as the derivatives of vasopressin, used in treating diabetes insipidus.

Administration of Drugs by the Enteral Route

Drugs are given most commonly by mouth. Absorption, in general, takes place along the whole length of the upper gastrointestinal tract, but the chemical properties of each drug determine whether it will be absorbed in the strongly acid stomach or in the nearly neutral small intestine.[38] Gastric absorption is often (but not always) favored by an empty stomach, in which the drug, in undiluted gastric juice, will have good access to the mucosal wall. When a drug is irritating to the gastric mucosa, it may be rational to administer it with or after a meal. The antibiotic griseofulvin is an example of a substance with poor water solubility, the absorption of which is aided by a fatty meal.[39] The rate of absorption of certain sustained-release oral theophylline preparations is dramatically increased if a high fat meal is ingested within hours of drug administration. The large surface area of the intestinal villi, the presence of bile, and the rich blood supply all favor intestinal absorption.

The presence of food can impair the absorption of drugs given by mouth. Suggested mechanisms include reduced mixing, complexing with substances in the food, and retarded gastric emptying. In experiments with rats prolonged fasting was shown to diminish the absorption of several drugs, possibly by deleterious effects upon the epithelium of intestinal villi.[40]

Drugs that are metabolized or extracted rapidly by the liver may not be effective when given by the enteral route because the portal circulation carries them directly to the liver. An example is lidocaine, already discussed for its value in controlling cardiac arrhythmias. This drug is absorbed well from the gut but is largely inactivated in a single passage through the liver.[41,42]

Drugs are occasionally administered by rectum, but most are not as well absorbed here as from the upper intestine. Rectal absorption, in part, avoids the portal circulation. The drug coats the rectal membranes upon melting of the suppository. Inert vehicles employed for suppository preparations include cocoa butter, glycerinated gelatin, and polyethylene glycol. Owing to erratic absorption, suppository formulations are rarely recommended for systemic drug delivery in adult medicine. Some use is still made of this route in pediatric medicine (e.g., for administration of analgesic-antipyretic drugs when oral dosing is difficult. Topical treatment of mild ulcerative colitis limited to the rectum or rectosigmoid is possible with corticosteroid retention enemas or foams. Systemic absorption of the active drug is in the range of 10 to 20 percent of the dosage instilled.

The principles governing the absorption of drugs from the gastrointestinal lumen are the same as for the passage of drugs across biologic membranes elsewhere. Low degree of ionization, high lipid/water partition coefficient of the nonionized form, and small atomic or molecular radius of water-soluble substances all favor rapid absorption. Water passes readily in both directions across the wall of the gastrointestinal lumen. Sodium ions are probably transported actively from lumen into blood. Magnesium ions are very poorly absorbed and therefore magnesium acts as a cathartic, retaining an osmotic equivalent of water as it passes down the intestinal tract. Ionic iron is absorbed as an amino acid complex, at a rate that is regulated by the body's need for iron. Glucose and amino acids are transported across the intestinal wall by specific carrier systems. Some compounds of high molecular weight (polysaccharides, neutral fats) cannot be absorbed *until* they are degraded enzymatically. Other substances are not absorbed *because* they are destroyed by gastrointestinal enzymes; insulin, epinephrine, and histamine are examples. Substances that form insoluble precipitates in the gastrointestinal lumen or that are not soluble either in water or in lipid obviously cannot be absorbed.

Absorption of Weak Acids and Bases

Gastric secretion is very acid (about pH 1), whereas the intestinal contents are nearly neutral (actually very slightly acid). The pH difference between plasma (pH 7.4) and the lumen of the gastrointestinal tract plays a major role in determining whether a drug that is a weak electrolyte will be absorbed into plasma or whether it will be excreted from plasma into the stomach or intestine. We may assume for practical purposes that the mucosal lining of the gastrointestinal tract is impermeable to the ionized form of a weak acid or base, but that the nonionized form equilibrates freely. The rate of equilibration of the nonionized molecule is directly related to its lipid solubility. If there is a pH difference across the membrane, then the fraction ionized may be considerably greater on one side than on the other. At equilibrium the concentration of the *nonionized* moiety will be the same on both sides, but there will be more *total* drug on the side on which the degree of ionization is greater. This mechanism is known as *ion trapping*. The energy for sustaining the unequal chemical potential of the acid or base in question is derived from whatever mechanism maintains the pH difference; in the stomach this mechanism is the energy-dependent secretion of hydrogen ions.

Consider how a weak electrolyte distributes across the gastric mucosa between plasma (pH 7.4) and gastric fluid (pH 1.0). In each compartment the Henderson-Hasselbalch equation gives the ratio of the concentrations [base]/[acid]. Here, and throughout the rest of this book, we shall designate the negative logarithm of the acid dissociation constant by the symbol pK_a.

$$pH = pK_a + \log \frac{[base]}{[acid]}$$

$$\log \frac{[base]}{[acid]} = pH - pK_a$$

$$\frac{[base]}{[acid]} = antilog\ (pH - pK_a)$$

For a weak acid with $pK_a = 3$, $pH - pK_a = 4.4$ in plasma and -2 in stomach. Thus, in plasma at equilibrium, log ([base]/[acid]) = 4.4, and [base]/[acid] = 25,000. In stomach, log ([base]/[acid]) = -2, and [base]/[acid] = 0.01. Now for a weak acid it is the acid moiety that is nonionized and is in free equilibrium in both compartments:

Plasma pH 7.4	Stomach pH 1.0
$H^+ + A^- \rightleftharpoons HA$	$HA \rightleftharpoons H^+ + A^-$
$25,000 \rightleftharpoons 1.0$	$1.0 \rightleftharpoons 0.01$

Total drug
(i.e., base + acid):

	Plasma	Stomach
	25,001	1.01
or:	24,800	1.0

For a weak base with the same pK_a, the fraction [base]/[acid] in each compartment will, of course, be exactly the same as above. The difference is that now the nonionized form, which has to be equated on both sides, is the base:

	Plasma		Stomach
$\dfrac{[base]}{[acid]}$	$\dfrac{25,000}{1}$	$\rightleftharpoons$	$\dfrac{0.01}{1}$

Rewriting these fractions to equate the numerators, we obtain

	Plasma		Stomach
	$\dfrac{1}{4 \times 10^{-5}}$	$\rightleftharpoons$	$\dfrac{1}{100}$

	Plasma	Stomach
Total drug concentration ratio	1	101

The conclusions are obvious. Weak acids are absorbed readily from the stomach. Weak bases are not absorbed well; indeed, they would tend to accumulate within the stomach at the expense of drug in the bloodstream. Naturally, in the more alkaline intestine, bases would be absorbed better, acids more poorly.

A simple general equation to describe the concentration ratios of a drug on both sides of a membrane at equilibrium, as determined by the ion-trapping mechanism, may be derived as follows[43]:

Let the two sides be at pH_I and pH_{II}. Then

$$pH = pK_a + \log \frac{[base]}{[acid]}$$

$$\log \frac{[base]}{[acid]} = pH - pK_a$$

$$\frac{[base]}{[acid]} = 10^{(pH - pK_a)}$$

and R, the ratio of total drug concentration on side I to that on side II, is given by

$$R = \frac{[\text{acid}_\text{I}] + [\text{base}_\text{I}]}{[\text{acid}_\text{II}] + [\text{base}_\text{II}]}$$

Substituting base = acid $\cdot 10^{(\text{pH} - \text{p}K_\text{a})}$, we obtain

$$R = \frac{[\text{acid}_\text{I}] (1 + 10^{\text{pH}_\text{I} - \text{p}K_\text{a}})}{[\text{acid}_\text{II}](1 + 10^{\text{pH}_\text{II} - \text{p}K_\text{a}})}$$

For acids, $(\text{acid}_\text{I}) = (\text{acid}_\text{II})$, so that

$$R = \frac{1 + 10^{\text{pH}_\text{I} - \text{p}K_\text{a}}}{1 + 10^{\text{pH}_\text{II} - \text{p}K_\text{a}}}$$

$$R = \frac{1 + \text{antilog} (\text{pH}_\text{I} - \text{p}K_a)}{1 + \text{antilog} (\text{pH}_\text{II} - \text{p}K_a)}$$

For bases,

$$[\text{acid}] = \frac{[\text{base}]}{10^{(\text{pH} - \text{p}K_\text{a})}} = [\text{base}] \cdot 10^{(\text{p}K_\text{a} - \text{pH})}$$

$$R = \frac{[\text{base}_\text{I}](1 + 10^{\text{p}K_\text{a} - \text{pH}_\text{I}})}{[\text{base}_\text{II}](1 + 10^{\text{p}K_\text{a} - \text{pH}_\text{II}})}$$

and since $(\text{base}_\text{I}) = (\text{base}_\text{II})$,

$$R = \frac{1 + 10^{\text{p}K_\text{a} - \text{pH}_\text{I}}}{1 + 10^{\text{p}K_\text{a} - \text{pH}_\text{II}}}$$

$$R = \frac{1 + \text{antilog} (\text{p}K_a - \text{pH}_\text{I})}{1 + \text{antilog} (\text{p}K_a - \text{pH}_\text{II})}$$

It should be realized that although the principles outlined here are correct, the system is dynamic, not static. Drug molecules that are absorbed across the gastric or intestinal mucosa are removed constantly by blood flow; thus, simple reversible equilibrium across the membrane does not occur until the drug is distributed throughout the body.

The volume of the stomach or intestine from which the drug is being absorbed is small with respect to the total body volume in which the drug is distributed. Moreover, drug that has crossed the membranes of the gastrointestinal tract is rapidly distributed away from the gut by the lymphatic and portal venous systems. Accordingly, drug absorption is more accurately treated as a rate of diffusion from a point source into a larger sink of far lower drug concentration. Under these circumstances the rate of drug absorption dQ/dt can be equated as follows for organic acids:

$$\frac{dQ}{dt} = D\,(\text{SA})(\text{PC}) \frac{1}{(1 + 10^{(\text{pH} - \text{p}K_\text{a})})} \left(\frac{dc}{dx}\right)$$

and for organic bases:

$$\frac{dQ}{dt} = D\,(\text{SA})\,(\text{PC}) \frac{1}{(1 + 10^{\text{p}K_\text{a} - \text{pH}})} \left(\frac{dc}{dx}\right)$$

where D is the diffusion coefficient of the drug, SA is the surface area of absorption, PC is the lipid/water partition coefficient, and dc/dx is the concentration gradient across the membrane.

While many of these parameters cannot be precisely determined, a knowledge of their relative magnitude illustrates the principles of drug absorption. The diffusion coefficient is influenced by the molecular radius of the drug, temperature, and viscosity. Most congeneric drugs have approximately the same molecular radius so this term will not show a large variance. The viscosity term is the viscosity in the membrane and also will not be highly variant. On the other hand, the viscosity of the luminal content may retard the rate at which drugs reach the membrane by diffusion and may be a primary factor in diminishing absorption from the colon.

The surface area term shows large differences. For example, owing to the microvillae, the surface area of the intestine is 1,000 times that of the stomach and is a primary factor in the increased absorption in the intestine. Also effective absorptive surface area will be increased by tablet disintegration and mixing of gastric contents. The partition coefficient can also vary substantially and accounts for the more rapid absorption of lipid-soluble drugs. The exponential pH and pK_a term accounts for the fraction of drug in the ionized state that will not diffuse across the membrane. Accordingly, this term will only serve to decrease the flux rate. Finally the dc/dx or concentration gradient term is largely influenced by the concentration in the gut since the diffusion distance is probably constant. Hence the higher the concentration, the greater the flux rate.

The above equations are not useful for measuring absolute rates of absorption but rather are valuable in comparing rates of absorption of closely related drugs. In such situations one may analyze the effect of partition coefficient and gastrointestinal tract pH on rates of drug absorption.

Absorption from the stomach, as determined by direct measurements, conforms, in general, to the principles outlined above. Organic acids are absorbed well since they are all almost completely nonionized at the gastric pH. Strong acids whose pK_a values lie below 1, which are ionized even in the acid contents of the stomach, are not absorbed well. Weak bases are absorbed only negligibly, but their absorption can be increased, as expected, by raising the pH of the gastric fluid. All this is shown in Table 3-4, the results of experiments in which drugs were placed in the ligated stomachs of rats and the residual amounts determined after 1 hour.[44] Especially interesting is the effect of changing the stomach pH by addition of sodium bicarbonate. Acids such as salicylic and nitrosalicylic acids, with pK_as well on the acid side of neutrality, were absorbed much more poorly when the gastric acidity had been neutralized, for they were then almost completely ionized. Very weak acids such as thiopental and phenol were but little affected by the same pH change, since even at pH 8 they remained almost wholly nonionized.

The three barbituric acid derivatives studied (Table 3-4, thiopental, barbital, secobarbital) are interesting because, although they have about the same pK_a, the extent of their gastric absorption differed considerably. This is related to the difference in lipid/water partition coefficients of their nonionized forms. Measurements in a number of organic solvents have revealed that thiopental has the highest partition coefficient, secobarbital a considerably smaller one, and barbital the smallest of all.

As for bases, only the weakest were absorbed to any appreciable extent (Table 3-4) at normal gastric pH, but their absorption could be increased substantially by neutralizing the stomach contents. The quaternary cations, however, which are charged at all pH values, were not absorbed at either pH.

The accumulation of weak bases in the stomach by ion trapping mimics a secretory

Table 3-4 Absorption of Organic Acids and Organic Bases from the Rat Stomach

	pK_a	Percent Absorbed in 1 hour	
		0.1 M HCl	NaHCO₃, pH8
Acid:			
5-Sulfosalicylic	(strong)	0 ± 0 (2)	0 ± 0 (2)
Phenolsulfonphthalein	(strong)	2 ± 2 (3)	2 ± 1 (2)
5-Nitrosalicylic	2.3	52 ± 3 (2)	16 ± 2 (2)
Salicylic	3.0	61 ± 7 (4)	13 ± 1 (2)
Acetylsalicylic	3.5	35 ± 4 (3)	—
Benzoic	4.2	55 ± 3 (2)	—
Thiopental	7.6	46 ± 3 (2)	34 ± 2 (2)
p-Hydroxypropiophenone	7.8	55 ± 3 (2)	—
Barbital	7.8	4 ± 3 (4)	—
Secobarbital	7.9	30 ± 2 (2)	—
Phenol	9.9	40 ± 5 (3)	40 ± 5 (3)
Base:			
Acetanilid	0.3	36 ± 3 (2)	—
Caffeine	0.8	24 ± 3 (2)	—
Antipyrine	1.4	14 ± 3 (4)	—
m-Nitroaniline	2.5	17 ± 0 (2)	—
Aniline	4.6	6 ± 4 (3)	56 ± 3 (2)
Aminopyridine	5.0	2 ± 2 (3)	—
p-Toluidine	5.3	0 ± 0 (2)	47 ± 4 (2)
α-Acetylmethadol	8.3	0 ± 0 (4)	—
Quinine	8.4	0 ± 0 (2)	18 ± 2 (2)
Dextrorphan, levorphanol	9.2	0 ± 2 (8)	16 ± 1 (2)
Ephedrine	9.6	3 ± 3 (2)	—
Tolazoline	10.3	7 ± 2 (4)	—
Mecamylamine	11.2	0 ± 0 (2)	—
Darstine	(cation)	0 ± 0 (2)	—
Procaine amide ethobromide	(cation)	0 ± 0 (2)	5 ± 1 (2)
Tetraethylammonium	(cation)	0 ± 1 (2)	—

The percent absorbed in 1 hour is expressed as mean ± range, followed by the number of experiments in parentheses.
(Modified from Schanker et al.,[44] with permission.)

process; if the drug is administered systemically, it accumulates in the stomach. Dogs were given various drugs intravenously by continuous infusion to maintain a constant drug level in the plasma, and the gastric contents were sampled by means of an indwelling catheter.[45] The results, representing concentrations after 30 to 60 minutes, are shown in Table 3-5. Both acids and bases behaved according to expectation. The stronger bases ($pK_a > 5$) accumulated in stomach contents to many times their plasma concentrations; the weak bases appeared in about equal concentrations in gastric juice and in plasma. Among the acids only the weakest appeared in detectable amounts in the stomach. It may be wondered why the strong bases, which are completely ionized in gastric juice and whose theoretical concentration ratios (gastric juice/plasma) are very large, should nevertheless have attained only about 40-fold excess over plasma. Direct measurements of arterial and venous blood showed that essentially all the blood flowing through the gastric mucosa was cleared of these drugs; obviously, no more drug could enter the gastric juice in a given time than was brought there by the circulation. Another limitation comes into play when the base pK_a exceeds 7.4; now, a major fraction of the circulating base is cationic and a decreasing fraction is nonionized, so that the effective concentration gradient for diffusion across the stomach wall is reduced.

The ion trapping mechanism provides a method of some forensic value for determining

Table 3-5. Gastric Secretion of Drugs in the Dog

	pK_a	Plasma Protein Binding (%)	Plasma Concentration (Total) (mg/L)	Gastric Juice Concentration (mg/L)	Gastric Juice/ Plasma Concentration Ratio	Ratio Corrected for Plasma Binding	Theoretical Ratio
Bases:							
Acetanilid	0.3	0	126	126	1.0	1.0	1.0
Theophylline	0.7	15	81	118	1.5	1.3	1.5
Antipyrine	1.4	0	230	938	4.1	4.2	4.2
Aniline	5.0	25	8.5	358	42		10^4
Aminopyrine	5.0	15	24	1010	42		10^4
Quinine	8.4	75	4.7	189	40		10^6
Levorphanol	9.2	50	0.2	8.3	42		10^6
Tolazoline	10.3	23	13.2	135	10		10^6
Acids:							
Salicylic	3.0	75	338	0	0	0	10^{-4}
Probenecid	3.4	75	14	0	0	0	10^{-4}
Phenylbutazone	4.4	90	195	0	0	0	10^{-3}
p-Hydroxypropiophenone	7.8	75	5.5	0.62	0.11	0.5	0.6
Thiopental	7.6	75	20	2.0	0.10	0.5	0.6
Barbital	7.8	0	254	152	0.6	0.6	0.6

Measurements were made 30 to 60 min after initiation of continuous intravenous drug infusion.
(From Shore et al.,[45] with permission.)

the presence of alkaloids (e.g., narcotics, cocaine, amphetamines) in cases of death suspected to be due to overdosage of self-administered drugs. Drug concentrations in gastric contents may be very high even after parenteral injection.

Absorption from the intestine has been studied by perfusing drug solutions slowly through rat intestine in situ and by varying the pH as desired. The principles that emerge from such studies are the same as those for stomach; the difference is that the intestinal pH is normally near neutrality. Some data are presented in Table 3-6. As the pH was increased, the bases were absorbed better, the acids more poorly.[46] Detailed studies with a great many drugs in unbuffered solutions revealed that in the normal intestine acids

Table 3-6. In Situ Intestinal Absorption of Drugs from Solutions of Various pH in the Rat

		Percent Absorbed			
		pH of Intestinal Solution			
	pK_a	3.6–4.3	4.7–5.0	7.2–7.1	8.0–7.8
Bases:					
Aniline	4.6	40 ± 7 (9)	48 ± 5 (5)	58 ± 5 (4)	61 ± 8 (10)
Aminopyrine	5.0	21 ± 1 (2)	35 ± 1 (2)	48 ± 2 (2)	52 ± 2 (2)
p-Toluidine	5.3	30 ± 3 (3)	42 ± 3 (2)	65 ± 4 (3)	64 ± 4 (2)
Quinine	8.4	9 ± 3 (3)	11 ± 2 (2)	41 ± 1 (2)	54 ± 5 (4)
Acids:					
5-Nitrosalicylic	2.3	40 ± 0 (2)	27 ± 2 (2)	< 2 (2)	< 2 (2)
Salicylic	3.0	64 ± 4 (4)	35 ± 4 (2)	30 ± 4 (2)	10 ± 3 (6)
Acetylsalicylic	3.5	41 ± 3 (2)	27 ± 1 (2)	—	—
Benzoic	4.2	62 ± 4 (2)	36 ± 3 (4)	35 ± 4 (3)	5 ± 1 (2)
p-Hydroxypropiophenone	7.8	61 ± 5 (3)	52 ± 2 (2)	67 ± 6 (5)	60 ± 5 (2)

The percent absorbed is expressed as mean ± range; figures in parentheses indicate number of animals.
(From Hogben et al.,[46] with permission.)

with $pK_a > 3.0$ and bases with $pK_a < 7.8$ are very well absorbed; outside these limits the absorption of acids and bases, respectively, fell off rapidly. This behavior leads to the conclusion that the "virtual pH" in the microenvironment of the absorbing surface in the gut is about 5.3; this is somewhat more acidic than is usually considered to be the pH in the intestinal lumen.

Absorption from the buccal cavity has been shown to follow exactly the same principles as described above for stomach and intestine.[47] The pH of saliva is usually about 6. The relationship between pH, pK_a, and lipid/water partition coefficient was studied in human subjects by the following simple procedure. A known amount of a drug, usually 1 mg, in 25 ml of buffer was placed in a subject's mouth. It was circulated by means of vigorous movements of the tongue and cheeks with care not to allow any to be swallowed. After 5 minutes, the whole volume was expectorated into a beaker, the mouth was rinsed several times with water, and the drug concentration was assayed. Absorption was taken to be the difference between the amount introduced and the amount remaining. These studies yielded remarkably consistent results for a given subject on different days, with more variability between subjects. The extent of absorption in 5 minutes varied from drug to drug as shown in Figure 3-5. Bases were absorbed only on the alkaline side of their pK_a (i.e., only in the nonionized form) (Fig. 3-5A). At normal saliva pH only chlorpheniramine, the weakest base tested, was absorbed to a significant extent. In a series of *n*-alkyl-substituted carboxylic acids (Fig. 3-5B), the inverse relationship was found; all were absorbed best on the acid side of the pK_a. In addition, absorption increased with the length of the alkyl chain, reflecting the increase in lipid/water partition coefficient. The efficient

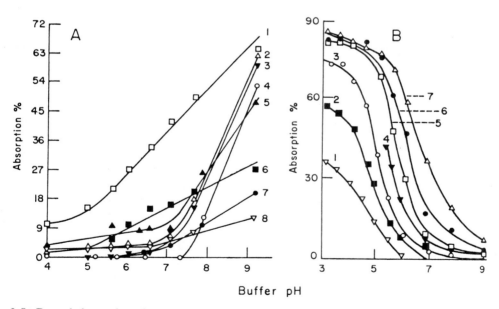

Fig. 3-5. Buccal absorption of organic acids and bases. The tests were performed on human subjects as described in text. (**A**) Basic drugs: 1, chlorpheniramine; 2, ephedrine; 3, methylephedrine; 4, ethylephedrine; 5, pseudoephedrine; 6, nicotine; 7, norpseudoephedrine; 8, norephedrine. (**B**) Congeneric series of *p-n*-alkylphenylacetic acids: 1, unsubstituted phenylacetic acid; 2, methyl; 3, ethyl; 4, propyl; 5, butyl; 6, pentyl; 7, hexyl. (From Beckett and Hossie,[47] with permission.)

buccal absorption of the lipid-soluble vasodilator nitroglycerin is made use of routinely in the treatment of angina pectoris; a pellet containing the drug is placed under the tongue.

Methods of Modifying Drug Delivery

Enteral Route: Drug Formulations, Bioavailability

As pointed out earlier, although the enteral route is very convenient, the numerous factors influencing absorption make it rather unpredictable. It is subject to variability from patient to patient and even in the same patient at different times. Considerable effort has therefore been expended, especially by the pharmaceutical industry, to develop drug formulations with better absorption characteristics.[48] Enteric coatings were introduced long ago to resist the action of gastric fluids and to disintegrate and dissolve after passage into the intestine. The purpose was to protect a drug that would be degraded in the stomach, to prevent nausea and vomiting caused by local gastric irritation, to achieve a high local concentration of a drug intended to act locally in the intestine, to produce a delayed drug effect, or to deliver a drug to the intestine for optimal absorption there. Enteric coatings are usually fats, fatty acids, waxes, shellac, or cellulose acetate phthalates. The major problem, however, is the great variability in gastric emptying time, especially on different diets; measurements in human subjects range from a few minutes to as long as 12 hours for passage of enteric-coated tablets through the pylorus.

More complex, laminated coatings have been introduced, which are *sustained-release* medications.[48] The drug may be applied in soluble form to the outside layer of a tablet containing an insoluble core. More of the same drug is trapped inside the core so that it can dissolve in intestinal fluid that gains access through pores in the matrix. Thus an initial dose is provided in the outer coating, followed by a delayed release from the core. A variation of this theme consists of tiny pellets of drug with different coatings subject to dissolution at different rates, so that the total drug dose is released over a prolonged period.

Several variables have been shown to affect the rate of release of drugs from sustained-release preparations in vitro[10,49]; for example, the size of the tablet determines the surface area for solution and the actual rate at which the drug will dissolve. The pore size of the inert matrix and its resistance to sloughing, the presence of water-soluble substances in the matrix, and the intrinsic solubility of the drug in an aqueous medium also affect the rate of release. Obviously the rate of movement of the preparation through the gastrointestinal tract can also affect the amount absorbed. If the intestinal contents move too rapidly, a portion of the drug may be wasted in the feces.

A clear danger of sustained-release preparations is that a larger dose than usual may be administered at one time on the assumation that the sustained release will yield a continuous slow rate of absorption. If the actual rate of release should be unexpectedly high, potentially toxic levels may result; if unexpectedly low, therapeutically inadequate levels may result. Either outcome might endanger the patient. The overdose danger has been demonstrated in the case referred to previously in which excessive abrupt absorption of a once a day dosage preparation of sustained-release theophylline occurred following a high fat meal. Furthermore, sustained-release preparations are often more expensive than ordinary dosage forms. So the choice of such preparations ought to be justified by some real need. Since the oral ingestion of a drug three or four times daily presents a potential compliance challenge for the patient, more reliable drug administration can be achieved by using a once a day regimen. Some drugs only need to be administered once daily in their ordinary dosage forms (e.g., digitalis glycosides); with these there is no justification for sustained-release preparations.

The difficulties associated with reliable administration of drugs by the enteral route have raised important questions about *bioavailability*.[49] Given that two formulations contain the same amount of a certain drug, will both actually yield the same amount at the same rate for absorption into the circulation? Two testing procedures are relevant. First, the rate of disintegration of the tablet or capsule can be measured in vitro in a medium simulating the gastric or intestinal contents. Here considerable variability has been found, attributable to differences in particle size, binders, compression of the tablet, or thickness of the capsule wall. Second, once disintegration has occurred, the rate of dissolution of the drug in the aqueous medium can be determined. Again variability has been observed, presumably related to the particle size and to the presence of substances capable of preventing the efficient wetting of drug particles. Major differences have been noted, not only between products of different manufacturers but also between lots by the same manufacturer. Clearly, dissolution tests are more relevant than disintegration tests, but even after dissolution, substances capable of complexing with drug molecules may interfere with their efficient passage across the intestinal wall. Thus, the most satisfactory test is to measure blood or plasma drug concentration (i.e., to determine bioavailability directly). This type of test has revealed important differences between formulations of aspirin, chloramphenicol, diphenylhydantoin, oxytetracycline, and other drugs.

Sometimes, of course, large variations in bioavailability are tolerable, but often the consequences of too slow or too rapid absorption or of greater or lesser total absorption can be serious for the patient. Figure 3-6 illustrates the remarkable differences in serum digoxin levels achieved with four preparations of this cardiac glycoside administered on different occasions to four volunteer subjects.[50] Relative total absorption of digoxin can be estimated from the individual areas under the serum concentration versus time curves. All the preparations were technically in conformance with the standards that regulate drug content, yet preparations B_2 and C were distinctly inferior to A and B_1. It may be argued that the dosage of a cardiac glycoside has to be titrated in the individual patient anyway, and the data presented in the figure certainly show significant subject to subject variability. It would seem desirable, however, for all preparations of a given drug to be as good as the best from the standpoint of bioavailability. An important lesson is the potential danger of switching preparations after a patient has been stabilized on any one preparation in view of the narrow therapeutic margin in this class of drugs.

Another example concerns the anticoagulant bishydroxycoumarin. A manufacturer of this drug increased the size of the tablet in order to facilitate breaking it into fractional doses. This was accomplished by increasing the amount of inert filler. It was found that inadequate therapeutic effects were then obtained, and the dosage had to be increased. To overcome this difficulty, the company dispersed the drug more finely. The result was excessive anticoagulant activity, and several patients suffered hemorrhagic reactions. As a result of all these findings, substantial effort is being accorded to the development of assay procedures for standardizing bioavailability and achieving better quality control over drug formulations for enteral use.

Sustained Release from Parenteral Depots

Long-term drug release from parenteral depots has been achieved by several means; (1) by modifying the drug in such manner that it is administered as a *prodrug*, which is slowly hydrolyzed or cleaved by enzymes to form the active drug; (2) by modifying the

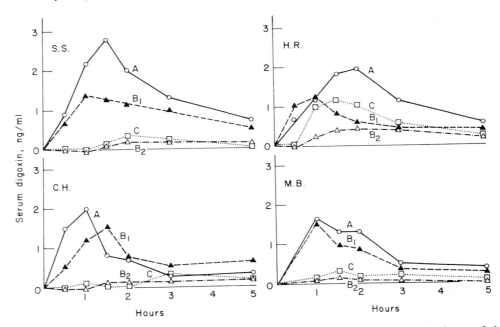

Fig. 3-6. Differences in absorption of four digoxin products in four subjects. Products of three manufacturers are designated A, B_1, B_2, and C. The four subjects are identified by initials, S.S., H.R., C.H., and M.B. Order of administration was varied. Interval between administrations to the same subject was 8 days to 4 weeks. All subjects received two 0.25 mg tablets of digoxin by mouth with 100 ml of water after an overnight fast. (From Lindenbaum et al.,[50] with permission).

drug or drug vehicle in such manner that it is slowly absorbed from the injection site (e.g., benzathine penicillin G); (3) by encasing the drug in a polymer matrix, from which it is slowly released at a controlled rate; (4) by encasing the drug in an ingestible or implantable mechanism, from which it is pumped at a constant rate.[10] In many cases the goal is to provide a long sustained, nearly zero-order absorption into the general circulation, simulating a slow, constant intravenous infusion. Often, however, a prolonged local release is desired, providing for drug action on tissues in the immediate vicinity, and avoiding significant systemic effects as the drug is diluted in the general circulation. Experimental approaches have been made to both these goals.[10,49]

A major advantage of certain sustained-release drug preparations is the assurance of patient compliance. One use of benzathine penicillin, for example, is to provide ensured prophylaxis against β-hemolytic streptococcal infection by administering a once monthly injection rather than relying on daily self-administration of oral penicillin by the patient. A repository preparation of cycloguanyl pamoate and acedapsone can be administered at 3-month intervals for prophylaxis of malaria.[13] These are examples of sustained-release preparations, the long half-life of which is due purely to a slow rate of drug absorption from the injection site. In most cases in which the chemical structure of a drug has been modified to achieve a longer duration of action, the prolonged drug effect is due to slower metabolism and/or excretion.

A technology that is being developed is to achieve a controlled rate of drug release by incorporating drugs into polymer matrices.[10,49] With such *controlled-release* formulations the rate of drug release from the polymer matrix may be determined either by diffusion or by biodegradation. In a diffusion-controlled system, the compound may be dispersed uniformly in the polymer medium (cat and dog flea collars are commercial examples of this method) or may be sandwiched in a reservoir between polymer membranes, through which it slowly diffuses. An ocular insert for 7-day delivery of pilocarpine and a 1-year intrauterine delivery system for contraception are examples of the membrane reservoir type of system that have been approved for human use. The earliest biodegradable systems were the oral dosage forms mentioned above in which the polymer coating slowly dissolves to release the drug. There is now considerable interest in the potential use of biodegradable polymers in parenteral formulations.[51] The drug would be incorporated throughout the matrix, with the rate of drug release being controlled by the rate of biodegradation of the polymer. Biodegradable systems would have a great advantage over nondegradable, diffusion-controlled systems in that they would not have to be retrieved from the implant site after release of the drug. At present biodegradable systems for injection or implantation are still experimental in human medicine.

The principle of slow drug release from a polymer matrix should be applicable to the administration of numerous drugs at a subcutaneous implantation site whenever very prolonged action is required. If the physical properties of the polymers can be standardized to yield zero-order release of drug over periods of weeks or months, this technique may have very wide applicability. Its advantages could include not only a more constant rate of drug delivery as compared with the enteral route but also ensured compliance. Such biodegradable implants may be used most often in underdeveloped areas of the world, where the patient population is seen infrequently by the treating physician. They may play an important role in regions where there is a great need for simplified and ensured methods of contraception. One can envision their potential usefulness in the treatment of aged patients for whom compliance may be a serious problem and controlled-release formulations represent an effective method of ensuring that a full course of treatment is received. The method might also have value in providing long-term protection against the effects of narcotics by continuous delivery of a narcotic antagonist (see Ch. 10).

New Techniques for Controlled Drug Administration

As indicated by the developments recounted above, there has been increasing recognition that the time-honored methods of administering drugs often fall short of the ideal, and a variety of new methods of drug delivery are being tested.[52] Major advances in controlled-drug delivery will come from the development of ingestible or implantable devices from which drugs can be pumped at a constant rate either into a local region or into the general circulation. Both osmotic and mechanical pumps have been designed for drug infusion.

Osmotic pumps have been developed for both oral administration and subcutaneous implantation. These systems may be shaped like either tablets or capsules, and they employ the force generated by an osmotic gradient to push the drug-containing infusion fluid out through a small hole at a controlled rate (Fig. 3-7). In the general design of these devices, the infusion fluid is separated by an elastic diaphragm from a chamber containing a solid salt, which acts as an osmotic attractant. The osmotic chamber is separated from the body fluid by a semipermeable membrane, and as water is imbibed from the surrounding medium, the chamber swells, forcing the infusion fluid out through a delivery port. In some osmotic devices, like the oral tablet shown in Figure 3-7, the medication

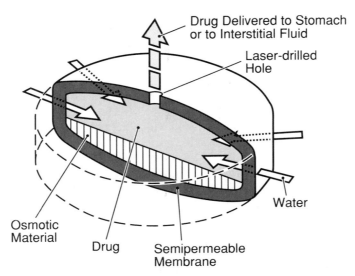

Fig. 3-7. Osmotic tablet for controlled drug delivery. In the stomach water passes through the semipermeable membrane, dissolving the drug and causing the osmotic attractant to swell and push the drug out through a small hole in the capsule.

is sandwiched with the osmotic agent, and the sandwich is coated with a semipermeable membrane. Water passes through the membrane, simultaneously putting the drug into solution and causing the osmotic material to swell.

The implantable mechanical pump is a disc-shaped device in which the vapor pressure of a fluorocarbon propellant provides the energy source for the infusion.[53] The pump is separated into two chambers by titanium bellows, the inner chamber containing the solution to be infused and the outer chamber containing the fluorocarbon liquid in equilibrium with its vapor phase (Fig. 3-8). The pump is placed beneath the skin, and the inner chamber is filled with drug by percutaneous injection through a self-sealing septum. As the infusion fluid is injected, the drug chamber expands, compressing the fluorocarbon vapor back to the liquid phase, thus simultaneously filling the pump and recharging the power source. As the fluorocarbon vaporizes at body temperature, the pressure drives the drug from the inner chamber into an outlet catheter, which may be placed in a vessel, in a body cavity, or in the subcutaneous space. Mechanical pumps such as this have been used to deliver anticancer drugs directly into the hepatic artery for treatment of tumors of the liver, and they have been used for both intraventricular and intra-arterial treatment of central nervous system tumors.[54] The concentration of drug achieved in the perfused region can be 100 to 1,000 times as high as the systemic concentration, thus permitting a better antitumor effect while lessening the chances of adverse drug reaction in the bone marrow or elsewhere in the body.[54]

Implanted mechanical pumps have also been used for intravenous and subcutaneous treatment of patients with diabetes.[55] By using external pumps for programmed drug delivery, it has been shown that intravenous infusion of insulin in appropriate amounts can dramatically improve glycemic control in patients with insulin-dependent diabetes mellitus.[56] Algorithms governing the rate of insulin delivery mimic the normal daily pattern, producing a basal infusion rate, with increased delivery rates before meals. These

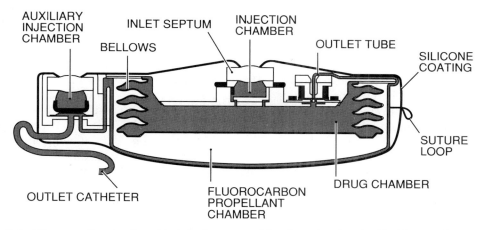

Fig. 3-8. Diagram of an implantable infusion pump. The drug chamber is filled by passing a needle through the patient's skin and through the inlet septum, releasing the drug into the injection chamber. As the drug chamber is filled, the bellows expands and the fluorocarbon propellant is compressed back to the liquid phase. As the fluorocarbon subsequently vaporizes, the pressure drives the drug solution through the outflow tube and catheter into the vessel. (Adapted from Ensminger and Gyves,[54] with permission.)

treatment regimens are complex and not devoid of complications; yet in carefully selected and highly motivated patients, near normoglycemia can be maintained by such insulin infusion.[56] Techniques are now being developed for continuous monitoring of plasma glucose concentration by means of implanted devices containing miniaturized circuitry, which could regulate the rate of infusion of mechanical pumps. With incorporation of such a sensor element, a totally implantable mechanism could possibly maintain a constant drug level by feedback regulation of the infusion rate or even adjust drug delivery to the physiologic state of the patient. A system that adjusted an insulin infusion to the blood sugar level could mimic the homeostatic mechanisms controlling secretion of that hormone from the normal pancreas. Similar systems combining chemical analysis and regulated infusion could be applied to the administration of other hormones and drugs in appropriate clinical situations.[57] Vigorous research and development along the lines outlined here may be expected in the coming years.

DRUG DISTRIBUTION

Apparent Volume of Distribution

The body water may be regarded as partitioned into several compartments that are functionally distinct. These are the vascular fluid, the extracellular (interstitial) fluid, and the intracellular fluid. In a normal lean 70-kg man, the whole body water comprises about 60 percent of the body weight, or about 42 L. The extracellular water is about one-third of the total, around 20 percent of the body weight, or approximately 14 L. Included in this is the volume of circulating plasma water, about 4 percent of body weight, or 3 L. The whole blood volume, including the intracellular water of the erythrocytes, is about twice the plasma volume, or about 6 L. These data are summarized in Figure 3-1. The volumes of the various compartments differ slightly between adult men and women. In obese people a larger fraction of the body weight is fat, so the fluid compartments all represent smaller percentages of the body weight. In infants the body water is a higher percentage of the body weight (as much as 77 percent), in part because the bony tissues are incompletely calcified and hence contribute less to body weight than in the adult.

The *apparent volume of distribution* (V_d) of a drug is the fluid volume in which it seems to be dissolved. The determination of V_d is simple in principle. A known amount of a drug is injected intravascularly, and after sufficient time for it to distribute, a sample of blood is taken and the drug's concentration in plasma water is determined. Suppose the drug were distributed ideally, without any metabolic degradation, without being eliminated from the body, and without any binding or sequestration. The situation would then be analogous to finding the volume of fluid in a flask by adding a known amount of dye, mixing, and then determining the resulting concentration.

Let x be the amount of dye added, and c the resulting concentration; then $c = x/V_d$, or $V_d = x/c$.

A high molecular weight dye, Evans blue, is almost wholly confined to the circulating plasma and therefore can be used in just this way to determine the total plasma volume (and the blood volume, if the hematocrit is also known). Several minutes are needed for complete mixing of the dye with the circulating plasma. During this time the plasma concentration falls to a plateau, which then remains unchanged, whence V_d is found. A significant fraction of the circulating blood is in tissues, where the blood flow is slow. The initial very fast mixing (about 1 minute) distributes the dye into the volume of blood that perfuses kidney, brain, liver, lungs, and the active musculature. Over the next several minutes, this solution will be diluted by mixing with dye-free blood from the more slowly perfused tissues (fat depots, skin, etc.). If 100 µg of Evans blue were injected, the plateau concentration would be about 33 µg/L, and $V_d = 100/33 = 3$ L.

Thus, the volume of distribution compares the plasma concentration of a drug with the quantity of drug administered. To normalize values for subjects of different weights, the dose is often expressed in milligrams per kilogram. Thus,

$$V_d = \frac{\text{dose}}{\text{plasma concentration}} = \frac{\text{mg/kg}}{\text{mg/L}} = \frac{\text{L}}{\text{kg}}$$

This value would be dimensionless if the body's specific gravity were 1.0, and it essentially expresses V_d as a percent of body weight. Thus, if a drug partitions into only extracellular space $V = 0.20$ L/kg, and if it distributes into the intracellular space, $V = 0.60$ L/kg. If there is extensive drug binding in the tissues, V will be greater than the 60 percent of body weight represented by the whole body water.

Many different substances distribute approximately into the extracellular fluid volume. Chloride and sodium ions, for example, are primarily extracellular, but a small fraction is always found within cell water; consequently, V_ds determined with isotopes of these ions (^{24}Na is often used) tend to be a little higher than the true volume of extracellular space. Stable or radioactive bromide salts, thiocyanate, radioactive iodide, sucrose, and inulin have been used to estimate the extracellular fluid, and each V_d differs slightly from the others. Actually, the ratio of extracellular fluid volume to tissue water differs from tissue to tissue, and so does the capillary permeability, so the differences in V_d probably reflect real differences in distribution. In general, with these substances the initial very rapid fall of the plasma level due to intravascular mixing blends into a further decline, reflecting distribution into the interstitial fluid. Thus a lower plateau is reached than with Evans blue. If 100 mg of bromide ion were injected (as NaBr), the ultimate plateau reached

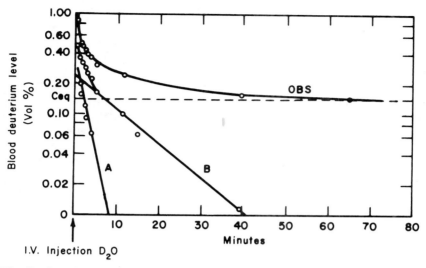

Fig. 3-9. Distribution of deuterium oxide into total body water. D_2O, 80 ml, was given intravenously to a human subject weighing 82 kg. Samples were taken from the femoral artery. Note logarithmic scale of ordinates. Upper curve (OBS): raw observations; lower curves (A and B): analysis into kinetic components, as described in the text. C_{eq} denotes the equilibrium concentration eventually attained. (Adapted from Schloerb et al.,[58] with permission.)

before significant excretion could occur would be about 8 mg/L, whence $V_d = 100/8 = 12$ L, which is slightly less than the volume of the extracellular fluid.

Finally, the volume of the total body water may be estimated by tracer water (D_2O or ^3H_2O) or some substances with high lipid/water partition coefficient, since these cross cell membranes readily. Here, 1 hour or more may be required for all the body tissues to come to equilibrium, and various fractions of the body water may be observed to equilibrate at different rates. In Figure 3-9 an experiment with heavy water is shown.[58] Here, 80 ml of D_2O was injected intravenously, and samples of blood from the femoral artery were analyzed for their deuterium content by means of a falling-drop density determination. The standard deviation of this determination is small, about 4 parts per 1,000; the final estimates of body water are accurate to within ±0.2 L. The upper curve represents the raw data, D_2O concentration (on a logarithmic scale) plotted against time. Equilibrium was attained in about 1 hour, at a plateau level of about 0.16 volume percent, or 1.6 g/L; thus $V_d = 80/1.6 = 50$ L, representing 61 percent of the body weight in this subject, who weighed 82 kg.

In this experiment the arterial concentration curve could be analyzed into two log-linear kinetic components. The procedure is as follows: The net rate of movement of D_2O out of the bloodstream should be proportional to the difference, at any moment, between the arterial concentration and the eventual concentration to be attained at equilibrium. The first step was, therefore, to subtract the equilibrium concentration (C_{eq}) from each point. This yielded the middle curve B. This curve seems to be composed of at least two processes going on at different rates. The final part is log-linear, so it was assumed that whatever process it represented had gone on from the start. An extrapolation was therefore made back to time zero. Now the extrapolated part of curve B was subtracted from the actual early points on curve B, yielding another straight line (A) with a much steeper slope. In other words, the observed course of decline of the arterial plasma level could be accounted for by two simultaneous exponential decay curves with different time constants.

Despite the alluring simplicity of analyses such as the above, they can be very misleading. The equilibration processes going on at such different rates, for example, could have nothing to do with actual body fluid compartments but might represent either the equilibration of two groups of tissues with very different vascularity or partitioning of the drug. Sometimes, the volume of distribution of the drug is determined experimentally and (as in this example) is found to correspond reasonably well with the actual volume of some fluid compartment. Thus, any drug with V_d approximately 14 L might be supposed to enter extracellular fluid but not to penetrate cells. Two factors may operate frequently to invalidate such direct and simple interpretations. On the one hand if as is commonly done, the drug concentration in total plasma is determined rather than that in plasma water, then a high degree of protein binding will make the observed concentration unduly high, and the estimate of V_d will therefore be falsely low. If a substantial fraction of the drug is bound to plasma proteins in the concentration range studied, this error can be very large. For example, in the hypothetical case just proposed, where $V_d = 12$ L, if the original dose is 100 mg, then the observed plasma concentration is about 8.0 μg/ml. If the drug is 70 percent bound at this total concentration, then the true equilibrium concentration in plasma water is only 2.4 μg/ml and the true volume of distribution is 42 L, a volume greatly in excess of the extracellular fluid and close to that of the total body water. On the other hand, binding or sequestration of drug at an extravascular site can withdraw so much from the circulation that V_d will appear to be very large. A drug that is stored in fat depots (e.g., cyclopropane, thiopental) may have an apparent volume of distribution very much greater than the entire fluid volume of the body.

A practical problem in estimating V_d is the fact that drugs do not often display kinetics of distribution in the body such that a plateau or constant plasma concentration is achieved. They are metabolized, excreted, or sequestered, so that no real distribution plateau is ever attained. The plasma concentration falls rapidly at first, more slowly later, and then continues to fall. What is needed is an estimate of what the plasma concentration would have been in the absence of the process responsible for the continuous decline. This estimate is obtained by extrapolating the eventual stable rate of decline back to the time of injection. Naturally, this has to be done on a semilogarithmic plot, it being assumed that the various phases of drug disappearance from plasma are all first-order. An illustration is presented in Figure 3-10. Antipyrine (1 g) was injected intravenously into four human subjects.[59] Inasmuch as the investigators were not interested in the kinetics of approach to equilibrium but only in estimating V_d, the first venous blood samples were drawn after 1 hour had elapsed. The rates of plasma level decline were nearly identical in the four subjects, corresponding to the rate of metabolism of antipyrine. The extrapolated values, 28 to 41 μg/ml, yielded values for V_d from 25 to 36 L. These volumes are rather low for total body water. In the subjects represented in Figure 3-10, D_2O gave slightly higher values of V_d. The D_2O estimates are usually somewhat too high because water in the gastrointestinal tract (usually not considered part of the body water) equilibrates with the heavy water; and more importantly, because deuterium partially exchanges with hydrogen in many compounds in the body tissues, so that part of the deuterium removed from the plasma is no longer in the form of water at all. The antipyrine estimates, on the other hand, are usually low because an appreciable fraction of the plasma antipyrine is bound to plasma protein; how this affects the estimate of V_d was explained earlier.

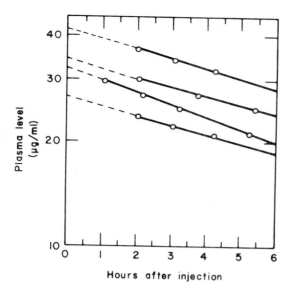

Fig. 3-10. Distribution of antipyrine into total body water. Antipyrine (1 g) was injected intravenously into four human subjects. Plasma levels are shown. The rapid fall of plasma level during the first hour (phase of distribution) was not measured. The slopes represent metabolism and excretion. (From Soberman et al.,[59] with permission.)

The Binding of Drugs to Plasma Proteins

The interactions between drugs and proteins were discussed in Chapter 1 from the standpoint of the molecular mechanisms responsible. Here we shall consider how interactions with plasma proteins influence the distribution of drugs in the body and their access to sites of action, of metabolism, and of excretion.[60,61]

Several kinds of plasma protein interact with small molecules (Fig. 3-11). The metal-binding globulins transferrin and ceruloplasmin interact strongly and specifically with iron and copper, respectively, and are essential to the transport of these ions in the body. The α- and β-lipoproteins account in large measure for the binding of lipid-soluble molecules, including those of physiologic importance, such as vitamin A and other carotenoids, vitamin D, cholesterol, and the steroid hormones. The antibody γ-globulins interact very specifically with antigens but negligibly with most drugs. Some steroid drugs are quite tightly bound by unique serum proteins (e.g., transcortin and the sex steroid-binding protein), which probably play a normal role in the physiology of the endogenously produced steroid hormones.

By far the most important contribution to drug binding is made by albumin, the principal protein of plasma (50 percent of the total). Its sequence is known and its physical properties have been well characterized, and because it reacts with a wide variety of drugs, it is used frequently in model investigations of drug binding. Its molecular weight is about 68,000, and at its isoelectric point (pH 5) it carries about 100 each of negative and positive charges.[63] At plasma pH (7.4) it has a net negative charge; nevertheless, organic anions primarily interact with serum albumin. Serum albumin is the natural carrier of free fatty acids in the plasma. As in the case of fatty acids, albumin contains several binding sites

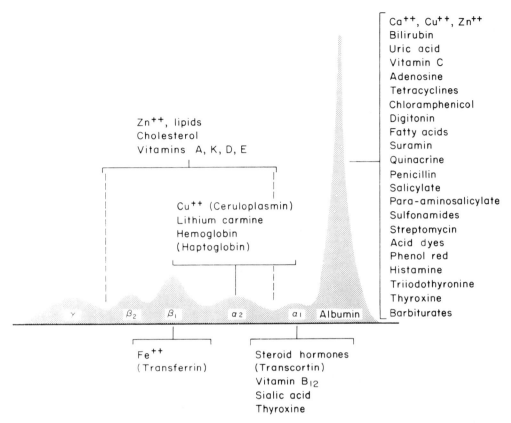

Fig. 3-11. Interactions with plasma proteins. Plasma proteins are depicted according to their relative amounts (*y* axis) and electrophoretic mobilities (*x* axis). Some representative interactions are listed. (Adapted from Putnam,[62] with permission.)

of varying affinity for drugs that are organic anions. Competition between the various drugs and between drugs and fatty acids can be demonstrated at these sites.

Although albumin is the primary serum protein responsible for drug binding, another protein has received considerable attention since 1983, namely, α_1-acid glycoprotein, an α_1-globulin with a molecular weight of 44,100, which contains a number of branching carbohydrate side chains.[64] In contrast to the multiple binding sites found in albumin, α_1-acid glycoprotein has only one high-affinity binding site and binds only basic drugs. α_1-Acid glycoprotein is an acute-phase reactant, which undergoes a severalfold rise in its plasma concentration after acute major injury, with the concentration falling to normal over several days (half-time 5.5 days). Despite the low number of binding sites relative to albumin, α_1-acid glycoprotein may influence the kinetics of some important drugs, such as the antiarrhythmic drug lidocaine.[65]

The reversible binding of drugs by proteins often requires that the native configuration of the protein be intact. This has important practical consequences for the assay of bound and free drug. Most routine procedures for determination of drug concentrations in plasma or other body fluids begin with a deproteinization step. This step is invariably a precipitation (e.g., with phosphotungstic or trichloroacetic acid), followed by removal of protein by filtration or centrifugation. In such procedures the analytical data will represent *total* drug concentrations because the protein-bound drug is released into the supernatant solution or filtrate. Most bioassay procedures, on the other hand, will be sensitive only to *free* (unbound) drug if whole plasma is used for the assay. Dilution of the plasma, however, favors dissociation because it reduces the concentration of free drug in equilibrium with the protein-bound moiety; therefore, the degree of binding will usually be underestimated if a dilution step precedes the assay.

If a drug is able to combine with a certain number of sites n on each protein molecule, if all these sites have the same affinity for the drug, and if there are no cooperative effects on affinity (i.e., the binding of a drug molecule to one site does not influence the affinity for the next site), then simple mass-law expressions describe the relationship between binding and the concentration of free drug at equilibrium. The total number of binding sites is nP, where P is the total protein concentration; so, as in the expression for receptor binding (Ch. 1), we have

$$\frac{[PX]}{nP} = \frac{[X]}{K + [X]}$$

where $[X]$ is the concentration of free drug, $[PX]$ is the concentration of drug-protein complex, and K is the dissociation constant. Let r be the ratio $[PX]/P$ (i.e., the moles of drug bound per mole of protein). Then

$$r = \frac{n[X]}{K + [X]}$$

and a plot of r against $[X]$ (Fig. 3-12A) yields a typical hyperbolic curve, identical to that of an adsorption isotherm. The same equation, in the familiar form of a log dose–response curve, is plotted in Figure 3-12B. The saturation of available sites (in this example, when $r = 10$) is evident.

The problem that concerns us in this chapter is not how many drug molecules can be bound to a molecule of plasma protein, but rather what *fraction* of the total drug molecules in the plasma are bound. We should like to know how the bound fraction β varies with

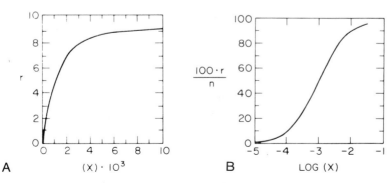

Fig. 3-12. Relationship between drug concentration (X) and moles bound per mole of protein (r), for a drug interacting with plasma albumin. (**A**) Typical hyperbolic curve; (**B**) a log dose-response curve.

drug concentration, protein concentration, maximum number of binding sites, and affinity constant. By definition,

$$\beta = \frac{[PX]}{[PX] + [X]} = \frac{1}{1 + [X]/[PX]}$$

But from the previous equation

$$\frac{[X]}{[PX]} = \frac{K + [X]}{nP}$$

so that

$$\beta = \frac{1}{1 + K/nP + [X]/nP}$$

This equation tells us that for a given protein concentration and a given number of binding sites per protein molecule, if the binding affinity is very high (K very low) and the drug concentration is very low, practically all the drug present will be bound (β approaches unity). As common sense suggests, if the total number of binding sites is reduced, a greater fraction of total drug tends to become free. An exact quantitative analysis, shown in Figure 3-13, illustrates some important principles. Here the individual curves are for chosen values of K/nP.

In plasma, P is fixed, and both n and K are determined by the particular drug whose distribution is under consideration; thus, nP is invariant and the whole expression K/nP is invariant. The horizontal scale becomes a measure of the logarithm of the free drug concentration. For a given drug, one particular curve (for one value of K/nP) will be relevant. We see that all drugs at high enough concentration saturate the binding sites. At still higher concentration the additional drug is all free, so that the fraction bound decreases toward zero. At high concentrations the maximum amount of drug is bound to

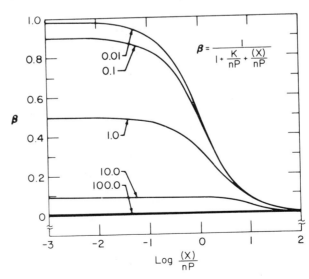

Fig. 3-13. Effect of drug concentration upon the fractional binding of a drug to plasma proteins. Axis of ordinates: fraction bound (β); axis of abscissas: relative scale of log concentration for a fixed protein concentration. See text for explanation. (From Goldstein,[66] with permission.)

the plasma proteins, but this maximum amount represents only a small fraction of total drug. As the drug concentration is progressively reduced (e.g., by elimination mechanisms in the body) the fraction bound tends to increase, but the extent of the increase may be negligibly small because some drugs have too low an affinity to be bound significantly even at very low concentrations. In those cases in which the fraction bound does increase at low drug concentration, a maximum fraction bound is always approached. If the affinity, the concentration of binding sites or both, are high enough, then this maximum fractional binding may approach unity (i.e., practically all the drug is bound), but it need not do so, and may drugs are only partially bound even under the most favorable conditions.

It follows that reports about the fractional binding of drugs in plasma (usually expressed as "percent of drug bound to plasma protein") are not useful unless qualified by a statement of the free drug concentration at the equilibrium actually measured. Interactions should be measured at therapeutic drug concentrations if conclusions relating to these concentrations are to be drawn; investigations carried out at higher concentrations may provide greater convenience or accuracy in the assay procedures, but the degree of fractional binding may be underestimated seriously.

The effects of protein binding upon drug distribution can be deduced readily from the same principles.[60,67] At equilibrium the concentration in the extravascular water will be the same as the concentration of unbound drug in plasma water (i.e., usually lower than the total plasma level). The difference in total drug concentration between plasma and cerebrospinal fluid (CSF) in patients led to the initial observation of reversible drug-protein interaction.[68] Several sulfonamide drugs were found to reach levels in CSF that were always below that in plasma, sometimes as low as one-quarter the plasma concentration. Yet the sulfonamides were very effective in bacterial meningitis, so the low concentrations were obviously adequate. It was found that the concentrations in cerebrospinal fluid were the same as in plasma water; these, indeed, were the true antibacterial concentrations.

Only free drug is available for glomerular filtration; therefore the persistence of a drug that is excreted in this way can be influenced by the fractional binding. Moreover, the rate of disappearance from the body tends to be self-limiting, at least through the range in which fractional binding increases with falling drug concentration; the lower the concentration, the smaller the fraction subject to filtration at the glomeruli.

On the other hand, active processes such as secretion at the renal tubules or carrier-mediated transport across other cell membranes are not restricted to free drug. The reversibility of the drug-protein interaction is so rapid that free drug molecules withdrawn from the water phase by one of these active processes are replaced instantly by more free drug derived by dissociation of the bound complex. Penicillin and β-aminohippuric acid (PAH) are examples; even at concentrations at which they are bound as much as 90 percent to plasma protein, they are cleared almost completely from the blood by renal secretory mechanisms during a single passage through the kidney.[69]

The rate of transfer of drug molecules from the bloodstream into the tissues by diffusion across capillary membranes depends upon the concentration gradient of free drug. Thus, protein binding can slow the disappearance of drug from the circulation and also provide a reservoir of bound drug, which will replenish (by dissociation) some of the drug that is lost by metabolism and excretion. A striking example is suramin, a polycyclic sulfonated compound used in the treatment and prophylaxis of trypanosomiasis. Suramin is a dye derivative that is bound very tightly to plasma proteins.[70] The slow release of drug from plasma protein results in long-term effective plasma levels, which permit it to be administered on a bimonthly basis for chemoprophylaxis of sleeping sickness.[13] Another example of retention by the plasma proteins is the dye Evans blue, mentioned earlier. It is useful in estimating the plasma volume only because the high fractional binding to plasma proteins minimizes the escape of dye at the capillaries.

Differences in the drug-binding capacity of plasma proteins are found between animal species. Such differences have also been noted occasionally among people (e.g., in the extent of binding of the antiepileptic drug phenytoin[71] or the antidepressant drug imipramine[72]) and in a few instances a genetic basis has been demonstrated (cf. Ch. 7). People vary greatly in the dosage of many drugs that is required to produce a therapeutic action. A part of this variability may be accounted for by differences in protein binding. Disease-induced changes in the quantity or properties of plasma proteins (particularly albumin and α_1-acid glycoprotein) are known to affect drug response in patients.[73] Paramount among these changes is hypoalbuminemia, which occurs in a variety of conditions, including liver disease, renal failure, nephrotic syndrome, and protein-wasting diseases such as cancer.

Competition between two drugs for the same binding sites on plasma proteins may lead to large increases in the free concentration of one of them in the plasma water, thus enhancing its therapeutic effect, producing unexpected toxicity, or increasing its rate of metabolism or excretion. Drug interactions due to competition for protein binding sites are much more likely to be clinically significant when the drug that is displaced is one that is highly (i.e., over 90 percent) bound to plasma protein and has a relatively small volume of distribution.[74] Consider the drugs warfarin, which is 97 percent bound (V_d 0.11 L/kg) and phenobarbital, which is 50 percent bound to plasma protein and has a much larger volume of distribution (V_d 0.54 L/kg). If 3 percent of warfarin is displaced from its plasma protein binding sites, the amount of free warfarin that can diffuse to the site of action is increased from 3 to roughly 6 percent, a twofold increase. If 3 percent of phenobarbital is displaced, however, the increase in free plasma phenobarbital is only from 50 to 53 percent, a change that is likely to be inconsequential. Administration of strongly displacing drugs, such as the anti-inflammatory agent phenylbutazone, to patients treated chronically with warfarin or other highly bound coumarin anticoagulants may lead to severe hypoprothrombinemia and bleeding as a consequence of increased drug action.[75]

In some cases the adverse reaction is not due to one drug competing for binding sites with another drug but is due to competition for binding sites with an endogenous ligand. The sulfonamide binding sites on plasma protein are also the binding sites for bilirubin,[76] and this forms the basis for a classic drug toxicity. In the presence of sulfonamides less bilirubin is bound, and more of the compound circulates in the free form. In newborn infants, who have decreased ability to conjugate bilirubin to the glucuronide, the concentration of unconjugated bilirubin increases rapidly in the presence of sulfonamides. The unconjugated bilirubin can pass across the blood-brain barrier of the newborn, where it becomes deposited in the basal ganglia and subthalamic nuclei of the brain, causing a toxic encephalopathy called kernicterus.[13]

Passage of Drugs across Blood Capillaries

Drug molecules are distributed throughout the body by means of the circulation of blood. The cardiac output (about 6 L min^{-1}) is equivalent to the whole volume of the vascular system. Thus, several minutes after a drug enters the bloodstream it is largely diluted into the total blood volume as a result of turbulent mixing and of flow through the various vascular beds. This initial phase of dilution (sometimes called the *distribution phase*) is best observed with a drug that passes only slowly, or not at all, out of the bloodstream. With such a drug the volume of distribution in the first few minutes should approach 6 L if the drug permeates erythrocytes freely, or about 3 L (the approximate plasma volume) otherwise. If a drug can leave the capillaries readily, its concentration may fall so fast that the initial phase of dilution is obscured, and a much larger volume of distribution is then approached.

The rate of entry of a drug into the various tissues of the body obviously depends upon the relative rates of blood flow through the respective capillary beds and the permeability of the capillaries for the particular drug molecules. Blood flow varies within wide limits, with capillary density varying among the tissues in accordance with their different physiologic roles and metabolic rates. For example, the frequency of capillaries per square millimeter is 2,000 in myocardium, 600 to 1,200 in skeletal muscle, 1,000 in brain cortex, and only 50 in skin and connective tissue.[77] Although the capillary bed contains only 8 percent of the blood volume, 1 ml of blood may be exposed to approximately 5,000 cm^2 of endothelial surface area for exchange processes.[77]

Blood flowing through the kidneys is ultrafiltered at the capillaries of the renal glomeruli, and most of the ultrafiltrate is reabsorbed by the renal tubules. Drug molecules, to the extent to which they are free in the plasma and filterable, will also appear in the glomerular filtrate, whence they may be reabsorbed or excreted in the urine. A small fraction of the cardiac output gives rise, at the choroid plexus of the brain, to CSF; and this protein-free solution, circulating over the tissues of the central nervous system, may contain some of the drug. The aqueous humor too may contain filterable drug derived from the blood. The bile may serve as a route for passage of drug out of the circulation into the intestinal tract, and drug molecules also pass directly from the blood across the gastrointestinal mucosa. At all the capillaries some ultrafiltration occurs, driven by high hydrostatic pressure at the arterial end, and there is some reabsorption of interstitial fluid at the venous end, driven primarily by the colloid osmotic pressure of plasma. Depending upon their molecular size and other properties, drug molecules may move with this bulk flow of solvent. Some of the drug in the interstitial fluid may remain in lymph and return to the circulation by way of the lymphatic channels. Since drug molecules that pass out of the circulation have first to traverse the capillary walls, we shall consider what is known about capillary permeability.

The functional anatomy of capillaries has been studied by direct microscopic observation of living tissue; the earliest reliable quantitative data about permeability were obtained by perfusion of isolated regions such as the cat hindlimb.[78-80] Blood was perfused through the femoral artery, and the rate of disappearance of various solutes was studied. One method was to measure the *osmotic transient* (i.e., the change in osmotic pressure as the solute passed into the interstitial fluid). This was accomplished by suspending the limb in a delicate balance and opposing the osmotic movement of fluid by adjustments of the hydrostatic venous and arterial pressures so as to maintain isogravimetric (constant weight) conditions. This procedure sufficed to measure a wide range of transfer rates with half-times from a few minutes to more than 1 hour. Another method was to measure directly the arteriovenous concentration difference; this method would be useful for transfer rates not much slower than the flow rates employed.

Lipid-soluble molecules such as urethane, paraldehyde, or triacetin left the blood almost instantaneously in its passage through the tissue, and so did gases of physiologic or pharmacologic interest (oxygen, carbon dioxide, nitrogen, and the anesthetic gases). For all the substances in this class, the most important determinant of the rate of transcapillary

Table 3-7. Permeability of Muscle Capillaries to Water-Soluble Molecules

	Molecular Weight	Radius of Equivalent Sphere (A)	Diffusion Coefficient	
			In Water, D $(cm^2/sec) \times 10^5$	Across Capillary, P $(cm^3/sec \cdot 100\ g)$
Water	18		3.20	3.7
Urea	60	1.6	1.95	1.83
Glucose	180	3.6	0.91	0.64
Sucrose	342	4.4	0.74	0.35
Raffinose	594	5.6	0.56	0.24
Inulin	5,500	15.2	0.21	0.036
Myoglobin	17,000	19	0.15	0.005
Hemoglobin	68,000	31	0.094	0.001
Serum albumin	69,000		0.085	<0.001

Data for radius of equivalent sphere are calculated from viscosity or diffusion measurements, taking into account the degree of hydration. The diffusion coefficient across the capillary is the rate of movement for unit molar concentration difference as given by the Fick equation, $dM/dt = (C_1 - C_2)P$.
(Data from Pappenheimer[78] and Renkin.[79])

movement was the lipid/water partition coefficient. The *partition coefficient* is the ratio of concentration in lipid phase to concentration in aqeuous phase when a substance is allowed to come to equilibrium in a two-phase system. The conditions of measurement (e.g., temperature, pH) must be specified. Glycerol derivatives, for example, passed through capillary walls at rates that varied with their lipid/water partition coefficients but in the opposite order to what would be expected from their aqueous diffusion coefficients. In the glycerol series increasing molecular size is achieved by increasing the length of hydrophobic substituents, so that partition coefficients and aqueous diffusion coefficients tend to vary inversely. The rapid rates of movement of all lipid-soluble compounds indicated that practically the entire capillary endothelial surface must be available for their diffusion.

For water-soluble molecules of various sizes, the results were quite different, as indicated in Table 3-7. Here the smaller the molecule, the more rapidly did it pass out of the capillary. Even the smallest molecules (including water itself) behaved as though only a very small fraction of the capillary wall (about 0.2 percent) were available for their filtration or diffusion. Moreover, the impediments to free diffusion (i.e., discrepancies between theoretical diffusion coefficients and transcapillary diffusion coefficients) were greater as molecular size increased. It appeared that a system of pores about 30 Å in radius (6 nm in diameter) must be present to account for the restricted diffusion as molecular radii approached 30 Å (corresponding to a molecular weight of approximately 60,000), and for the sharp cutoff above this.

Improved quality and special staining techniques have revealed electron microscopic evidence consistent with the existence of pores, but the pores themselves have not been directly visualized.[81] The physiologic experiments indicate the presence of two types of pores—small pores of about 10 nm and large pores of 50 to 70 nm diameter.[77] Only the small pores restrict diffusion with increasing size of the solute. The existence of the large pores is inferred by directly visualizing the passage of large molecular probes of known diameter (e.g., dextrans of diameter 5 to 20 nm and glycogens of diameter 25 to 30 nm) from the luminal side of the capillary endothelium to the interstitial side. The small pores have been studied indirectly by passage of small molecules, such as horseradish peroxidase (diameter 5 nm) or cytochrome c (diameter 3.3 nm), which can be detected by histochemical reaction. There are several regions in which transepithelial passage could occur. The capillary membrane is composed of an interlocking mosaic of endothelial cells with *junctions* between them that could function as the postulated pores. Some capillaries also contain endothelial cells possessing discrete disc-shaped regions called *fenestrae*, through which diffusion apparently occurs. In addition, a system of vesicles continuous with the inner and outer surfacs of the capillary membrane transports larger molecules at slow rates by a process called *transcytosis*.[77] The junctions were once the obvious candidates for the small pore system with the fenestrae and vesicles serving as the equivalent of the large pore system. The location of the small pores is, however, unclear, and structures not yet visualized by electron microscopy are thought likely to contain the pores that discriminate between small solutes of various sizes.[81]

The relatively small water-soluble molecules traverse the capillary membrane largely by diffusion in aqueous medium; their rates of movement are nearly independent of the perfusion pressure but are directly proportional to the concentration gradient across the capillary. Molecules the size of proteins penetrate only very slowly, and their rate of movement is strongly dependent upon the pressure difference between the arterial and venous ends of the capillary. There is still doubt about the precise mechanism whereby macromolecules traverse the capillary endothelium. Large tracer molecules are taken up from the luminal side of the endothelial cell by a process of membrane invagination and fluid engulfment called *endocytosis*. The resulting vesicles traverse the cytoplasm, bypassing the lysosomal apparatus, and discharge their contents by *exocytosis* at the interstitial surface. This shortcut, which directly couples endocytosis to exocytosis, is transcytosis,[77] mentioned above. Molecules can be carried across the endothelium in quanta via discrete vesicles, or the vesicles may fuse to form transient channels that traverse from the luminal to the interstitial side of the endothelial cell. This vesicular system discriminates in favor of anionic proteins, such as most plasma proteins, and is probably responsible for most of the protein in the lymphatic fluid draining from the capillary bed.

It follows from all the above that the rate at which a drug leaves the bloodstream will depend upon its lipid solubility, its molecular weight, and its physical state of aggregation. If it is bound to macromolecules, then its rate of transcapillary passage will be determined by that of the protein or other substance to which it is bound. Capillaries differ widely in their permeability characteristics; those of the glomeruli, for example, are very much more permeable to molecules of all sizes than are those of the muscles (hindlimb). The sinusoidal capillaries of the liver appear to lack any endothelial wall and therfore permit the passage of large molecules quite readily. Thus, capillaries in the various organ systems display wide variation in their permeability to drugs. Nevertheless, all the capillaries except those of the brain permit drugs to pass with relative ease as compared with cell membranes, and thus all drugs of small or intermediate molecular size that are free in the circulation gain access readily to the interstitial fluid. In brain, on the other hand, permeability to water-soluble molecules of all sizes is drastically reduced.

The capillaries are not rigid tubes with invariant properties. They, too, are subject to the actions of drugs as well as to effects of tissue metabolites and hormones.[82] Capillary permeability can be enhanced by such agents as histamine and estrogens and by decreased tissue pH associated with lactic acid production. Humoral agents such as norepinephrine affect the passage of substances across capillaries by constricting arterioles, thus reducing capillary blood flow and hydrostatic pressure in the capillary lumen.

Passage of Drugs across Cell Membranes

Membrane Structure

Cell membranes[83,84] are of importance in pharmacology for two principal reasons. First, many drugs owe their pharmacologic effects to a primary action at the outer membrane surface. Second, drugs that act inside cells must obviously pass through the cell membrane first. An adequate picture of cell membrane structure therefore not only must account for the known bioelectric properties and biochemical functions but also must include surface receptors and mechanisms for the passage of drugs to the cell interior. For secretory cells and neurones the movement of substances out of the cell must also be explained.

The basic structure of cell membranes is the phospholipid bilayer, a sheet consisting of two layers of phospholipid molecules aligned so that their polar heads face the adjacent aqueous mileu while the fatty acid chains form a continuous hydrophobic internal core (Fig. 3-14). Integral (or intrinsic) protein molecules are embedded in the lipid bilayer by interaction of one or more of their regions with fatty acyl chains in the hydrophobic core. Most integral proteins span the bilayer and are called *transmembrane proteins*. Peripheral membrane proteins are associated with the membrane by specific lipid-protein or protein-protein interactions. Oligosaccharides are linked mainly to proteins and to a lesser degree to membrane lipids. Proteins are visualized as moving freely within the lateral plane of the bilayer—the fluid mosiac model of biologic membranes.[85] This membrane structure

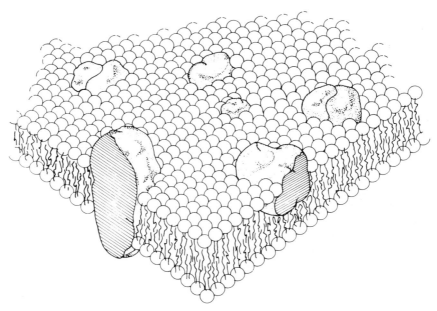

Fig. 3-14. A general model of the structure of biologic membranes. A phospholipid bilayer constitutes the basic structure. The circles represent ionic and polar head groups of the phospholipid molecues. Wavy lines represent the fatty acid chains. Solid bodies with stippled surfaces represent the integral proteins, which have one or more of their regions embedded in the lipid bilayer, interacting with the fatty acyl chains in the hydrophobic cores. (From Singer and Nicholson,[85] with permission.)

is remarkably suited to its functions—transportation of drugs or other small molecules into or out of cells, transduction of signals from hormones or drugs acting at receptor sites on the exterior of the membrane to systems in the interior of the cell, anchoring of cytoskeletal elements and components of the extracellular matrix, and enzymatic catalysis of metabolic reactions.

Membranes of different cells vary considerably in structural detail and in function. For example, liver and pancreas cells, because they produce proteins for use elsewhere in the body, require a mechanism for secreting macromolecules. This is accomplished by packaging the proteins in vesicles that become confluent with the cell membrane; the contents are thus extruded and enter the extracellular spaces or gland ducts by exocytosis. At the synaptic terminals of neurones a similar mechanism operates to release neuro-transmitters from storage vesicles into the synaptic cleft.

The entry of drugs into cells depends upon many of the same mechanisms already considered for transcapillary movement.[86] Very small water-soluble molecules and ions (e.g., K^+, Cl^-) evidently diffuse through aqueous channels of some kind. Lipid-soluble molecules of any size diffuse freely through the cell membranes. Water-soluble molecules and ions of moderate size, including the ionic forms of most drugs, cannot enter cells readily except by specific transport systems, which mediate the translocation of naturally occurring substrates. Finally, cholesterol, iron, and some peptide hormones enter cells by a process of *receptor-mediated endocytosis*.

Diffusion

Rates of diffusion of substances across biologic membranes can be measured in many ways. The most reliable method is to sample the solutions on both sides of the membrane at intervals and thus to determine the concentrations of a substance as it diffuses into the cell from the medium. In 1933 an elegant series of experiments was performed on the penetration of nonelectrolytes into the large cells of the marine plant *Chara ceratophylla*.[87] The findings turned out to be generally relevant to penetration of other kinds of cells by nonelectrolytes.

The entrance rates conformed to the diffusion equation of Fick (i.e., they were proportional to the concentration gradients). However, a distinctive diffusion coefficient had to be assigned to each substance because the membrane (as in the case of capillaries) offered different degrees of resistance to the passage of each substance. There was no polarity; diffusion rates were the same for influx and efflux of a given substance.

There was a good correlation between partition coefficients (olive oil/water) and penetrating ability. This is shown in Figure 3-15, where molecular size is indicated by the size of the symbol used for each compound. Except for very small or very large molecules, there was a fairly direct proportionality between the rate of penetration (permeability constant) and the partition coefficient. Molecules below about 15 Å in radius penetrated faster than their partition coefficients would lead one to predict. Very large molecules with high partition coefficients were retarded somewhat. Later studies with red cell membranes have refined these principles. The ether/water partition coefficient was found to correlate better with permeability constants than did other solvent/water partition coefficients. Lipophilic molecules capable of forming hydrogen bonds were found to interact in this way during passage through the membrane.[88-91]

For weak acids and bases the ionized and nonionized forms have completely different lipid/water partition coefficients. The ionized groupings (usually $-COO^-$ or $-NR_2H^+$)

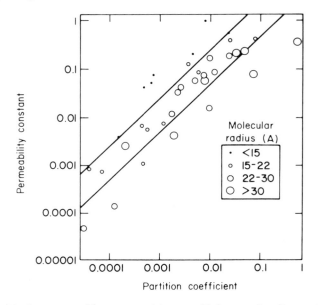

Fig. 3-15. Relationship between oil/water partition coefficient and cell membrane permeability. Abscissas: partition coefficient, olive oil/water; ordinates: permeability rate constant in *Chara ceratophylla*. Each circle represents a single compound; radius of circle symbolizes the molecular radius, in angstroms, as indicated. (From Collander and Bärlund,[87] with permission.)

interact strongly with water dipoles and consequently penetrate only poorly or not at all into the lipoidal cell membranes. Thus, drugs that are partially ionized at body pH enter cells at rates that are strongly pH-dependent. For all practical purposes the diffusion rate can usually be ascribed to the concentration gradient for the nonionized form alone.

Figure 3-16 shows this typical pH dependence for an acridine dye with a pK_a of 9.65. Here, the rate of entry into cultured human conjunctival cells was measured by a quantitative fluorescence technique.[92] At pH 8.5 about 8 percent of the dye is in the nonionized form, the remainder having a proton associated to a nitrogen atom in the acridine ring. At the more acidic pH values an ever smaller fraction is nonionized. The penetration rates are seen to vary as though only the nonionized form crossed the cell membrane.

The same phenomena occur in the whole animal and profoundly influence the distribution of drug between plasma and interstitial fluid on the one hand and intracellular water on the other.[93] Figure 3-17 shows experiments in which phenobarbital, a weak acid, was administered to dogs. When the plasma pH was lowered by CO_2 inhalation, there was a drop in the plasma drug level. This could be attributed to the fact that a greater fraction of the total phenobarbital in the blood assumed the nonionized acid form. The plasma concentration of undissociated diffusible phenobarbital was thus increased, and a larger amount of the drug moved across the cell membranes and into cells, where the pH remains relatively stable. Plasma alkalosis produced the opposite shift. These shifts occurred in all the tissues studied, including brain, where the depth of anesthesia paralleled the tissue concentrations. In other words, administration of acid deepened the anesthesia, while alkalosis lightened it. To promote just such a shift of drug out of the tissues (and also for a similar effect at the kidneys) alkalosis is induced therapeutically in the treatment of barbiturate poisoning.

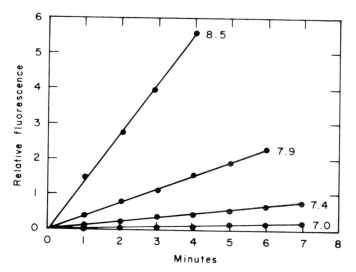

Fig. 3-16. Effect of pH on entry of an acridine dye into cultured human conjunctival cells. Intracellular dye concentration was measured by a fluorometric technique. The dye, proflavin, has pK_a = 9.65. The pH value of the surrounding medium is given on each curve. (After Robbins,[92] with permission.)

Membrane Transport

Substances that are insoluble in the cell membrane pass into the cell interior by forming a complex with a specific carrier protein.[94,95] It was formerly thought that the drug-carrier protein complex then traversed the membrane, the drug being released on the other side. It is now quite clear, however, that carrier proteins span the membrane from its inner to its outer surface. Most hydrophilic drugs that act inside the cell are structural analogs of natural substrates normally transported into the cell by a limited number of carrier proteins, each with a specific binding site that recognizes a narrow range of structurally similar compounds. When the carrier sites are saturated, the rate of transport is maximal. The high specificity of the binding sites and the fact that there is a maximal rate of passage distinguish this method of drug uptake from passive diffusion.

In *facilitated diffusion* the carrier protein facilitates transfer of the solute across the

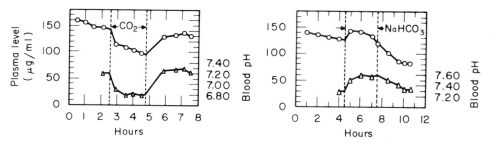

Fig. 3-17. Effects of acidosis and alkalosis on phenobarbital plasma levels in dogs. Phenobarbital concentrations are designated by circles, blood pH values by triangles. (From Waddell and Butler,[93] with permission.)

membrane in a manner that is energy-independent and that proceeds only in the direction from high to low solute concentration. *Active transport* is also a selective and saturable process, but it requires energy and can move molecules "uphill" against a concentration gradient. Examples of active transport are: the secretion of H^+ into the stomach and into the renal tubular urine; the accumulation of iodide ions in the thyroid gland; the generation of the membrane potential by the sodium-potassium pumps; the absorption of glucose and amino acids in the intestine and their reabsorption in the kidney; and the secretion of numerous organic anions and cations by the proximal renal tubules.

It is difficult to find examples in which drugs pass across membranes by facilitated diffusion. Most hydrophilic drugs that act inside cells enter via active transport; thus their entry can be prevented by inhibitors of energy metabolism as well as by competition from compounds of similar structure. Almost all the anticancer drugs, for example, enter both cancer cells and normal cells by active transport.[96] Alteration of transport systems leading to decreased drug entry is a common mechanism by which cancer cells become resistant to these drugs. One method that has been used successfully to treat such resistant cancers is administration of lipophilic drug analogs that enter by passive diffusion, thus bypassing the defective transport mechanism. In many cases drugs may also be transported from the inside of cells back into the interstitial fluid, and resistance can arise as a result of increased drug efflux (Ch. 9). In this type of resistance the gene for a carrier protein that transports several drugs becomes amplified, and the cancer cells become resistant to multiple drugs because of their increased ability to transport the drugs out of the cell, thus keeping the drug concentration inside the cell too low to be effective. Active transport also plays an important role in the distribution of drugs across membranes that separate body fluid spaces (e.g., choroid plexus, synovium). As will be discussed in a subsequent section of this chapter, active transport across renal tubular cells and hepatocytes is critical for eliminating many drugs from the body.

Active transport of solutes is dependent upon a source of energy; this may involve ATP hydrolysis by the carrier proteins themselves, or transport may be driven by the co-transport of Na^+ or H^+ down its electrochemical gradient. The carrier proteins behave like membrane-bound enzymes in that they bind solute to a specific binding site which is analogous to the substrate binding site on an enzyme, and they then carry out an energy-dependent transfer of the solute molecule across the lipid bilayer. As with enzymes, each carrier protein has a characteristic binding constant (K_M) for its solute, and when the carrier is saturated, the rate of transport is maximal (V_{max}). Despite the fact that the carrier protein may hydrolyze adenosine triphosphate (ATP) in deriving energy for the transfer of the solute, the analogy with an enzyme is limited because there is no covalent modification of the solute by the carrier protein. This implies that the site for ATP hydrolysis is spatially separate from the pathway for solute translocation, the linkage between the processes being mediated by the protein.

It is inherent to the concept of active transport that the pathway of solute transfer must never be simultaneously accessible from both sides of the membrane because it must permit energetically uphill movement.[95] The most viable model for how this occurs is the *alternating access model* of transfer, diagrammed in Figure 3-18, which shows the carrier protein in two conformational states, and in each case the solute binding site has unrestricted access to the adjacent aqueous medium. The protein could have one or multiple solute binding sites, and examples of both situations exist. Energy provided by ATP hydrolysis or by an ion gradient is required to convert the carrier protein from one conformation to another. The change from the uptake to the discharge conformation is ac-

Uptake

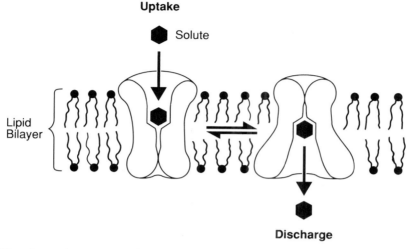

Discharge

Fig. 3-18. The alternating access model of translocation. Although only one solute-binding site is shown, there may be two or more binding sites, permitting the passage of several ions with a single change in the conformation of the carrier protein. Different binding sites may exist on each surface of the carrier so that transport of one ion across the membrane may be accompanied by counter-transport of another ion in the opposite direction. In the case of Na^+-K^+ ATPase, for example, there are three Na^+ sites at the inner membrane surface of the carrier and two K^+ sites at the outer surface. Thus, for each three Na^+ that are transported out, two K^+ are transported in. In the case of facilitated diffusion, transfer occurs only down an ion concentration gradient in an energy-independent manner.

companied by a reduction in the affinity of the binding site for the transported solute. The simplest model is to assume that the carrier protein (or protein complex) has only two conformational states and that the change in the accessibility of the solute binding site from one side of the membrane to the other occurs only with ATP hydrolysis. In the case of a number of transport proteins, ATP hydrolysis is accompanied by phosphorylation of the carrier protein itself. One clear requirement for such a system is that the reaction pathway must be unable to catalyze the uncoupled hydrolysis of ATP (i.e., ATP hydrolysis must yield the conformational change in the carrier).

Membrane Potential and the Na^+-K^+ ATPase

Microelectrode techniques have established the presence of a potential difference across cell membranes, generally around 60 to 90 mV. The inside of the cell is negative with respect to the outside. The Gibbs-Donnan equilibrium predicts an unequal distribution of other ions when any ion is prevented from equilibrating across the membrane. The resulting concentration gradients produce a potential difference whose magnitude is given by the Nernst equation. Analysis of the ion concentrations in intracellular and interstitial fluids of mammalian muscle cells reveals that whereas K^+ and Cl^- are in equilibrium with the membrane potential, Na^+ is not. The observed excess of external over internal Na^+ concentration would be in equilibrium with a membrane potential of $+65$ mV, in contrast to the actual -90 mV. Thus, the membrane behaves as though it is largely impermeable to Na^+ but freely permeable to the other small ions. The great excesses of

Table 3-8. Comparison of Cation Fluxes and Na^+-K^+ ATPase Activities

Tissue	Temperature (°C)	Cation Flux (10^{-14} mole cm^{-2} sec^{-1})	Na^+-K^+ ATPase Activity (10^{-14} mole cm^{-2} sec^{-1})	Ratio
Human erythrocytes	37	3.87	1.38 (± 0.36; 4)	2.80
Frog toe muscle	17	985	530 (± 94; 4)	1.86
Squid giant axon	19	1200	400 (± 79; 5)	3.00
Frog skin	20	19,700	6640 (± 1100; 4)	2.97
Toad bladder	27	43,700	17,600 (± 1640; 15)	2.48
Electric eel, noninnervated membrane	23	86,100	38,800 (± 4160; 3)	2.22

Standard error of the mean and the number of determinations are given in parentheses.
(From Bonting,[97] with permission.)

internal over external K^+ and of external over internal Cl^- are seen as the expected consequence of the Na^+ impermeability, as predicted by the Gibbs-Donnan equilibrium. Studies with radioactive Na^+, however, revealed that this ion does indeed cross the membrane, at a sufficient rate so that equal concentrations would soon be established inside and outside the cell unless Na^+ were being extruded continually. The conclusion is that a *sodium-potassium pump* operates to exclude Na^+ from the cell interior. This, of course, is tantamount to making the membrane selectively impermeable to Na^+.

The physical basis of the sodium-potassium pump is a sodium- and potassium-activated ATPase, widely distributed in cell membranes, and especially abundant in secretory cells and excitable tissue such as nerve and muscle.[97] The good correlation between the activity of this enzyme and the cation flux in a variety of tissues is shown in Table 3-8. The Na^+-K^+ ATPase has been isolated from a variety of cells and species. Within the membrane it consists of two subunits, each containing two polypeptides, one a 50,000-dalton glycoprotein (β subunit) and the other a 100,000-dalton nonglycosylated polypeptide (α subunit), which contains the catalytic site for ATP hydrolysis.[98] Regions of the Na^+-K^+ ATPase are exposed at both faces of the membrane. The region facing into the cell has one ATP binding site and three high-affinity sites for binding Na^+ ions. Externally the ATPase has two high-affinity binding sites for K^+ ions as well as a binding site for ouabain. As binding of Na^+ and K^+ ions on the opposite faces occurs independently, the protein does not move across or rotate within the membrane. Rather it seems likely that with the protein in one conformational state, three sodium ions and ATP bind to their respective sites on the inner side of the membrane. Bound ATP is hydrolyzed with phosphorylation of the enzyme, producing a conformational change, with extrusion of the Na^+ ions to the exterior. Two K^+ ions bind to their specific sites on the external surface, allowing dephosphorylation of the protein, a return to the original conformation, and release of the K^+ ions within the cell.

The connection between the sodium-potassium pump and the Na^+-K^+ ATPase was made when it was observed that ouabain and other cardiac glycosides that inhibit cation transport also inhibit Na^+-K^+-activated ATPase.[99] The nearly perfect quantitative agreement between these two effects of ouabain is shown in Figure 3-19. The transport of Na^+ was inhibited only when the drug was added to the external, serosal surface of the membrane; there was no effect at the mucosal surface. The cardiac glycosides thus act by combining with a receptor on the outer surface of the cell membrane.

Further evidence implicating the ouabain-sensitive Na^+-K^+ ATPase as the essential

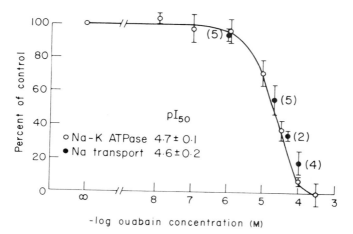

Fig. 3-19. Effect of ouabain on Na^+-K^+ ATPase activity and short circuit current (Na^+ transport) in toad bladder. Enzyme activity (open circles) was determined in homogenates; short-circuit current (solid circles) was measured with ouabain added to the serosal side of the chamber containing the toad bladder. Number of experiments indicated in parentheses. (From Bonting,[97] with permission.)

element in the sodium pump was obtained with sheep red blood cells.[100] Most sheep have erythrocytes with low K^+ concentration, about 13 mM (called LK cells), but in some the concentration is about 80 mM (HK cells), more like the usual value in other mammalian species. These two phenotypes are determined by two alleles at a single genetic locus. For complete inhibition of the sodium flux, HK cells have to bind about six times as many ouabain molecules as do LK cells. The normal ratio of Na^+ fluxes or of K^+ concentrations in the two cell types is about 6:1. It appears, therefore, that the essential difference between HK and LK cells is the number of Na^+-K^+ ATPase molecules per cell; as judged by the number of ouabain molecules bound, there are 42 and 8 pump sites, respectively, per square micron of membrane surface. The value for HK cells is about one-half that reported for human red cells. A given site, whether HK or LK, transported about 50 to 60 ions sec^{-1}.

It was established beyond all doubt that Na^+-K^+ ATPase is responsible for maintaining membrane potential when the purified enzyme was inserted into liposomes and demonstrated to direct the transport of Na^+ and K^+ against a gradient in a manner dependent upon ATP hydrolysis.[101] Ouabain inhibits the Na^+-K^+ ATPase by inhibiting the dephosphorylation of the enzyme that occurs when the K^+ site is occupied. Thus, the enzyme cannot return to its original sodium-binding conformation. The relationship between inhibition of the Na^+-K^+ ATPase and increase in myocardial contractility seen with the cardiac glycosides is considered in Chapter 2.

Drugs That Act as Carriers

Ionophores are antibiotics that act by facilitating the passage of ions across membranes. Some ionophores, such as the cyclic peptide valinomycin, form a three-dimensional cage around a cation and act via a carrier-type of mechanism as shown in Figure 3-20. Valinomycin binds K^+ at the membrane surface via ion-dipole interactions that replace the

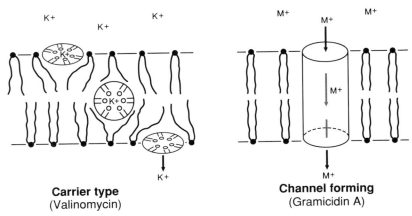

Carrier type
(Valinomycin)

Channel forming
(Gramicidin A)

Fig. 3-20. Schematic models of the mechanisms by which the carrier and the channel-forming type of ionophore antibiotics facilitate the passage of cations across biologic and artificial membranes. The solid circles oriented at the membrane surface represent the polar head groups of the phospholipids, and the wavy lines denote the hydrophobic fatty acid chains. Valinomycin (an antibiotic not used clinically) is used as an example of the carrier type. In general, the carrier ionophores are much more specific with regard to the ions with which they interact, valinomycin being quite selective for potassium (K^+). The channel formers are less selective, and in the case of gramicidin A, a variety of monovalent metal cations (M^+) are able to diffuse through the pore formed in the center of the antibiotic channel. (Adapted from Pratt and Fekety,[13] with permission.)

water of hydration normally surrounding the ion. The exterior of the antibiotic cage is quite hydrophobic; thus the ion-antibiotic complex is lipid-soluble and able to diffuse to the opposite membrane surface, where the cation is released. Carrier-type ionophores are highly selective and can be moderately efficient; one antibiotic molecule can facilitate the passage of several thousand ions per second.[102]

Another group of antibiotics act as channel-forming ionophores (Fig. 3-21). These antibiotics are able to form tubes with hydrophilic interiors that span from one surface of the membrane to the other. An example is the antibacterial drug gramicidin A,[103,104] shown in Figure 3-21. Ions enter the antibiotic channel at one membrane surface and diffuse through the hydrophilic interior of the channel to the other side. The channel formed by gramicidin A permits passage of univalent cations but completely excludes anions and polyvalent cations.[105] The channels are not static; they are constantly forming and disappearing. The channel-forming ionophores are more efficient than the carrier ionophores; one antibiotic molecule can facilitate the passage of up to 10^7 ions per second. The enhanced rate is a consequence of the ion remaining partially hydrated as it traverses the membrane. Additional energy is required to remove all the water of hydration from an ion; hence transport is slower with the carrier-type ionophore.

In some cases channel-forming antibiotics can facilitate the passage of other drugs through cell membranes. Amphotericin B is a channel-forming antibiotic used to treat fungal infections. By mechanisms that are not well defined, amphotericin B facilitates the entry of some other antibiotics into the fungal cell. Thus amphotericin B can potentiate the antifungal effects of 5-fluorocytosine,[106] and for this reason the two drugs are often used together in therapy of fungal infection.[13] The ability of amphotericin B to potentiate the antifungal effect of rifampin is demonstrated in Figure 9-1. Amphotericin B has been

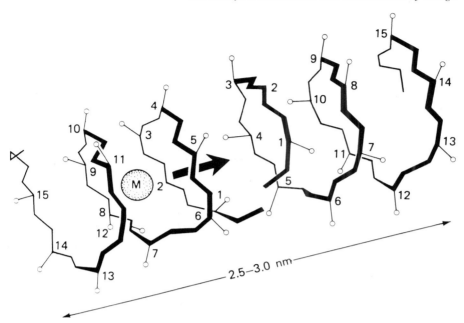

Fig. 3-21. Schematic presentation of the gramicidin A channel proposed by Urry et al.[103] A helical dimer is formed by head-to-head (formyl end to formyl end) association of two gramicidin monomers. The structure is stabilized by intra- and intermolecular hydrogen bonds. The π^6 (L,D)-helix has a diameter of about 0.4 nm and is lined with peptide C-O moieties. The hydrophobic moieties lie on the exterior surface of the helix. The arrow indicates the center of the helix, which allows the passage of monovalent metal cations (M). (From Pratt and Fekety,[13] after Ovchinnikov,[104] with permission.)

shown to permit the entry of the anticancer drug dactinomycin into cancer cells that are dactinomycin-resistant because of decreased drug uptake (or possibly because of increased drug efflux as described above). In the presence of amphotericin B, the resistant cells were readily killed by dactinomycin.[107] This raises the possibility of future combined drug therapeutic protocols in which one drug is present solely to facilitate the passage of the second drug across the membrane of the target cells.

Receptor-Mediated Endocytosis

The binding of some peptide hormones, growth factors, antibodies, and other substances to their receptors on the cell surface can trigger a process of endocytosis that brings both the ligand and the receptor into the cell. This method of transfer across cell membranes is called *receptor-mediated endocytosis*.[108,109] The process was first described for the passage of low-density lipoprotein (LDL) into the cell.

The generic term *endocytosis* refers to the nonspecific engulfment of extracellular fluid and its contents into the cell, whereas receptor-mediated endocytosis is a more selective uptake process. After certain cell surface receptors have bound their ligands, the receptors become clustered in specialized depressions in the cell membrane called *coated pits*. These coated pits comprise about 2 percent of the surface of some cells (e.g., hepatocytes, fibroblasts); they become pinched off from the cell surface to form *coated vesicles* (Fig.

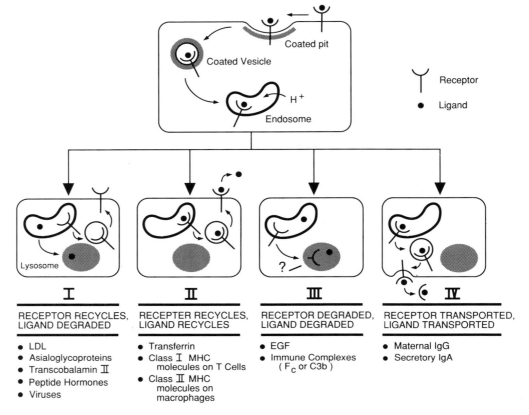

Fig. 3-22. Fates of receptors and ligands in different pathways of receptor-mediated endocytosis. The initial steps (clustering of receptors in coated pits, internalization of coated vesicles, and fusion of vesicles to form endosomes) are common to all pathways. After entry into the acidic endosomes, receptor ligand complexes follow one of the four pathways indicated. (From Goldstein et al.,[108] with permission.)

3-22). The structures are called coated pits because the inner membrane surface has an electron-dense coating that is detectible by electron microscopy. The coating is made up of a protein called *clathrin,* which polymerizes and somehow pinches off the receptor-containing vesicle. This process is quite dynamic; it has been calculated that the half-life of a coated pit is about 1 minute.[110] After internalization, the vesicles shed their clathrin coats as the result of the action of a clathrin-depolymerizing enzyme, and they then fuse with one another to form larger vesicles called *endosomes.* The endosomes are maintained at pH 5 on the inside by an ATP-dependent proton pump.

It is not clear how the process of receptor-mediated endocytosis is initiated. In some cases, as with epidermal growth factor, the receptor is distributed diffusely on the cell surface and only becomes clustered in coated pits after it is bound by the ligand. In the case of LDL, transferrin, and insulin, however, the receptors spontaneously move to coated pits and enter the cells continuously even in the absence of ligand. Thus the ligand moves through the membrane by "hitching a ride" on a normal dynamic process involved in the turnover of membrane proteins and lipids. Despite differences in the way receptors enter the endocytotic process, it appears that all receptors that are endocytosed enter cells in the same coated pits and are delivered to the same acidified endosomes.

After the receptor and ligand have followed a common route to the formation of acidified endosomes, they may take four different paths, depending upon the receptor involved. The first pathway shown in Figure 3-22 is of particular importance because it is the classic pathway described for LDL, insulin, luteinizing hormone, and some other peptide hormones. In this pathway the receptor is recycled and the ligand is degraded. In the low pH environment of the endosome, the ligands dissociate from their receptors, and the receptors are recycled to the cell surface through small vesicles that apparently pinch off from the endosomes. Thus, the receptors participate in several internalization cycles; the LDL receptor, for example, can go through 150 such cycles without losing its function. After dissociation from the receptor, the ligand is transferred to lysosomes and degraded. The principal role of this pathway may be to permit rapid control of receptor number (down-regulation, desensitization), as discussed in Chapter 1, and it may play a physiologically significant role in the removal of a hormone or growth factor from the circulation.

In the second pathway, both the receptor and the ligand are recycled. From the viewpoint of the pharmacologist, the major ligand of interest that follows this pathway is the iron-transferrin complex. The main site of iron storage in the body is the liver, and iron is carried throughout the bloodstream in combination with the serum glycoprotein transferrin. Under most physiologic conditions, iron exists in its oxidized state, and as most Fe^{3+} salts are hydrolyzed at neutral pH to insoluble ferric hydroxide, any ferric ions in excess of 25 nM are insoluble.[111] Vertebrates have solved this problem through the evolution of high-affinity iron-binding serum proteins. Transferrin has two high-affinity binding sites for ferric iron (K_d = 6nM at neutral pH), and the iron-transferrin complex binds to transferrin receptors located on virtually all cells. Hemoglobin-synthesizing reticulocytes have a particularly large requirement for iron, and they have approximately 300,000 transferrin receptors on the cell surface and can internalize over 1 million atoms of iron per minute.[111] The iron-transferrin/receptor complex is internalized by the common mechanism, but its fate in the acidic environment of the endosome is quite different from that of ligand-receptor complexes that follow the other pathways. At pH 5 the Fe^{3+} dissociates from the transferrin and is somehow transferred to the cytoplasm, where it is utilized. In contrast to the dissociation of ligand and receptor described above for the first pathway, the iron-free apotransferrin remains bound to the transferrin receptor in the acidic environment of the endosome and the apotransferrin-receptor complex is recycled to the cell surface. Once on the cell surface and again at neutral pH, the apotransferrin dissociates.

The pH dependence of binding of transferrin to its receptor is critical to this cycle. The iron-transferrin complex has a high affinity for the receptor at neutral pH, thus permitting uptake; the iron-free apotransferrin binds tightly to the receptor at pH 5, permitting recycling of the unit to the cell surface, but the binding affinity for apotransferrin at neutral pH is very low, permitting dissociation from the receptor after recycling. The apotransferrin is now free to bind more iron in the liver or intestine, and the receptor is free to bind another iron-transferrin complex and repeat the cycle. The entire process of receptor binding, internalization, iron release, and return of apotransferrin to the medium takes place within 15 to 30 seconds.[111]

In the third pathway, both the receptor and the ligand are degraded. This pathway has been described in greatest detail for epidermal growth factor (EGF).[112] Like substances following the first pathway, EGF dissociates from its receptor in the acidic environment of the endosome, but in the case of the third pathway both components are degraded. The pathway is not absolute, as in some cells a portion (20 percent) of the EGF receptors continues to bind, internalize, and degrade EGF with kinetics that suggest recycling. It is possible that internalization of the receptor is necessary for the mitogenic effect of EGF.[109] It has been speculated that some of the receptor that is internalized finds its way to the nucleus, where the tyrosine kinase activity, which is normally contained in the cytoplasmic domain of the receptor, may associate with nuclear structure and form the mitogenic stimulus.[113] From this point of view, the receptor would not be in the membrane to be activated by the ligand or to permit the passage of the ligand through the membrane; rather, the ligand would permit the receptor to be transfered from the plasma membrane to its site of mitogenic action inside the cell.

In the fourth pathway both the receptor and the ligand are transported to another cell surface. This pathway has been most extensively described for the transport of immunoglobulins (IgA and IgM) across liver cells for excretion into the bile and across mammary epithelia for excretion into the milk.[114] In this pathway the receptor mediating transfer across the membrane must be located on a specific surface of the cell. For example, the receptor that carries immunoglobulin in the liver appears on the sinusoidal surface of the hepatocyte, where it is internalized after binding IgA dimer. At some time after internalization, the receptor is cleaved and thereby dissociated from the vesicle membrane. The IgA-containing vesicle migrates to the canalicular surface of the hepatocyte, where it fuses with the cell membrane and discharges its contents into the bile duct.

With respect to its general properties, receptor-mediated endocytosis resembles active transport in that both processes of membrane transfer require energy, both are highly specific, and both have a maximal rate that is determined by occupancy of a limited number of binding sites in the membrane. Receptor-mediated endocytosis is a much more versatile process, however, in that it can direct the passage of moderate-size to very large molecules and even polymolecular structures such as viruses into the cell. A new field of drug development is evolving that is based on exploiting the process of receptor-mediated endocytosis to selectively deliver drugs to certain cells.

Site-Specific Drug Delivery

Since Paul Ehrlich conceived of therapeutic drugs as "magic bullets" that could specifically attack invading organisms or cancer cells, medicinal chemists and pharmacologists have focused on the achievement of greater and greater degrees of selective drug action. One mechanism of achieving *selective toxicity* is to modify a drug so as to alter its distribution and "target" its delivery to a specific organ or cell type. Similarly, if a compound with a particular affinity for a specific target can be radiolabeled, then one can develop diagnostic agents to better resolve specific structures by nuclear scanning. The classic example of such *site-specific drug delivery*[115–118] is the use of radioiodine, both as a diagnostic agent for detecting thyroid tumors and as a treatment for hyperthyroidism.

Several approaches have been used to package drugs in phospholipid or lipoprotein structures that will be cleared from the circulation by specific cell types. One of the first of these approaches involved the packaging of insoluble hydrophobic drugs in phospholipid vesicles called *liposomes*.[119] Liposomes are prepared by sonicating aqueous suspensions containing phosphatidyl choline, phosphatidyl glycerol, and other phospholipids. Upon sonication the lipids come together to form vesicles with various properties dictated both by the chemical composition of the lipids and by the conditions of sonication. When the sonication is carried out in the presence of a drug, the drug becomes trapped within a vesicle defined by a single phospholipid layer or within a multilamellar vesicle containing multiple concentric phospholipid layers. The free drug can be separated from the liposome-entrapped drug (e.g., by passing the mixture through a molecular sieving column) and the liposome suspension can be administered to experimental animals or to patients. When liposome-entrapped drug was administered to animals, it was found that the drug became concentrated in the highly phagocytic reticuloendothelial cells of the liver and spleen and that there was reduced drug uptake in the heart and kidney.[120] The first observation led to the use of liposome-entrapped antiparasitic drugs to fight infections such as leishmaniasis, in which the microorganisms reside within the cells of the reticuloendothelial system. Enhanced therapeutic action in test animals infected with *Leishmania* is observed as a result of enhanced drug entry into the target cells of the reticuloendothelial system.[121] The second observation (decreased cardiac and renal uptake) led to the administration of the cardiotoxic anticancer drug doxorubicin in liposome-entrapped form. When liposome-entrapped doxorubicin is administered to animals bearing tumors, there is reduced cardiotoxicity without a decrease in antitumor effect.[122] The examples with liposomes show that when drug distribution is altered so as to produce selective uptake by a target tissue or selective decrease in uptake by a tissue in which there is major drug toxicity, the *therapeutic index* (the ratio of the therapeutic dose to the toxic dose) is thereby increased.

In the particular case of the anticancer drugs, which often have a rather limited biochemical basis for selective action on a tumor cell versus a normal cell, it would be highly desirable to obtain more specific delivery to tumor cells. Of the several approaches to tumor-specific delivery that are being tried, one of the most promising will surely be the coupling of drugs to monoclonal antibodies directed against tumor-specific surface antigens.[118] Drugs may also be targeted by linking them to lectins and other compounds that bind to specific, cell surface receptors that mediate endocytosis. If the drugs are coupled in such a way that they can be hydrolyzed and released after endocytosis, then even greater selective antitumor effect should be obtained. Drugs, toxins, or even liposome-drug complexes can be linked to antibodies that recognize surrface antigens specific for normal cell types, such as thymic lymphocytes or bone marrow-derived lymphocytes, thus enhancing specificity of drug action against T-cell or B-cell leukemias that still express the normal surface antigen.[123]

Viruses also recognize cell surface receptors and enter cells via endocytosis, and the development of site-directed therapy based upon viral vectors is approaching reality. Two properties of viruses are particularly important: (1) they often have an affinity for specific cell types (tissue tropism), which is based upon their recognition by specific cell surface receptors, and (2) the retroviruses have the ability to transfer new genetic information into the genome of the cell. In the future we may see treatment that is based on site-directed therapy involving highly specific and efficient gene transfer via specially designed viral vectors.

Passage of Drugs into the Central Nervous System

Blood Flow to the Brain

The brain constitutes only 2 percent of the body weight, yet receives about 16 percent of the cardiac output.[124–126] The average blood flow is about 0.5 ml g^{-1} min^{-1}, which is 10 times greater than the blood flow in resting muscle. There is considerable variation in blood flow to different regions of the central nervous system (CNS). In general, blood flow is greater in gray matter than in white matter. In the rat, for example, the cerebral gray matter receives more than 1.3 ml g^{-1} min^{-1}, compared with approximately 0.4 ml g^{-1} min^{-1} in white matter.[127] The differences in blood flow from one brain region to another correlate with differences in capillary density. In the rat the capillary surface area per unit volume in high-flow gray matter is estimated to be 15 mm^2 mm^{-3}, compared with 4.1 mm^2 mm^{-3} in low-flow white matter.[128] The technique of positron emission tomography was used with various radionuclides to obtain estimates of blood flow in human brain ranging from 0.39 to 0.65 ml g^{-1} min^{-1} for gray matter and from 0.19 to 0.26 ml g^{-1} min^{-1} for white matter.[129] As the average blood flow in brain is high with respect to most other organs, one might expect, therefore, that drugs would equilibrate very rapidly between blood and brain. And indeed some do, but many substances enter brain tissue only very slowly, and some practically not at all.[125]

The Blood-Brain Barrier

A drug may gain access to the tissues of the central nervous system by two distinct routes; the capillary circulation and the cerebrospinal fluid (CSF). A drug entering via the capillary circulation must pass across the capillary endothelial cells, through the brain interstitial fluid, and into the brain cells. The so-called blood-brain barrier[125,126] is made up of brain microvessel endothelial cells, which are far less permeable than capillaries in other organs, such as the kidney, liver, and muscle. In contrast to the permeable capillaries found elsewhere in the body, the brain capillaries are characterized by continuous tight endothelial junctions, the absence of fenestrations, and markedly diminished transendothelial vesicle movement.[126] The brain capillary endothelium forms a very effective barrier to the diffusion of polar compounds. The barrier is illustrated in Figure 3-23. Radiolabeled histamine was injected into a mouse, which was sacrificed 30 minutes later by quick freezing in liquid nitrogen, and the distribution of histamine was determined by autoradiography. Figure 3-23 shows a saggital section in which the drug is present in all the mouse tissues except brain and spinal cord.[130]

It appears that the unique permeability features of the brain capillary system are induced

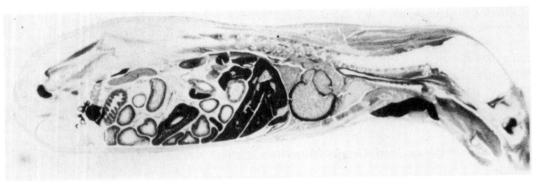

Fig. 3-23. Autoradiogram of a sagittal section of a mouse killed 30 minutes after intravenous injection of [^{14}C]histamine. Histamine is a small molecule that readily passes through capillaries in organs such as the viscera (*left and center*) but does not pass through the blood-brain barrier. Thus, there is no radioactivity in the brain (*clear area at top right*) or in the spinal cord. (From Pardridge,[130] with permission.)

by factors secreted by the brain itself during development. This is suggested by experiments in which embryonic quail brain was transplanted into embryonic chick gut prior to vascularization.[131] The quail brain subsequently became vascularized by vessels that were of chick gut origin but demonstrated the unique properties of cerebral capillaries with a normal blood-brain barrier. Conversely, when embryonic quail gut was transplanted to embryonic chick brain, the gut was vascularized by vessels of chick brain origin that lacked the usual permeability restrictions of the brain microvasculature. Thus, there appear to be trophic factors produced by embryonic brain cells that induce the expression of endothelial cell genes determining the diminished permeability of the blood-brain barrier. The permeability properties of the brain microvessels are being studied in primary endothelial culture systems that will permit detailed examination of the molecular basis for the blood-brain barrier in vitro.[132]

It is generally thought that the blood-brain barrier evolved in order to provide the brain with a fluid environment with a low concentration of potassium.[125] Reduced potassium levels are needed for nerve impulse conduction. Although the term *blood-brain barrier* implies a general impermeability, the barrier should be considered to be selectively permeable. The endothelial cells of the barrier permit the passage of water and lipid-soluble molecules, but the composition of the ultrafiltrate, the brain interstitial fluid, differs strikingly from that of interstitial fluid elsewhere by the nearly complete absence of protein. The brain microvessel endothelial cells restrict the passage of most small polar molecules (e.g., histamine, catecholamines, small peptides) and macromolecules (e.g., proteins) from the cerebrovascular circulation to the brain.[125,133] The endothelial cells transport small, polar essential nutrients such as glucose and amino acids from the blood to the brain interstitial fluid,[134] and they transfer essential polypeptides such as insulin, insulin-like growth factors, and transferrin by receptor-mediated endocytosis.[130] A saturable carrier-mediated system capable of blood to brain transport of small peptides containing an N-terminal tyrosine may also transport enkephalins into the brain.[135] Despite the fact that the brain endothelial cells act as a barrier to the entry of polar drugs, the capillary circulation is the major route by which drugs pass from the blood to brain cells.

The Blood-CSF Barrier

The interstitial space surrounding the individual cellular elements of the brain is in direct anatomic continuity with the large CSF cavities encircling the brain and spinal cord.[136] The CSF is formed both as a result of "lymphatic-like" drainage of the interstitial fluid from the brain and by ultrafiltration of plasma, which occurs primarily at the *choroid plexus* and to a lesser extent at other circumventricular organs, such as the median eminence and the area postrema in the roof of the fourth ventricle (containing the chemoreceptor trigger zone, an important site of drug action). The choroid plexus and the other small circumventricular organs are perfused by porous, fenestrated capillaries, which are much more permeable than the capillaries that make up the blood-brain barrier system. These capillaries form the blood-CSF barrier. The surface area of the blood-brain barrier is more than 5,000 times as great as the surface area of the blood-CSF barrier.[130] Thus, the major barrier that limits the movement of drug molecules from blood into the brain interstitial fluid is located at the endothelial cells of the capillaries forming the blood-brain barrier and not in the choroid plexus.

The choroid plexus is the main source of CSF, which then flows out through the ventriculocisternal system, bathing the surface of the brain and spinal cord. The CSF leaves the CNS by flowing into the venous blood sinuses through a system of large channels and valves in the arachnoid villi.[136] In humans the rate of CSF formation is about 3 ml min^{-1}, and its total volume is about 200 ml, so the rate of turnover is approximately 10 percent per hour. Because of the deep convolutions of the human brain surface, no brain cells are more than 0.5 to 1.0 cm away from the major CSF-containing space. These distances are quite large for diffusional movement of molecules, however, and intrathecal administration of drugs allows only for delivery of drug to the meningeal surfaces of the brain.[137] The intrathecal route of drug administration (injection of drug directly into the subarachnoid space) is employed in treating conditions involving primarily the meninges, such as infectious meningitis and CNS leukemia. Because the CSF surrounding the spinal cord flows in a caudal direction,[138] however, intralumbar injection of a drug is not very beneficial if one wishes the drug to have an effect in the ventricles and at the meninges surrounding the brain.[139] In an effort to circumvent this problem, investigators have delivered drug directly into the ventricular CSF by injection into a subcutaneous dome of siliconized rubber (Ommaya reservoir) with an outlet catheter that extends via a burr hole in the cranium into the lateral cerebral ventricle. This procedure is accompanied by a high incidence of complications due to infections and plugging of the catheter, and another method that is both safer and easier has been used in the treatment of fungal meningitis with amphotericin B. The drug is dissolved in a solution of 10 percent dextrose, which is injected by the intralumbar route, and the patient is then placed in the Trendelenburg position (the body at a 30 degree tilt with the head downward). The specific gravity of the dextrose solution is greater than that of the CSF, and it migrates downhill to the cisterna magna, carrying the drug with it.[140]

The CSF is formed by a combined process of ultrafiltration and secretion. In addition to its almost complete lack of protein, CSF differs from plasma water by having lower concentrations of K^+, Ca^{2+}, and phosphate and a higher Cl^- concentration.[136] The glucose level is lower, but this is not necessarily remarkable in view of the rapid metabolic utilization of glucose by the brain cells. The pH of the CSF is about 0.05 unit lower than that of plasma.[141] These differences in ionic concentrations require the presence of active transport mechanisms.[136] In addition, in many species the CSF is normally 2 to 5 mV electropositive with respect to plasma. However, these differences vary with plasma pH and with different CSF sampling sites. At present, interpretation of the potential difference and its effect on ionic fluxes between CSF and plasma is unclear.

Drugs may enter the CSF by diffusion, transport, or transcytosis directly across the capillaries into the interstitial fluid or by way of the choroid plexus. Drugs may leave the CSF by bulk flow into the venous sinuses, by diffusion back into the capillaries, by absorption at the choroid plexus, or by diffusion into the neuronal cells. One consequence for drug equilibration is that brain cells, brain interstitial fluid, and CSF may come to equilibrium with plasma water at quite different rates. It is even possible for a drug entering the CSF to be "washed out" continually by the bulk flow of water, so that equilibrium between its concentration in plasma water and in CSF is never attained. Let us begin with no drug in CSF and abruptly establish a constant plasma level of drug. Then the net rate of entry of drug into CSF is given by $Q(c_p - c_c)$, where Q is a constant with the dimensions of clearance (milliliters of plasma water cleared of drug per minute), determined by the permeability for the drug; c_c is the drug concentration in CSF; and c_p is the drug concentration in plasma water. The rate of exit of drug from CSF is given by Fc_c, where F is the bulk flow rate. Then

$$\frac{dc_c}{dt} = \frac{1}{V}[Q(c_p - c_c) - Fc_c]$$

where V is the volume of CSF. This equation can be integrated to give the exponential approach of c_c to its steady-state level. The steady state itself is found directly by setting $dc_c/dt = 0$, whence

$$\frac{c_c}{c_p} = \frac{Q}{(Q + F)} = \frac{1}{(1 + F/Q)}$$

Evidently, the ratio of drug concentration in CSF to that in plasma water approaches unity (true equilibrium) as the rate of bulk flow becomes small relative to the clearance of drug from blood into brain, but the steady-state ratio can become indefinitely low at the other extreme.

The diagram in Figure 3-24 summarizes the pathways of drug entry and exit from the CNS.[142] Special note can be made of two mechanisms of exit from the CSF, transport and bulk flow. A number of acidic drugs and radiocontrast agents are transported from the CSF to the blood by an organic acid transport system similar to the renal and hepatic organic acid transport systems that participate in elimination of a wide variety of organic acids from the body. Penicillins, for example, are actively transported from the CSF to the blood.[143] Although the concentrations of penicillins achieved in the CSF are normally low, in the presence of meningeal inflammation concentrations adequate to treat meningitis are achieved.[13] When the meninges are inflamed, active transport of penicillins from the CSF to the blood is impaired.[144] It has been shown in animal experiments that administration of probenecid, another organic acid carried by the same transport system, de-

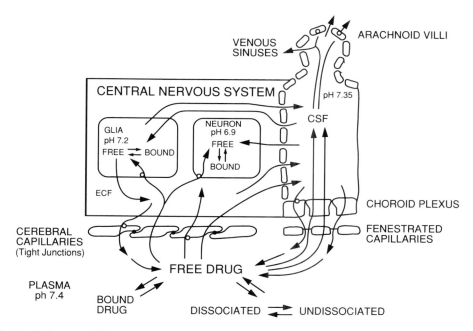

Fig. 3-24. Pathways of drug entry, distribution, and exit from the central nervous system. Drugs may enter and exit by passive diffusion of the undissociated (nonionized) form or by transport of the dissociated (ionized) form. Transport is indicated by open circles with arrows in membranes of various cells. ECF denotes the brain interstitial fluid (extracellular fluid). Bulk flow of CSF is indicated by arrows extending out of the brain interstitial fluid to the CSF and into the venous sinuses. (From Woodbury,[142] with permission.)

creases the rate of efflux of penicillin from the CSF.[145] In animals given penicillin intravenously, pretreatment with probenecid increases the concentration of penicillin achieved in the CSF. Part of this effect may reflect the higher blood level of penicillin that is achieved as a result of competition for renal tubular secretion of the drug, but some of the increased CSF concentration is due to competition for outward transport from the CSF. Drugs that cannot exit the brain by the specific mechanisms mentioned above can leave the brain by diffusion from interstitial fluid into CSF and then by bulk flow of the CSF into the venous circulation. This bulk flow mechanism serves as a sink for drugs entering the CSF from brain, ensuring low concentrations in CSF.[142]

Factors that Determine Rates of Drug Penetration into Brain and CSF

Evidence has been amassed[125,146] that provides the basis for understanding how the physical properties of each drug determine how readily it will cross the blood-brain or blood-CSF barrier. In order to obtain valid data in this field one must, of course, be able to measure drug concentrations in blood, CSF, and brain at short time intervals and accurately. Ideally, one would also like to measure drug concentrations in the brain interstitial fluid and compare values from different brain regions. This technology is being developed. The method of determination has to be specific, distinguishing the drug from any of its metabolic products. Otherwise, one might measure drug plus metabolite in plasma and drug alone in brain or CSF and thus arrive at completely false relative concentrations. In addition, the criteria discussed below have to be satisfied.

Protein Binding. Since only free drug molecules pass across the membranes under study, the drug concentrations should ideally be measured in the water phase of all tissues. Determination of drug concentration in whole brain (the common procedure) presupposes that a negligible fraction is bound, but instances are known in which binding to cellular sites is considerable. Certainly the degree of binding to plasma proteins must be ascertained; because the rate of diffusion across a membrane is proportional to the *free* drug concentration, the measured rates will be determined by this concentration and not by the total drug concentration in plasma. At equilibrium the concentration of lipid-soluble drugs in CSF will be equal to the free drug concentration in plasma (i.e., in plasma water). CSF contains practically no protein, so corrections do not have to be made for free drug concentrations in this fluid. Since the fraction of drug that is bound to protein depends upon the drug concentration, the relevant information is the fraction bound at the concentration actually studied in the experiment. If the plasma drug level falls during an experiment, the fraction bound may increase, and it is therefore best to maintain a constant plasma level throughout the whole experimental period. Obviously, binding to plasma protein should be measured at normal plasma pH and, if possible, at normal body temperature.

Ionization. For drugs that are weak electrolytes, the pK_a must be known so that the degree of ionization at pH 7.4 can be computed from the Henderson-Hasselbalch equation. The permeability of membranes to the nonionized form of a weak electrolyte is so much greater than to the ionic form that for all practical purposes the latter may be considered not to penetrate at all. This major influence of ionization is illustrated by a study[147] in which sulfonamides were injected intraperitoneally into rats. One hour later the animals were decapitated and the concentrations of drug compared in brain and in whole blood. Despite the fact that no corrections were made for protein binding or binding to brain tissue, there is a clear-cut result. For 12 different sulfonamides with pK_as in the range of 2.9 to 7.8, the brain/blood ratio at 1 hour was approximately 0.1 and actually may have been 0 since blood trapped in the brain was included in the brain drug analyses. With pK_a greater than 7.8, there was a systematic increase in the brain/blood ratio to nearly unity at pK_a 10.4. Inasmuch as the plasma pH is 7.4 and sulfonamides dissociate as acids, those compounds whose pK_a values lay below 7.4 would be largely ionized as anions at plasma pH. Sulfonamides with pK_a values much above 7.4 would be almost completely nonionized at plasma pH. Thus, the results are tantamount to saying that the sulfonamide anion did not penetrate into brain at all, even in 1 hour, so that the rate of transfer from plasma to brain was proportional to the concentration of the nonionized moiety. Ideally, the pH should be measured, not only in plasma but in all the compartments under study, since relatively small pH differences on the two sides of a membrane may appreciably influence the distribution ratio through an ion trapping effect.

Partition Coefficient. The lipid solubility of a drug plays a major role in determining the rate at which it penetrates into brain and CSF. Because the only meaningful measurement here is that for the nonionized form of the drug, the determination of a solvent/water partition coefficient should be performed with a strongly acid aqueous phase when the drug is an acid and a strongly alkaline aqueous phase when the drug is a base. If (as is frequently done) partition coefficients are measured at pH 7.4, relationships between drugs may be obscured by simultaneous changes in the degree of ionization and in the partition coefficient of the nonionized form. Unfortunately, there is no way to decide which organic solvent most resembles cell membranes. In general, when compounds are ranked according to their partition coefficients in one solvent, there is approximate correspondence with the rank order in a different solvent, although minor discrepancies do occur. Good correlations with rates of passage across biologic membranes are obtained with nonpolar solvents such as *n*-heptane or benzene, but ether has also proved useful.[88] The absolute values of the partition coefficients have not proved useful; it is the rank order in a series of compounds that one tries to relate to the rates of penetration into brain or CSF.

Figure 3-25 presents the results of a series of experiments in which rates of drug entry

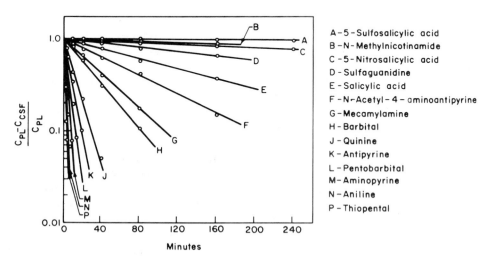

A – 5 – Sulfosalicylic acid
B – N – Methylnicotinamide
C – 5 – Nitrosalicylic acid
D – Sulfaguanidine
E – Salicylic acid
F – N – Acetyl – 4 – aminoantipyrine
G – Mecamylamine
H – Barbital
J – Quinine
K – Antipyrine
L – Pentobarbital
M – Aminopyrine
N – Aniline
P – Thiopental

Fig. 3-25. Kinetics of entry of various drugs into CSF. C_{PL} is concentration of drug in plasma water. C_{CSF} is concentration in cerebrospinal fluid. The drug level in plasma was held constant. Note that the ordinate scale is logarithmic. (From Brodie et al.,[148] with permission.)

into CSF were measured in dogs.[148] The plasma drug levels were held constant by means of a continuous intravenous infusion. The data are plotted with a logarithmic ordinate as the difference between the plasma level and the CSF level divided by the plasma level at each sampling. For plasma levels the free drug concentrations in plasma water were used. A penetration process that was exponential (as expected from the Fick equation) would yield a family of straight lines with slopes representing the penetration rate constant for each drug. Conformity to the expectation is obvious in Figure 3-25. According to Fick's law, the rate of diffusion is proportional to the concentration gradient. Thus, the rate at which the concentration *difference* $c_p - c_c$ decreases is proportional to that difference.

$$\frac{d(c_p - c_c)}{dt} = -P(c_p - c_c)$$

Here P is a penetration rate constant with the dimension of reciprocal time. If the drug level in plasma water is held constant, as by a continuous infusion, we may divide both sides of the equation by c_p, as follows:

$$\frac{d(c_p - c_c)/c_p}{(c_p - c_c)/c_p} = -P\,dt$$

and integrating, we obtain

$$\ln\left(\frac{c_p - c_c}{c_p}\right) = -Pt$$

The constant of integration is 0, since when $t = 0$, $c_c = 0$, and $\ln[(c_p - c_c)c_p] = 0$.

It follows that semilogarithmic plots of $[(c_p - c_c)/c_p]$ against time should yield a family of straight lines whose negative slopes are the penetration (permeability) rate constants. The dimensions of P are min^{-1}, and the half-times to equilibrium are given by $t_{1/2} = 0.693/P$.

From experiments of this kind the penetration rate constants for many drugs have been obtained. Table 3-9 presents such data for the drugs included in Figure 3-25. The tabulation includes all three parameters that should influence the rate of drug penetration if that process is purely a physical diffusion of nonionized drug through a lipid barrier, namely, the fraction bound to plasma protein, the nonionized fraction, and the *n*-heptane/water partition coefficient of the nonionized moiety. In column (f) an effective partition coefficient has been computed by multiplying together the fraction not ionized and the partition coefficient. The observed values of P, the penetration rate constant, were obtained by considering only that fraction of drug in the plasma that is not bound to protein; the actual data showing fraction bound are given in column (b). The semiquantitative agreement between the rank orders in columns (f) and (g) is noteworthy.

Some prototype data in Table 3-9 may be examined profitably. Compounds such as thiopental and aniline penetrate into CSF very quickly because they are largely nonionic at plasma pH and have very high partition coefficients. Pentobarbital, although it is even less ionized than thiopental, has a very much lower partition coefficient and therefore penetrates more slowly. Barbital, although its nonionized fraction is about the same as that of thiopental and although it is much less bound to plasma protein, has so low a partition coefficient that its penetration is very slow. Sulfaguanidine is the extreme example of a compound whose very poor lipid solubility retards its penetration into CSF. Salicyclic acid is largely bound to plasma protein, and the free fraction is nearly all ionized;

Table 3-9. Correlation of Physical Properties of Weak Electrolyte Drugs with Their Rates of Penetration into Cerebrospinal Fluid

(a) Drug	(b) Fraction Bound to Plasma Protein at pH 7.4	(c) pK_a	(d) Fraction Nonionized at pH 7.4	(e) Partition Coefficient n-Heptane/Water of Nonionized Form	(f) Effective Partition Coefficient $(d) \times (e)$ $(\times 10^3)$	(g) Penetration Rate Constant P (min^{-1})	(h) Penetration Half-Time (min)
Thiopental (A)	0.75	7.6	0.613	3.3	2000	0.50	1.4
Aniline (B)	0.15	4.6	0.998	1.1	1100	0.40	1.7
Aminopyrine (B)	0.20	5.0	0.996	0.21	210	0.25	2.8
Pentobarbital (A)	0.40	8.1	0.834	0.05	42	0.17	4.0
Antipyrine (B)	0.08	1.4	>0.999	0.005	5.0	0.12	5.8
Barbital (A)	<0.02	7.5	0.557	0.002	1.1	0.026	27
Mecamylamine (B)	0.20	11.2	0.016	>400	>4.8	0.021	32
N-Acetyl-4-aminoantipyrine (B)	<0.03	0.5	>0.999	0.001	1.0	0.012	56
Salicyclic acid (A)	0.40	3.0	0.004	0.12	0.48	0.006	115
Sulfaguanidine (A)	0.06	>10.0	>0.998	<0.001	<1.0	0.003	231

The penetration rates into CSF were determined in dogs as in Figure 3-25. Data for plasma protein binding may not always have been obtained at the same concentrations used in the in vivo experiments on penetration rate. The entries in column (f) are obtained by multiplying the nonionized fraction (d) by the n-heptane/water partition coefficient (e). The letters A and B after drug names indicate *acid* and *base*, respectively.

Data from Brodie et al.[148] and Hogben et al.[46]

it would hardly penetrate at a measurable rate were it not for the fact that the partition coefficient of its nonionic form is so high. Similar considerations apply to mecamylamine. Its nonionized form has a much higher partition coefficient than any other compound listed, so on these grounds alone it would be expected to penetrate extremely fast. However, it is a basic compound with pK_a well above the physiologic range, so that a negligibly small fraction is nonionic at pH 7.4. The diffusion gradient for the lipid-soluble form of the drug is therefore extremely small compared with the total drug concentration present in plasma. The unfavorable ionization effectively cancels out the highly favorable partition coefficient to yield a moderately low rate constant of penetration.

Pharmacologic Consequences of the Diverse Rates of Entry of Different Drugs into the CNS

The most obvious consequence of the very slow rate of entry of water-soluble and ionized drugs into the brain and spinal cord is that systemic administration of such substances may be useless if the intended site of action is the CNS. The converse proposition is also true. Drugs that act upon the CNS after systemic administration must obviously have a suitable combination of those properties that confer ready penetration, namely, low ionization at plasma pH, low binding to plasma protein, and fairly high lipid/water partition coefficient. These correlations of physicochemical properties with entry into brain can be taken advantage of. Atropine, for example, is a tertiary amine that penetrates brain moderately well, and at higher doses it has significant pharmacologic actions there; its quaternized derivative, atropine methyl sulfate, is effectively excluded from the CNS, yet it produces the same anticholinergic effects in the periphery as does atropine. Neostigmine, a quaternary ammonium cholinesterase inhibitor, acts only peripherally and is effective in the treatment of myasthenia gravis. In contrast, physostigmine, a tertiary amine that is a cholinesterase inhibitor, crosses the blood-brain barrier and is used to treat the central anticholinergic syndrome produced by intoxication with anticholinergic drugs.[149] Dopamine and other amine neurotransmitters are unable to enter the brain when administered intravenously in tolerated doses, but the amino acid L-dihydroxyphenyla-lanine (levodopa), the precursor of dopamine, does pass across the blood-brain barrier via a transport carrier and is effective in the treatment of Parkinson's disease.

Some drugs are virtually excluded from the CNS when they are administered systemically but have striking actions when injected directly into the CSF.[150] Often these central effects are unlike any peripheral effects produced by the same drugs, and sometimes they are quite opposite. Penicillin, which rarely produces toxicity by the usual routes of administration (except in allergically sensitized individuals), causes convulsions if brought into direct contact with spinal cord or brain.[13] Intravenous epinephrine has cardiovascular and hyperglycemic actions and it also produces arousal; injected into a lateral ventricle, on the other hand, it brings about a sleeplike state. Tubocurarine has been studied thoroughly. In the periphery this drug causes paralysis through neuromuscular blockade. When injected into a lateral ventricle in the cat, it initiated a symptom complex that strikingly resembled an epileptic seizure in humans: tremor, myoclonic contractions, loud calling, and generalized convulsions associated with spiking activity in the electroencephalogram. These effects did not occur when the drug was injected into the cisterna magna, whence the CSF flows into the subarachnoid space, indicating that the drug acts on deep structures, not surface ones bathed by subarachnoid fluid. Moreover, the discharge was most pronounced on the side of the injection, suggesting a local action on areas in the vicinity of the lateral ventricles. Other experiments localized this effect of tubocurarine to the hippocampus. Acetylcholine, which certainly cannot enter brain from the capillaries (both because it is a quaternary ammonium cation and because it is hydrolyzed so rapidly by plasma and tissue cholinesterases), caused a curious catatonic stupor when injected intraventricularly in cats. Cholinesterase inhibitors evoked the same symptom complex when administered by the same route.

An interesting consequence of the relationship between ionization and penetration into brain is the effect of acidosis or alkalosis upon the distribution of drugs between brain and plasma. The general effect, insofar as it applies to all body tissues, has already been discussed. Here, the practical importance is that toxic amounts of such CNS depressants as the barbiturates can be removed from the brain by establishing a pH gradient, as illustrated earlier in Figure 3-17. If the plasma is made temporarily more alkaline than the CSF (as by sodium bicarbonate infusion), the fraction of ionized barbiturate in plasma increases and the nonionized fraction decreases. A concentration gradient is thus established for the diffusible (nonionized) form of the drug, and a net movement ensues from brain to plasma. Were the drug not excreted or metabolized, this shift would eventually be reversed as the CSF itself became more alkaline or the plasma alkalosis was compensated. A second and important effect of the alkalosis, however, is to promote renal excretion of the drug, since ionized compounds are reabsorbed very poorly from the tubular urine. As the urine as well as the blood becomes alkaline, an enhanced urinary output results from the ion trapping effect. Obviously, for all drugs whose range of ionization is near pH 7.4, alkalosis will favor the removal of acidic ones from the CNS and passage of basic ones into the central nervous system; acidosis will have the opposite effects.

A dramatic result of the rapid penetration of lipid-soluble substances into the brain is the quick onset of anesthesia caused by gases such as cyclopropane and nitrous oxide, which diffuse very readily through lipid membranes. A less apparent instance of high lipid solubility affecting the onset and duration of drug action is the behavior of thiopental as an intravenous anesthetic agent. Thiopental is unique among the commonly used barbiturates in its very high partition coefficient and extremely rapid passage into the brain.[151] Its oxygen homolog, pentobarbital, has a lower partition coefficient and therefore enters brain somewhat more slowly (Table 3-9). The structures and physical constants for these two drugs are given in Table 3-10. A single intravenous injection of thiopental can produce an almost instantaneous state of anesthesia that lasts for only about 5 minutes, followed by rapid and complete recovery. If the single dose is made very much larger, the anesthesia will be too deep, and respiratory arrest will occur. Pentobarbital has about the same potency as thiopental (i.e., approximately the same concentration in brain is required to produce anesthesia), but no dose can be found that will mimic the ultrashort duration of action of thiopental. If the same intravenous dose is given that was effective in the case of thiopental, no anesthesia results. If the dose is raised, any desired depth of anesthesia can be attained, but the onset will be slow (several minutes) and the duration long (1 hour or more).

At first the ultrashort duration of thiopental action was ascribed to a rapid rate of metabolism, since the drug disappeared eventually from the blood without being accounted for in the urine. Then it was found that thiopental becomes localized in the fat depots, so that after several hours practically all of a single dose is found there. This manifestation of the drug's high lipid/water partition coefficient was then made responsible for its ultrashort duration of action. However, the blood supply to the fat depots is insufficient to

Table 3-10. Comparison of Structures and Properties of Thiopental and Pentobarbital

	Thiopental	Pentobarbital
Structure		
pK_a	7.6	8.1
Fraction nonionized at pH 7.4	0.61	0.83
Partition coefficient of nonionized form (heptane/water)	3.3	0.05

transfer more than a fraction of the total body thiopental there within the 5-minute period that concerns us. What data are available show clearly that the rate of sequestration of thiopental in fat is relatively slow, extending over a period of hours. What, then, is the real explanation of thiopental's ultrashort duration of action?

Experiments were performed by administering thiopental or pentobarbital to rats intravenously and decapitating them at 30 seconds and periodically thereafter.[152] The results, shown in Figure 3-26, were quite clear. Thiopental entered the brain extremely rapidly while the blood level was still very high shortly after the injection. Then, as the blood level fell rapidly as a result of the distribution of thiopental into all the tissues, the drug moved rapidly out of the brain to maintain equilibrium. The time course of this inflow and outflow of thiopental corresponded with the course of onset and offset of anesthesia. In contrast, because pentobarbital equilibrated with brain relatively slowly, the rapid fall in the plasma level was already complete by the time equilibrium was attained, for during the few minutes that the brain concentration was rising, the plasma level was falling fast. Finally, after equilibration the rates of fall of the brain concentration and the plasma concentration were determined by the rate of metabolism and excretion of pentobarbital.

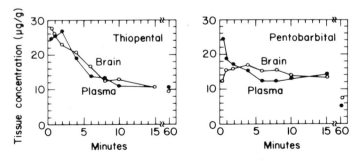

Fig. 3-26. Plasma and brain concentrations of thiopental (**A**) and pentobarbital (**B**) after intravenous injection in rats. The dose for both drugs was 15 mg kg^{-1}. The threshold anesthetic concentration for both drugs was about 20 μg g^{-1} of brain tissue. Each point represents the mean value for four male rats. (From Goldstein and Aronow,[152] with permission.)

Here, since the doses of the two drugs were the same, the rats receiving pentobarbital were not anesthetized. The significant point here is the time course of the changes in brain concentration; these show why a higher dose (as compared with thiopental) would be needed to produce anesthesia, why the onset of anesthesia would be slow, and why the duration of anesthesia would be protracted. Thiopental eventually, of course, becomes localized in fat depots, but this has little influence upon the duration of anesthesia after a single small dose. If multiple doses of thiopental are administered, however, or a continuous infusion of the drug is given, then equilibrium may be attained between an anesthetic concentration in the brain and the same concentration throughout the body fluids. Under these conditions thiopental has an extremely long duration of action, and the drug effect is terminated primarily by its sequestration in fat depots, its subsequent very low rate of metabolism, and the consequent gradual lowering of the concentration in all the body tissues, including the brain. The ultrashort duration of action of thiopental, therefore, is a consequence of its high lipid solubility but only because this confers upon it the ability to enter and leave brain tissue very rapidly.

Finally, the rate of onset of barbital anesthesia presents an illustrative contrast. Although the rate of penetration of thiopental was shown to be much faster than that of pentobarbital, the latter enters brain considerably faster than many other drugs. Table 3-9 indicates that barbital has an extremely unfavorable partition coefficient and that it penetrates very much more slowly than either thiopental or pentobarbital. This is reflected very well in its slow onset of action, which renders the drug useless as an anesthetic or hypnotic agent in humans; even after intravenous administration of an anesthetic dose to experimental animals, many minutes elapse before any effects are seen.

Passage of Drugs across the Placenta

Structure and Function of the Placenta

The mature placenta[153] contains a network of maternal blood sinuses into which protrude villi carrying the fetal capillaries (Figure 3-27). These villi are covered with a trophoblastic layer, beneath which are a layer of mesenchymal tissue and finally the capillary endothelium. There is also a close apposition of the fetal amnion to the chorionic membrane of the uterine wall. Isolated human amniotic membrane has been shown to be permeable to such diverse substances as Na^+, Cl^-, I^-, creatinine, quinine, and serum albumin. In the early stages of gestation the passage of substances directly into the amniotic sac may be significant, but later the amniotic fluid is only in contact with the fetal epidermis. The exchange of nutrients, oxygen and carbon dioxide, and drugs must occur primarily across the placenta, from the maternal arterial supply by way of the intervillous spaces into the fetal capillaries in the villi, and thus into umbilical venous blood.

The membranes separating fetal capillary blood from maternal blood in the intervillous spaces resemble cell membranes elsewhere in their general permeability behavior. Lipid-soluble substances diffuse across readily, water-soluble substances increasingly less well the greater their molecular radii, and large organic ions very poorly or not at all.[155] Very few detailed and systematic quantitative measurements have been made at various times throughout gestation. It is known that the tissue layers interposed between the fetal capillaries and maternal blood become progressively thinner, from about 25 μm early in pregnancy to only 2 μm at term. Permeability to sodium ions has been found to increase greatly over the same period of time, and it is likely that comparable changes in permeability to other substances also occur.[156]

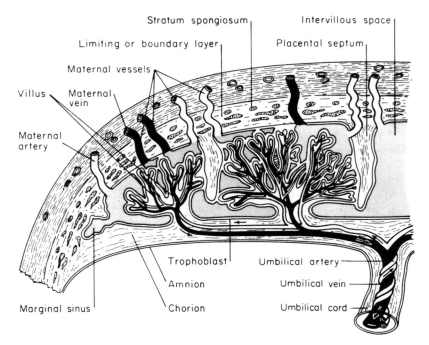

Stratum spongiosum

Limiting or boundary layer

Maternal vessels

Intervillous space

Placental septum

Villus

Maternal vein

Maternal artery

Trophoblast

Amnion

Chorion

Marginal sinus

Umbilical artery

Umbilical vein

Umbilical cord

Fig. 3-27. Scheme of placental circulation. (From Gray,[154] with permission.)

The mature placenta is far more than a semipermeable membrane, and molecules pass across it by all the mechanisms discussed previously.[156,157] Glucose moves down a maternal to fetal concentration gradient by facilitated diffusion.[158] Amino acids are actively transported from the maternal to the fetal circulation by systems that are stereospecific for L-amino acids, and in general, the concentration of an amino acid is higher in the fetal blood than in the maternal blood.[159] Calcium and phosphate both move across the placenta into the fetus by active transport against a gradient,[156] and in some species (e.g., sheep) vitamin D is necessary to maintain the gradient.[160] Although it is of obvious importance for fetal growth, the transfer of vitamins is not well understood. Receptor-mediated endocytosis is an important mechanism of transfer across the placenta. For example, the placenta contains transferrin receptors and transfers iron from the maternal to the fetal side.[161] In general, maternal proteins do not pass across the placenta, but all classes of IgG readily cross the human placenta.[162] IgG is the principal immunoglobulin involved in the passive transfer of immunity to the fetus, and its selective passage into the fetal circulation must involve receptor-mediated endocytosis (described previously in this chapter).

Monoamine oxidase, cholinesterase, and other enzymes are present in the placenta; these may play a role in protecting the fetus against substances for which fetal tissues have not yet developed metabolic pathways. Throughout pregnancy the placenta synthesizes gonadotropins, estrogens, progesterone, and other steroid hormones.[163] It also metabolizes both maternally and fetally derived steroids. Steroid hormone precursors are synthesized in the fetus and utilized by placental biosynthetic hormones, the resulting products appearing in the maternal circulation. Moreover, a wide variety of drugs can be metabolized by placental tissue,[164] and the placental microsomal drug-metabolizing system appears to be similar or identical to that in liver. The drug-metabolizing capacity of placenta is increased by administration of certain drugs to the mother,[165] as described in Chapter 5 for the liver.

Transplacental Passage of Various Drugs

Study of the transplacental passage of drugs[166,167] has been hampered by a number of special circumstances. Kinetic data are difficult to obtain because the fetal concentration can usually only be measured once—at the moment the fetus is delivered or (in an experimental situation) removed surgically. No methods have been developed yet for cannulating the fetal circulation in utero in small animals in a nondestructive way so that measurements can be made over a long time. Ideally, one would wish to establish a constant plasma level in the maternal arterial blood and then perform serial determinations of concentrations in the fetal blood.

Recently a technique was developed in which ultrasound waves are used to guide a needle through the maternal abdominal wall and into the umbilical vein of the human fetus. To date, the technique has been used only for fetal transfusion in humans, but it will permit careful studies of transplacental drug kinetics in large animals. Basic processes of drug passage can be studied by perfusion of human placental tissue postpartum,[168] but this in vitro experimental system does not include most of the variables that determine rates of drug passage into the fetus, and meaningful kinetic data cannot be obtained.

The typical study in the human entails administration of drug to the mother just prior to delivery, then determination of drug concentrations in maternal and cord blood at the moment of delivery. Thus, information about rates of equilibration has to be pieced together from a great many separate experiments. A good example is shown in Figure 3-28. Here, the equilibration of two sulfonamide drugs between maternal and cord blood was studied. The same dose was given to all the mothers intravenously. Whenever delivery occurred, the maternal and cord blood samples were taken simultaneously. Thus, each point on the curve represents one mother and her infant. Despite the scatter it is apparent that these sulfonamides require about 2 hours to reach complete equilibrium.

A critical comment is in order about the practice of sampling cord blood without distinguishing between umbilical venous and umbilical arterial blood and then supposing that the concentration found represents that in the fetal tissues. When the fetus has come into complete equilibrium with maternal blood this will be true, but at all earlier times it will be false. At the outset only the umbilical vein carries any drug at all, and the umbilical artery is essentially drug-free. If the sample is taken from the cut end of the cord with placenta still in situ, it is likely to be pure umbilical venous blood at the placental drug concentration, regardless of the amount of drug in the fetus. In general, at any time during the equilibration process, the highest levels will be found in cord venous blood, the next highest in fetal arterial blood (including cord arterial blood) and the lowest in the fetal tissues as a whole, especially those tissues with a poor blood supply. The importance of this point is illustrated by a study of the distribution of lidocaine administered to mothers just before delivery (Figure 3-29). During the first 30 minutes but especially during the first 15 minutes, the umbilical venous blood contained considerably more drug than did the umbilical arterial blood, reflecting the dilution of the drug in the fetal circulation and the uptake of lidocaine by fetal tissues.

The necessity of distinguishing between a drug and its metabolite is shown in Table 3-11. Here, sulfanilamide was administered to rabbits near term, and the fetal and maternal

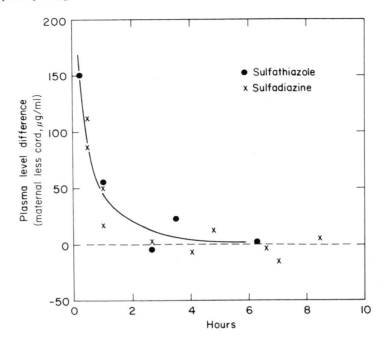

Fig. 3-28. Maternal-fetal equilibration of two sulfonamides in the human. Sulfonamide, 5 g, was given to mothers intravenously as the sodium salt at zero time. Maternal and cord blood was drawn for analysis at delivery. Each point represents one subject mother and infant. Data are for unconjugated drug. (Data from Speert,[169] with permission.)

blood samples were obtained several hours later. The total sulfanilamide concentrations give the impression that equilibrium has not yet been established, but the concentrations of unconjugated sulfanilamide are seen to be about the same in maternal and fetal blood. The experiment did not reveal why the conjugated (acetylated) product was in excess in maternal blood. It might have crossed the placenta more slowly than the parent drug because of its more polar structure; thus free sulfanilamide (the therapeutically active drug) would have attained equilibrium earlier than the acetylated derivative. If a metabolic transformation proceeds rapidly in the mother but not in the fetus and if the metabolic product crosses the placenta very slowly, the product might not equilibrate until after all the parent drug has been metabolized.

An important measurement, without which transplacental transfer rates cannot be assessed meaningfully, is the degree of binding to plasma proteins. Obviously, only free drug is able to cross membranes, and only the free drug concentration need be the same on both sides of a membrane at equilibrium. The free drug may be measured directly (as by analyzing an ultrafiltrate), or the total (free plus bound) concentration may be measured and a correction then applied for the fraction bound as determined independently. The extent of binding to plasma proteins is generally assumed to be the same in maternal and fetal blood inasmuch as the protein composition of plasma appears to be the same, at least in the mature fetus. The binding of a substantial fraction of a drug to maternal plasma proteins will reduce the concentration gradient of free drug molecules and thereby diminish the rate of their passage across the placenta. It may be argued that only free drug matters anyway, since that is the pharmacologically active form, but every unit of free drug trans-

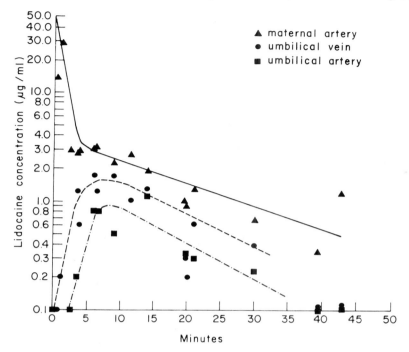

Fig. 3-29. Lidocaine concentrations in maternal arterial, umbilical venous, and umbilical arterial plasma at delivery. Data from human subjects following a single intravenous injection of lidocaine (2 mg kg^{-1}) in 16 mothers just before delivery. (From Shnider and Way,[170] with permission.)

ferred to the fetus will itself undergo binding in the same proportions as in maternal blood. The fetal plasma proteins act as a sink for the drug molecules after they cross the placenta; therefore a relatively large amount of drug may have to be transferred, at a relatively low concentration gradient, in order to establish maternal-fetal equilibrium. Thus, protein binding can considerably retard the passage of drugs across the placenta.

Table 3-11. Maternal-Fetal Equilibration of Sulfanilamide and Acetylsulfanilamide in Rabbits

Rabbit Number	[a]Total Sulfanilamide		Unconjugated Sulfanilamide	
	Maternal	Fetal	Maternal	Fetal
1	26.5	18.1	15.7	14.6
2	24.7	16.7	13.7	12.1
3	21.0	12.5	2.6	2.7
4	29.2	—	9.8	6.2
5	35.2	10.3	6.3	6.4
6	11.5	7.3	4.4	3.1
7	22.0	20.0	20.3	16.9

[a] Sulfanilamide was administered to rabbits near term in a single oral dose, and the fetal and maternal blood were sampled about 3.5 to 5.5 hours later. Total sulfanilamide includes unchanged drug and the acetylated derivative. Figures represent milligrams per 100 ml plasma.
(From Lee et al.,[171] with permission.)

This analysis is valid for drugs whose permeability across the placenta is rate-limiting. The degree to which rate of drug passage across the placenta is retarded will be less if the extent of binding to plasma protein is less in fetal blood than in maternal blood.[172] Analysis of rat sera obtained at different stages of gestation demonstrates that fetal plasma protein concentration rises nearly twofold as the animals approach term.[173] Thus, early in gestation the transfer of hydrophilic drugs across the placenta may be faster than late in gestation.

Substances that are very lipid-soluble (e.g., the anesthetic gases) diffuse across the placental membranes so rapidly that their overall rates of equilibration are limited only by the placental blood flow.[153] Inasmuch as dissociation of the complexes between drugs and plasma proteins is practically instantaneous, equilibration rate would not be affected significantly by protein binding in this group of substances. For drugs transferred at moderate rates or slowly, however, diffusion is rate-limiting, and protein binding can play a role.

Consider two drugs, X and Y, both therapeutically effective at the same *free* concentrations $[X]$, $[Y]$. Drug X is 90 percent bound to plasma protein (i.e., its total concentration is $10[X]$); Y is not bound at all. Since the volume of maternal body water is so much greater than that of the fetus, we may assume, roughly, that after equilibration the maternal plasma level remains unchanged. The net transfer of Y will be $[Y]$ times the volume of fetal body water, and initially this will take place at a concentration gradient $[Y] - 0 = [Y]$. As for X, at equilibrium the fetus will contain $[X]$ times the volume of fetal body water; in addition, there will be a bound component, $9[X]$ times the fetal plasma volume. The initial concentration gradient is $[X] - 0 = [X]$, so that relative to the total amount that has to be transferred, the transfer rate will be much lower than it was for Y.

This dependence of the rate of equilibration of free drug upon plasma protein binding is probably unique for transplacental transfer; elsewhere (e.g., brain, renal glomeruli) the fluid on the other side of the membrane contains very little protein, so the sink effect is not operative.

Studies on fetal drug levels at various times during gestation are obviously out of the question in the human, with a few exceptions. Occasionally data have been obtained at the time of delivery of a nonviable deformed fetus (e.g., an anencephalic monster) or a fetus killed by a drug taken suicidally by the mother, and rarely, advantage has been taken of a therapeutic abortion, usually in the first trimester, to gain information about passage of a drug into the early embryo. Under such conditions it was shown[174] that caffeine, which distributes freely into all the body water, also equilibrated with the fetal tissues when it was administered to women at the seventh or eighth week of gestation.

Despite the difficulties cited above, considerable qualitative and semiquantitative information has been obtained in human and animal studies about which drugs cross readily into the fetal circulation and which do not.[166,167] Among drugs that enter the fetus at all, two extreme equilibration rates are indicated in Table 3-12. Tubocurarine, a quaternary ammonium compound that is excluded completely from the brain, had barely reached a detectable level in fetal blood at 9 minutes. In contrast, thiopental, which equilibrates with brain as fast as the blood delivers it, had attained about half-equilibration with fetal blood at 9 minutes, and had reached a considerable concentration earlier than 5 minutes. The wide range of transplacental transfer rates is reminiscent of the kinetics of equilibration between blood and brain (or CSF). The principles, indeed, are the same except that the placental membranes are obviously more permeable to water-soluble molecules and ions than are the brain capillaries. Moreover, as discussed in detail below, the fastest

Table 3-12. Maternal-Fetal Equilibration of Tubocurarine and Thiopental in Humans

Time after Drug Administration (min)	[a]Tubocurarine		[a]Thiopental	
	Maternal	Fetal	Maternal	Fetal
5	3	0	8.5	5.5
5	2.4	0		
6	3.2	0	8.0	3.5
9	1.1	0.1	4.8	2.5
10			1.9	1.1
11	2.1	0.1	2.0	1.2
12			3.0	2.0

[a] Thiopental, 125 mg, was given as single rapid intravenous injection. Tubocurarine was given intravenously over a 1-minute period, usually a total dose of 30 to 36 mg. Blood values are in micrograms per milliliter of plasma.
Data from Cohen.[175]

equilibrium possible between maternal and fetal blood is a great deal slower than that between blood and brain, primarily because the blood flow to the placenta limits the rate of delivery of drug to the fetal circulation.

Of the agents (besides thiopental) that would be expected to equilibrate at the maximum rate, trichloroethylene attained nearly equal concentration in fetal and maternal blood within 16 minutes; other anesthetics (ether, cyclopropane, halothane) equilibrated in about the same time. Data showing unequal distribution of nitrous oxide even after 30 minutes are difficult to accept at face value in view of the universal finding that this gas equilibrates rapidly and completely in other tissues, including brain. Oxygen and carbon dioxide, the lipid-soluble respiratory gases, also pass rapidly across the placenta.

Narcotic analgesics have been found at near equilibrium values in fetal blood plasma after several hours, but rates of transfer are not available. Some effects of morphine (e.g., depressed respiration, pinpoint pupils) have been observed in newborn infants of mothers given morphine during labor; and the occurrence of withdrawal symptoms in infants born of addicted mothers makes it plain that morphine and heroin have free access to the fetus during gestation. The tranquilizers of the phenothiazine and reserpine classes evidently cross the placenta, as judged by typical drug effects observed in newborn infants.

Steroids, as might be expected, cross the placenta readily (e.g., cholesterol, progesterone, estradiol, estriol), but the more water-soluble glucuronides of these compounds penetrate at much reduced rates. Antibiotics, including penicillin, chloramphenicol, tetracyclines, streptomycin, and erythromycin, all appear in fetal blood, but rather slowly and at very different rates. Penicillin attains near equilibrium in about 10 hours, streptomycin in about 18 hours. The tetracyclines cross the placenta into the fetus, where they are incorporated into the structure of fetal bones and teeth.

Teratogenic agents of diverse chemical structure obviously cross the placenta; numerous studies have implicated a direct action of such drugs on the tissues undergoing embryogenesis (Ch. 13). Of especial concern is the ease with which hazardous products of nuclear fission (e.g., ^{137}Cs, ^{45}Ca, ^{90}Sr, ^{131}I) cross the placental membranes and localize in vulnerable fetal tissues. Not only viruses (e.g., the teratogenic rubella virus, HIV virus) but cellular pathogens (e.g., spirochetes) may cross the placenta and infect the fetus.

It is an obvious clinical fact that a mother deeply anesthetized with a barbiturate can give birth to a fairly alert infant who scores well on the Apgar test, a crude but rapid and exceedingly useful scoring system for evaluating several vital indices immediately after birth. Unfortunately, follow-up has often been haphazard, so that no reliable data are to be found on the longer-lasting and delayed effects of maternal medication on the infant. If adequate records were available, a relationship might even be sought between the extent of drug use at delivery and the overall neonatal mortality. It is clear that infants of mothers who were delivered under deep anesthesia often show depression over the next 24 hours compared with those delivered without benefit of drugs or with short-acting volatile anesthetics. Leif[176] has stated:

> Although the youngster at birth cries vigorously and, it is true, has an arterial plasma level of thiopental lower than the mother, there is still enough drug within the child for 12 and possibly 24 hr to make this newborn infant much more drowsy than the other child. We feel that the observations at birth and at delivery do not tell the entire story. . . . Although you can arouse the child, the newborn can readily go back into drowsiness and practically not move for several hours.

The unmedicated infant, although born with a respiratory acidosis caused by CO_2 accumulation, rapidly eliminates the excess CO_2 by vigorous respiration, and the plasma pH rises to a normal level with the first hour. In the infant of the medicated mother this may not occur. With many drugs the difficulty imposed upon the infant by the unwanted drug effect and by acidosis is compounded by the absence of drug-metabolizing enzymes and by poor renal function in the neonatal period.

That a wakeful infant should be born of an anesthetized mother is not surprising when one considers what is known and can be calculated about the rates of equilibration of maternal and fetal tissues with respect to an anesthetic drug. What is confusing and difficult to interpret are findings indicating that fetal and maternal blood have the same concentration of a barbiturate (or other anesthetic agent) at the time of delivery, and yet the mother is anesthetized, the newborn awake. Everything we know indicates that infants should be *more* depressed than adults at a given barbiturate concentration and should be in still further trouble because of their immature liver microsomal drug-metabolizing system. As shown in the next section, data indicating complete equilibration of secobarbital in 3 to 5 minutes, of pentobarbital in 1 minute, of thiopental in 3 minutes, and even of barbital (usually the slowest to penetrate cell membranes) in 4 minutes must be discounted. The most likely source of error would be that the analyses were done principally on umbilical venous blood carrying a drug concentration nearly the same as that in the placenta but greatly in excess of that in fetal brain and body water.

Theory of Maternal-Fetal Equilibrium Rates

The kinetics of equilibration of the fetal tissues with drugs in the maternal circulation depend upon the rates of delivery of drug to the placenta and of its removal and circulation on the fetal side, as well as upon the rate of permeation at each membranous interface in the system. We shall compute *maximum* rates by assuming instantaneous equilibration at every membrane, as might nearly be true of such agents as thiopental or the anesthetic gases. We shall assume at the outset that a constant drug concentration is maintained in the maternal plasma water. Later we shall postulate various rates of decline of the maternal drug level.

The plan of the fetal circulation is presented in Figures 3-30 and 3-31. Blood from the placental villi, which are bathed in the intervillous maternal blood, enters the fetus by

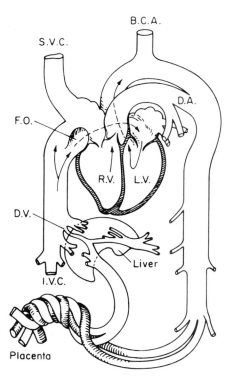

Fig. 3-30. Plan of the fetal circulation. I.V.C., Inferior vena cava; R.V., right ventricle; D.V., ductus venosus; D.A., ductus arteriosus; S.V.C., superior vena cava; L.V., left ventricle; F.O., foramen ovale; B.C.A., brachiocephalic artery (in humans the common carotid artery). (Adapted from Dawes,[177] with permission.)

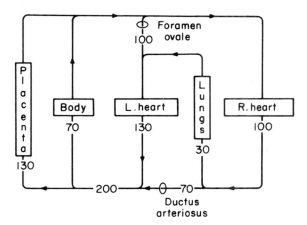

Fig. 3-31. Schematic view of fetal lamb circulation. This shows that both sides of the fetal lamb heart work in parallel. Approximate data for blood flow (milliliters per kilogram per minute) are shown in each portion of the circuit. (From Dawes,[177] with permission.)

way of the umbilical vein, is mixed with the venous return from the lower body of the fetus, and enters the inferior vena cava through the ductus venosus. Most of this blood, instead of entering the right heart (as it will do after birth), passes directly through the foramen ovale in the atrial septum and into the left heart. The left cardiac output supplies the fetal brain and upper extremity; a part of this blood passes into the aorta to supply the remaining fetal tissues, and a part returns to the placenta via the umbilical artery. Blood returning from the head in the superior vena cava enters the right heart. Some passes through the inactive lungs and back to the left atrium, but most bypasses the pulmonary circulation through the ductus arteriosus and enters the aorta directly. The unusual feature of this circulation is, as shown schematically in Figure 3-31, that both sides of the heart work in parallel rather than in series.

Using the best estimates available for the blood flows and blood volumes in the human, Avram Goldstein has derived expressions for the changes to be expected in each compartment at successive 1-second intervals. These expressions were then evaluated by an iterative process on a digital computer to obtain the time course of drug transfer. The following diagram is a schematic representation of the placental and fetal circulations.

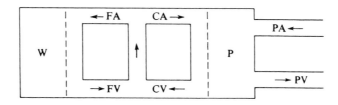

The symbols in the diagram and in the calculations below have the following meanings:

PA = drug concentration in maternal arterial blood to the placenta; flow = 8.33 ml sec^{-1}

P = drug concentration in placental intervillous blood; volume = 250 ml

PV = drug concentration in maternal venous blood draining the placenta, assumed to be equilibrated with P

CA = drug concentration in umbilical artery; flow = 8.33 ml sec^{-1} = 57 percent of fetal cardiac output

CV = drug concentration in umbilical vein, assumed to be equilibrated with P

FA = drug concentration in fetal arterial blood; flow = 6.28 ml sec^{-1} = 43 percent of fetal cardiac output

FV = drug concentration in fetal venous return other than umbilical vein, assumed to be equilibrated with W

W = drug concentration in fetal body water; volume = 77 percent of 3.5 kg fetal weight = 2700 ml

t = time in seconds

k = rate constant (sec^{-1}) for decline in maternal arterial drug level, so that $PA_t = PA_{t-1} - k \cdot PA_{t-1}$

For our purposes we may consider 1 second to be an infinitesimally small Δt. We shall solve for concentration increments in successive 1-second periods and sum these to obtain the desired time courses.

In P the net increment in total drug in 1 second is the input less the output, 8.33 ($PA - PV$) + 8.33 ($CA - CV$). Since $PV = CV = P$, and the volume of dilution is 250 ml,

$$P_t = P_{t-1} + \frac{8.33(PA + FA - 2P_{t-1})}{250}$$

Since FA and CA are derived from the mixing of CV and FV in proportion to their respective flows, and since $FV = W$,

$$FA = \frac{(8.33P_t + 6.28W)}{(8.33 + 6.28)}$$

Finally, the increment in W is given by 6.28($FA - FV$)/2700, so that

$$W_t = W_{t-1} + \frac{6.28(FA - W_{t-1})}{2700}$$

When $t = 0$, then $PA = 1$ and all other concentrations are 0. The above equations were evaluated for all values of t until attainment of 95 percent equilibration, when $W_t = 0.95PA_t$. Solutions were obtained for selected values of k. Flow rates and volumes were taken from Dawes,[177] Martin,[178] and Reid[179] and fetal body water from Edelman et al.[180] Uncertainty about the precise volume of the intervillous space has little effect; all time courses computed for 125 ml intervillous blood are identical to those for 250 ml except within the first minute.

The results of these calculations are graphically represented in Figure 3-32. The curves show the course of equilibration of the cord venous blood (in equilibrium with placental intervillous blood), of the fetal arterial blood (such as would bathe the fetal brain), and of the fetal tissue water in general. All the assumptions on which the calculations were based would lead to an overestimate of the speed of equilibration. For example, no permeability barrier was assumed to be present in the placenta, so substances whose rates of transfer are diffusion-limited may equilibrate very much more slowly than shown. Also, the entire tissue water in the fetus has been supposed to equilibrate as a homogeneous mass, with the whole of the blood traversing the nonplacental circuit, while in fact the poorly perfused components of the fetal tissue mass will come to equilibrium more slowly. With these qualifications we may examine the theoretical course of drug transfer.

Consider first what happens if the maternal arterial drug concentration remains constant (Fig. 3-32A). Half-equilibration of the fetal tissues (shown by the curve FW) requires at least 13 minutes; 90 percent equilibration would take about 40 minutes. Throughout the equilibration process but especially in the first few minutes, cord venous blood contains a much higher concentration than fetal arterial blood, and the drug concentration in fetal tissue water lags well behind that in the fetal arteries. If an infant were delivered a few minutes after establishment of a constant maternal drug level, the cord venous blood would only poorly reflect the fetal drug concentration; even mixed cord blood would give a very false impression. Moreover, as long as the drug concentration in fetal arterial blood exceeds that in fetal tissue water, interruption of the cord at delivery would lead to a rapid redistribution of drug within the fetus; drug would leave organs having a rich blood supply (such as the brain), which have equilibrated rapidly, and enter those of greater mass and poorer blood supply, which are still far from equilibrium. It is obvious, then, why anesthetic drugs can affect the mother and not the fetus in many common circumstances.

If the maternal blood level is falling rather than constant, then fetal equilibration is

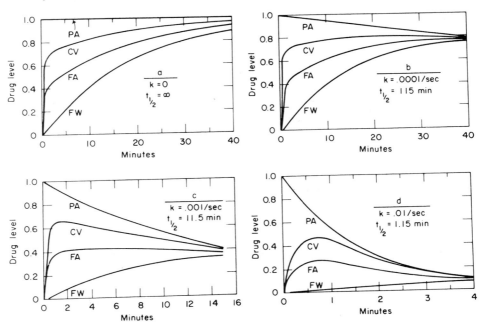

Fig. 3-32. Kinetics of equilibration of maternal and fetal tissues. Theoretical curves, computed as described in the text. Four time courses are shown representing four different elimination rate constants (k) and the corresponding biologic half-lives ($t_{1/2}$) in maternal plasma. In each case are shown the drug levels in maternal (placental) arterial blood (PA), cord venous blood (CV), fetal arterial blood (FA), and fetal body water (FW). Note change in time scale in c and d. All drug levels are expressed as fractions of the initial maternal arterial level. Absorption and distribution in the maternal circulating blood are assumed to be instantaneous.

speeded, but the more rapid the disappearance of drug from maternal blood, the lower will be the actual drug level attained in the fetus at equilibrium. Figures 3-32B to D show this effect quite clearly (note change of time scale in C and D). Figure 3-32C could nearly represent the administration of thiopental to a mother at delivery. During the course of the intravenous injection the arterial blood (to brain and to placenta) carries a high enough drug concentration to anesthetize the mother. Immediately after the injection is completed, thiopental leaves the circulation, equilibrating rapidly with the maternal body water, with a half-time probably not too different from the 11.5 min represented in the diagram. Suppose the infant is delivered 5 to 10 minutes later. The figure shows that although the mother's brain is still exposed to more than half the original anesthetic concentration, the fetal brain never was (and never will be) exposed to an anesthetic drug level. Moreover, the fetal tissue water, still lagging far behind, will accept thiopental from the fetal brain as soon as the cord is cut; very shortly, then, the thiopental concentration in the fetal brain will have been reduced to the lower level.

Although not shown in Figure 3-32, it is true that when the maternal drug concentration is falling rapidly, the fetal levels may eventually exceed those in the maternal blood.[181] This overshoot simply reflects the sluggishness of the fetal equilibration mechanisms; it is followed, of course, by a reverse flow of drug from fetus to mother. This effect is small and of no practical consequence, but occasional experiments have confirmed that it may indeed occur.

In summary, it may be concluded that the fastest equilibration possible between fetal tissues and a *constant maternal blood level* of a drug would require at least 40 minutes for 90 percent equilibration. This makes it understandable that drugs whose passage across the placental membranes is impeded by their size, water solubility, ionization, or protein binding should require hours for equilibration; many such examples have been presented. Equilibration with a *falling maternal blood level* is, of course, faster, but if the initial drug concentration in the mother was at an appropriate therapeutic level, then the fetus is not likely ever to experience an effective blood level, since the equilibrium concentration will be considerably lower. More systematic kinetic studies in animal fetuses in utero are badly needed, as well as more critical quantitative data and long-term follow-up in humans.

DRUG ELIMINATION: THE MAJOR ROUTES

Metabolism, storage, and excretion are the three mechanisms whereby drugs are ultimately removed from their sites of action. Drug metabolism will be considered in detail in another chapter. Deposition and storage of drugs in fat depots and in the reticuloendothelial system play significant roles in the removal of lipid-soluble agents and colloidal substances, respectively; examples of each process were presented earlier in this chapter. Excretion at the kidneys, biliary system, intestine, and sometimes the lungs accounts for most drug elimination, and renal excretion is by far the most important of those routes. An additional route of elimination must be considered in the case of nursing mothers. Some drugs are secreted into the milk in sufficient concentration to present a risk to the nursing infant.[182]

Renal Excretion of Drugs

The kidney is admirably suited to the task of drug elimination.[183] About 130 ml of plasma water is filtered each minute (190 L/day) through the glomerular membranes. Of this volume only about 1.8 L is excreted as urine, the remainder is reabsorbed in the renal tubules.[184] A drug will be filtered if its molecular size is not excessively large; since even some plasma albumin appears in the filtrate, most drugs, being smaller, will encounter no difficulty if they are not bound tightly to plasma proteins. The glomerular capillaries are composed of a particularly thin endothelium, which is very rich in fenestrae, and filtration constants derived experimentally reveal the glomerulus to be far more permeable to solutes than are the capillaries of muscle. Only free drug in plasma water (not drug that is bound to plasma proteins) can be filtered. The principles governing passage back from the glomerular filtrate across the tubular epithelium into the blood (reabsorption) are the familiar ones that relate to any transmembrane passage. Drugs with high lipid/water partition coefficients will be reabsorbed readily as the solute in the lumen of the tubule becomes concentrated; polar compounds and ions will be unable to diffuse back and therefore will be excreted unless reabosrbed by a carrier transport system.

The kidney receives a very large blood supply (25 percent of the cardiac output) through wide, short renal arteries that permit blood to enter the tissue with but little drop in hydrostatic pressure. The afferent arterioles bring blood to the glomeruli for filtration; the efferent arterioles carry about four-fifths of the same blood (one-fifth having been filtered) to the tubules and thence to the venous collecting system. The epithelial cells of the proximal tubules are rich in mitochondria and are supplied with a "brush border" of very large area lining the tubular lumen. These epithelial cells carry on active energy-dependent reabsorption. About 80 percent of the NaCl and water is isosmotically reabsorbed here, as are glucose and amino acids. The proximal tubule is also the site of active secretion of various metabolites and drugs from plasma into the tubular urine. Further down the nephron the loop of Henle, together with its adjacent blood vessels, is the site of the countercurrent mechanism generating the hypertonic gradient in the renal medulla that allows concentration of urine by water reabsorption at the distal tubules and collecting ducts, subject to control by the pituitary hormone vasopressin. The distal tubular epithelium is also the site of urine acidification and of potassium excretion.

The renal excretory mechanisms (glomerular filtration, tubular reabsorption, tubular secretion, or any combination thereof) have the net effect under most conditions of removing a constant fraction of the drug presented to the kidneys by the renal arterial blood. A simplified nomenclature has grown up describing the quantitative aspects of the excretory process in terms of a hypothetical clearance of a certain volume of plasma each minute. Let c be the concentration of a drug in the plasma water, U its concentration in urine, V_u the volume of urine, and t the time of urine collection in minutes. Then UV_u/t is the *amount* of drug excreted per minute, and obviously UV_u/tc is the volume of plasma in which this amount of drug was contained. We may imagine, then, that such a volume of plasma water was actually cleared of its drug per minute, and so we speak of the term UV_u/tc as the *clearance* of a drug; its units are milliliters per minute. The symbol P is often used to denote the plasma drug concentration in clearance calculations. For consistency in this book we use c for drug concentrations in plasma. Clearance is usually stated to be UV/P rather than UV_u/tc, UV being defined as the urinary excretion *per minute*.

The polymeric carbohydrate inulin (in the dog, also creatinine) is not bound appreciably to plasma proteins; it is filtered at the glomeruli and neither reabsorbed nor secreted at the tubules. Its clearance is therefore a measure of the glomerular filtration rate, about 130 ml min^{-1} in humans. The clearance of glucose under normal conditions is zero since it is completely reabsorbed in the tubules. If there were a substance so vigorously secreted by the tubules that the renal arterial plasma could be completely cleared in a single passage through the kidney, that substance would serve as a measure of the renal plasma flow. Penicillin and p-aminohippurate (PAH) approach this ideal; their clearance is about 650 ml min^{-1}. Since the plasma volume is about one-half the blood volume, the renal blood flow through both kidneys, as estimated from the PAH clearance, would be about 1,300 ml min^{-1}, or 25 percent of the cardiac output. Of course, drugs that are actively secreted are also filtered. However, since secretion is so much more effective than filtration, it is customary to say that a certain drug is "excreted by tubular secretion" even though it is understood that a certain fraction (the *filtration fraction*, about one-fifth) is removed from the blood by filtration before that blood is even presented to the tubules.

The clearance can be related to the amount of a drug x that is excreted into the urine per minute, as follows:

$$\frac{dx}{dt} = \text{clearance} \times c = (\text{ml min}^{-1}) \times (\text{mg ml}^{-1}) = \text{mg min}^{-1}$$

However, it tells us nothing about the extent to which the plasma drug concentration is decreased by the renal excretory process. For this we have to know the apparent volume of distribution V_d. Clearly, for a given renal clearance the greater the volume of distribution, the more total drug will have to be eliminated from the body, and the more slowly will the plasma drug level fall.

The relationship between renal clearance and the overall elimination rate, for various values of V_d, is of general interest. Let k_e be the rate constant of elimination, defined by the first-order equation $dc/dt = k_e c$. The units of k_e are reciprocal time (e.g., min^{-1}). Then

$$k_e = \frac{clearance}{V_d}$$

and since the half-time of an exponential process is given by $0.693/k$, the elimination half-time for a drug excreted by the kidneys will be

$$t_{1/2} = 0.693 \frac{V_d}{clearance}$$

The general relationships between clearance, rate constant of elimination, and elimination half-time are shown in Table 3-13 for several possible volumes of distribution. The shortest possible elimination half-time would be for a drug that was wholly contained in the plasma water and was cleared by tubular secretion; half the amount of the drug would be eliminated in 3 minutes. More usual values would lie between 13 and 44 minutes, depending upon the degree to which the drug had entered into body cells. The corresponding range of half-times for a drug cleared by glomerular filtration alone is seen to be 64 to 219 minutes (i.e., 1 to 4 hours). There is no upper limit on elimination half-times, since renal clearances may be as low as zero, and apparent volumes of distribution can exceed the body water volume if extensive tissue binding occurs. The first line of the table represents an arbitrarily selected illustration of partial reabsorption; a clearance of 30 ml min^{-1} is assumed, but any clearance between 0 (complete reabsorption) and 650 ml min^{-1} is possible.

The dependence of the elimination rate constant upon the volume of distribution is illustrated nicely by a study on the adrenergic blocking agent tolazoline, a tertiary amine, in the dog.[185] This drug was shown in renal clearance studies to be secreted actively by the renal tubules, at a rate practically identical to that of PAH, which is cleared completely from the plasma passing through the kidney. The very high pK_a of tolazoline means that at body pH it is almost entirely present as the ionized moiety, and it is therefore possible that it is confined to the extracellular space, that is, to about 18 percent of the body weight. We can see from Table 3-13 that a drug with these properties should be eliminated with a half-life of about 13 minutes. The experiment depicted in Figure 3-33, on the

Table 3-13. Relationships Between Clearance, Rate Constant of Elimination, and Elimination Half-Time for a Drug Eliminated by the Renal Route

Clearance	[a]Drug Distributed in:		
	Plasma Water (3,000 ml)	Extracellular Fluid (12,000 ml)	Body Water (41,000 ml)
Partial reabsorption (e.g., 30 ml min^{-1})	1.00×10^{-2} (69 min)	2.50×10^{-3} (277 min)	7.32×10^{-4} (947 min)
Glomerular filtration 130 ml min^{-1}	4.33×10^{-2} (16 min)	1.08×10^{-2} (64 min)	3.17×10^{-3} (219 min)
Tubular secretion 650 ml min^{-1}	2.17×10^{-1} (3 min)	5.42×10^{-2} (13 min)	1.59×10^{-2} (44 min)

[a] Entries are values for k_e, the rate constant of elimination (units = min^{-1}); parenthetic entries are corresponding values of the elimination half-time. The clearance given under "partial reabsorption" is arbitrary; any clearance between 0 (complete reabsorption) and 650 ml min^{-1} is possible.

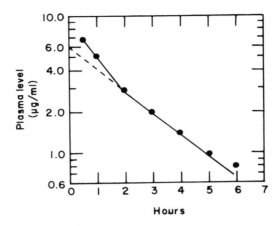

Fig. 3-33. Plasma levels of tolazoline after intravenous administration. The drug was given as a single injection (13 mg kg^{-1}) to a dog, and plasma levels were measured periodically. (From Brodie et al.,[185] with permission.)

contrary, shows a measured half-life of nearly 2 hours. The discrepancy is accounted for by the fact that a large fraction of the administered drug (as shown by tissue analyses) was sequestered in liver, spleen, kidney, and other organs. The high lipid solubility of the nonionized moiety favors entry into cells, leading to a high tissue/plasma concentration ratio, by a principle similar to that explained for ion trapping. Thus, the apparent V_d of such a drug is much larger than the extracellular space, and it accounts well for the surprisingly long half-life. The actual magnitude of the apparent V_d cannot be determined by extrapolation of the slow phase back to zero time in Figure 3-33 as could be done with the simple equilibration of a virtually closed system (cf. Fig. 3-9). Here, where material is being excreted from the body at a rapid rate, extrapolation leads to serious overestimation of V_d.[186] Extrapolation of the fast phase yields a V_d of 1.44 L/kg, which reflects the distribution of drug into tissue.

The availability of a drug for glomerular filtration is strictly dependent upon its concentration in plasma water. Meaningful clearance values can therefore not be obtained unless the degree of protein binding is determined at the relevant drug concentrations. For drugs cleared by tubular secretion, however, it makes no difference what fraction is bound to plasma protein provided that the binding is reversible. All the drug, bound as well as free, becomes available for active secretion. Then as free drug is removed by the tubular cells, bound drug dissociates very rapidly to maintain the equilibrium with plasma water.

The tubular secretory process handles organic anions and cations by separate transport mechanisms. The group of anions has been studied most thoroughly.[187,188] The process is energy-dependent and is blocked by metabolic inhibitors. The secretory transport capacity can be saturated at high concentrations of the anions, and so each substance has its characteristic maximum secretion rate, called *tubular maximum* (T_m). The anionic group is often a carboxylate or sulfonate group, but sulfones (such as phenol red or chlorothiazide) carrying partial negative charges are transported equally well. The various anionic compounds compete with one another for secretion, and this can be put to practical use. Thus, probenecid will block the otherwise rapid renal secretion of penicillin and thereby prolong its duration of action in the body. Evidently, the same (or a similar) mechanism mediates the tubular reabsorption of the uric acid anion, for this is also blocked by probenecid; the uricosuric action finds some therapeutic use in gout, since uric acid excretion is thereby promoted. A striking feature of organic anion secretion is the variety of chemical structures that are transported. In contrast to the highly selective transport systems discussed earlier in this chapter, the steric arrangement of chemical groupings in the substrates does not seem to be critical in the renal anion transport system. Thus, there may be multiple modes of attachment to the carrier site, or possibly there are subsystems with somewhat different specificities. PAH is the compound that has been classically used to study the properties of the anion transport system, and a number of commonly administered drugs are excreted by this mechanism (e.g., salicylate, phenylbutazone, penicillins, cephalosporins, and most of the potent diuretics). The normal function of the anion secretion system is apparently to eliminate from the body metabolites that have been conjugated with glycine, with sulfate, or with glucuronic acid.

Organic cations are secreted by a different pathway, also energy-dependent and stereospecific.[188,189] The organic cations compete with each other but not with anions. N-methylnicotinamide and tetraethylammonium ion have been used as prototype compounds to study this cation transport system in the same manner that PAH has been used to study the anion transport system. Natural substrates include neurotransmitters, such as acetylcholine, dopamine, histamine, and serotonin, and metabolic products such as creatinine. Although the molecules secreted by the organic cation transport mechanism vary widely in chemical structure, all contain a nitrogen atom and carry a net positive charge at physiologic pH. The cation transport mechanism is important in the elimination of many drugs from the body (e.g., atropine, hexamethonium, isoproterenol, neostigmine, and meperidine). An unmodified drug and its metabolite may be preferentially transported by different secretory systems. Morphine, for example, is transported by the organic cation system,[189] but the glucuronide and sulfate conjugates, which are excreted to a great extent by glomerular filtration, may also be transported by the organic anion system.[187]

In newborn infants, especially premature infants, the renal tubular secretory mechanisms are imcompletely developed and inefficient.[190,191] Confusion is often introduced by the practice of "correcting" the clearance values on the basis of surface area. From the standpoint of drug elimination, the relevant measure is the actual clearance relative to the volume of distribution of the drug. Experimental data on clearances in infants are presented in Table 3-14. The elimination half-time for inulin (glomerular filtration) is about three times as long in the infant as in the adult because of a smaller renal blood flow relative to the body water volume. More striking is the deficiency in PAH excretion

Table 3-14. Comparison of Newborn and Adult Renal Clearances

	Average Infant	*Average Adult*
Body weight (kg)	3.5	70
Body water		
(%)	77	60
(liters)	2.7	42
Inulin clearance		
(ml·min^{-1})	approx. 3	130
k(min^{-1})	3/2,700 = 0.0011	130/42,000 = 0.0031
$t_{1/2}$(min)	630	224
PAH clearance		
(ml·min^{-1})	approx. 12	650
k(min^{-1})	12/2,700 = 0.0044	650/42,000 = 0.015
$t_{1/2}$(min)	160	45

[a] Computations are for a drug distributed in the whole body water, but any other V_d would give the same relative values.
(Data for average infant from West et al.[192])

(tubular secretion); here, the elimination half-time is nearly four times as long as in the adult.

It has been shown in several species (including humans) that the ability of renal cortical cells to transport organic anions increases during the first few weeks after birth.[191] The increase is associated with an increase in the apparent maximal velocity for PAH transport, which suggests that an increased number of carrier protein molecules becomes available for anion transport. Interestingly, it was found that administration of penicillin to pregnant animals leads to the birth of offspring with a fully developed renal PAH transport system.[193] It is thought that penicillin, as well as some other anions carried by the anion transport system, induce the synthesis either of the carrier protein itself or of other proteins that are required for the organic anion secretory process. It is possible that in utero the concentration of substrates that would promote induction is normally low because they are carried to the placenta and efficiently eliminated by the mother's kidneys.[194] Exposure to organic anions, either in utero or after birth, induces the transport system to higher activity. The activity of the organic cation transport system is also decreased at birth and matures during the first few weeks thereafter, but the induction phenomenon defined for the organic anion transport system does not seem to occur when the fetus is exposed to organic cations in utero.[194]

The effects of such immaturity of a major renal excretory pathway will depend upon the circumstances of drug administration. Suppose a drug that is excreted by tubular secretion is given to a premature infant intravenously or by another route with fast absorption. If the dosage is appropriate, then the usual initial drug level will be established; the only effect of the renal secretory deficiency will be to make the slope of the elimination curve less steep than in the adult. This in itself might be beneficial inasmuch as the duration of action of the single dose is extended. Difficulties ensue, however, with repeated dosage, for the residual drug level just before each successive dose will be higher than would have been expected in the adult. Succeeding doses may therefore build up the drug concentration to excessive levels. The likelihood of accumulation to toxic levels will be greatly increased if the drug is one that is usually given by a slow absorption route. Here, the customary magnitude and spacing of the doses takes into account both the absorption rate and the elimination rate. If the usual dosage schedule is employed but the elimination rate is substantially diminished, cumulative buildup to potentially toxic levels will be inevitable. Although several of the recently discovered drug toxicity syndromes in infants have been attributed to defective drug metabolism, it is clear that inefficient renal secretory mechanisms are also involved.

The acidity of the urine is maintained within fairly strict limits, usually pH 4.5 to 8.0. The acidification of urine, which takes place in the distal tubules and collecting ducts, may have a profound effect upon the rate of drug excretion. Since the nonionized form of a weak acid or base tends to diffuse readily from the tubular urine back across the tubule cells, it should be obvious that acidification will increase the reabsorption (and thus diminish the excretion) of weak acids whose pK_a is in the neutral range and promote the excretion of weak bases with pK_a in the same range. What is not so obvious is that the same effects will occur even when the ionization ranges are several pH units away. This seems surprising. Salicylic acid, for example, with $pK_a = 3$, is more than 99.9 percent ionized at pH 7.4 and still 99 percent ionized at pH 5.0. One might suppose, therefore, that acidification of the distal tubular urine to pH 5.0 could have only negligible effect. On the contrary, the rate of reabsorption is greatly enhanced, as is shown in the following illustration.

At pH 7.4 the ratio of base (ionized) to conjugate acid (nonionized) is calculated from

$$7.4 = 3.0 + \log \frac{[A^-]}{[HA]}$$

$$\frac{[A^-]}{[HA]} = \frac{25,000}{1} = \frac{1,000}{0.04}$$

At pH 5.0,

$$5.0 = 3.0 + \log \frac{[A^-]}{[HA]}$$

$$\frac{[A^-]}{[HA]} = \frac{100}{1} = \frac{990}{9.9}$$

	Plasma	Urine
Proximal tubule	pH 7.4 $\frac{1,000}{0.04}$	$\rightleftharpoons$ pH 7.4 $\frac{1,000}{0.04}$
Distal tubule	pH 7.4 $\frac{1,000}{0.04}$	$\leftarrow$ pH 5.0 $\frac{990}{9.9}$

With respect to the diffusible, nonionized form, acidification of the urine creates a very large diffusion gradient from urine to plasma. Consequently, the excretion of salicylate (or other weak acid) is promoted in an alkaline urine, retarded in acid urine. The opposite relationship holds for weak bases. These effects of urine pH have significant practical applications. For example, the elimination of barbiturates may be hastened by administering bicarbonate to alkalinize the urine.

From the above one can appreciate how drug elimination can be affected in a variety of ways in the patient with compromised renal function.[195] Both acute and chronic renal failure are accompanied by changes in the rates of glomerular filtration and tubular secretion, the latter leading to an inability to appropriately regulate urine pH. Renal failure may lead to marked changes in extracellular fluid volume, thus changing the plasma concentrations of drugs, such as the aminoglycoside antibiotics, that distribute largely or solely in the extracellular fluid compartment.[13] Because of both the hypoalbuminemia and the accumulation of aromatic acids such as hippurate in the blood, the extent of plasma binding of several acidic drugs (e.g., salicylate, sulfonamides, phenytoin, furosemide) is profoundly decreased in uremic patients.[194] This leads to higher levels of unbound drug, further potentiating the risk of toxicity. Given all these possible changes that can affect free drug concentrations, it is clear why the physician must exert special care in administering drugs to the patient with diminished renal function. Rational guidelines are available for reducing drug dosage according to the degree of renal functional impairment.[196] Patients must be carefully monitored for signs of drug toxicity, and frequent serum drug assays may be necessary to ensure that drug concentrations are within the appropriate therapeutic range.

Extracorporeal Dialysis

The "artificial kidney" is now widely used for the long-term maintenance of patients with chronic renal failure or for the support of such patients until renal transplantation can be carried out. Another application is in the treatment of drug overdosages. The patient's blood is made to flow across membranes permeable to water and to solutes of low molecular weight. The membranes are bathed on the other side by an aqueous solution of the same ionic composition as plasma water. Thus, by simple diffusion, an artificial process resembling glomerular filtration is established. Frequent changes of the dialysate bath hasten the elimination of drug from the plasma. The capacity of the apparatus depends upon the surface area of the membranes, the hydrostatic pressure difference across the membranes, the pore size, and the particular solute being removed.[197] Substances that ordinarily are largely reabsorbed by back diffusion may be eliminated very effectively in the artificial kidney. Thus, a urea clearance of 140 ml min^{-1} can be achieved, about twice the normal value in humans.

As many patients on chronic extracorporeal dialysis receive drugs on fixed dosing regimens, the effect of dialysis on drug elimination must be taken into consideration when planning drug doses and dosing intervals.[198,199] In the case of those drugs that are efficiently eliminated by dialysis, a replacement dosage must be administered at the end of each dialysis session to return drug plasma concentrations to the effective therapeutic range. The endogenous aromatic acids that accumulate in uremic patients are efficiently removed by hemodialysis. Since these aromatic acids compete for drug binding sites, the binding of some acidic drugs to serum protein may increase during dialysis, and the therapeutic effectiveness of a given drug dosage may be decreased.[183]

Extracorporeal dialysis is used to treat drug overdose, a procedure that has intrinsic limitations. A major fraction of the drug must be free in the plasma, and that portion of the total drug that is in tissues must be able to diffuse sufficiently rapidly into the plasma. The reason is that only the concentration gradient of free drug in a given extracorporeal dialysis unit determines the rate of removal from the circulation. Thus, a drug with high fractional binding to plasma proteins is a poor candidate for this method. For the same reason significant storage of the drug in tissue depots diminishes the usefulness of the procedure. For drugs that are rapidly metabolized so that metabolic disposition plays the major role in their removal, the artificial kidney is unlikely to accelerate the removal rate significantly. Salicylates, bromides, and the poorly metabolized barbiturates (e.g., phenobarbital) are examples of good candidates, but only if the poisoning is so severe that other methods of supportive treatment will not suffice. Ethanol and methanol poisoning are very well handled by extracorporeal dialysis; considerable acceleration of the removal rates is possible, and in the case of methanol this can prevent accumulation of the dangerously toxic metabolite formaldehyde.

When the effectiveness of hemodialysis in the poisoned patient is limited by the physical properties of the offending agent (e.g., poor aqueous solubility, extensive plasma protein binding), hemoperfusion has been successfully employed.[198] In this procedure the patient's blood is cleansed by direct perfusion through columns containing sorbents (e.g., activated charcoal) or exchange resins to which the compound binds with high affinity.

In the absence of equipment for extracorporeal dialysis or hemoperfusion, peritoneal lavage may be employed.[200] This technique consists of washing out the peritoneal cavity with isotonic solutions in order to remove metabolites or drugs that can diffuse readily across the peritoneal membranes. It is a relatively simple procedure, but it is much less efficient than extracorporeal dialysis.

Biliary Excretion of Drugs

A drug may be excreted by the liver cells into the bile and thus pass into the intestine.[201,202] The vascular system of the liver is uniquely modified to facilitate the clearance of compounds from the blood. The blood from the hepatic artery and the portal vein flows into the hepatic sinusoids, which are lined by a discontinuous matrix of porous, highly fenestrated endothelial cells lacking complete basal laminae. Also present are numerous phagocytic Kupffer cells, which remove particulate matter from the blood. Drugs that are administered orally are absorbed from the gastrointestinal tract into the portal venous system and must pass through the liver before reaching the general systemic circulation. With some drugs a substantial portion may be removed from the blood during this first pass through the liver. This removal is called the *first pass effect* or *presystemic hepatic elimination*. The β-adrenergic blocking drug propranolol provides an example. As much as 90 percent of a low dose of propranolol is cleared from the blood in a single pass through the liver. This hepatic clearance mechanism appears to be saturable; after a propranolol dose of 0.8 mg/kg, virtually no drug is found in systemic blood, but with higher doses there is a linear increase in the systemic blood concentration.[203] The antiarrhythmic drug lidocaine is also rapidly cleared by this mechanism; this accounts for the poor efficacy of lidocaine when given orally.

After passage across the endothelium of the sinusoids, compounds that are actively secreted in the bile must pass across the luminal surface of the hepatic parenchymal cells to the cell interior, where they may be modified by metabolism. The drug and/or its metabolites then pass across the canalicular portion of the cell membrane into the bile canaliculus. Two physical properties influence biliary excretion namely, polarity and molecular weight. The presence of a polar group augments excretion. The polar group may be part of the parent molecule or it may be acquired by biotransformation. Many drugs are first conjugated in the parenchymal cells and pass into the bile as glucuronide, sulfate, glycinate, or glutathione conjugates. Conjugation adds a polar group, which allows a molecule to exist at physiologic pH as a water-soluble anion, facilitating secretion by an anion transport system. Conjugation may also significantly increase a compound's molecular weight, the second property that increases biliary excretion. In general, compounds that are efficiently secreted by the renal tubules have low molecular weights (200 to 400) whereas chemicals excreted into the bile are larger. The threshold molecular weight for biliary excretion in the rat is about 300, and in the human it is about 500. Above the threshold there is no relationship between the extent of biliary excretion and the molecular weight.

Chemicals are secreted into the bile by four different mechanisms specific for anions, bile acids, cations, and neutral organic compounds, respectively. Several findings show four distinct and independent carrier-mediated active transport processes. First, secretion into bile occurs against a high concentration gradient; bile/plasma concentration ratios of 50:1 and higher are not unusual. Second, if the drug concentration in plasma is raised progressively, a limiting rate of drug secretion (transport maximum) is reached, which cannot be exceeded (Fig. 3-34). Third, various members of the same class (anion, bile acid, cation, nonionized molecule) compete, one depressing the biliary excretion of another, but there is no competiton between members of different classes.

The organic anions that are excreted well in bile include phenol red, fluorescein, and penicillin. The prototype of this group is sulfobromophthalein (Bromsulphalein, BSP), which is excreted in the bile predominantly as the glutathione conjugate and was used extensively at one time as a test of liver function. In the normal subject after an intravenous dose of 5 mg kg^{-1}, 90 to 100 percent of the dye is removed from the blood within 30 minutes. The maximum rate of removal of such a dye may be depressed in liver damage, and return to normal as other aspects of liver function recover. Bile acids such as taurocholate are anions, but they are excreted by a different carrier than that used for hepatic anion secretion.[202]

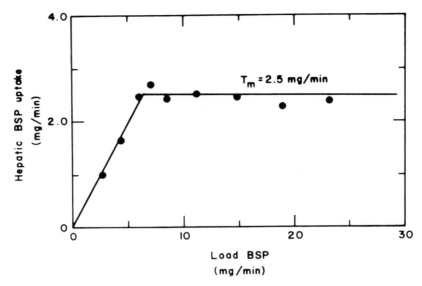

Fig. 3-34. Saturation of the biliary excretory system for sulfobromophthalein. Sodium sulfobromophthalein (Bromsulphalein, BSP) was infused intravenously in a 26-kg dog. Plasma levels and hepatic uptake of dye were measured, and hepatic blood flow was also determined. Hepatic uptake is shown as function of varying rates of BSP presentation to liver. Transport maximum at about 2.5 mg min^{-1} is evident. (From Combes et al.,[204] with permission.)

Drugs are transported into hepatocytes on the same carriers utilized by naturally occurring substances such as bilirubin and bile acids. The uptake process can be quite efficient even though most anionic drugs are bound to serum albumin. Efficient extraction is possible since the sinusoidal capillaries surrounding the hepatocyte are discontinuous, which enables albumin-bound drug to enter the space of Disse and come into direct contact with the hepatocyte surface. Some evidence indicates that it is not only free drug that is rapidly taken up by the hepatocyte; in addition, the drug-albumin complex may interact with a receptor on the membrane, which facilitates dissociation of the drug or transfer to the plasma membrane carrier. Once in the hepatocyte, the drug binds to cytoplasmic carrier proteins, principally the ligandins and the Z proteins. Both these protein types may facilitate transfer of drug to the endoplasmic reticulum for oxidation or conjugation. These proteins may also have a storage function, which minimizes efflux back into the plasma. Interestingly, ligandin also has a catalytic function in that it is a glutathione-*S*-transferase and conjugates glutathione with activated substrates. Transport from the hepatocyte into the canaliculi seems to be a slower and sometimes rate-limiting process. Secretion into the bile is an active transport mechanism, and the process is particularly efficient for the glucuronide conjugates of the drugs and bilirubin.

There is a distinct mechanism for the biliary excretion of organic cations. The structural requirements for transport by the organic cation pathway are a basic amino group on one side of the molecule and one or more nonpolar groups on the other side, making the molecule amphipathic. Procaine amide ethobromide, a quaternary derivative of procaine amide, is a good example. The secretion of this drug is competitively depressed by other quaternary ammonium compounds (mepiperphenidol, benzomethamine, oxyphenonium, N^1-methylnicotinamide), and these drugs are themselves secreted into the bile. Tubocurarine is also secreted by this mechanism, but not all quaternary ammonium derivatives are.

The biliary secretion of large nonionized compounds is not thoroughly understood. Some molecules of this type can be conjugated to anions such as glucuronate or sulfate in the hepatic cells, then transported into the bile ducts by the anion transport mechanism. In these instances conjugation has been shown to be essential for secretion. Thus, inhibition of the conjugation enzymes blocks biliary secretion, and animals with deficient conjugating systems secrete such drugs poorly or not at all. Many drugs and hormones, on the other hand, are secreted into the bile unchanged despite the fact that they contain no ionizing groups. Some of the cardiac glycosides are typical. Here biliary secretion is favored by a molecular asymmetry with respect to hydrophilic and lipophilic groups (e.g., a large steroid nucleus attached to sugar moieties at one position). Little is known about the mechanism of secretion of the nonionized molecules.

Metals are usually eliminated from the body more slowly than most organic compounds, and many of them (e.g., manganese, mercury, copper, zinc, cadmium) are excreted into the bile to a greater extent than into the urine. Bile to plasma ratios of 10:1 to 20:1 are common after toxic metal exposure, and the existence of apparent transport maxima suggests that metals undergo active biliary transport. It has been proposed that reduced glutathione is the carrier molecule for mercury, copper, silver and zinc. Glutathione is present in high concentration in bile, and the metal-glutathione binding constants are very high. Pretreatment of rats with compounds that deplete glutathione has been shown to inhibit biliary excretion of these metals.[202]

Biliary secretion of some peptide hormones may occur via receptor-mediated transcytosis. As discussed previously, IgA dimers bind to receptors located on the sinusoidal surface of the parenchymal cell and are subsequently discharged from the canalicular surface into the bile. It is well established that receptors for hormones such as insulin, growth hormone, and prolactin exist on the sinusoidal plasma membrane,[205] and it may be that some transcytosis with excretion at the canalicular surface can occur.

When hepatic function is impaired, excretion of drugs that are eliminated by the hepatic route may be severely decreased.[206] Unfortunately, the kinds of guidelines that exist for dosage adjustment in renal failure are not available to guide dosage adjustment in patients with compromised hepatic function. Several factors impede the systematic study of the effects of hepatic failure on drug elimination. First, hepatic failure may involve the parenchymal cells, the biliary tree, and the vascular supply to different degrees, depending upon the cause. Second, studies of drug elimination are limited to patients, as animal models of different types of liver disease are either difficult to establish or simply not available. Third, although it is usually easy to collect and analyze urine for the presence of a drug and its metabolites, it is not possible to collect bile unless the patient has a patent biliary fistula. Last, precise tests of hepatic function that reflect drug excretory capacities have not been developed. The physician faced with treatment of a patient with compromised hepatic function must therefore take special care to titrate the drug dosage to the patient's clinical response and to monitor plasma drug levels. There is a clear need for more precise indicators of hepatic drug-eliminating capacity upon which to base a less empirical approach to dosage adjustment.

Enterohepatic Cycling

If the properties of a drug or its metabolite happen to be favorable for intestinal absorption, an *enterohepatic cycle*[207] may result. This is a cycle in which biliary secretion and intestinal reabsorption continue until renal excretion finally eliminates the drug from the body. This process enables the body to conserve endogenous substances such as the bile acids, vitamins D_3 and B_{12}, folic acid, pyridoxine, and estrogens. Sometimes the enterohepatic cycle may be responsible for a drug's long persistence in the body, and a major fraction of the total drug may be trapped in this circuit. Enterohepatic cycling is partly responsible for the long half-lives of some cardiac glycosides, for example. Administration of the binding resin cholestyramine to patients receiving digitoxin has been shown to decrease the serum half-life of the drug from 11.5 to 6.6 days by interfering with enterohepatic reabsorption.[208] Some drugs are glucuronidated in the liver, secreted into the bile as the β-glucuronide, and then hydrolyzed in the small intestine by β-glucuronidase. Hydrolysis yields the unconjugated original compound or a polar metabolite, which again is subject to intestinal absorption.

REFERENCES

1. Wagner JG: Fundamentals of Clinical Pharmacokinetics. Drug Intelligence Publications, Inc. Hamilton, Ont., 1975
2. Ritschel WA: Handbook of Basic Pharmacokinetics. Drug Intelligence Publications, Inc. Hamilton, Ont., 1986
3. Gibaldi M, Perrier D: Pharmacokinetics. 2nd Ed. Marcel Dekker, New York, 1982
4. Gibaldi M: Biopharmaceutics and Clinical Pharmacokinetics. Lea & Febiger, Philadelphia, 1984
5. Ames MM, Powis G, Kovach JS: Pharmacokinetis of Anticancer Agents in Humans. Elsevier, New York, 1983
6. Gibaldi M, Prescott L. (eds): Handbook of Clinical Pharmacokinetics. ADIS Health Science Press, Sydney, 1983
7. Eckman WW, Patlak CS, Fenstermacher JD: A critical evaluation of the principles governing the advantages of intra-arterial infusions. J Pharmacokinet Biopharm 12:257, 1974
8. Gianelly R, von der Groeben JO, Spivack AP, Harrison DC: Effect of lidocaine on ventricular arrhythmias in partients with coronary heart disease. N Engl J Med 277:1215, 1967
9. Bederka J, Takemori AE, Miller JW: Absorption rates of various substances administered intramuscularly. Eur J Pharmacol 15:132, 1971
10. Baker R: Controlled Release of Biologically Active Agents. John Wiley & Sons, New York, 1987
11. Schou J: Subcutaneous and intramuscular injection of drugs. Ch. 4. In Brodie BB, Gillette JR (eds): Handbook of Experimental Pharmacology. Springer-Verlag, Berlin, 1971
12. Koivisto VA, Felig P: Alterations in insulin absorption and in blood glucose control with varying insulin injection sites in diabetic patients. Ann Intern Med 92:59, 1980
13. Pratt WB, Fekety FR: The Antimicrobial Drugs. Oxford University Press, New York, 1986
14. Bishop PMF, Folley SJ: Implantation of testosterone in cast pellets. Lancet 1:434, 1944
15. Scheuplein RJ, Blank IH: Permeability of the skin. Physiol Rev 51:702, 1971
16. Katz M, Poulsen BJ: Absorption of drugs through the skin. Ch. 7. In Brodie BB, Gillette JR (eds): Handbook of Experimental Pharmacology. Berlin, Springer-Verlag, 1971
17. Stoughton RB, Fritsch W. Influence of dimethylsulfoxide (DMSO) on human percutaneous absorption. Arch Dermatol 90:512, 1964
18. Barry BW: Dermatological Formulations: Percutaneous Absorption. Marcel Dekker, New York, 1983
19. Schuman RM, Leech RW, Alvord EC: Neurotoxicity of hexachloraphene in the human. I. A Clinicopathological study of 248 children. Pediatrics 54:689, 1974
20. Chien YW, Siddiqui O, Sun Y, et al: Transdermal iontophoretic delivery of therapeutic peptides/proteins. p. 32. In Biological Approaches to the Controlled Delivery of Drugs, Juliano RL (ed): Ann NY Acad Sci 507:32, 1987

21. Shaw JE, Chandrasekaran SK: Controlled topical delivery of drugs for systemic action. Drug Metab Rev 4:223, 1975
22. Breimer DD: Rationale for rate-controlled drug delivery of cardiovascular drugs by the transdermal route. Am Heart J 108:196, 1984
23. Price NM, Schmitt LG, McGuire J, et al: Transdermal scopolamine in the prevention of motion sickness at sea. Clin Pharmacol Ther 29:414, 1981
24. Moren F, Newhouse MT, Dolovich MB (eds): Aerosols in Medicine: Principles, Diagnosis and Therapy. Elsevier, Amsterdam, 1985
25. Clark SW, Pavia D (eds): Lung Mucociliary Clearance and the Deposition of Aerosols. Chest, suppl 81, 1981
26. Brain JD, Valberg PA: Deposition of aerosol in the respiratory tract. Am Rev Respir Dis 120:1325, 1979
27. Morrow PE: Aerosol characterization and deposition. Am Rev Respir Dis 110(6:Part 2):88, 1974
28. Hatch TF, Gross P: Pulmonary Deposition and Retention of Inhaled Aerosols. Academic Press, Orlando, FL, 1964
29. Goldsmith JR, Hexter AC: Respiratory exposure to lead: Epidemiological and experimental dose-relationships. Science 158:132, 1967
30. Ter Haar GL, Bayard MA: Composition of airborne lead particles. Nature 232:553, 1971
31. Kehoe RA: The metabolism of lead in man in health and disease. I. The normal metabolism of lead. J R Inst Public Health 24:81, 1961
32. Stopps GJ: Symposium on air quality criteria—lead. J Occup Med 10:550, 1968
33. Bellinger D, Leviton A, Waternaux C, et al: Longitudinal analyses of prenatal and postnatal lead exposure and early cognitive development. N Engl J Med 316:1037, 1987
34. Sterk PJ, Plomp A, van der Vate JF, Quanjer PH: Physical properties of the aerosols produced by several jet and ultrasonic nebulizers. Bull Eur Physiopathol Respir 20:65, 1984
35. Dolovich MB, Ruffin RE, Roberts R, Newhouse MT: Optimal delivery of aerosols from metered dose inhalers. Chest 80, suppl. 6:911, 1981
36. Newhouse MT, Dolovich MB: Control of asthma by aerosols. N Engl J Med 315:870, 1986
37. Inman WHW, Adelstein AM: Rise and fall of asthma mortality in England and Wales in relation to use of pressurized aerosols. Lancet 2:279, 1969
38. Forth W, Rummel W (eds): Pharmacology of Intestinal Absorption: Gastrointestnal Absorption of Drugs. Pergamon Press, New York, 1975
39. Khalafalla N, Elgholm ZA, Khalil SA: Influence of high fat diet in gastrointestinal absorption of griseofulvin tablets in man. Pharmazie 36:692, 1981
40. Doluisio JT, Tan GH, Billups NF, Diamond L: Drug absorption. II. Effect of fasting on intestinal drug absorption. J Pharm Sci 58:1200, 1969
41. Boyes RN, Scott DB, Jebson PJ, et al: Pharmacokinetics of lidocaine in man. Clin Pharmacol Ther 12:105, 1971
42. Stenson RE, Constantino T, Harrison DC: Interrelationships of hepatic blood flow, cardiac output, and blood levels of lidocaine in man. Circulation 43:205, 1971
43. Jacobs MH: Some aspects of cell permeability to weak electrolytes. Cold Spring Harbor Symp Quant Biol 8:30, 1940
44. Schanker LS, Shore PA, Brodie BB, Hogben CAM: Absorption of drugs from the stomach. I. The rat. J Pharmacol Exp Ther 120:528, 1957
45. Shore PA, Brodie BB, Hogben CAM: The gastric secretion of drugs: A pH partition hypothesis. J Pharmacol Exp Ther 119:361, 1957
46. Hogben CAM, Tocco DJ, Brodie BB, Schanker LS: On the mechanism of intestinal absorption of drugs. J Pharmacol Exp Ther 125:275, 1959
47. Beckett AH, Hossie RD: Buccal absorption of drugs. Ch. 3. In Brodie BB, Gillette JR (eds): Handbook of Experimental Pharmacology. Springer-Verlag, Berlin, 1971
48. Smolen VF, Ball L (eds): Controlled Drug Bioavailability. John Wiley & Sons, New York, 1984

49. Roseman TJ, Mansdorf SZ (eds): Controlled Release Delivery Systems. Marcel Dekker, New York, 1983
50. Lindenbaum J, Mellow MH, Blackstone MO, Butler VP Jr: Variation in biologic availability of digoxin from four preparations. N Engl J Med 285, 1344, 1971.
51. Heller J: Biodegradable polymers in controlled drug delivery. Crit Rev Ther Drug Carrier Syst 1:39, 1984
52. Ihler GM (ed): Methods of Drug Delivery. Pergamon Press, New York, 1986
53. Blackshear PJ, Rohde TD: Artificial devices for insulin infusion in the treatment of patients with diabetes mellitus. In Bruck SD (ed): Controlled Drug Delivery, Vol. 2, Clinical Applications. CRC Press, Boca Raton, FL, 1983
54. Ensminger WD, Gyves JW: Regional chemotherapy of neoplastic diseases. Ch. 10. In Ihler GM (ed): Methods of Drug Delivery. Pergamon Press, New York, 1986
55. Buchwald H, Barbosa J, Varco RL, et al: Treatment of a type II diabetic by a totally implantable insulin infusion device. Lancet 1:1233, 1981
56. Rizza RA: New modes of insulin administration: Do they have a role in clinical diabetes? Ann Intern Med 105:126, 1986
57. Urquhart J, Fara J, Willis KL: Rate controlled delivery systems in drug and hormone research. Annu Rev Pharmacol Toxicol 24:199, 1984
58. Schloerb PR, Friis-Hansen BJ, Edelman IS, et al: The measurement of total body water in the human subject by deuterium oxide dilution. J Clin Invest 29:1296, 1950
59. Soberman R, Brodie BB, Levy BB, et al: The use of antipyrine in the measurement of total body water in man. J Biol Chem 179:31, 1949
60. Jusko WJ, Gretch M: Plasma and tissue protein binding of drugs in pharmacokinetics. Drug Metab Rev 5:43, 1976
61. Vallner JJ: Binding of drugs by albumin and plasma protein. J Pharm Sci 66:447, 1977
62. Putnam FW: Structure and function of the plasma proteins. Ch. 14. In Neurath H (ed): The Proteins, 2nd Ed. Vol. III. Academic Press, Orlando, FL, 1965
63. Tanford C, Swanson SA, Shore WS: Hydrogen ion equilibria of bovine serum albumin. J Am Chem Soc 77:6414, 1955
64. Paxton JW: Alpha$_1$-acid glycoprotein and binding of basic drugs. Methods Find Exp Clin Pharmacol 5:635, 1983
65. Svensson CK, Woodruff MN, Lalka D: Influence of protein binding and use of unbound (free) drug concentrations. p. 187. In Evans WE, Schentag JJ, Jusko WJ (eds): Applied Pharmacokinetics. Principles of Therapeutic Drug Monitoring, Applied Therapeutics Inc., Spokane, 1986
66. Goldstein A: The interactions of drugs and plasma proteins. Pharmacol Rev 1:102, 1949
67. Keen P: Effect of binding to plasma proteins on the distribution, activity and elimination of drugs. Ch. 10. In Brodie BB, Gillette JR (eds): Handbook of Experimental Pharmacology. Springer-Verlag, Berlin, 1971
68. Davis BD: The binding of sulfonamide drugs by plasma proteins. A factor in determining the distribution of drugs in the body. J Clin Invest 22:753, 1943
69. Craig WA, Welling PG: Protein binding of antimicrobials: Clinical pharmacokinetic and therapeutic implications. Clin Pharmacokinet 2:252, 1977
70. Hawking F: Suramin: With special reference to onchocerciasis. Adv Pharmacol Chemother 15:289, 1978
71. Porter RJ, Layzer RB: Plasma albumin concentration and diphenylhydantoin binding in man. Arch Neurol 32:298, 1975
72. Glassman AH, Hurwic MJ, Perel JM: Plasma binding of imipramine and clinical outcome. Am J Psychiatry 130:1367, 1973
73. Tillement JP, Lhoste F, Giudicelli JF: Diseases and drug protein binding. Clin Pharmacokinet 3:144, 1978
74. Shinn AF, Shrewsbury RP: Basic principles of drug interaction. Ch. 1. In Shinn AF, Shrewsbury RP (eds): Evaluations of Drug Interactions, 3rd Ed. CV Mosby, St Louis, 1985

75. Koch-Weser J, Sellers EM: Drug interactions with coumarin anticoagulants. N Engl J Med 285:487, 547, 1971

76. Anton AH: Increasing activity of sulfonamides with displacing agents: A review. Ann NY Acad Sci 226:273, 1973

77. Simionescu N, Simionescu M: The cardiovascular system. Ch. 9. In Weiss L (ed): Histology, Cell and Tissue Biology. 5th Ed. Elsevier, New York, 1983

78. Pappenheimer JR: Passage of molecules through capillary walls. Physiol Rev 33:387, 1953

79. Renkin EM: Transport of large molecules across capillary walls. Physiologist 7:13, 1964

80. Crone C: Capillary permeability—techniques and problems. Ch. 1. In Crone C, Lassen NA (eds): Capillary Permeability. Academic Press, Orlando, FL, 1970

81. Bundgaard M: Transport pathways in capillaries—in search of pores. Ann Rev Physiol 42:325, 1980

82. Mortillaro NA (ed): The Physiology and Pharmacology of the Microcirculation, Vols. 1 and 2. Academic Press, Orlando, FL, 1983

83. Darnell J, Lodish H, Baltimore D: The plasma membrane. Ch. 14. In Molecular Cell Biology. Scientific American Books, New York, 1986

84. Finean JB, Coleman R, Mitchell RH (eds): Membranes and Their Cellular Functions. Blackwell Scientific Publications, Oxford, 1984

85. Singer SJ, Nicolson GL: The fluid mosaic model of the structure of cell membranes. Science 175:720, 1972

86. Friedman MH: Principles and Models of Biological Transport. Springer-Verlag, Berlin, 1986

87. Collander R, Barlund H: Permeabilitätsstudien an *Chara ceratophylla*. II. Die Permeabilität für Nichtelektrolyte. Acta Bot Fenn 11:1, 1933

88. Sha'afi RI, Gary-Bobo CM, Soloman AK: Permeability of red cell membranes to small hydrophilic and lipophilic solutes. J Gen Physiol 58:238, 1971

89. Overton E. Studien über die Narkose zugleich ein Beitrag zur allgemeinen Pharmakologie. Gustav Fischer, Jena, 1901, p. 101

90. Meyer KH, Hemmi H: Beiträge zur Theorie der Narkose. III. Biochem Z 277:39, 1935

91. Ferguson J: The use of chemical potentials as indices of toxicity. Proc R Soc B127:387, 1939

92. Robbins E: The rate of proflavin passage into single living cells with application to permeability studies. J Gen Physiol 43:853, 1960

93. Waddell WJ, Butler TC: The distribution and excretion of phenobarbital. J Clin Invest 36:1217, 1957

94. Darnell J, Lodish H, Baltimore D: Transport across cell membranes. Ch. 15. In Molecular Cell Biology. Scientific American Books, New York, 1986

95. Tanford C: Mechanism of free energy coupling in active transport. Annu Rev Biochem 52:379, 1983

96. Goldman ID (ed): Membrane Transport of Antineoplastic Agents. Pergamon Press, Oxford, 1986

97. Bonting SL: Sodium-potassium activated adenosine triphosphatase and cation transport. Ch. 8. In Bittar EE (ed): Membranes and Ion Transport. Vol. 1. Wiley-Interscience, New York, 1970

98. Cantley LC: Structure and mechanism of the (Na,K)-ATPase. Curr Top Bioenerget 11:201, 1981

99. Skou JC: Further investigations on a Mg^{2+} + Na^+-activated adenosine triphosphatase, possibly related to the active, linked transport of Na^+ and K^+ across the nerve membrane. Biochim Biophys Acta 42:6, 1960

100. Dunham PB, Hoffman JF: Active cation transport and ouabain binding in high potassium and low potassium red blood cells of sheep. J Gen Physiol 58:94, 1971

101. Goldin SM: Active transport of sodium and potassium ions by the sodium and potassium ion-activated adenosine triphosphatase from renal medulla. J Biol Chem 252:5630, 1977

102. Bakker EP: Ionophore antibiotics. p. 67. In Hahn FE (ed): Antibiotics. Vol. 1. Springer-Verlag, New York, 1979

103. Urry DW, Goodall MC, Glickson JD, Mayers DF: The gramicidin A transmembrane channel: Characteristics of head-to-head dimerized helices. Proc Natl Acad Sci USA 68:1907, 1971

104. Ovchinnikov YA: Physicochemical basis of ion transport through biological membranes: Ionophores and ion channels. Eur J Biochem 94:321, 1979

105. Urry DW: Molecular perspectives of monovalent cation selective transmembrane channels. Int Rev Neurobiol 21:311, 1979

106. Medoff G, Kobayashi GS, Kwan CN, et al: Potentiation of rifampicin and 5-flurocytosine as antifungal antibiotics by amphotericin B. Proc Natl Acad Sci USA 69:196, 1972

107. Medoff J, Medoff G, Goldstein MN, et al: Amphotericin B-induced sensitivity to actinomycin D in drug-resistant HeLa cells. Cancer Res 35:2548, 1975

108. Goldstein JL, Brown MS, Anderson RGW, et al: Receptor-mediated endocytosis: Concepts emerging from the LDL receptor system. Annu Rev Cell Biol 1:1, 1985

109. Hopkins CR: Uptake and intracellular processing of cell surface receptors: Current concepts and prospects. Ch. 18. In Poste G, Crooke ST (eds): New Insights Into Cell and Membrane Transport Processes. Plenum, New York, 1986

110. Pearse BMF, Bretscher MS: Membrane recycling by coated vesicles. Ann Rev Biochem 50:85, 1981

111. Newman R, Schneider C, Sutherland R, et al: The transferrin receptor. Trends Biochem Sci 7:397, 1982

112. Carpenter G, Cohen S: Epidermal growth factor. Ann Rev Biochem 48:193, 1979

113. Mroczkowski B, Mosig G, Cohen S: ATP-stimulated interaction between epidermal growth factor receptor and supercoiled DNA. Nature 309:270, 1984

114. Solari R, Kraehenbuhl JP: Biosynthesis of the IgA antibody receptor: A model for the transepithelial sorting of a membrane glycoprotein. Cell 36:61, 1984

115. Juliano RL (ed): Biological Approaches to the Controlled Delivery of Drugs. Ann NY Acad Sci Vol. 507, 1987

116. Tomlinson E, Davis SS (eds): Site-Specific Drug Delivery: Cell Biology, Medical and Pharmaceutical Aspects. Wiley, New York, 1986

117. Borchardt RT, Repta AJ, Stella VJ: Directed Drug Delivery: A Multidisciplinary Approach. Humana Press, Clifton, NJ, 1985

118. Order SE (ed): International Symposium on Labeled and Unabeled Antibody in Clinical Diagnosis and Therapy. NCI Monogr No. 3, 1987

119. Poznansky MJ, Juliano RL: Biological approaches to the controlled delivery of drugs: a critical review. Pharmacol Rev 36:277, 1984

120. Papahadjopoulos D, Gabizon A: Targeting of liposomes to tumor cells in vivo. Ann NY Acad Sci 507:64, 1987

121. New RRC, Chance ML, Heath S: Antileishmanial activity of amphotericin and other antifungal agents entrapped in lysosomes. J Antimicrob Chemother 8:371, 1981

122. Gabizon A, Dagan A, Goren D, et al: Liposomes as in vivo carriers of Adriamycin: Reduced cardiac uptake and preserved antitumor activity in mice. Cancer Res 42:4734, 1982

123. Edwards DC, McIntosh DP: Targeting potential of antibody conjugates. Ch. 5. In Ihler GM (ed): Methods of Drug Delivery. Pergamon Press, New York, 1986

124. Eisenberg HM, Suddith RL (eds): The Cerebral Microvasculature: Investigation of the Blood-Brain Barrier. Plenum, New York, 1979

125. Cornford EM: The blood-brain barrier, a dynamic regulatory interface. Mol Physiol 7:219, 1985

126. Pardridge WM, Oldendorf WH, Cancilla P, Frank HJL: Blood-brain barrier: Interface between internal medicine and the brain. Ann Intern Med 105:82, 1986

127. Sakurada O, Kennedy C, Jehle J, et al: Measurement of local cerebral blood flow with iodo(^{14}C)antipyrine. Am J Physiol 234:H59, 1978

128. Fenstermacher JD, Sposito NM, Nornes SE, et al: Relationship of capillary density to glucose utilization and blood flow in white and gray matter of the rat brain. Microvasc Res 29:219, 1985

129. Mazziotta JC, Phelps ME: Positron emission tomography studies of the brain. Ch. 11. In Phelps ME, Mazziotta JC, Schelbert HR (eds): Positron Emission Tomography and Autoradiography. Principles and Applications for the Brain and Heart. Raven Press, New York, 1986
130. Pardridge WM: Receptor-mediated peptide transport through the blood-brain barrier. Endocr Rev 7:314, 1986
131. Stewart PA, Wiley MJ: Developing nervous tissue induces formation of blood-brain barrier characteristics in invading endothelial cells: A study using quail-chick transplantation chimeras. Dev Biol 84:183, 1981
132. Audus KL, Borchardt RT: Bovine brain microvessel endothelial cell monolayers as a model system for the blood brain barrier. Ann NY Acad Sci 507:9, 1987
133. Bodor N, Brewster ME: Problems of delivery of drugs to the brain. Ch. 8. In Ihler GM (ed): Methods of Drug Delivery. Pergamon Press, New York, 1986
134. Pardridge WM, Oldendorf WH: Transport of metabolic substrates through the blood brain barrier. J Neurochem 28:5, 1977
135. Banks WA, Kastin AJ, Fischman AJ, et al: Carrier-mediated transport of enkephalins and N-tyr-MIF-1 across blood-brain barrier. Am J Physiol 251:E477, 1986
136. Milhorat TH, Hammock MK: Cerebrospinal fluid as reflection of internal milieu of the brain. Ch. 1. In Wood JH (ed): Neurobiology of Cerebrospinal Fluid, Vol. 2. Plenum, New York, 1983
137. Collins JM, Dedrick RL: Distributed model for drug delivery to CSF and brain tissue. Am J Physiol 245:R303, 1983
138. Dichiro G, Hammock MK, Bleyer WA: Spinal descent of cerebrospinal fuid in man. Neurology 26:1, 1976
139. Poplack DG, Bleyer WA, Horowitz ME: Pharmacology of antineoplastic agents in cerebrospinal fluid. Ch. 39. In Wood JH (ed): Neurobiology of Cerebrospinal Fluid. Vol. 1. Plenum, New York, 1981
140. Alazraki NP, Fierer J, Halpern SE, Becker RW: Use of a hyperbaric solution for administration of intrathecal amphotericin B. N Engl J Med 279:1025, 1968
141. Lensen RI, Weyne JJ, Demeester GM: Regulation of acid base equilibrium of cerebrospinal fluid. Ch. 2. In Wood JH (ed): Neurobiology of Cerebrospinal Fluid. Vol. 2. Plenum, New York, 1983
142. Woodbury DM: Pharmacology of anticonvulsant drugs in cerebrospinal fluid. Ch. 38. In Wood JH (ed): Neurobiology of Cerebrospinal Fluid. Vol. 2. Plenum, New York, 1983
143. Dixon RL, Owens ES, Rall DP: Evidence of active transport of benzyl-^{14}C-penicillin from the cerebrospinal fluid to the blood. J Pharm Sci 58:1106, 1969
144. Spector R, Lorenzo AV: Inhibition of penicillin transport from the cerebrospinal fluid after intracisternal inoculation of bacteria. J Clin Invest 54:316, 1974
145. Spector R, Lorenzo AV: The effects of salicylate and probenecid on the cerebrospinal fluid transport of penicillin, aminosalicylic acid and iodide. J Pharmacol Exp Ther 188:55, 1974
146. Rapoport SI: Blood Brain Barrier in Physiology and Medicine. Raven Press, New York, 1976
147. Goldsworthy PD, Aird RB, Becker RA: The blood-brain barrier—the effect of acidic dissociation constant on the permeation of certain sulfonamides into the brain. J Cell Physiol 44:519, 1954
148. Brodie BB, Kurz H, Schanker LS: The importance of dissociation constant and lipid-solubility in influencing the passage of drugs into the cerebrospinal fluid. J Pharmacol Exp Ther 130:20, 1960
149. Aquilonius SM: Physostigmine in the treatment of drug overdose. p. 817. In Jenden DJ (ed): Cholinergic Mechanisms and Psychopharmacology. Vol. 24. Plenum, New York, 1977
150. Feldberg W: A Pharmacological Approach to the Brain, from Its Inner and Outer Surface. Williams & Wilkins, Baltimore, 1963
151. Stanski DR: Pharmacokinetics of barbiturates. Ch. 6. Prys-Roberts C, Hug CC Jr (eds): Pharmacokinetics of Anesthesia, Blackwell Scientific Publications, Oxford, 1984

152. Goldstein A, Aronow L: The durations of action of thiopental and pentobarbital. J Pharmacol Exp Ther 128:1, 1960

153. Faber JJ, Thornburg KL: Placental Physiology. Structure and Function of Fetomaternal Exchange. Raven Press, New York, 1983

154. Gray H: Anatomy of the Human Body. 30th Ed. Clemente CD (ed). Lea & Febiger, Philadelphia, 1985. Figure 2-71

155. Schneider H, Sodha RJ, Progler M, Young MPA: Permeability of the human placenta for hydrophilic substances studied in the isolated dually in vitro perfused lobe. Contrib Gynecol Obstet 13:98, 1985

156. Dancis J: Placental physiology. Ch. 1. In Kretchmer N, Quilligan EJ, Johnson JD (eds): Prenatal and Perinatal Biology and Medicine. Vol. 1. Harwood, New York, 1987

157. Chamberlain GVP, Wilkinson AW (eds): Placental Transfer. Pitman Publishing, London, 1979

158. Schneider H, Challier JC, Dancis J: Transfer and metabolism of glucose and lactate in the human placenta studied by a perfusion system in vitro. Placenta 2, suppl:129, 1981

159. Schneider H, Mohlen KH, Dancis J: Transfer of amino acids across in vitro perfused human placenta. Pediatr Res 13:236, 1979

160. Ross R, Care AD, Taylor CM, et al: The transplacental movements of vitamin D in the sheep. p. 341. In Norman AW, Schaefer K, Herrath D, et al (eds): Vitamin D, Basic Research and its Clinical Application. Gruyter, Berlin, 1979

161. Brown PJ, Johnson PM: Isolation of a transferrin receptor structure from sodium deoxycholate solubilized human placental syncytiotrophoblast plasma membrane. Placenta 2:1, 1981

162. Pitcher-Wilmott RW, Hindocha P, Wood CBS: The placental transfer of IgG subclasses in human pregnancy. Clin Exp Immunol 41:303, 1980

163. Sanfilippo JS, Stoelk EM: Endocrinology of the placenta. Ch. 11. In Lavery JP (ed): The Human Placenta. Aspen Publishers, Rockville, MD, 1987

164. Juchau MR: Drug biotransformation reactions in the placenta. Ch. 2. In Mirkin BL (ed): Perinatal Pharmacology and Therapeutics. Academic Press, Orlando, FL, 1976

165. Welch RM, Harrison YE, Gommi BW, et al: Stimulatory effect of cigarette smoking on the hydroxylation of 3,4-benzpyrene and the N-demethylation of 3-methyl-4-monomethylaminoazobenzene by enzymes in human placenta. Clin Pharmacol Ther 10:100, 1969

166. Ward RM, Singh S, Mirkin BL: Fetal clinical pharmacology. Ch. 3. In Avery GS (ed): Drug Treatment. ADIS Health Science Press, Sydney, 1980

167. Waddell WJ, Marlowe C: Transfer of drugs across the placenta. Pharmacol Ther 14:375, 1981

168. Schneider H, Dancis J (eds): In Vitro Perfusion of Human Placental Tissue. Karger, Basel, 1985

169. Speert H: Placental transmission of sulfathiazole and sulfadiazine and its significance for fetal chemotherapy. Am J Obstet Gynecol 45:200, 1943

170. Shnider SM, Way EL: The kinetics of transfer of lidocaine across the human placenta. Anesthesiology 29:944, 1968

171. Lee HM, Anderson RC, Chen KK: Passage of sulfanilamide from mother to fetus. Proc Soc Exp Biol Med 38:366, 1938

172. Green TP, O'Dea RF, Mirkin BL: Determinants of drug disposition and effect in the fetus. Annu Rev Pharmacol Toxicol 19:285, 1979

173. Tam PPL, Chan STH: Changes in the composition of maternal plasma, fetal plasma and fetal extraembryonic fluid during gestation in the rat. J Reprod Fertil 51:41, 1977

174. Goldstein A, Warren R: Passage of caffeine into human gonadal and fetal tissue. Biochem Pharmacol 11:166, 1962

175. Cohen EN: Thiopental-curare-nitrous oxide anesthesia for cesarean section, 1950–1960. Anesth Analg (Cleve) 41:122, 1962

176. Leif P: Discussion, p. 243, following Villee C: Placental transfer of drugs. Ann NY Acad Sci 123:237, 1965

177. Dawes GS: Changes in the circulation at birth. Br Med Bull 17:148, 1961

178. Martin CB Jr: Uterine blood flow and placental circulation. Anesthesiology 26:447, 1965
179. Reid DE: A Textbook of Obstetrics. WB Saunders, Philadelphia, 1962
180. Edelman IS, Haley HB, Schloerb PR, et al: Further observations on total body water. I. Normal values throughout the life span. Surg Gynecol Obstet 95:1, 1952
181. Anderson DF, Phernetton TM, Rankin JH: Prediction of fetal drug concentrations. Am J Obstet Gynecol 137:735, 1980
182. Wilson JT: Determinants and consequences of drug excretion in milk. Drug Metab Rev 14:619, 1983
183. Brenner BM, Rector FC (eds): The Kidney. 3rd Ed. Vol. 1. WB Saunders, Philadelphia, 1986
184. Vander AJ, Sherman JH, Luciano DS: Regulation of water and electrolyte balance. Ch. 13. In Human Physiology. The Mechanisms of Body Function. McGraw-Hill, New York, 1985
185. Brodie BB, Aronow L, Axelrod J: The fate of benzazoline (Priscoline) in dog and man and a method for its estimation in biological material. J Pharmacol Exp Ther 106:200, 1952
186. Riggs DS: The Mathematical Approach to Physiological Problems. Williams & Wilkins, Baltimore, 1963, Ch. 8.
187. Moller JV, Sheikh MI: Renal organic anion transport system: Pharmacological, physiological, and biochemical aspects. Pharmacol Rev 34:315, 1983
188. Ross CR, Holohan PD: Transport of organic anions and cations in isolated renal plasma membranes. Annu Rev Pharmacol Toxicol 23:65, 1983
189. Rennick BR: Renal tubule transport of organic cations. Am J Physiol 240:F83, 1981
190. Hook JB, Bailie MD: Perinatal renal pharmacology. Annu Rev Pharmacol Toxicol 19:491, 1979
191. Roberts RJ: Drug Therapy in Infants. Philadelphia, WB Saunders, 1984
192. West JR, Smith HW, Chasis H: Glomerular filtration rate, effective renal blood flow, and maximal tubular excretory capacity in infancy. J Pediatr 32:10, 1948
193. Hirsch GH, Hook JB: Maturation of renal organic acid transport. Substrate stimulation by penicillin. Science 165:909, 1969
194. Grantham JJ, Chonko AM: Renal handling of organic anions and cations; metabolism and excretion of uric acid. Ch. 17. In Brenner BM, Rector FC (eds): The Kidney. 3rd Ed. Vol. 1. WB Saunders, Philadelphia, 1986
195. Fabre J, Balant L: Renal failure, drug pharmacokinetics and drug action. p. 212. In Gibaldi M, Prescott L (eds): Handbook of Clinical Pharmacokinetics. ADIS Health Science Press, Sydney, 1983
196. Bennett WM, Arnoff GR, Morrison G, et al: Drug prescribing in renal failure: dosing guidelines for adults. Am J Kidney Dis 3:155, 1983
197. Gibson TP, Nelson HA: Drug kinetics and artificial kidneys. Clin Pharmacokinet 8:301, 1983
198. Maher JF: Pharmacological aspects of renal failure and dialysis. Ch. 39. In Drukker W, Parsons FM, Maher JF (eds): Replacement of Renal Function by Dialysis. 2nd Ed. Martinus Nijhoff Publishers, Boston, 1983
199. Golper TA, Bennett WM: Drug usage in dialysis patients. Ch. 23. In Nissenson AR, Fine RN, Gantile DE (eds): Clinical Dialysis. Appleton-Century-Crofts, E. Norwalk, CT, 1984
200. Golper TA: Drugs and peritoneal dialysis. Dial Transplant. 8:41, 1979
201. Rollins DE, Klaassen CD: Biliary excretion of drugs in man. Clin Pharmacokinet 4:368, 1979
202. Klaassen CD, Watkins JB: Mechanisms of bile formation, hepatic uptake, and biliary excretion. Pharmacol Rev 36:1, 1984
203. Routledge PA, Shand DG: Clinical pharmacokinetics of propanolol. Clin Pharmacokinet 4:73, 1979
204. Combes B, Wheeler HO, Childs AW, Bradley SE: The mechanisms of bromsulfalein removal from the blood. Trans Assoc Am Physicians 69:276, 1956
205. Evans WH: Membrane traffic at the hepatocyte's sinusoidal and canalicular surface domains. Hepatology 1:452, 1981
206. Roberts RK, Desmond PV, Shenker S: Drug prescribing in hepatobiliary disease. Drugs 17:198, 1979

207. Carey MC: The enterohepatic circulation. Ch. 27. In Arias I, Popper H, Schachter D, Shafritz DA (eds): The Liver: Biology and Pathobiology. Raven Press, New York, 1982
208. Caldwell JH, Bush CA, Greenberger JJ: Interruption of the enterohepatic circulation of digitoxin by cholestyramine. II. Effect on metabolic disposition of tritium-labeled digitoxin and cardiac systolic intervals in man. J Clin Invest 20:2638, 1971

4

The Time Course of Drug Action

Richard R. Neubig

The previous chapters have considered the effects of drugs on isolated systems and described processes that determine a drug's access to and elimination from its site of action. Here we will integrate those concepts and examine how we can predict the time course of drug action. Such predictions are necessary to optimize the efficacy and safety of drug therapy. Two advances have been particularly important in optimizing drug delivery. The first is the development of sensitive methods of assaying the concentrations of drugs and their metabolites in blood plasma and other body fluids. The second is the recognition that both the therapeutic and the toxic effects of drugs are in most cases closely related to the concentration of the drug in the plasma (or serum).[1,2]

The study of drug and metabolite concentrations in the blood and body fluids constitutes the discipline of *pharmacokinetics*. The value of measurement of plasma drug concentrations is greatest in the case of those drugs for which there is only a small difference between the concentration required to produce a therapeutic effect and that producing toxic effects. The cardiac glycoside digoxin and the aminoglycoside antibiotic gentamicin are good examples of drugs possessing such a "narrow therapeutic window." The monitoring of plasma drug concentrations is also particularly important when there are great differences among individuals in drug absorption, metabolism, or elimination, resulting in unpredictable relationships between the dose administered and the plasma concentration achieved. An example is the anticonvulsant phenytoin, which will be discussed later in this chapter. Some exceptions to the generalization that pharmacologic effects are directly related to plasma drug concentration will be presented, and the importance of drug tissue interactions (*pharmacodynamics*) in modifying drug effects[3] will be discussed (Fig. 4-1).

RATE OF DRUG ABSORPTION

The rate of drug absorption is generally either constant and independent of the amount of drug to be absorbed (*zero-order kinetics*) or diminishing and always in proportion to the amount of drug still to be absorbed (*exponential*, or *first-order kinetics*). If a drug is injected intravascularly, one cannot really speak of absorption, although in a formal sense

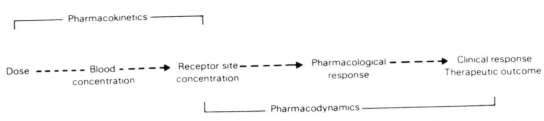

Fig. 4-1. Factors that determine a drug response. (Adapted from Sheiner et al.,[3] with permission.)

we may regard the entire dose as being "absorbed" into the bloodstream instantaneously. As we shall see later in this chapter, it is convenient to analyze *the kinetics of elimination* under these conditions because no simultaneous absorption process complicates matters.

The most straightforward example of constant-rate absorption is that seen with a continuous intravenous infusion, in which the rate of entry of the drug into the vascular system is fixed and maintained at will. Two types of apparatus are employed. The simplest is a gravity-flow intravenous drip, commonly used at the bedside in hospitals. The apparatus is employed to administer blood, plasma, physiologic saline solutions, glucose, and other nutrients. It is a simple matter to add a drug in appropriate concentration. The flow rate is maintained approximately constant by a simple adjustable clamp on the tubing, and the rate is monitored by counting drops in a glass bulb designed for the purpose. A more precise apparatus is the infusion pump, calibrated to deliver solution at a constant rate. The method of continuous infusion has been used for administration of oxytocin at term to induce labor and for administration of sodium nitroprusside, which has a rapid and profound blood pressure lowering effect. In these cases the exact regulation of dosage is of critical importance. As will be discussed, if a constant-rate infusion delivers new drug at a rate that just replaces drug eliminated from the body, a steady-state constant drug concentration will be maintained throughout the volume of distribution in the body.

Constant-rate absorption may be approximated by various techniques for sustained-release medication. As already shown in Chapter 3, a subcutaneous pellet in the shape of a flat disk may release drug into solution at a practically constant rate until it is nearly all dissolved. If the dissolution of the drug can be made the rate-limiting process for absorption (i.e., if the rate of absorption is fast compared with the rate of solution), then the overall absorption rate will be practically constant. The same principle applies to some extent to any insoluble drug in a subcutaneous or intramuscular depot during an initial period, before the total surface area exposed to solution diminishes by much. Protamine zinc insulin and procaine penicillin are examples of drugs whose absorption from depots may proceed at a nearly constant rate for some time after their administration. In sustained-release medications for oral administration, the aim of the manufacturing process is to achieve a nearly constant rate of liberation into the gastrointestinal lumen (cf. Fig. 3-7). Generally, for any situation in which a supply (or reservoir) of available drug can replace what is absorbed, a constant rate of absorption may be expected. An example would be the transdermal drug delivery system described in Chapter 3. Another example is found in the administration of anesthetic gases. Here, drug absorbed into the pulmonary blood at the alveoli during each breath is replaced at the next breath from the unlimited supply maintained in the anesthetist's breathing bag.

Except for the rather special cases cited above, both for enteral and parenteral routes of administration, most drug absorption follows first-order kinetics (i.e., a constant fraction of the total drug present is absorbed in each equal interval of time). After subcutaneous or intramuscular injection of a drug solution, for example, the probability that a given drug molecule will enter a nearby capillary in a given short period of time depends upon the intrinsic vascularity of the tissue (i.e., how near the capillary is), the permeability of the capillaries to the drug, the local blood flow, and the diffusion rate of the drug. The rate of absorption (molecules per minute) will be the product of this probability times the total number of drug molecules present. As the total amount of drug diminishes, the rate of absorption will obviously decrease proportionately, and the time course of the absorption process can be described by the following equations:

$$\frac{dM}{dt} = -k_a M$$

$$M = M_0 e^{-k_a t}$$

$$\ln \frac{M}{M_0} = -k_a t$$

$$\ln M = \ln M_0 - k_a t$$

$$\log M = \log M_0 - \frac{k_a t}{2.30}$$

where M_0 is the amount of drug placed initially at the absorption site, M is the amount remaining at the absorption site at time t, and k_a is the rate constant for absorption. The last two equations give straight lines, so if the amount of unabsorbed drug is plotted against time on semilogarithmic coordinates, a line should be obtained with the negative slope $k_a/2.30$ and intercept M_0 on the y axis. In this treatment back-diffusion from the blood into the depot is neglected. Figure 4-2 presents a good example. Radioactive sodium, as NaCl, was injected intramuscularly in a human subject, and the residual radioactivity was determined for 25 minutes with a Geiger counter at the skin surface. The exponential course of the absorption is clearly demonstrated by the data. Incorporation of epinephrine into the injection markedly reduced the absorption rate (by reducing the local blood flow), but the residual absorption was still first-order.

The rate constant of absorption tells us the instantaneous rate of absorption as a fraction of the amount still present. For the experiment of Figure 4-2, this rate constant, k_a, was 0.064 min^{-1} in the control resting muscle, meaning that the remaining sodium ions were absorbed at a rate of 6.4 percent per minute.

Another useful measure, directly related to k_a, is the *absorption half-time*, $t_{1/2}$, the time when the drug content of the depot has been reduced to half its initial value. As shown above,

$$\ln \frac{M}{M_0} = -k_a t$$

Substituting $M/M_0 = \frac{1}{2}$, we obtain

$$\ln \frac{1}{2} = -k_a t_{1/2}$$

$$t_{1/2} = \frac{0.693}{k_a}$$

For sodium absorption, where $k_a = 0.064$ min^{-1}, $t_{1/2} = 11$ minutes.

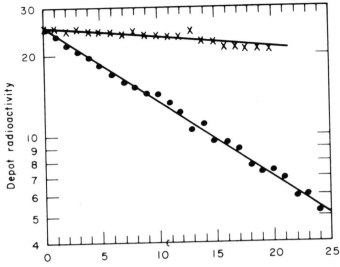

Fig. 4-2. Absorption of $^{24}Na^+$ from an intramuscular depot in man. The radioisotope (5 μCi) was injected deep into the gastrocnemius muscle. Residual radioactivity was determined by a Geiger counter at the skin. The ordinate represents counts per minute on logarithmic scale, but the scale factor (which is irrelevant to the purpose of the graph) is not given. The slope is a measure of k_a, the fraction removed per minute. Lower curve, control resting muscle, $k_a = 0.064$ min^{-1}; upper curve, epinephrine incorporated in the injection, $k_a = 0.010$ min^{-1}. (From Kety,[4] with permission.)

Very similar results were obtained in rats with several radioactive compounds.[5] Here the method was to excise the injection site at various times in different animals and assay the remaining drug by liquid scintillation counting. The substances chosen for study were ouabain, benzylpenicillin, hexamethonium, glucose, urea, and water. Despite a 30-fold range in molecular weights and a 5-fold range in diffusion coefficients and considerable differences in ionic state and lipid solubility, the absorption rates were virtually the same— about 0.16 min^{-1} (half-time 4.4 min). This result, like that with $^{24}Na^+$, suggests that the blood flow at the injection site is the rate-limiting factor for absorption. Confirmatory evidence was a marked slowing of absorption by epinephrine (as seen also in Fig. 4-2) and a speeding of absorption by the vasodilator prostaglandin E_2.

RATE OF DRUG ELIMINATION

Elimination refers to all the processes that operate to reduce the effective drug concentration in the body fluids. Depending upon the mechanism of elimination, the course of disappearance of a drug from the body (or the decay of its plasma level) may be zero-order (constant rate) or first-order (exponential). First-order elimination is the general rule, but if an elimination mechanism can become saturated, then at drug concentrations above the saturation level the elimination will be zero-order. An excellent example already discussed is the renal tubular secretion of drugs, for which there is a maximum transport capacity (T_m). If the plasma level of a drug is so high that T_m is reached, zero-order kinetics will obtain until the concentration falls below the saturation level, and then subsequently the elimination rate will decrease with decreasing concentration; at a low enough concentration the elimination will always be first-order (i.e., proportional to the concentration).

First-Order Elimination

Most elimination mechanisms are approximately first-order; a constant fraction of the drug in the body disappears in each equal interval of time. Typical is the excretion of drugs by glomerular filtration at the kidneys, as discussed in Chapter 3. Also, most drug metabolism occurs at concentrations below saturation, where the kinetics are first-order (see next section for discussion of nonsaturated Michaelis-Menton clearance). Another first-order process is the elimination of volatile drugs at the lungs. Both processes are first-order because every drug molecule has a fixed probability of being excreted within a given time; the total rate of excretion is therefore equal to that probability times the total number of drug molecules present.

For first-order (exponential) elimination the familiar equations apply, where X denotes total amount of drug in the body at time t, X_0 the amount of drug present at time zero, and k_e the rate constant for elimination:

$$X = X_0 e^{-k_e t}$$

$$\log X = \log X_0 - \frac{k_e t}{2.30}$$

$$t_{1/2} = \frac{0.693}{k_e}$$

The half-time for elimination is also called the *biologic half-life*. The meaning of $t_{1/2}$ is easily grasped, but the first-order rate constants (both for absorption and elimination) may be misunderstood. Consider a drug that is eliminated with $k_e = 0.5$ day^{-1}. This does not mean that half the initial amount will be present after 1 day. The rate constant, k_e, describes the instantaneous rate of elimination at any time. Thus, initially, the elimination is at such a rate that if the absolute rate continued, one-half of the drug would be gone in 1 day. But that absolute rate does not continue. It starts to diminish immediately, as soon as the total amount of drug starts to decrease, and it continues to diminish. Thus, the biologic half-life of such a drug is not 1 day, but rather $0.693/0.5 = 1.39$ days, and the fraction of drug eliminated in 1 day is $1 - e^{-k_e t}$, which is equal to 0.393 (or 39.3 percent).

Figure 4-3 shows a typical first-order elimination curve after intravenous injection of penicillin into a dog. The decline in the plasma concentration is almost perfectly linear on semilogarithmic coordinates (i.e., a constant fraction was eliminated in each equal interval of time). The biologic half-life is found by measuring the time required for a given plasma concentration to decline by one-half, here 25 minutes. The elimination rate constant k_e equals $0.693/25 = 0.028$ min^{-1}, or about 3 percent per minute. The elimination rate is consistent with the renal tubular secretion of a drug whose V_d is somewhat larger than the extracellular fluid volume (cf. Table 3-13 for comparable data in humans), and the first-order kinetics indicate that even at the highest concentration observed here, 8 units ml^{-1}, the T_m was not reached.

Zero-Order Elimination

Saturated elimination mechanisms are characterized by a constant *amount* of drug being excreted per unit time rather than a constant *fraction* as in first-order mechanisms. Renal tubular secretion and secretion of drugs into the bile are both saturable processes with a T_m value for each drug.

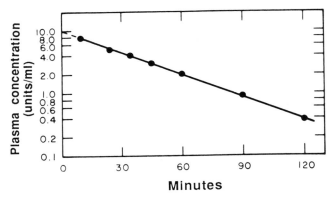

Fig. 4-3. First-order elimination of penicillin from plasma. Penicillin G (50,000 units, 30 mg) was injected intravenously at time zero in a dog weighing about 18 kg. Plasma concentrations of penicillin were determined periodically, as shown. (Adapted from Beyer et al.,[6] with permission.)

Substrates for drug-metabolizing enzymes may be degraded or conjugated at a constant rate when their concentrations are above saturation levels or when a coupled reaction is rate-limiting. As with renal tubular and biliary transport systems at concentrations between half saturation and saturation, complex kinetics apply. At low saturation of enzyme (i.e., when 80 percent or more of the enzyme is not in combination with substrate) the reaction becomes first-order. From the Michaelis-Menten equation (see Ch. 1)

$$v = \frac{dS}{dt} = \frac{S}{(K + S)} V_{max}$$

and when $S \ll K$, so that $v \ll V_{max}$, we have approximately

$$\frac{dS}{dt} = \frac{V_{max}}{K} S$$

which is obviously the equation of a first-order process, since V_{max}/K is a constant. Initially, therefore, the metabolic elimination of drugs may be zero-order or first-order, depending upon the drug concentration and the affinity of the particular drug for its metabolizing enzymes. Eventually, as the drug concentration falls, its metabolism will become first-order.

Figure 4-4 presents an example of metabolic elimination in the same species by different kinetics. In both cases the metabolic reaction under study was the conjugation of a substituted benzoic acid with glycine. For curve A the drug was anisic acid (*p*-methoxybenzoic acid), and a large excess of glycine was administered simultaneously. The excretion of glycine conjugate in the urine followed a typical exponential course; the rate declined progressively as the level of unconjugated drug in the body declined. For curve B the drug was *p*-fluorobenzoic acid, and no exogenous glycine was furnished. The rate of conjugation of this compound is very much faster than that of anisic acid, but it proceeds at a constant rate (zero-order) until very little unconjugated drug remains. This occurs because endogenous glycine cannot be made available at a sufficient rate; thus, the glycine supply is rate-limiting, and the overall conjugation rate remains constant. When exogenous glycine was administered simultaneously with *p*-fluorobenzoic acid (not shown in the figure), the initial rate of conjugation was much faster, but it slowed progressively according to first-order kinetics.

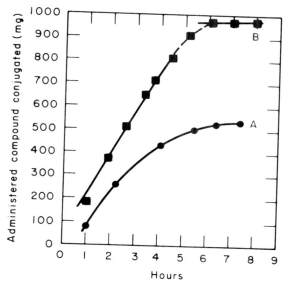

Fig. 4-4. Examples of zero-order and first-order kinetics in drug metabolism. Urinary excretion of glycine conjugates was followed in the rabbit after administration of 1-g doses of two different compounds: Curve *A:* anisic acid + glycine (4 g); Curve *B: p*-fluorobenzoic acid. Curve *A* is exponential because excess glycine is supplied. The incomplete excretion occurs because the drug is also metabolized by other pathways. The initial part of curve *B* is linear because the endogenous glycine supply is rate-limiting, nearly to the end of the reaction. (From Bray et al.,[7] with permission.)

An interesting example of zero-order metabolism is the oxidation of ethanol in humans and other animals. Three hepatic enzymes appear to play a role in ethanol metabolism in vivo; alcohol dehydrogenase, catalase, and a microsomal ethanol oxidizing system.[8,9] Alcohol dehydrogenase normally predominates, but the microsomal ethanol oxidizing system is induced following chronic ethanol ingestion and may play a greater role in ethanol metabolism in chronic alcoholics.[9] Ethanol is converted to acetaldehyde by the liver alcohol dehydrogenase in an NAD-coupled reaction:

$$CH_3CH_2OH + NAD^+ \rightleftharpoons CH_3CHO + NADH + H^+$$

The acetaldehyde is further metabolized to acetic acid by aldehyde dehydrogenase. The equilibrium for the oxidation of ethanol to acetaldehyde lies far to the left; with equal concentrations of NAD^+ and NADH, the equilibrium ratio of ethanol to acetaldehyde will be more than 1,000:1. Only the continuous removal of acetaldehyde forces the reaction to completion.

Except at very low concentrations, the metabolism of ethanol in humans is essentially constant (about 10 ml hr^{-1} on the average) regardless of concentration; the rate, however, differs considerably from person to person.[10] Alcohol dehydrogenase has been studied extensively, the human liver enzyme has been crystallized, and all the equilibrium constants and reaction rates have been determined.[11,12] The dissociation constant for the interaction of ethanol with the enzyme-NAD^+ complex is 1.2×10^{-3} M. The blood ethanol concentration associated with mild intoxication is about 1 mg ml^{-1} (2×10^{-2} M), or 17 times the dissociation constant. Thus, the enzyme would be 94 percent saturated even at this pharmacologically low level of ethanol, and saturation would be virtually

304 • *Principles of Drug Action*

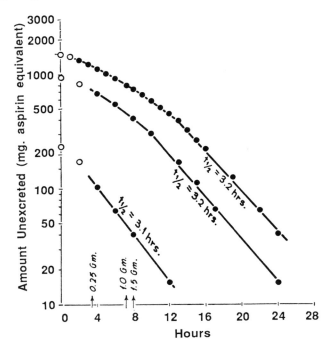

Fig. 4-.5. Elimination of salicylate by a healthy human subject as a function of dose. Vertical arrows indicate the time necessary to eliminate 50 percent of each dose. (From Levy,[13] with permission.)

complete at higher levels in the intoxicating range. However, enzyme alone is not the main determinant of limited ethanol metabolism. The cofactor NAD^+ is consumed stoichiometrically by the reaction, and the rate of reoxidation of NADH to NAD^+ limits the conversion of ethanol to acetaldehyde.[8,9]

Some well-known facts about drinking are logical consequences of the zero-order kinetics and slow rate of ethanol metabolism. To achieve an intoxicating level of 1 mg ml^{-1} (0.1 mg percent) throughout 42 L of body water (the volume of distribution for ethanol) will require an intake of about 42 g (56 ml) of absolute ethanol. Most strong liquor contains 40 to 50 percent ethanol, so the required intake of whiskey, gin, vodka, or similar drink will be approximately 120 ml, or 4 ounces. This "priming" amount is often ingested quite rapidly in order to obtain the desired effect. However, the maximum that can be metabolized is 10 ml hr^{-1}, so that 5 hours would be required to eliminate the 56 ml taken at the outset. It follows that continuation of the same dosing rate would very soon lead to progressively higher and more toxic blood levels. The safe maintenance dose (after priming), to maintain a constant level of mild intoxication, will be just 10 ml of ethanol (about 20 to 25 ml of liquor) per hour.

Another commonly used drug that has a saturable elimination mechanism is aspirin.[13] Aspirin is rapidly deacetylated by the liver to form salicylate, which is then eliminated by three mechanisms: (1) by conjugation with glycine; (2) by glucuronide formation; and (3) to a small degree, by renal excretion of unchanged salicylate. After low doses of aspirin (e.g., 250 mg), salicylate is rapidly eliminated by first-order kinetics with a half-time of 3.1 hours (bottom curve in Fig. 4-5). At higher doses of 1,000 or 1,500 mg (equivalent to two or three extra-strength aspirin tablets), the fraction of drug eliminated in a given time is initially reduced, as indicated by the decreased slope on the semilogarithmic plot. As the amount of drug remaining in the body decreases to approximately 250 mg, the elimination again becomes first-order, with the same half-time observed at the lower dose. This is the behavior predicted for a saturable clearance mechanism. In the case of aspirin, as for benzoic acid derivatives, it is the glycine conjugation reaction that is saturated at high drug concentrations. The arrows at the bottom of Figure 4-5 show the time required to eliminate half of the administered dose. Because the kinetics are not first-order (except at the lowest dose), this should not be called a half-time. Indeed, the time required to eliminate half of the drug increases with the dose administered and may be as long as 20 hours. This has grave implications in aspirin poisoning (see discussion later in this chapter).

Duration of Drug Action after Single Doses

First-Order Elimination

For a first-order elimination, *the duration of a therapeutically effective drug concentration increases as the logarithm of the amount of drug in the body fluids.* In many instances this means simply that the duration of action increases as the logarithm of the dose. This would be true, for example, if the dose were given intravenously, and it would be nearly true whenever the drug is absorbed very rapidly in comparison with its rate of elimination. It is easy to see from the schematic diagram of Figure 4-6 why this relationship should hold. Let x^* be the threshold concentration for therapeutic effect, established by the distribution of a just effective dose X^* in its volume of distribution V_d. Let x_1 and x_2 be plasma concentrations established by the doses X_1 and X_2. Since V_d is independent of dose, $X_1 = x_1 V_d$, $X_2 = x_2 V_d$, and $X^* = x^* V_d$. The durations of effective concentrations of the two doses are t_1 and t_2, and the slopes of the elimination curves, also independent of dose, are $-k_e/2.30$. If the ordinates are natural logarithms, $\ln x$, the slopes are simply $-k_e$. If logarithms to the base 10 are used, the slope becomes $-k_e/2.30$ because $\log x = (\ln x)/2.30$.

The fundamental equation for first-order elimination and the geometry of Figure 4-6 yield equations describing the relationship between duration of effective concentration

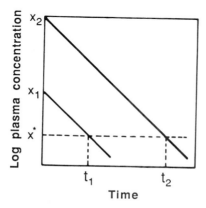

Fig. 4-6. Schematic first-order elimination curves for two doses. Concentration x* is the threshold concentration for therapeutic effect; x_1 and x_2 are the initial concentrations established by the two doses. It is assumed that absorption is very rapid or that the doses were administered intravenously.

and dose. First we find t^*, the time required for the concentration to fall from any initial level x_0 to the threshold level x^*, as follows:

$$\log \frac{x^*}{x_0} = -\frac{k_e t^*}{2.30}$$

and, substituting $x = X/V_d$, cancelling V_d, and inverting, we obtain

$$t^* = \frac{2.30}{k_e} \log \frac{X_0}{X^*}$$

Also, obviously, for the ratio of effective times after the two doses,

$$\frac{t_2}{t_1} = \frac{\log X_2 - \log X^*}{\log X_1 - \log X^*}$$

These equations, especially the one that gives t^* as a function of dose, have practical importance. The duration of a therapeutic level of a drug depends upon the *ratio of administered dose to the just-effective dose*, and also upon the rate constant of elimination. Evidently, the longer the biologic half-life (i.e., the smaller the value of k_e), the longer the duration for a given dose ratio. Whatever the duration may be at a particular ratio X_1/X^*, geometric increments in the dose will produce only linear increments in the duration of effective drug levels. Suppose, for example, that doubling the threshold dose would result in an effective drug level for 1 hour (i.e., the biologic half-life is 1 hour). Then the dose would have to be doubled again to achieve an effective level for 2 hours and doubled yet again to achieve a 3-hour duration. The tolerable limit of geometric increases in drug dosage will be determined by the dose-related toxicity of the particular drug.

Figure 4-7 presents a graphic summary of these relationships for realistic ranges of dose ratio and of k_e. Whatever a just effective dose may be, it is unlikely, as a general rule, that a dose more than five times as great can be given without grave danger of toxicity; certainly few drugs have this large a margin of safety, although penicillin, propranolol, and some of the water-soluble vitamins are notable exceptions. Usually one would be restricted to a smaller, perhaps only two- or threefold, excess over the just effective level. Dose ratios X/X^* greater than 5 are therefore not considered here. Values of k_e spanning four orders of magnitude are indicated on the curves. Values in the range 0.01 to 0.001 min^{-1} are encountered frequently (biologic half-lives about 1 to 10 hours), since so many drugs are eliminated primarily at the kidneys without significant tubular reabsorption. Figure 4-7 is shown as a double logarithmic plot in order to encompass the wide range of durations and dose ratios. Note that if twice the just effective dose is administered (vertical broken line), the duration of therapeutic level will be simply the biologic half-life. This leads to a useful and practical rule: If a drug's effect is to last several hours, then that drug must be one whose biologic half-life is at least several hours (i.e., it must not be metabolized rapidly or secreted by the renal tubules).

Zero Order Elimination

In the case of a drug with zero-order elimination kinetics, *the duration of a therapeutically effective drug concentration increases linearly with the amount of drug in the body fluids.* This can be seen in the schematic diagram in Figure 4-8. For a drug with zero-order kinetics, a constant amount rather than a constant fraction is eliminated in a given

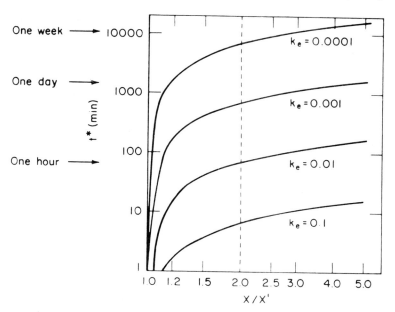

Fig. 4-7. Relationship between duration of effective therapeutic levels and dose. Administered dose X is assumed to be absorbed very rapidly or to be administered intravenously; X' is the just-effective dose; t^* is the time (in minutes) during which the drug concentration in the body fluids exceeds the threshold level. Each curve is for a different value of the rate constant of elimination, as indicated; biologic half-lives are (from top to bottom) 6,930, 693, 69, 6.9 minutes. Note that both axes have logarithmic scales.

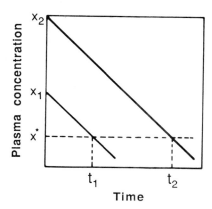

Fig. 4-8. Schematic zero-order elimination curves for two doses of drug. Concentration x^* is the threshold concentration for the therapeutic effect; x_1 and x_2 are the initial concentrations established by the two doses.

time period. Thus, the ordinate scale in Figure 4-8 is linear rather than logarithmic as in Figure 4-6. If the minimum therapeutic drug concentration is x^*, then the total amount of drug present in the body would be $X^* = x^* V_d$. As long as the drug concentration is high enough to keep the elimination mechanism saturated, the amount of drug eliminated per unit time is V_{max} (or T_m). If the amount of drug in the body starts at X_0, then at time t it would be

$$X = X_0 - V_{max}t$$

By substituting X^* for X, we can see that the duration of the therapeutically effective drug concentration would be

$$t^* = (X_0 - X^*)/V_{max}$$

This relationship implies that an n-fold increase in the dose of a drug cleared by zero-order kinetics would result, *at minimum*, in an n-fold increase in the duration of the therapeutic effect. This might seem to be advantageous, but as will be seen later in this chapter, very small changes in the dose rate of drugs with zero-order kinetics produce large changes in the steady-state plasma concentrations. Consequently, such drugs are generally not practical for routine clinical use. There are, however, clinically useful drugs (e.g., aspirin and phenytoin) for which the metabolism or elimination becomes saturated at plasma concentrations above the usual therapeutic range. Thus, for overdoses or poisonings involving drugs with zero-order kinetics, the above considerations have serious practical implications. While a 10-fold higher dose of a drug with first-order clearance would only result in approximately a threefold increase in the duration of action, a drug with zero-order elimination kinetics would have a more than 10-fold increase in duration of action, with the attendant increased risk of toxic complications.

ZERO-ORDER ABSORPTION, FIRST-ORDER ELIMINATION: THE PLATEAU PRINCIPLE

Drugs are seldom given in single isolated doses; most often, a sustained therapeutic effect is desired, so the drug is given either as a continuous infusion or as intermittent parenteral or oral doses. For drugs eliminated by first-order kinetics, the fundamental pharmacologic concept of *drug clearance* allows us to predict the steady state drug concentration during continuous therapy. Also, drug clearance is inversely proportional to the *elimination half-time*, which is important for determining the time course of drug action. In this section we will develop these concepts as we show the derivation of an elementary principle about steady states, the *plateau principle*, which has direct application to the kinetics of drug accumulation in the body as well as much broader application to fundamental biologic, chemical, and physical processes.

Steady-State Plasma Concentrations: Drug Clearance

If the rate of input into a system is constant and the rate of output from the system is proportional to the amount of drug present (i.e., exponential or first-order elimination), then the amount of drug in the system (here designated by X) will accumulate until a steady state is reached:

$$\xrightarrow{k_{in}} X \xrightarrow{k_{out}}$$

Constant input rate $= k_{in}$

Output rate $= k_{out}X$

At the steady state, X will have increased to X', a level at which the output rate is equal to the input rate:

$$k_{out}X' = k_{in}$$

$$X' = \frac{k_{in}}{k_{out}}$$

Let us examine the case of constant infusion. Let V_d be the volume of distribution of a drug (ml); Q a constant rate of infusion of the drug (mg·min^{-1}); k_e the first-order rate constant for elimination of the drug (min^{-1}), the rate of change of concentration being given by $k_e x$, where x is the drug concentration in plasma (mg·ml^{-1}); and t the elapsed time (min) from the start of the infusion.

Since the elimination rate is expressed in terms of the plasma concentration of the drug rather than of the total drug in the body, k_{in} is represented by Q/V_d, the rate of input per volume of body fluid. Then the equation describing the change in x with time is

$$\frac{dx}{dt} = \frac{Q}{V_d} - k_e x$$

The change in x from the start of the infusion ($x = 0$, $t = 0$) is given by

$$x = \frac{Q}{k_e V_d} (1 - e^{-k_e t})$$

This equation shows that with a constant infusion a plasma plateau is eventually reached; for when t becomes infinite, $1 - e^{-k_e t}$ becomes unity, and at the steady state

$$x' = Q/k_e V_d$$

Since $k_e V_d$ equals clearance (cf. Ch. 3),

Steady-state plasma concentration = dose rate/clearance

Rearranging the steady-state equation, we have $k_e(x' V_d) = Q$. Here, $x' V_d$ is the total amount of drug in the body; therefore $k_e(x' V_d)$ is the elimination rate, which is equal to the infusion rate Q, which must be the case at steady state.

The fundamental importance of clearance lies in the fact that it is the proportionality constant between dose rate Q and the steady-state drug concentration in plasma. Clearance is constant and is therefore a useful concept only when elimination is first-order. Since the goal of optimal drug therapy is to maintain a "therapeutic" plasma concentration, knowing a drug's clearance is a major step toward that goal. If drug clearance changes owing to a pathologic alteration such as renal insufficiency or to inhibition or induction of a metabolic pathway, then the dose rate must be changed proportionately to maintain a constant plasma concentration.

The concept of clearance is also useful in understanding the pharmacokinetics of drugs that are eliminated by multiple routes. This is true because clearances, like exponential rate constants, are additive. Let us assume, in our first-order system, that there are two routes of elimination represented by k_{out_1} and k_{out_2}.

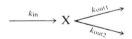

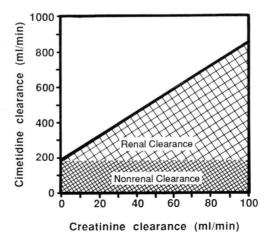

Fig. 4-9. Predicted cimetidine clearance for different degrees of renal insufficiency. Total cimetidine clearance for any value of creatinine clearance is indicated by the solid line. The nonrenal and renal components of cimetidine clearance are indicated by the finely and coarsely hatched areas respectively. (According to equations by Dettli.[15])

The change in X is

$$\frac{dX}{dt} = k_{in} - k_{out_1}X - k_{out_2}X$$

or

$$\frac{dX}{dt} = k_{in} - (k_{out_1} + k_{out_2})X$$

and the overall elimination rate constant k_e equals $k_{out_1} + k_{out_2}$. We saw in Chapter 3 that the k_e is proportional to clearance. In this case

$$\text{Total clearance} = k_e V_d$$
$$= (k_{out_1} + k_{out_2})V_d$$
$$= k_{out_1} V_d + k_{out_2} V_d$$
$$= \text{clearance}_1 + \text{clearance}_2$$

As an example, cimetidine, a histamine H_2 blocker used to treat peptic ulcers, is eliminated with a clearance of 650 ml min^{-1} by renal tubular secretion and with a clearance of 200 ml min^{-1} by hepatic metabolism.[14] It is reasonable to talk about a clearance value for hepatic elimination of cimetidine because no saturation occurs over the usual range of plasma concentrations, and first-order kinetics are followed.

The additivity of clearances makes it easy to predict the pharmacokinetics of cimetidine in patients with varying degrees of renal insufficiency[15] (Fig. 4-9). Since the apparent V_d for cimetidine is 150 L (note: this is three times total body water), the k_e is normally 850 ml min^{-1}/150,000 ml, or 0.0057 min^{-1}, with a $t_{1/2}$ of 122 minutes (2.0 hours). For half normal renal function, the predicted clearance is 200 + ½ × 650, or 525 ml min^{-1}, with a $t_{1/2}$ of 3.3 hours. In the absence of any renal function, only metabolic elimination occurs, and clearance is 200 ml min^{-1}, with a $t_{1/2}$ of 8.7 hours. In practice, the dose of cimetidine must be reduced significantly in renal insufficiency.

Time Course of Approach to Steady State: Key Role of Elimination Rate Constant

In our simple first-order model (Eq. 1), the steady state can be altered by changing the input rate k_{in} or by changing the output rate constant k_{out}, or both. Any such change will cause a *shift* to a new steady state.

According to the plateau principle, regardless of how a shift is brought about from one steady state to another, *the time course of the shift* (i.e., the rate at which the new plateau concentration is reached) *is determined solely by* k_{out}, the first-order rate constant of the output process that is operative during the shift. Thus, if the shift is caused by an abrupt alteration of k_{in} without change in k_{out}, the sole determinant is the unchanged k_{out}. If the shift is caused wholly or in part by a change in k_{out}, then the sole determinant is the *new* value of k_{out}. In any case, *the rate constant for the shift is equal to* k_{out}, *so the shift half-time is identical to the half-time of the output process*, $0.693/k_{out}$. The same principle applies when the initial value of X is zero and k_{in} is abruptly changed from zero to some finite value; then the shift is simply the establishment of a steady state. And the principle also applies when a steady-state value of X is in effect and k_{in} is abruptly changed to zero (i.e., the input is stopped); then the shift is simply the exponential disappearance of X, resulting in the new "steady state" at which $X = 0$.

The plateau principle is fundamental to understanding constant infusions, drug accumulation, dosage regimens, chronic toxicity by drug accumulation, and enzyme induction. We shall derive it first, then show its specific applications. For the change in X

$$\frac{dX}{dt} = k_{in} - k_{out}X$$

and at the initial steady state

$$X'_1 = \frac{k_{in_1}}{k_{out_1}}$$

Now change k_{in_1} to a new value k_{in_2}, and also change k_{out_1} to a new value k_{out_2}, and consider the time course of the change in X from X'_1 to its new steady-state value X'_2. Accordingly,

$$\frac{dX}{dt} = k_{in_2} - k_{out_2}X$$

and at the new steady state

$$X'_2 = \frac{k_{in_2}}{k_{out_2}}$$

To find X as a function of time after the shift, rearrange the differential equation to

$$\frac{dX}{k_{in_2} - k_{out_2}(X)} = dt$$

which is equivalent to

$$-\frac{1}{k_{out_2}} \frac{d[k_{in_2} - k_{out_2}(X)]}{[k_{in_2} - k_{out_2}(X)]} = dt$$

and integrating, we obtain

$$\ln[k_{in_2} - k_{out_2}(X)] = -k_{out_2}t + C$$

When $t = 0$, $X = X'_1$, and the constant of integration C is found to be

$$C = \ln[k_{in_2} - k_{out_2}(X'_1)]$$

Then, substituting and taking antilogarithms,

$$\frac{k_{in_2} - k_{out_2}(X)}{k_{in_2} - k_{out_2}(X'_1)} = e^{-k_{out_2}t}$$

Now we are concerned with the *shift* from one steady state to the other. The total extent of the shift is $(X'_2 - X'_1)$, and the amount by which X has changed from its initial steady state value is given by $(X - X'_1)$. Thus, the fraction f of the total shift that has been accomplished at any value of X is given by

$$f = \frac{(X - X'_1)}{(X'_2 - X'_1)}$$

and

$$X = fX'_2 + X'_1 - fX'_1$$

Substituting this value of X into the equation obtained above and substituting for k_{in_2} its equivalent value $k_{out_2}(X'_2)$, we obtain

$$\frac{X'_2 - fX'_2 - X'_1 + fX'_1}{X'_2 - X'_1} = e^{-k_{out_2}t}$$

which simplifies to

$$1 - f = e^{-k_{out_2}t}$$

This equation makes it evident that the kinetics of the shift are the exponential kinetics of a process with rate constant k_{out_2}. The half-time of the shift is found by setting $f = 0.5$:

$$\ln(0.5) = -k_{out_2}t$$

$$t_{1/2} = \frac{-\ln(0.5)}{k_{out_2}} = \frac{0.693}{k_{out_2}}$$

Simply, $t_{1/2}$ is the half-time of the output process.

It may seem paradoxical for the time course of the establishment of a steady state or of a shift from one steady state to another to be determined by the output rate constant and to be independent of the input rate. A physical analogy may help to clarify this relationship. Consider a water reservoir with outlet at bottom and outflow rate proportional to the outlet size and the head of water pressure. What are the conditions for establishing a specified steady-state water level? Since the inflow and outflow rates will be equal at the steady state, the inflow rate cannot be chosen at will; only one particular inflow rate will yield the specified level at steady state. A higher inflow rate will, of course, produce a faster rise of the water level, but then the specified level will be exceeded. A slower inflow rate will produce a slower rise, but then the specified level will not be attained. Only if the outlet size is changed will it become possible to alter the inflow rate so that the specified steady state is approached at a different rate, and clearly, the larger the outlet, the more rapidly can the specified steady state be approached.

The same principle applies when no particular steady-state level has been specified. With a given outlet the actual rate of rise of the water level will obviously be greater at high than at low inflow rate, but the steady-state level to be attained will also be proportionately higher. The *relative* rate of rise, measured as fraction of the ultimate level approached (f, as defined earlier), will be the same for all inflow rates. In a given reservoir this relative rate of approach to any steady state will be directly proportional to the outlet size, which is analogous to the rate constant of the drug output process.

In the example of a constant infusion considered previously, k_{out_2} is simply the elimination rate constant k_e. Thus, the kinetics of attaining the plateau concentration, of shifting from one plateau to another, or of the die-away when the infusion is stopped, are given by the general expression

$$f = 1 - e^{-k_e t}$$

where, in the general case

$$f = \frac{x - x'_1}{x'_2 - x'_1}$$

For starting an infusion ($x'_1 = 0$)

$$f = \frac{x}{x'_2}$$

and for stopping an infusion ($x'_2 = 0$)

$$f = 1 - \frac{x}{x'_1}$$

In summary, regardless of the means by which a steady state is changed (e.g., if the rate of a constant infusion is increased or decreased, if an infusion is started or stopped, or if the elimination rate constant is increased or decreased), *the half-time of the shift to the new steady state is the new elimination half-time (i.e., the biologic half-life of the drug).* For discontinuance of an infusion, the time course of the shift is the normal die-away curve of drug concentration. As for all exponential processes, if we know the half-time (or k, from which we can calculate the half-time), it is easy to predict the extent of approach to steady state. Substituting $\ln 2/t_{1/2}$ for k_e

$$f = 1 - e^{-(\ln 2/t_{1/2})t}$$
$$= 1 - 2^{-t/t_{1/2}}$$
$$= 1 - 0.5^{t/t_{1/2}}$$

Thus, the process is 50 percent complete for $t = t_{1/2}$, 75 percent for $2t_{1/2}$, 93.75 percent for $4t_{1/2}$, and 97.875 percent for $5t_{1/2}$. A usual rule of thumb is that exponential processes are virtually complete by four or five half-times.

The plateau principle can be applied to experimental constant infusions in order to gain information about the way a drug is disposed of in the body. The rate of infusion is set by the investigator. By periodic determinations of the drug plasma level, the rate of attaining a plateau can be found, and this rate yields an estimate of the elimination rate constant k_e. The actual concentration at the plateau is $Q/k_e V_d$, as we have seen, from which V_d can also be estimated. By exploring a range of infusion rates leading to widely differing plateau concentrations, it is possible to see whether or not the overall elimination follows first-order kinetics, and it is also possible to see what different mechanisms play the major roles in elimination at different drug concentrations. For example, any exper-

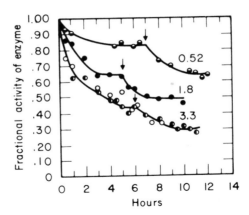

Fig. 4-10. Constant intravenous infusions of neostigmine in dogs. Vertical scale is activity of plasma cholinesterase, used as a measure of the concentration of neostigmine, an inhibitor of that enzyme. Since the relationship between inhibitor concentration and observed enzyme activity is complex, curves may only be interpreted semiquantitatively. Each curve represents a different infusion rate; values given are to be multiplied by 10^{-10} moles kg^{-1} min^{-1}. Renal artery and vein were ligated at times shown by arrows. (From Goldstein et al.,[16] with permission.)

imental procedure that alters k_e will change the plateau level during a constant infusion. If renal excretion is a significant mechanism and the renal arteries are clamped, the plasma drug level will promptly rise, and if other first-order mechanisms are present, a new plateau will be attained. By the plateau principle the time course of the shift gives an estimate of the *new* k_e, as does also the new plateau concentration (provided V_d did not change). If all elimination pathways are blocked or saturated, then continuing the infusion will cause the plasma drug level to rise without limit until toxicity and then death supervene.

An application of this technique is illustrated in Figure 4-10. Here, neostigmine, a cholinesterase inhibitor, was given to dogs by constant infusion. The plasma neostigmine levels were measured periodically by a method that makes use of the degree of inhibition of the plasma cholinesterase—a given depression of enzyme activity signifies a certain concentration of neostigmine, although the relationship is not one of simple proportionality. The data shown on the figure are measurements of enzyme activity, plotted as fractions of the initial uninhibited activity. We see that plateau levels were established at three different infusion rates into the femoral vein. The effect of tying the renal vessels indicates that the kidneys play a significant role in the overall elimination. The investigators used the difference between the two plateau levels, with and without the kidneys functioning, to obtain a quantitative estimate of the rate constant of renal excretion. This corresponded to a renal clearance for neostigmine of about 100 ml min^{-1}, a value consistent with elimination by glomerular filtration in the dog. The renal clearance estimate was confirmed directly by measurements of neostigmine in the urine.

Neostigmine was also administered by constant infusion to human patients suffering from myasthenia gravis, a disease for which it is the drug of choice. Figure 4-11 shows the relationship between the rate of drug infusion at the steady state (equal to the rate of elimination at the steady state) and the neostigmine concentration at the steady state. The data from the experiments with dogs are also shown on the graph. If the elimination is first-order throughout the range examined, the relationship between the logarithm of the

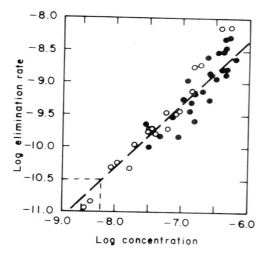

Fig. 4-11. Relationship of elimination rate to the steady-state plasma level of neostigmine. *Solid circles:* myasthenia gravis patients, for whom neostigmine is the drug of choice. *Open circles:* dogs. Note that this is log-log plot. Broken line has a slope of 1. Elimination rate (which at steady-state equals the infusion rate) is expressed as moles, per kilogram per minute, neostigmine concentration as moles per liter. (From Goldstein et al.,[16] with permission.)

infusion rate (or of the elimination rate) and the logarithm of the concentration should be linear, and the slope of the line should be unity. We see from Figure 4-11 that this seems to be true of neostigmine in both dogs and humans, within the limits of the experimental errors. Since all the points fall approximately on the same line, it follows that the neostigmine clearance is about the same in both species. The elimination rate constant is also the same if we assume the same manner of distribution into the body fluids. This k_e can be found by applying to Figure 4-11 the equation $x' = Q/k_e V_d$, then taking the values at the dotted lines $Q = $ antilog $(-10.5) = 3 \times 10^{-11}$ moles kg^{-1} min^{-1} and $x' = $ antilog $(-8.2) = 6.3 \times 10^{-9}$ moles L^{-1}, and assuming that neostigmine, a quaternary ammonium derivative, is confined to the extracellular fluid ($V_d = 0.20$ L kg^{-1}):

$$k_e = Q/x'V_d$$

$$= \frac{3 \times 10^{-11} \text{ mole kg}^{-1} \text{ min}^{-1}}{6 \times 10^{-9} \text{ moles L}^{-1} \times 0.20 \text{ L kg}^{-1}}$$

$$= 0.025 \text{ min}^{-1}$$

Thus, a little less than 3 percent is eliminated per minute, and

$$t_{1/2} = \frac{0.693}{0.025} = 28 \text{ min}$$

Dosage Regimens

The plateau principle also provides a fundamental basis for understanding the rationale of dosage schedules and of drug accumulation in the body. When we give a drug we are attempting to establish a certain therapeutic concentration in the body fluids or a certain total amount of drug in the body. This *effective drug concentration* (EDC) is a characteristic biologic property of the drug, over which we have no control. If the drug level is much below this EDC, the desired drug actions will not occur. If the level is much higher, toxic effects may well become manifest.

Although the EDC has been defined here as a concentration, the argument to follow would apply equally well if EDC were the total amount of drug in the body or the amount of drug fixed at some site of action, assuming of course that equilibration is quickly established between the site of action and the plasma.

Dosage schedules entail two variables: the magnitude of the single dose and the frequency with which that dose is repeated, usually expressed as a *dosing interval*. For any given dose, the extent to which the drug level in the body will fluctuate within a dosing interval is determined by several factors. For a given rate of elimination, the faster the absorption, the greater the fluctuation. With rapid absorption the bulk of the drug will enter the circulation rapidly, and the drug level will be high at first, then fall relatively fast, whereas with slower absorption, the buildup to a peak will be less rapid and the drug level more sustained, as seen with sustained-release medications. For a given rate of absorption, the fluctuation is obviously greater the more rapid the elimination. No generalization will reliably answer the question of just how much the drug level may be permitted to fluctuate above and below the desired level; this will depend entirely upon the particular drug. Detailed analysis of the kinetics of the establishment and decay of drug levels after single doses will be deferrred to a later section.

Here, we shall begin by ignoring the fluctuations. We assume, as a first approximation, that the absorption of a dose proceeds at a practically constant rate throughout each dosing interval and that it is complete at the end of the dosing interval. In other words, we suppose that the conditions are practically equivalent to those of a constant infusion. Our aim is to establish and maintain the EDC as a steady state. Obviously, if the individual dose were large enough and the dosing interval short enough, the EDC would be reached quickly, but the drug concentration would continue to increase. There must be some lower rate of drug input that would just establish but not exceed the desired EDC; this rate is defined as the *maintenance dose rate*.

A good illustration is found in the use of digitoxin to maintain cardiac compensation in a patient with congestive heart failure; the dose of about 0.1 mg daily, given day after day indefinitely, is the maintenance dose rate for this drug. What determines the maintenance dose rate of a drug, in general? The familiar equation for a constant infusion provides the answer:

$$Q = \text{maintenance dose rate} = k_e V_d (\text{EDC})$$

Since $(k_e V_d)$ is the total clearance, we may write

$$Q = (\text{total clearance})(\text{EDC})$$

The equations show that the maintenance dose rate will have to be higher the greater the clearance.

The time required to establish the EDC with any drug, under the conditions specified, is given by the plateau principle; the half-time will simply be the elimination half-time. Thus, a drug with short biologic half-life can come to the EDC quickly when the maintenance dose is administered from the start, but a drug that is eliminated slowly will necessarily achieve its EDC slowly. If k_e is known, then the whole time course of approach to the EDC is simply that predicted for an exponential process, as described previously.

Once it has been decided to administer a drug, rapid onset of the therapeutic effect is

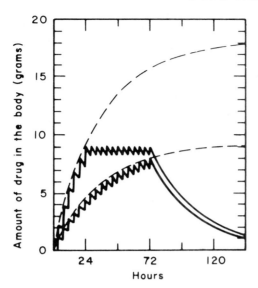

Fig. 4-12. Curves of accumulation with repeated dosage at constant intervals. Elimination constant $k_e = 0.0289$ hr^{-1}, elimination half-time = 24 hours, dosing interval = 4 hours. In lower curve, dose is 1 g; in upper curve, 2 g for the first six doses, then 1 g. Solid curves are computed from the given parameters; zigzag portions represent fluctuations during period of drug administration. Broken curves indicate course of continued accumulation if drug administration were continued. Drug stopped at 72 hours. Elimination curve is seen to be identical to accumulation curve, but inverted. (From Gaddum,[17] with permission.)

usually desired, certainly within a few hours. Yet this is impossible if the drug's half-life is longer than a few hours. The solution to the dosage problem for drugs that are eliminated slowly is to administer relatively large doses intially in order to establish the EDC quickly, and then to continue with the maintenance dose rate thereafter. The large initial doses are called *priming doses or loading doses.* Note especially that if the priming dose rate were continued, the EDC would be greatly exceeded, at the risk of serious toxicity. A theoretical illustration of this principle is shown in Figure 4-12. Here, the fluctuations due to the individual doses are shown also; clearly, the fluctuations can be minimized by subdividing the doses and administering them more frequently, the limit of such dose fragmentation being a constant infusion. In practice it is inconvenient to administer medication more often than once every few hours, and the desirability of uninterrupted sleep at night further demands that the dosing interval be as long as possible. A certain amount of fluctuation is therefore inevitable, and it will be more extreme the more rapidly the drug is eliminated.

Let us now undertake a rigorous theoretical treatment of repeated drug administration leading to attainment of the EDC.[17] Whereas our application of the plateau principle entailed the assumption that drug absorption is continuous, this approach takes into account the fluctuations resulting from drug elimination during the intervals between doses. It assumes, however, that each single dose is absorbed instantaneously. Let M_0 be the dose of a drug, X_0 the resulting drug level in the body (X_0/V_d would be the plasma concentration), and t^* the dosing interval. Now we give M_0, at $t = 0$, repeat after t^*, $2t^*$,

$3t^*, \ldots, nt^*$. At $t = 0$, just after the first dose, $X = X_0$. At $t = t^*$, just before the second dose

$$X = X_0 e^{-k_e t^*}$$

because of the exponential elimination of the drug during the interval t^*. To simplify the algebra, denote $e^{-k_e t^*}$ by the symbol p. Then just before the second dose, at $t = t^*$

$$X = X_0 p$$

and just after the instantaneous absorption of the second dose, still at $t = t^*$

$$X = X_0 + X_0 p = X_0(1 + p)$$

At $2t^*$, just before the third dose

$$X = X_0(1 + p)p$$

and just after the third dose

$$X = X_0 + X_0(1 + p)p = X_0(1 + p + p^2)$$

Just after the nth dose

$$X_n = X_0(1 + p + p^2 + \cdots + p^{n-1})$$

Solving the series, we obtain

$$X_n = X_0 \frac{(1 - p^n)}{(1 - p)}$$

and eventually, as $n \to \infty$, $p^n \to 0$, since $p < 1$

$$X_\infty = X_0/(1 - p).$$

Here X_∞ is the peak drug level established immediately after each dose at steady state. As shown in Figure 4-12, the "plateau" established in this model is a fluctuating one, but the peak levels do become constant when steady-state conditions have been attained. For attainment of a certain fraction of the eventual plateau

$$f = \frac{X_n}{X_\infty} = \frac{X_0(1 - p^n)}{(1 - p)} \cdot \frac{(1 - p)}{X_0} = (1 - p^n)$$

$$f = 1 - e^{-k_e t^* n}$$

Since t^*n, the dosing interval times the number of doses, is the same as the total time t, this equation is identical to Equation 2, derived previously in connection with the plateau principle.

Suppose we wish to compute how many doses will be required at a certain dosing interval to attain a given fraction of the eventual plateau drug level. Rewriting the equation to solve for n, we obtain

$$n = \frac{\ln(1 - f)}{-k_e t^*} = \frac{2.3 \log(1 - f)}{-k_e t^*}$$

As an example, suppose $k_e = 0.1 \text{ hr}^{-1}$, $t^* = 4$ hours, and we wish to calculate the number of doses needed to achieve 90 percent of the plateau. Then

$$n = \frac{2.3 \log(1 - 0.9)}{(-0.1)(4)} = 6 \text{ doses}$$

which requires 24 hours, or 3.5 times the half-time of 6.9 hours.

Suppose we wish to fix the level of drug in the body and maintain that level. Obviously there will be a direct relationship between the dosing interval and the maintenance dose required. Since the maintenance dose has to replace drug that was eliminated during the dosing interval, the longer the interval, the greater the required dose and the greater also the fluctuation. As shown above

$$X_\infty = \frac{X_0}{(1 - p)}$$

$$\frac{X_0}{X_\infty} = 1 - e^{-k_e t^*}$$

This expression gives the fraction of total drug in the body that has to be replaced in each dosing interval. Thus, immediately after the maintenance dose is given (assuming instantaneous absorption), the plateau level is restored. Just before the next dose, the fraction $(1 - e^{-k_e t^*})$ has been eliminated and must be replaced. This fraction therefore represents the maximum fluctuation below the plateau level. Evidently, the smaller the value of k_e and the shorter the dosing interval t^*, the smaller will be the fluctuation.

As an example, suppose we wish to establish and maintain a plasma level of 10 µg ml^{-1} with a drug whose volume of distribution is the extracellular fluid and whose elimination rate constant is 0.001 min^{-1}. If the dosing interval is to be 3 hours, what maintenance dose is required, how long will it take to attain 90 percent of the desired EDC, and what will be the maximum fluctuation below the EDC?

$$V_d = 12 \times 10^3 \text{ ml}$$

$$X_\infty = V_d(\text{EDC}) = 12 \times 10^3 \times 10 = 120 \text{ mg}$$

$$k_e = 0.001 \text{ min}^{-1}$$

$$t^* = 3 \times 60 = 180 \text{ min}$$

$$\frac{X_0}{X_\infty} = 1 - e^{(-0.001)(180)} = 1 - 0.835 = 0.165$$

$$X_0 = 20 \text{ mg}$$

The EDC will fluctuate 16.5 percent below its appropriate level, in other words, from 10 µg ml^{-1} to 8.4 µg ml^{-1} in each 3-hour interval.

The time required to attain 90 percent of the EDC if the maintenance dose is administered from the beginning is found readily from the number of doses needed at the fixed 3-hour interval:

$$n = \frac{2.3 \log(1 - 0.9)}{(-0.001)(180)} = \frac{-2.3}{-0.18} = 13 \text{ doses}$$

and the time required to administer these doses is 39 hours. This is an undesirably long time. Obviously, the preferable procedure would be to administer the total amount required in the body (120 mg) as a single priming dose or a series of closely spaced priming doses and then continue with the 20-mg maintenance dose.

The use of priming doses to overcome the otherwise slow buildup to the EDC with drugs that have long biologic half-lives is exemplified by the procedure known as *digitalization*. Digitoxin, one of the digitalis glycosides, is eliminated very slowly from the body, at a rate of approximately 10 percent per day; half-life is about 7 days. Then if the

Table 4-1. Distribution of Amiodarone and its Primary Metabolite Desethylamiodarone in Postmortem Tissues

Tissue	Amiodarone $(mg\ kg^{-1})$	Desethylamiodarone $(mg\ kg^{-1})$
Liver	496	2,400
Lung	197	945
Skeletal muscle	23	57
Fat	310	76
Serum	~2	~2

The greatest accumulations of drug and metabolite are in liver and lung. Fat selectively accumulates the parent compound.
(Data from Holt et al.[20])

daily maintenance dose were given from the start, the EDC would not nearly be achieved for weeks, an intolerable situation for a drug whose rapidity of action in congestive heart failure is potentially life-saving. Moreover, drugs of this class have a very narrow range between therapeutic and toxic levels, so that large fluctuations cannot be tolerated. Digitalization consists of giving priming doses until the electrocardiographic and clinical signs confirm that the EDC is just being reached and then continuing with the much smaller maintenance dose rate.

Another drug for which loading doses are very important is amiodarone.[18,19] This drug is effective against life-threatening cardiac arrhythmias that can not be controlled by other drugs. Amiodarone binds very extensively to tissues, especially liver, lung, fat, and muscle[20] (see Table 4-1). Because of tissue binding, the apparent volume of distribution is 1000 to 10,000 L. This enormous V_d, along with a relatively small clearance, results in an elimination half-time of 5 to 8 weeks. Obviously one cannot wait the 15 to 40 weeks required for plasma concentrations to approach steady-state levels in this life-threatening condition. In fact, in early studies of amiodarone, patients were often hospitalized for many weeks while the drug took effect. The use of loading doses has greatly improved this situation. In a controlled trial the time required for arrhythmia suppression was reduced from 18 days without loading doses to 10 days with oral loading doses.[19] Times as short as 1 or 2 days have been reported for the onset of arrhythmia suppression following intravenous loading doses.

Amiodarone has significant adverse effects, which are partly related to its tissue binding. First, the very long elimination half-life of the drug makes any adverse effects (as well as the therapeutic effect) quite prolonged. In the rare cases in which amiodarone causes the arrhythmia to become worse (as can happen with all antiarrhythmic drugs), management of this serious adverse effect is complicated by the long duration of drug action. A rare but potentially life-threatening side effect of amiodarone therapy is pulmonary fibrosis. The accumulation of amiodarone in lung tissue likely accounts for the unique effect of this drug on the lung. Finally, amiodarone has been found to reduce the elimination of many other drugs.[21] Effects of amiodarone on hepatic drug metabolism play a role in some of these drug interactions, and accumulation of amiodarone in the liver may contribute to the large number of drug interactions seen with this drug.

In situations in which life-threatening disorders are being treated with drugs that have potentially serious side effects, the rational application of pharmacokinetic principles becomes even more important to the safety and well-being of patients. Now let us specify more rigorously a rational dosage schedule that can be applicable to all drugs regardless of their rates of elimination. We begin by determining the *dosing interval t**. This is dependent upon the amount of fluctuation that is tolerable once the steady state has been established. For illustrative purposes let us limit the range of fluctuation to 10 percent of the EDC, a fairly narrow range. This means that t^* must be equal to the time in which one-tenth of the drug amount will be eliminated. From the equation $f = (1 - e^{-k_e t})$, when $f = 0.1$, $k_e t \cong 0.1$, $t^* \cong 0.1/k_e$. Also, since $t_{1/2} = 0.693/k_e$, it follows that t^* is almost exactly one-seventh of the elimination half-time, $0.1/0.693$. Now the maintenance dose rate is given by M/t^*, where M is the single dose, and thus

$$\frac{M}{t^*} = (EDC)V_d k_e$$

$$M = (EDC)V_d k_e t^* = (EDC)\frac{V_d}{10}$$

This means that if no priming dosage is employed but the maintenance dosage is used from the start, then the plateau level ultimately established will be 10 times that attained during the first dosing interval. For oral or parenteral sustained-release medication, the "single dose" will mean the amount of drug that is absorbed in the interval t^* even though the nominal dosing interval may be longer.

On this dosage schedule we may also estimate how many doses will be required to attain 90 percent of the EDC without priming dosage. For $f = 0.9$ we find $k_e t = 2.3$, $t = 2.3/k_e$. But, as shown above, $1/k_e = 10t^*$; therefore $t = 23t^*$, and 24 doses will be required. If priming dosage is to be used, then, of course, the priming doses have to furnish the total amount of drug needed in the body at the EDC [i.e., $(EDC)V_d$]. Therefore, in the present example the total drug given as priming doses will have to be 10 times the maintenance dose.

It is interesting to examine the customary dosage schedules for drugs in common use to see whether or not they conform to these rational principles, and if not, to consider why not. Clinical experience alone has served to shape a very suitable dosage schedule for the digitalis glycosides. Digoxin is the most widely used drug of this family. Here $k_e = 0.50$ day^{-1}, one-third of the amount present is eliminated each day, and $t_{1/2} = 1.4$ days. As shown above, if the fluctuation is to be held within 10 percent of the EDC, the rational dosing interval t^* will be $0.1/k_e$, which is equal to 5 hours. Also, as shown above, 24 doses (5 days) would be required to attain 90 percent of the EDC if priming dosage were not used. A typical procedure for rapid digitalization with digoxin in a normal 70-kg man employs 1.0 mg I.V. initially for priming, followed by a maintenance dose of 0.25 to 0.50 mg. In practice the priming dose is administered in several portions at 4 hour intervals with careful clinical evaluation of the patient's status before each administration. Also, the maintenance dose can be given as a single daily dose rather than a divided dose (i.e., greater fluctuation of the plasma level can be tolerated than the 10 percent assumed above).

Now let us consider a hypothetical drug that is eliminated primarily by glomerular filtration, without extensive tissue binding. If the drug is distributed in body water, $k_e = (0.13 \text{ L·min}^{-1})/42 \text{ L} = 0.0031 \text{ min}^{-1}$. Applying the same criteria as before, that fluctuation is to be held to 10 percent of the EDC, we find $t^* = 0.1/0.0031 = 32$ minutes. Now as a practical matter, such a drug would not be given parenterally every half hour, but more likely every 4 hours. Thus, as in the previous example, a far greater degree of fluctuation is tolerated for the sake of convenience, a dosing interval shorter than several hours for parenteral administration being regarded as impractical. This means either that larger fluctuations are tolerable because the EDC can safely be exceeded by a large amount, or that the EDC is simply not maintained continuously and some of the therapeutic effect is sacrificed. Such a drug could, however, be given orally or in a sustained-release form parenterally if the absorption could be smoothed out over several dosing intervals. Thus, the nominal dose interval might be 4 hours and the nominal dose would contain eight times as much medication as was required in each 30-minute dosing interval; then if the total administered dose were absorbed evenly over the whole 4 hours, the desired dose rate would be achieved.

There is a limit to the usefulness of periodic dosing. When k_e becomes much larger than 0.003 min^{-1} and $t_{1/2}$ is less than 4 hours (e.g., when the drug is rapidly metabolized), then no dosing interval is practical, and the method of constant infusion must be adopted. A good example is the administration of the polypeptide hormone oxytocin to induce labor at term; this drug is destroyed by a peptidase in the blood. Another example is succinylcholine, a neuromuscular blocking agent used in anesthesia. This drug is hydrolyzed rapidly by plasma and liver cholinesterases. Its elimination rate in vivo can be estimated from the increment in duration of effect that is produced by logarithmic dose increments. Thus, for example, in a large number of patients[22] an intravenous dose of 1,000 mg caused apnea by paralyzing the muscles of respiration for 17.8 minutes on the average. A dose of 500 mg caused apnea for only 11.9 minutes. The difference, 5.9 min, represents the time required for 1,000 mg to be decreased by metabolism to only 500 mg (i.e., it is the biologic half-life). Then $k_e = 0.12$ min^{-1}, a much faster rate of elimination than even renal secretory mechanisms could accomplish. Drugs are metabolized at widely varying rates, some even faster than succinylcholine. In all such cases the EDC will be established very soon after starting a constant infusion and can be maintained readily, and the drug effect will disappear within minutes after discontinuing the infusion. Complete elimination of fluctuation and excellent control are the two important advantages gained by the constant infusion of drugs with high k_e values.

Drug Accumulation and Toxicity

The plateau principle also explains why cumulative toxicity sometimes occurs. If a drug's elimination rate is slow and one attempts nevertheless to achieve a therapeutic effect with a constant dosage schedule (i.e., without priming doses), toxicity is the likely outcome. The reason for this is that if one seeks to obtain the therapeutic action quickly and the dose rate is chosen to give that result, then the eventual steady state will greatly exceed the EDC. How can we determine how much additional accumulation of a drug will occur? The fractional approach to steady state $f = (1 - e^{-k_e t})$ is useful in answering this question. Obviously if one-tenth of the steady-state value has been achieved (i.e., $f = 0.1$), then the final steady-state value will be $1/f$, or 10 times as high.

To illustrate, suppose a drug with a half-life of 5 days is given at a dose rate that gives one-half the EDC in 16 hours (0.67 days). Then $kt_1 = (0.693/5)(0.67) = 0.0929$, and $f = 0.09$. Therefore the level reached at this dose rate in 16 hours is only 0.09 of the eventual plateau, which will be 0.5·EDC/0.09, or six times the EDC. The half-time of cumulation to this probably toxic level will, of course, be 5 days.

A very good example of cumulative toxicity with repeated drug administration is seen with bromide ion in humans. Bromide used to be relied upon heavily in the chronic treatment of epilepsy, and it was also used as a mild sedative. It is still found in sedative preparations sold over the counter to the general public. The EDC for this drug is about

12 mEq L^{-1}. Psychotic symptoms and neurologic signs occur at concentrations above 20 mEq L^{-1}. The bromide ion is distributed in approximately the same volume as the chloride ion, a volume somewhat greater than that of the extracellular fluid, or about 15 L in the average man. It is handled at the kidneys in much the same way as chloride— filtered at the glomeruli and largely reabsorbed in the tubules. Bromide is actually reabsorbed somewhat more efficiently than chloride; the chloride clearance is about 1.2 L daily, the bromide clearance about 0.9 L daily.[23] From the clearance and the volume of distribution we find k_e = 0.9/15 = 0.06 day^{-1}; thus, half-life = 0.693/0.06 = 12 days. An experimental investigation using radioactive ^{82}Br in 10 human subjects and measuring plasma levels twice daily gave exactly this theoretical value for the half-life.[24]

Two conclusions may be drawn from k_e and the half-life. The half-time for achieving the steady state on a constant daily dosage of bromide will be 12 days, and the steady-state level will be about 1/0.06 (or about 16) times the level established on the first day. To use the drug properly, one would compute the maintenance dosage as follows:

$$EDC = 12 \text{ mEq } L^{-1}$$

$$V_d = 15 \text{ L}$$

$$k_e = 0.693/t_{1/2} = 0.058 \text{ day}^{-1}$$

$$Clearance = k_e V_d = 0.87 \text{ L/day}$$

The maintenance dosage is designated by Q, and

$$Q = k_e V_d(EDC)$$

$$Q = 0.87 \times 12 = 10 \text{ mEq day}^{-1} \text{ or about 0.8 g day}^{-1}$$

This dose could be given daily for an indefinite period without harm, but it will require 12 days to attain half the EDC, and 40 days (3.3 times the half-time) to achieve 90 percent of the EDC. Alternatively, the required 180 mEq (15 g) could be given within the first few days as a priming dose to establish the EDC, followed by the maintenance dosage thereafter. The reason why toxicity develops so frequently and so insidiously with this drug is that dosage sufficient to produce any sedation at all within a day or two must necessarily be higher than the maintenance dose rate, and so it will inevitably, if continued, produce plasma bromide levels much higher than the EDC.

The bromide half-life can be shortened to 3 or 4 days by chloride administration at about 200 mEq day^{-1} in excess of normal intake. The reason for this is simply that chloride and bromide are treated very much alike at the renal tubules. Increasing the chloride level in the plasma and glomerular filtrate leads to a diminution in the fraction of chloride plus bromide that is reabsorbed and thus to an increased bromide clearance.

For the same reasons cumulative toxicity may develop insidiously with various substances that are not employed therapeutically but to which people may be exposed chronically. Often such poisons are bound tightly at specialized sites in the body. This accumulation in vulnerable tissues causes toxic manifestations, and the low elimination rate associated with extensive binding is responsible for the slow time course of the accumulation. Poisoning by heavy metals follows this pattern. Lead, for example, is present in the urban environment as a result of the combustion of leaded gasoline, and city dwellers breathe it constantly. Because lead is stored in many tissues and deposited in bones, it has a very long half-life in the body. When a human subject was given 2 mg day^{-1} of a soluble lead salt, the blood concentration of lead increased from 0.29 μg ml^{-1} to 0.72 μg ml^{-1} with a half-time of about 2 months.[25] The blood level then remained fairly constant for 2 years, during which the daily intake was maintained. Despite the steady state in the blood and body fluids, a continuous accumulation went on during the whole period of the experiment, as indicated by a persistent small discrepancy between daily intake and daily output (positive lead balance). When the daily dose was discontinued after 2 years, the blood level fell, with a half-time of 2 months, but an elevated urine output persisted for much longer. Clearly we are dealing here with complex kinetics. Tissue binding and deposition in bone continue after the fluid compartments are at a steady state, and loss of lead from its sites of very tight binding or deposition continues after the body fluids have nearly eliminated their lead. The symptoms of lead poisoning are, initially at least, rather vague; irritability and other mood changes predominate in the early stages, frank psychosis and encephalopathy later. The long biologic half-life results in so slow a buildup of toxic levels in the body that no connection may seem evident between the beginning of exposure to a chronically noxious environment and the development and progression of the symptoms of lead poisoning.

Hazards of cumulative toxicity involving a combination of radioactivity and long biologic half-life are presented by the fallout of debris from nuclear explosions. For example, ^{90}Sr is handled like calcium by the body: it is deposited in bone, and only a minute fraction of the total is excreted daily. Therefore, with constant exposure there is a slow buildup of the body burden. Once the element is stored in the bones, its radioactive decay subjects the erythroblastic tissues and the bone cells to continuous bombardment. The accident that occurred with the nuclear reactor at Chernobyl in the Ukraine resulted in the release of substantial quantities of radionuclides, including ^{131}I and ^{134}Cs, into the atmosphere. The ^{131}I was detected in vegetables and also in milk from cows that grazed on pasture in regions of Europe lying downwind that had received rain in the few days after the accident. ^{131}I is concentrated in the thyroid gland by an active transport mechanism and is there incorporated into thyroid hormone. The uptake and incorporation are responsible for the long biologic half-life of iodine, and again the combination of radioactivity, accumulation, and tissue storage intensifies the risk of serious toxicity. For these reasons the potential hazard in the use of ^{131}I for the diagnosis and treatment of thyroid disease is still a matter of controversy among clinicians. Extreme hazards, for similar reasons, are presented by ^{14}C and ^{3}H in chemical forms that permit their incorporation into nucleic acids. A molecule of DNA containing ^{14}C atoms may persist without turnover throughout a person's life, while the radioactivity of this isotope barely diminishes in a human lifetime. If the DNA in question is contained in the germinal cells, mutations resulting from the radioactive disintegrations will present a threat to that person's progeny. Radioactive carbon or tritium present in drugs, intermediate metabolites, or even proteins is far less hazardous because of the relatively short biologic half-lives of these substances as compared with that of DNA.

Slow accumulation of drugs and poisons is also seen in the fat depots of the body. The lipid-soluble insecticide DDT has been found regularly in human fat at autopsy, even in persons who had no known direct contact with it. This is typical of the environmental contamination that affects everyone in cases in which continuous exposure can cause slow accumulation over a period of years. Likewise, estrogenic compounds used to promote weight gain in beef cattle have been found in human fat depots at autopsy.

Kinetics of Changes in Enzyme Levels

The enzyme content of an animal tissue is maintained at its normal level by equal rates of enzyme synthesis and enzyme degradation. A drug may increase this steady-state amount of enzyme by speeding its production or by slowing its breakdown. Continuous

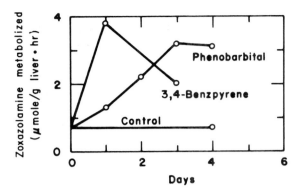

Fig. 4-13. Stimulation of zoxazolamine metabolism by benzpyrene and phenobarbital. Weanling rats were injected once with 3,4-benzpyrene (25 mg kg^{-1}) or with phenobarbital (38 mg kg^{-1}) twice daily for the duration of the experiment. Zoxazolamine metabolism by liver was determined in vitro at the times shown. (From Conney et al.[28] with permission.)

protein synthesis is essential for both these mechanisms. Therefore, if an enzyme "induction" is abolished by blocking protein synthesis, it cannot be concluded that increased synthesis rather than stabilization was responsible (although activation of existing enzyme can be ruled out as the mechanism of drug action). The apparent induction of tryptophan pyrrolase by its substrate, for example, is prevented by puromycin, ethionine, and other inhibitors of protein synthesis, but it is now clear that tryptophan stabilizes the enzyme rather than increasing its rate of synthesis.[26]

The time course of a shift from one steady-state level of enzyme to another is given by the plateau principle; its half-time is simply the turnover half-time (half-life) of the enzyme. Consequently, if an enzyme is to respond quickly to regulatory influences, it must be degraded rapidly. The more rapidly degraded it is, the more rapidly can its level change in response to changes in either the synthesis rate or the degradation rate.[27]

Much confusion has resulted from failure to recognize this application of the plateau principle. Consider enzymes A and B, both subject to regulation by steroid hormones. Enzyme A is rapidly degraded, B is quite stable. Suppose that both rates of synthesis are increased fivefold by hormone treatment. Then both enzyme activities will also have increased fivefold when the new steady state is reached, since

$$X' = \frac{k_{in}}{k_{out}}$$

and we have increased k_{in} by a factor of 5 in both cases. But the rates of increase in enzyme activity will be very different for A and for B. One day after hormone administration is begun, A may already have increased nearly fivefold whereas B may have changed but little. If the enzyme determinations are performed at this time, therefore, the false conclusion may be drawn that steroid hormones have a much greater effect upon the synthesis of A than upon the synthesis of B. One should always refrain from drawing negative conclusions unless sufficient data are available to be certain that the shift from one steady state to another has been completed.

If a drug that causes an increase or decrease in the steady-state level of an enzyme is given as a single injection, interpretation is usually impossible, because there is no way to assess whether or not new steady states have been reached. Figure 4-13 presents an illustrative example. The capacity of rat liver to metabolize zoxazolamine was followed after injections of 3,4-benzpyrene or phenobarbital. The rats that received benzpyrene had a single injection, but those that were given phenobarbital had two injections daily for the duration of the experiment. Evidently, the enzyme activity was stimulated by phenobarbital to about a fourfold increase over the starting level, and a new plateau was reached. The half-time of this shift was about 40 hours, whence it may be concluded that in the presence of phenobarbital the half-time of enzyme degradation was 40 hours. There is no way to decide, from these data alone, whether phenobarbital increases the rate of enzyme synthesis or decreases the rate of enzyme degradation. One might also be tempted to conclude that benzpyrene stimulates the increase in enzyme activity faster than phenobarbital does, but that would not be justified on the basis of the limited data shown. Continuous administration of benzpyrene might have increased the activity to a much higher level, so the shift half-time could well be identical to that produced by phenobarbital. Interpretation of these data in terms of a simple kinetic model is also complicated by the fact that the P450 proteins involved in this metabolism are a family of enzymes each member of which presumably has a different rate of turnover (see Ch. 5 and Ch. 6).

The plateau principle can be used as a practical test to distinguish between increased enzyme synthesis and decreased enzyme breakdown as mechanisms underlying a drug-induced increase in enzyme level, assuming that enzyme activation has been ruled out. The following preconditions must be established: The inducing drug must become fully effective quickly and must remain present continuously until the new steady-state enzyme level is clearly established, and the inducing action must cease quickly when drug administration is discontinued. Then the half-time of the initial shift is the degradation half-time of the enzyme in the presence of the drug. The half-time of return to the original steady state after the drug is withdrawn is the degradation half-time of the enzyme in the absence of drug. If these two time courses are the same, the drug did not stabilize the enzyme but must have acted by increasing the rate of enzyme synthesis. If the rise is slower than the fall, the drug must have acted, at least in part, by stabilizing the enzyme. The quantitative contributions of the two mechanisms may be estimated from the relationship between the initial and elevated enzyme levels, E'_1 and E'_2, respectively, as follows:

$$\frac{E'_2}{E'_1} = \frac{Q_2}{Q_1} \cdot \frac{k_1}{k_2}$$

where Q_1 and Q_2 are the respective rates of enzyme synthesis (analogous to k_{in} in Eq. 1), and k_1 and k_2 are the degradation rate constants in the absence and presence of the drug, respectively.

The plateau principle has been applied in the manner described above to the problem of analyzing the mechanism whereby continuous administration of phenobarbital increases the amount of liver microsomal barbiturate-oxidizing enzyme.[29] Phenobarbital was administered daily to rats in dosage sufficient to produce a maximal and sustained shift of the enzyme level. Then the drug was withdrawn, and the enzyme was permitted to return to the original level. The half-time of the shift up was 2.2 days, that of the shift down was 2.6 days. Thus, the enzyme turnover was essentially unaffected by the drug; the main cause of the increase in enzyme level was therefore increased rate of synthesis.

MIXED FIRST- AND ZERO-ORDER ELIMINATION: SATURABLE CLEARANCE MECHANISMS

Since many processes contributing to drug elimination involve enzymes or transport mechanisms, it is actually surprising how many drugs follow first-order kinetics. As described previously, one explanation of this paradox may be that under conditions of low drug concentrations these saturable processes behave as if they were first-order. There are, however, several important examples of drugs that do follow concentration-dependent "Michaelis-Menten" kinetics of elimination. We will now see how certain aspects of the plateau principle can be applied to these drugs.

The rate of drug elimination v for a simple saturable process is

$$v = \frac{V_{\max} \cdot x}{K_{\mathrm{m}} + x}$$

where x is the plasma drug concentration, $V_{\max}$ is the maximal rate of elimination, and K_{m} is the drug concentration at which half the maximal elimination is achieved. If we look at our simple system for input and output, assuming a constant input and saturable elimination

$$\xrightarrow{Q} X \xrightarrow{v}$$

a steady state will result whenever the rate of input Q is less than $V_{\max}$. If Q is greater than $V_{\max}$, the amount X of drug in the body, will increase without bound, and toxicity and death will ensue.

It is easy to determine the steady-state plasma concentration x' that will result for any given input rate because at steady state

$$Q = \frac{V_{\max} \cdot x'}{K_{\mathrm{m}} + x'}$$

and rearranging

$$x' = K_{\mathrm{m}} \cdot \frac{Q}{(V_{\max} - Q)}$$

When Q equals one-half of $V_{\max}$, x' equals K_{m}. As Q increases toward $V_{\max}$, the denominator ($V_{\max} - Q$) approaches zero, and x' increases dramatically. It is convenient to think of a plot of steady-state plasma concentration versus dose rate as a rectangular hyperbola plotted against the y axis rather than against the x axis as is usual in enzyme kinetics.

One of the best examples of saturable clearance is the anticonvulsant phenytoin. Several studies of plasma concentration versus dose rate have shown precisely the type of behavior expected for a drug following saturable elimination kinetics (Fig. 4-14). The K_{m} and $V_{\max}$ values have been determined for large numbers of patients. The wide range of dose rates required to achieve the EDC in different patients is due to substantial interindividual differences in $V_{\max}$ and K_{m}. Since the typical K_{m} for phenytoin is 5 to 8 mg L^{-1}, which is below the EDC, the function relating drug concentration and dose rate is quite steep, and the range of dose rates producing acceptable plasma concentrations is quite narrow. For example, in one patient represented in Figure 4-14, dose rates between 225 and 275 mg day^{-1} were required to maintain the plasma concentration between 10 and 20 mg L^{-1}. For a drug cleared by first-order elimination, a twofold change in dose rates (e.g., 225 to 450 mg day^{-1}) would be needed to double the plasma concentration. Thus drugs with saturable clearance mechanisms must be titrated very carefully when the plasma concentration is above the K_{m}.

What generalizations can be made about the time course of approach to steady state for drugs with saturable clearance mechanisms? The differential equation describing the total body elimination of the drug is

$$\frac{dX}{dt} = -\frac{V_{\max} \cdot x}{K_{\mathrm{m}} + x}$$

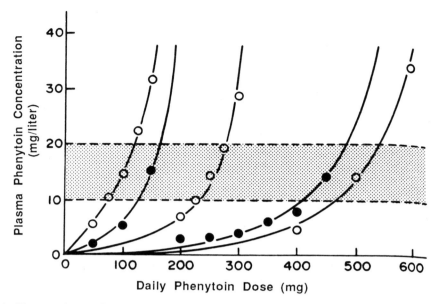

Fig. 4-14. Plasma phenytoin concentration as a function of dose rate. Phenytoin was administered to five patients at the indicated dose rate until steady-state plasma concentrations were achieved. The lines represent the predicted values based on Michaelis-Menten parameters estimated for each patient. The shaded area indicates the usual therapeutic concentration range for phenytoin of 10 to 20 mg L^{-1}. (Adapted from Richens et al.[30] with permission.)

To express the equation in terms of plasma drug concentration x we can divide by V_d to get

$$\frac{dx}{dt} = -\frac{(V_{max}/V_d) \cdot x}{K_m + x}$$

When x is much less than K_m, the equation reduces to

$$\frac{dx}{dt} = -\frac{V_{max}}{K_m \cdot V_d} \cdot x$$

which is the equation for a first-order process, as discussed previously. The k_e can be seen by inspection to be $V_{max}/(K_m V_d)$. Let us apply this result to our example, phenytoin. Average values for the parameters are $K_m = 5.7$ mg L^{-1}, $V_{max} = 7.5$ mg kg^{-1} day^{-1}, and $V_d = 0.65$ L kg^{-1}. Thus

$$k_e = \frac{7.5}{5.7 \times 0.65} = 2.0 \text{ day}^{-1}$$

$$t_{1/2} = \frac{0.693}{2.0} = 0.34 \text{ day or } 8.2 \text{ hours}$$

The K_m and V_{max} values were estimated for phenytoin elimination in a group of 12 patients.[31] Calculations using those data of the $t_{1/2}$ for the low concentration limit ranged from 1.7 to 22 hours. Thus there is considerable variability in phenytoin handling by different patients.

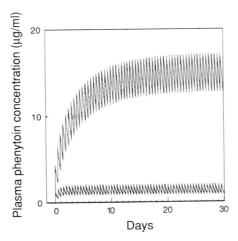

Fig. 4-15. Computer simulation of time course of phenytoin accumulation. Michaelis-Menten parameters are $V_{max} = 525$ mg day^{-1}, $K_m = 5.7$ mg L,$^{-1}$ $V_d = 45.5$ L. In the lower curve, dosage is 50 mg every 12 hours and in the upper curve 200 mg every 12 hours. (Data from Neubig.[32])

How can we apply these $t_{1/2}$ values to normal therapeutic situations when the EDC for phenytoin is 10 to 20 mg L^{-1}, which is greater than the K_m? The $t_{1/2}$ value at low concentrations, as seen for the example of aspirin, will represent a minimum time for elimination of half of the drug. Since the fractional rate of change of drug concentration in the body [i.e., $V_{max}/V_d(K_m + x)$] continuously decreases as x increases, the fractional rate of approach to equilibrium also decreases. Figure 4-15 shows a computer simulation of phenytoin accumulation using the population average K_m and V_{max}. For a 70-kg person the maximal elimination rate is 7.5 mg kg^{-1} day^{-1} × 70 kg, which equals 525 mg day^{-1}. At a low dose rate of 100 mg day^{-1}, the steady-state plasma drug concentration is 1.3 mg L^{-1}, and the accumulation is nearly first-order, reaching 90 percent of steady state in about 24 hours as predicted from the $t_{1/2}$ of 8 hours for low drug concentrations. For a higher dose rate of 400 mg day^{-1}, the peak steady-state plasma concentration is near the predicted value of 18 mg L^{-1} but nearly 10 days are required to reach 90 percent of the steady-state value. Note that a fourfold change in dose rate increased steady-state plasma concentrations 14-fold. For drugs with saturable clearance, the time to reach steady-state increases with the dose, while the plateau principle shows that first-order drugs have the same half-time regardless of dose. As the dose rate approaches the V_{max}, extremely long equilibration times are seen, making dosage adjustment difficult. An understanding of the complex kinetics of drugs such as phenytoin is essential to their safe and effective clinical use.

FIRST-ORDER ABSORPTION, FIRST-ORDER ELIMINATION: KINETICS OF DRUG LEVELS AFTER SINGLE DOSES

We have examined the kinetics of elimination after a drug is introduced intravenously and the time course of attaining a plateau when a drug is administered at a constant rate. We considered the constant rate to be achieved either rigorously, by a constant infusion, or approximately, by the repetition of a dose at regular intervals. In the latter case we assumed that relative to the whole time course under consideration no serious error would be introduced by ignoring fluctuations due to rapid absorption just after drug administration and progressively slower absorption between doses. Now we shall examine the detailed kinetics of the rise and fall of drug plasma levels after single doses. As is usually found to be the case, we assume the absorption process to be first-order, and we again assume overall elimination to be first-order.

Let M_0 be the dose of a drug (i.e., the amount of drug placed at the site of administration at time zero), and let k_a be the rate constant of absorption. Then at any time t thereafter, the drug remaining at the site of administration is:

$$M = M_0 e^{-k_a t}$$

Now let X be the amount of drug that is present in the body and let k_e be the rate constant of elimination; then

$$\frac{dX}{dt} = k_a M - k_e X$$

and, substituting for M

$$\frac{dX}{dt} + k_e X = k_a M_0 e^{-k_a t}$$

This linear first-order differential equation yields the following solution for the case $k_a \neq k_e$, as first shown many years ago in a classical theoretical study of this problem.[33]

$$X = \frac{k_a M_0}{(k_e - k_a)} [e^{-k_a t} - e^{-k_e t}]$$

And for the case $k_a = k_e$, the following equation is obtained:

$$X = k_e M_0 t e^{-k_e t}$$

and for the purpose of graphing, as in Figure 4-16

$$\frac{X}{M_0} = \frac{1}{(k_e/k_a) - 1} [e^{-k_e t/(k_e/k_a)} - e^{-k_e t}]$$

Figure 4-16 presents a generalized plot of these equations. Certain normalizing procedures have been followed in order to make a single graph represent all possible relationships between dose administered, rate constant of absorption, and rate constant of elimination. The vertical scale shows X/M_0 rather than X (i.e., regardless of what the actual dose may be, we are following the fractional absorption of that dose into the body tissues from the site of administration). The above equations, showing that the time course of absorption is independent of the dose M_0, justify this procedure. The equations have been solved for various chosen values of the ratio of rate constants k_e/k_a, and the time scale has consequently been generalized to include one of the rate constants.

For any given drug the transformed scale of time, although not reading directly in minutes, is nevertheless proportional to actual time. Some important conclusions about the kinetics of drug levels in the body may be drawn from inspection of this diagram. The curve for $k_a = \infty$ depicts the limiting case of intravenous injection, "absorption" being instantaneous. This shows the usual exponential decay of the drug level. As absorption becomes slower (k_a smaller) relative to elimination, curves are obtained that rise to a peak and then fall again. The slower the absorption relative to elimination, the later is the peak attained and the lower is its actual value.

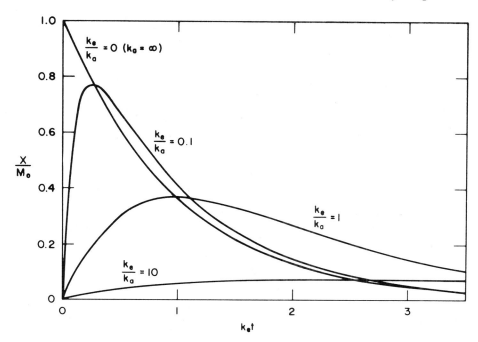

Fig. 4-16. Kinetics of first-order absorption and first-order elimination. This graph shows the amount of drug in the body (X) as fraction of total drug (M_0) placed at an absorption site at time zero. The family of curves is for different ratios of the rate constant of elimination (k_e) to the rate constant of absorption (k_a). The scale on the x axis includes k_e; to convert its values to actual time t, divide by k_e. See text for complete description.

In order to transform the time scale to real time, it is only necessary to divide the values by the elimination rate constant k_e. An example will serve to illustrate how Figure 4-16 can be used to predict real behavior of drugs. Suppose a drug is absorbed from a subcutaneous depot at a rate of 0.1 min^{-1} and eliminated by excretion and metabolism at a rate of 0.01 min^{-1}. Then $k_e/k_a = 0.1$, and every value on the $k_e t$ scale has to be divided by 0.01 (so that the scale will read 100, 200, 300 minutes, etc.). We see that the peak circulating drug level will be attained in about 25 minutes, and at that time about 75 percent of the dose will be distributed into whatever its V_d may be.

Differentiation of the equations yields expressions for the time at which the maximum drug level is attained. For $k_a \neq k_e$,

$$t_{max} = \frac{2.30}{k_a - k_e} \log \frac{k_a}{k_e}$$

and for $k_a = k_e$,

$$t_{max} = \frac{1}{k_e}$$

These equations show that the time in which the maximum drug level is achieved is the same regardless of what dose is administered. Substitution of the values of t_{max} into the original equations yield solutions for the maximum amount of drug in the body. For $k_a \neq k_e$, the peak level is given by

$$\frac{X_{max}}{M_0} = \left[\frac{k_a}{k_e}\right]^{k_e/(k_e - k_a)}$$

and for $k_a = k_e$

$$\frac{X_{max}}{M_0} = e^{-1} = 0.368$$

(i.e., when the rate constants for absorption and elimination are equal, the peak level in the body is 37 percent of the dose).

In this analysis we have assumed that all the drug is eventually absorbed into the body, regardless of how slowly absorption takes place. In reality if a drug is absorbed very slowly (e.g., $k_a = 0.0005$, $t_{1/2} \approx 24$ hours) then some of the drug may pass through the small intestine without being absorbed. Consequently the total amount of drug reaching the bloodstream will not be M_0 but will be some fraction thereof (e.g., $F \times M_0$). The fraction F reaching the bloodstream is called the *bioavailability* of the drug. In addition to slow absorption, metabolism of a drug during the "first pass" through the hepatic portal system (cf Ch. 3) can reduce the amount of active drug reaching the systemic circulation, thus reducing the bioavailability. An interesting property of the equations just derived provides a common method for determining the bioavailability of an orally administered drug. The same property has a bearing on the total exposure of the body to drug.

Let us consider the plasma drug concentration after administration of a drug governed by first-order absorption and first-order elimination kinetics. Since the drug will be distributed in a volume V_d, the plasma concentration at any given time will be

$$x = \frac{X}{V_d}$$

Let us first evaluate the specific case in which the drug is absorbed completely and instantaneously, as in an intravenous injection. The initial plasma concentration will be $x_0 = M_0/V_d$, and the time course will be

$$x = \frac{M_0}{V_d} e^{-k_e t}$$

What is the total exposure of the body to the drug? One measure of this is the integral of the plasma concentration versus time curve, or the *area under the curve* (AUC) of a plot of plasma concentration versus time. This is simply determined by integration

$$AUC = \int_0^\infty \frac{M_0}{V_d} e^{-k_e t} dt$$

$$= -\frac{M_0}{V_d k_e} (e^{-k_e t}) \Big|_0^\infty$$

$$= -\frac{M_0}{V_d k_e} (0 - 1)$$

$$= \frac{M_0}{V_d k_e}$$

What happens if absorption is not instantaneous but is complete and governed by the first order rate constant k_a as above?

$$x = \frac{X}{V_d}$$

$$= \frac{k_a M_0}{(k_e - k_a) \cdot V_d} [e^{-k_a t} - e^{-k_e t}]$$

Integrating once again

$$AUC = \int_0^\infty \frac{k_a M_0}{(k_e - k_a) V_d} (e^{-k_a t} - e^{-k_e t}) dt$$

$$= \frac{k_a}{(k_e - k_a)} \cdot \frac{M_0}{V_d} \left(\int_0^\infty e^{-k_a t} dt - \int_0^\infty e^{-k_e t} dt \right)$$

$$= \frac{k_a}{(k_e - k_a)} \cdot \frac{M_0}{V_d} \left[-\frac{1}{k_a} (e^{-k_a t}) + \frac{1}{k_e} (e^{-k_e t}) \right] \Big|_0^\infty$$

$$= \frac{k_a}{(k_e - k_a)} \cdot \frac{M_0}{V_d} \left(\frac{1}{k_a} - \frac{1}{k_e} \right)$$

$$= \frac{k_a}{(k_e - k_a)} \cdot \frac{M_0}{V_d} \frac{k_e - k_a}{k_e \cdot k_a}$$

$$= \frac{M_0}{V_d k_e}$$

Thus delayed absorption lowers the peak plasma drug concentration reached, but the integrated exposure of the body to drug (i.e., the AUC) is the same as for instantaneous absorption. If the body's response is directly proportional to the drug concentration, the cumulative effect of drug would not depend on the rate of absorption but would be inversely related to the rate of excretion. Unfortunately, as we will see in the next section, such linear responses to drugs do not commonly occur, so we must look at the overall plasma concentration versus time curve to predict cumulative responses.

The AUC, however, has been used extensively to study the bioavailability of orally administered drugs. This is done most commonly by comparing the AUC for an intravenous injection of the drug with that for oral administration. If drug is absorbed exponentially but only a fraction F reaches the bloodstream intact, then $AUC_{oral} = F \cdot M_0/V_d k_e$. Then the bioavailability is determined from

$$F = \frac{AUC_{oral}}{AUC_{IV}}$$

Wagner[2] has discussed the determination of oral drug bioavailability in detail.

These basic equations, transformed in various ways, are routinely used to develop rational approaches to dosage regimens or to examine how closely observation and theory conform in experimental animals or humans.[2,34] An illustration of unusual interest concerns the precursor-product relationship for drugs that are metabolized. If a precursor W is transformed metabolically to a product X, which in turn is further transformed or excreted, then we have

$$W \to X \to elimination$$

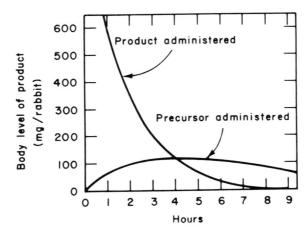

Fig. 4-17. Kinetics of precursor-product relationship in drug metabolism. Theoretical diagram of the body level of a product, *p*-methoxyphenol, in the rabbit, when its precursor, anisole, is administered, and when it is administered itself in equimolar amount. For the *O*-methylation, $k = 0.11$ hr^{-1}. Subsequent conjugation with sulfate proceeds with $k = 0.54$ hr^{-1}. (From Bray et al.,[35] with permission.)

with a rate constant $k_{w \rightarrow x}$ for the first-order transformation reaction, and a rate constant k_e for the first-order elimination of X. Then the kinetics of the rise and fall of X are formally identical to those of sequential first-order absorption and first-order elimination. The same equations apply, and the same characteristic family of curves will be found as in Figure 4-16. This is illustrated in Figure 4-17 for anisole (methoxybenzene) transformed to its hydroxylation product *p*-methoxyphenol in the rabbit. It can be seen that administration of the precursor will have the same effect as though the product itself had been given by a slow-absorption technique. The curve labeled "Precursor administered" is determined by the relative rate constants, 0.11 hr^{-1} for the hydroxylation and 0.54 hr^{-1} for the elimination (here actually a sulfate conjugation). The curve is simply that predicted by Figure 4-16 for $k_e/k_a = 5$, and time in hours is $k_e t/0.54$.

Ideally, every drug should be given in such a way as to establish its EDC very rapidly and then maintain it with as little fluctuation as possible. Rapid establishment of the EDC, as we have seen, requires priming dosage if the rate constant of elimination is low. Practically speaking, if the drug level rises quickly and falls quickly, fluctuation can only be smoothed by repeating the dose very frequently, and this may be considered too inconvenient. Patients do not welcome parenteral administration more often than every few hours, and even oral medication is unlikely to be taken reliably more often than that, especially by ambulatory patients. Thus, if a considerable "overshoot" above the EDC is tolerable, fluctuations may be preferred to an inconvenient dose schedule. To what extent it may be safe to exceed the EDC periodically cannot be stated as a general rule; this will depend upon the range between EDC and toxic levels for each particular drug. It is absurd, therefore, to administer all drugs on arbitrary fixed schedules (e.g., with each meal, every 4 hours). Appropriate dosage schedules need to be developed for each drug determined on the basis of its k_a, its k_e, its EDC, and the level at which its toxic effects manifest themselves. If it is important to obtain a drug's maximum benefit, then it may also be important to override considerations of convenience and to administer doses as often as necessary to maintain an effective drug level and at the same time minimize fluctuations.

PHARMACODYNAMICS: ROLE OF DRUG DISTRIBUTION AND TISSUE RESPONSIVENESS

We have referred to the duration of effective therapeutic concentration of a drug in plasma as though it were identical to duration of action. Often it is, but there are many factors that can modify the relation between plasma drug concentrations and responses. First, there may not be rapid equilibration of drug in plasma with the target tissue. Second, the time course of tissue response may not precisely follow the time course of drug concentration even at the site of action. There are instances in which a drug's therapeutic action may far outlast its presence in the body fluids. Also a drug's action may be briefer than its presence in blood. Certain bactericidal drugs kill pathogenic organisms rapidly and then need not be present at all for a certain interval during which the pathogens are unable to recover. Alkylating agents usually produce their irreversible chemical effects very quickly, and they may also be quickly destroyed, so that they are not present at all during the subsequent period when the biologic effects develop. Organic phosphate cholinesterase inhibitors are degraded rapidly, but the consequences of their irreversible alkylation of the enzyme persist until new enzyme is synthesized. Barbiturates and other centrally acting agents may produce typical actions at a certain threshold concentration, but recovery from these actions may occur at a different concentration; thus, the duration of drug action and the time during which drug concentrations exceed the original threshold may not be the same.

Drug Concentrations in Plasma and Tissue: Multicompartment Kinetics

The distribution of drugs within the body does not occur instantaneously. Following intravenous injection of a strongly tasting compound such as saccharin into the antecubital vein in the arm, a delay of approximately 9 to 10 seconds occurs before the subject tastes the saccharin. This delay represents the time required for blood to circulate from the arm vein through the right side of the heart, the lungs, and the left side of the heart and out to the arterial supply of the tongue. Given a typical cardiac output of 5 L min^{-1} and a typical blood volume of approximately 6 L, a drug would be expected to distribute evenly in blood and well perfused tissues in a few minutes. Thus, although equilibration of a drug with blood can take a measurable amount of time, in practice it does not significantly delay the onset of drug action.

The movement of a drug from blood to other tissues can significantly affect the time course and extent of drug action. An extreme example is the nearly complete exclusion of some drugs from brain tissue by the blood-brain barrier (cf. Ch. 3). More generally, the movement of a drug into tissues may be limited by transfer across the capillary endothelium, by slow diffusion in the extracellular space, or by low blood flow, which limits the amount of drug supplied to the tissue. In poorly perfused tissues, such as resting muscle, fat, and skin, very long times may be required for a drug to accumulate to its steady-state level, especially if extensive binding to the tissue increases the amount of drug that must be delivered.

The transfer of several antibiotics from blood to tissue was examined in an ingenious experiment.[36] Perforated pieces of Silastic tubing were implanted subcutaneously in a

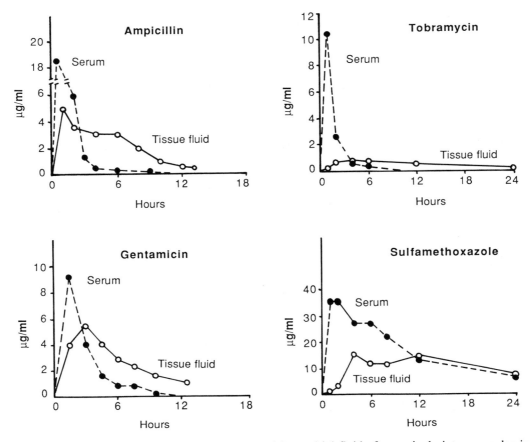

Fig. 4-18. Antibiotic concentrations in serum and interstitial fluid after a single intramuscular injection in dogs. The animals were injected with antibiotic at time zero, and samples of blood serum and interstitial fluid (tissue fluid) were obtained periodically thereafter. (From Chisholm et al.,[36] with permission.)

dog. Fluid withdrawn from the tubing had the composition expected for extracellular fluid (i.e., low protein and slightly alkaline pH). Following intramuscular injection of four antibiotics, the concentration of the drug was determined in samples of serum and tissue fluid (Fig. 4-18). There was a substantial delay in the appearance of drug in tissue fluid as compared with serum. For the aminoglycoside antibiotic tobramycin, the peak serum level occurred at 1 hour, while the tissue fluid peak was much lower and did not occur until 4 hours. If the infection and thus the site of action of the antibiotic were in the tissue, the effect would be much less than predicted from the peak serum concentration of 10 μg ml^{-1} and would be delayed.

Two-Compartment Model

When we analyzed first-order elimination of drugs previously, we assumed that the drug equilibrated instantaneously throughout its entire volume of distribution. As we have just seen, distribution is not always instantaneous. To account for this fact, somewhat more

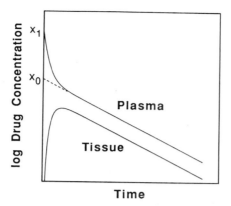

Fig. 4-19. Simulated plasma and tissue drug concentrations in a two-compartment pharmacokinetic model. Logarithms of the concentration of drug in the central compartment (plasma) and peripheral compartment (tissue) were simulated. Distribution is 30 times faster than elimination; x_1 is the plasma drug concentration immediately after injection, and x_0 is the zero-time concentration determined by extrapolation of the elimination curve (dashed line). The V_d (extrapolated) is determined from x_0 as described in the text.

complex models of drug distribution and elimination have been used. In the two-compartment open model, the drug in the body is considered to be in one of two pools or compartments.

$$\xrightarrow{k_{in}} X_1 \underset{k_{21}}{\overset{k_{12}}{\rightleftarrows}} X_2$$
$$\xrightarrow{k_{out}}$$

The drug is administered into the central compartment X_1, which is usually considered to include the blood and highly perfused tissues such as heart, brain, and kidney. The drug in the peripheral compartment X_2 can be thought of as being in tissue fluid or poorly perfused tissues. It should be noted that the exact anatomic location of the two compartments cannot be identified, since they are only mathematical constructs to account for the time course of drug concentrations in blood. In fact, in most circumstances one can only measure the drug concentration in the plasma (i.e., central compartment) while the concentration in the peripheral compartment (tissue) is estimated from the mathematical model. The drug is considered to enter (k_{12}) and leave (k_{21}) the peripheral compartment by first-order processes with their corresponding rate constants.

This model was first proposed in 1937 by Teorell.[33] To understand the time course of action of drugs that follow two-compartment kinetics we must know the time course of drug concentrations in the two compartments. When a bolus of drug X_0 is administered into the central compartment, which we will assume has a volume of V_1, a high initial concentration $x_1 = X_0/V_1$ is obtained (Fig. 4-19). The concentration of drug in the central compartment falls rapidly as drug is distributed to the peripheral compartment. This rapid fall is called the *distribution* or α phase of the plasma concentration versus time curve. The slower fall in drug concentration is called the *elimination* or β phase. If distribution of the drug is very fast compared with its elimination, it is useful to examine the plasma drug concentration immediately after distribution. At that time the drug will be in an apparent volume of distribution V_d, which can be thought of as the sum of the volumes of the central and peripheral compartments, and the concentration will be $x_0 = X_0/V_d$. This calculation assumes, of course, that no drug has been eliminated during the time of distribution. Since there will always be at least some elimination, these results must be considered only approximations. A better estimate of V_d is obtained by extrapolating the linear portion of the log plasma concentration during the β phase back to zero time (Fig. 4-19). This approximation, which is called V_d (extrapolated), is most accurate when distribution is very fast relative to elimination. Following the distribution of the drug, there is a parallel decline in the concentration of drug in the plasma and tissue compartments. Thus, the ratio of drug in the two compartments remains nearly constant during the β phase. We can calculate the ratio just after distribution by noting that the amount of drug in the central compartment is x_0V_1, while the amount of drug in the body is x_0V_d. Consequently, the fraction of drug in the central compartment is V_1/V_d. As with the extrapolated estimate of V_d, this ratio is an approximation. Exact solutions to the equations describing this model are beyond the scope of this discussion but they have been presented in detail elsewhere for the interested reader.[2,37] Modern computer methods make simulations of such models relatively easy.

Site of Drug Action: Effect Compartment

The time required for equilibration of a drug between the central and peripheral compartments can vary greatly. The neuromuscular blocking drug atracurium has a half-time for distribution of 2 minutes, while that for digoxin is 35 minutes, and for amiodarone many hours are required for distribution to the deep tissue compartment. As we have seen in Figure 4-19, the concentration of drug in the central compartment falls while that in the peripheral compartment is rising. This fact has significant implications for the time course of drug action. If the receptors responsible for the drug effect are in equilibrium with drug in the central compartment, the effect will peak rapidly and decline in a manner similar to the plasma drug concentration. If the receptors are in equilibrium with drug in the peripheral compartment, one would expect a delay in the onset of the response.

The cardiac glycoside digoxin has provided a useful model with which to examine this question. Its distribution is relatively slow, and its positive inotropic effect can be monitored quickly and noninvasively by recording the time required for blood to be ejected from the left ventricle. The change in this left ventricular ejection time index (LVETI) yields a measure of digoxin's effect. Although measured plasma concentrations peak and decline rapidly, the effect of digoxin requires hours to develop (Fig. 4-20). When the time course of drug concentrations in the plasma and tissue compartments is calculated from the pharmacokinetic model, the response closely follows the time course calculated for the tissue compartment. This has been explained by noting that a major site of distribution for digoxin is skeletal muscle and digoxin's effect is produced on cardiac muscle. The two types of muscle might be expected to follow a similar time course of drug distribution.

In the case of the antiarrhythmic drug lidocaine, both the toxic effects on the central nervous system and the cardiac electrophysiologic effects correlate best with the concentration of drug in the central compartment.[39,40] In fact, distribution of the drug from the central to the peripheral compartment results in the rapid disappearance of the response to a single bolus of lidocaine. Thus for different drugs (digoxin and lidocaine), even those affecting the same tissue (the heart), receptors may appear to be in equilibrium with either the peripheral or central compartment.

The two-compartment model of pharmacokinetics is obviously a simplification but it

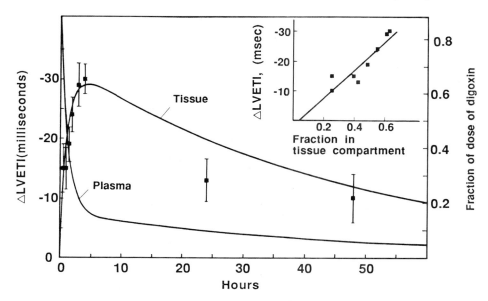

Fig. 4-20. Time course of digoxin distribution and response. A single dose of digoxin was administered intravenously to six normal volunteers. The fraction of the dose remaining in plasma and tissue compartments was calculated from a two-compartment pharmacokinetic model (solid lines) and compared with the time course of the decrease in left ventricular ejection time index (Δ LVETI), indicated by the solid squares with standard error bars. The inset shows the correlation between the amount of drug in the tissue compartment (expressed as a fraction of the dose) and the degree of digoxin response. (From Reuning et al.,[38] with permission.)

allows prediction of plasma drug concentrations and in some cases prediction of drug responses. The body is actually composed of many different organs with different perfusion rates and capacities to retain drug. Thus, one can not reasonably expect the drug concentration in the target tissue to follow the same time course as that in the bulk of the body tissues, which determines the plasma pharmacokinetics. For example, the effect of an oral hypoglycemic drug to increase insulin release will depend on its concentration in the extracellular fluid of the pancreas. Because of the small mass of that organ, it is unlikely that the whole body pharmacokinetics will reflect pancreatic uptake. A more general approach has been taken to identifying the site of drug action kinetically. Several investigators have suggested the addition of an *effect compartment* to the standard pharmacokinetic models.[41,42] The time of equilibration of drug into the effect compartment is not tied to any of the parameters determining overall drug distribution. Instead, the entry of drug into the effect compartment is determined by observing the onset of the pharmacologic effect. More complete descriptions of these models and their application are available.[43,44]

The synthetic opiates fentanyl and alfentanil are given intravenously to supplement nitrous oxide anesthesia, and the time courses of their actions have been studied by using the effect compartment model. The opiate effect on the central nervous system can be monitored continuously by observing the drug-induced slowing of electroencephalographic (EEG) signals. The EEG signal is broken down into different frequencies by Fourier analysis, and the frequency below which 95 percent of the signal occurs is called

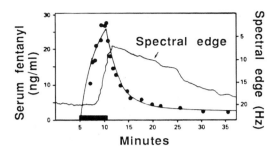

Fig. 4-21. Time course of serum fentanyl concentration and EEG response. Fentanyl was infused during surgery at a rate of 150 μg min^{-1}. The solid bar indicates the duration of the infusion. Serum fentanyl concentrations (solid circles) and spectral edge frequency (wavy line) were measured. The smooth curve shows calculated serum fentanyl concentrations based on pharmacokinetic parameters determined for that patient. (From Scott et al.,[45] with permission.)

the *spectral edge*. Following therapeutic doses of either fentanyl (shown in Fig. 4-21) or alfentanil the spectral edge frequency decreases from 20 to approximately 5 Hz.[45] During continuous infusion of the drug there is a delay between the increase in plasma drug concentration and the change in spectral edge frequency. In contrast to the situation with digoxin, the delay in onset of this opiate response cannot be related to the time course of bulk tissue distribution. This is most clearly illustrated by comparing fentanyl and alfentanil. Distribution of fentanyl,[46] determined from the plasma drug concentrations ($t_{1/2} = 4.5$ minutes), is slightly faster than the onset of response ($t_{1/2} = 6.4$ minutes) while for alfentanil, distribution ($t_{1/2} = 6.2$ minutes) is slower than response ($t_{1/2} = 1.1$ minutes). This can be explained by postulating that entry of alfentanil into the target site (effect compartment) is faster than that of fentanyl, even though both are distributed with similar kinetics into the peripheral tissues that determine the plasma concentration curves. The difference between the two drugs is unlikely to be due to slow activation of receptors since both drugs have a very rapid onset of action in vitro.

Nonlinear Concentration Effect Relations

Once the drug has arrived at its site of action, we need to know how large a response will be produced by any given concentration of drug. This is easiest to understand for drugs producing rapid effects that remain constant as long as the drug concentration is constant. This is true for many drugs, and the biologic basis for such responses has been discussed extensively in Ch. 1. We will defer to the next section the more complex cases in which there is a delay in response or a decrease in response with time (i.e., desensitization or tolerance).

For most responses that are mediated by specific receptors, the dependence of response on drug concentration follows the characteristic Langmuir equation (see Ch. 1) or the more general Hill equation

$$R = \frac{R_{max} \cdot x^n}{EC_{50}{}^n + x^n}$$

where R is the magnitude of the response, R_{max} is the maximum response attainable, x is the concentration of drug at the effect site, EC_{50} is the concentration of drug producing a half-maximal response, and n is the slope factor describing the steepness of the response

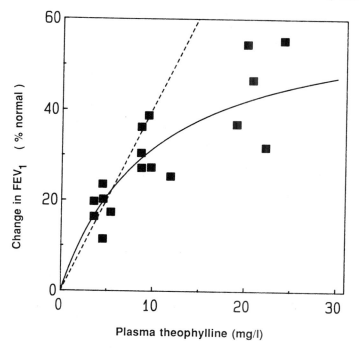

Fig. 4-22. Steady-state theophylline plasma concentration and response. Six patients were given various doses of theophylline until plasma concentrations reached steady state. The change in forced expiratory volume (FEV$_1$), expressed as a percentage of the normal value, is plotted against plasma theophylline concentration on a linear scale. The solid curve represents a saturating response function with an R_{max} of 63 percent and an EC$_{50}$ of 10 mg L^{-1}. The dashed line shows the response expected for a linear response based on the lowest dose for each patient. (Adapted from Holford et al.,[43] and after Mitenko et al.,[47] with permission.)

function. For many drugs the slope factor is unity, in which case the Hill equation reduces to the Langmuir equation and the response is said to be hyperbolic. Such saturating responses are seen with in vivo drug treatments as well as in a number of systems extensively studied in vitro. One example of a saturating response in vivo is the increase in forced expiratory volume produced by the bronchodilator theophylline. As shown in the experiment of Figure 4-22, the response to theophylline does not increase linearly with plasma drug concentration, but rather it begins to saturate at higher concentrations. When the concentration-response data were fitted to a hyperbolic response function, R_{max} was a 63 percent increase in normalized forced expiratory volume, and a plasma concentration of 10 mg L^{-1} resulted in the half-maximal increase.[43]

The effect of a saturating response function on the time course of drug responses has been analyzed by evaluating three regions of the drug concentration range.[2,43] In the saturation range, which corresponds to drug concentrations x producing more than 80 percent of the maximal response (i.e., x > EC$_{80}$), very large changes in drug concentration result in only small changes in response. For example, a fivefold decrease in concentration from 20 times EC$_{50}$ to 4 times EC$_{50}$ will reduce the response only 15 percent (from 95 to 80 percent of R_{max}). In the middle range of concentrations (EC$_{80}$ > x > EC$_{20}$), an exponentially decreasing drug concentration results in a nearly linear decrease in response.[48]

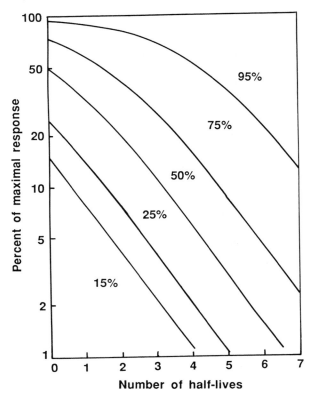

Fig. 4-23. Time course of simulated effect. The response to a drug with first-order elimination kinetics and a hyperbolic response function was simulated and shown on a semilogarithmic scale. Initial responses were (top to bottom) 95, 75, 50, 25, and 15 percent of the maximal response. The time axis represents the number of elimination half-times. (From Wagner,[49] with permission.)

At the lowest concentrations ($EC_{20} > x$), the response is essentially a linear function of drug concentration, and the time course of response will parallel the time course of drug concentration.

The most important implication of these observations is that for drugs that have a large therapeutic index (e.g., the β blocker propranolol) effects of relatively long duration can be achieved despite a short half-time of elimination if doses in the saturation range are given. A theoretical study (Fig. 4-23) has shown that five elimination half-times are required for the response to decrease from 95 to 50 percent of R_{max}.[49] Thus, a drug with a 2-hour elimination half-time may have an effective half-time of 10 hours if doses that produce 95 percent of R_{max} can be tolerated.

These saturating response functions have been used by many investigators to develop comprehensive pharmacokinetic-pharmacodynamic models. The models have been most successful in analyzing responses that can be monitored continuously, such as neuromuscular blockade and the central nervous system effects of anesthetics such as thiopental and the opiate fentanyl (see above). The individual factors that determine responses, such as plasma pharmacokinetics, transfer of drug to the effect compartment, R_{max}, and EC_{50}, can be identified, and differences between individuals in pharmacologic response may be localized to the specific pharmacokinetic or pharmacodynamic factor.[44]

Time Dependence of Responses

Delayed Response

We have mentioned several examples of responses that require substantial time to develop. Many of them involve inhibition of enzymes or effects on complex cellular processes. The anticoagulant warfarin exerts its effect by inhibiting the synthesis of the vitamin K–dependent clotting factors prothrombin and factors VII, IX, and X. The extent of warfarin's effect is measured clinically by determination of the time required for blood to clot in vitro (prothrombin time). As discussed in the section on the plateau principle, if warfarin were to immediately reduce the synthesis rate of the clotting factors, the rate of approach to the new steady state would be determined by the rate of degradation of the clotting factor. Since prothrombin has a degradation half-time of 0.5 to 1 day, the response would be expected to be half-maximal by approximately 12 to 24 hours, and that is what was observed. The delayed appearance of warfarin's effect initially resulted in some confusion regarding the relation between plasma warfarin concentrations and the pharmacologic effect. By considering the effect to be a decrease in the rate of prothrombin synthesis rather than the change in measured prothrombin time, it is possible to account quantitatively for the dose and time dependence of warfarin's response.[50,51]

Drugs acting on intracellular receptors often regulate gene expression, a relatively slow process, which results in substantial delay in the pharmacologic response. Induction of the hepatic enzyme tyrosine aminotransferase (TAT) by glucocorticoids is one example. For this system an attempt has been made to integrate pharmacokinetics, transfer of drug to the effect compartment, and subsequent time-dependent responses into a comprehensive model.[52] A single dose of the glucocorticoid prednisolone was given to rats, and the total and free concentrations of drug in plasma were measured. Parallel measurements of drug concentration, unoccupied glucocorticoid receptors, and TAT activity were performed on samples of liver obtained at various times. The receptor measurements provided a unique method of characterizing the appearance of drug in the effect compartment. The principle of this approach depends on the fact that prednisolone bound to the receptors in vivo prevents subsequent measurement of the receptor under cell-free conditions in hepatic cytosol, both because the bound prednisolone does not dissociate from the receptor during the cell-free assay and because it induces translocation of the receptor out of the cytosolic fraction and into the nuclear fraction of the cell.

It is interesting that the concentration of drug in the plasma accounted for the time course of receptor occupation better than did the liver content of steroid. This points out the difficulty in identifying the exact anatomic location of the site of action of the drug. It is likely that drug may accumulate at sites in the liver that are sequestered away from the receptors in hepatocyte cytosol. In fact, the appearance of drug in the effect compartment is quite fast, since loss of measurable receptors occurs by the first time point (Fig. 4-24). The induction of TAT was significantly delayed as compared with the time course of prednisolone concentrations in plasma or receptor occupation.

The time course of increases in TAT activity was accounted for by a model in which there was an initial lag of 1.7 hours before increased synthesis began and the increased rate of synthesis was maintained for 3.6 hours. The lag time in this pharmacokinetic model is similar to results seen in in vitro experiments when drug concentrations are precisely defined and the rate of protein synthesis is measured directly. The precise relation between receptor occupation and the amount and duration of enzyme synthesis was not included in this model; however, the combination of careful pharmacokinetic modeling with mea-

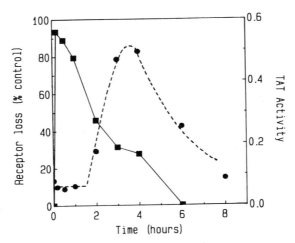

Fig. 4-24. Time course of steroid receptor occupancy and steroid-induced enzyme activity. The squares indicate the decrease in measurable cytosolic glucocorticoid receptor in rat liver following a single dose of prednisolone (5 mg kg^{-1} IV). The decrease in receptor concentration in hepatic cytosol in vitro is an indicator of receptors occupied in vivo. Activity of the enzyme tyrosine aminotransferase (TAT) is shown in arbitrary units (solid circles). The dashed line for TAT activity is a theoretical prediction based on a pharmacokinetic-pharmacodynamic model. (Modified from Boudinot et al.,[52] with permission.)

surements of receptor binding and response provides a rational approach to the study of in vivo drug responses.

Acute Desensitization

Another pharmacologic process that can modify the time course of drug action is the decrease in tissue responsiveness that occurs in the presence of a constant concentration of drug. This phenomenon has been termed variously desensitization, tolerance, and tachyphylaxis. The term *desensitization* usually refers to a specific loss of receptor responsiveness, while *tolerance* and *tachyphylaxis* define whole animal responses. Tachyphylaxis (literal meaning, "rapid protection") typically shows a more rapid onset than tolerance. The biochemical mechanisms for some forms of receptor desensitization have been discussed in Chapter 2, and tolerance at the level of the whole organism is discussed in Chapter 10. They are most commonly observed with drugs acting on the central nervous system, but peripheral tissues including heart, blood cells, and smooth muscle also exhibit desensitization of responses. One of the most dramatic demonstrations of these phenomena is the loss of response to continuous administration of opiates. Based on the brain concentration of the drug, one would expect nearly a constant response, but instead there is a slow diminution of the response to zero.[53] Since the decreased responsiveness is a complex property of the biologic system, it is not possible to predict a priori the time course of the decrease in response.

Although tolerance is usually associated with prolonged administration of drugs, there are many examples in which a rapid loss of responsiveness can occur. Following intranasal administration of cocaine in "experienced" volunteers, the peak of euphoria occurred before the peak plasma concentration.[54] This is illustrated in a plot of effect versus plasma

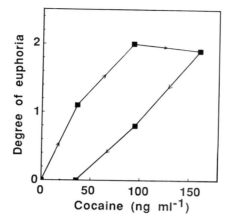

Fig. 4-25. Hysteresis loop indicating acute tolerance to cocaine. The subjective response to a single intranasal dose of cocaine is plotted against the plasma concentration determined at the same times. The arrowheads indicate the time sequence of the measurements. (Modified from Holford et al.,[43] after data of van Dyke et al.[54])

drug concentration at various times (Fig. 4-25). The arrows indicate the direction of increasing time. A clockwise hysteresis loop is observed as more drug is required for the same effect at later times. In contrast, a counterclockwise hysteresis loop is observed when there is a delay between the appearance of drug in the blood and the effect. As discussed in the previous sections, this could be due to delayed access to the site of action (effect compartment), to metabolic activation of the drug, or simply to a slow onset of response after receptor binding.[43]

KINETICS OF THE UPTAKE AND DISTRIBUTION OF DRUGS ADMINISTERED BY INHALATION

The administration of gases, especially anesthetic gases, is characterized by two interesting new features, as compared with the drugs discussed earlier in this chapter.[55] First, the rate of entry is controlled by a cyclic process, the respiration, so that the drug is presented for absorption at the alveoli in an interrupted fashion about 20 times per minute. Second, many of these agents are not metabolized or excreted to any significant extent by the usual routes. They are eliminated almost entirely at the lungs, the site of their absorption. Thus, the eventual plateau at the "steady state" is really an equilibrium. The net transfer rate from alveoli to blood is rapid at first, then progressively slower as the blood concentration builds up, until finally, at the plateau blood level, the rate of transfer from blood to alveoli equals the rate of transfer from alveoli to blood.

At equilibrium, the concentration in blood (x'_b) is related to the concentration in alveolar air (x'_a) by the expression

$$\frac{x'_b}{x'_a} = S$$

where S is simply the solubility of the gas in blood. The solubility of a gas in a fluid is defined as the ratio of the concentration of dissolved gas to the concentration in the gas phase, at equilibrium. This solubility is also known as the *Ostwald coefficient*. The defi-

Table 4-2. Properties of Volatile Anesthetics

	Molecular Weight	(S) Soubility in Blood at 38°C	(x'_b) mM Blood at III_{2-3}	(x'_a) mM Alveolar Air at III_{2-3}	(p) mmHg at III_{2-3}	mg ml^{-1} Blood at III_{2-3}	(S_L) Oil/Water Partition Coefficient
(Ethanol)	46	1100	88	0.080	1.5	4.0	—
Ether	74	15	20	1.3	25	1.5	3.2
Chloroform	119	7.3	1.8	0.25	4.8	0.21	100
Ethyl chloride	64	2.5	4.6	1.8	35	0.29	—
Halothane	197	2.3	1.0	0.43	8.3	0.21	220
Vinyl ether	70	1.5	2.6	1.7	33	0.18	41
Acetylene	26	0.82	22	27	520	0.57	—
Cyclopropane	42	0.47	4.1	8.7	170	0.17	34
Nitrous oxide	44	0.47	29	61	1200	1.3	3.2
Propylene	42	0.22	4.8	22	420	0.20	—
Ethylene	28	0.14	5.7	41	790	0.16	14

The data of this table are approximate; they are assembled from several sources, and obtained by methods of differing reliability. The expression III_{2-3} means stage III, plane 2–3 anesthesia, a typical depth for abdominal surgery. Most of the data are summarized in Larson et al.[56]

nition of solubility is often confusing to the student, but it should be remembered that, unlike solids, gases distribute themselves between a fluid and a gas phase so that the amount dissolved increases without limit (theoretically, at least) as the concentration in the gas phase is increased. The only reasonable way to define solubility is therefore to relate the amount of gas dissolved in a given volume of fluid to the gas phase concentration required to hold it in solution.

Anesthetic gases vary widely in their solubilities, as shown in Table 4-2. Since the solubility is a ratio of concentrations, it does not matter in what units these are expressed provided they are the same for both phases. The solubility equation $x'_b = S(x'_a)$ is simply another way of stating Henry's law, which relates the concentration of dissolved gas to the partial pressure in the gas phase at equilibrium. The transformation of gas concentration to partial pressure is accomplished most simply by means of the ideal gas law

$$pV = nRT$$

If the concentration is expressed as moles per liter (n/V), and the partial pressure p is to be obtained in millimeters of mercury, then the gas constant R has the value 62 L·mmHg·(mol·K)$^{-1}$, the temperature T being in kelvins.

Example. What is the partial pressure exerted by a gas at 38°C (311 K) whose concentration is 8.70 millimoles L^{-1}?

$$p = (n/V)RT = (8.7 \times 10^{-3})(62)(311) = 168 \text{ mmHg}$$

For present purposes we will not distinguish between vapors and gases. Any substance in the gaseous state obeys the gas laws sufficiently well, regardless of whether its boiling point is above or below room temperature. The principal difference arises from the fact that while the concentration of a gas in the inspired air can be varied at will up to 100 percent, the maximum concentration of a vapor is limited by its vapor pressure at ambient temperature. As this vapor pressure is by definition the partial pressure in equilibrium with the liquid, it follows that no higher partial pressure can exist, any tendency to further evaporation being balanced by re-entry of vapor molecules into the liquid phase. If a liquid is to be a useful volatile anesthetic, it must therefore be potent enough, or volatile enough, so that surgical anesthesia can be produced with a partial pressure (in the inspired air) below its vapor pressure at room temperature. Throughout this section, *surgical anesthesia* means stage III, plane 2–3 anesthesia, a suitable level for major surgery without adjuvant muscle relaxants. In actual practice it is common to use many different levels of anesthesia, supplemented by the use of preanesthetic medications, muscle relaxants, and pain-relieving drugs. The reader is referred to textbooks of anesthesiology for details.

Example. The vapor pressure of ether at 20°C is 442 mmHg. This is the maximum partial pressure of ether vapor that could be attained, but the partial pressure required to produce surgical anesthesia is only about 25 mmHg; thus, establishing a sufficient alveolar ether concentration presents no problem.

Equilibrium in Clinical Anesthesia

The various stages of anesthesia are associated with definite concentrations of each anesthetic agent in the brain and (provided equilibrium has been attained) with definite concentrations in the circulating blood. With a number of anesthetic agents the concentrations in blood and in whole brain have been found to be approximately equal. Because of the precise relationship between depth of anesthesia and blood anesthetic concentration and because it is impractical to measure the anesthetic concentration in the brain, we shall concern ourselves with blood anesthetic concentration. We shall further limit the discussion by considering that particular blood concentration which, at equilibrium, will produce surgical anesthesia. For any given anesthetic agent there is one and only one such blood concentration, namely, the EDC (effective drug concentration). If the agent is very potent, this required blood concentration will be low; if it is not very potent, the required blood concentration will be high. Anesthesiologists sometimes think of potency in connection with the effective concentration in the alveolar air, but this is a very restricted meaning. Rigorously defined, potency refers to the effective molecular concentration of a drug at its site of action, and we use the word in this sense. Low or high, the EDC is determined by the physicochemical properties of the agent on the one hand and the behavior of the central nervous system on the other, both of which are beyond the control of the anesthesiologist.

At equilibrium there will be a predictable relationship between this concentration in blood (the EDC) and that in the alveolar air, a relationship defined by the solubility of the agent, already discussed above. Because the solubility of any agent in blood at body temperature is a fixed physical property, also beyond the control of the anesthesiologist, it follows that the concentration of anesthetic required in the alveolar air in order to just reach and then maintain surgical anesthesia is also absolutely fixed and beyond control. If a lower concentration is used, we shall not achieve surgical anesthesia when equilibrium is reached; if a higher concentration is employed, we shall exceed the safe levels of surgical anesthesia and cause respiratory paralysis. The situation is exactly the same as that described previously for dosage regimens in general.

When equilibrium has been reached, the partial pressure of anesthetic in the alveolar air will obviously be the same as that in the inspired air (for example, in the breathing bag). The concentration in the inspired air in equilibrium with the EDC in blood is called the *safe anesthetic gas concentration*. If the anesthesiologist employs this concentration from the start, then at equilibrium a safe depth of anesthesia will be reliably achieved, and there will be no danger of exceeding this depth. In most of the subsequent discussion we shall assume that the anesthesiologist makes use of the safe anesthetic concentration from the beginning of the anesthesia, even though for some agents (as we shall see) such a procedure would be impractical.

Example 1. The solubility of ether at 38°C is 15. If the concentration in the alveolar air is kept constant at 1.3 mM, what will be the concentration in blood at equilibrium?

$$S = 15$$

$$x'_a = 1.3 \text{ m}M$$

$$x'_b = S(x'_a) = 15 \times 1.3 = 20 \text{ m}M$$

Example 2. At equilibrium, the concentration of halothane is found to be 1.0 mM in blood (38°C), with partial pressure 8.3 mmHg in the inspired air (20°C). What is the solubility of halothane?

The partial pressure exerted by a gas in a mixture does not change with temperature, provided the sum of all the partial pressures remains the same (i.e., 760 mmHg at sea level). Thus, $p = 8.3$ mmHg also at 38°C in alveolar air, and

$$\frac{n}{V} = \frac{p}{RT} = \frac{8.3}{62 \times 311} = 0.43 \text{ m}M$$

$$S = x'_b/x'_a = \frac{1.0}{0.43} = 2.3$$

Example 3. At equilibrium, the concentration of cyclopropane in the inspired air (20°C) is found to be 9.2 mM, and its solubility is 0.47. What is the blood concentration?

$$p = (n/V)RT = (9.2 \times 10^{-3})(62)(293) = 167 \text{ mmHg}$$

In the alveoli, at 38°C this same partial pressure exists, but because of expansion with increased temperature the concentration of all gases is lower than in the inspired air. Here

$$\frac{n}{V} = \frac{p}{RT} = \frac{167}{(62)(311)} = 8.7 \text{ m}M$$

or, more simply,

$$\frac{n}{V} = (9.2)\frac{293}{311} = 8.7 \text{ m}M$$

whence

$$x'_b = S(x'_a) = (0.47)(8.7) = 4.1 \text{ m}M$$

Rate of Equilibration of Blood and Body Water

Equilibration at the Blood-Alveolar Membrane

Let us now consider the factors determining the rate at which the EDC is attained when the anesthetic in the inspired air is maintained at the safe anesthetic gas concentration from the start. As the gaseous anesthetics are all relatively small molecules, they diffuse very rapidly from the blood into all the tissues of the body. As the surface area is large and the anesthetics are lipid-soluble, they are able to cross cell membranes rapidly and distribute themselves in intracellular as well as extracellular fluid. Thus, for an average-sized man (70 kg) we shall have to consider the equilibration not of 6 L of circulating blood but of 42 L of total body water.

Gas in the alveoli equilibrates almost instantaneously with blood passing through the pulmonary capillary bed. This has been established by careful physiologic studies, most recently by the use of radioactive gases. Let us assume for the moment that it were possible by some kind of special pump to maintain the safe anesthetic concentration in the alveolar air (i.e., to replace continuously all anesthetic that passes over into the pulmonary blood). In that case, all the blood coming from the lungs would continuously carry an equilibrium concentration of anesthetic, namely, the EDC, which will be reached ultimately in all the body water. The entire cardiac output passes through the pulmonary capillary bed, so if the cardiac output is 5 L min^{-1} and the body water is 42 L, it follows, as a first approximation, that the total body water could be brought to equilibrium in about 8 minutes. Actually, this is an underestimate of the time, since the approach to equilibration is asymptotic. As soon as blood returning to the lungs contains some anesthetic, blood leaving the lungs will begin to contribute less toward equilibration of the total body water, because the anesthetic brought to the lungs by blood will simply be carried away again, and the net transfer of anesthetic will be diminished by this amount.

The asymptotic nature of the equilibration process can perhaps best be understood in relation to the total amount of anesthetic needed to bring the body water to equilibrium. If the equilibrium concentration to be achieved is x'_b and the body water amounts to 42 L, then $42x'_b$ is the amount of anesthetic that must be transferred from the alveoli into the blood in order to reach equilibrium. At the start, when no anesthetic is yet in the blood, the net transfer will be at the rate of $5x'_b$ min^{-1}, as stated above. But now suppose the concentration in the blood and body water has already reached $0.1x'_b$. This will be the concentration in blood arriving at the lungs, while the blood leaving the lungs will always contain the concentration x'_b. The net transfer rate at this point is therefore no longer $5x'_b$ but $5(x'_b - 0.1x'_b)$, or $4.5x'_b$ min^{-1}. Obviously then, the approach to equilibrium will continue to slow down as greater fractions of equilibrium are achieved. Complete equilibrium is only achieved in an infinite time; we can only measure the attainment of a specified *fraction* of equilibrium. The correct estimate of the time required to attain 90 percent equilibration of body water under these hypothetical conditions is approximately 21 minutes instead of our rough estimate of 8 minutes. The derivation of equations describing this rather complex process is an interesting exercise in the application of mathematics to physiologic problems.[57–60]

Lung Washout

We assumed above that it was somehow possible to establish at once and then to maintain the safe anesthetic concentration in the alveoli. As a matter of fact, respiration is a cyclic process. The amount of anesthetic inhaled in the first breath will be diluted in a considerable lung volume containing no anesthetic whatsoever. The alveolar ventilation is about 0.3 L. The total effective lung volume after normal inspiration is equal to this volume plus the functional residual capacity and end-expiratory volume, amounting in all to some 2.8 L.

Now suppose the inspired gas mixture contains x'_a, the alveolar concentration in equilibrium with the EDC (i.e., x'_b). Anesthetic taken into the lungs at the first breath ($0.3x'_a$) is diluted immediately so that the alveolar concentration during the interrespiratory pause is only $(0.3/2.8)x'_a$, or $0.11x'_a$. Some of the alveolar anesthetic passes into the blood and is carried away, while the rest remains in the lungs to be added to the amount inhaled during the next breath. If very little passes into the blood at each breath, the alveolar concentration will quickly build up in stepwise fashion toward x'_a. But if nearly all the anesthetic in the alveoli passes into the blood at each breath, the alveolar concentration after the second, third, and subsequent breaths will not be appreciably greater than after the first breath.

In general, the repeated addition of air carrying an anesthetic concentration x'_a to the total lung volume containing a lower concentration causes anesthetic to accumulate in the alveoli with each successive breath. Soon, however, each inspiration replaces exactly the amount of anesthetic that passed into the blood during the previous breath. When this state is reached, the alveolar concentration would have risen but little higher than $0.11x'_a$ in the case of an agent of very high S, since nearly $0.3x'_a$ passes into the blood during each breath, and $0.3x'_a$ is the most that can be replaced by a normal inspiration. However, the steady-state alveolar concentration would be nearly x'_a in the case of an agent of very low S, where very little passes into the blood during each breath. The process whereby the alveolar anesthetic concentration reaches a steady state is termed *lung washout*. It is virtually complete within less than 2 minutes.

Agents of Very Low Solubility

We have seen that with an agent of very low solubility the alveolar concentration at the end of the washout period is practically the same as that of the inspired air (namely, the safe anesthetic concentration x_a). This anesthetic will distribute itself instantaneously and continuously between alveoli and blood in accordance with its solubility. For example, the anesthetic in 1 ml of alveolar air will bring the same volume of blood to equilibrium without appreciable change in the alveolar concentration. As shown in Figure 4-26, an agent of solubility 0.1 will have accomplished this when only one-eleventh of the total anesthetic in the given volume of alveolar air has passed into an equal volume of blood.

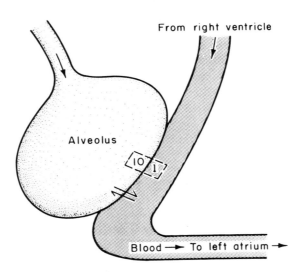

Fig. 4-26. Diagram showing momentary equilibrium between equal volumes of blood and air at blood-alveolar membrane for an anesthetic agent of solubility 0.1.

The blood flowing through the lungs during each breath (respiratory rate 20 min^{-1}) is one-twentieth of the cardiac output, or 0.25 L. All this blood leaves the lungs in equilibrium with the alveolar concentration, which is practically x'_a. The blood, therefore, carries away a concentration $x'_b = S(x'_a)$, or an amount equal to $(0.25)(S)(x'_a)$ per breath. For an agent of solubility 0.1, this would be $0.025x'_a$ per breath, or less than 1 percent of the total anesthetic in the lungs, an amount that can readily be replaced at the next inspiration.

Because the blood is already carrying all the anesthetic it can, increasing the respiratory rate or minute volume could not significantly increase the transfer of anesthetic into the blood and therefore could not shorten the equilibration time significantly. On the other hand, increasing the cardiac output would markedly increase the rate of removal of anesthetic from the lungs. In fact, doubling the cardiac output would nearly double the rate of removal and thereby nearly halve the equilibration time. Thus, for agents of very low solubility the cardiac output (and not the respiration) is the major physiologic factor limiting the rate of equilibration. At each breath only a small fraction of the anesthetic in the lungs is removed, and after 3 seconds even this is replenished at the next inspiration. The alveoli continuously contain nearly the safe anesthetic gas concentration, the arterial blood ejected from the left ventricle contains the corresponding x'_b (the EDC), and the situation is very much like the hypothetical one discussed earlier, in which 21 minutes was shown to be a reasonable estimate of the time required to bring the body water to nine-tenths of its equilibrium anesthetic concentration.

Agents of Very High Solubility

We have already seen that with an agent of very high solubility so much is transferred to the blood during each breath that little if any remains in the alveoli just before the next inspiration (cf. Fig. 4-26, as it would apply to an agent of solubility 10). The alveolar concentration established at the first inspiration ($0.11x'_a$) is re-established again and again (without appreciable increment) at every succeeding inspiration and falls practically to zero before the next breath. The arterial anesthetic concentration closely reflects this fluctuating pattern, never exceeding $0.11x'_b$ initially and falling off nearly to zero during every breath. Naturally, the time required to equilibrate the body water with the inspired air will be very much longer than with low-solubility agents. Assuming that the lungs are wholly depleted at each breath, we have $0.3x'_a \times 20$, or $6x'_a$ entering the blood every minute. Since $S = 10$, this is equal to $0.6x'_b$ min^{-1}, and it would take 68 minutes (at the very least) to carry away from the lungs the $42x'_b$ needed to equilibrate 42 L of body water. This calculation also ignores the asymptotic nature of the process and is therefore a considerable underestimate, as in the similar example given previously.

The mean alveolar anesthetic concentration (and consequently the arterial concentration) begins to rise only as blood returning from the body tissues to the lungs carries more and more anesthetic. Slightly less is removed from the alveoli during each breath (for the reasons explained before), and the remainder gradually accumulates. With an agent of high solubility, the mean alveolar anesthetic concentration approaches that of the inspired air (x'_a) at essentially the same rate as the venous blood approaches equilibrium.

Here, respiration is the principal factor that limits attainment of equilibrium. Because the blood is already removing virtually all anesthetic from the lungs, increasing the cardiac output could not materially shorten the equilibration time, but equilibration can be very substantially hastened by furnishing anesthetic to the alveoli more rapidly (i.e., by increasing the respiratory rate or depth). This is precisely what is accomplished by inhalation of CO_2 or by increasing the rate of controlled respiration, procedures primarily useful in accelerating equilibration (and de-equilibration) of agents with *high solubility* such as ether and chloroform (Table 4-2).

The Transition Zone Between Low- and High-Solubility Behavior

We have said a good deal about agents of "very low" and "very high" solubility. But what values of S are we justified in regarding as high or low in this connection? As S determines the relative roles of respiratory minute volume and cardiac output in limiting the equilibration rate, it follows that at an intermediate value of S these physiologic parameters will have equal importance. This critical solubility, which proves to be about 1.2, marks the center of a transition zone between the two types of extreme behavior described. Actually, this zone is fairly broad, but as S becomes much smaller or much greater than 1.2, the behavior of the anesthetics will approach more closely that of the prototype low- and high-solubility agents examined in the foregoing discussion. It should be noted that the value $S = 1.2$ is arrived at on the basis of average physiologic data; namely, respiratory rate 20 min^{-1}, alveolar ventilation 0.3 L, cardiac output 5 L min^{-1}. A substantial change in any of these values will shift the transition zone toward higher or lower solubilities.

Figure 4-27 shows an arrangement of volatile and gaseous anesthetics according to solubility, on a scale indicating their behavior with respect to equilibration rate. As S

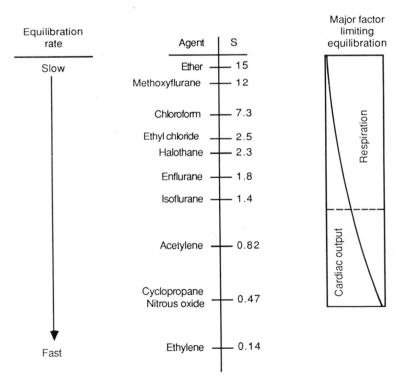

Fig. 4-27. Relation of solubility S to equilibrium rate, showing relative limitation by respiration and cardiac output.

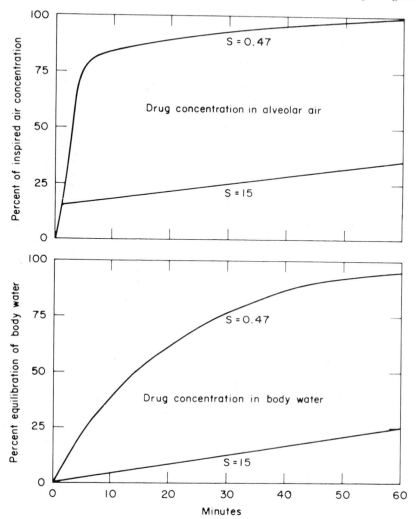

Fig. 4-28. Theoretical course of equilibration with nitrous oxide ($S = 0.47$) and ether ($S = 15$).

increases, the equilibration time becomes longer, without limit. As S decreases, however, a minimum equilibration time is approached (approximately 21 minutes for 90 percent equilibration as shown earlier). Thus, agents of very low solubility do not differ materially among themselves in their rates of equilibration.

Figure 4-28 represents the calculated course of equilibration with two agents of different solubility. The change in alveolar anesthetic concentration is plotted in the upper half, the change in anesthetic concentration in body water (or venous blood) in the lower half.

It should follow from the above discussion and from Figure 4-28 that the rate of equilibration is independent of the concentration of the anesthetic agent; however, at very high concentrations this is not so. Rather, the rate of approach of alveolar concentration to inspired concentration is faster, the higher the inspired concentration. This phenomenon is called the *concentration effect*.[61,62] The principle is apparent if one imagines a con-

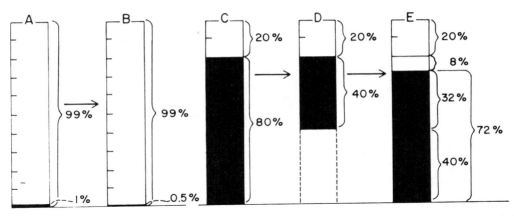

Fig. 4-29. The concentration effect. **(A & B)** The change in alveolar concentration when one-half of a 1.0 percent concentration is taken up. The decrease in concentration is proportional to the amount taken up. **(C–E)** The change when one-half of an 80 percent concentration is taken up. The reduction is to 40/(20 + 40) = 67 percent, which is not proportional to the amount taken up. When more gas is added at the same concentration, the final concentration (at *E*) is 72 percent. Were the reduction proportional to uptake, the final concentration would be 40 percent. (From Eger,[61] with permission.)

centration of 100 percent of an anesthetic gas in the inspired air. Regardless of how much passes across the alveoli, the remaining concentration will still be 100 percent, and the gas drawn in to replace the volume of anesthetic agent that passes into the blood at each breath will also contain 100 percent. Thus, even with a high-solubility agent, the alveolar concentration will approach 100 percent very quickly. The concentration effect will be significant whenever the anesthetic agent constitutes a significant fraction of the total inspired gas volume, as illustrated in Figure 4-29. Theoretical curves for nitrous oxide and for ether are given in Figure 4-30. As would be expected, the concentration effect is theoretically greatest for agents of high solubility. As a practical matter, however, only nitrous oxide ($S = 0.47$) is used at concentrations high enough to account for a major fraction of the total gas volume.

An interesting corollary of the concentration effect is the *second gas effect*. If an agent such as halothane, used at low concentration, is present in a gas mixture with another agent such as nitrous oxide at high concentration, the additional inflow of gas mixture to replace the absorbed nitrous oxide will also raise the alveolar concentration of halothane. This effect is small but significant, and it has been demonstrated in vivo.[63]

De-equilibration

If the anesthetic intake is abruptly stopped, after the EDC has been established, anesthetic begins to be eliminated from the blood into the lungs. The factors affecting de-equilibration of the body water are the same as those already considered in connection with equilibration. An agent of very low solubility can be eliminated almost as fast as the blood delivers it to the lungs. The elimination of an agent of very high solubility is limited by the respiratory rate and minute volume, only a small fraction being removed from the blood during a single passage. Obviously, increasing respiration will be effective in has-

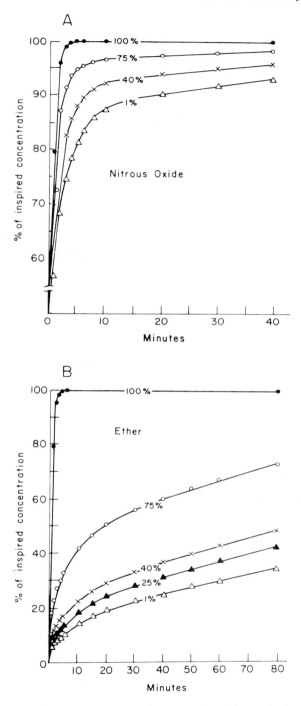

Fig. 4-30. The concentration effect for nitrous oxide and ether. Theoretical curves for approach of alveolar concentration to inspired concentration in humans. (**A**) Nitrous oxide ($S = 0.47$). (**B**) Ether ($S = 15$). (From Eger,[62] with permission.)

tening de-equilibration of high-S agents, but will be of no use for this purpose with low-S agents. The curves of de-equilibration are essentially inverted equilibration curves.

Potency and the Availability of Oxygen

The potency of an anesthetic is inversely proportional to the EDC. Table 4-2 shows that potency varies widely, and quite independently of solubility. There is a relationship, which is the basis of the Overton-Meyer hypothesis, between potency and *lipid solubility*.[64,65] Anesthetics of high potency (i.e., those that act at low EDC) are generally very soluble in lipid, so that the effective concentrations of all volatile anesthetics in the lipid material of the central nervous system are thought to be approximately the same.

Potency has no bearing on the rates of equilibration or de-equilibration, which depend on S alone. This is a point about which the student is often confused. We can only reasonably compare rates of equilibration when the safe anesthetic gas concentration is consistently employed with all agents. Under these conditions S represents the relation between how much anesthetic must be transferred into a given volume of blood (i.e., x'_b) and what "driving force" is available to accomplish the transfer (i.e., x'_a). Naturally, if we arbitrarily increase the alveolar anesthetic concentration, we can force anesthetic into the blood as fast as we wish, but the patient will be dead if we persist. The following hypothetical summary will illustrate why, when the safe anesthetic gas concentration is used, potency is irrelevant to the rate of equilibration.

	EDC = x'_b	S	$x'_a (= x'_b/S)$
Gas A	1	1	1
Gas B	1	10	0.1
Gas C	10	1	10

Gas A and gas B are equipotent. Yet, because B is 10 times more soluble than A, the "driving force" available for achieving the same x'_b is 10 times lower with B than with A, and the rate at which x'_b is approached must obviously be considerably lower.

Gas C is 10 times less potent than gas A, so the x'_b to be attained is 10 times higher. Yet, because S is the same, the "driving force" of C is just 10 times greater than that of A, and equilibrium will be reached at the same rate.

The potency of a gaseous anesthetic is immaterial except in one respect that has nothing to do with equilibration rate. If the potency is very low relative to the solubility, the safe anesthetic gas concentration may be so high that there is no room (at ordinary atmospheric pressure) for sufficient oxygen. The minimum oxygen requirement in the inspired air is about 15 percent, or 114 mmHg. It follows that the partial pressure of an anesthetic gas may not exceed 646 mmHg (33.5 mM at 38°C). Reference to Table 4-2 will show that by this criterion neither ethylene nor nitrous oxide is a suitable agent for producing surgical anesthesia (although either may be useful for lesser degrees of anesthesia), since both require partial pressures greater than 646 mmHg. The only way to induce surgical anesthesia with either of these agents alone is to employ *total* pressures greater than 760 mmHg, thereby incorporating oxygen at a partial pressure of at least 114 mmHg. To the extent that it may be thought desirable to furnish oxygen in excess of the minimum 114 mmHg, other agents may also be found deficient. Acetylene, for example, permits only about 25 percent of oxygen in the anesthetic mixture. In contrast, anesthesia can be produced with a mixture of 0.7 percent chloroform and 99.3 percent oxygen.

If follows from the above discussion that after discontinuation of anesthesia with an agent such as nitrous oxide, which has a relatively low solubility and is used at high concentration, a very large amount of the gas will be delivered to the alveoli from the blood. This may result in *diffusion anoxia* (i.e., the alveoli are effectively filled with nitrous oxide diffusing from the blood, and the alveolar oxygen tension is reduced). Suppose the blood has been equilibrated with a mixture of 80 percent nitrous oxide and 20 percent oxygen. If the anesthesia is simply discontinued and the patient is allowed to breathe air, the alveoli will, for some time, contain 80 percent nitrous oxide, the concentration in equilibrium with the blood perfusing the lungs, and the remaining 20 percent (even ignoring carbon dioxide and water vapor), since it is air, will provide only one-fifth the adequate amount of oxygen. Especially in conditions of marginally sufficient oxygenation, therefore, significant hypoxemia may result unless pure oxygen is administered during the early recovery phase.[66]

Influence of Body Fat

The Anesthetic Content of the Body at Equilibrium

Up to this point we have examined the equilibration of body water as though the anesthetic did not dissolve appreciably in other components of the body. However, some agents are quite soluble in lipid, and fat constitutes an important fraction of the body weight. In an average person, without prominent fat depots, the fat of the organs and subcutaneous tissues amounts to not less than 15 percent of the body weight, while it is obvious that in very obese people this fraction may be much higher.[67]

The solubility of an anesthetic in lipids (often estimated approximately from measurements with a vegetable oil) is expressed as a partition coefficient between lipid and blood at 38°C:

$$S_L = \frac{x_L}{x_b}$$

To distinguish between lipid solubility and blood solubility in this section, we shall use the symbol S_b instead of S to denote the latter and S_L to denote lipid solubility.

When the blood and body water attain their equilibrium concentration x'_b, fat will contain $x'_L = S_L(x'_b)$. What volume of blood will contain the same amount of anesthetic as a given volume of fat? Obviously this "blood equivalent" of fat is simply S_L. Suppose, for example, $S_L = 10$. This means that any volume of fat at equilibrium will contain 10 times as much anesthetic as the same volume of blood, or, in other words, 1 L of fat is the equivalent of 10 L of blood. The effect of body fat is, therefore, to increase the apparent volume of distribution of an anesthetic agent to an extent that depends on S_L and the volume of fat and thus to increase the total amount of anesthetic in the body at equilibrium. An agent of very high lipid solubility may be distributed largely in the fat depots at equilibrium, and the total anesthetic content of obese patients may be surprisingly high.

Example. The blood concentration of enflurane during surgical anesthesia is 1.1 mM; molecular weight = 167, $S_L = 81$. What weight of the gas is contained in a 90-kg man, of whom 20 kg is fat?

Approximately 20 L fat is equivalent to (20 × 81) L blood. Total blood equivalent = 1620 L blood + 50 L body water = 1,670 L. Then the weight of gas is: 1.1 mM × 1,670 = 1.78 moles, or (1.78 × 167) g = 298 g. Note that of this total weight of enflurane, 1620/1670, or 97 percent, is in the fat.

Rate of Uptake of Anesthetic by Fat Depots

Let us assume that all the arterial blood arriving at a fat depot contains x'_b, that the fat contains no anesthetic, and that S_L is high. A high S_L means that a great deal of anesthetic has to be transferred from blood to fat, relative to the concentration available in blood. Consequently the blood will be practically depleted of anesthetic in the proximal portion of the capillaries, and equilibration will be prolonged until, with the arrival of more and more blood carrying x'_b, enough is finally transferred to bring the whole fat depot to its equilibrium concentration x'_L. This process will be reflected in the anesthetic content of venous blood draining the fat depot; initially containing practically no anesthetic, its concentration will gradually increase to x'_b when the fat depot has reached equilibrium. The word *saturate* is very often misused in this connection. There is never any question of "saturating" the body or fat depots with anesthetic but only of equilibrating with a given alveolar anesthetic concentration.

Effect of Depot Fat Upon Rates of Equilibration and De-equilibration of Body Water

The rate of uptake of anesthetic by fat depots is of little interest in itself, but the question is naturally raised of whether fat depots modify the rate of equilibration (or de-equilibration) of blood and body water. The maximum effect of depot fat would be observed under circumstances such that all the blood flowing through all the fat depots was cleared of anesthetic in a single passage. This would be the case initially, as has already been noted, with agents of high S_L. However, the blood flow through all the fat depots represents so small a fraction of the cardiac output (approximately 3 percent) that the anesthetic concentration in mixed venous blood would not be substantially lowered even in this extreme case. This conclusion is confirmed by experimental data on nitrogen elimination, showing that the fat depots do not appreciably influence the main course of de-equilibration but only come into the picture as a slow component after the concentration in mixed venous blood has fallen to a low level.[68,69]

Whatever amount of anesthetic is transferred in a given breath from lungs to blood must be distributed to various organs and tissues in proportion to their respective blood flows. Thus, the rate of uptake by fat cannot exceed a small fraction of the rate of entry from lungs into blood, except in very obese patients, in whom a larger fraction of the cardiac output flows through fat. The blood, brain, and body water reach near equilibrium while fat is still far from equilibrium. Anesthetic is then transferred slowly from arterial blood to fat, and replaced at the same rate in the pulmonary capillary blood, without appreciable change in the blood concentration. Thus, once the blood and body water have been practically equilibrated, the anesthesiologist will be supplying anesthetic to the fat depots by way of the alveoli and blood, whose anesthetic concentrations remain essentially constant (x'_a, and x'_b, respectively).

When the anesthetic is discontinued, fat depots have just as little influence on the main course of de-equilibration and for the same reason (anesthetic flow from fat to blood being similarly limited by the total blood flow through fat). However, after the blood and body water have been largely cleared of anesthetic, we should expect a continued leakage from the fat depots, slowest and most prolonged in the case of agents with high S_L. Mixed venous blood should show traces of anesthetic long after the body water is essentially de-equilibrated. Such persistence in the venous blood is observed with cyclopropane (S_b

0.47, S_L 34) and chloroform (S_b 7.3, S_L 100), but not, apparently, with nitrous oxide (S_b 0.47, S_L 3.2) or ether (S_b 15, S_L 3.2).

Speed of Induction and Recovery in Clinical Anesthesia

Induction

The progressive deepening of anesthesia reflects the increasing concentration of anesthetic agent at the sites of action in the brain. By measuring the rate of increase of the concentration in internal jugular (venous) blood as it approaches that of common carotid (arterial) blood, it has been found that when the anesthetic concentration of arterial blood is kept constant, the brain reaches 90 percent of equilibrium in about 7 minutes. The rate of blood supply to brain tissue is reported[70] to be 350 ml kg^{-1} min^{-1}, while the mean figure for the rest of the body water is approximately 100 ml L^{-1} min^{-1}. One would therefore expect an equilibration rate about 3.5 times faster for brain than for body water as a whole. This conclusion based on the blood flow/volume ratio agrees fairly well with the theoretical prediction of 21 minutes for 90 percent equilibration of body water and the observed time of about 7 minutes for the same fraction of equilibrium in brain, both for agents of low solubility.

The relative rates of equilibration for both the brain and body water should be the same, regardless of the blood solubility of the anesthetic agent (i.e., regardless of whether the equilibration rate is slow or fast). The rate of induction of anesthesia is therefore determined by the same factors that govern the equilibration of body water, but it is faster. A patient will reach surgical anesthesia while the venous blood and body water are still far from equilibrium, and the fat depots farther still. Thereafter, anesthetic leaves the brain at the same rate it arrives, and the patient remains at the same depth of anesthesia while the venous blood and body water (and ultimately the fat depots) come to equilibrium. If a perfect, closed system is being used, one will find that early in anesthesia new anesthetic has to be furnished at a considerable rate. As time goes on, however, less and less has to be added to the system until, eventually, no new anesthetic is required. When the whole body is at equilibrium, the patient can rebreathe the same anesthetic gas while O_2 is supplied and CO_2 is absorbed.

Practical Induction with High-Solubility Agents

For agents of high solubility, such as ether and methoxyflurane, the theoretical induction time on our premise of maintaining the safe anesthetic gas concentration from the start would be so long (as shown earlier) that even the use of increased respiration would not make it a practical proposition. One alternative is to induce with higher gas concentrations (i.e., concentrations that are unsafe in the sense that continued administration would invariably lead to respiratory paralysis and death). At an appropriate time the concentration in the inspired air must be reduced to the safe anesthetic concentration. What the procedure accomplishes is to force large amounts of anesthetic rapidly into the arterial blood and thus establish a desired level of clinical anesthesia quickly. The rest of the body can then equilibrate over a long period of time while the depth of anesthesia is held constant. The procedure is exactly analogous to the use of priming doses; it is illustrated diagrammatically in Figure 4-31.

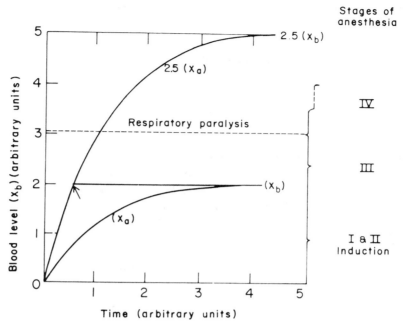

Fig. 4-31. Approach to equilibrium in stage III ($x_b = 2$) when safe anesthetic gas concentration is employed from start is shown by curve x_a. By using $2.5\ x_a$, the upper curve would theoretically be obtained, approaching $x_b = 5$, but respiratory failure would occur. If at arrow the anesthetic concentration in the inspired air is reduced to x_a, blood level $x_b = 2$ can be maintained. Thus, induction time can be reduced greatly.

Recovery

The speed of recovery from surgical anesthesia to full consciousness, reflecting the progressive de-equilibration of the brain, will be influenced by the same factors that determine the speed of induction. When a low-S agent is discontinued, the arterial blood concentration falls very quickly as venous blood is almost completely cleared of anesthetic at the lungs. A steep concentration gradient is thus provided, which, with the high blood flow/brain volume ratio, favors rapid transfer of brain anesthetic to the cerebral capillary blood, and consciousness is quickly regained.

When a high-S agent is discontinued after equilibration of the body water, the arterial concentration falls only slowly, and the de-equilibration of the brain tends to be limited by the rate of elimination of anesthetic from the whole of the body water. The way to accelerate the otherwise slow recovery from prolonged anesthesia with a high-S agent is to stimulate the respiration by administering CO_2 or to increase the rate of controlled respiration.

An excessive concentration of a high-S anesthetic in the blood, causing too deep an anesthesia, has very different implications depending upon the circumstances. If anesthesia has just been induced with concentrations greater than the safe anesthetic gas concentration and the anesthetic is stopped abruptly as soon as the condition is recognized (e.g., by depressed respiration), there will be a rapid outflow of drug from the brain into the blood, whose concentration is still much lower. Because the bulk of the brain is so small compared with the body water, such a redistribution will readily reduce the danger; indeed, the patient may return toward consciousness with surprising speed. This ability of the body water to act as a "sink" for anesthetic before equilibrium is established serves as a useful safety factor. For the same reason, however, it complicates induction because the depth of anesthesia responds quickly to transient fluctuations in the alveolar anesthetic concentration (e.g., those caused by breath-holding). On the other hand, as the blood and body water approach equilibrium, recovery takes ever longer. Control of the depth of anesthesia becomes easier, but respiratory paralysis late in anesthesia presents a far more serious problem, since now the whole of the body water acts as a buffer opposing outflow of anesthetic from the brain.

REFERENCES

1. Koch-Weser J: Serum drug concentrations as therapeutic guides. N Engl J Med 287:227, 1972
2. Wagner JG: Fundamentals of Clinical Pharmacokinetics. Drug Intelligence Publications, Hamilton, Ont., 1975
3. Sheiner LB, Tozer TN: Clinical pharmacokinetics: The use of plasma concentrations of drugs. Ch. 3. In Melman KL, Morelli AF (eds): Clinical Pharmacology; Basic Principles in Therapeutics. Macmillan, New York, 1978
4. Kety SS: Measurement of regional circulation by the local clearance of radioactive sodium. Am Heart J 38:321, 1949
5. Bederka J Jr, Takemori AE, Miller JW: Absorption rates of various substances administered intramuscularly. Eur J Immunol 15:132, 1971
6. Beyer KH, Russo HF, Tillson EK, et al: "Benemid," *p*-(di-*n*-propylsulfamyl)-benzoic acid: Its renal affinity and its elimination. Am J Physiol 166:625, 1951
7. Bray HG, Humphris BG, Thorpe WV, et al: Kinetic studies on the metabolism of foreign organic compounds. 6. Reactions of some nuclear-substituted benzoic acids, benzamides and toluenes in the rabbit. Biochem J 59:162, 1955
8. Goldstein DB: Pharmacology of Alcohol. Oxford University Press, New York, 1983
9. Pirola RC: Drug Metabolism and Alcohol. University Park Press, Baltimore, 1978
10. Holford NHG: Clinical pharmacokinetics of ethanol. Clin Pharmacokinet 13:273, 1987
11. Von Wartburg JP, Bethune JL, Vallee BL: Human liver alcohol dehydrogenase. Kinetic and physicochemical properties. Biochemistry 3:1775, 1964
12. Mourad N, Woronick CL: Crystallization of human liver alcohol dehydrogenase. Arch Biochem Biophys 121:431, 1967
13. Levy G: Pharmacokinetics of salicylate elimination in man. J Pharm Sci 54:959, 1965
14. Schentag JJ, Carra FB, Calleri GM, et al: Age, disease and cimetidine disposition in healthy subjects and chronically ill patients. Clin Pharmacol Therap 29:737, 1981
15. Dettli L: Individualization of drug dosage in patients with renal disease. Med Clin North Am 58:977, 1974
16. Goldstein A, Krayer O, Root MA, et al: Plasma neostigmine levels and cholinesterase inhibition in dogs and myasthenic patients. J Pharmacol Exp Ther 96:56, 1949
17. Gaddum JH: Repeated doses of drugs. Nature 153:494, 1944
18. Siddoway LA, McAllister CB, Wilkinson GR, et al: Amiodarone dosing: A proposal based on its pharmacokinetics. Am Heart J 106:951, 1983
19. Rakita L, Sobol SM, Mostow N: Amiodarone treatment for refractory arrhythmias: Dose-ranging and importance of high initial dosage. p. 143. In Breithardt G, Loogen F (eds): New Aspects in the Medical Treatment of Tachyarrhythmias. Urban & Schwarzenberg, Munich, 1983
20. Holt DW, Tucker GT, Jackson PR, Storey GCA: Amiodarone pharmacokinetics. Am Heart J 106:840, 1983

21. Gillis AM, Kates RE: Clinical pharmacokinetics of the newer antiarrhythmic agents. Clin Pharmacokinet 9:375, 1984

22. Kalow W, Gunn DR: The relation between dose of succinylcholine and duration of apnea in man. J Pharmacol Exp Ther 120:203, 1957

23. Palmer JW, Clarke HT: The elimination of bromides from the blood stream. J Biol Chem 99:435, 1933

24. Söremark R: The biological half-life of bromide ions in human blood. Acta Physiol Scand 50:119, 1960

25. Kehoe RA, Cholak JC, Hubbard OM, et al: Experimental studies on lead absorption and excretion and their relation to the diagnosis and treatment of lead poisoning. J Ind Hyg Toxicol 25:71, 1943

26. Schimke RT, Sweeney EM, Berlin CM: The roles of synthesis and degradation in the control of rat liver tryptophan pyrrolase. J Biol Chem 240:322, 1965

27. Berlin CM, Schimke RT: Influence of turnover rates on the responses of enzymes to cortisone. Mol Pharmacol 1:149, 1965

28. Conney AH, Burns JJ: Factors influencing drug metabolism. Adv Pharmacol 1:31, 1962

29. Arias IM, De Leon A: Estimation of the turnover rate of barbiturate side chain oxidation enzyme in rat liver. Mol Pharmacol 3:216, 1967

30. Richens A, Dunlop A: Serum phenytoin levels in the management of epilepsy. Lancet 2:247, 1975

31. Ludden TM, Allen JP, Valutsky WA, et al: Individualization of phenytoin dosage regimens. Clin Pharmacol Ther 21:287, 1977

32. Neubig RR: PHARMKIN: A Pharmacokinetics Teaching Simulation. University of Michigan Software, Ann Arbor, 1987

33. Teorell T: Kinetics of distribution of substances administered to the body. I. The extravascular modes of administration. II. The intravascular modes of administration. Arch Int Pharmacodyn Ther 57:205, 226, 1937

34. Gibaldi M, Prescott L (eds): Handbook of Clinical Pharmacokinetics. ADIS Health Science Press, Sydney, 1983

35. Bray HG, Thorpe WV, White K: Kinetic studies of the metabolism of foreign organic compounds. 5. A mathematical model expressing the metabolic fate of phenols, benzoic acids and their precursors. Biochem J 52:423, 1952

36. Chisholm GD, Waterworth PM, Calnan JS, Garrod LP: Concentration of antibacterial agents in interstitial tissue fluid. Br Med J 1:569, 1973

37. Welling PG: Pharmacokinetics; Process and Mathematics. American Chemical Society, Washington, 1986, Ch. 14

38. Reuning RH, Sams RA, Notari RE: Role of pharmacokinetics in drug dosage adjustment. I. Pharmacologic effect, kinetics and apparent volume of distribution of digoxin. J Clin Pharmacol 13:127, 1973

39. Benowitz NL: Clinical applications of the pharmacokinetics of lidocaine. Cardiovasc Clin 6:77, 1974

40. Thomson AH, Elliott HL, Kelman AW, et al: The pharmacokinetics and pharmacodynamics of lignocaine and MEGX in healthy subjects. J Pharmacokinet Biopharm 15:101, 1987

41. Hull CJ, Vanbeem HBH, McLeod K, et al: A pharmacodynamic model for pancuronium. B J Anaesth 50:1113, 1978

42. Sheiner LB, Stanski DR, Vozeh S, et al: Simultaneous modeling of pharmacokinetics and pharmacodynamics. Applications to *d*-tubocurarine. Clin Pharmacol Ther 25:358, 1979

43. Holford NHG, Sheiner LB: Understanding the dose-effect relationship: Clinical application of pharmacokinetic-pharmacodynamic models. Clin Pharmacokinet 6:429, 1981

44. Swerdlow BN, Holley FO: Intravenous anesthetic agents: Pharmacokinetic-pharmacodynamic relationships. Clin Pharmacokinet 12:79, 1987

45. Scott JC, Ponganis KV, Stanski DR: EEG quantitation of narcotic effect: The comparative pharmacodynamics of fentanyl and alfentanil. Anesthesiology 62:234, 1985

46. Bower S, Hull CJ: Comparative pharmacokinetics of fentanyl and alfentanil. Br J Anaesth 54:871, 1982
47. Mitenko PA, Ogilvie RI: Rational intravenous doses of theophylline. N Engl J Med 289:600, 1973
48. Levy G: Relationship between rate of elimination of tubocurarine and rate of decline of its pharmacological activity. Anaesthesia 36:694, 1964
49. Wagner JG: Relations between drug concentration and response. J Mond Pharm 14:279, 1971
50. Nagashima R, O'Reilly RA, Levy G: Kinetics of pharmacologic effects in man: The anticoagulant effect of warfarin. Clin Pharmacol Ther 10:22, 1969
51. Powers WF, Abbrecht PH, Covell DG: Systems and microcomputer approach to anticoagulant therapy. IEEE Trans Biomed Eng 27:520, 1980
52. Boudinot FD, D'Ambrosio R, Jusko WJ: Receptor-mediated pharmacodynamics of prednisolone in the rat. J Pharmacokinet Biopharm 14:469, 1986
53. Goldstein A, Judson BA, Sheehan P: Cellular and metabolic tolerance to an opioid narcotic in mouse brain. Br J Pharmacol 47:138, 1973
54. Vandyke C, Jatlow P, Ungerer J, et al: Oral cocaine: Plasma concentration and central effects. Science 200:211, 1978
55. Attia RR, Grogno AW, Domer FR: Practical Anesthetic Pharmacology. Appleton-Century-Crofts, E. Norwalk, CT, 1987
56. Larson Jr CP, Eger II EI, Severinghaus JW: Ostwald solubility coefficients for anesthetic gases in various fluids and tissues. Anesthesiology 23:686, 1962
57. Riggs DS: The Mathematical Approach to Physiological Problems. Williams & Wilkins, Baltimore, 1963
58. Riggs DS, Goldstein A: Equation for inert gas exchange which treats ventilation as cyclic. J Appl Physiol 16:531, 1961
59. Kety SS: The physiological and physical factors governing the uptake of anesthetic gases by the body. Anesthesiology 11:517, 1950
60. Kety SS: The theory and applications of the exchange of inert gas at the lungs and tissues. Pharmacol Rev 3:1, 1951
61. Eger EI: Effect of inspired anesthetic concentration on the rate of rise of alveolar concentration. Anesthesiology 24:153, 1963
62. Eger EI: Applications of a mathematical model of gas uptake. Ch. 8. In Papper EM, Kitz RJ (eds): Uptake and Distribution of Anesthetic Agents. McGraw-Hill, New York, 1963
63. Epstein RM, Rackow H, Salanitre E, Wolf GL: Influence of the concentration effect on the uptake of anesthetic mixtures: The second gas effect. Anesthesiology 25:364, 1964
64. Overton E: Studien über die Narkose zugleich ein Beitrag zur allgemeinen Pharmakologie. Gustav Fischer, Jena, 1901, p. 101
65. Meyer KH, Hemmi H: Beiträge zur Theorie der Narkose. III. Biochem. Z. 277:39, 1935
66. Fink BR: Diffusion anoxia. Anesthesiology 16:511, 1955
67. Schloerb PR, Friis-Hansen BJ, Edelman IS, et al: The measurement of total body water in the human subject by deuterium oxide dilution. J Clin Invest 29:1296, 1950
68. Jones HB: Respiratory system: Nitrogen elimination. Med Phys 2:855, 1950
69. Robertson JS, Siri WE, Jones HB: Lung ventilation patterns determined by analysis of nitrogen elimination rates; use of the mass spectrometer as a continuous gas analyzer. J Clin Invest 29:577, 1950
70. Kety SS: Quantitative determination of cerebral blood flow in man. Methods Med Res 1:204, 1948

5

Pathways of Drug Metabolism

Alvito P. Alvares
William B. Pratt

After their entry into the body, most drugs are substrates for chemical reactions that change their physical properties and biologic effects.[1-3] These metabolic conversions, which usually affect the polarity of the compound, profoundly alter the way in which drugs are distributed in and excreted from the body. In some cases metabolism of the drug is required for the therapeutic effect. This is often seen with anticancer drugs of the antimetabolite class, for example, which must be converted to their active forms after they are transported into the cancer cell. In most cases, metabolism is accompanied by some loss in therapeutic activity, and often a single metabolic conversion renders a drug therapeutically inactive, either because it no longer occupies the receptor site or because it no longer reaches its site of action. In addition to affecting clinically desirable drug responses, metabolism may result in the generation of toxic forms of a drug or lead to its detoxification. We will consider the subject of drug metabolism in three stages. In this chapter we will discuss many of the ways in which drugs are chemically altered and provide examples of how the alterations affect drug distribution and elimination. In Chapter 6 we will discuss the biochemistry of the microsomal drug-metabolizing system, the genes encoding the enzymes in the system, and the mechanisms through which the activity of the system is regulated by a variety of factors, including other drugs. In Chapter 7 we will review a variety of ways in which genetic differences between individuals determine therapeutically significant differences in the way they metabolize drugs.

Since most drugs undergo metabolic transformation, the biochemical reactions that have to be considered under the heading of drug metabolism are numerous and diverse. The main site of drug metabolism is the liver, although other tissues may also participate. A feature characteristic of nearly all these transformations is that the metabolic products are more polar than the parent drugs. This has an important consequence for renal and biliary excretion, and it may also have evolutionary significance. Substances with high lipid/water partition coefficients, which pass easily across membranes, also diffuse back readily from the tubular urine through the renal tubular cells into the plasma, and such substances therefore tend to have a very low renal clearance and a long persistence in the body. If such a drug is metabolized to a more polar compound, one with a much lower partition coefficient, its tubular reabsorption will be reduced greatly. Moreover, as we have seen in Chapter 3, the specific secretory mechanisms for anions and cations in the proximal renal tubules and in the parenchymal liver cells operate upon highly polar substances. Oxidation of a methyl group to carboxyl, for example, could make a drug suitable for the renal or biliary secretory pathway; that single metabolic alteration could reduce the biologic half-life of the drug from many hours to a few minutes. Conjugation of a relatively nonpolar drug with sulfate anion could have a similar effect. The evolutionary implication is that drug metabolizing systems have developed as adaptations to terrestrial life. Fish and other marine organisms do have some of the microsomal drug-metabolizing systems found in mammals, but they can also excrete lipid-soluble exogenous and endogenous compounds directly into the surrounding water across the gill membranes.

Decreased lipid solubility of a drug metabolite does not necessarily mean increased water solubility. The antibacterial sulfonamides, for example, are metabolized to more polar, less lipid-soluble acetyl derivatives, but some of these are less water-soluble than their parent compounds. Sulfathiazole, for example, is transformed to acetylsulfathiazole, which is much less soluble in water than sulfathiazole itself:

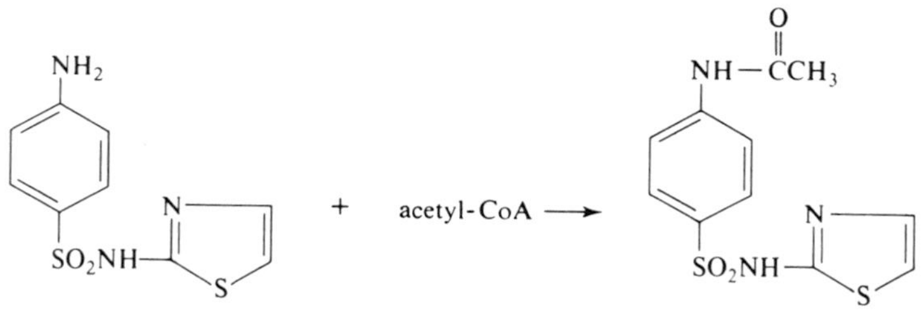

sulfathiazole   acetylsulfathiazole

At pH 5.5 the water solubility of sulfathiazole is 960 μg ml^{-1}, that of the acetylated derivative only 60 μg ml^{-1}. The reduced water solubility of acetylsulfathiazole led to such serious toxicity from precipitation in the renal tubules that sulfathiazole was abandoned in favor of sulfonamides with more favorable properties.

A comment is in order concerning the representation of drug metabolic pathways in this chapter. All intermediates, even if they are known, will not necessarily be shown. For the sake of simplicity, weak electrolytes will be represented in their nonionized forms; it will be understood that, depending on their pK_a values, they may actually be ionized to a substantial degree at physiologic pH.

Sometimes a polar drug yields a less polar product. An example is the deacetylation of acetanilid to aniline, to be discussed shortly. Another example is the reduction of the hypnotic drug chloral hydrate to the pharmacologically active trichloroethanol:

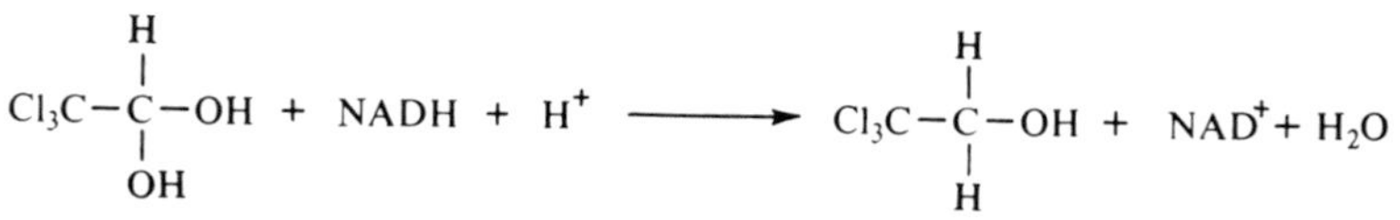

chloral hydrate   trichloroethanol

Usually, however, the same enzyme (alcohol dehydrogenase) would mediate the oxidation of an alcohol to a more polar aldehyde, passing electrons to NAD^+, the reverse of the reaction shown here.

Some typical and atypical features of drug metabolism are illustrated in Figure 5-1. Phenacetin (acetophenetidin) and acetanilid are mild analgesic and antipyretic agents that were in clinical use for over half a century. Studies of their metabolism have revealed that both compounds are transformed in the body to a more polar metabolite, *p*-hydroxyacetanilid (acetaminophen), which is widely used as an analgesic and antipyretic drug today.[4,5] As shown in the figure, acetanilid undergoes hydroxylation at the para position on the benzene ring, whereas phenacetin undergoes *O*-dealkylation.

Since the major metabolite, acetaminophen, is an antipyretic analgesic in its own right, it seemed possible that this metabolite was the only active compound, and that the two

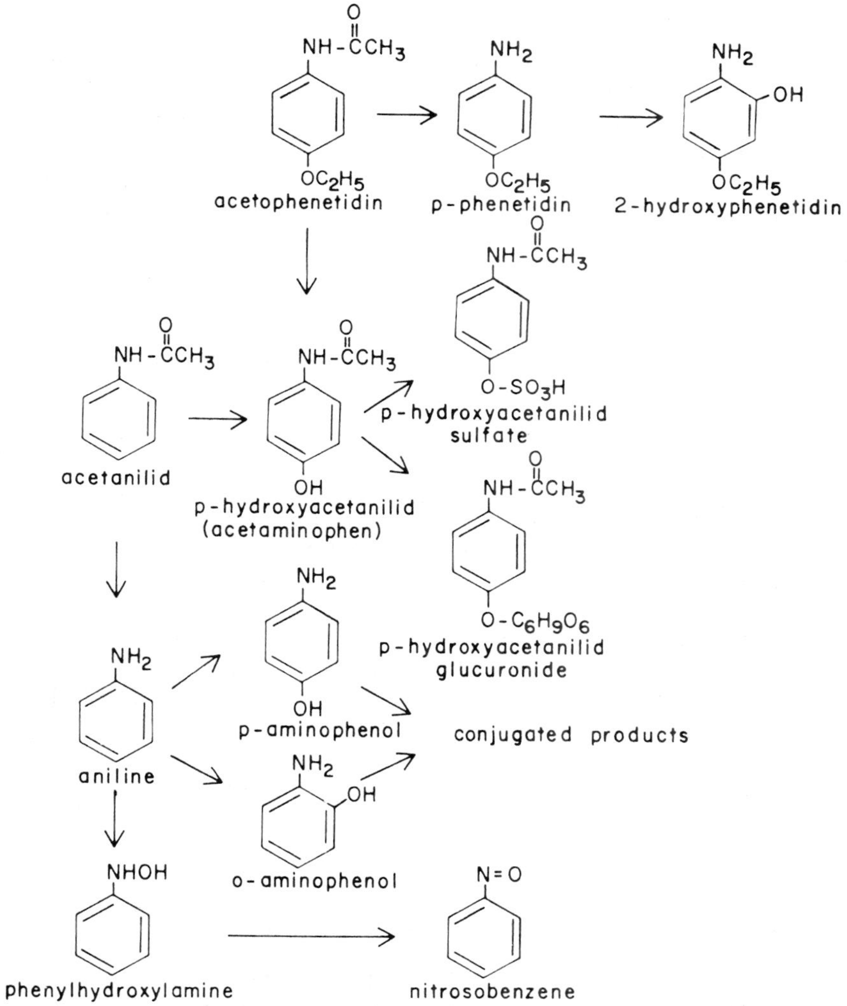

Fig. 5-1. Metabolism of acetanilid and phenacetin.

older, established drugs were inert. This has been tested by inhibiting the metabolism of phenacetin by means of SKF 525A (to be discussed in detail later in this chapter). The results indicated that the unmetabolized phenacetin did have antipyretic activity.[6]

The further metabolism of acetaminophen entails typical conjugation reactions, yielding a sulfate ester and a glucuronide, both highly polar compounds. The conjugates appear in the urine and are pharmacologically inert. When a dose of acetanilid is given to a person, the successive metabolites peak and decay in the plasma sequentially. During the first hour, acetanilid is the principal plasma component. In the second hour, as the acetanilid level falls, the acetaminophen concentration reaches a peak. Finally, after a few hours the principal plasma component is conjugated acetaminophen. This sequence illustrates the importance of determining separately the plasma concentrations of a drug and of all its metabolites if meaningful information is to be obtained, since some metabolites may be pharmacologically active and some may be inert.

Both phenacetin and acetanilid are also metabolized to a minor extent by deacetylation of the amino group, yielding aniline derivatives, which may then be further transformed to aminophenols (which are eventually conjugated) or to phenylhydroxylamine.

The well-known toxic effect of acetanilid on red blood cells affords an excellent illustration of how the main pharmacologic action of a drug and its apparent toxicity may inhere in different chemical entities, the one a metabolic product of the other. After ordinary doses of acetanilid a small amount of methemoglobinemia is often seen, and after large doses of the drug there may be extensive methemoglobin formation and destruction of erythrocytes. This toxic action is not caused by acetanilid itself or by acetaminophen but by aniline produced metabolically in the body. Aniline itself does not produce methemoglobin in vitro, but its metabolites, phenylhydroxylamine and nitrosobenzene (Fig. 5-1), can do so.[7]

The principal aim in studies of drug metabolism is to identify the pathways by which drugs are transformed in the body and to ascertain quantitatively the importance of each pathway and intermediate. To define a pathway such as that shown in Figure 5-1, each of the metabolites must be separated from the others and then accurately identified and quantitated. The most useful methods for separating metabolites are based on differences in their polarities and charges. The unchanged drug and its metabolites in blood serum, urine, feces, or a body fluid or tissue extract are most commonly separated from each other by gas chromatography or high-pressure liquid chromatography. Fractions separated by chromatography are then submitted to multiple analytical procedures, such as spectrophotometry, fluorometry, mass spectrometry, and nuclear magnetic resonance spectrometry, to identify and quantitate each species. Radioactive forms of drugs are also used extensively to study drug metabolism. Regions of a drug are often labeled with an isotope such as carbon 14 or tritium, and the radiolabeled compound is administered to animals or humans. The appearance of radioactivity in various metabolites isolated from blood, feces and urine, or in the case of animals in extracts from specific tissues, permits integration of both metabolic and pharmacokinetic data to yield a very sophisticated and dynamic view of how the body handles the compound.

PHASE I REACTIONS OF DRUG METABOLISM

The reactions involved in drug metabolism are often classified into two groups (Table 5-1). Phase I (or functionalization) reactions consist of oxidative and reductive reactions that alter and create new functional groups and hydrolytic reactions that cleave esters

Table 5-1. Classification of Pathways of Drug Metabolism

Phase I reactions (functionalization reactions):

Oxidation via the hepatic microsomal P450 system
    Aliphatic oxidation
    Aromatic hydroxylation
    N-Dealkylation
    O-Dealkylation
    S-Dealkylation
    Epoxidation
    Oxidative deamination
    Sulfoxide formation
    Desulfuration
    N-Oxidation and *N*-hydroxylation
    Dehalogenation

Oxidation via nonmicrosomal mechanisms
    Alcohol and Aldehyde oxidation
    Purine oxidation
    Oxidative deamination (monoamine oxidase
      and diamine oxidase)

Reduction
    Azo and nitro reduction

Hydrolysis
    Ester and amide hydrolysis
    Peptide bond hydrolysis
    Epoxide hydration

Phase II reactions (conjugation reactions):

Glucuronidation

Acetylation

Mercapturic acid formation

Sulfate conjugation

N-, *O*-, and *S*-methylation

Trans-sulfuration

and amides to release masked functional groups. These changes are usually in the direction of increased polarity. The phase II reactions are conjugation reactions in which the drug, or most often a metabolite, is coupled to an endogenous substrate such as glucuronic acid, acetic acid, or sulfuric acid. In this section we will discuss the phase I reactions, beginning with the oxidative reactions, which are by far the most common. The oxidative reactions are listed in Table 5-1, and the detailed pathways and mechanisms will be presented later. First we shall consider the properties and characteristics of the microsomal drug-metabolizing system that catalyzes the oxidative transformations.[8]

The Liver Microsomal Drug-Metabolizing System

The oxidative metabolism of many drugs and also of steroid hormones is mediated by enzymes located in the microsomal fraction of mammalian liver, consisting of fragments of endoplasmic reticulum.[8] Liver is homogenized, and the homogenate is centrifuged at 9,000 to 12,000 g for 30 minutes. Then the supernatant solution is centrifuged at 105,000 g for 1 hour, and the sediment is collected. The microsome fraction thus obtained contains a family of closely related hemoproteins known as cytochromes P450, which act as terminal oxidases for a variety of oxidative reactions that drugs undergo. The term P450 refers to the ability of the reduced (ferrous) form of the hemoprotein to react with carbon monoxide, yielding a complex with an absorption peak at 450 nm.

In an in vitro system containing liver microsomes, various drugs can be oxidized provided NADPH and O_2 are present. The requirement for reduced pyridine nucleotide and for molecular oxygen categorizes the enzyme system as a mixed-function oxidase (also called monooxygenase). One molecule of O_2 is consumed for each molecule of substrate oxidized; one atom of O is introduced into the substrate, and the other is reduced to form H_2O. The overall reaction may be formulated as follows, where A is the oxidized form and AH_2 is the reduced form of cytochrome P450.

1. $NADPH + A + H^+ \rightarrow AH_2 + NADP^+$
2. $AH_2 + O_2 \rightarrow$ "active oxygen complex"
3. "active oxygen complex" + drug substrate $\rightarrow$ oxidized drug + A + H_2O

$$NADPH + O_2 + \text{drug substrate} + H^+ \rightarrow NADP^+ + \text{oxidized drug} + H_2O$$

The electron flow pathway has been partially worked out, and a simplified scheme is seen in Figure 5-2. Here NADPH is oxidized by the flavoprotein NADPH-cytochrome P450 reductase, forming $NADP^+$ and resulting in transfer of an electron through the flavoprotein to the oxidized form of cytochrome P450, which has already interacted with the drug substrate. The flavoprotein is able to transfer electrons to cytochrome c or other electron acceptors (methylene blue, menadione) if they are added to the incubation mixture. Such electron acceptors therefore inhibit drug oxidations while leaving NADPH oxidation unaffected or even accelerating it.

The solubilization, separation, and partial purification of microsomal NADPH-cytochrome P450 reductase and cytochrome P450 in 1968 by Lu and Coon[9] permitted for the

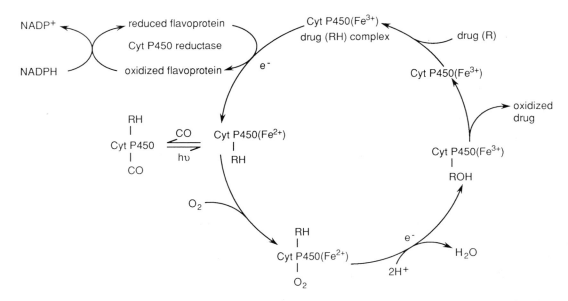

Fig. 5-2. Electron flow pathway in the microsomal drug-oxidizing system.

first time the reconstitution of the cytochrome P450-mediated monooxygenase system. The requirement for NADPH-cytochrome P450 reductase in reconstituting maximal hydroxylation activities for various substrates demonstrated the role for this flavoprotein in cytochrome P450-mediated reactions. The reductase was originally called *NADPH-cytochrome c reductase*; however, since cytochrome *c* is not present in microsomes and plays no role in drug oxidations, the name *NADPH-cytochrome P450 reductase* is more appropriate and is the one that will be used here. Purified rat liver cytochrome P450 reductase contains 1 mole of flavin mononucleotide (FMN) and 1 mole of flavin adenine dinucleotide (FAD) per mole of apoprotein and has a molecular weight of 78,000 daltons.

The only other component necessary for activity in reconstituted systems is a phospholipid, phosphatidylcholine. The phospholipid is not directly involved in electron transfer but appears to be involved in the coupling of the reductase and P450 and in the binding of the substrate to the cytochrome. The reconstituted system has been used to demonstrate that the substrate specificity of the liver monooxygenases is determined primarily by cytochrome P450. NADPH-cytochrome P450 reductase and microsomal lipids from a variety of microsomal sources are generally interchangeable. Although some studies have shown that the metabolism of some substrates can be enhanced by the presence of cytochrome b_5, cytochrome P450 is by far the most important factor in determining substrate specificity.

In contrast to the liver, in the adrenal gland monooxygenase system electrons are transferred from the flavoprotein, termed *NADPH-adrenodoxin reductase*, to cytochrome P450 through an iron sulfide protein termed adrenodoxin. The adrenal monooxygenase system localized in the mitochondria appears to metabolize only endogenous substrates, such as 11-deoxycorticosterone and cholesterol. NADPH-adrenodoxin reductase isolated from bovine adrenal mitochrondria has been shown to be immunologically distinct from liver microsomal NADPH-cytochrome P450 reductase.[10]

Multiple cytochrome P450 isoenzymes have been purified from animal and human livers. Each of the cytochrome P450 isoenzymes from rat liver microsomes has its own characteristic but often overlapping substrate specificity for the metabolism of different xenobiotics (Table 5-2).[11,12] Thus, the relative rates of detoxification and metabolic activation of diverse foreign chemicals will depend on the relative amounts of the various P450 isoenzymes that are present in an organism.

The active site of cytochrome P450 has long been known to contain a single iron protoporphyrin IX prosthetic group. Studies on the events leading up to substrate oxidation have resulted in general acceptance of the catalytic cycle depicted in Figure 5-2. The salient features of the catalytic cycle involve an initial binding of the substrate to the oxidized (Fe^{3+}) state of P450 to give a P450-drug complex. The complex then undergoes a one-electron reduction, the electron being derived from NADPH via cytochrome P450 reductase. The reductase reaction is considered to be rate-limiting; reductase activity is enhanced by adding many substrates. Molecular oxygen then binds to give a reduced (Fe^{2+}) cytochrome P450-dioxygen complex. This is followed by a transfer of a second electron from cytochrome P450 reductase or of an electron from NADH via cytochrome b_5 to the complex. Next, cleavage of the oxygen-oxygen bond occurs concurrently with incorporation of an oxygen atom into a molecule of water, the transfer of the second oxygen atom to the substrate, and the dissociation of the oxidized product.

Oxycytochrome P450, $O_2 \cdot P450(Fe^{2+}) \cdot RH$, can dissociate to give a superoxide anion, $O_2^{\cdot-}$, concomitantly with regeneration of the ferric hemoprotein $P450(Fe^{3+}) \cdot RH$. Dioxygen (O_2) is thought to be toxic to tissues because of its ability to generate free radicals.[13]

Table 5-2. Metabolism of Xenobiotics and Steroids by Purified Cytochrome P450 Isozymes
from Rat Liver Microsomes

Substrate	P450a	P450b	P450c	P450d	P450e	P450f	P450g	P450h	P450i	P450j
					$(nmol \cdot min^{-1} \cdot nmol\ P\text{-}450^{-1})$					
Benzphetamine	2.3	132.5	6.7	3.9	19.8	1.3	4.9	52.1	2.8	5.5
Hexobarbital	<0.5	42.7	0.9	<0.5	8.2	<0.5	<1.1	22.6	1.0	<0.5
Benzo[a]pyrene	0.2	0.4	23.4	0.3	0.1	<0.1	<0.1	1.8	<0.1	<0.1
Zoxazolamine	0.9	3.3	60.8	21.1	1.1	0.9	<0.5	7.4	0.7	3.4
Estradiol-17β	<0.5	<0.5	1.7	13.8	0.9	0.5	0.6	8.0	1.3	0.8
7-Ethoxycoumarin	0.6	9.6	97.1	0.6	2.0	<0.5	1.1	0.9	0.7	1.2
p-Nitroanisole	<0.5	1.8	21.6	0.7	<0.5	<0.5	<0.5	1.5	<0.5	1.6
Aniline	<0.5	1–2	1–2	9.6	<0.5	<0.5	<0.5	1–2	<0.5	12.7
5α-Androstane-3α,17β-diol-3,17-disulfate	<0.1	<0.1	<0.1	<0.1	<0.1	<0.1	<0.1	<0.1	4.8	<0.1

Catalytic activity was determined under conditions such that metabolism was proportional to hemoprotein concentration and time of incubation. A high substrate concentration, saturating NADPH–cytochrome c reductase concentration, and optimal dilauroylphosphatidylcholine concentrations were used in all experiments. The reactions measured were: benzphetamine N-demethylation, hexobarbital 3-hydroxylation, benzo[a]pyrene 3- and 9-hydroxylation, zoxazolamine 6-hydroxylation, estradiol 2-hydroxylation, 7-ethoxycoumarin O-deethylation, p-nitroanisole O-demethylation, aniline 4-hydroxylation, and 5α-androstane 3α,17β-diol-3,17-disulfate 15β-hydroxylation.
(Adapted from Ryan et al.[11] and Conney,[12] with permission.)

Dioxygen readily undergoes one-electron reduction in biologic systems, resulting in formation of O_2^-. This reaction may occur nonenzymatically, or it may be catalyzed by numerous enzymes such as NADPH–cytochrome P450 reductase, xanthine oxidase, and several mitochondrial enzymes. Once formed, superoxide may produce further reduction products known collectively as *reactive oxygen* or *oxyradicals*. Superoxide may damage mammalian cells and tissues either directly (i.e., by inactivating enzymes) or indirectly by stimulating lipid peroxidation. The sequential four-electron reduction of dioxygen may be depicted as:

$$O_2 \xrightarrow{e^-} O_2^- \xrightarrow{e^-} H_2O_2 \xrightarrow{e^-} \cdot OH \xrightarrow{e^-} H_2O$$

Superoxide, hydrogen peroxide, and especially the highly reactive hydroxyl radical (·OH) are individually and collectively toxic to tissues and cells. Normally, tissues have defense mechanisms that can protect them against the toxic effects of oxyradicals. Among these are superoxide dismutase, catalase, and glutathione peroxidase. However, when these defenses are overwhelmed, as in oxygen toxicity or paraquat poisoning, toxic levels of various oxyradicals accumulate in tissues.

Association of substrate to oxidized cytochrome P450 can be followed spectrophotometrically.[14] This association will for some compounds produce a type I difference spectrum (Fig. 5-3), which shows a trough at about 420 nm and a peak at 385 nm, or a type II difference spectrum, which shows a trough at about 394 nm and a peak at about 430 nm.[15] Type I ligands are believed to bind at a hydrophobic site in the protein in close proximity to the heme iron, whereas type II ligands interact directly with the heme iron. Some drugs, such as hexobarbital and ethylmorphine, yield a type I difference spectrum, whereas others, such as aniline and acetanilid, yield a type II difference spectrum. In some cases the rate of metabolism has been shown to be proportional to the binding of the substrate to microsomal cytochrome P450. However, similarities between the spectral

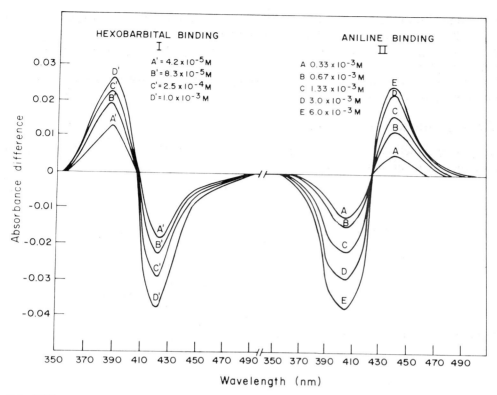

Fig. 5-3. Difference spectra for binding of drugs to P450. Spectra represent differences in absorption at each wavelength between ligand-free and ligand-bound cytochrome P450 at various drug concentrations. Type I binding spectra are typified by hexobarbital (at left), type II by aniline (at right). (From Mannering,[15] with permission.)

dissociation constant and the Michaelis constant K_m for the oxidation of the substrate appear not to be the general rule.

Although the liver is the major site of cytochrome P450–mediated oxidations, such biotransformations can also occur in extrahepatic tissues. The sites of extrahepatic drug metabolism are often the portals of entry or excretion of xenobiotics (e.g., the lung, kidney, skin, and intestinal mucosa). Even though extrahepatic metabolism may not be important in all phases of drug disposition, metabolism in these tissues can play an important role in determining target organ toxicity. Toxicity may be mediated in extrahepatic tissues by the parent compound or by a chemically reactive metabolite that is either generated directly in the target organ or in the liver followed by transport of the toxic metabolite to the target organ. Within a tissue itself, there may be differences in cellular or subcellular distribution of monooxygenases. In the adrenal cortex the mitochondrial fractions catalyze side-chain cleavage, and 11β-hydroxylation and 18-hydroxylation of cholesterol, while the microsomal fractions are responsible for 17α-hydroxylation and 21-hydroxylation of steroid hormones (see Fig. 7-14).

A number of xenobiotics, including some drugs, would remain in the body indefinitely were it not for phase I and phase II enzymes of biotransformation. As indicated previously, during phase I metabolism one or more polar groups (e.g., hydroxyl, carboxyl, or amino) are introduced into the parent molecule, thereby presenting phase II enzymes (e.g., glucuronosyltransferases) with a substrate. The oxidative biotransformations catalyzed by liver microsomal enzymes are the most important enzymic reactions involved in phase I metabolism of drugs.

Now we shall examine typical examples of the oxidative transformations catalyzed by the liver microsomal enzyme system.

Side-Chain (Aliphatic) Oxidation

The principal metabolites of pentobarbital in dogs and humans are alcoholic derivatives, formed by side-chain oxidation:

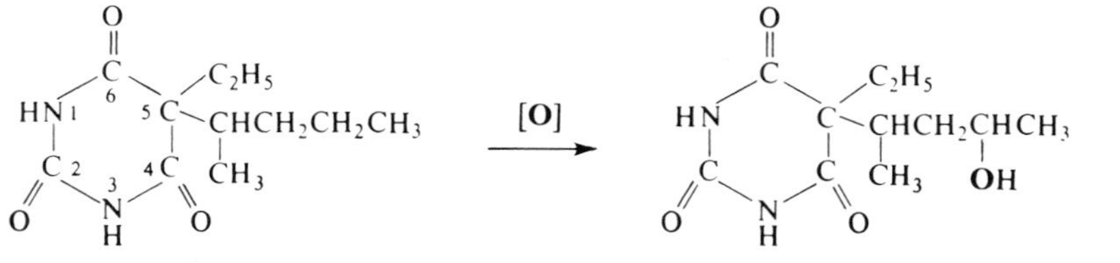

pentobarbital

[O]

5-ethyl-5-(3'-hydroxy-1'-methylbutyl) barbituric acid

Carboxylic acids may also occur as minor metabolites:

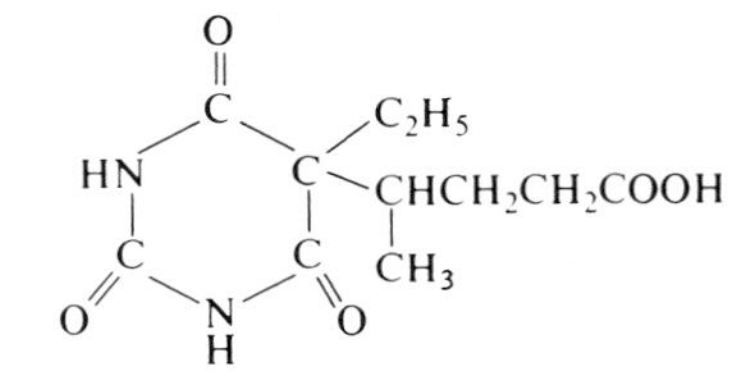

5-ethyl-5-(3'-carboxy-1'-methylpropyl) barbituric acid

In aliphatic oxidations the products of the microsomal system are alcohols. Further oxidation to aldehydes and carboxylic acids requires the soluble enzymes alcohol dehydrogenase and aldehyde dehydrogenase.

Side-chain oxidation of a slightly different kind is seen with the N_1-methylated barbiturate hexobarbital. This compound, which has a cyclohexenyl ring attached to position 5, is oxidized to a keto derivative:

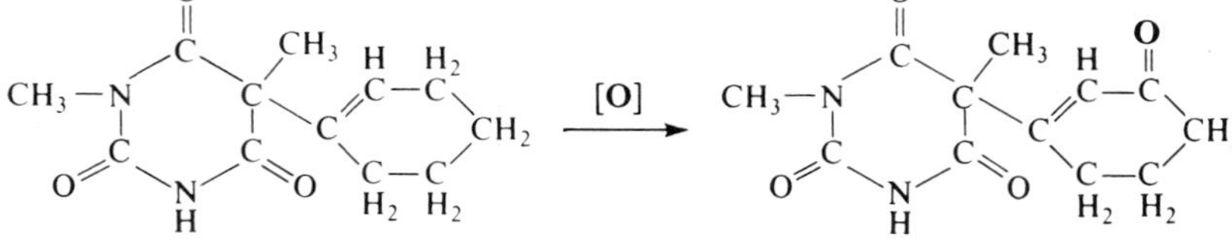

hexobarbital

[O]

5-(3'-oxocyclohexen-1'-yl)-1, 5-dimethylbarbituric acid

Aromatic Hydroxylation

The conversion of acetanilid to *p*-hydroxyacetanilid illustrates hydroxylation in the aromatic ring:

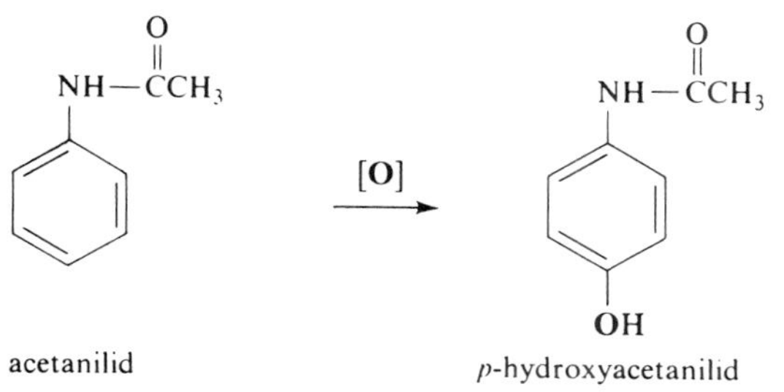

acetanilid   *p*-hydroxyacetanilid

The reaction occurs through the formation of an epoxide intermediate. The P450-catalyzed reaction forms the epoxide, which then spontaneously (nonenzymatically) forms the corresponding aromatic hydroxide. Steroid hormones such as testosterone and estradiol-17β are also hydroxylated by a liver microsomal system requiring NADPH,[16] probably the same system that oxidizes drugs. Hydroxylations of non-lipid-soluble metabolic intermediates (e.g., phenylalanine, tyrosine) are carried out by entirely different enzyme systems.

N-Dealkylation

N-Methyl, *N*-ethyl, and *N*-alkyl groups in general can be removed oxidatively and converted to aldehydes (formaldehyde, acetaldehyde, etc.). The initial oxidative step forms a hydroxyalkyl congener, which spontaneously breaks down to form the corresponding noralkyl compound and an aldehyde. The reactions are clearly different from the usual single-carbon transfers in intermediary metabolism, which involve either *S*-adenosylmethionine or a folic acid derivative. The conversion of ethylmorphine to norethylmorphine illustrates this reaction:

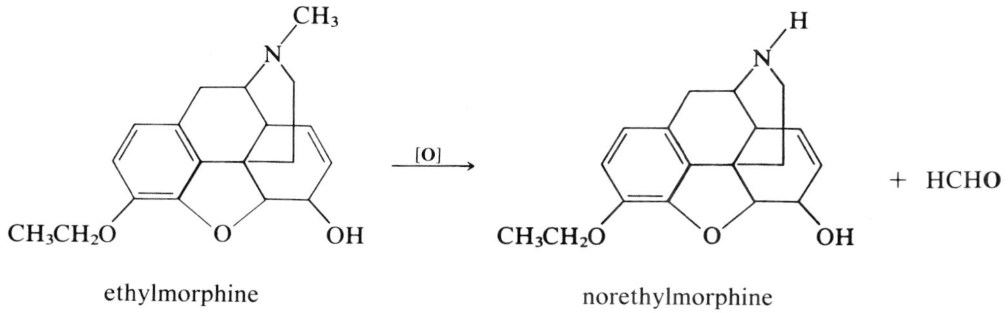

ethylmorphine   norethylmorphine

The prefix *nor* referring to products of *N*-dealkylation, comes from the German *N ohne Radikal* ("nitrogen without a radical"), meaning a primary amine derived from *N*-alkyl.

O-Dealkylation

Aromatic ethers are cleaved as in the following reaction:

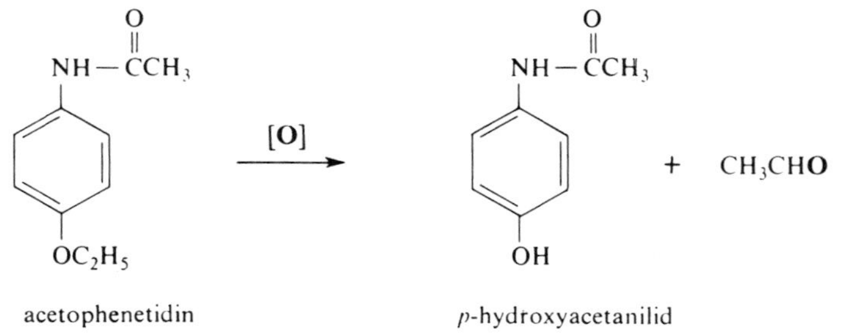

acetophenetidin   *p*-hydroxyacetanilid

S-Demethylation

An oxidative reaction similar to *N*- or *O*-demethylation occurs with certain methyl thioethers:

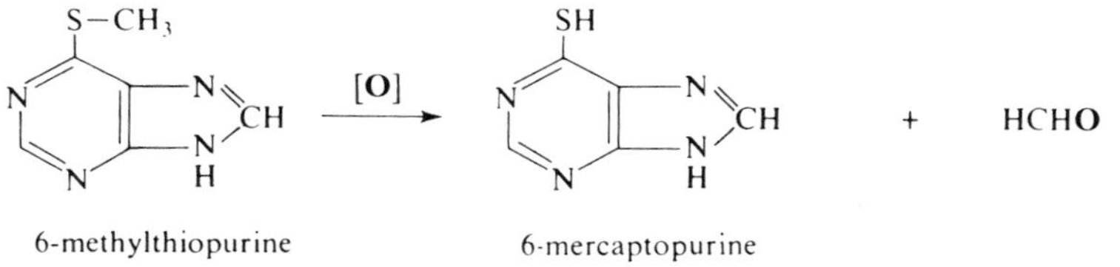

6-methylthiopurine   6-mercaptopurine

Epoxidation

Many aromatic or olefinic compounds are metabolized to arene or alkene oxides. The carcinogenic polycyclic hydrocarbon benzo[a]pyrene is metabolized to several epoxides. For simplicity, only the metabolism of the hydrocarbon at the 4,5 (K region) and 7,8 (non-K region) double bonds is shown:

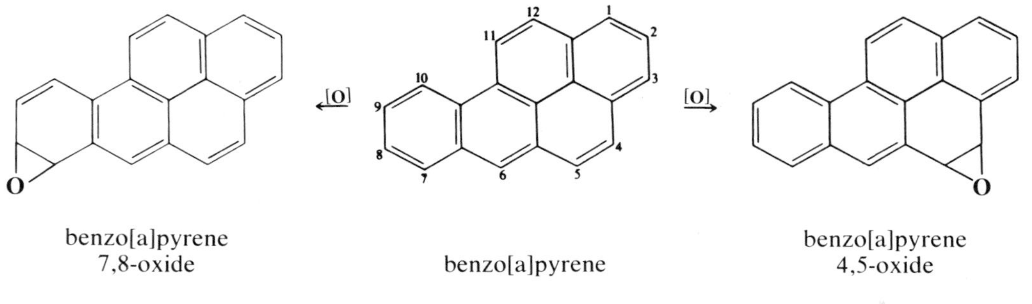

benzo[a]pyrene
7,8-oxide   benzo[a]pyrene

benzo[a]pyrene
4,5-oxide

Arene oxides can be hydrated enzymatically by microsomal epoxide hydrolase, or they can undergo nonenzymatic isomerization to phenols, be conjugated with glutathione, and also react with DNA, RNA, and proteins to form covalently bound products (see Figure 12-7 and discussion in Chapter 12 for mechanism of reaction with DNA).

Oxidative Deamination

The metabolism of amphetamine to phenylacetone by rabbit liver is an example of oxidative deamination:

amphetamine   phenylacetone

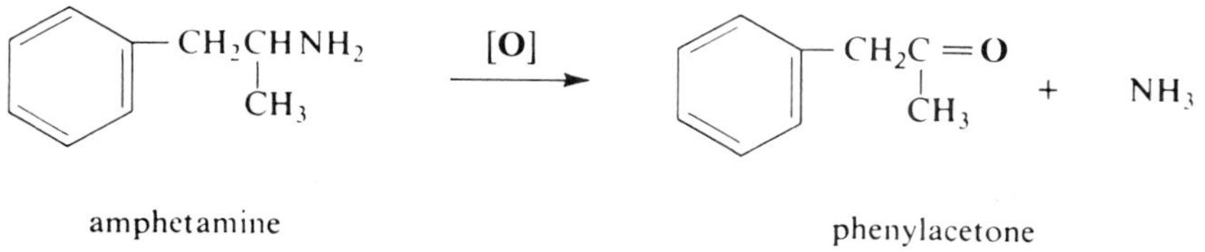

In the dog and rat, however, amphetamine undergoes *p*-hydroxylation of the benzene ring rather than deamination.

Sulfoxide Formation

Thioethers in general are oxidized to sulfoxides, as shown below:

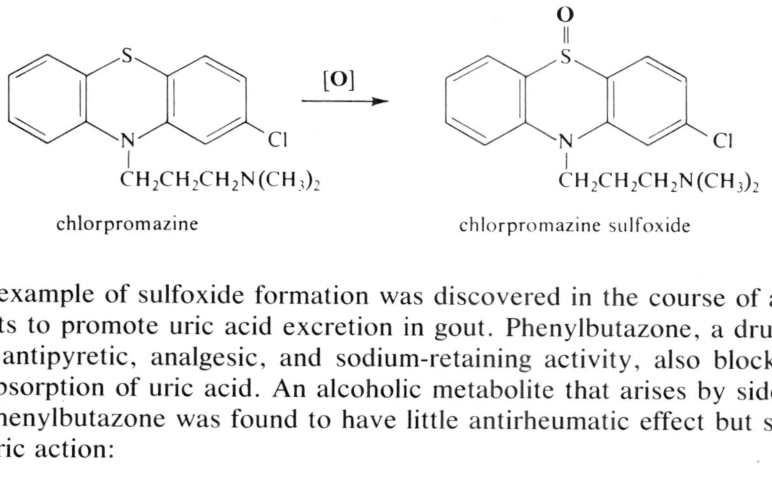

chlorpromazine   chlorpromazine sulfoxide

Another example of sulfoxide formation was discovered in the course of a search for better agents to promote uric acid excretion in gout. Phenylbutazone, a drug with anti-rheumatic, antipyretic, analgesic, and sodium-retaining activity, also blocks the renal tubular reabsorption of uric acid. An alcoholic metabolite that arises by side-chain oxidation of phenylbutazone was found to have little antirheumatic effect but still retained the uricosuric action:

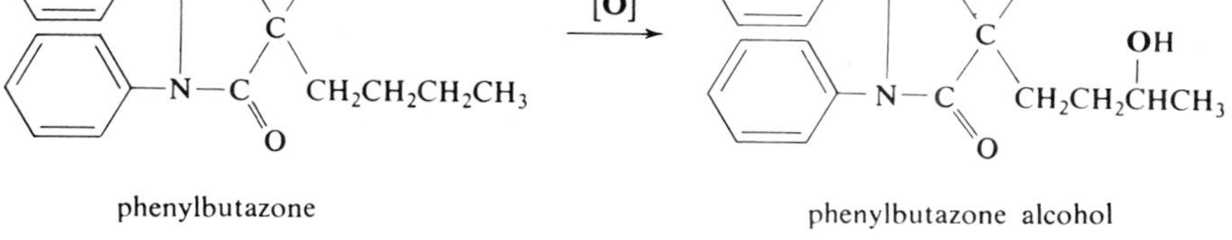

phenylbutazone   phenylbutazone alcohol

Manipulations of the side chain of phenylbutazone alcohol led to the discovery that sulfur-containing derivatives had marked uricosuric action. One of these, the 4-phenylthioethyl analog of phenylbutazone, was found to be metabolized by sulfoxide formation to yield an even more potent uricosuric drug, sulfinpyrazone[17]:

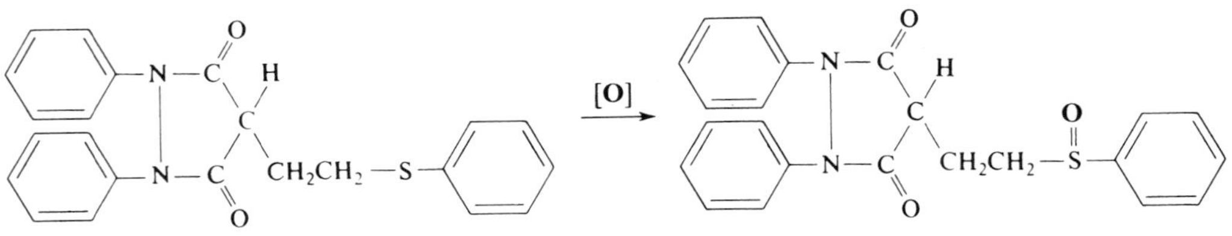

phenylbutazone thio derivative   sulfinpyrazone

Sulfinpyrazone came into therapeutic use as a selectively uricosuric drug, practically devoid of antirheumatic, analgesic, and sodium-retaining activity. It is also used as an antiplatelet drug.

Desulfuration

An example of desulfuration is the conversion of parathion to its oxygen analog, par-aoxon. Parathion is used as an insecticide, but it is biologically inert; it depends for its effectiveness upon oxidative desulfuration in the insect, and for its toxicity to mammals upon oxidative desulfuration in the liver:

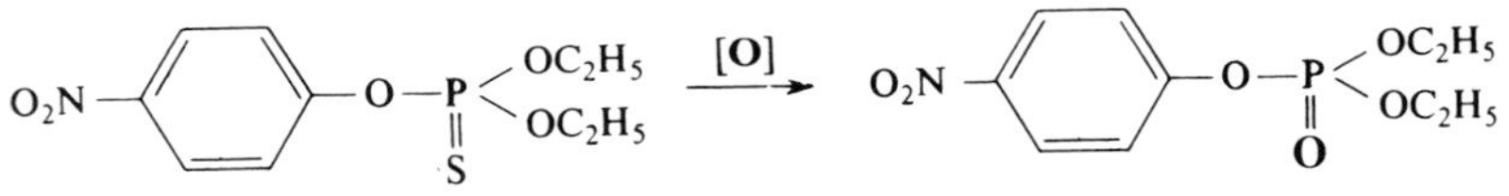

parathion   paraoxon

In this reaction the specificity of the pyridine nucleotide remains uncertain. In contrast to the widely accepted belief that NADPH is the preferred cofactor, several workers have reported NADH to be equal to or even more efficient than NADPH in desulfuration of thionate insecticides. Otherwise, it resembles the usual drug oxidations; the system is found in microsomes and requires oxygen.

N-Oxidation and *N*-Hydroxylation

N-Oxidation is exemplified by the oxidative conversion of trimethylamine to its *N*-oxide:

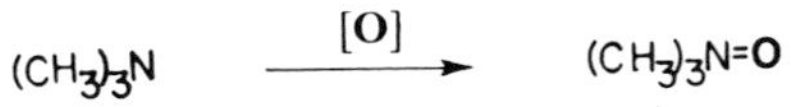

$$(CH_3)_3N \xrightarrow{[O]} (CH_3)_3N{=}O$$

trimethylamine   trimethylamine *N*-oxide

Secondary and tertiary amines are oxidized by microsomal enzymes that require NADPH and molecular oxygen, but it is becoming clear that there is a special amine oxidase present (a flavoprotein distinct from NADPH-cytochrome *c* reductase), which is responsible for these oxidations.[18] The amine oxidase is a mixed-function oxidase, and cytochrome P450 appears not to be involved. Secondary amines are converted to hydroxylamines and tertiary amines to amine oxides.

When the carcinogenic compound 2-acetylaminofluorene is administered to rats or other animal species in which it produces cancer, an *N*-hydroxy metabolite is formed:

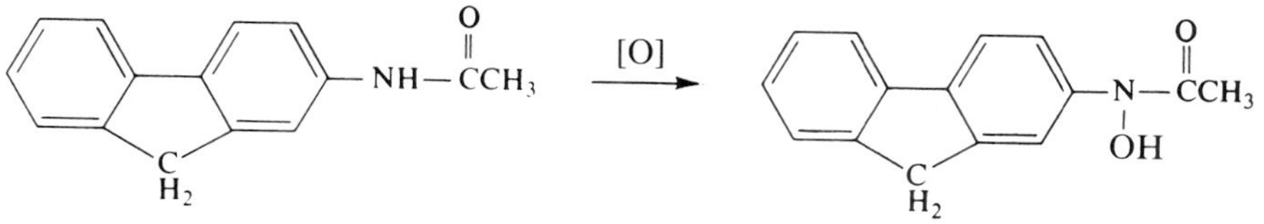

2-acetylaminofluorene   *N*-hydroxy derivative of
2-acetylaminofluorene

N-Hydroxy-2-acetylaminofluorene is not itself, nor is the parent compound, an ultimate carcinogen. A sulfate ester of the *N*-hydroxy metabolite is an intermediate in the formation of the ultimate carcinogen, ester formation being catalyzed by a cytoplasmic sulfotransferase.[19] Accordingly, 2-acetylaminofluorene is not a hepatic carcinogen in the guinea pig, a species with a very low sulfotransferase activity.

Dehalogenation

Certain halogenated insecticides, anesthetics, and other compounds can undergo dehalogenation in the animal body. Halogenated aliphatic hydrocarbons possess pharmacologically useful properties in the case of the anesthetic agents. Humans may also be exposed to halogenated aliphatic hydrocarbons through environmental contamination, and some of these compounds, such as carbon tetrachloride, are important toxicants.

The dehalogenation of carbon tetrachloride to chloroform has been shown to involve the cytochrome P450 monooxygenase system. Carbon tetrachloride is thought to undergo a cytochrome P450-catalyzed one-electron reduction to yield a trichloromethyl radical. In the endoplasmic reticulum the trichloromethyl radical may abstract a hydrogen atom from the lipid membrane to yield chloroform and initiate oxygen consuming lipid peroxidation.

$$CCl_4 + e^- \xrightarrow[\text{NADPH}]{\text{P450}} \cdot CCl_3 + Cl^-$$
carbon tetrachloride

$$\cdot CCl_3 + RH \longrightarrow CHCl_3 + R\cdot$$
chloroform

Alternatively, the trichloromethyl radical may react with oxygen to form a trichloromethyl peroxy radical (CCl_3–O–O·), which may be converted to phosgene.

$$\cdot CCl_3 + O_2 \rightarrow CCl_3\text{-O-O}\cdot$$
trichloromethyl peroxy radical

$$CCl_3\text{-O-O}\cdot \rightarrow COCl_2 + \text{electrophilic Cl}$$
phosgene

The CCl_3–O–O· radical may also initiate lipid peroxidation. The findings that chloroform formation from carbon tetrachloride is inhibited by cobaltous chloride[20] and that phenobarbital administration markedly enhances the acute toxicity of carbon tetrachloride[21] strongly suggest that cytochrome P450 is the site of its bioactivation.

The halogenated anesthetics, such as halothane, fluroxene, and methoxyflurane, have been shown to be metabolized to a significant extent in humans and experimental animals. Generally the carbon-fluorine bond has been found to be more stable than the carbon-

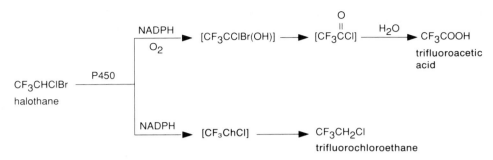

Fig. 5-4. In vivo metabolism of halothane by P450.

chlorine bond. Nevertheless, substantial amounts of the free fluoride ion have been found in humans and experimental animals after methoxyflurane administration, sufficient to implicate the fluoride ion in cases of renal toxicity (polyuric renal inefficiency).[22]

Halothane is metabolized in vivo by cytochrome P450 via both oxidative (approximately 90 percent) and reductive (approximately 10 percent) pathways (Fig. 5-4).[23] About 15 percent of halothane that is not exhaled undergoes biotransformation. Oxidative metabolism of halothane proceeds by insertion of oxygen into the carbon-hydrogen bond to generate an unstable dihalocarbinol, which collapses to trifluoroacetyl chloride via dehydrobromination. Subsequent reaction of the intermediate acyl chloride with water yields trifluoroacetic acid. Reductive carbon-bromine bond rupture is proposed to yield 1,1,1-trifluoro-2-chloroethyl radical ($CF_3\dot{C}HCl$), which undergoes reduction to yield 1,1,1-trifluoro-2-chloroethane (see review by MacDonald[23]).

Drug Oxidations That Are Not Mediated by the Liver Microsomal System

Alcohol and Aldehyde Oxidation

Alcohol dehydrogenase and aldehyde dehydrogenase are rather nonspecific enzymes found in the soluble fraction of liver, which catalyze several important oxidative transformations. The substrates include some compounds normally found in the body, for example, the alcohol vitamin A and the aldehyde retinene. Ethyl alcohol and its metabolite acetaldehyde are oxidized by this pair of enzymes, as are a variety of other alcohols and aldehydes.

$$C_2H_5OH + NAD^+ \xrightarrow{\text{alcohol dehydrogenase}} CH_3CHO + NADH + H^+$$
Ethanol $\qquad\qquad\qquad\qquad\qquad\qquad\qquad$ Acetaldehyde

$$CH_3CHO + NAD^+ + H_2O \xrightarrow{\text{aldehyde dehydrogenase}} CH_3COOH + NADH + H^+$$
Acetaldehyde $\qquad\qquad\qquad\qquad\qquad\qquad\qquad$ Acetic acid

Alcohol dehydrogenase, located in the liver cytosol, catalyzes the conversion of ethanol to acetaldehyde in a reaction that requires NAD as a cofactor. The acetaldehyde produced in the reaction is further converted to acetate by aldehyde dehydrogenase. Alternate pathways for ethanol oxidation are the cytochrome P450–dependent microsomal ethanol-oxidizing system (MEOS)[24] and the catalase present in various cell fractions, including peroxisomes and microsomes. The quantitative role of these alternate pathways is probably small under normal conditions. However, there is an adaptive increase of the MEOS during chronic ethanol consumption.[25] The MEOS is localized in the endoplasmic reticulum and utilizes NADPH and oxygen.

Regular drinkers tolerate large amounts of alcoholic beverages, mainly because of central nervous system adaptation. In addition, alcoholics develop increased rates of blood ethanol clearance, so-called metabolic tolerance. Chronic treatment of rabbits with ethanol results in the induction of a unique new isoenzyme of cytochrome P450, termed *P450 3a*. This isoenzyme displays the highest activity of all rabbit isoenzymes in the oxidation of ethanol to acetaldehyde.[26] Isolation and purification of this form of cytochrome P450 have provided strong support for a microsomal pathway distinct from the reactions catalyzed by alcohol dehydrogenase and catalase. A variety of observations indicate that the 3a form of P450 is a unique gene product, but it is not yet possible to evaluate the relative physiologic significance of the MEOS in alcohol disposition. The MEOS may play a significant role in chronic ethanol consumption (see Chapter 10 for discussion of ethanol tolerance).

Purine Oxidation

Several purine derivatives (e.g., 6-mercaptopurine, theophylline, caffeine) are known to undergo oxidation in vivo. A major pathway for metabolism of mercaptopurine involves the enzyme xanthine oxidase, which oxidizes it to 6-thiouric acid, a noncarcinostatic metabolite. Theophylline is metabolized in humans primarily to 1,3-dimethyluric acid, 1-methyluric acid, and 3-methylxanthine.[27]

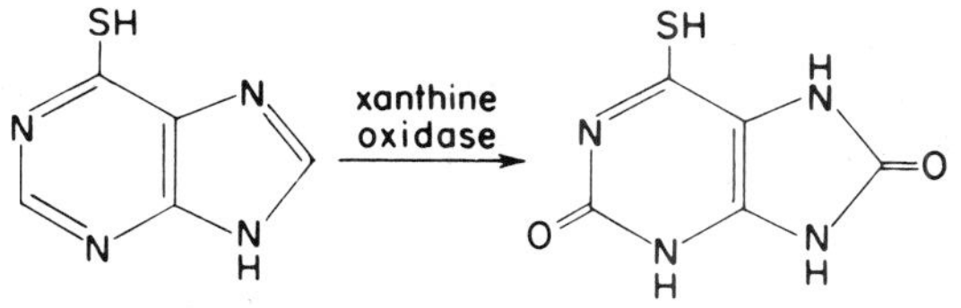

6-mercaptopurine → (xanthine oxidase) → 6-thiouric acid

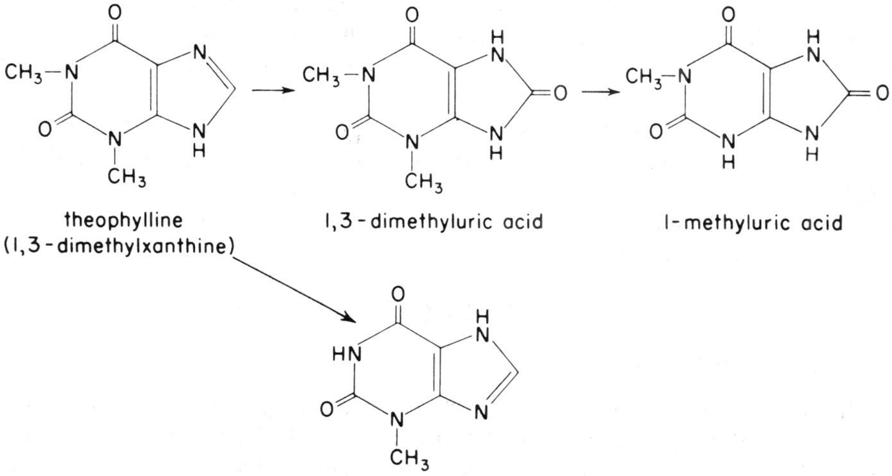

theophylline (1,3-dimethylxanthine) → 1,3-dimethyluric acid → 1-methyluric acid

3-methylxanthine

The oxidative metabolism of theophylline can be affected by inducers and inhibitors of cytochrome P450–mediated oxidations, which indicates a major role for this enzyme system in theophylline metabolism, possibly through *N*-demethylation of theophylline to 3-methylxanthine. While some monomethylxanthines are substrates for xanthine oxidase, it seems well established that dimethylxanthines and caffeine are not oxidized by this enzyme.

Monoamine Oxidase (MAO) and Diamine Oxidase (DAO)

The similar enzymes monoamine oxidase (MAO) and diamine oxidase (DAO)[28,29] oxidatively deaminate several naturally occurring amines as well as a number of drugs. The reaction products are aryl or alkyl aldehydes, which are usually oxidized further by other enzymes to the corresponding carboxylic acids. MAO is a mitochondrial enzyme found especially in liver, kidney, intestine, and nervous tissue; its substrates include phenylethylamine, tyramine, catecholamines (dopamine, norepinephrine, epinephrine), and tryptophan derivatives (tryptamine, serotonin):

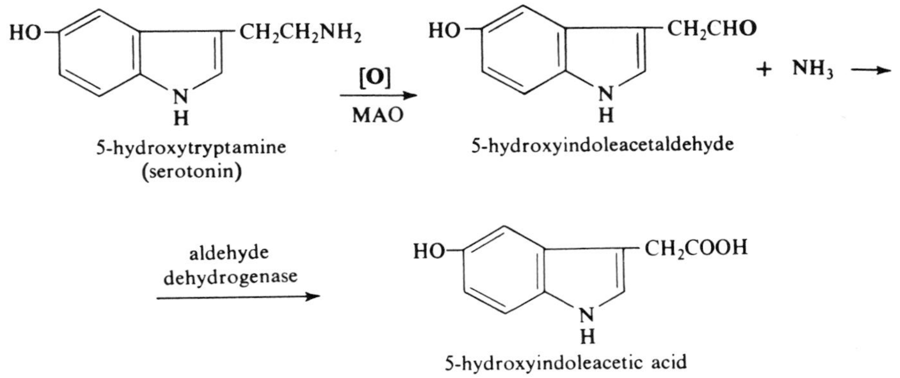

5-hydroxytryptamine
(serotonin)

5-hydroxyindoleacetaldehyde

aldehyde
dehydrogenase

5-hydroxyindoleacetic acid

Other simple amines, both aryl and alkyl, are attacked by MAO, a relatively nonspecific enzyme, but not all amines are good substrates. Amphetamine, for example, and any other phenylethylamine derivative carrying a methyl group on the α carbon atom, are not oxidized well.

DAO also converts amines to aldehydes in the presence of oxygen. Its substrate specificity overlaps that of MAO. Good substrates include histamine and polymethylene diamines, $H_2N-(CH_2)_n-NH_2$. In the latter series the most rapid oxidation is seen at $n = 4$ (putrescine) and $n = 5$ (cadaverine). The enzyme is found in bacteria and higher plants and in the soluble cell fractions of liver, intestine, and placenta.

Reduction

Azo and Nitro Reduction

Azo reduction is illustrated by an important historical example. The era of specific antibacterial chemotherapy began with the introduction of Prontosil, an azo dye, for the treatment of streptococcal and pneumococcal infections. Subsequently it was discovered that the active drug was not Prontosil itself but a metabolite, sulfanilamide (*p*-amino-benzenesulfonamide):

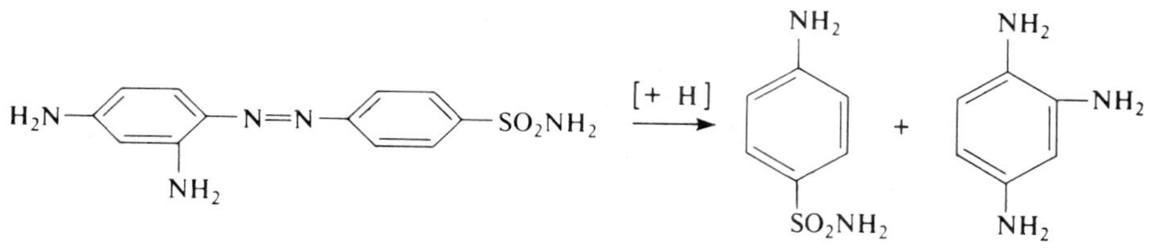

prontosil   sulfanilamide

Nitro reduction is also illustrated well by an antibacterial agent, the antibiotic chloramphenicol, which is transformed in part to an amine by bacterial and mammalian nitro reductase systems:

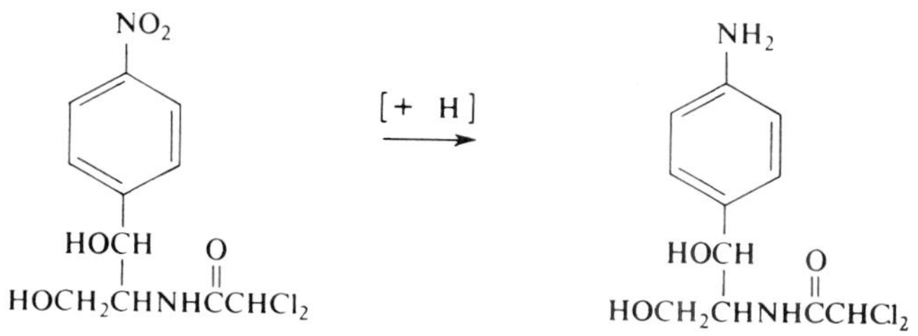

chloramphenicol   chloramphenicol reduction product

The subcellular distribution of nitrobenzene reductase activity indicates the existence of two different enzyme systems, one localized in the endoplasmic reticulum and the other in the cytosol of liver cells.[30] The activity in the cytosol is mainly attributable to xanthine oxidase, which converts nitrobenzene to its hydroxyamino derivative, and this reaction is inhibited by allopurinol. Studies with antibodies to NADPH-cytochrome *c* reductase and cytochrome P450, using reconstitution systems, showed that the reduction of nitrobenzene to an intermediate, possibly nitrosobenzene or phenylhydroxylamine, is catalyzed by NADPH-cytochrome *c* reductase, whereas the conversion of this intermediate to aniline requires cytochrome P450. These reactions were carried out under anaerobic conditions. To what extent reductive reactions occur in vivo is not known.

Oxygen tension in the liver may not be uniform, and under certain conditions (e.g., anesthesia) the oxygen tension may even be lower than normal. The capacity for reductive reactions may be rather weak in mammalian tissues, and in instances in which extensive reduction does occur (e.g., with Prontosil), intestinal anaerobic bacteria appear to be largely responsible.

Hydrolysis

Hydrolysis of Esters and Amides

Drug metabolism by hydrolysis occurs with esters and amides. The numerous hydrolytic enzymes (esterases and amidases) are found in blood plasma and other tissues, including the liver. After cell fractionation by differential centrifugation, the esterases that hydrolyze carboxyl and amide esters are localized primarily in the microsomal fraction of tissues such as liver, kidney, and brain. Occasionally, the bulk of liver carboxylesterase activity is found in the soluble fraction. This has been attributed to autolysis, which readily solubilizes the membrane-bound carboxylesterases.[32] Enzymes prepared from different tissues or different species can have widely differing substrate specificities. The hydrolysis of the local anesthetic procaine by liver and plasma cholinesterase is illustrative:

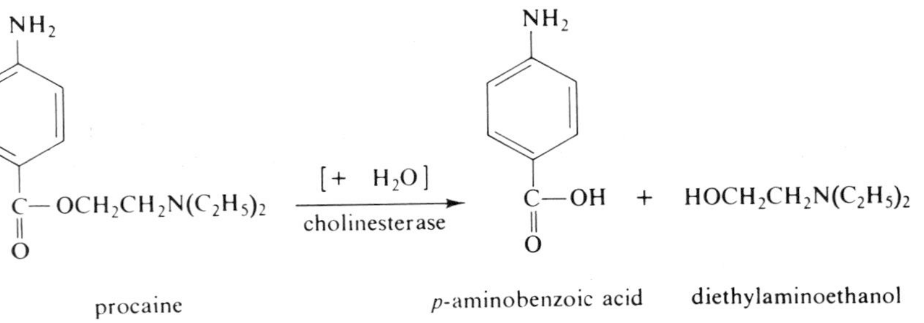

procaine → p-aminobenzoic acid + diethylaminoethanol

$$\xrightarrow[\text{cholinesterase}]{[+\ H_2O]}$$

When the amide bond –CONH– is hydrolyzed, an acid and an amine are formed instead of an acid and an alcohol (as in the hydrolysis of an ester). Procainamide, the amide analog of procaine, is hydrolyzed in the tissues much more slowly than procaine, and not at all in plasma. Most amides are hydrolyzed more slowly than the corresponding esters.

Not all esters undergo hydrolysis in the body. Atropine, for example, is hydrolyzed to an insignificant extent in mice and humans. Enzymes responsible for hydrolysis of esters include acetylcholinesterase, plasma cholinesterase, and even carbonic anhydrase, which has been shown to catalyze the hydrolysis of esters of α- and β-naphthol in addition to its better known role in the hydration of CO_2. The hydrolysis of succinylcholine by plasma cholinesterase is an important example of rapid termination of drug effect by metabolic cleavage; some interesting examples of genetic variation in plasma cholinesterase, leading to altered drug responses, will be discussed in Chapter 7.

Hydrolysis of Peptide Bonds

Although peptides such as insulin and growth hormone have been administered as drugs for many years, recombinant DNA technology has permitted introduction of a variety of human peptide hormones and growth factors into therapy. Once inside the body, peptides are subject to hydrolysis by a wide range of *peptidases*,[32,33] each with its own substrate specificity.

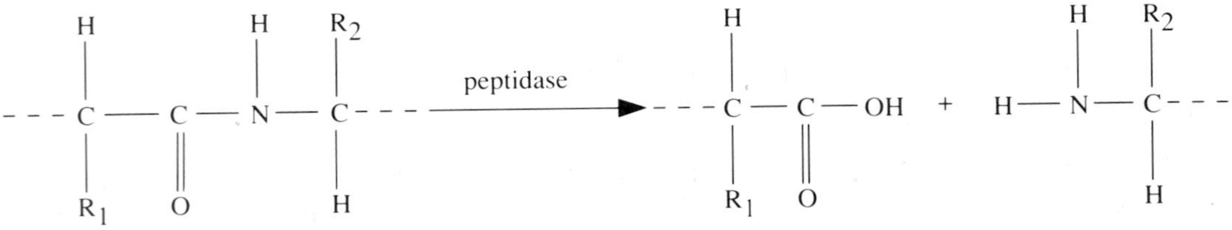

Table 5-3. Specificity of Some Common Peptidases[a]

Enzyme	Substrate Site
	↓
Aminopeptidases	NH_2-L-amino acid—X – – –
Carboxypeptidases	– – – X—XCOOH
Chymotrypsin	– – – Phe or Tryp or Tyr—X – – –
Elastase	– – – Ala or Gly—X – – –
Thrombin	– – – Arg—Gly – – –
Trypsin	– – – Arg or Lys—X – – –

[a] Aminopeptidases cleave at L-amino acids except for proline. Chymotrypsin is specific for those peptide linkages in which the carbonyl function is contributed by aromatic amino acid residues, such as phenylalanine, tryptophan, or tyrosine. The vertical arrow points to the peptide bond that is cleaved, and X represents any amino acid.

Some examples of peptidases are given in Table 5-3. Cleavage may occur only at one terminus of the peptide, as with aminopeptidases and carboxypeptidases, or it may occur internally (endopeptidases). As peptide hormones must reach their sites of action on surface receptors of target cells, peptidases located in the plasma (e.g., aminopeptidases), at the vascular endothelium (e.g., angiotensin-converting enzyme), in the interstitial fluid (e.g., aminopeptidases), and at cell surfaces (e.g., aminopeptidases and carboxypeptidases) are the most important in terms of the immediate drug effect. After a peptide is taken either into target cells or into the cells of a major organ of clearance, such as liver or kidney, the endopeptidases in the lysosomes play the major role in metabolism (see Chapter 3 for discussion of receptor-mediated endocytosis and the fate of internalized peptides).

Considerable effort is being devoted to attempts to modify peptides so as to minimize their hydrolysis at extracellular sites and thereby increase both efficacy and duration of action. Several approaches may be taken. If a major site of cleavage has been identified, then amino acid substitutions may be made that will result in a decreased hydrolysis rate with retention of receptor-binding activity. Many peptidases do not cleave peptide bonds when one of the adjacent amino acid units is in the D configuration or when it is a proline; therefore, common strategies in the design of more stable peptide hormones and growth factors include replacement of L with D amino acids, replacement with proline, and N-methylation at the peptide nitrogen. The incorporation of D-Ala[2], MeTyr[1], and MePhe[4] in Met-enkephalin, for example, increases stability. Together with introduction of a chiral sulfoxide group, these modifications increase the oral activity of Met-enkephalin from a negligible level to a level that is nearly equivalent to that of morphine.[34] Substitution of the amino terminus of a peptide (e.g., by acylation or alkylation) or alteration of its carboxy terminus (e.g., by reduction or amide formation) hinders attack by exopeptidases. The effect of terminus modification is seen with an analog of the tripeptide thyrotropin-releasing hormone in which a cyclized N-terminal pyroglutamic acid residue and a C-terminal amide hinder attack by exopeptidases[35] while substitution of the proline ring with two methyl groups prevents attack by an amidase.[36] Obviously, the genetic engineers and medicinal chemists who are designing such analogs must achieve a favorable balance between metabolic stability and potential impairment of intrinsic potency at the level of the receptor such that the modified drug is therapeutically better than the original hormone or growth factor.

Epoxide Hydration

Many drugs, mutagens, and environmental carcinogens are aromatic or olefinic compounds that can be oxidized by the cytochrome P450 enzymes to biologically active epoxides (Fig. 5.5). These reactive epoxides and arene oxides can be hydrated enzymatically to transdihydrodiols. The hydration of epoxides is catalyzed by epoxide hydrolase (epoxide hydrase, epoxide hydratase). The substrate specificity of the hydrolase is very broad. The purified rat enzyme can hydrate a variety of alkene oxides, such as styrene 7,8-oxide, as well as arene oxides of polycyclic aromatic hydrocarbons, such as benzo[a]pyrene. The role of epoxide hydrolase can be either beneficial or harmful depending on the particular metabolic pathways involved and whether the resulting oxide intermediates are substrates for the enzyme. For example, the presence of epoxide hydrolase effectively eliminates the mutagenicity of benzo[a]pyrene 4,5-oxide by catalyzing its transformation to a relatively nonmutagenic product, benzo[a]pyrene 4,5-dihydrodiol. In this case, the role of epoxide hydrolase is to inactivate a harmful product. On the other hand, the hydration of benzo[a]pyrene 7,8-oxide by the enzyme results in the formation of benzo[a]pyrene 7,8-dihydrodiol, which, like the 7,8-oxide, is weakly mutagenic. Benzo[a]pyrene 7,8-dihydrodiol is, however, the substrate for a second monooxygenation step, resulting in the formation of the 7,8-diol-9,10-epoxide with the epoxide oxygen in the so-called bay region of the hydrocarbon (see Fig. 12-7). As we discuss later in Chapter 12, this bay region diol epoxide is highly mutagenic and carcinogenic.[37,38] The role of epoxide hydrolase in this case is one of activation to a potentially harmful product, which is the precursor of an ultimately formed carcinogen.

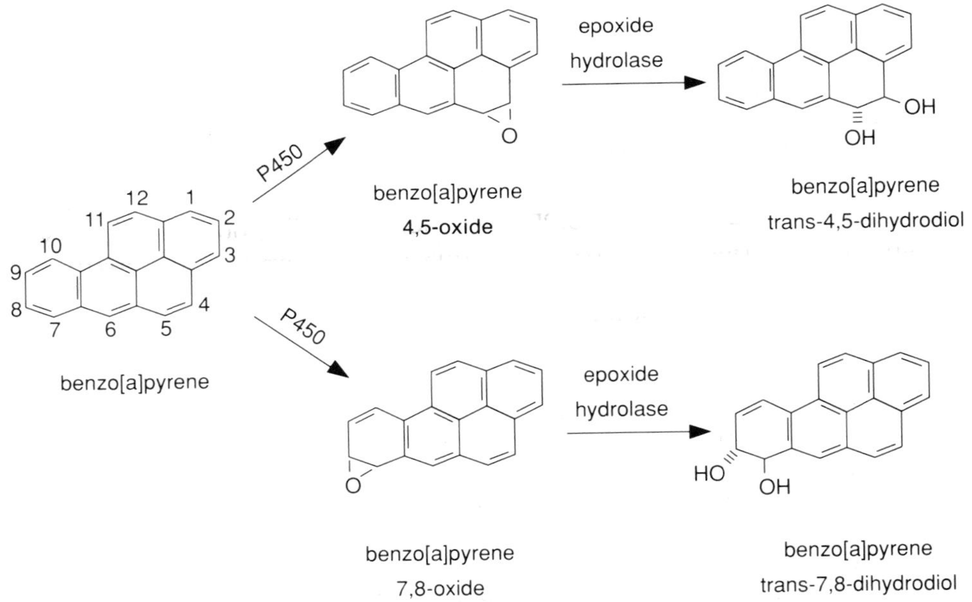

Fig. 5-5. Oxidation of benzo[a]pyrene to biologically active epoxides by P450 and subsequent hydration of these epoxides by epoxide hydrolase.

In the liver the purified microsomal epoxide hydrolases have a relative molecular mass (M_r) of approximately 50,000, and the catalytic function does not require the presence of any prosthetic groups. The enzyme is readily inducible by phenobarbital, whereas it is only weakly induced by 3-methylcholanthrene. Multiple forms of epoxide hydrolase exist in rat and human livers. These forms have broad and overlapping substrate specificities.[39] A unique form of microsomal epoxide hydrolase with a high specificity for cholesterol 5α,6α-oxide has been detected.[40] Epoxide hydrolase activity is present in essentially all organs and tissues of rats. A cytosolic form of epoxide hydrolase has also been detected.[41]

PHASE II REACTIONS OF DRUG METABOLISM

Several kinds of small molecules normally present in the body can react with drugs or with drug metabolites. Glucuronic acid combines with phenols, alcohols, aromatic amines, and carboxylic acids to form the corresponding glucuronides. Addition of ribose and phosphate converts purine and pyrimidine analogs to nucleosides and nucleotides. Amines and carboxylic acids can be acylated. Other examples are syntheses of mercapturic acids and of sulfuric acid esters, trans-sulfurations, and methylations.

Synthesis of Glucuronides

The soluble fraction of liver contains enzymes that catalyze the synthesis of uridine diphosphate-glucuronic acid (UDPGA):

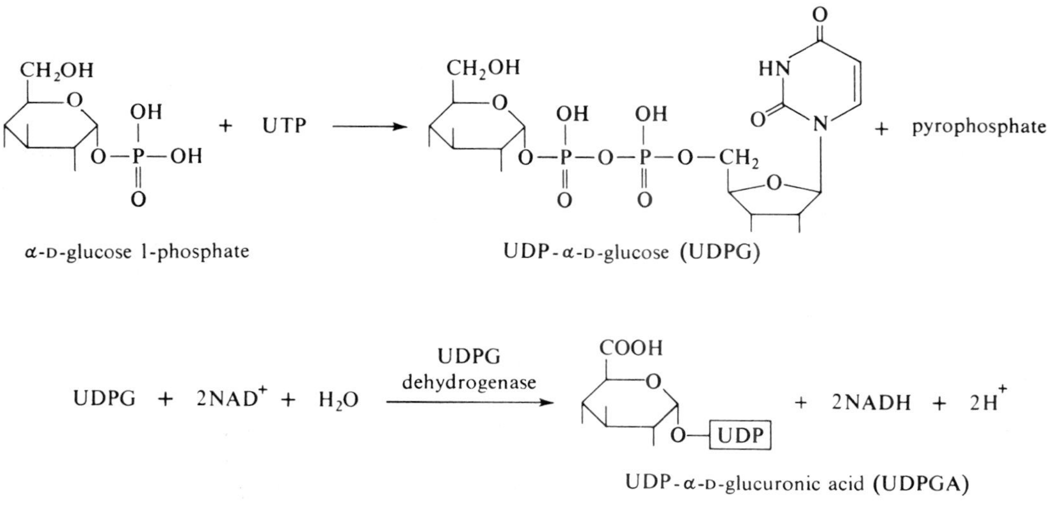

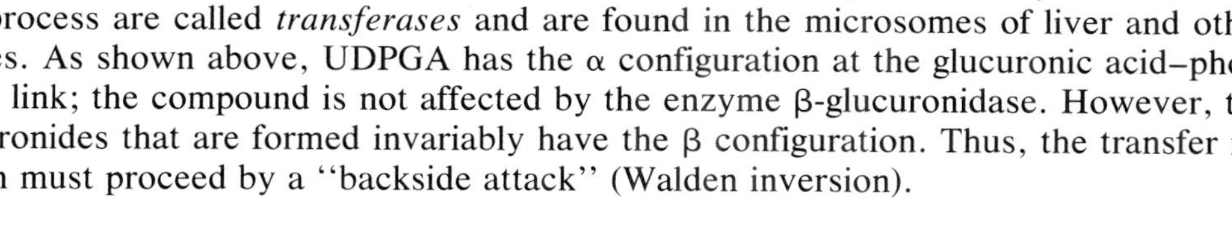

α-D-glucose 1-phosphate   +   UTP ⟶   UDP-α-D-glucose (UDPG)   +   pyrophosphate

UDPG + 2NAD$^+$ + H$_2$O $\xrightarrow{\text{UDPG dehydrogenase}}$ + 2NADH + 2H$^+$

UDP-α-D-glucuronic acid (UDPGA)

UDPGA serves as a donor of glucuronic acid to various acceptors.[42] Enzymes mediating this process are called *transferases* and are found in the microsomes of liver and other tissues. As shown above, UDPGA has the α configuration at the glucuronic acid–phosphate link; the compound is not affected by the enzyme β-glucuronidase. However, the glucuronides that are formed invariably have the β configuration. Thus, the transfer reaction must proceed by a "backside attack" (Walden inversion).

The hydroxyl group in phenols and aliphatic alcohols is conjugated with glucuronic acid to form a hemiacetal glucuronide. Compounds of this type are often called *ether glucuronides*:

UDPGA   *p*-hydroxyacetanilid   *p*-hydroxyacetanilid glucuronide

Carboxylic acids are conjugated through the carboxyl group to form *ester glucuronides*:

benzoic acid   benzoyl glucuronide

In all these reactions, there is a nucleophilic attack by the electron-rich atom (oxygen, nitrogen, or sulfur) at the C-1 position of the glucuronic acid in UDPGA. Glucuronides of naturally occurring compounds (e.g., steroid alcohols, thyroxine, bilirubin) appear to be formed by the same pathways as glucuronides of exogenous compounds. Aromatic amines and even occasionally a sulfhydryl group can be conjugated. The nitrogen and sulfur glucuronides are acid-labile, in contrast to the oxygen-linked glucuronides.

The capacity to glucuronidate a large variety of structurally unrelated substances is attributable in part to the existence of several forms of the transferase, which are differentially regulated and appear to be specific for different sets of substrates. Two major groups of glucuronosyltransferases have been purified from rat liver.[43] One of the forms is inducible by phenobarbital and preferentially catalyzes the glucuronidation of morphine, while the other form is preferentially induced by 3-methylcholanthrene and catalyzes the conjugation of 1-naphthol and *p*-nitrophenol. Endogenous substrates, such as bilirubin, bile acids, and steroid hormones, may be glucuronidated by only one or by both forms of the enzyme. In Gunn rats, a mutant strain in which bilirubin glucuronidation cannot be detected, glucuronidation of a variety of other substrates appears to be unaffected,[44] which provides further evidence in support of the multiplicity of this family of transferases. Since primary sequence data are not yet available on the individual enzyme forms, structural differences between forms that govern the choice of an aglycone are unknown. The cDNA encoding a phenobarbital-inducible form of rat liver UDP-glucuronosyltransferase has been isolated, sequenced, and expressed to yield a catalytically active enzyme.[45]

Glucuronides tend to be biologically and chemically less reactive than the parent compound, but certain conjugates of *N*-hydroxylarylamines induce the formation of tumors in the urinary bladder. *N*-Glucuronides of arylamines formed in the liver can be hydrolyzed by acidic urine to form the *N*-hydroxy derivative of the arylamine, which in turn is converted to the electrophilic arylnitrenium ion and other electrophilic derivatives[46] (see Fig.

12-8). As discussed in Chapter 12, these electrophiles can then covalently bind to DNA, RNA, and protein of the bladder epithelium and lead to tumor formation. In this example, glucuronidation generates the proximate carcinogen in the liver. The glucuronide is then converted to its ultimate carcinogen in the target organ, the bladder.

Conjugation With Other Sugars

Certain carbohydrates other than glucuronic acid can participate in synthetic reactions with foreign compounds. Ribonucleosides and ribonucleotides are formed with analogs of purines and pyrimidines by the same enzyme systems (in the soluble fraction of the cell) responsible for synthesizing nucleosides and nucleotides of the naturally occurring purines and pyrimidines. Many analogs of these compounds, of interest as anticancer agents, have been studied, and in almost every instance the biologically active compounds are the phosphorylated ribonucleoside derivatives.[47] This type of reaction is exemplified by conversion of 6-mercaptopurine to a ribonucleotide by reaction with phosphoribosyl-pyrophosphate (PRPP) catalyzed by a purine phosphoribosyl transferase:

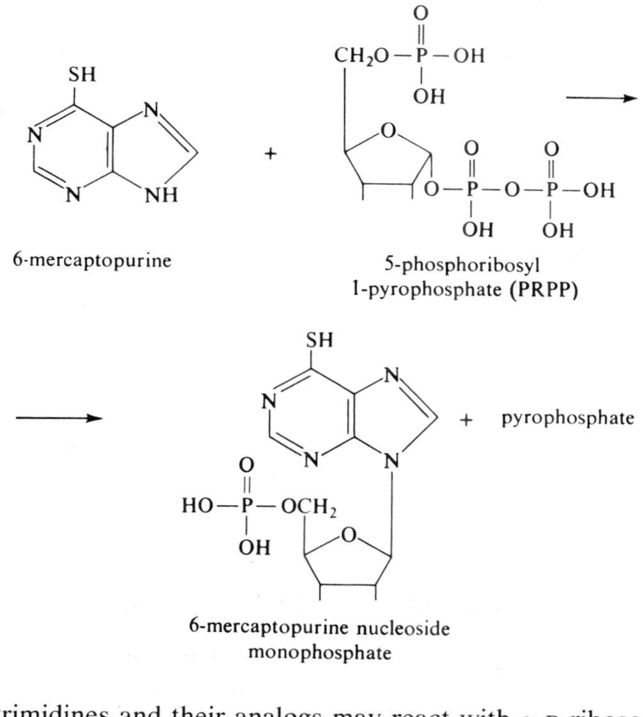

6-mercaptopurine

5-phosphoribosyl
1-pyrophosphate (PRPP)

6-mercaptopurine nucleoside
monophosphate

Alternatively, pyrimidines and their analogs may react with α-D-ribose 1-phosphate; the phosphate group is split out and a ribonucleoside results. This type of reaction is catalyzed by a nucleoside phosphorylase.

Acetylation Reactions

Acetylation of compounds containing amino, hydroxyl, and sulfhydryl groups occurs in animals and humans.[48] Acetylation is the major route of arylamine metabolism, for example. Coenzyme A (CoA), through its free sulfhydryl group, reacts with an activated form of a carboxylic acid to form the acyl-CoA derivative, and the acyl group is then transferred to a suitable acceptor, such as an aromatic amine as shown below for acetylation of sulfanilamide.

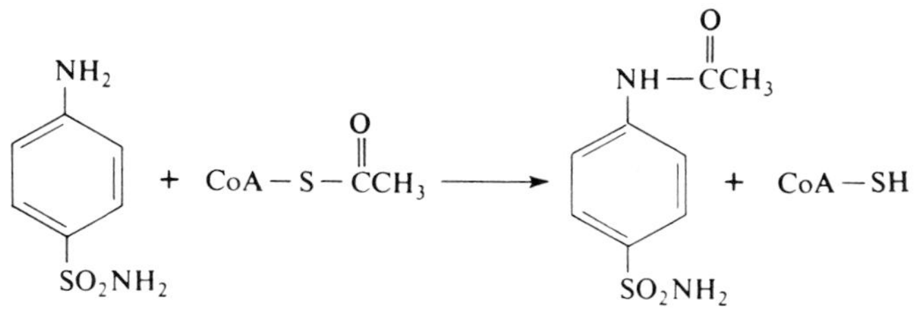

sulfanilamide   acetyl-CoA N_4-acetylsulfanilamide

Developmental and genetic factors play an important role in acetylation reactions. Individuals of both human and rabbit species can be classified as "rapid" or "slow" acetylators of isoniazid. This genetic polymorphism will be discussed in detail in Chapter 7.

Enzymatic *N*-acetylation of drugs proceeds according to a "ping-pong Bi-Bi"[49,50] reaction mechanism. This reaction sequence may be depicted, from left to right, as follows:

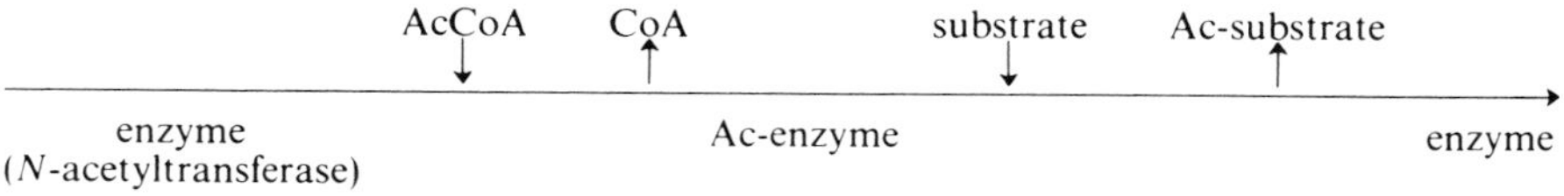

The overall reaction can be written in conventional form as follows:

$$\text{enzyme} + \text{AcCoA} \rightleftharpoons \text{Ac-enzyme} + \text{CoA}$$
$$\underline{\text{Ac-enzyme} + \text{substrate} \rightleftharpoons \text{Ac-substrate} + \text{enzyme}}$$
$$\text{AcCoA} + \text{substrate} \xrightarrow{\text{enzyme}} \text{Ac-substrate} + \text{CoA}$$

N-Acetyltransferase is a cytosolic enzyme found in many tissues, such as liver, small intestine, blood, and kidney. In mammals extrahepatic tissues contribute significant amounts of activity to the total acetylating capacity of the body, particularly in the genetically slow acetylator.

Mercapturic Acid Formation

A variety of electrophiles conjugate with the nucleophilic tripeptide glutathione (GSH). The products of GSH conjugation undergo further metabolism to yield mercapturic acids as the final urinary elimination products.[51,52] Substrates such as halo- and nitroalkanes and halo- and nitrobenzenes may be sufficiently electrophilic to directly conjugate with GSH. A second group of substrates, which includes arene oxides and aliphatic epoxides, are reaction products of cytochrome P450–mediated oxidations. The likely reaction mechanism for naphthalene as substrate is shown in Figure 5-6. Naphthalene is converted by the microsomal monooxygenases to an epoxide, which reacts with GSH in the presence of cytosolic glutathione *S*-transferase. The renal proximal tubule cells and jejunal epithelial cells contain high γ-glutamyltransferase activity, which removes the γ-glutamyl residue.

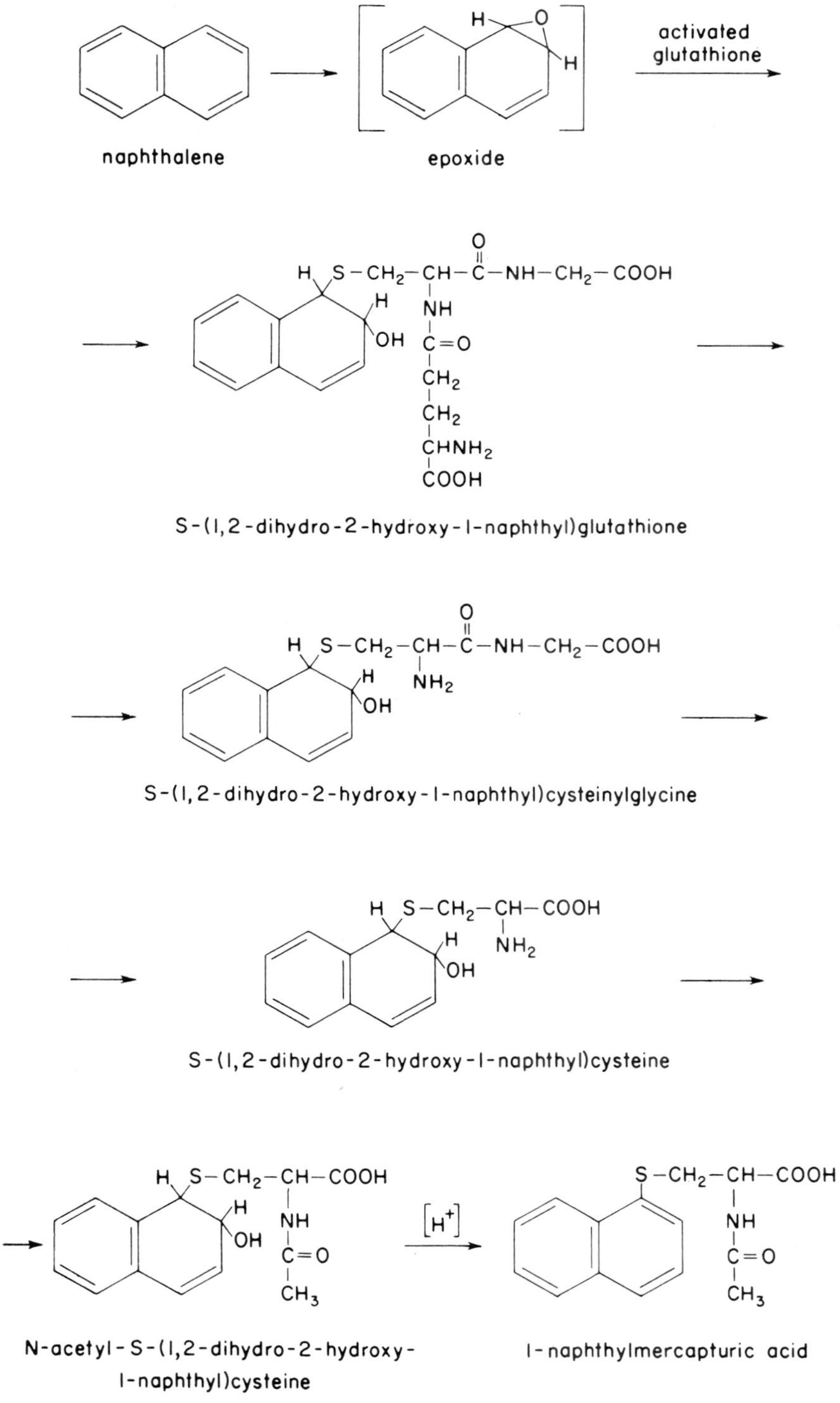

Fig. 5-6. Mercapturic acid formation.

This is followed by removal of the glycyl residue by cysteinyl glycinase. The cysteine derivative is subsequently *N*-acetylated. All the 2-hydroxynaphthyl intermediates undergo spontaneous dehydration at acid pH, yielding the corresponding mercapturic acids.

Glutathione *S*-transferases are widely distributed in the animal kingdom, and the mammalian cytosolic enzymes are encoded by three multigene families.[53,54] The enzymes are composed of two subunits with molecular weights in the range of 24,000 to 27,500. Both homodimers and heterodimers exist, but only subunits that are members of the same family can hybridize.[55] Each of the glutathione *S*-transferases is active on a distinct spectrum of electrophiles, and the different isoenzymes appear to perform different selective roles in detoxification of carcinogens and other environmental pollutants.[56,57] Induction of glutathione *S*-transferase has been most thoroughly documented following phenobarbital administration, although 3-methylcholanthrene and tetrachlorodibenzo-*p*-dioxin are also inducers. Of particular interest is the effect of the common food antioxidant BHA [2(3)-*tert*-butyl-4-hydroxyanisole], which is a transferase inducer in mice and rats, and whose anticarcinogenic properties in these animals is significant.[58]

Sulfate Conjugation

Sulfate conjugation is an important pathway in the biotransformation of phenolic and aliphatic hydroxyl groups and of certain neurotransmitters, bile acids, and organic hydroxylamines. The enzymes responsible for sulfate conjugation are collectively known as *sulfotransferases*. Aryl, or phenol, sulfotransferase is the most important of the enzymes that catalyze the sulfate conjugation of drugs and neurotransmitters. The sulfate donor for the reaction is an activated form of the sulfate known as 3'-phosphoadenosine-5'-phosphosulfate (PAPS) which is generated from inorganic sulfate by a two-step process, following which the sulfate group is transferred to a phenolic acceptor (e.g., *p*-hydroxyacetanilid) in the presence of the sulfotransferase:

adenosine 5'-phosphosulfate (APS)

3'-phosphoadenosine 5'-phosphosulfate (PAPS)

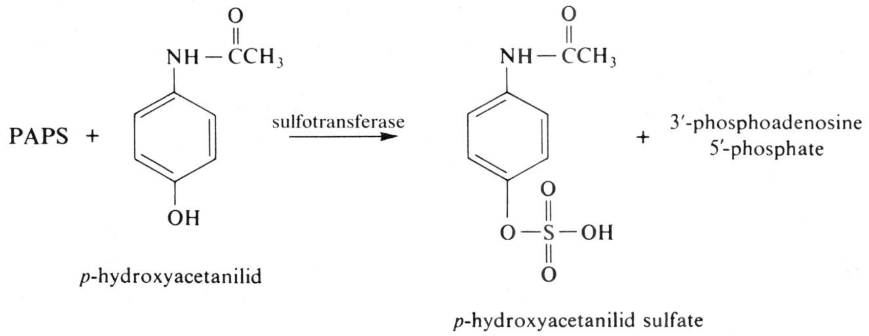

p-hydroxyacetanilid sulfate

All human tissues that have been studied in detail contain at least two forms of phenol sulfotransferase,[59] one of which is thermolabile and catalyzes the sulfate conjugation of dopamine and other phenolic monoamines, whereas the other form is thermostable and catalyzes the sulfate conjugation of simple phenols such as *p*-nitrophenol. The widely used analgesic medication acetaminophen is a substrate for both forms of the enzyme. The two forms of sulfotransferase have been physically separated and partially purified from several human tissues, including an easily accessible tissue, the blood platelet. Both forms are found in the soluble fraction of tissues such as liver, brain, and small intestine.

N-, *O*-, and *S*-Methylation

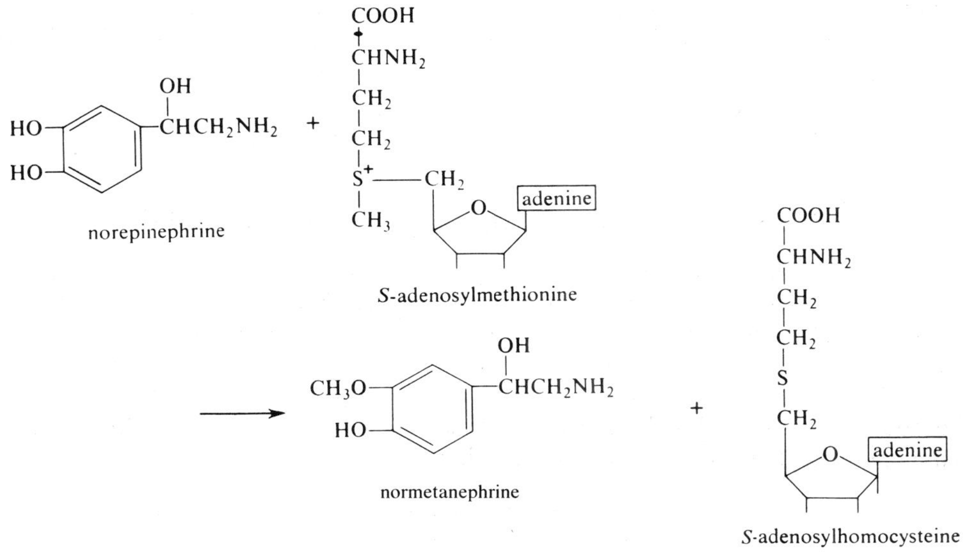

Methylations proceed by a pathway in which *S*-adenosylmethionine serves as methyl donor. There are a number of methyltransferase enzymes, one of which, catechol *O*-methyltransferase (COMT), is found in the soluble supernatant fraction of rat liver and other tissues and can catalyze the transfer of a methyl group to a phenolic –OH of epinephrine, norepinephrine, and other catechol derivatives (e.g., dihydroxyphenylethylamine and dihydroxybenzoic acid). Methylation occurs in the meta position. The reaction is dependent upon magnesium ions; *S*-adenosylmethionine is required, but ATP and methionine can substitute, in which case *S*-adenosylmethionine is formed in the presence of rat liver supernatant fraction.

COMT activity is found in all species and is widely distributed in mammalian tissues. This enzyme is involved in the physiologic inactivation of the adrenergic neurotransmitter norepinephrine, as well as of other cathecholamines, whether of endogenous or exogenous origin.

N-Methylation of numerous amines has been reported. A highly specific enzyme methylates histamine. Another enzyme, phenylethanolamine *N*-methyltransferase (PNMT), methylates phenylethanolamine derivatives and is responsible for the conversion of norepinephrine to epinephrine:

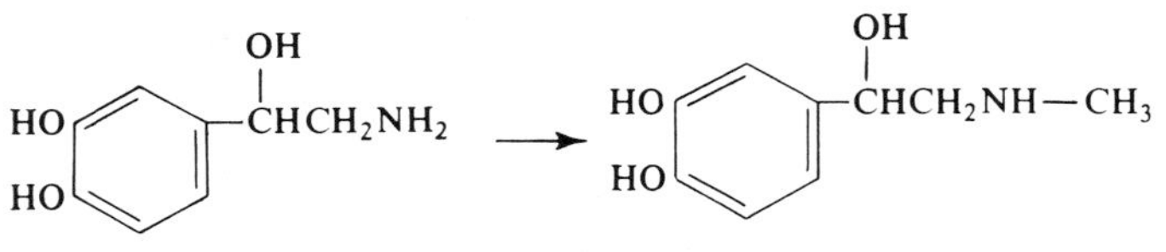

norepinephrine   epinephrine

PNMT is abundant in the soluble fraction of the adrenal medulla, and it is also found in small amounts in heart and brain.

PNMT can methylate phenylethanolamines but not phenylethylamines. Endogenous substrates include norepinephrine, normetanephrine, epinephrine, metanephrine, and octopamine. Exogenous compounds metabolized by the enzyme include phenylethanolamine, phenylephrine, norephredrine, and para- and dihydroxynorephedrine.

Only a few methylated sulfur-containing compounds have been identified in the urine after injection of sulfhydryl compounds. *S*-Methyltransferases have been implicated in the metabolism of dialkyldithiocarbamates, such as Antabuse,[60] and of thio-substituted purines and pyrimidines, including the antithyroid drugs 2-thiouracil and 6-propyl-2-thiouracil.[61] An in vitro system has been described[62] that methylates such sulfhydryl compounds as 2-mercaptoethanol, *N*-acetylcysteine, and hydrogen sulfide. The enzyme has been found in rat liver, kidney, and lung microsomes and also requires *S*-adenosylmethionine.

$$HS-CH_2CH_2OH \xrightarrow{\textit{S-adenosylmethionine}} CH_3-S-CH_2CH_2OH$$

mercaptoethanol   *S*-methylmercaptoethanol

Trans-sulfuration and the Metabolism of Cyanide

Millions of people ingest cassava as a major staple in their diet. Cassava contains cyanogenic glycosides, and chronic cyanide toxicity has been directly implicated in the widespread ataxic neuropathy, and indirectly implicated in the prevalence of goiter and a variety of other ills, in these populations.[63] Cyanide is a potent inhibitor of cytochrome oxidase, the terminal respiratory enzyme in aerobic organisms. Cyanide is metabolized in the body by the mitochondrial enzyme rhodanase (thiosulfate sulfurtransferase). The enzyme catalyzes the following overall reaction:

$$CN^- + S_2O_3^{2-} \dashrightarrow CNS^- + SO_3^{2-}$$

cyanide thiosulfate   thiocyanate   sulfite

However, a more complex chemical mechanism for its action has been proposed.[64] Rhodanase is found in liver, kidney, and other tissues.

Another sulfurtransferase in liver, kidney, and blood cells utilizes β-mercaptopyruvic acid as sulfur donor:

$$CN^- + HS\!-\!CH_2\!-\!\overset{\overset{\displaystyle O}{\|}}{C}\!-\!COOH \rightarrow CNS^- + CH_3\!-\!\overset{\overset{\displaystyle O}{\|}}{C}\!-\!COOH$$

β-mercaptopyruvic acid   pyruvic acid

β-Mercaptopyruvate is believed to arise metabolically from cysteine by transamination. In the liver cell this enzyme occurs primarily in the mitochondria, but some occurs in the cytosol as well. Several compounds besides cyanide can serve as sulfur acceptors for β-mercaptopyruvate sulfurtransferase. For example, when sulfite is the acceptor substrate, thiosulfate is generated.

In cyanide poisoning the immediate removal of cyanide is achieved by administration of nitrites or aminophenols, which allow some of the cyanide to be bound temporarily with methemoglobin. The subsequent conversion of cyanide to the nontoxic thiocyanate is promoted by administration of thiosulfate. Mercaptopyruvate has been found to be an effective antidote in some mammals but not in others.

INHIBITION OF DRUG METABOLISM
SKF 525A

As with substrates for other enzymes, drugs that are substrates for a particular P450 can compete with other drugs and inhibit their metabolism. This competitive inhibition is the basis for a number of clinically important drug interactions. Certain classes of drugs and xenobiotics, however, are potent inhibitors of P450-mediated drug metabolism because they form inactive complexes with the hemoprotein. Many of these inhibitors are nitrogenous compounds, and they include a number of drugs that are in routine clinical use[65,66] (Table 5-4). One of the most thoroughly investigated of these substrate inhibitors of drug metabolism is 2-diethylaminoethyl diphenylpropylacetate, more usually known

Table 5-4. Examples of Drugs and Xenobiotics that Inhibit Drug Metabolism by Forming Metabolic Intermediate Complexes with Cytochrome P450

Nitrogenous Compounds	*Nonnitrogenous Compounds*
Amphetamine	Isosafrole
Cimetidine	Piperonyl alcohol
Dapsone	Piperonyl butoxide
2-Diethylaminoethyldiphenylpropyl acetate (SKF 525A)	Safrole
2,5-Dimethoxy-4-methylamphetamine	
Diphenhydramine	
Fenfluramine	
Methadone	
Methamphetamine	
Nortriptyline	
Sulfanilamide	

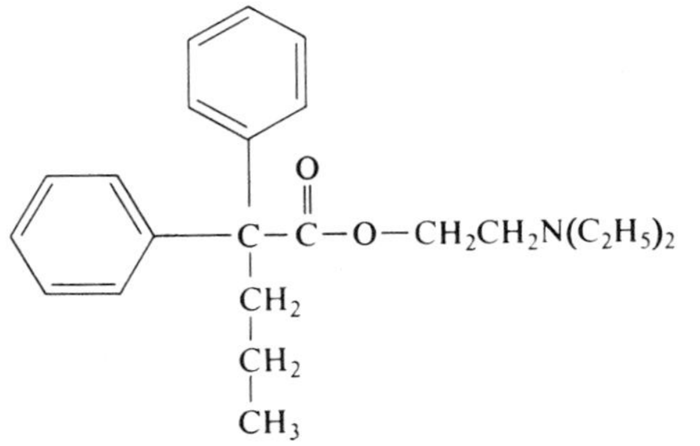

$$C-C-O-CH_2CH_2N(C_2H_5)_2$$

SKF 525A

by its commercial code number SKF 525A. The action of this compound upon microsomal drug oxidations was discovered in the course of routine studies of its pharmacologic properties. The compound had little pharmacologic effect of its own, but when administered prior to hexobarbital, it caused a dramatic prolongation of the hypnotic action. The plasma half-life of hexobarbital was greatly increased, whereas the intrinsic sensitivity of the brain to hexobarbital (measured as the plasma level at the moment of awakening) remained unchanged. Moreover, when animals that had received hexobarbital alone were given SKF 525A at the instant of awakening, they did not go back to sleep, as they ought to have done if SKF 525A had made them more sensitive to the barbiturate.[67] SKF 525A affects the metabolism of many drugs in the same way as it does that of hexobarbital; for example, the durations of action and biologic half-lives of other barbiturates, amphetamine, numerous analgesics, and aminopyrine are also prolonged. In every such case the rate of metabolism in vitro by a liver microsomal preparation is also inhibited.

Oxygen and NADPH are essential for inhibition of metabolism by SKF 525A and the other nitrogenous inhibitors listed in Table 5-4. The compounds are metabolized by cytochrome P450 with formation of a metabolic intermediate that forms a tight but reversible complex with the hemoprotein. This intermediate complex exhibits an absorbance maximum in the Soret region between 448 and 456 nm when the heme iron is in the reduced (ferrous) state. Once it is formed, the complex inhibits oxidations by the affected P450 in a noncompetitive manner.[65]

Inhibition of P450-mediated oxidations should not be regarded solely from the viewpoint of mechanistic interest or as a basis for explaining certain clinical drug interactions. Indeed, it is possible that inhibition of selective P450s will prove to be a useful avenue of drug development. An example exists with the aromatase enzyme that converts androgen precursors to estrogens.[68] The aromatase is a unique P450 system located in placental, ovarian, brain, and adipose tissue,[69,70] and drugs that act as aromatase inhibitors (e.g., aminoglutethamide) have proved useful in the treatment of estrogen-dependent tumors.[71,72]

Cimetidine

Cimetidine is an antagonist of histamine at the H_2 receptor; it is used to treat peptic ulcer and other states in which gastric acidity should be minimized.

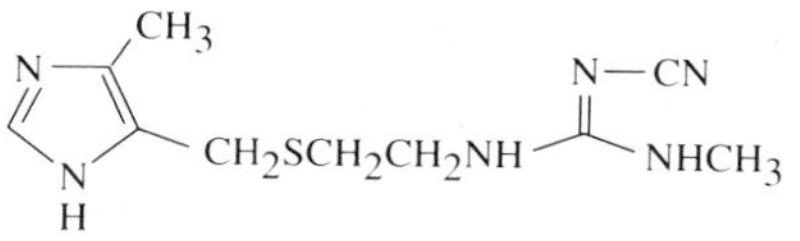

Cimetidine 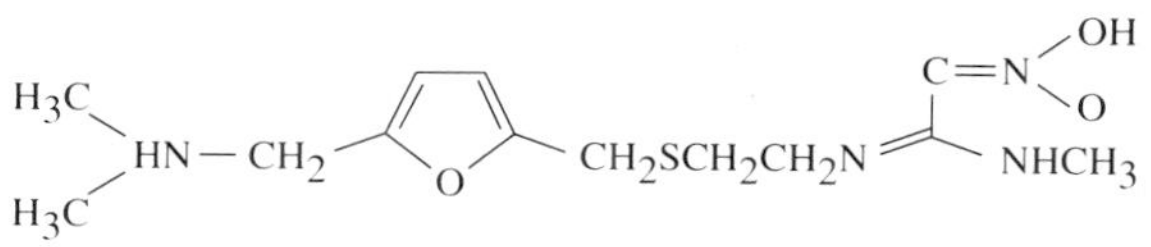   Ranitidine

Cimetidine inhibits the P450-mediated metabolism of a variety of drugs, including warfarin, benzodiazepines, phenytoin, and morphine.[73] The interaction between cimetidine and diazepam is of major clinical importance because both drugs are widely prescribed medications. In a study in which cimetidine was administered to patients receiving long-term diazepam therapy at a constant daily dose for the treatment of anxiety, tension, or insomnia, cimetidine increased the plasma concentration of diazepam and its active metabolite desmethyldiazepam by 62 and 54 percent, respectively.[74] During the cimetidine treatment period, patients fell asleep significantly faster and slept more soundly. In a similar interaction, significant lengthening of prothrombin times has been reported in patients receiving both cimetidine and the anticoagulant drug warfarin.[75]

Cimetidine interferes with the elimination of these drugs, both by inhibiting hepatic cytochrome P450-mediated oxidations and by reducing hepatic blood flow. Cimetidine binds to the hemin iron of cytochrome P450 with its imidazole and cyano groups.[76] Ranitidine, another H_2-receptor blocker, differs from cimetidine in both potency and chemical structure. The fact that ranitidine has a furan ring instead of an imidazole ring may explain the clinical and experimental observations that ranitidine impairs drug metabolism much less than cimetidine. Although it is not required for H_2-receptor antagonism, the imidazole ring confers the capacity to inhibit drug oxidation in humans. Spectroscopic studies have shown that although the interactions of cimetidine and ranitidine with cytochrome P450 are qualitatively similar, cimetidine binds to P450 much more strongly than does ranitidine. In addition, cimetidine is only one-third to one-fifth as potent as ranitidine at H_2-receptor blockade. Based on these facts ranitidine might be expected to have a much lower potential than cimetidine for interaction with drugs that are extensively metabolized in the liver. Both drugs, however, have similar abilities to reduce portal blood flow.

Disulfiram

Disulfiram (tetraethylthiuram disulfide, Antabuse) is an inhibitor of drug metabolism with a unique therapeutic application in the treatment of alcoholism[77]:

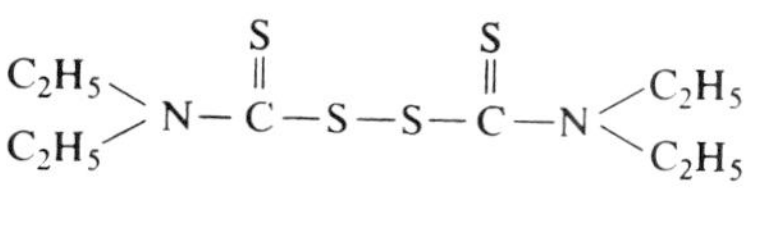

disulfiram

This compound has virtually no pharmacologic effects of its own. If, however, ethyl alcohol is ingested after its administration, a violently unpleasant syndrome develops, including flushing, dyspnea, nausea, vomiting, and hypotension. These remarkable effects are specific for alcohol, and they occur even a day or two after disulfiram is taken. The drug was introduced for the treatment of chronic alcoholism. Alcoholics take disulfiram regularly; thus, their resolve to abstain from alcohol is reinforced by the knowledge of how ill they will inevitably become if they drink. If they drink nevertheless, serious toxicity may ensue. The hypotension may be severe enough to produce shock, and myocardial damage has been reported. These potentionally dangerous effects limit the use of disul-firam to selected patients under strict medical supervision, who are also usually receiving psychotherapy.[77]

Disulfiram inhibits aldehyde dehydrogenase, the enzyme that normally oxidizes ace-taldehyde to acetic acid in the pathway.

$$CH_3CH_2OH \underset{\text{dehydrogenase}}{\overset{\text{alcohol}}{\rightleftharpoons}} CH_3CHO \overset{\text{aldehyde}}{\underset{\text{dehydrogenase}}{\longrightarrow}} CH_3COOH$$

ethanol   acetaldehyde   acetic acid

The consequent accumulation of acetaldehyde is thought to be responsible for the char-acteristic physiologic disturbances in humans, since the syndrome can be reproduced, at least in part, by acetaldehyde infusion. Also, administration of sodium metabisulfite, a compound that reacts with acetaldehyde, controls the symptoms of the disulfiram reaction in alcoholics who ingest ethanol.[77] When ethanol is ingested under normal conditions, the acetaldehyde level does not exceed a few micrograms per milliliter. This level is virtually independent of the dose of ethanol, since the alcohol dehydrogenase, which catalyzes formation of acetaldehyde, is saturated at ethanol concentrations in the mildly intoxicating range. When an identical dose of ethanol is given after disulfiram pretreatment, the ethanol blood level curve is the same, but acetaldehyde concentrations reach levels 5- to 10-fold higher.

Figure 5-7 shows how the relationship between blood ethanol concentration and blood

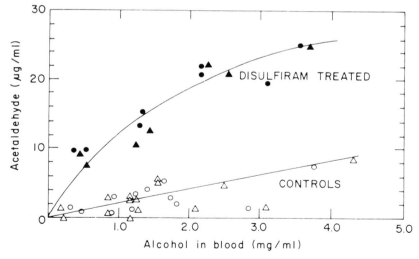

Fig. 5-7. Effect of disulfiram on relationship between blood alcohol and acetaldehyde concentra-tions in rabbits. Groups of rabbits were given ethanol after pretreatment with disulfiram; others were given the same dose of alcohol without pretreatment. At 1 hour (circles) and again at 2 hours (triangles), blood ethanol and acetaldehyde levels were determined. Each point represents a single animal. (Modified from Hald et al.,[78] with permission.)

acetaldehyde concentration is changed by disulfiram in rabbits. At any given concentration of ethanol, the corresponding acetaldehyde level was increased severalfold by disulfiram.

Aldehyde dehydrogenase is recovered in both mitochondrial and cytosolic fractions of the cell, but it has not yet been determined if the enzyme exists in one or more than one form. Initially, disulfiram interacts reversibly with aldehyde dehydrogenase in a manner that is competitive with NAD^+ but noncompetitive with respect to the substrate.[79] This interaction is converted to a permanent inhibition of the enzyme, apparently through a disulfide interchange reaction with essential thiol groups located in or near the active center of the enzyme, as has been demonstrated for disulfiram inhibition of D-amino acid oxidase.[80] Administration of disulfiram to rats decreases aldehyde dehydrogenase activity in the liver. Recovery of the enzyme's activity is very slow (half-time about 24 hours), and it is prevented by cycloheximide, which suggests that new enzyme has to be synthesized.[81]

Monoamine Oxidase Inhibitors

Research on synthetic antibacterial agents led to the introduction of iproniazid, a hydrazide, for the chemotherapy of tuberculosis:

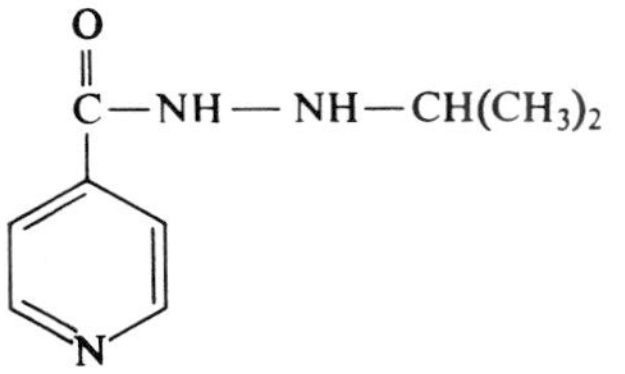

iproniazid

Unexpectedly, mood-elevating effects (euphoria) and other stimulatory actions on the central nervous system were seen. Iproniazid and related compounds were found to be monoamine oxidase (MAO) inhibitors. Since amines (e.g., norepinephrine, serotonin) are normally present in the brain, it was thought that inhibition of their metabolism might underlie the psychopharmacologic actions of these drugs. Related hydrazides (e.g., phenelzine and isocarboxazid) were introduced for the treatment of severe depressions:

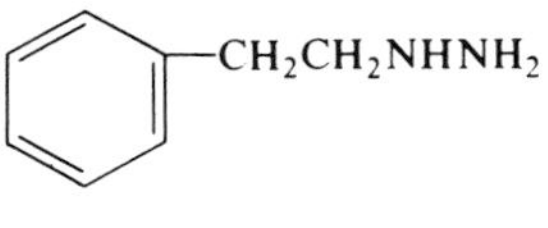

phenelzine

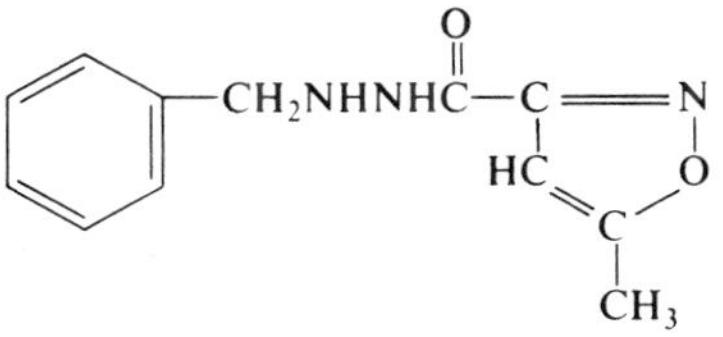

isocarboxazid

Several nonhydrazide inhibitors of MAO, such as tranylcypromine and pargyline, have also been developed.

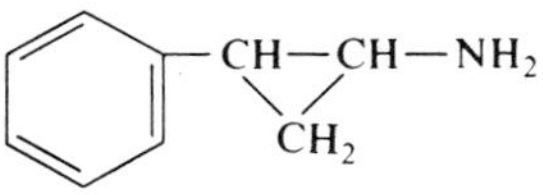

tranylcypromine

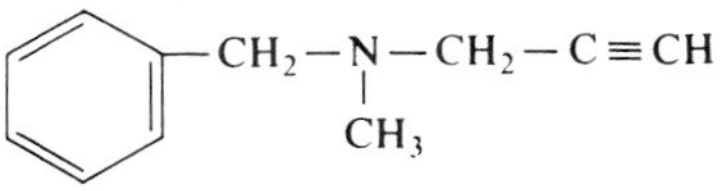

pargyline

All these MAO inhibitors act in vitro as well as in vivo. The administration of iproniazid (5×10^{-5} moles kg^{-1}) to rats resulted in complete inhibition of their liver mitochondrial MAO for 24 hours, and normal activity did not return for 5 days.[82] In vitro, the onset of the inhibition by iproniazid (5×10^{-5} M) takes about 10 minutes. Tyramine, a substrate, can protect the enzyme and delay the development of inhibition, but once inhibition develops, it is practically irreversible.

The MAO inhibitors that are used clinically interact initially with the enzyme in a reversible manner but then form covalent adducts. MAO is a flavin-containing enzyme, and depending on the nature of the inhibitor, adducts are formed between the inhibitor and the flavin or between the inhibitor and the apoprotein near the flavin site[83]; thus, they are *site-directed* enzyme inhibitors (see Ch. 2). Reversible MAO inhibitors have been developed, but their clinical usefulness has not been defined.[84]

The MAO inhibitors have complex pharmacologic actions, which are not thoroughly understood.[84] They certainly cause elevations in the norepinephrine and serotonin levels in the central nervous system, but exactly how this action is related to their mood-elevating action is uncertain. They also may produce a variety of toxic effects, including hypotension, liver damage and jaundice, nausea, vomiting, constipation, dry mouth, and psychic disturbances (delusions or hallucinations).

The MAO inhibitors have little or no potentiating action upon the cardiovascular effects of the natural catecholamines, presumably because O-methylation and tissue uptake rather than oxidative deamination are primarily responsible for terminating their peripheral actions. However, MAO inhibitors do potentiate the cardiovascular effects of simple phenylethylamines such as tyramine. For example, patients receiving tranylcypromine who also took drugs of the phenylethylamine class showed exaggerated hypertensive effects, including fatal cerebral hemorrhages. Even foods can become dangerous in the presence of MAO inhibitors. A remarkable incident of cheese toxicity[85,86] that came to light in the 1960s highlights the unexpected dangers that may be associated with any new drug. Some cheeses (Camembert, Brie, Stilton, New York cheddar) are rich in tyramine. Ordinarily harmless because it is oxidized so rapidly by MAO, tyramine was markedly toxic in patients who had received tranylcypromine. Hypertensive crises and, in a few instances, fatal cerebral hemorrhage occurred. Consequently, tranylcypromine was removed from the market by the Food and Drug Administration, but eventually it was admitted to use again provided appropriate warnings were included on the label and in the promotional literature.

Inhibitors of Aromatic L-Amino Acid Decarboxylase

Drugs that inhibit the peripheral metabolism of levodopa (L-3,4-dihydroxyphenylalanine) have greatly improved the usefulness of this drug in the treatment of Parkinson's disease. The parkinsonian syndrome, which is characterized by tremor, bradykinesia, and rigidity, results from a deficiency of the neurotransmitter dopamine in the striatal region of the brain. Since dopamine does not pass the blood-brain barrier, parkinsonism is treated with large doses of levodopa, the immediate precursor of dopamine. Levodopa is converted to dopamine by the enzyme aromatic L-amino acid decarboxylase.

After oral administration of levodopa, more than 95 percent of the drug is decarboxylated by this enzyme in the periphery, largely by first-pass metabolism in the liver. As a result, very little unchanged drug reaches the cerebral circulation. Carbidopa is an aromatic L-amino acid decarboxylase inhibitor that does not penetrate into the central

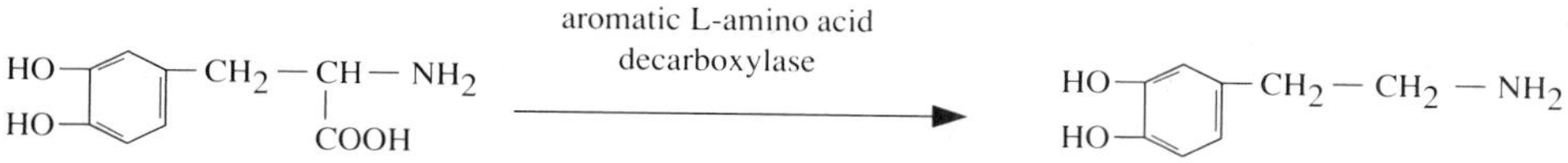

aromatic L-amino acid
decarboxylase

Levodopa

Dopamine

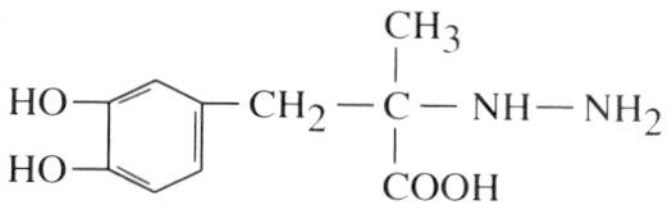

Carbidopa

nervous system, and concurrent administration of carbidopa with levodopa results in a longer half-life and higher plasma concentrations of levodopa than administration of levodopa alone.[87] Clinically, administration of carbidopa permits a reduction in the optimal dosage of levodopa, with a decrease in side effects and an improvement in the control of symptoms.[88]

Xanthine Oxidase Inhibitors

Xanthine oxidase[89] catalyzes the oxidation of hypoxanthine to xanthine and of xanthine to uric acid (see Fig. 7-10). It also acts upon drugs that are analogs of the naturally occurring xanthines, such as 6-mercaptopurine. The desire to improve the efficacy of 6-mercaptopurine in cancer therapy by blocking its metabolism to 6-thiouric acid led to the synthesis and testing of allopurinol.[90–92]

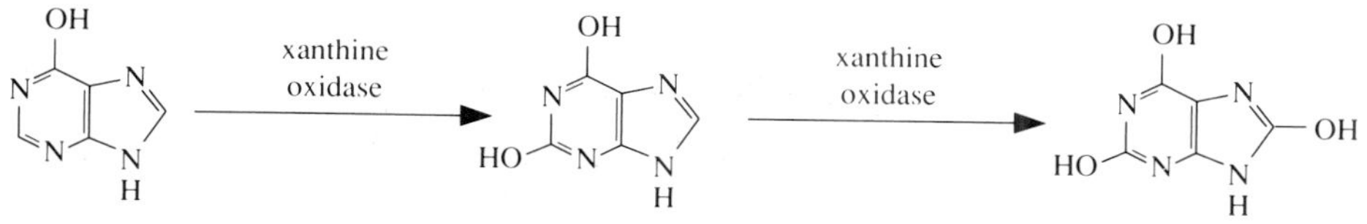

Hypoxanthine   xanthine oxidase   Xanthine   xanthine oxidase   Uric acid

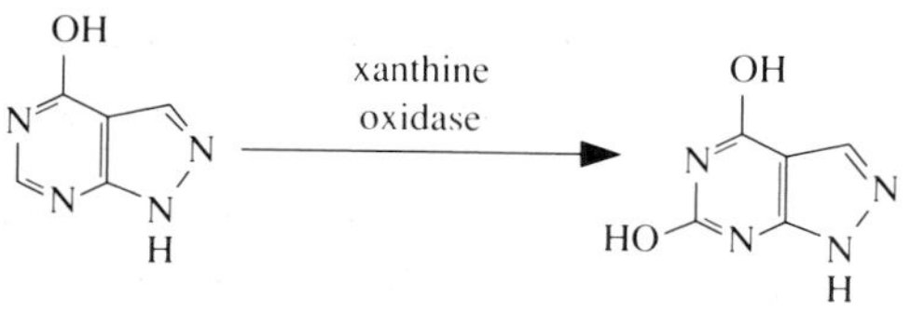

Allopurinol   xanthine oxidase   Oxipurinol

This drug proved to be an effective xanthine oxidase inhibitor in vivo, and it did enhance both the therapeutic and toxic actions of 6-mercaptopurine. The effect of greatest clinical significance, however, turned out to be its efficacy in the treatment of gout. The rate of production of uric acid in this disease is excessively high, and since the urates are poorly soluble in water, urate crystals deposit in kidney, joints, and various soft tissues. Allopurinol, by inhibiting xanthine oxidase, decreases the rate of urate synthesis and consequently the steady-state urate level, permitting gouty deposits to redissolve.[93]

The action of allopurinol in inhibiting xanthine oxidase would in itself be expected to raise hypoxanthine and xanthine levels (since these are the precursors of uric acid) but not necessarily to alter the total rate of synthesis and excretion of all the purines. Purine biosynthesis, however, is under feedback regulation, as shown in Figure 7-10. Blocking xanthine oxidase tends to increase the levels of hypoxanthine and guanine. In the presence of normal activity of hypoxanthine guanine phosphoribosyltransferase, levels of the corresponding nucleotides, inosinic and guanylic acids, increase. These, in turn, inhibit the first step in purine biosynthesis, the combination of PRPP with glutamine. The result of this mechanism is that allopurinol not only reduces the rate of uric acid formation from xanthine but also indirectly decreases the rate of biosynthesis of the purines. Allopurinol itself is converted to a nucleotide by hypoxanthine guanine phosphoribosyltransferase, and this allopurinol derivative acts directly as a feedback inhibitor of the PRPP-glutamine reaction.[93]

Xanthine oxidase is a metalloflavoenzyme that is found mainly in the liver and in the small intestinal mucosa, although some activity is also present in the kidney, spleen, and heart.[83] Allopurinol, a structural analog of hypoxanthine, is both a substrate for and an inhibitor of xanthine oxidase. The affinity of the enzyme for allopurinol is actually 10 to 40 times as great as for xanthine.[93] The initial interaction of allopurinol with xanthine oxidase is competitive, but incubation with the enzyme for several minutes leads to enzyme inactivation. The product of the allopurinol oxidation is oxypurinol, which complexes with partially reduced xanthine oxidase in which the molybdenum is in the tetravalent state.[92,94] The binding of oxypurinol to the enzyme is very tight, and extensive dialysis or oxidation of the enzyme is required to dissociate the complex. The clinical effect of allopurinol must in large measure be due to its oxypurinol metabolite, both because oxypurinol produces xanthine oxidase inhibition of long duration and because it persists in the body fluids.[93]

Peptidase Inhibitors

As mentioned previously in this chapter, recombinant DNA technology permits the synthesis of a variety of human peptides for use as drugs. In addition to the approach mentioned earlier of modifying peptides to make them more resistant to hydrolysis by peptidases, coadministration of compounds that inhibit specific peptidases responsible for drug inactivation may both lengthen the duration of peptide hormone action and increase the concentration of the hormone or growth factor in the relevant body fluid. An example of this approach is seen in the coadministration of cilastatin with the β-lactam antibiotic imipenem.

When imipenem is administered alone, the concentration of the unaltered, antibacterially active drug in the urine is low because the β-lactam ring is cleaved by a dipeptidase, dehydropeptidase-I, located on the brush border of the proximal renal tubular cells.[95] Since the dipeptidase cleaves the drug after it has been excreted into the tubular lumen, the phenomenon is called *postexcretory metabolism*. Cilastatin is one of several inhibitors of the dehydropeptidase, and it was chosen for the drug combination because its pharmacokinetic properties are similar to those of imipenem. Coadministration of the inhibitor results in consistently higher concentrations of the unaltered drug in the urine, with improvement in therapeutic activity against urinary tract infections.[96]

Imipenem (N-formimidoyl thienamycin)

Inactive product with cleaved β-lactam ring

Cilastatin

INDUCTION OF DRUG METABOLISM

The phenomenon of hepatic enzyme induction was first reported in the late 1950s by Drs. James and Elizabeth Miller and their associates at the University of Wisconsin, who found that administration of the carcinogen 3-methylcholanthrene and other polycyclic aromatic hydrocarbons increased the levels of liver enzymes that metabolize aminoazo dyes to noncarcinogenic products by *N*-demethylation and reduction of the azo bond.[97,98] In these early studies the investigators found that ethionine blocked induction of aminoazo dye and benzo[a]pyrene metabolism, and that this block was prevented by methionine.[97,98] At about the same time, Remmer demonstrated a stimulatory effect of barbiturates and other drugs on drug metabolism.[99] Although the enhanced metabolism of foreign chemicals that occurs after exposure of an organism to a chemical is often an adaptive response that enhances the detoxification and elimination of the compound from the organism, some chemicals are metabolized to toxic products, and the induction of microsomal enzymes may increase the toxicity of these chemicals. Several hundred synthetic and naturally occurring compounds with diverse structures are now known to increase the levels of microsomal enzymes when administered to experimental animals. Examples of inducers of microsomal monooxygenases include drugs, steroids, industrial chemicals, pesticides, herbicides, polycyclic aromatic hydrocarbons, and normally occurring constituents in our diet.

The ability of benzpyrene to induce its own metabolism in rats is illustrated in Figure 5-8. The animals were treated with benzpyrene at two different doses, and then the benzpyrene hydroxylase activity of their livers was tested in vitro at intervals for 6 days.[100] At the higher dose a sevenfold stimulation was seen, with a half-time of about 6 hours. At 6 days (144 hours), the stimulation caused by both doses had subsided. Similar results were obtained with another carcinogen, 3-methylcholanthrene. Activity toward azo dyes (reduction and demethylation) was also stimulated by these hydrocarbons.

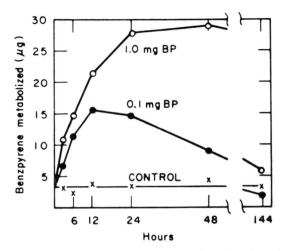

Fig. 5-8. Stimulation of benzpyrene-metabolizing activity of rat liver by administration of benzpyrene. Weanling rats were given a single intraperitoneal injection of benzpyrene at the doses indicated. Animals were sacrificed periodically, and benzpyrene-metabolizing activity of liver samples was measured for a 12-minute period. Each point is the average from two rats. (From Conney et al.,[100] with permission.)

The magnitude of the changes in rate of metabolism and duration of action of a drug that may occur after enzyme induction is illustrated by the example of rats given zoxazolamine after pretreatment with compounds that act as inducers of drug metabolism.[101] Zoxazolamine is a muscle relaxant drug, which is metabolized by hepatic microsomal enzymes to the pharmacologically inactive compound 6-hydroxyzoxazolamine.

Zoxazolamine   6-Hydroxyzoxazolamine

Administration of benzpyrene to rats rapidly stimulated hepatic zoxazolamine hydroxylase activity, with maximum activity being achieved in 24 hours. When phenobarbital was administered to the rats, maximum stimulation of hydroxylase activity was not obtained unless the animals were treated for 3 to 4 days. Increased hepatic microsomal zoxazolamine hydroxylase activity of animals treated with phenobarbital or benzpyrene was associated with an accelerated rate of zoxazolamine metabolism in vivo. The half-life of zoxazolamine was 9 hours in control rats, 48 minutes in phenobarbital-pretreated rats, and only 10 minutes in benzpyrene-pretreated rats (Figure 5-9).[102] The dramatic changes in zoxazolamine half-life were paralleled by changes in the drug's duration of action. Control rats given a high dose of zoxazolamine were paralyzed for 730 minutes whereas rats pretreated with phenobarbital were paralyzed for 102 minutes and rats pretreated with benzpyrene were paralyzed for only 17 minutes. Subsequent studies showed that treatment of rats with polycyclic aromatic hydrocarbons such as 3-methylcholanthrene

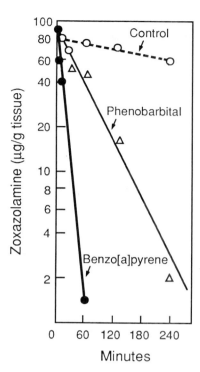

Fig. 5-9. In vivo metabolism of zoxazolamine in rats pretreated with phenobarbital or benzpyrene. Immature male rats were given intraperitoneal injections of sodium pentobarbital (37 mg/kg) twice daily for 4 days or benzpyrene (25 mg/kg) 24 hours prior to an intraperitoneal injection of zoxazolamine (100 mg/kg). Total body homogenates were made at various times after the injection of zoxazolamine and the amount of zoxazolamine per gram of tissue was assayed. (From Conney,[102] with permission.)

caused the appearance of a microsomal hemoprotein with spectral properties that were different from those of cytochrome P450.[103,104]

Stimulation of drug metabolism may produce a state of apparent drug tolerance. For example, rabbits pretreated with pentobarbital for 3 days slept a much shorter time after an intravenous test dose than did controls (Table 5-5). Inasmuch as the blood concentrations of pentobarbital were about the same in both groups at the moment of awakening, all the effect is accounted for by an increased rate of metabolism; there was no significant change in the animals' sensitivities to given drug concentrations.

Table 5-5. Effect of Pentobarbital Pretreatment on Duration of Pentobarbital Action[a]

Pretreatment	Sleeping Time (min)	Plasma Level of Pentobarbital on Awakening (μg ml^{-1})	Pentobarbital Half-Life in Plasma (min)
None	67 ± 4	9.9 ± 1.4	79 ± 3
Pentobarbital	30 ± 7	7.9 ± 0.6	26 ± 2

[a] Rabbits were pretreated with three daily doses of pentobarbital (60 mg kg^{-1}) subcutaneously, then given a single challenging dose of 30 mg/kg^{-1} intravenously. Sleeping times and pentobarbital levels in plasma were measured. (Data from Remmer.[105])

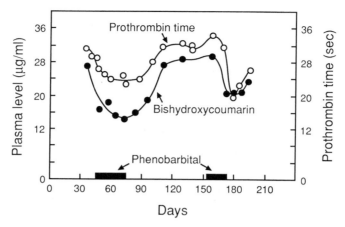

Fig. 5-10. Effect of phenobarbital on plasma levels of bishydroxycoumarin. A human subject was treated with bishydroxycoumarin (75 mg daily). Drug plasma levels and prothrombin times were determined periodically. Phenobarbital was administered (65 mg once daily) during periods indicated by heavy marks on abscissal axis. (From Cucinell et al.,[106] with permission.)

If the drug-metabolizing system is depressed, excessive responses or prolonged responses to ordinary doses of drugs may occur. On the other hand, should a suitable maintenance dose be instituted under these abnormal conditions, it might prove inadequate later on when the rate of drug metabolism increases to normal. Or conversely, a patient using barbiturate sedatives regularly is likely to have an unusually high activity of the drug-metabolizing enzymes, as discussed already; if another drug is given simultaneously, at customary dosages, it may prove wholly ineffective. If an appropriately higher dosage of the second drug is established for this patient, the drug levels may become excessive later on, should the barbiturate be discontinued. Figure 5-10 illustrates effects of this sort in a human subject.[106] The patient was on a maintenance dosage of 75 mg daily of the anticoagulant drug bishydroxycoumarin. Plasma levels of the drug were followed, as well as prothrombin time, a measure of the drug effect in delaying blood clotting. During periods of regular phenobarbital administration the plasma level of bishydroxycoumarin fell, and the therapeutic action of the drug was significantly diminished. This illustration points up dramatically how drugs may interact.

Inducers of hepatic monooxygenases have been categorized into two main groups. One group, of which phenobarbital is a prototype, enhances the metabolism of a large variety of substrates. This group of inducers causes a marked proliferation of the smooth endoplasmic reticulum and increases the synthesis of cytochrome P450 in liver cells. Polycyclic aromatic hydrocarbons such as benzo[a]pyrene and 3-methylcholanthrene comprise a second major group of enzyme inducers. This group induces the synthesis of cytochrome P448, which differs in its catalytic properties from the cytochrome P450 present in untreated rats or in rats pretreated with phenobarbital. Phenobarbital is a potent inducer of benzphetamine N-demethylase and testosterone 16α-hydroxylase activities in liver microsomes, whereas aryl hydrocarbon (e.g., benzo[a]pyrene) hydroxylase, zoxazolamine hydroxylase, and 7-ethoxycoumarin O-dealkylase activities are preferentially induced by polycyclic aromatic hydrocarbons in experimental animals as well as in human tissues. Purified forms of rat liver cytochromes P450 and P448 have been termed *cytochromes*

Table 5-6. Catalytic Activity of Various Purified Forms of Rat Liver Cytochrome P450[a]

Substrate	Phenobarbital		3-Methylcholanthrene	
	P450a	P450b	P450a	P450c
Benzphetamine	2.2	216.6	2.6	5.0
Benzo[a]pyrene	0.04	0.2	0.3	24.5
7-Ethoxycoumarin	0.2	13.9	1.1	67.5
Zoxazolamine	0.5	2.2	2.0	29.7
Testosterone:				
7α-OH	4.1	<0.1	5.4	<0.1
16α-OH	<0.05	1.9	<0.05	<0.05
6β-OH	<0.1	<0.1	<0.1	0.36

[a] Male Long-Evans rats were treated intraperitoneally with phenobarbital 75 mg/kg or 3-methylcholanthrene 25 mg/kg daily for 4 days. Cytochrome P450 forms were purified, and the catalytic activity of each heme protein was assayed. Metabolic activities are expressed as nanomoles of product formed per minute per nanomole of cytochrome P450. (Data from Ryan et al.[139])

P450b and *P450c*, respectively. Differences in substrate specificities of these purified hemoproteins and a third form of cytochrome P450 termed *P450a* are shown in Table 5-6. Other environmentally derived chemicals, such as 2,3,7,8-tetrachlorodibenzo-*p*-dioxin (TCDD), can induce other distinct forms of these hemoproteins.

The long-lived environmental pollutants called polychlorinated biphenyls (PCBs) have been used as a biologic tool to induce various forms of cytochromes P450. PCBs have been categorized as a "mixed" type of inducer, because in rats they possess the inducing properties of both the phenobarbital class and the 3-methylcholanthrene class of inducers. When the PCB mixture called Aroclor 1254 was administered to rabbits, however, the animals did not exhibit the nonspecific induction previously reported in rats.[106,107] Pretreatment of rabbits with Aroclor 1254 resulted in effects that were highly tissue-dependent[108] (Fig. 5-11). In liver the PCB mixture caused a significant increase in cytochrome P450 content and ethylmorphine *N*-demethylase activity, but there was little or no significant induction of benzpyrene hydroxylase activity. In kidney the Aroclor 1254 pretreatment resulted in stimulation of all three activities, and the factor by which activity was increased relative to nonpretreated controls was considerably higher than in liver. In lung, however, PCB treatment had the opposite effect, producing significant decreases both in cytochrome P450 content and in monooxygenase activities.

The example shown here with the PCBs demonstrates that it is not possible to extrapolate inducing effects observed in one organ to another. Such differences in microsomal enzyme induction may account for target organ toxicities exhibited by certain environmentally derived toxins. The action of Aroclor 1254 on pulmonary monooxygenases is clearly species-dependent. In rats treated with this PCB mixture, pulmonary cytochrome P450 content was increased by 34 percent, and benzpyrene hydroxylase activity was enhanced fourfold.[109] Thus, microsomal enzyme induction by either drugs or environmentally derived chemicals can be species-specific as well as tissue-specific.

An abundance of evidence demonstrates that the stimulation of activity of microsomal enzymes involves new protein synthesis. The stimulating agents are without effect in vitro; animals have to be pretreated, and a period of time has to elapse that corresponds to known rates of protein synthesis. Phenobarbital, which stimulates a great many enzyme activities, produces a detectable increase in the amount of microsomal protein per gram of liver, but 3-methylcholanthrene, which stimulates fewer enzymes, does not. Electron micrographs show that after phenobarbital treatment there is an increase in the amount of smooth endoplasmic reticulum in liver cells, and it will be recalled that the microsomal

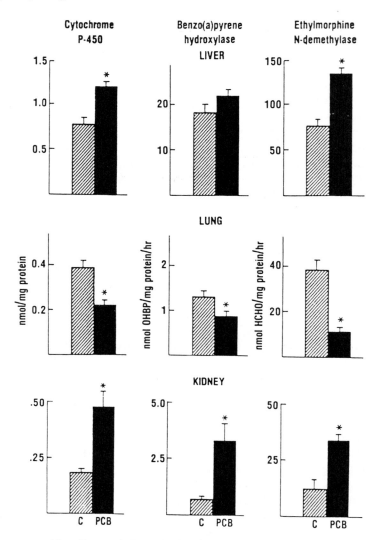

Fig. 5-11. Tissue-specific effects of the polychlorinated biphenyl (PCB) mixture Aroclor 1254 on monooxygenase activities in rabbit liver, lung, and kidney. Aroclor 1254 (100 mg/kg) was administered intraperitoneally to rabbits on days 1 and 4, and the rabbits were killed on day 7 (C = control rabbits; PCB = rabbits given Aroclor 1254; each bar represents mean ± S.E. for tissue obtained from four rabbits). Asterisks represents values significantly different from the respective controls ($P < 0.05$). (From Alvares et al.,[108] with permission.)

drug-metabolizing enzymes are associated with this structure. It has also been found that the kinetic properties (substrate affinities, etc.) of the various drug-metabolizing enzymes after phenobarbital stimulation are indistinguishable from those of control enzymes.

In the 1960s it was shown that both inhibitors of protein synthesis (e.g., puromycin) and inhibitors of RNA synthesis (e.g., actinomycin D) prevent induction of benzpyrene hydroxylase activity in rat liver.[110] It is now firmly established that the regulation of cytochrome P450 induction resides primarily at the level of gene transcription, and the mechanisms that regulate the induction process are being determined at the molecular level. The structure of the P450 genes and the molecular basis for the regulation of their expression will be considered in detail in Chapter 6.

It is a legitimate question to ask why the microsomal monooxygenases are inducible in the first place. Enzyme induction appears to be an adaptive response by the organism living in (or having previously lived in) an environment containing a wide variety of chemical substances that may be harmful to the individual. The question of whether induction of microsomal P450 isoenzymes is good or bad requires a complex answer, which depends on the isoenzymes that are induced and the available substrates. Although induction of P450 isozymes with phenobarbital, for example, is associated with an increased toxicity of bromobenzene, the induction of a different profile of P450 isoenzymes by 3-methyl-cholanthrene is associated with protection of rats from the hepatotoxicity of bromobenzene.[111] Similarly, induction of P450 isoenzymes that metabolize polycyclic hydrocarbons present in cigarette smoke to their ultimate carcinogens may enhance the risk of lung cancer in smokers. In this case, smokers who are genetically less competent with respect to induction of pulmonary P450s may not be at as high risk of developing lung cancer as those who have a high capacity for induction. It is clear that the oxidative P450 enzymes also metabolize endogenous substrates, such as steroid hormones, sterols, fatty acids, and prostaglandins, as well as xenobiotics; thus, microsomal inducers can stimulate the metabolism of these normal body constituents.

SPECIES AND SEX DIFFERENCES IN DRUG METABOLISM

Investigations into the phylogenetic aspects of drug metabolism suggest that drug-metabolizing systems may have developed in response to the special needs of terrestrial life. In fish, lipid-soluble compounds can pass readily across the gills into the aquatic environment. Although early reports suggested that fish lacked the ability to oxidatively metabolize foreign compounds, cytochrome P450-dependent monooxygenase activities have subsequently been demonstrated in several varieties of both freshwater and marine fish.[112,113] The requirements for oxidation by the liver microsomes of fish appear to be similar to those for mammalian liver microsomes. Two forms of cytochrome P450 have been partially purified from hepatic microsomes of little skate and rainbow trout.[113,114] Reptiles, birds, and mammals have the necessary enzymic machinery for increasing the polarity of lipid-soluble compounds and thus achieving their more rapid excretion. Insects have evolved a remarkable spectrum of enzymatic capabilities that provide biochemical defenses, in varying degrees, against the potentially toxic effects of a large number of naturally occurring and synthetic chemicals. Both oxidative and conjugative reactions have been characterized in various insect species.

Species Differences in Metabolism

Among the mammals there are wide differences in drug metabolism by different species. Rates of metabolism may differ even when the pathways are the same, and different species may also have entirely different metabolic pathways for dealing with the same drug. An example of variation in metabolic rate is afforded by the antirheumatic agent phenylbutazone. The biologic half-life of this drug is only 3 hours in the rabbit and less than 6 hours in the rat, guinea pig, and the dog, yet its half-life in humans is 3 days. Striking interspecies differences have been well documented for conjugation reactions as well as for drug oxidation by hepatic monooxygenases.

Table 5-7. Species Differences in Metabolism of Hexobarbital[a]

	Sleeping Time (min)	Hexobarbital Half-Life (min)	Enzyme Activity ($\mu g/g \cdot hr$)
Mice (12)	12 ± 8	19 ± 7	598 ± 184
Rabbits (9)	49 ± 12	60 ± 11	196 ± 28
Rats (10)	90 ± 15	140 ± 54	134 ± 51
Dogs (8)	315 ± 105	260 ± 20	36 ± 30
Humans	—	360 (approx.)	—

[a] Dose of barbiturate 100 mg kg^{-1} (50 mg kg^{-1} in dogs). Figures in parentheses refer to number of animals in each species. Data are given $\pm$ standard deviation. The half-life in humans is a crude estimate. (Data from Quinn et al.[115])

The metabolism of hexobarbital was shown to be responsible for species differences in its duration of action (Table 5-7). Determinations of plasma levels at various times following intravenous administration of the compound permitted estimation of the biologic half-life in each species. There was a direct relationship between duration of action (sleeping time) and biologic half-life. In addition, the in vitro activity of microsomes prepared from livers of these animals correlated well with the drug metabolism rate in vivo. Thus, mice with the shortest sleeping time and shortest barbiturate half-life had the highest liver microsomal enzyme activity. Presumably, these species all metabolized hexobarbital by aliphatic side-chain oxidation, although direct proof of this is lacking.

Species differences in the metabolism of foreign compounds may also be considered in terms of differences in individual metabolic pathways. For example, the hepatic micro-

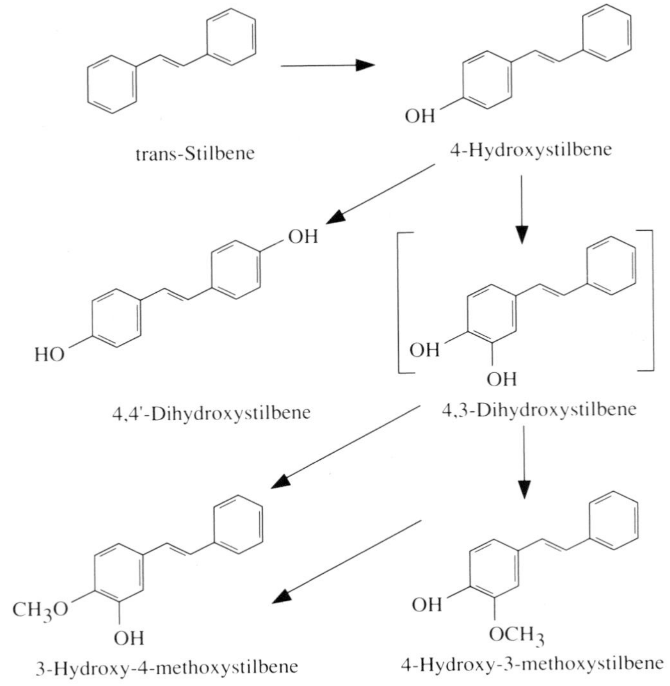

trans-Stilbene → 4-Hydroxystilbene

4,4'-Dihydroxystilbene   4,3-Dihydroxystilbene

3-Hydroxy-4-methoxystilbene   4-Hydroxy-3-methoxystilbene

somal enzyme coumarin 7-hydroxylase, which is responsible for a high proportion of coumarin hydroxylation in cats, guinea pigs, hamsters, rabbits, and humans, is absent from the livers of ferrets, mice, and rats.[116] In humans 7-hydroxycoumarin is the principal metabolite (68 to 92 percent), but in rats and rabbits 3-hydroxycoumarin and its degradation products predominate. Thus, the ratio of the two metabolites is species-dependent. The metabolism of *trans*-stilbene is another example of a species difference in metabolic pathways. This compound is metabolized in vivo differently by mouse and rabbit.[117] In the rabbit biotransformations into 4-hydroxy-, 4,4'-dihydroxy-, 3-hydroxy-4-methoxy-, and 4-hydroxy-3-methoxystilbene occur. In the mouse, however, the only hydroxylated product is a limited amount of 4,4'-dihydroxystilbene.

Species differences in both cytochrome P450 content and NADPH-cytochrome P450 reductase activity have been reported in mice, rats, and cats.[118] Mice have the highest cytochrome P450 content and NADPH-cytochrome P450 reductase and aminopyrine *N*-demethylase activities, and cats have the lowest levels of each. The species differences observed in liver microsomal preparations do not necessarily exist in extrahepatic tissues. For example, rat and rabbit livers have similar cytochrome P450 contents, but rabbit lung contains seven to eight times as much cytochrome P450 as rat lung. In addition to quantitative differences, qualitative differences in composition of cytochrome P450 isoenzymes can determine the organ-specific toxicity of certain environmentally derived chemicals. Several distinct P450 isoenzymes differing in amino acid sequence as well as spectral and catalytic properties have been purified from hepatic microsomes of female rats.[119] The existence of multiple P450s provides considerable room for species differences in microsomal oxidative capacity.

A variety of species differences in metabolic conjugation capacity have also been documented.[120] The best described differences are defects of glucuronidation in the cat and related feline species and of *N*-acetylation in the dog. It is important to note that these defects are not absolute; rather, they must be qualified with reference to the substrate in question. For example, the cat is unable to conjugate simple, relatively water-soluble phenols and carboxylic acids, but conjugation of complex, lipid-soluble substrates proceeds to the same extent in the cat as in other species. Similarly, dogs are unable to *N*-acetylate aromatic amino groups and hydrazides, but they do acetylate the *S*-substituted cysteines that are the penultimate intermediates in the conversion of glutathione conjugates to mercapturic acids. Guinea pigs, on the other hand, apparently cannot *N*-acetylate these substituted cysteines, but they do acetylate a variety of other amines.

The problems posed by species differences for the development and screening of new drugs are considerable; yet a knowledge of the metabolism of a new chemical agent is fundamental to its safety evaluation in humans. A fairly detailed metabolic pathway for a new biologically actve agent should be elucidated in at least two animal species. Validation in humans of the metabolic pathway determined for a compound in animals depends on finding a similarity in rates of excretion and plasma kinetics after administration of comparable doses and on the detection of a similar profile of metabolic products in the urine.

In addition to species differences in the rates of drug metabolism, strain differences also exist. Because of the complexity of their genetic makeup, strain differences in drug metabolism would be expected to be particularly evident in humans, and a number of specific examples are presented in Chapter 7. A good example of a strain difference in drug metabolism in animals is provided by the Gunn strain of Wistar rat. The Gunn rat cannot form *O*-glucuronides of bilirubin and of most exogenous organic compounds, but

Table 5-8. Strain Differences in Duration of Action of Hexobarbital in Mice[a]

Strain	Mean Sleeping Time ± Standard Deviation (min)
A/NL (25)	48 ± 4
BALB/cAnN (63)	41 ± 2
C57L/HeN (29)	33 ± 3
C3HfB/HeN (30)	22 ± 3
SWR/HeN (38)	18 ± 4
Swiss (noninbred) (47)	43 ± 15

[a] Male mice, 70–80 days old, given hexobarbital (125 mg kg^{-1}) intraperitoneally. Figures in parentheses are number of mice in each strain. (Data from Jay.[122])

it does form *N*-glucuronides, for example of aniline. This defect is due to a deficiency of *O*-glucuronyl transferase, but not all *O*-glucuronyl transferases are absent–the Gunn rat is able to form *O*-glucuronides of *p*-nitrophenol but not of *o*-aminophenol.[121]

Table 5-8 illustrates pronounced strain differences in the oxidative metabolism of hexobarbital in mice.[122] The data are sleeping times after a single dose of hexobarbital, but it is well known that in mice the duration of action of this drug is determined by the rate of its oxidation. Besides the highly significant differences between strains, another point is evident: the one strain that was not inbred had a much greater variability between animals (as measured by the standard deviation) than did the inbred strains. This is just what one would expect for a trait under genetic control.

Sex Differences in Metabolism

In rats although strain differences are not usually very great, sex differences in drug metabolism are very prominent; they are not normally found in guinea pigs, rabbits, dogs, or humans, and while some strains of mice do show sex differences, these are not as generalized as in rats. Sex differences in hepatic drug metabolism appear with the onset of puberty in rats and are maintained throughout the adult life of the animals.[123] Male rats metabolize certain drugs at faster rates than females, and these differences occur not only in the oxidative pathways but also with glucuronide and glutathione conjugation of certain substrates. Among the oxidative reactions, the sex differences observed depend both on the substrate and on the reaction measured. For example, the well-known sex difference in the rate of *N*-dealkylation of ethylmorphine in mature rats was not observed with *O*-dealkylation of the same substrate, nor did *O*-dealkylase activity increase as male rats reached maturity, as does *N*-dealkylase activity.[124] Adult male and female rats do not show sex differences in the aromatic hydroxylation of substrates such as aniline and zoxazolamine. Some sex differences are specific only to certain tissues. Male rat liver microsomes show significantly higher benzphetamine *N*-demethylase, benzpyrene hydroxylase, and UDP-glucuronyl transferase activities than do microsomes from female rat livers. However, no significant differences in these activities are observed with lung microsomes from adult male and female rates.[125]

The increased levels of cytochrome P450 measured in livers of adult male rats versus female rats do not match the much higher rates of hepatic metabolism seen with certain substrates, such as ethylmorphine, in the male compared with the female. This disparity reflects qualitative differences in the cytochrome P450 isoenzyme composition of male and female rat liver microsomes. Studies in which four cytochromes P450 isoenzymes from untreated adult rats were purified and characterized have shown that cytochrome P450*f* is present in both males and females, cytochrome P450*i* is a female-specific iso-enzyme, and cytochromes P450*g* and P450*h* are male-specific proteins.[126,127] Several studies have shown that sex hormones, especially androgens, play an important role in defining the differences in cytochrome P450 composition of male and female rats.[123] Enzyme activity is decreased by castration in the male, and administration of androgens to castrated animals increases the activity of the sex-dependent enzymes. Administration of anabolic steroids to female rats also increases the drug-metabolizing enzyme activities of the females. Some aspects of these sex differences are attributed to androgen imprinting during the neonatal period, although the exact site of androgen imprinting has not yet been determined. These sex-dependent differences persist for life even if the adult male rat is deprived of androgenic steroids via castration for a prolonged time. The higher levels of cytochrome P450*i* in female rats suggest that estrogenic hormones may play a role in its regulation. Male rats who are neonatally castrated have decreased levels of the P450*h* isoenzyme. In contrast to these sex-dependent cytochrome P450s isolated from rat liver, no significant sex differences characterize the several other forms of cytochromes P450 from rat livers.

EFFECTS OF AGE ON DRUG METABOLISM

The levels of hepatic microsomal monooxygenase activity are very low during the fetal development of most mammals, but they increase rapidly soon after birth. It has become clear that, unlike the fetuses of common laboratory species, the human fetus is able to metabolize drugs and other foreign compounds. The differences in fetal enzyme activities observed between animals and humans may result from differences in gestation periods, differences in the maturity of fetuses of various species, and dietary differences, as well as exposure to environmental chemicals that may cross the placental barrier. Unlike humans, experimental animals are bred and housed in rather carefully controlled environments, and they may not be exposed to the variety of chemical inducers that reach the human fetus.

Figure 5-12 presents an idealized scheme of the development of drug-metabolizing activity in the human and the rat.[128,129] Curve A represents the development of a number of oxidizing activities in human liver. The activities develop during the first trimester and then remain at a plateau until birth. After birth, the drug-metabolizing activity rises gradually until adult levels are achieved. Curve B is typical of several drug-metabolizing activities in the rat and other common laboratory animals. Curve C represents the so-called late fetal group of UDP-glucuronyl transferase activities in the rat, and curve D represents the development of aryl hydrocarbon hydroxylase activity in the perinatal rat liver.

Various factors that influence the development of drug-oxidizing activity also influence the metabolism of endogenous substrates such as steroid hormones. Figure 5-13 shows the development of three hepatic enzymes in male rats that hydroxylate testosterone in the 6β, 7α, and 16α positions.[130] It is clear that there are different patterns of development for the three different hydroxylase reactions. The 16α-hydroxylation of testosterone is low at birth and remains low for 4 weeks, but it then increases markedly over the next several weeks. The 6β-hydroxylation activity is seen to increase during the first week of life, to remain at a plateau during the next 6 weeks, and to undergo a second increase during weeks 8 through 10. The 7α-hydroxylation activity increases rapidly after birth but then decreases between 4 and 7 weeks of age.

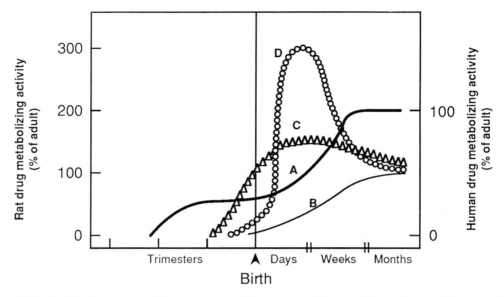

Fig. 5-12. Idealized patterns of development of drug-metabolizing activity in livers of humans (A) and rats (B, C, and D). The curves are described in the text. (From Mannering,[128] after Pelkonen,[129] with permission.)

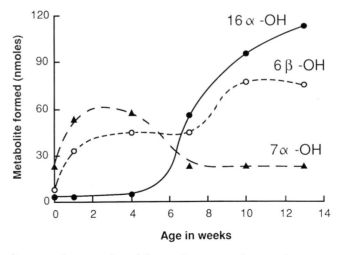

Fig. 5-13. Effect of age on the capacity of liver microsomes from male rats to carry out the 6β-, 7α-, and 16α-hydroxylation of testosterone. The ordinate represents nanomoles of product formed from testosterone C14 by rat liver microsomes incubated at 37°C with an NADPH-generating system. Rats of mixed sex were used for newborn data and male rats only were used for all other data points. (From Conney et al.,[130] with permission.)

Of the conjugation reactions, glucuronide formation has been studied most extensively.[43] The pattern of development observed for the glucuronidation pathway depends somewhat upon the species, strain, and substrate used for the study. In general, it can be said that most conjugation pathways are poorly developed in the fetus. Bilirubin UDP-glucuronyl transferase activity, in particular, is low in the human fetus and neonate. In premature infants the conjugating system responsible for coupling bilirubin with glucuronic acid is deficient. This metabolic deficiency can lead to a prolonged and elevated level of unconjugated bilirubin, which can pass across the blood-brain barrier and cause kernicterus. As we have discussed in Chapter 3, the situation is aggravated when drugs, such as sulfonamides, that can displace bilirubin from its plasma-binding sites are administered.

The tragic experience with chloramphenicol in newborn infants[131] highlights the serious consequences that can result from deficient drug metabolism. The therapeutic or prophylactic use of chloramphenicol in hospital nurseries led to cases of cyanosis ("gray syndrome"). Some deaths occurred, especially in premature infants, after cardiovascular and respiratory collapse. In the adult human about 90 percent of a dose of chloramphenicol is excreted as the monoglucuronide derivative, about 8 percent as free drug, and traces as the hydrolyzed deacetylated derivative. In newborn infants (and in cats) a small amount of a dehalogenated product is also found. In premature infants and during the first week or two of life in normal infants, the mechanism for glucuronide conjugation is grossly deficient. At the same time renal function (both glomerular filtration and tubular secretion) is also very inefficient. Consequently, an ordinary dose of chloramphenicol leads to a high and prolonged plasma level of the free drug. Plasma glucuronide levels also increase because of the defective tubular secretory mechanism, but, at least in the adult, chloramphenicol monoglucuronide is nontoxic. Repeated doses at intervals that would be suitable in the older infant cause a progressive buildup of the plasma level of chloramphenicol into the range of severe hematologic toxicity.

Although comprehensive human data regarding age-related differences in oxidative metabolism are not available for a large spectrum of drugs, clear differences have been established for a few drugs. It is known, for example, that children metabolize certain drugs (e.g., diazoxide, phenobarbital, antipyrine, and phenylbutazone) at a faster rate than adults. In children ranging in age from 1 to 8 years, for example, the mean antipyrine half-life was found to be 6.6 hours compared with a mean of 13.6 hours in adults, and the mean phenylbutazone half-life was 1.7 days versus 3.2 days in adults[132] (Fig. 5-14). As both these drugs are metabolized primarily through oxidative pathways, it is likely that these differences reflect differences in oxidative capacity. Studies of theophylline administration to asthmatic patients show that children eliminate this bronchodilating drug at a considerably faster rate than adults[133]; therefore, higher doses are required to achieve therapeutic theophylline concentrations in children.[134]

Studies of metabolism in old rats show that aging is accompanied by a decline in the rate of metabolism of a number of xenobiotics.[135] Although systematic studies have not been carried out with humans, several clinical studies have provided indirect evidence for reduced oxidative metabolic activity in the elderly. Again, antipyrine and phenylbutazone provide useful examples.[136,137] The mean plasma half-lives of antipyrine (Fig. 5-15) and phenylbutazone were found to be 45 and 29 percent greater in geriatric patients than in adults 20 to 50 years old. The lower metabolic activity of the liver in geriatric patients may be due both to lower hepatic enzyme activity and to decreased hepatic blood flow. Since the liver has a substantial reserve of cell mass and functional capacity when

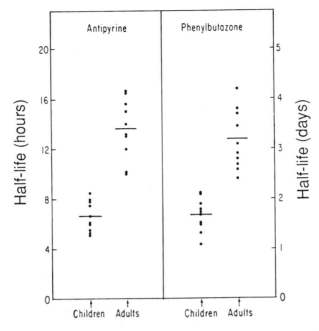

Fig. 5-14. Antipyrine and phenylbutazone half-lives in children and adults. Antipyrine (18 mg/kg) or phenylbutazone (6 mg/kg) was administered orally, and plasma drug levels were assayed. The horizontal bar represents the mean value for 10 children aged 1 to 8 years or 10 adults aged 25 to 42 years. For both drugs the difference in the mean plasma half-life between children and adults is significant ($P < .001$). (From Alvares et al.,[132] with permission.)

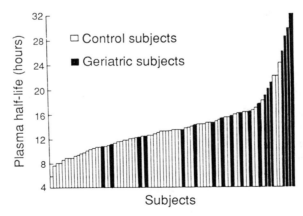

Fig. 5-15. Individual plasma antipyrine half-life values in control and geriatric patients. The mean plasma antipyrine half-life in control patients (open bars) 20 to 50 years old was 12 ± 3.5 hours, and in geriatric patients (solid bars) 70 to 100 years old the mean half-life was 17.4 ± 6.8 hours. The difference between the two groups is significant at the $P < 0.01$ level. (From O'Malley et al.,[136] with permission.)

adulthood is achieved, the normal loss of liver mass that occurs with advanced age probably does not play a significant role in decreased drug metabolism. Drugs with a high hepatic clearance, such as propranolol, remain in their unmetabolized state in the bloodstream longer in elderly than in younger patients. Such age-related decreases in hepatic metabolism have been documented in humans with at least 17 drugs.[138] The decline in hepatic metabolism that occurs with aging principally involves the cytochrome P450 system.

REFERENCES

1. Jenner P, Testa B (eds): Concepts in Drug Metabolism. Marcel Dekker, New York, 1980
2. Gibson GG, Skett P: Introduction to Drug Metabolism. Chapman & Hall, New York, 1986
3. Benford DJ, Bridges JW, Gibson GG (eds): Drug Metabolism—from Molecules to Man. Taylor & Francis, London, 1987
4. Brodie BB, Axelrod J: The fate of acetanilide in man. J Pharmacol Exp Ther 94:29, 1948
5. Brodie BB, Axelrod J: The fate of acetophenetidin (phenacetin) in man and methods for the estimation of acetophenetidin and its metabolites in biological material. J Pharmacol Exp Ther 97:58, 1949
6. Conney AH, Sansur M, Soroko F, et al: Enzyme induction and inhibition in studies on the pharmacological actions of acetophenetidin. J Pharmacol Exp Ther 151:133, 1966
7. Kiese M: Relationship of drug metabolism to methemoglobin formation. Ann NY Acad Sci 123:141, 1965
8. Schenkman JB, Kupfer D (eds): Hepatic Cytochrome P-450 Monooxygenase System. Pergamon Press, Oxford, 1982
9. Lu AYH, Coon MJ: Role of hemeprotein P-450 in fatty acid ω-hydroxylation in a soluble system from liver microsomes. J Biol Chem 243:1331, 1968
10. Masters BSS, Baron J, Taylor WE, et al: Immunochemical studies on electron transport chains involving cytochrome P-450. I. Effects of antibodies to pig liver microsomal triphosphopyridine nucleotide-cytochrome c reductase and the non-heme iron protein from bovine adrenocortical mitochrondria. J Biol Chem 246:4143, 1971
11. Ryan DE, Ramanathan L, Iida S, et al: Characterization of a major form of rat hepatic microsomal cytochrome P-450 induced by isoniazid. J Biol Chem 260:6385, 1985
12. Conney AH: Induction of microsomal cytochrome P-450 enzymes. Life Sci 39:2493, 1986
13. Digiuseppi J, Fridovich I: The toxicity of molecular oxygen. CRC Crit Rev Toxicol 12:315, 1984
14. Remmer H, Schenkman J, Estabrook RW, et al: Drug interaction with hepatic microsomal cytochrome. Mol Pharmacol 2:187, 1966
15. Mannering GJ: Microsomal enzyme systems which catalyze drug metabolism. In LaDu BN, Mandel HG, Way EL (eds): Fundamentals of Drug Metabolism and Drug Disposition. Williams & Wilkins, Baltimore, 1971
16. Schulster D, Burstein S, Cooke BA: Molecular Endocrinology of the Steroid Hormones. John Wiley & Sons, London, 1976
17. Burns JJ, Yu TF, Ritterband A, et al: A potent new uricosuric agent, the sulfoxide metabolite of the phenylbutazone analogue, G-25671. J Pharmacol Exp Ther 119:418, 1957
18. Ziegler DM, Mitchell CH: Microsomal oxidase. IV. Properties of a mixed function amine oxidase isolated from pig liver microsomes. Arch Biochem Biophys 150:116, 1972
19. Debaum JR, Miller EC, Miller JA: N-Hydroxy-2-acetylaminofluorene sulfotransferase: Its probable role in carcinogenesis and protein-methion-S-yl binding in rat liver. Cancer Res 30:577, 1970
20. Suarez KA, Bhonsle P: The relationship of colbaltous chloride-induced alterations of hepatic microsomal enzymes to altered carbon tetrachloride hepatotoxicity. Toxicol Appl Pharmacol 37:23, 1976

21. Garner RC, McLean AEM: Increased susceptibility of carbon tetrachloride poisoning in the rat after pretreatment with oral phenobarbital. Biochem Pharmacol 18:645, 1969

22. Mazze RI, Trudell JR, Cousins MF: Methoxyfurane metabolism and renal dysfunctions. Anesthesiology 35:247, 1971

23. MacDonald TL: Chemical mechanisms of halocarbon metabolism. CRC Crit Rev Toxicol 11:85, 1983

24. Lieber CS, Decarli LM: Hepatic microsomal ethanol oxidizing system: In vitro characteristics and adaptive properties in vivo. J Biol Chem 245:2505, 1970

25. Ishii H, Joly JG, Lieber CS: Effect of ethanol on the amount and enzyme activities of hepatic rough and smooth microsomal membranes. Biochim Biophys Acta 291:411, 1973

26. Koop DR, Morgan ET, Tarr GE, Coon MJ: Purification and characterization of a unique isozyme of cytochrome P-450 from liver microsomes of ethanol-treated rabbits. J Biol Chem 257:8472, 1982

27. Jenne JW, Nagasawa HT, Thompson RD: Relationship of urinary metabolites to serum theophylline levels. Clin Pharmacol Ther 19:375, 1976

28. Blaschko H: Amine oxidase. p. 337. In Boyer PD, Lardy H, Myrbäck K (eds): The Enzymes. Vol. 8. 3rd Ed. Academic Press, Orlando, FL, 1973

29. Zeller EA: Diamine oxidases. p. 313. In Boyer PD, Lardy H, Myrbäck K (eds): The Enzymes. Vol. 8. 3rd Ed. Academic Press, Orlando, FL, 1973

30. Harada N, Omura T: Participation of cytochrome P-450 in the reduction of nitrocompounds by rat liver microsomes. J. Biochem (Tokyo) 87:1539, 1980

31. Heymann E: Carboxylesterases and amidases. p. 291. In Jakoby WB (ed): Enzymatic Basis of Detoxification. Vol. 2. Academic Press, Orlando, FL, 1980

32. Humphrey MJ, Ringrose PS: Peptides and related drugs: A review of their adsorption, metabolism, and excretion. Drug Metab Rev 17:283, 1986

33. McMartin C: Delivery, distribution, clearance and degradation: Key factors in the design and development of peptide and protein drugs. p. 604. In Benford DJ, Bridges JW, Gibson GG (eds): Taylor & Francis, London, 1987

34. Roemer D, Pless J: Structure-activity relationships of orally active enkephalin analogues as analgesics. Life Sci 24:621, 1979

35. Yokohama S, Yamashita K, Toguchi H, et al: Intestinal absorption mechanisms of thyrotropin-releasing hormone. J Pharm Dyn 7:445, 1984

36. Brewster D, Humphrey MJ, Wareing MV: Metabolism and pharmacokinetics of TRH and an analog with enhanced neuropharmacological potency. Neuropeptides 1:153, 1981

37. Wislocki PG, Wood AW, Chang RL, et al: High mutagenicity and toxicity of a diol epoxide derived from benzo[a]pyrene. Biochem Biophys Res Commun 68:1006, 1976

38. Kapitulnik J, Wislocki PG, Levin W, et al: Tumorigenicity studies with diol-epoxides of benzo[a]pyrene which indicate that (±)-trans-7β,8α-dihydroxy-9α,10α-epoxy-7,8,9,10-tetrahydrobenzo(a)pyrene is an ultimate carcinogen in newborn mice. Cancer Res 38:354, 1978

39. Guengerich FP, Wang P, Mitchell MB, Mason PS: Rat and human liver microsomal epoxide hydratase: Purification and evidence for the existence of multiple forms. J Biol Chem 254:12248, 1979

40. Oesch F, Timms CW, Walker CH, et al: Existence of multiple forms of microsomal epoxide hydrolases with radically different substrate specificities. Carcinogenesis 5:7, 1984

41. Ota K, Hammock BD: Cytosolic and microsomal epoxide hydrolases: Differential properties in mammalian liver. Science 207:1479, 1980

42. Dutton GJ: Glucuronidation of Drugs and Other Compounds. CRC Press, Boca Raton, FL, 1980

43. Bock KW, von Clausbruch UC, Kaufmann R, et al: Functional heterogeneity of UDP-glucuronyl-transferase in rat tissues. Biochem Pharmacol 29:495, 1980

44. Schmid R: Hyperbilirubinemia. p. 1141. In Stanbury JB, Wyngaarden JB, Frederickson DS (eds): Metabolic Basis of Inherited Disease. 3rd Ed. McGraw-Hill, New York, 1972

45. Mackenzie PI: Rat liver UDP-glucuronosyltransferase. Sequence and expression of a cDNA encoding a phenobarbital-inducible form. J Biol Chem 261:6119, 1986
46. Kadlubar FF, Miller MA, and Miller EC: Hepatic microsomal N-glucuronidation and nucleic acid binding of N-hydroxylarylamines in relation to urinary bladder carcinogenesis. Cancer Res 37:805, 1977
47. Pratt WB and Ruddon RW: The Anticancer Drugs. Ch. 6. Oxford University Press, New York, 1979
48. Weber WW: The Acetylator Genes and Drug Response. Ch. 4. Oxford University Press, New York, 1987
49. Weber WW: Acetylation of drugs. p. 249. In Fishman WH (ed): Metabolic Conjugation and Metabolic Hydrolysis. Vol. 3. Academic Press, Orlando, FL, 1973
50. Weber WW: Acetylator genes in animals. In The Acetylator Genes and Drug Response Ch. 6. Oxford University Press, New York, 1987
51. Bakke J and Gustafsson JA: Mercapturic acid pathway for metabolites or xenobiotics: Generation of potentially toxic metabolites during enterohepatic circulation. Trends Pharmacol Sci 5:517, 1984
52. Chassaud LF: The role of glutathione and glutathione S-transferases in the metabolism of chemical carcinogens and other electrophilic agents. Adv Cancer Res 29:175, 1979
53. Mannervik B, Alin P, Guthenberg C, et al: Identification of three classes of cytosolic glutathione transferase common to several mammalian species: Correlation between structural data and enzymatic properties. Proc Natl Acad Sci USA 82:7202, 1985
54. Hayes JD, McLellan LI, Stockman PK, et al: Human glutathione S-transferases. p. 82. In Benford DJ, Bridges JW, Gibson GG (eds): Drug Metabolism—from Molecules to Man. Taylor & Francis, London, 1987
55. Hayes JD: Purification and physical characterization of glutathione S-transferase K. Biochem J 233:789, 1986
56. Glatt H, Friedberg T, Grover PL, et al: Inactivation of a diol-epoxide and a K-region epoxide with high efficiency by glutathione transferase X. Cancer Res 43:5713, 1983
57. Coles B, Meyer DJ, Ketterer B, et al: Studies on the detoxication of microsomally-activated aflatoxin B_1 by glutathione and glutathione transferases *in vitro*. Carcinogenesis 6:693, 1985
58. Benson AM, Batzinger RP, Ou SL, et al: Elevation of hepatic glutathione S-transferase activities and protection against mutagenic metabolites of benzo[a]pyrene by dietary antioxidants. Cancer Res 38:4486, 1978
59. Weinshilboum RM: Phenol sulfotransferase in humans: Properties, regulation, and function. Fed Proc 45:2223, 1986
60. Cobby J, Meyersohn M, Selliah S: Methyl diethyldithiocarbamate, a metabolite of disulfiram in man. Life Sci 21:937, 1977
61. Weisiger RA, Jakoby WB: S-methylation: Thiol S-methyl-transferase. p. 131. In Jakoby WB (ed): Enzymatic Basis of Detoxication. Vol. 2. Academic Press, Orlando, FL, 1980
62. Weisiger RA, Jakoby WB: Thiol S-methyltransferase from rat liver. Arch Biochem Biophys 196:631, 1979
63. Wilson J: Cyanide and human disease. p. 121. In Nestel B, MacIntyre R (eds): Chronic Cassava Toxicity. Monogr. IDRC-010e. Int Dev Res Cent, Ottawa, 1973
64. Schlesinger P, Westley J: An expanded mechanism for rhodanese catalysis. J Biol Chem 249:780, 1974
65. Franklin MR: Inhibition of mixed-function oxidases by substrates forming reduced cytochrome P-450 metabolic-intermediate complexes. In Schenkman JB, Kupfer D (eds): Hepatic Cytochrome P-450 Monooxygenase System, Pergamon Press, New York, 1982
66. Murray M: Mechanisms of the inhibition of cytochrome P-450-mediated drug oxidation by therapeutic agents. Drug Metab Rev 18:55, 1987
67. Axelrod J, Reichenthal J, Brodie BB: Mechanism of the potentiating action of β-diethyl-aminoethyl diphenylpropylacetate. J Pharmacol Exp Therap 112:49, 1954

68. Siiteri P: Review of studies on estrogen biosynthesis in the human. Cancer Res suppl. 42:3269s, 1982

69. Mendelson CR, Wright EE, Evans CT, et al: Preparation and characterization of polyclonal and monoclonal antibodies against human aromatase cytochrome P-450 (P-450$_{AROM}$), and their use in its purification. Arch Biochem Biophys 243:480, 1985

70. Tan L, Muto N: Purification and reconstitution properties of human placental aromatase. A cytochrome P-450-type monoxygenase. Eur J Biochem 156:243, 1986

71. Harvey HA, Lipton A, Santen RJ (eds): Conference on Aromatase: New Perspectives for Breast Cancer. Cancer Res suppl. 42:No. 8, 1982

72. Brodie AMH: Aromatase inhibition and its pharmacologic implications. Biochem Pharmacol 34:3213, 1985

73. Sedman AJ: Cimetidine-drug interactions. Am J Med 76:109, 1984

74. Greenblatt DJ, Abernethy DR, Morse DS, et al: Clinical importance of the interaction of diazepam and cimetidine. N Engl J Med 310:1639, 1984

75. Serlin MJ, Sibeon RG, Mossman S, et al: Cimetidine: Interaction with oral anticoagulants in man. Lancet 2:317, 1979

76. Rendic S, Kajfez F, Ruff HH: Characterization of cimetidine, ranitidine, and related structures' interaction with cytochrome P-450. Drug Metab Dispos 11:137, 1983

77. Kitson TM: The disulfiram-ethanol reaction. J Stud Alcohol 38:96, 1977

78. Hald J, Jacobsen E, Larsen V: Formation of acetaldehyde in the organism in relation to dosage of Antabuse (tetraethylthiuramidisulphide) and to alcohol concentration in blood. Acta Pharmacol Toxicol 5:179, 1949

79. Kitson TM: The effect of disulfiram on the aldehyde dehydrogenases of sheep liver. Biochem J 151:407, 1975

80. Neims AH, Coffey DS, Hellerman L: Interaction between tetraethylthiuram disulfide and the sulfhydryl groups of D-amino acid oxidase and of hemoglobin. J Biol Chem 241:5942, 1966

81. Dietrich RA, Erwin VG: Mechanism of inhibition of aldehyde dehydrogenase in vivo by disulfiram and diethyldithiocarbamate. Mol Pharmacol 7:301, 1971

82. Zeller EA, Barsky J, Berman ER: Amine oxidases. XI. Inhibition of monoamine oxidase by 1-isonicotinyl-2-isopropylhydrazine. J Biol Chem 214:267, 1955

83. Singer TP: Active site-directed, irreversible inhibitors of monoamine oxidase. p. 7. In Singer TP, von Korff RW, Murphy DL (eds): Monoamine Oxidase, Structure, Function, and Altered Functions. Academic Press, Orlando, FL, 1979

84. Tipton KF, Dostert P, Strolin Benedetti M (eds): Monoamine Oxidase and Disease. Prospects for Therapy with Reversible Inhibitors. Academic Press, Orlando, FL, 1984

85. Asatoor AM, Levi AJ, Milne MO: Tranylcypromine and cheese. Lancet 2:733, 1963

86. Blackwell B: Tranylcypromine. Lancet 2:414, 1963

87. Bianchine JR, Shaw GM: Clinical pharmacokinetics of levodopa in Parkinson's disease. Clin Pharmacokinet 1:313, 1976

88. Calne DB: Progress in Parkinson's disease. N Engl J Med 310:523, 1984

89. Fox IH: Degradation of purine nucleotides. In Kelley WN, Weiner IM (eds): Uric Acid. Handbuch der Experimentellen Pharmakologie. Vol. 51: Springer-Verlag, Berlin, 1978

90. Elion GB, Callahan S, Rundles RW, Hitchings GH: Relationship between metabolic states and antitumor activities of thiopurines. Cancer Res 23:1207, 1963

91. Rundles RW, Wyngaarden JB, Hitchings GH, Elion GB: Drugs and uric acid. Annu Rev Pharmacol 9:345, 1969

92. Spector T, Johns DG: Stoichiometric inhibition of reduced xanthine oxidase by hydroxypyrazolo[3,4-*d*]pyrimidines. J Biol Chem 245:5079, 1970

93. Elion GB: Allopurinol and other inhibitors of urate synthesis. In Kelley WN, Weiner IM (eds): Uric Acid. Handbuch der Experimentellen Pharmacologie. Vol. 51. Springer-Verlag, Berlin, 1978

94. Massey V, Komai, H, Palmer G, and Elion GB: On the mechanism of inactivation of xanthine oxidase by allopurinol and other pyrazolo[3,4-*d*]pyrimidines. J Biol Chem 245:2837, 1970

95. Kahan FM, Kropp H, Sundelof JG, and Birnbaum J: Thienamycin: Development of imipenem-cilastin. J Antimicrob Chemother 12: suppl. D, 1, 1983

96. Barza M: Imipenem: First of a new class of beta-lactam antibiotics. Ann Intern Med 103:552, 1985.

97. Conney AH, Miller EC, Miller JA: The metabolism of methylated aminoazo dyes. V. Evidence for induction of enzyme synthesis in the rat by 3-methylcholanthrene. Cancer Res 16:450, 1956

98. Conney AH, Miller EC, Miller JA: Substrate-induced synthesis and other properties of benzpyrene hydroxylase in rat liver. J Biol Chem 228:753, 1957

99. Remmer H: Die Beschleunigung der Evipanoxydation und der Dimethylierung von Methy-laminoantipyrin durch Barbiturate. Arch Exp Pathol Pharmakol 237:296, 1959

100. Conney AH, Miller EC, Miller JA: Substrate-induced synthesis and other properties of benzpyrene hydroxylase in rat liver. J Biol Chem 228:753, 1957

101. Conney AH, Davison C, Gastel R, Burns JJ: Adaptive increases in drug-metabolizing enzymes induced by phenobarbital and other drugs. J Pharmacol Exp Ther 130:1, 1960

102. Conney AH: Induction of microsomal enzymes by foreign chemicals and carcinogenesis by polycyclic aromatic hydrocarbons. Cancer Res 42:4875, 1982

103. Alvares AP, Schilling G, Levin W, Kuntzman R: Studies on the induction of CO-binding pigments by phenobarbital and 3-methylcholanthrene. Biochem Biophys Res Commun 29:521, 1967

104. Sladek NE, Mannering GJ: Evidence for a new P-450 hemoprotein in hepatic microsomes from methylcholanthrene treated rats. Biochem Biophys Res Commun 24:668, 1966

105. Remmer H: Drugs as activators of drug enzymes. p. 235. In Brodie BB, Erdös EG (eds): Metabolic Factors Controlling Duration of Drug Action. Proceedings of First International Pharmacological Meeting. Vol. 6. Macmillan, New York, 1962

106. Cucinell SA, Conney AH, Sansur M, Burns JJ: Drug interactions in man. I. Lowering effect of phenobarbital on plasma levels of bishydroxy coumarin (dicumarol) and diphenylhydantoin (Dilantin), Clin Pharmacol Ther 6:420, 1965

107. Alvares AP, Kappas A: Heterogeneity of cytochrome P-450s induced by polychlorinated biphenyls. J Biol Chem 252:6363, 1977

108. Alvares AP, Ueng T-H, Eiseman JL: Polychlorinated biphenyls (PCBs) inducible monooxygenases in rabbits and mice: Species and organ specificities. Life Sci 30:747, 1982

109. Ueng T-H, Eiseman JL, Alvares AP: Inhibition of pulmonary cytochrome P-450 and benzo(a)pyrene hydroxylase in rabbits by polychlorinated biphenyls (PCBs). Biochem Biophys Res Commun 95:1743, 1980

110. Gelboin HV: Mechanisms of induction of drug-metabolizing enzymes. In Brodie BB, Gillette JR (eds): Concepts in Biochemical Pharmacology. Handbuch der Experimentellen Pharmacologie. Vol. 28, Part 2: Springer-Verlag, New York, 1971

111. Zampaglione N, Jollow DJ, Mitchell JR, et al: Role of detoxifying enzymes in bromobenzene-induced liver necrosis. J Pharmacol Exp Ther 187:218, 1973

112. Pohl RJ, Bend JR, Guarino AM, Fouts JR: Hepatic microsomal mixed-function oxidase activity of several marine species from coastal Maine. Drug Metab Dispos 2:545, 1974

113. Arinc E, Adali O: Solubilization and partial purification of two forms of cytochrome P-450 from trout liver microsomes. Comp Biochem Physiol 76B:653, 1983

114. Ball LM, Elmamlouk TH, Bend JR: Metabolism of benzo[a]pyrene in little skate mixed-function oxidase systems. p, 1203. In Coon MJ, Conney AH, Estabrook RW, et al (eds): Microsomes, Drug Oxidations and Chemical Carcinogenesis. Vol. 2. Academic Press, Orlando, FL, 1980

115. Quinn GP, Axelrod J, Brodie BB: Species, strain and sex differences in metabolism of hexobarbitone, amidopyrine, antipyrine, and aniline. Biochem Pharmacol 1:152, 1958

116. Kaighen M, Williams RT: The metabolism of [3-^{14}C]coumarin. J Med Pharm Chem 3:25, 1961
117. Sinshimer JE, Smith RV: Metabolic hydroxylations of trans-stilbene. Biochem J 111:35, 1969
118. Kato R: Characteristics and differences in the hepatic mixed function oxidases of different species. Pharmacol Ther 6:41, 1979
119. Imaoka S, Kamataki T, Funae Y: Purification and characterization of six cytochromes P-450 from hepatic microsomes of immature female rats. J Biochem 102:843, 1987
120. Caldwell J: Conjugation mechanisms of xenobiotic metabolism: Mammalian aspects. p. 2. In Paulson GD, Caldwell J, Hutton DH, Menn JM (eds): Xenobiotic Conjunction Chemistry, American Chemical Society, Washington, 1986
121. Van Leusden HAIM, Bakkeren JAJM, Zilliken F, Stolte LAM: p-Nitrophenylglucuronide formation by homozygous adult Gunn rats. Biochem Biophys Res Commun 7:67, 1962
122. Jay GE Jr: Variation in response of various mouse strains to hexobarbital (Evipal). Proc Soc Exp Biol Med 90:378, 1955
123. Waxman DJ: Interactions of hepatic cytochromes P-450 with steroid hormones. Regioselectivity and stereoselectivity of steroid metabolism and hormonal regulation of rat P-450 enzyme expression. Biochem Pharmacol 37:71, 1988
124. Nerland DE, Mannering GJ: Species, sex, and developmental differences in the O- and N-dealkylation of ethylmorphine by hepatic microsomes. Drug Metab Dispos 6:150, 1978
125. Chabra RS, Fouts JR: Sex differences in the metabolism of xenobiotics by extrahepatic tissue in rats. Drug Metab Dispos 2:375, 1974
126. Ryan DE, Iida S, Wood AW, et al: Characterization of three highly purified cytochromes P-450 from hepatic microsomes of adult male rats. J Biol Chem 259:1239, 1984
127. Ryan DE, Dixon R, Evans RH, et al: Rat hepatic cytochrome P-450 isozyme specificity for the metabolism of the steroid sulfate 5α-androstane-3α, 17β-diol-3,17-disulfate. Arch Biochem Biophys 233:636, 1984
128. Mannering GJ: Drug metabolism in the newborn. Fed Proc 44:2302, 1985
129. Pelkonen O: The differentiation of drug metabolism in relation to developmental toxicology. p. 165. In Snell K (ed): Developmental Toxicology. Praeger, New York, 1982
130. Conney AH, Levin W, Jacobson M, et al: Specificity in the regulation of the 6β-, 7α- and 16α-hydroxylation of testosterone by rat liver microsomes. p. 279. In Gillette JR, Conney AH, Cosmides GJ, et al (eds): Microsomes and Drug Oxidations. Academic Press, Orlando, FL, 1969
131. Pratt WB, Fekety R: Bacteriostatic inhibitors of protein synthesis. In The Antimicrobial Drugs. Oxford University Press, New York, 1986
132. Alvares AP, Kapelner S, Sassa S, Kappas A: Drug oxidation in normal children, lead-poisoned children, and normal adults. Clin Pharmacol Ther 17:179, 1975
133. Ellis EF, Koysooko R, Levy G: Pharmacokinetics of theophylline in children with asthma. Pediatrics 58:542, 1976
134. Hendles L, Weinberger M: Improved efficacy and safety of theophylline in the control of airway hyperreactivity. Pharmacol Ther 18:91, 1982
135. Kato R, Takanaka A: Metabolism of drugs in old rats: Activities of NADPH-linked electron transport and drug-metabolizing enzyme systems in liver microsomes of old rats. Jpn J Pharmacol 18:381, 1968
136. O'Malley K, Crooks J, Duke E, Stevenson IH: Effect of age and sex on human drug metabolism. Br Med J 3:607, 1971
137. Vestal RE, Norris AH, Tobin JD, et al: Antipyrine metabolism in man: Influence of age, alcohol, caffeine, and smoking. Clin Pharmacol Ther 18:425, 1975
138. Roberts J, Tumer N: Age and diet effects in drug action. Pharmacol Ther 37:111, 1988
139. Ryan DE, Thomas PE, Korzeniowski D, Levin W: Separation and characterization of highly purified forms of liver microsomal cytochrome P-450 from rats treated with polychlorinated biphenyls, phenobarbitol and 3-methylcholanthrene. J Biol Chem 254:1365, 1979

6

Molecular Aspects of Regulation and Structure of the Drug-Metabolizing Enzymes

Robert H. Tukey
Eric F. Johnson

Chapter 5 reviewed the many ways in which drugs and other foreign chemicals are transformed to diminish their biologic effects and to speed their elimination from the body. It is remarkable that we and other mammalian species have evolved with the capacity to metabolize such a diverse array of chemical substances. Many of these compounds did not exist until this century, and the capacity to metabolize them reflects not only the ability of individual enzymes to metabolize a range of structurally distinct substrates but also the multiplicity and diversity of enzymes that constitute the cytochrome P450 monooxygenases, the glucuronosyl transferases, and the glutathione transferases. The distinct properties of the individual forms of these enzymes together with their differential regulation lead to differences in drug metabolism between species, individuals, and tissues as well as at different ages. Moreover, inducing chemicals can alter the expression of individual enzymes, leading to selective increases in the capacity to metabolize drugs. The mechanism of induction in relation to cellular transcriptional and translational events is considered in this chapter; the consequences of induction are detailed in Chapter 5. Regulation of the drug-metabolizing enzymes has important consequences in carcinogenesis (Ch. 12) and teratogenicity (Ch. 13) and is often a determinant of pharmocogenetic differences in drug response (Ch. 7).

The techniques of molecular biology have greatly expanded our knowledge of the identity and structures of the multiple forms of the cytochrome P450 monooxygenases as well as of the glucuronosyl transferases and the glutathione transferases. In addition, these techniques are now employed to define the mechanisms by which drugs and other foreign compounds regulate the expression of the genes that encode the drug-metabolizing enzymes. This chapter will introduce this approach to studying the structure and regulation of the families of enzyme systems controlling the metabolism of drugs.

THE CYTOCHROME P450 MONOOXYGENASES

The forms of cytochrome P450 that metabolize foreign compounds are membrane proteins generally associated with the endoplasmic reticulum. A single form of the microsomal NADPH–cytochrome P450 reductase supports the reactions catalyzed by the different forms of cytochrome P450.

Cytochrome P450 proteins have molecular weights ranging roughly between 45 and 60 kDa. Each enzyme contains one molecule of heme, which functions in the reduction of oxygen and in the subsequent oxidation of the organic substrate. Because these enzymes are heme proteins, they absorb light in the visible region of the spectrum. As discussed in Chapter 5, a characteristic feature of all cytochrome P450 enzymes is that carbon monoxide binds to the iron of the heme when the latter is in its reduced state, Fe(II). This complex exhibits an absorption maximum near 450 nm, a feature incorporated into the generic name for these proteins, cytochrome P450. Different forms of cytochrome P450 exhibit small differences in the wavelength for maximum spectral absorption, which led to early attempts to distinguish and name cytochrome P450 proteins by the wavelength of maximum absorption (e.g., cytochrome P448, cytochrome P450, and cytochrome P452). It is now apparent that this procedure cannot distinguish each of the many forms of cytochrome P450 and that it is inadequate as a basis for a systematic nomenclature.

Individual forms of cytochrome P450 proteins can differ greatly (i.e., by over 70 percent) in their amino acid sequences. This structural diversity was first evident from peptide mapping studies, which demonstrated that different purified forms of cytochrome P450 did not exhibit common peptide fragments when digested with sequence-specific proteases.[1] Differences were also apparent from the limited sequence information that could be determined directly by Edman degradation of the protein, which sequentially cleaves amino acids from the NH_2 terminus of the polypeptide chain. This approach indicated that the NH_2-terminal amino acid sequences of different cytochrome P450 proteins are often distinct.[2]

These early studies suggested that the various cytochrome P450 enzymes could differ substantially in their amino acid sequences and thus that they likely are encoded by distinct genes. This has been confirmed by comparisons of the complete amino acid sequences of over 71 forms of cytochrome P450 and of the nucleotide sequences of their corresponding cDNAs and of several genes.[3,4] Sequence comparisons indicate that the amino acid sequence identity between different cytochrome P450 proteins ranges from less than 30 percent to greater than 95 percent in a single animal species.

Nomenclature

Ideally, it would be desirable to identify and name cytochrome P450 enzymes by the reactions they catalyze, as is generally done for other enzymes. Because each protein catalyzes several reactions and because these reactions are often catalyzed by two or more forms of cytochrome P450, it is not possible to uniquely identify cytochrome P450 enzymes in this manner.

Investigators have often identified cytochrome P450s by nomenclatures developed in their own laboratories. As a result, the same protein might be named according to its relative order of elution from a specific ion-exchange column used during its purification, according to its relative electrophoretic mobility, or according to the chronology of its isolation in a particular laboratory. For instance, the protein identified as P450c in Table 5-2 has been designated as BNF-b, P448, P446, P447, MC-1, form 5, and MC-B by various investigators. The correspondences between purified preparations of cytochrome P450 from different species has been reviewed.[4-6]

In 1987 a uniform system of nomenclature was proposed based on the extensive accumulation of protein sequence information derived largely from the nucleotide sequences of cDNAs.[7] The amino acid sequences of cytochrome P450 enzymes uniquely define them. Moreover, the similarities and differences between these sequences are likely to reflect evolutionary determinants of structure and function.

The uniform system of nomenclature employs a two-tiered system of classification for different forms of cytochrome P450. A roman numeral is used to designate broad classes of cytochrome P450s, where the amino acid sequences in one class differ by more than about 70 percent from other classes. The proteins within each broad class are further grouped together in subclasses denoted by a letter when their amino acid sequences exhibit roughly 70 percent or greater similarity. A given subclass includes cytochrome P450 enzymes from several mammalian species.

Each form of cytochrome P450 is designated by a combination of a roman numeral and a letter corresponding to its specific class and subclass, respectively, and an identifying arabic numeral (e.g., IIA1, IIB3). Table 6-1 lists the designations for different forms of cytochrome P450 that are known to constitute classes I through IV, as listed in a 1989 update of this nomenclature.[3] These classes comprise the cytochrome P450s that are known to mediate the phase I reactions of drug metabolism, discussed in Chapter 5. Because our knowledge of the extent of cytochrome P450 diversity is incomplete, this list will undoubtedly grow as additional forms of cytochrome P450 are identified.

When the cytochrome P450 enzymes that constitute the different classes and subclasses listed in Table 6-1 exhibit diverse functions across species, they are each given identifying numbers that are unique to that species. On the other hand, when cytochrome P450 enzymes serve the same functions in several species, they are given a single designation

Table 6-1. Cytochrome P450 Enzymes of Classes I–IV of Rat, Rabbit and Human

	I	II						III	IV	
	A	A	B	C	D	E	F	A	A	B
Rat	IA1	IIA1	IIB1	IIC6	IID1	IIE1		IIIA1	IVA1	IVB1
	IA2	IIA2	IIB2	IIC7	IID2			IIIA2	IVA2	
		IIA3	IIB3	IIC11	IID3				IVA3	
				IIC12	IID4					
				IIC13	IID5					
Rabbit	IA1		IIB4	IIC1		IIE1		IIIA6	IVA4	IVB1
	IA2		IIB5	IIC2		IIE2			IVA5	
				IIC3					IVA6	
				IIC4					IVA7	
				IIC5						
				IIC14						
				IIC15						
Human	IA1	IIA3	IIB6	IIC8	IID6	IIE1	IIF1	IIIA3		IVB1
	IA2		IIB7	IIC9	IID7			IIIA4		
			IIB8	IIC10	IID8			IIIA5		

for all species. This is best illustrated by the biosynthetic enzymes, namely, the cholesterol side-chain cleavage enzyme P450XIA1; the steroid 11β-hydroxylase P450XIB1; the sterol 26-hydroxylase P450XVIA1; the adrenal deoxycorticosterone synthetase P450XXIA1; the steroid 17α-hydroxylase/lyase P450XVIIA1; and the aromatase (estrogen synthetase) P450XIXA1. In each case the enzyme provides the same function in several species, and in each species the enzyme sequence is more closely related to that of the enzyme catalyzing the same reaction in the other species than to the sequences of other forms of cytochrome P450.

Selected Attributes of the Different Classes of Cytochrome P450

It is not possible in the context of this chapter to review all that is known regarding the function and regulation of each of the cytochrome P450 enzymes. For more detailed descriptions, the reader is referred to a monograph on this subject.[8] However, several attributes of the different enzymes will be highlighted in the next sections.

Class IA

Benzo[a]pyrene and other polycyclic aromatic hydrocarbons induce P450IA1, which efficiently metabolizes these compounds in many species.[9] In contrast, rat[10,11] and rabbit[12] P450IA2 exhibit very low benzo[a]pyrene hydroxylase activities when compared with P450IA1. Like the latter enzyme, P450IA2 is induced in the liver by polycyclic aromatic hydrocarbons, but in contrast to P450IA1, it is not expressed or induced in rat or rabbit kidney or lung.[13–15]

Class IIA

P450IIA1 is also induced by 3-methylcholanthrene in rat liver, although it is induced to lower levels than P450IA1.[16] P450IIA1 catalyzes the 7α-hydroxylation of testosterone.[17] In the mouse and rat additional members of class IIA catalyze the 15α-hydroxylation of testosterone,[18,19] and another catalyzes the hydroxylation of coumarin and is induced by pyrazole in mice.[20]

Class IIB

The predominant enzymes induced by phenobarbital in the liver are of class IIB. Members of this class are also expressed in the lung and constitute a major fraction of cytochrome P450 in pulmonary microsomes.[21,22] Several variants of these enzymes, which exhibit high (above 95 percent) amino acid identity, are seen in both rabbit and rat.

Class IIC

The enzyme that catalyzes the 4-hydroxylation of S-mephenytoin in humans is a member of class IIC.[23] Roughly 20 percent of the Japanese population exhibits a genetic deficiency of this enzyme. In rats, P450IIC13 and P450IIC11 have been shown to be male-specific,[24,25] whereas P450IIC12 is female-specific.[26] These three rat enzymes exhibit regiospecific differences in the metabolism of steroid substrates, and they also catalyze the oxidation of foreign compounds. Examples are shown in Table 5-2, where they are designated as g, h, and i, respectively. Rabbit P450IIC3 and P450IIC5 have been linked to genetic polymorphisms affecting the 6β- and 21-hydroxylation of progesterone, respectively.[27,28]

The metabolism of benzo[a]pyrene by liver microsomes prepared from untreated rabbits is also affected by genetic differences in the expression of the P450IIC5 enzyme.[29] P450IIC6 is induced by phenobarbital in rat liver,[30] while P450IIC2 and P450IIC1 are induced by phenobarbital in rabbit liver.[31] P450IIC2 is expressed in the kidney and has been demonstrated to catalyze the (ω-1)-hydroxylation of lauric acid.[32-34] Southern blotting experiments suggest that there is considerable genetic diversity in class IIC, and the characterization of the enzymes of this class is not complete.[35]

Class IID

Roughly 10 percent of the British population exhibits a genetic deficiency for the metabolism of debrisoquine.[36] This deficiency, which impairs the metabolism of other drugs, is discussed in greater detail in Chapter 7. The enzymes catalyzing debrisoquine 4-hydroxylation have been identified in humans and rats as members of this class.[37,38] Additional class IID enzymes catalyze steroid hydroxylations and are expressed in a sex-dependent manner in rats and some strains of mice.[39,40]

Class IIE

Ethanol, acetone, imidazole, isoniazid, and pyridine induce P450IIE1 in rats and rabbits.[41-46] This enzyme is associated with the oxidation of ethanol and the metabolism of the carcinogen dimethylnitrosamine.[47-49]

Class IIF

A cDNA encoding the founding member of class IIF was cloned from nasal epithelium.[50] The NH_2-terminal sequence predicted from the human cDNA exhibits a high similarity to that of a cytochrome P450 protein isolated from rabbit nasal tissue.[51] This enzyme does not appear to be expressed in the liver of either species. Specific functional attributes that might be related to the unusual tissue distribution of P450IIF have not been identified.

Class IIIA

Dexamethasone, erythromycin, and troleandromycin induce class IIIA enzymes in rabbits and rats,[52] whereas rifampicin induces class IIIA enzymes in rabbits[52] and humans[53] but not in rats.[52] Pregnenolone 16α-carbonitrile induces P450IIIA1 in rats but does not induce P450IIIA6 in rabbits.[52] Class IIIA enzymes often catalyze the 6β-hydroxylation of steroids. They also form metabolic intermediate complexes when they metabolize erythromycin or other antibiotics containing aminoglycoside residues.[54,55] In humans, these enzymes are linked to variations among individuals in their capacity to metabolize nifedipine,[56] and a class IIIA enzyme is one of the principal forms of cytochrome P450 expressed in human fetal liver.[57] This class is heterogeneous in humans and rats, with constituents in each species exhibiting very similar amino acid sequences.

Class IVA

Fatty acid ω-hydroxylases that are induced by clofibrate and other hypolipidemic agents are constituents of class IVA.[58,59] In rabbits, P450IVA4 is elevated in the lung during pregnancy, where it catalyzes the ω-hydroxylation of prostaglandins.[60,61]

Class IVB

P450IVB1 is found in the lungs of all species that have been examined. It constitutes 40 percent of the pulmonary cytochrome P450 in nonpregnant rabbits, and it is known to catalyze the conversion of aromatic amines to intermediates that are mutagenic[62] (see Ch. 11). It is expressed in other tissues of some species, including rabbits, in which it can be induced by phenobarbital.[63]

Evolution of the P450 Gene Families

The systematic nomenclature is based on the likely evolutionary origins of the structural and functional diversity exhibited by these proteins. It is thought that complex multicellular organisms evolved from simple unicellular organisms. This theory is consistent with the temporal appearance of new species as recorded in the fossil record. The repertoire of genes in each species is thought to have increased in complexity by the duplication of individual genes and the subsequent divergence of each of the duplicated genes through mutation and genetic recombination. As a result, the size of the genome has expanded in complex organisms to provide genes that encode additional proteins with distinct functions.

By comparing the extent of the differences in amino acid sequences of homologous proteins from different species that once shared the same gene in a common ancestor, a rate can be predicted for the accumulation of mutations in different gene families. This information can in turn be used to generate a phylogenetic tree called a *dendrogram*, which indicates when various forms of cytochrome P450 may have last shared a common ancestral gene. A dendrogram generated from a large number of cytochrome P450 sequences is shown in Figure 6-1.

Nelson and Strobel[64] have suggested that substrates for some of the earliest known P450s must have been compounds rich in carbon, such as cholesterol and fatty acids, which are incorporated into cellular membranes. Two P450 families, XI and IV, which comprise enzymes for the metabolism of cholesterol and fatty acids, respectively, may have diverged at this early time, more than 1,300 million years ago, to provide additional enzymes for the metabolism of lipids. These authors speculate that a duplication event about 900 million years ago led to distinct ancestral genes for the steroid-synthesizing enzymes and for the foreign compound-metabolizing monooxygenases.

The emergence of the P450I and II gene families marked the acquisition of a new function for P450, the metabolism of lipid-soluble foreign compounds. This event was followed about 400 million years ago by the rapid expansion of the class II genes into the six distinct classes that now account for more than half of the known cytochrome P450 genes. This expansion may have coincided with the colonization of land by animals.

The development of detoxification pathways would have been highly advantageous to the first species to colonize land. The increased diversity of the class II enzymes may have permitted these first land animals to consume a wide variety of plants containing an array of foreign compounds. The complexity seen within each subclass appears to have arisen during the last 100 million years during the rapid speciation of mammals and may reflect the adaptation of each mammalian species to different habitats and diets.

Because many of the cytochrome P450s listed in Table 6-1 appear to have arisen after lagomorphs (rabbits), rodents, and primates last shared a common ancestor, different numbers of enzymes are seen in the different categories for the three species shown. Moreover, as indicated earlier, the members of each category often exhibit distinct en-

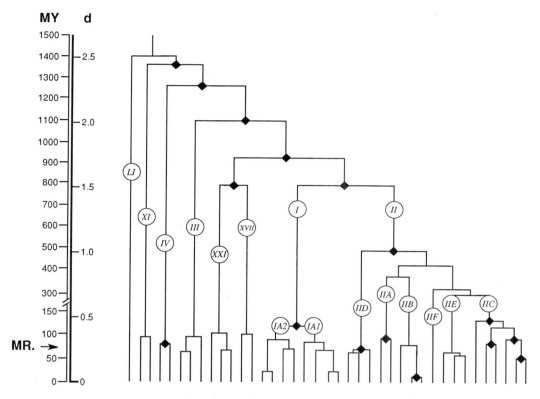

Fig. 6-1. A dendrogram of cytochrome P450 proteins. A phylogenetic tree of 39 cytochrome P450 proteins is shown. Black diamonds indicate gene duplication events because the genes on both sides of the branch point occur in the same species. Unmarked branch points represent species divergences. One scale expresses millions of years before the present (MY), and the other scale is based on the unit of evolutionary distance (d). Mammalian radiation (MR) occurred approximately 75 MY. Gene families and subfamilies are circled. (Adapted from Nelson et al.,[64] with permission).

zymatic capacities. Because of these differences, most of the entries for different mammalian species in Table 6-1 display unique arabic numeral identifiers within each classification. The same designation is used in different species only when the different enzymes within a classification are regulated in a similar manner and share similar enzymatic properties (e.g., P450IA1) or when the classification contains a single entry (e.g., P450IVB1). Similarities and differences in the enzymatic properties of the multiple forms of cytochrome P450 and in their regulation will be discussed in later sections.

Cytochrome P450 Gene Organization

The organization of the genes encoding cytochrome P450s differs among the major classes. Genes encoding class IV enzymes possess 11 to 12 introns. The two class I genes of mice, rats, and humans contain seven exons and six introns. All the class II genes that have been characterized are divided into nine exons by eight introns. The location of the introns within the genes of each class is conserved.[4]

It is not surprising then, considering that the various classes diverged long ago, to find

Table 6-2. Chromosome Locations of P450 Genes

Gene Family or Subfamily	Locus Symbol	Chromosome (Ref.)	
		Human	Mouse
I	Cyp1A	15	9
IIA	Cyp2A	19	7
IIB	Cyp2B	19	7
IIC	Cyp2C	10	19
IID	Cyp2D	22	15
IIE	Cyp2E	10	7
III	Cyp3A	7	6
IV	Cyp4A	1	4
XIA	Cyp11A	15	ND[a]
XIB	Cyp11B	8	ND
XVII	Cyp17A	10	ND
XIX	Cyp19A	15	ND
XXI	Cyp21A	6	17

[a] ND = not determined.
(Adapted from Gonzalez,[4] with permission.)

that genes in the different classes of cytochrome P450 are most often localized on different chromosomes. Table 6-2 summarizes the chromosomal assignments of the different P450 gene classes in mice and humans. Genetic loci are denoted by Cyp and alphanumeric designation corresponding to the name given to the enzyme in the uniform nomenclature.[3]

Gene Duplication

As discussed above, the major classes and subclasses of cytochrome P450 are thought to have originated from gene duplication and divergence. These events occurred before the radiation of mammals, when primates, rodents and lagomorphs split from their common ancestor and evolved separately. After this time, gene duplication led to different numbers of genes in each species for any given enzyme classification. For instance, two P450IIE genes have been identified in rabbits, whereas only one is known in rat or human (Table 6-1).

The initial effect of gene duplication is to provide two identical copies of the gene. Although the increase in protein capacity generated by the expression of two identical genes may be of some advantage, gene duplication events are thought to be of paramount importance for the generation of diversity. This process may have led to the extensive heterogeneity of cytochrome P450 genes and consequently to the capacity to metabolize an almost limitless range of lipid-soluble foreign compounds, since once mutational or recombinational events have altered one of the duplicated genes, a new gene is created, which can evolve independently to serve in a new capacity.

Some cytochrome P450 sequences are highly similar, which suggests that they may have originated recently on the evolutionary time scale and have since acquired distinct functions. For this reason, many of the cytochrome P450 enzymes listed in Table 6-1 are identified with a unique arabic numeral rather than sharing a common designation with an enzyme characterized in another species.

Although gene duplication and divergence create diversity in the cytochrome P450 system, nonreciprocal recombination events may have decreased the differences between two related genes after their divergence.[4,65] This process, termed *gene conversion*, leads to the duplication of a portion of one gene within another. For example, P450IIB1 and P450IIB2 exhibit 97 percent identity in the nucleotide sequences of their cDNAs. The clustering of these differences in two discrete segments of the gene suggests that the divergent sequence in one of the genes was derived from a third gene by gene conversion.[65] This is a single event that alters a localized region of the gene. Alternatively, these differences could have accumulated over time as the result of independent mutations. The recombinational nature of gene conversion requires that another gene donate the sequence. An examination of class IIb genes in the rat has identified a potential donor gene containing a segment closely matching the divergent segment of the recipient gene.

The identification of segments of identical nucleotide sequence in different cytochrome P450 genes suggests that gene conversion events may have created the identical sequences in otherwise divergent genes. Such gene conversion events have been suggested as having given rise to segments of identical sequences in each of the P450IA, P450IIA, P450IID, P450IIIA, and P450IVA subfamilies.

General Features of Mammalian Microsomal Enzymes

The protein sequence alterations that have occurred as a result of genetic evolution must preserve the basic features that distinguish these proteins as cytochrome P450s. This may require that some amino acids be conserved among all P450s and that substitutions at other positions and changes in the distance between critical residues due to insertions and deletions of sequence be consistent with the requirement that the linear polypeptide chain be able to fold into a compact structure that will support the function of the enzyme.

Heme Binding

A fundamental aspect of the cytochrome P450 enzymes is that they are heme proteins. The way in which the heme prosthetic group is bound in a protein can determine both its physical and its chemical properties as well as its function in the protein. One of the basic factors affecting the redox properties of the heme and the nature of the reactions that it catalyzes is the identity of the amino acids that form coordinate bonds with the iron atom of the heme at its axial positions.[66] (The four equatorial positions are occupied by the pyrrole nitrogens of the protoporphyrin IX moiety of the heme.)

The cytochrome P450 enzymes are distinct from most other heme proteins in that the heme iron is coordinated at the fifth axial position with the lone pair electrons of the sulfur atom of a cysteine. This cysteine residue is conserved in all of the more than 71 sequences of cytochrome P450 enzymes that have been characterized from a wide range of life forms.[67] The coordination with the sulfur of the cysteinyl anion contributes to the low redox potential of these proteins, that is, the preference of the iron to be in the Fe(III) rather than the Fe(II) state.

The axial ligand at the sixth position is generally water when this site is occupied, although it can be vacant[66] (Fig. 6-2). When an organic substrate binds to the Fe(III), or oxidized form of cytochrome P450, the water molecule, if present, may be displaced, leading to the changes in spin state of the iron that are reflected by the spectral changes that were termed *type I* in Chapter 5.[68] The displacement of water, as well as the changes in protein conformation elicited by the substrate when it binds to the cytochrome P450, can also raise the redox potential of the enzyme, thereby facilitating the reduction of the cytochrome by the flavoprotein that initiates the reaction cycle depicted in Figure 6-2.

When the enzyme is reduced, molecular oxygen can bind to the sixth ligation position of the iron.[66,69] A second reduction step leads to the combination of the reduced oxygen species with two protons to form a molecule of water, leaving a residual oxygen atom

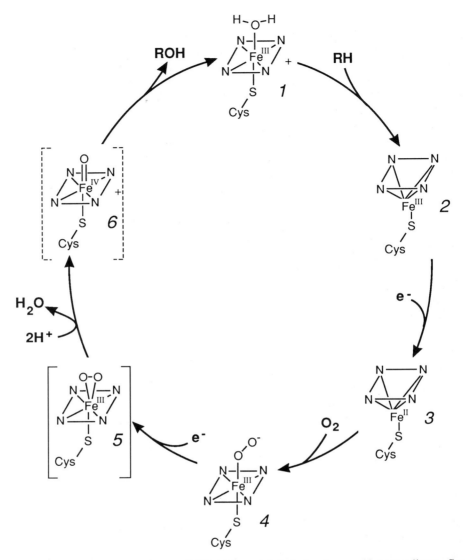

Fig. 6-2. Catalytic cycle of cytochrome P450 with postulated structures of intermediates. Structure 4 is displayed as a complex of the superoxide anion with Fe(III), but it could also be described as a complex of neutral oxygen with Fe(II). Structures 5 and 6 are hypothetical intermediates. The porphyrin is represented by the four nitrogens of the pyrrole rings. The net charge of structures 2, 3, and 6 is 0; that of structures 3 and 4 is −1; and that of structure 5 is −2. (Adapted from Dawson,[66] with permission.)

bound to the heme iron. This complex is highly reactive, and its oxygen atom can react with various organic substrates, which are thought to bind in close proximity to the heme-oxo complex in the protein. The selectivity of the different cytochrome P450 enzymes is derived from the way the proteins that harbor the heme cofactor limit the access of potential substrates to the highly reactive heme-oxo complex (Fig. 6-2; structure 6).

The binding and orientation of the substrate in a cytochrome P450 protein has been determined by x-ray diffraction for a non-membrane-bound form of the enzyme isolated from the bacterium *Pseudomonas putida*.[70] Although this enzyme is only distantly related to the mammalian microsomal enzymes, the basic features of the catalytic site are likely to serve as a prototype for the mammalian cytochrome P450 enzymes. Plate 6-1 shows three views of the catalytic site, where most of the protein residues are rendered invisible, so that the specific residues that interact with the substrate and the heme can be clearly seen.[71] Various amino acid residues contact the substrate and position it above the heme iron. This bacterial enzyme shows a high degree of selectivity for the hydroxylation of camphor in the 5-exo position, which is oriented directly toward the iron of the heme and the site where the reactive heme-oxo complex is formed.

When the heme is viewed from the edge (Plate 6-1), the coordination of the cysteinyl sulfur to the iron of the heme can be clearly seen. This cysteine residue is located on a portion of the polypeptide that forms one of the outer surfaces of the molecule, adjacent to helix L, and the side chain of the amino acid points inward from the surface so that the heme is located within the interior of the protein (Fig. 6-3). A second helix (I) runs across the opposite surface of the heme adjacent to the site where oxygen binds. Figure 6-3 also shows how the secondary structural elements formed by the amino acid chain fold to create the overall structure of the enzyme. The specific residues that mediate the binding of the camphor in the catalytic site are scattered along the length of the polypeptide chain, as indicated by the numbering in Figure 6-3. Thus, the close proximity of these amino acids to the substrate requires the folding of the polypeptide chain into the structure shown in Figure 6-3.

It is likely that the heme cofactor of the mammalian cytochrome P450 enzymes is bound in the interior of these proteins in a similar manner and that the substrates of these enzymes are oriented so that the site of oxidation is positioned for chemical reaction with the iron-bound oxo intermediate. However, the identity and position of the amino acid residues that perform this role in the mammalian enzymes will differ among the various P450s. The folding of the polypeptide chain is also likely to differ among enzymes so as to provide catalytic sites that can accommodate different substrates.

Membrane Anchorage

The NH_2-terminal region of the microsomal enzymes is thought to anchor the cytochrome P450 protein to the endoplasmic reticulum. Each of the microsomal enzymes exhibits a segment of hydrophobic amino acids at the NH_2 terminus, although the actual sequences differ markedly. These sequences are similar to the signal sequences found on secretory proteins.[72] This signal sequence is recognized by a complex of proteins and RNA called the *signal recognition particle*,[73] which functions to bind the nascent polypeptide and its associated ribosome to the endoplasmic reticulum during translation of the mRNA and synthesis of the protein. In this manner, the newly formed peptide is directly inserted into the membrane during the course of its synthesis.

Several experiments have demonstrated that the NH_2-terminal sequences found for microsomal cytochrome P450s can direct the insertion of unrelated proteins into microsomal membranes during translation. In these experiments the portion of the cDNA of the cytochrome P450 that codes for the NH_2 terminus was spliced to the coding region of the other protein. This chimeric cDNA was then transcribed, and the mRNA was translated to yield a hybrid protein.[74,75] When two basic amino acids were introduced

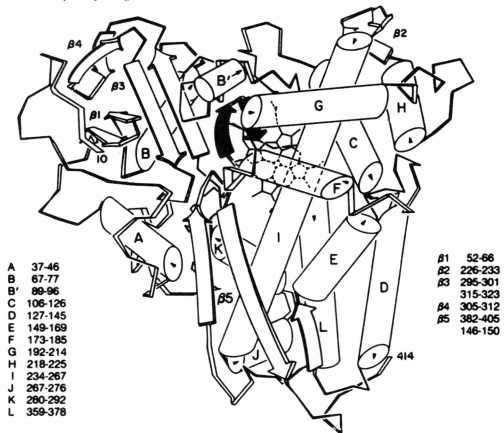

A	37-46
B	67-77
B'	89-96
C	106-126
D	127-145
E	149-169
F	173-185
G	192-214
H	218-225
I	234-267
J	267-276
K	280-292
L	359-378

β1	52-66
β2	226-233
β3	295-301
	315-323
β4	305-312
β5	382-405
	146-150

Fig. 6-3. A representation of cytochrome $P450_{cam}$. Helices are represented by cylinders and β structures are depicted by arrows. An antiparallel β region and bulge that contains the axial heme ligand C357 is shaded. The residue numbers for each segment of secondary structure are shown. (Adapted from Poulos et al.[70] with permission.)

into the NH_2 terminus of P450IIC2 by site-specific mutagenesis, the resulting protein was translocated through the endoplasmic reticulum into the lumen.[76,77] This demonstrates how the NH_2 terminus can determine whether the protein is inserted into the endoplasmic reticulum and can also determine that other sequences that might halt the translocation process are not present in the sequence of the enzyme. The mitochondrial cytochrome P450 enzymes exhibit different sequences at the NH_2 terminus that direct the incorporation of these enzymes into mitochondrial membranes. These presequences are then removed by proteolysis.[78]

It is clear that the hydrophobic NH_2-terminal sequence can reside in the lipid bilayer,[79] but it is not known whether additional portions of the protein also reside in the lipid bilayer. The bulk of each of the microsomal cytochrome P450 proteins is thought to reside on the cytoplasmic surface of the endoplasmic reticulum.[79,80]

The cytochrome P450 reductase is also anchored to the endoplasmic reticulum by a segment of hydrophobic residues at its NH_2 terminus.[81] The reductase supports the reactions catalyzed by each of the microsomal forms of cytochrome P450. Specific structural

Plate 6-1. Active site structure of cytochrome P450$_{cam}$. **(A)** An edge-on view of the heme (in red) and the substrate camphor (in green). The heme Fe is shown in yellow. The amino acids (in blue) cysteine 357 (the axial thiolate ligand), tyrosine 96, and valine 396 of the protein are shown. **(B)** The same perspective of the active site in the absence of the substrate camphor. A cluster of water molecules occupies the active site in the absence of the substrate. (*Plate continues.*)

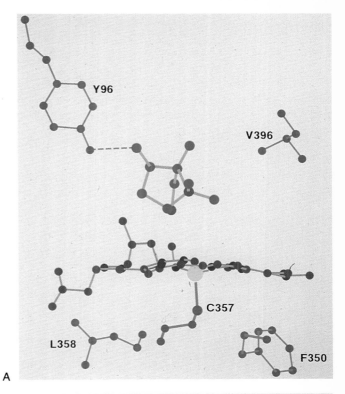

A

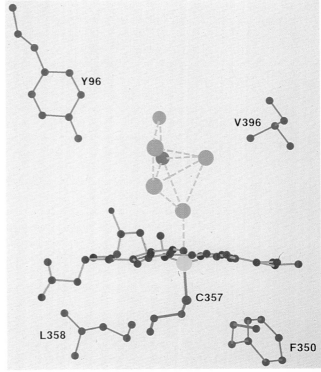

B

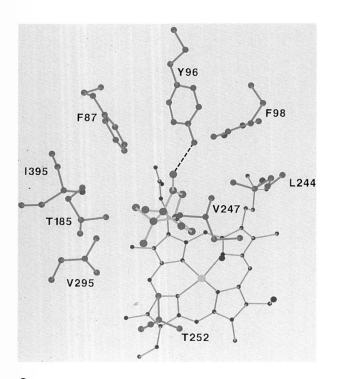

Plate 6-1 (*Continued*). **(C)** A view from above the active site. Phenylalanine 87 and leucine 244 also contact the substrate. Tyrosine 96 forms hydrogen bonds with the carbonyl oxygen of camphor. The other interactions are nonpolar. (Adapted from Atkins et al.,[71] with permission.)

C

features that might be required for a common mode of interaction with the reductase molecule have not yet been defined.

Induction of Cytochrome P450s

The selective induction of a subset of the reactions catalyzed by the cytochrome P450 monooxygenases suggested that distinct forms of cytochrome P450 are induced by specific inducers. Historically, this has been an impetus for the isolation and characterization of these enzymes. The compounds that induce cytochrome P450 enzymes can be grouped into five distinct categories based on the major enzyme affected by their action, as is shown in Table 6-3.

The effect of the inducer is to increase the microsomal concentration of the cytochrome P450 protein. This increase underlies the increased rate of metabolism catalyzed by microsomes isolated from animals treated with the inducer. The concentrations of the protein can be determined independently of estimates based on catalytic activity by the use of antibodies to the protein. This is shown in Figure 6-4, where a greater than 10-fold increase in the liver microsomal concentration of P450IIIA6 is seen by the Western blotting technique 24 hours following administration of the antibiotic rifampicin to an immature rabbit.[82] In this example, the principal, induced enzyme may account for more than 50 percent of the total microsomal content of cytochrome P450 forms following induction.

Although a single form of cytochrome P450 can often account for most of the microsomal cytochrome P450 after induction by a prototypic inducer, the expression of other forms of cytochrome P450 may also be affected. Examples of these secondary targets of induction are shown in Table 6-3. These secondary targets represent a smaller fraction of the total cytochrome P450 than the major form following induction. Although they are expressed in smaller amounts, the induction of these enzymes can significantly affect the rates of the reactions they catalyze in microsomes.

The major inducible forms of cytochrome P450 are often members of families that exhibit multiple forms of P450. Other enzymes of the same class may not respond to the inducer

Table 6-3. Classification of Inducers of Various Classes of Cytochrome P450s

	Enzyme Class	
Prototype Inducer	Predominant	Secondary
TCDD	IA	P450IIA
3-MC		
B (+) P		
Phenobarbital	IIB	P450IIC
		P450IIIA
		P450IVB
Imidazole	IIE	
Ethanol		
Fasting		
Pregnenolone 16α-Carbonitrile	IIIA	
Dexamethasone		
Troleandromycin		
Erythromycin		
Rifampicin		
Clofibrate	IVA	
Diethyl 2-hexylphthalate		

TCDD = tetrachlorodibenzo-*p*-dioxin; 3-MC = 3-methylcholanthrene; B (+) P = benzo[a]pyrene.

UNT   RIF

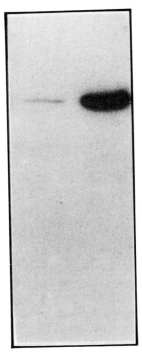

Fig. 6-4. Western blot analysis of P450IIIA6. Liver microsomes were prepared from 7-day-old rabbits 24 hours following administration of a single dose of rifampicin, as well as from untreated 7-day-old rabbits and 10 μg of protein was subjected to electrophoresis in the presence of sodium dodecyl sulfate (SDS). Following transfer of the proteins to a nitrocellulose sheet, P450IIIA6 was detected by reaction with a P450IIIA6 monoclonal antibody. The differences in the concentration of the P450IIIA6 protein in the microsomal preparations from the untreated and treated rabbits can be determined from the differences in intensity seen in the figure. (From Potenza et al.,[82] with permission.)

in the same way, and they may also exhibit significant differences in enzymatic capacity. For instance, P450IA1 and P450IA2 are both induced by tetrachlorodibenzo-*p*-dioxin (TCDD) (see Ch. 7) in adult rabbit and rat liver, but only P450IA1 is induced in kidney and lung. Moreover, the rat and rabbit P450IA2 enzymes exhibit very low rates of benzo[a]pyrene hydroxylation, a reaction that is catalyzed efficiently by P450IA1 and that is generally induced by TCDD in many species.

The duplication and divergence of genes within a family can lead to regulatory pathways that are not conserved among all species—for instance, clofibrate induces the class IVA enzymes that catalyze the ω-hydroxylation of fatty acids found in both rats and rabbits.[83] However, an additional class IVA enzyme is found in rabbits, but not in rats, which is elevated in the lung during pregnancy. It catalyzes the ω-hydroxylation of prostaglandins E_1 and $F_{2\alpha}$.[60,84]

Mechanisms for the Induction of Cytochrome P450s

As a general rule, the term *induction* is restricted to the stimulation of the synthesis of the protein in question. It is important to remember that the concentration of the protein is determined by the rate of its synthesis relative to its rate of degradation. Thus, the

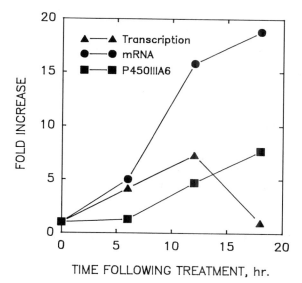

Fig. 6-5. Time course of induction of cytochrome P450IIIA6 by rifampicin. Young rabbits (7 days old) were treated with a single dose of the macrolide antibiotic rifampicin. At 6, 12, and 18 hours following treatment, the microsomal concentration of P450IIIA6 protein, the concentration of corresponding mRNA, and the transcriptional activity of the CypIIIA6 gene were measured. The amounts of P450IIIA6 protein were quantitated by Western blot analysis with a P450IIIA6 monoclonal antibody. The levels of RNA were determined by hybridization of the cDNA to total liver RNA by slot blot analysis. The amounts of specific CypIIIA6 transcripts were determined following nuclear run-on analysis and hybridization of the labeled nuclear RNA to the P450IIIA6 cDNA. (From Potenza et al.,[82] with permission.)

change in the steady-state concentration of the protein effected by the inducer could reflect alterations in either process. With few exceptions, inducers of the cytochrome P450 enzymes have been shown to stimulate de novo synthesis of the protein. The rate of protein synthesis depends on the concentration of mRNAs encoding the protein, which in turn will reflect the rate of transcription of the gene as well as the rate of degradation of the mRNA. In most cases, the induction of cytochrome P450 enzymes by prototypic inducers involves an increase in the rate of gene transcription.

The relationship between these events is illustrated in Fig. 6-5. This example depicts changes in the rate of transcription of the Cyp3A6 gene following treatment of 7-day-old rabbits with a single injection of the antibiotic rifampicin. A transient increase in the rate of transcription occurs within 24 hours of administration of this antibiotic, the maximum transcriptional activity being seen at about 12 hours. As the rate of transcription rises, the concentration of mRNA also rises. However, the mRNA is degraded relatively slowly, so that mRNA accumulates and remains elevated following the return of transcription to basal levels by 18 hours.

In this example the concentration of P450IIIA6 in the microsomes rises slowly following the elevation of mRNA concentrations. By 24 hours, 10- to 15-fold increases in the level of the enzyme are seen (Fig. 6-5). As discussed in Chapter 4, the time required for a protein to reach a new steady-state concentration following an increase in the rate of its synthesis is determined by its rate of degradation.[85] The degradation of cytochrome P450 proteins is generally described as a first-order process with a half-life of 8 to 30 hours, depending on the protein. Thus, the increase in the concentration of P450IIIA6 in the microsomes will lag behind the rise in synthesis due to increases of mRNA.

If the inducing agent decreases the rate of protein degradation, the concentration of the protein in the microsomes will increase more rapidly. Several examples of decreases in protein degradation rate following treatment with inducers have been reported.[86–88] The macrolide antibiotics erythromycin and troleandromycin extend the apparent half-life of P450IIIA1 by 10 to 14 hours to more than 60 hours.[87] These two compounds are metabolized by P450IIIA1 and A2 to form metabolic intermediate complexes (cf. Ch. 5) in which the product of the reaction remains bound to the enzyme, which leads to speculation that these complexes may be more stable than the enzyme alone. In a sense, the capacity of substrates and inhibitors to stabilize cytochrome P450 proteins can be considered a mechanism for selective induction of these enzymes.

Changes in the Concentrations of Specific mRNAs during Induction

Increases of the concentrations of mRNAs encoding specific forms of cytochrome are generally seen during the course of enzyme induction in which changes in de novo synthesis occur. Changes in the concentrations of mRNAs have been followed by two procedures. The first employs specific antibodies to characterize the synthesis of protein from mRNA by in vitro translation. This procedure was used in early studies, when antibodies to the inducible forms of cytochrome P450 were first developed following the purification of the enzymes.

The second method, Northern blot analysis, employs cDNA probes to monitor the concentration of mRNAs directly. Many of the cytochrome P450 subfamilies contain multiple genes with closely related nucleotide sequences. This requires the use of selected portions of the cDNA for probes in Northern blotting experiments to discriminate between the mRNA species corresponding to each gene. The Northern blots shown in Figure 6-6B demonstrate this point.

The rabbit cDNA clones that encode P450IA1 and P450IA2 were used as probes in this example. Figure 6-6A shows the coding and noncoding regions of the cDNA. Nucleic acid sequence analysis of the two cDNA clones indicates that P450IA1 and IA2 share 80 percent identity within the coding regions, with little or no nucleotide identity in the noncoding regions.[89] The Northern blot, hybridized with the P450IA1 cDNA, Fig. 6-6B, shows the induction of both P450IA1 and IA2 mRNAs by TCDD. Because of the high nucleotide sequence identity between the P450IA1 and P450IA2 over the region spanned by the probe, both mRNAs are detected in the blot. The P450IA2 mRNA is 2.0 kilobases in length, while the P450IA1 mRNA is 2.4 kilobases long.

When the blot is hybridized with a portion of the 3′ noncoding region of P450IA1, only the 2.4-kilobase RNA species corresponding to this enzyme is detected. This reflects the low nucleotide sequence similarity between P450IA1 and P450IA2 mRNAs in their noncoding portions. The Northern blot on the right, which was probed with a 3′ noncoding portion of the P450IA2 cDNA, shows hybridization with only the 2.0-kilobase mRNA species.

The induction of both mRNAs can be seen by comparing the intensity of the blot for the lanes containing mRNAs isolated from TCDD-treated rabbits with those from untreated rabbits. This difference of intensity reflects the relative abundance of the mRNA species from treated and untreated animals.

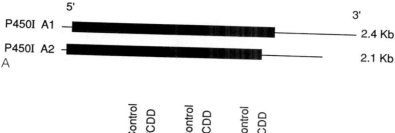

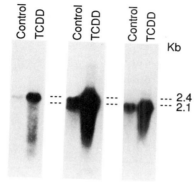

Fig. 6-6. Analysis of rabbit P450IA1 and P450IA2 mRNA. **(A)** Line drawing of P450IA1 and P450IA2 cDNAs. The solid bar represents the coding region, and the thinner lines represent the 5′ and 3′ noncoding portions of the mRNA. The coding regions display 80 percent nucleic acid sequence similarity, while the noncoding regions share little sequence homology. **(B)** Blot hybridization analysis. Preparations of rabbit liver mRNA from untreated or TCDD-treated animals were electrophoresed in 0.8 percent agarose gels and transferred to nitrocellulose paper. Each filter was hybridized with ^{32}P-labeled inserts, and 3′ noncoding portions of the P450IA1 and IA2 cDNA inserts were hybridized to the filters on the left and right. An insert containing the coding portion of the P450IA1 cDNA is shown in the middle panel. (From Okino et al.,[89] with permission.)

When an animal has several closely related genes, it may be necessary to use synthetic oligonucleotides to measure the induction of specific mRNAs. Computer alignments of highly similar sequences can identify short regions of nucleotide divergence. Oligonucleotides can then be made corresponding to these regions and used as probes to identify each of the corresponding mRNAs.

This approach has been used to monitor mRNAs corresponding to rat P450IIB1 and IIB2, which are 97 percent similar in their sequences.[90] By using oligonucleotides, it was shown that P450IIB2 is expressed in liver, whereas mRNAs for P450IIB1 are expressed in lung.[91] Following treatment of the animal with phenobarbital, mRNAs for both enzymes are greatly induced in the liver, P450IIB1 being the major component.

Four of the five major classes of inducers are seen to elicit increased mRNA abundance for their principal target enzymes—TCDD for IA1 and IA2; phenobarbital for IIB1; pregnenolone 16α-carbonitrile (PCN), or macrolide antibiotic for IIIA; and clofibrate for IVA (Table 6-4). In contrast, changes in mRNA corresponding to P450IIE1 have not been detected when this enzyme is induced by ethanol, which suggests that the increase in protein concentration arises by a different mechanism.[92] This could reflect changes in the rate of translation of existing mRNAs or the stabilization of the protein by ethanol or acetone.

Table 6-4. Cytochrome P450 mRNAs Induced by Various Compounds

Gene Family	Inducer	Specific mRNA
IA	Arochlor 1254	P450IA1
	Isosafrole	IA1
	α-Naphthoflavone	IA1/IA2
	3-Methylcholanthrene	IA1/IA2
	TCDD	IA1/IA2
IIA	3-Methylcholanthrene	P450IIA1
IIB	Phenobarbital	P450IIB1/B2
	R-Chlordane	IIB1/B2
	2-Acetylaminofluorene	IIB1/B2
IIC	Phenobarbital	P450IIC1/IIC2
IIIA	Phenobarbital	IIIA1/IIIA2
	Pregnenolone 16α-carbonitrile	IIIA1
	Dexamethasone	IIIA1/IIIA2/IIIA6
	Rifampicin	IIIA6
	Troleandomycin	IIIA6
IVA	Clofibrate	P450IVA1
	Progesterone	P450IVA4

Transcriptional Activation

TCDD, phenobarbital, clofibrate, pregnenolone 16α-carbonitrile, and rifampicin have each been shown to stimulate the transcription of genes encoding cytochrome P450 enzymes. The rate of transcription reflects the number of RNA polymerase II molecules that bind to the gene and initiate new transcripts rather than the rate at which the gene is transcribed by the polymerase. Several polymerase molecules may be bound to the gene as they proceed along its length, extending their transcripts. Assuming that the rate of RNA polymerase II-catalyzed elongation of the transcripts is similar for all genes, the number of polymerase II molecules and consequently the number of initiated transcripts bound to a gene reflect the rate of gene transcription.

The RNA polymerase II molecules that are already associated with the genes will remain bound to the gene when nuclei are isolated from tissues, and they can elongate their transcripts when the nuclei are supplemented with nucleotide triphosphates (Fig. 6-7). Uridine triphosphate ^{32}P is included so that transcripts are labeled when transcription resumes. Initiation of transcription does not appear to take place in nuclei that have been isolated from tissues. Transcripts of specific genes are then detected by their hybridization with the corresponding cDNA, which has been adsorbed onto a nitrocellulose membrane. This procedure is known as nuclear run-on analysis.

If an inducer increases the transcription of a cytochrome P450 gene, a greater number of the gene transcripts will be elongated, and these will anneal to the cDNA clones. The amount can be quantitated by liquid scintillation counting or densitometry following autoradiography. A list of the inducers and the P450 genes that have been shown experimentally to be transcriptionally activated when animals are exposed to the various inducers is presented in Table 6-5. Asterisks are used in the table to designate those genes that are highly similar to several other identified genes. The cDNA used in the assay is likely to hybridize with transcripts from each of the related genes, and it is not possible in these cases to distinguish between the rates of transcription of the individual genes.

For example, Southern blot analysis using the P450IIB2 cDNA as a probe indicates that at least six related structural genes are constituents of this subfamily,[93] and at least

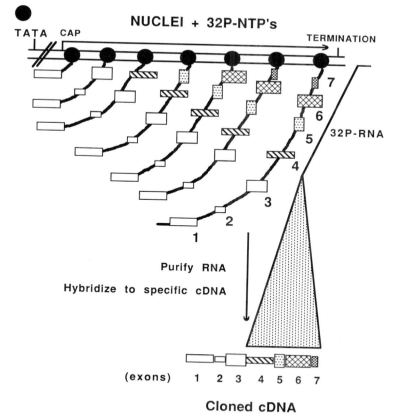

Fig. 6-7. Generation of radioactively labeled nuclear RNA by "nuclear run-on" experiments. Nuclei are isolated from cells or tissues. The RNA polymerase molecules are caught in the act of transcription and will faithfully continue to elongate when incubated in the presence of nucleotide triphosphates. When labeled nucleotides are included, a highly radioactive sample of the cell's transcribed sequences can be obtained. The boxes in the figure represent nuclear RNA that encodes the exon portions of the mRNAs, and the shaded boxes represent exon sequences that contain the incorporated radioactive nucleotides. The nuclear RNA is purified and hybridized to P450 cDNAs. The nuclear exonic sequences that are labeled will anneal to the complementary exonic sequences of the cDNAs. The greater the level of transcription, the more intense will be the signal following hybridization.

three full-length cDNA clones corresponding to three of these genes have been identified and characterized for the rat class IIB (Table 6-1). The cDNAs that encode the phenobarbital-inducible P450IIB1 and P450IIB2 are 97 percent similar in their nucleic acid sequence. This implies that a cDNA encoding either class IIB enzyme will detect transcripts from both the P450IIB1 and the P450IIB2 gene following phenobarbital treatment. Additional genes in this subfamily could also have contributed to the observed increase in the number of transcripts elicited by phenobarbital. The results of Northern blotting experiments using oligonucleotide probes to distinguish liver mRNAs for IIB1 and IIB2 indicate that mRNAs for both are elevated in response to phenobarbital, which suggests that both genes are affected.

Table 6-5. P450 Genes Transcriptionally Increased with Inducers

P450 Gene	Inducer
Cyp1A1	TCDD
Cyp1A2	
*Cyp2B1/B2	Phenobarbital
*Cyp3A1/A2	Dexamethasone
Cyp3A6	
*Cyp3A1/A2	Pregnenolone 16α-carbonitrile
Cyp3A6	Rifampicin
Cyp4A1	Clofibrate

* Differences between members of this subclass cannot be distinguished by this analysis.

In a similar manner, the P450IIIA1 cDNA was used to monitor the expression of P450IIIA genes in rats following treatment with dexamethasone and PCN.[94] The rat P450IIIA1 and IIIA2 cDNAs share 90 percent nucleotide similarity, which indicates that one or both of the corresponding genes could have been affected. However, when mRNA was analyzed with sequence-specific oligonucleotides,[95] dexamethasone and PCN were found to induce only those mRNAs that encoded P450IIIA1.

In the rabbit the P450IIIA subfamily is thought to consist of a single gene. This is based upon Southern blot analysis using the rabbit P450IIIA6 cDNA as a probe. Therefore, the identity of increased gene transcripts with the P450IIIA6 cDNA is likely to reflect the activation of a single Cyp3A gene by dexamethasone and rifampicin.

The long, divergent 3′ untranslated regions of the respective cDNAs for the Cyp1A1 and 1A2 genes were employed for nuclear run-on assays to discriminate between the effects of polycyclic aromatic hydrocarbons on the transcriptional rates of these genes in rats. The extent of transcriptional activation of the Cyp1A1 gene was much greater than that of the Cyp1A2.[96,97]

Mechanisms of Transcriptional Activation by Inducers

Information regarding the mechanism by which inducers alter the transcription of specific cytochrome P450 genes is largely derived from studies of the induction of Cyp1A1 genes by TCDD and related inducers. In 1973 Poland and Glover[98] proposed that these compounds induced benzo[a]pyrene hydroxylase activity by combining with an "induction receptor."[98] This hypothesis was based on the distinct structure versus activity relationships for induction of the enzyme by halogenated dibenzo-*p*-dioxins. It was also demonstrated that 3-methylcholanthrene and TCDD produced parallel log dose versus response curves for the induction of P450IA1-mediated monooxygenase activities. However, the dose required to elicit a maximal induction of this hydroxylase was 30,000-fold greater with 3-methylcholanthrene than with TCDD.

Evidence for a receptor mediation of the induction of P450IA1 was derived from studies using strains of mice that differ in their response to 3-methylcholanthrene.[99] Induction of P450IA1 by 3-methylcholanthrene was not seen in certain strains of mice such as DBA/2. This nonresponsiveness was inherited in an autosomal recessive manner when genetic crosses were made with a responsive strain such as C57BL/6. However, TCDD was able to induce P450IA1 in the strains that did not respond to 3-methylcholanthrene.[100] This result demonstrated that the nonresponsive mice contained the necessary regulatory components and structural genes for the induction of P450IA1, but that they only responded to the more potent inducer.

Binding studies with tritiated TCDD ([³H]-TCDD) indicated that hepatic cytosol contained a high-affinity, low-capacity receptor for TCDD and that the apparent affinity of the receptor for TCDD was much lower in DBA/2 than in C57BL/6 mice. The receptor in the responsive strain bound TCDD reversibly with high affinity (K_d = 0.27 nM) and with a capacity of 84 femtomoles per milligram of cytosolic protein.[101] Moreover, competitive binding experiments indicated that the binding affinities of the receptor for 23 halogenated dibenzo-*p*-dioxins and dibenzofurans correlated closely with the potencies of these compounds as inducers of the hydroxylase. In addition, polycyclic aromatic hydrocarbons competed with the [³H]-TCDD for binding, demonstrating that both 3-methylcholanthrene and TCDD bound to the same receptor. This receptor has been termed the *dioxin receptor* or the *Ah receptor*, because it mediates induction of P450IA1 by *aromatic hydrocarbons*.

Several experiments strongly implicate the accumulation of the receptor-ligand complex in the nucleus with the induction of the P450IA genes. First, when [³H]-TCDD is administered intravenously to mice, the extent of accumulation of cytoplasmic P450IA1 mRNA in liver is directly proportional to the accumulation of the [³H]-TCDD receptor complex in the nuclei.[102] The accumulation of the receptor-TCDD complex in the nucleus preceded the rise in cytoplasmic RNA. Second, several types of mutant hepatoma cell lines were defined in which the translocation of the receptor to the nucleus was absent and the induction was blocked.[103-105] One type of mutant cell line was unable to form a significant number of dioxin receptor complexes, most likely because of a defect in the ligand binding region of the receptor. When these cells were treated with TCDD, they accumulated little P450IA1 mRNA. The other type of mutant cell line exhibited normal levels of cytosolic dioxin receptor, measured by binding studies with [³H]-TCDD, but the ligand-receptor complex was not translocated to the nucleus. Again, when these cells were treated with TCDD, they accumulated little P450IA1 mRNA.[106] Fusion of these cell lines yielded hybridomas, which responded to TCDD in the same manner as the wild-type mouse hepatoma cells. Cell fusion permits genes from each cell line to mix, and as a result the mutant genes of each are complemented by the functional genes of the other.

These studies suggested that the site of action of the receptor-TCDD complex is in the nucleus, where it may interact directly with the Cyp1A1 gene. The accumulation of dioxin receptor in the nucleus is temperature-dependent, which suggests that a conformational change in the receptor occurs after binding, which is important for its translocation into the nucleus.[102,103,107] This process is similar to the temperature-dependent activation of steroid receptors, which also leads to accumulation of the receptors in the nucleus. Similarities between the TCDD receptor and the glucocorticoid receptor have been noted in their physical properties.[108] Both receptors interact with polyanions, such as heparin,[109] which can transform the receptors to DNA-binding forms.[110] The cytosolic forms of each receptor are also found complexed with the 90-kDa heat shock protein (hsp90).[111,112] A supergene family appears to encode a diverse family of proteins that are related to the steroid receptors,[113] and it is possible that the TCDD receptor is a member of this protein family.

Specific recognition sequences control the transcription of many genes that respond to steroid hormones[113,114] (see Also Ch. 2). These recognition sequences specify a site for physical interaction between the steroid receptor and the gene. Specific recognition sequences also mediate the induction of the mouse[115] and rat[116] Cyp1A1 genes by TCDD.

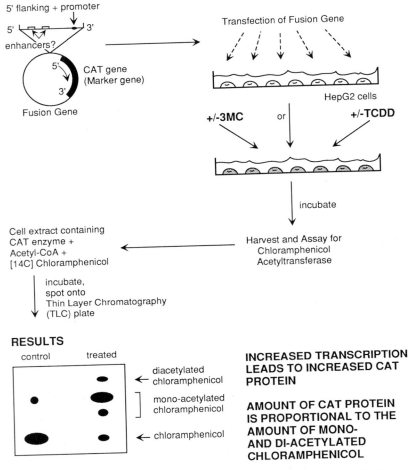

RESULTS

INCREASED TRANSCRIPTION
LEADS TO INCREASED CAT
PROTEIN

AMOUNT OF CAT PROTEIN
IS PROPORTIONAL TO THE
AMOUNT OF MONO-
AND DI-ACETYLATED
CHLORAMPHENICOL

Fig. 6-8. Analysis of the P450 gene promoter activity by the chloramphenicol acetyltransferase (CAT) expression assay. A P450 gene fragment containing the promoter is subcloned into a plasmid that contains the prokaryotic CAT gene. This fusion gene is transfected into eukaryotic cells, in this example human HepG2 cells, and the cells are treated with 3MC or TCDD. The cells are then harvested, and the cell extract is used as the enzyme source to measure CAT activity. If the portion of the P450 gene contains the appropriate *cis*-acting elements, shown here as enhancers, an increase in the levels of transcription will be observed when the cells are exposed to the inducer. The increase in rate of transcription will be reflected by an increase in CAT activity, as determined from the increase in mono- and diacetylated chloramphenicol.

Identification of Regulatory Elements of the Cyp1A1 Gene

Gene transfer experiments have identified a small regulatory element governing the induction of P450IA1 gene-transcription by TCDD (Fig. 6-8). In these experiments portions of the 5′ flanking regions of the P450IA1 gene were placed upstream of the coding region of the bacterial chloramphenicol acetyltransferase (CAT) gene. These constructs contained the promoter region of the Cyp1A1 gene. The RNA polymerase II promoter is the region on the gene that contains the DNA sequences required to initiate RNA synthesis.

The CAT gene is not expressed in eukaryotic cells, and any activity that is detected following its transfection into the host cell line can be attributed to transcription driven by the promoter and regulatory sequences derived from the Cyp1A1 gene. When this construct was transfected into hepatoma cells and the cells were then treated with TCDD or 3-methylcholanthrene, a large increase in CAT activity was observed. This response was not observed, however, if cells that were deficient in the dioxin receptor served as a host. This indicated that the 5′ flanking portion of the Cyp1A1 gene contains regulatory sequences that respond to the actions of the dioxin receptor.

By removing segments of the construct that were derived from the P450IA1 gene, a

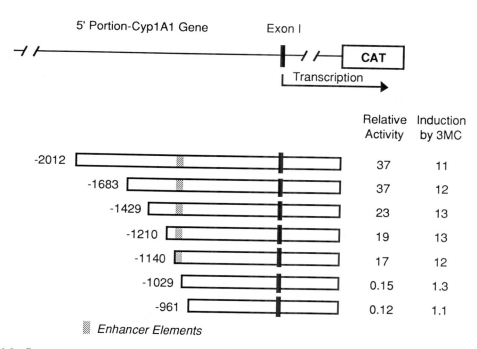

Fig. 6-9. Structure and activity of rat Cyp1A1 chloramphenicol acetyltransferase (CAT) chimeric genes. A DNA fragment from the 5′ end of the rat Cyp1A1 gene was used to construct hybrid plasmids, and deletions were introduced as shown. Nucleotide positions of the 5′ flanking sequence are assigned negative numbers from the mRNA start site. The first exon of the Cyp1A1 gene, which contains only untranslated DNA, is shown as a bar. The CAT coding sequence is represented by the box. Each construct was transfected into mouse hepa 1 cells, and the cells were treated with 3-methylcholanthrene. The relative CAT activity is shown, followed by the fold induction. (From Sogawa et al.,[117] with permission.)

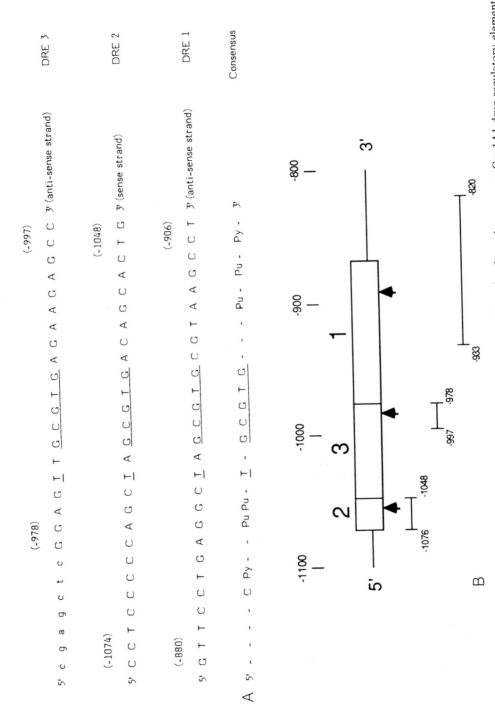

Fig. 6-10. Nucleotide sequences and nuclear protein-binding properties of domains from three mouse Cyp1A1 drug regulatory elements (DREs). (A) DNA sequences from three DREs (upper case letters). The numbers indicate the ends of the DNA fragments in nucleotides relative to the transcription start site. The common ''core'' sequence is underlined. (Pu = purine; Py = pyrimidine). (*Figure continues.*)

TCDD: − + + + + +

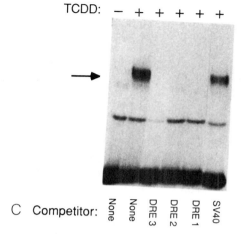

C Competitor: None None DRE 3 DRE 2 DRE 1 SV40

Fig. 6-10 (*Continued*). (**B**) DREs upstream of the cytochrome Cyp1A1 gene. The large numbers indicate the three known DREs, while the arrows indicate the positions of the core DNA sequences within the DREs. The brackets and small numbers indicate the location of the fragments used as competitors in the studies described below in Fig. C. (**C**) Competition experiments. The fragment containing DRE 3 (see Fig. A) was labeled with phosphorus 32, mixed with nuclear extracts from untreated or TCDD-treated cells, and analyzed by a gel retardation assay. An SV40 DNA fragment was used as a nonspecific competitor. The arrow indicates the position of the TCDD-inducible protein-DNA complex. The fact that each DRE competed with labeled DRE 3 indicates that the dioxin receptor recognizes each of the DRE elements. (Adapted from Denison et al.,[121] with permission.)

small segment was defined that controlled the transcription of the CAT gene in response to TCDD or 3-methylcholanthrene. As shown in Figure 6-9, transcription is supported in the presence of TCDD or 3-methylcholanthrene until roughly 1,100 bases remain upstream of the cap site (the site where transcription is initiated). Shorter segments did not support the induction of CAT activity by TCDD, suggesting that a regulatory control element is located in the portion of the gene between the shortest active construct and the longest inactive construct.[117] This segment was then tested for its capacity to support the induction of CAT activity by TCDD or 3-methylcholanthrene when the CAT gene was linked to a heterologous promoter such as the SV40 early promoter. Heterologous promoters, or foreign gene promoters, are used in place of endogenous promoters to ascertain whether foreign gene elements can support transcription. The SV40 promoter alleviated the requirement for the Cyp1A1 promoter in the constructs, so that small segments of the Cyp1A1 region of interest could be tested. Several small fragments supported TCDD-induced CAT activity regardless of their orientation in the vector or their distance from the SV40 promoter.[117–120] Regulatory sequences with these properties are termed *enhancer sequences*. These enhancer sequences were localized to three 15- to 20-nucleotide regions between −900 and −1100 bases from the cap site of the rat P450IA1 gene. These elements have been called *xenobiotic regulatory elements* (XRE) or *drug regulatory elements* (DRE). The DNA sequences of the P450IA1 enhancers are shown in Figure 6-10.

Interaction of the Dioxin Receptor Complex with XREs

Binding studies indicate that the dioxin receptor complex interacts directly with XREs.[119,121,122] In these experiments double-stranded DNA containing the enhancer sequence was labeled and incubated with nuclear extracts obtained from untreated cells or from cells treated with TCDD or 3-methylcholanthrene. The formation of DNA-protein complexes was then examined by electrophoresis in polyacrylamide gels. In the absence of binding, the labeled DNA migrates in the gel according to its length. When a protein binds to the labeled DNA, the migration of the DNA is retarded (Fig. 6-10C). This technique demonstrated that a specific XRE-protein complex was formed when TCDD was added to the cultured cells. When labeled TCDD was employed, it was found in association with the protein-enhancer complex. The formation of this complex was not detected when the nuclear proteins were derived from cells deficient in the dioxin receptor.

Induction of the P450IA2 Gene

Polycyclic aromatic hydrocarbons induce P450IA2 as well as P450IA1 in responsive mice but not in nonresponsive mice.[123] This implicates the dioxin receptor in the induction of P450IA2 as well as P450IA1. However, the expression of P450IA2, unlike that of P450IA1, is not seen in lung or kidney. In addition, the increase in transcriptional activity elicited by administration of polycyclic aromatic hydrocarbons is much less for P450IA2 than for P450IA1.[96,97]

In HepG2 human hepatoma cells, the human P450IA2 promoter and approximately 3,700 bases 5' to the cap site drive the transcription of CAT in a 3-methylcholanthrene-dependent manner.[124] When portions of the 5' flanking DNA were tested to determine if any could function as an enhancer element, a fragment of DNA located −3,202 to −1,595 bases from the cap site supported CAT activity following treatment of the cells with 3-methylcholanthrene. This enhancer was not active, however, when the MCF-7 human breast carcinoma cell line was transfected (Fig. 6-11). In contrast, the dioxin-responsive enhancer of the Cyp1A1 gene was active in both the hepatoma and the breast carcinoma cell lines, which indicates that the enhancer elements controlling the induction of the two genes differ and may control tissue differences in the expression of the two genes. When the nucleic acid sequence of the 5' flanking region of the Cyp1A2 gene was examined, XRE sequences were not seen.

THE GLUTATHIONE S-TRANSFERASES

The glutathione S-transferases catalyze the conjugation of glutathione with a variety of electrophilic compounds, as described in Chapter 5. They can also be considered as a class of non-selenium-requiring glutathione peroxidases, for they reduce organic hydroperoxides to the corresponding alcohols. The isolation and characterization of soluble glutathione S-transferases from rat tissues indicates that these enzymes are composed of either identical or nonidentical subunits with molecular weights of roughly 25,000 to 27,000 Da, which associate in dimers to form the catalytically competent enzyme.

Nomenclature

The distinct sizes of some of these subunits led Bass et al.[125] to designate rat subunits as Y with a letter subscript reflecting relative electrophoretic mobilities in the presence of sodium dodecylsulfate, which dissociates the subunits and allows their molecular

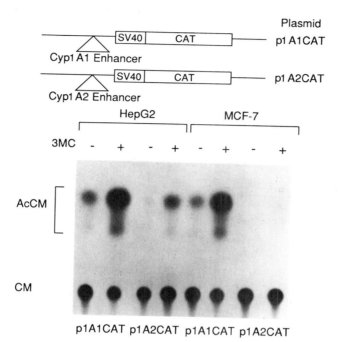

Fig. 6-11. Expression of 3-methylcholanthrene-responsive regions within the human P450IA1 and P450IA2 genes in HepG2 and MCF 7 cells. The constructs, shown at the top of the figure, were transfected into both the human-derived hepatoma cell line HepG2 and the human-derived breast carcinoma cell line MCF-7. Chloramphenicol acetyltransferase (CAT) activities were measured in extracts from untreated (−3MC) and 3-methylcholanthrene-treated (+3MC) cells. Analysis of acetylated chloramphenicol (AcCM) shows that the Cyp1A1 enhancer responds to 3-methylcholanthrene in both cell lines, whereas the Cyp1A2 enhancer is active only in the liver-derived cell line. (From Quattrochi et al.,[124] with permission.)

weights to be estimated from their electrophoretic mobilities. Not all the transferases can be distinguished by electrophoresis, and a numerical superscript is often added to distinguish one electrophoretically similar subunit from another.

More recently, Jakoby et al.[126] proposed a nomenclature that is also widely used. Each of the rat subunits is designated numerically in order of their discovery. Because heterodimers as well as homodimers form glutathione S-transferases, the enzymes are designated by a combination of two numbers describing the two subunits that constitute the enzyme. For example, the homodimers formed by subunits 1 and 2 are designated as 1-1 and 2-2, whereas the heterodimer is identified as 1-2. In the other widely used nomenclature they are designated, YaYa, YcYc, and YaYc.

As illustrated in Table 6-6, distinct catalytic activities are evident for glutathione S-transferases formed from different subunits. In general, the individual subunits are determinants of these differences, and heterodimeric forms display catalytic properties associated with each subunit.[127] Moreover, as was apparent in the other families of drug-metabolizing enzymes discussed in this chapter, there is a substantial overlap of function among the different glutathione S-transferases.

Mannervik et al.[128] have reviewed the relation between catalytic activity, inhibitor

Table 6-6. Activities[a] of Rat Glutathione S-Transferases towards Several Substrates

| | Enzymes by Class | | | | | | | |
| | α | | | μ | | | π | Unassigned |
Substrate	1-1	2-2	8-8	3-3	4-4	6-9	7-7	5-5
1-Chloro-2,4-dinitrobenzene	40.0	38.0	10.0	50.0	20.0	190.0	20.0	<0.15
1,2-Dichloro-4-nitrobenzene	0.15	0.15	0.12	8.4	0.7	2.4	<0.05	nil
trans-4-Phenyl-3-buten-2-one	0.1	0.1	0.1	0.1	1.2	0.2	0.02	<0.001
1,2-Epoxy-3-(*p*-nitrophenoxy)-propane	0.7	0.9	ND[b]	0.2	0.9	<0.5	1.0	25.5
Ethacrynic acid	0.3	2.1	18.0	0.4	1.0	(<0.5)	4.0	nil
4-Hydroxynon-2-enal	2.6	0.7	170.0	2.7	6.9	ND	ND	ND
Cumene hydroperoxide	1.4	3.0	1.1	0.1	0.4	0.04	0.01	12.5
Linoleate hydroperoxide	3.0	1.6	0.2	0.2	0.2	0.06	1.5	5.3
Δ^5-Androstene-3,17-dione	0.23	0.07	ND	0.02	0.002	ND	<0.001	ND

[a] Activities are expressed in micromoles per minute per milligram (μmol/min/mg).
[b] ND = not determined.
(From Ketterer et al.,[176] with permission.)

sensitivity, and immunoreactivity and have suggested that the transferase subunits of both human and rat can be grouped into three broad classes, α, μ, and π. These assignments are listed in Table 6-6 for several rat glutathione S-transferases.

In general, antibodies directed toward a subunit in one class do not cross-react with subunits of another class as judged by double diffusion immunoprecipitation assays. These antibodies will often react with other subunits in the class and with subunits of that class derived from other species.[128]

There is also a significant association between catalytic activity and inhibitor specificity for each class in different species as determined by pattern recognition analysis, a statistical treatment based on analysis of variance.[128] Clearly, however, a broad range of activities and inhibitor sensitivities is exhibited by members of each class, and these overlap with the properties exhibited by members of the other two classes. Distinct "marker" activities characteristic for specific subunits have not emerged from the characterization of these enzymes.

Sequence Relationships

Peptide mapping studies indicated that the amino acid sequences of the glutathione S-transferase subunits differ substantially over their length,[129] which strongly suggests that the subunits are encoded by distinct genes. Amino acid sequence analysis of the N-terminal portions of several subunits[130] further support and sequence data obtained from cDNA clones for several of the rat glutathione S-transferase subunits confirm this hypothesis.

Comparisons of the nucleotide sequences for cDNAs encoding the glutathione transferases as well as the amino acid sequences predicted from them indicate that some subunits exhibit close similarities while others are quite distant. Rat subunits 1 and 2 exhibit 68 percent amino acid sequence identity,[131] whereas when either is compared with subunit 3 or with subunit 4 they exhibit little similarity.[132,133] These similarities and differences may explain why subunits 1 and 2 form heterodimeric glutathione S-transferases but neither combines with subunit 3. Subunit 3 forms a heterodimer with subunit 4, and these two subunits exhibit an amino acid sequence identity of 79 percent.[134] Subunit 7 exhibits less than 33 percent sequence identity with subunits 1, 2, 3, and 4. Thus, the sequences of these five subunits can be divided into three groups, which fall into the three broad classifications discussed earlier (i.e., α, subunits 1 and 2; μ, subunits 3 and 4; and π, subunit 7). A comparison of the amino acid sequences derived from cDNAs for human α,[135] μ,[136] and π[137] subunits with their rat counterparts indicates a high degree (about 80 percent) of sequence conservation. Although the overall sequence conservation is low among the three classes, a number of conserved residues can be identified scattered throughout the length of each subunit. However, none of the conserved amino acids has been implicated in substrate recognition or catalysis.[135]

Microheterogeneity

Southern blot analysis of restriction fragments from rat genomic DNA indicates that there are a minimum of five subunit 1-like genes and subunit 2-like genes that hybridize with the cDNAs encoding the respective subunits.[138] Three distinct cDNAs have been isolated encoding subunit 1-like proteins[138–140] that diverge in their untranslated regions. The three cDNAs also differ in the coding regions, leading to several differences of amino acid sequence. Two closely related human α-class cDNAs have also been described that encode proteins that are 95 percent similar.[141] In addition, multiple sequences of rat μ-class subunits are evident.[142] It is not known at this time whether this genetic diversity underlies differences of function and of expression in different tissues. Based on the developments in characterization of the genetic diversity of cytochrome P450 enzymes, it seems likely that the genetic diversity of the glutathione S-transferases will also contribute to their capacity to metabolize a wide range of substrates.

Gene Structure and Organization

Portions of the rat and human genomes harboring genes encoding the different subunits have been characterized. The number of exons and the locations of introns differ among classes, whereas this number is conserved for each class across this limited number of examples. The rat subunit 1 gene (α class) exhibits seven exons,[143] as do both the rat[144] and human[145] π-class genes, whereas eight exons are found in the rat μ-class gene.[142] The location of introns is conserved between the rat and human π-class genes. Inspection of the amino acid sequence alignment reported by Lai et al.[146] indicates that the rat π-class gene also appears to share most intron locations with the μ-class gene, but the latter contains an additional intron splitting the last exon of the π gene into two exons in the μ-class gene. None of these locations are shared between the α-class gene and the genes of the other two classes. Human α-class genes have been mapped to chromosome 6 and μ-class genes to chromosome 1 by in situ hybridization techniques,[136,147] which indicates that these families are dispersed in the human genome, as was seen for the cytochrome P450 superfamily of genes.

Induction by Xenobiotics

Glutathione S-transferases are induced by phenobarbital and 3-methylcholanthrene, the prototype inducers of the cytochrome P450 enzymes, as well as other compounds. Constituents of both the α and μ classes are induced by each compound. Increases in mRNA concentrations have been shown to underlie the increases in subunit protein concentration,[148] and these in turn appear to reflect an increase in the rate of gene transcription in response to either compound. The time course of induction for α-gene transcription by 3-methylcholanthrene suggests that induction is delayed relative to the μ gene. Maximal values are seen at 16 hours, whereas for the μ genes maximal values are reached at 12 hours. The latter time is similar to that reported for response of P450IA1 genes to this inducer.

It is not clear whether these temporal differences reflect mechanistic differences such as direct versus indirect regulation by the dioxin receptor. In the latter case, TCDD might induce a protein that in turn regulates the expression of the α gene. It has been suggested that P450IA1 might serve this function by its capacity to increase the production of substrates for the glutathione S-transferases and the NADPH-quinone oxidoreductase from their precursors.[149] These substrates might then induce their respective enzymes. Transfection of receptor-competent and negative cell lines with the α-gene promoter and 5'-flanking region linked to the CAT indicator gene suggests that the TCDD receptor is required for induction of CAT transcription by β-naphthoflavone.[150] In addition, a comparison of the activities of constructs from which portions of the flanking region were deleted has localized the responsive element to a region more than 600 base pairs upstream of the promoter. The sequence of this responsive element has not been reported, and it is not known whether it is similar to that for the Cyp1A1 or that for the Cyp1A2 genes.

UDP–GLUCURONOSYLTRANSFERASE

The excretion of biologic end products and the elimination of drugs and other xenobiotics follows biotransformation of these products to water soluble metabolites. As described in Chapter 5, one of the predominant reactions is the addition of glucuronic acid to the aglycones, catalyzed by the microsomal uridine diphosphate–glucuronosyltransferases (UDPGT). The reaction scheme is

$$\text{UDPGA} + \text{R—OH} \xrightarrow{\text{UDPGT}} \text{UDP} + \text{R—O—Glucuronide}$$

The enzymatic transfer of the carbohydrate moiety from UDP-glucuronic acid can occur with compounds that contain —OH, —NH$_2$, —COOH, or —SH groups.

UDPGTs are integral membrane proteins located in the endoplasmic reticulum and depend upon the phospholipid matrix for catalysis. Treatment of microsomes with reagents or procedures that remove phospholipids inactivates the enzymes.[151-153] It is felt that the membrane lipids help to solubilize and concentrate the substrates, thus serving to transport the aglycones to the enzyme in a manner that facilitates catalysis.

One of the more unusual properties of the UDPGTs is their ability to be "activated" by agents that permeate the membrane. For example, treatment of microsomes with detergents or chaotropic agents results in dramatic increases in activity. Permeation of the microsomes by these agents increases the fluidity of the membranes, facilitating access of the aglycones and UDP-glucuronic acid to the enzyme. Studies of this nature have suggested that the UDPGT is associated tightly with the membrane, possibly with its active sites buried in the membrane or on the luminal surface of the microsomes. Disruption of the membrane increases availability to the enzyme of cofactors and substrates. As will be discussed later, information about the structure of the enzyme has been helpful in predicting how the UDPGTs are associated with the membrane.

The UDPGTs are a family of related enzymes. Enzyme heterogeneity was suggested by studies indicating that activities were differentially expressed as a function of the age of the animal and of the ability of the prototypic inducers, phenobarbital and 3-methylcholanthrene, to enhance differentially specific enzyme activities. The purification of the different UDPGTs has demonstrated that these enzymes are part of a multigene family.

Enzyme Purification

Solubilization of microsomes with nonionic detergents such as Emulgen 911 and Lubrol WX, followed by ion-exchange chromatography, demonstrated that proteins with different activities could be separated and partially purified. More efficient separation of the different enzymes has been accomplished by chromatofocusing, which separates the proteins on the basis of their isoelectric points.

Further purification of UDPGTs has been accomplished by passing the partially purified preparations over a UDP-hexanolamine-Sepharose column. Uridine diphosphate, which is an end product of the reaction, binds in a competitive fashion with the cofactor (UDP-glucuronic acid) binding site on the enzyme. Elution of the proteins from the resins is accomplished by addition of the cosubstrate UDP-glucuronic acid, which participates in an exchange for the active site based upon its greater affinity for the enzyme.

Purified UDPGT preparations have been obtained from human,[154] rat,[155-160] mouse,[161] and rabbit tissues.[162] It is unknown how many isozymes exist in these species, but a list of the purified preparations obtained from hepatic tissues is shown in Table 6-7, along with some of the physical properties that characterize the individual forms.

Many of the enzyme preparations possess multiple substrate specificities, yet also exhibit a degree of substrate selectivity. For example, the 3-methylcholanthrene-inducible, rat liver *p*-nitrophenol glucuronosyltransferase (PNP-GT) conjugates *p*-nitrophenol, 4-methylumbelliferone, and 1-naphthol,[155-157] while the 17β-hydroxysteroid UDPGT (17-OH-GT) conjugates testosterone as well as *p*-nitrophenol and 1-naphthol but not 4-methylumbelliferone.[157] The rat liver UDPGT that glucuronidates morphine is not active toward substrates used to characterize the other enzymes,[158] whereas a form purified from mouse

Table 6-7. Purification of Liver UDP-Glucuronosyltransferases

	Substrates	*Physical Properties*	
		Mol. Wt. (kDa)	*pI[a]*
Rat UDPGT			
PNP-GT	*p*-Nitrophenol, 1-naphthol, 4-methylumbelliferone	56–59	—
3-OH-GT	Androsterone, etiocholanolone, testosterone	52	7.8
17-OH-GT	Testosterone, β-estradiol, *p*-nitrophenol, 1-naphthol	50	8.5
4-OH-biphenyl-GT	4-Hydroxybiphenyl	ND	5.5
Morphine-GT	Morphine	56	7.9
Dt-1-GT	Digitoxigenin-monodigitoxoside	ND	10.0
Bilirubin-GT	Bilirubin	54	
Mouse UDPGT			
GT$_{m1}$	1-Naphthol, testosterone, morphine, *p*-nitrophenol, 4-methylumbelliferone	51	6.7
GT$_{m2}$	4-Nitrophenol, 3-OH-benzo[a]pyrene	54	8.5
Human UDPGT			
PNP-GT$_1$	*p*-Nitrophenol, 4-methylumbelliferone, α-naphthylamine, 4-aminobiphenyl	53	7.4
PNP-GT$_2$	*p*-Nitrophenol, 4-methylumbelliferone, α-naphthylamine, 4-aminobiphenyl	54	6.2
Rabbit UDPGT			
PNP-GT	*p*-Nitrophenol	57	6.8
Estrone-GT	Estrone	57	7.6

[a] Isoelectric point.

Table 6-8. UDPGT Full-Length cDNA Clones

Species	cDNA Clone	[a]UDPGT Family	Enzyme	Inducers of mRNA
Rat	4NP	GT-IA1	PNP-GT	3-MC
Human	HLUGP1	GT-IA2	Phenol-GT	
Rat	UDPGT$_{r1/r4}$	GT-IIA1	3-OH-GT	
	[b]RLUG23			
Rat	UDPGT$_{r3}$	GT-IIA2	17-OH-GT	
	[c]RLUG38			
Mouse	UDPGTm1	GT-IIA3		Pb/BP
Rat	UDPGT$_{r2}$	GT-IIB1	4-OH-Biphenyl-GT	Pb
Human	HLUG25	GT-IIB2		

[a] Based on the criteria outlined for the P450 nomenclature.
[b] Similarity in sequence to UDPGT$_{r1/r4}$ is 98 percent or greater.
[c] Similarity in sequence to UDPGT$_{r3}$ is 98 percent or greater.

liver (GT$_{m1}$) that utilizes morphine as a substrate also accepts the substrates 1-naphthol, *p*-nitrophenol, 4-methylumbelliferone.[161] Differences are also seen between enzymes for the positional conjugation of steroids, as evident from the separation and purification of a 3α-(3-OH-GT) and a 17β-hydroxysteroid (17-OH-GT).[163]

UDPGT Heterogeneity and Nomenclature

A number of rat,[161,164,165] mouse,[166] and human[167,168] full-length cDNA clones have been characterized (Table 6-8). It is not known how many different isoenzymes exist for UDPGTs, but their genetic diversity may be similar to that of the cytochrome P450s. A consensus nomenclature for the different UDPGTs does not exist at present. Many of the them have been named on the basis of substrate specificities, but this may not be appropriate since different enzymes are known to glucuronidate the same substrates.

An example of how the UDPGTs could be identified by gene family is shown in the third column of Table 6-8. Applying the same rules used to classify the cytochrome P450 enzymes, the UDPGTs can be divided into two classes based on the relative amino acid similarity between the enzymes. A comparison of the predicted amino acid similarities derived from the different cDNAs is shown in Table 6-9.

Table 6-9. Predicted Amino Acid Similarities Derived from the UDPGT cDNA Clones[a]

	IA2 (HLUGP1)	IIA1 (UDPGTr4)	IIA2 (UDPGTr3)	IIA3 (UDPGTm1)	IIB1 (UDPGTr2)	IIB2 (HLUG25)
IA1 (4NP)	79	40	42	41	41	42
IA2 (HLUGP1)		41	41	40	42	42
IIA1 (UDPGTr4)			84	83	62	65
IIA2 (UDPGTr3)				88	61	67
IIA3 (UDPGTm1)					63	67
IIB1 (UDPGTr2)						70

[a] The trivial names of the UDPGT cDNA clones are shown in parenthesis. The designated gene family name is shown above the name of each cDNA clone.

Gene Family UDPGT-I

The UDPGT-I gene family would encompass the rat PNP-GT[164] and its related homologs in other species, such as the human phenol-GT.[167] These UDPGTs are distantly related in amino acid sequence similarity (less than 50 percent) to the other enzymes and could be grouped into a separate family. The human and rat proteins, named UDPGT-IA1 and IA2, are 80 percent similar in amino acid sequence. This percent identity between species has been shown in the P450 gene family to indicate that the two proteins are orthologs, maintaining the same functional characteristics. This may be the case for UDPGT-IA1 and IA2 because they both catalyze the glucuronidation of phenols.

Gene Family UDPGT-II

The other UDPGTs could be categorized into the second gene family, UDPGT-II, since they are more than 50 percent related in amino acid sequence. The 3-OH-GT,[165,169] 17-OH-GT,[169,170] and the protein encoded by the mouse $UDPGT_{M1}$ cDNA[166] could be placed into a separate subfamily, UDPGT-IIA, since they exhibit more than 70 percent similarity. Likewise, the 4-OH-biphenyl-GT[171] and the proteins encoded by the human HLUG25 cDNA[168] could be classified as UDPGT-IIB since they are more related (over 70 percent) in amino acid sequence to each other than to the other UDPGTs.

As more cDNAs are cloned and characterized and their amino acid sequences are predicted, a uniform numbering system may be helpful to identify the different enzymes.

Identification of cDNA Clones

As indicated in Table 6-8, several full-length cDNA clones have been characterized for UDPGTs. However, an analysis of the proteins that they encode and a comparison with the previously purified UDPGTs have not been presented. To associate the catalytic activities of each of the purified UDPGTs with the proteins encoded by the characterized cDNA clones, results from several different laboratories were compiled; the comparisons are presented in Table 6-8. Based on these comparisons, we can speculate on which purified protein corresponds to a cDNA. The way in which these comparisons were made may be summarized briefly as follows:

1. When transfected into monkey kidney COS cells, each clone, $UDPGT_{r1}$, $UDPGT_{r2}$, $UDPGT_{r3}$,[171,172] and HLUGP1[167], expressed the enzyme activity associated with rat 3-OH-GT, 17-OH-GT, 4-OH-biphenyl-GT, or human phenol-GT, respectively, as shown in Table 6-7.

2. The N-terminal 38 amino acid sequence of the purified 17-OH-GT (17β-hydroxy-steroid UDPGT) was identical to the amino acid sequence predicted from the rat RLUG38 cDNA.[173]

3. A strain difference in the 3α-glucuronidation of androsterone, catalyzed by the 3-OH-GT, helped to identify the enzyme encoded by the cDNA clone RLUG23.[165] A genetic deficiency in certain strains of Wistar rat has been noted, with some animals expressing high (HA) and others expressing low (LA) androsterone UDPGT activities.[174] This difference between strains reflects differences of enzyme concentration.[175] When mRNA from HA and LA Wistar rats was analyzed by Northern blot with the ^{32}P-labeled RLUG23 cDNA, a 2.7-kilobase mRNA was detected in the HA mRNA but not in the LA mRNA. The differences in protein concentration between

the strains reflects the relative concentrations of specific mRNA, demonstrating that the cDNA clone used to detect the mRNA differences encoded the 3-OH-UDPGT.

4. The identity of the cDNA encoding the 3-methylcholanthrene-inducible PNP-GT was confirmed by comparison of the predicted amino acid sequence of the 4-NP clones with the amino acid sequence of the N-terminal and several internal tryptic fragments generated from the purified PNP-GT.[164]

At present, the cDNA clones that encode the rat liver morphine-GT, Dt-1-GT, and bilirubin-GT (Table 6-7) have not been identified.

Induction of the Glucuronosyltransferases

Different inducers have been shown to increase microsomal UDPGT activities. For example, phenobarbital induces 4-hydroxybiphenyl UDPGT activity, while 3-methylcholanthrene induces many of the phenol UDPGT activities. However, since several enzymes conjugate the same substrates, it has been difficult to accurately identify the specific isoenzyme induced.

The use of cDNAs as probes has helped to identify which UDPGTs are induced. Northern blot analysis of mRNA isolated from untreated and 3-methylcholanthrene-treated rats indicates that the polycyclic aromatic hydrocarbon induces the formation of mRNA for PNP-GT.[164] However, 3-methylcholanthrene did not induce the synthesis of mRNAs that encode the 3-OH-GT, 17-OH-GT, or 4-OH-biphenyl-GT enzymes.[161] This result suggests that the increase in *p*-nitrophenol UDPGT activity following 3-methylcholanthrene treatment results from the induction of PNP-GT and not the 17-OH-GT, although the latter has been shown to have *p*-nitrophenol UDPGT activity (see Table 6-7).

Administration of phenobarbital to rats increases UDPGT activity toward testosterone, 4-methylumbelliferrone, 4-hydroxybiphenyl, and other substrates. Some of these activities are catalyzed by more than a single enzyme. When mRNA levels that encode the different enzymes were analyzed following phenobarbital treatment, only the 4-OH-biphenyl mRNA level was increased. The lack of induction observed for other UDPGT mRNAs suggests either that the 4-OH-biphenyl GT exhibits multiple substrate specificities, or that other UDPGTs, not yet identified, contribute to the induced activities.

UDP-Glucuronosyltransferase Structure and Function

Analysis of the secondary structure as predicted from the cDNA sequences has revealed the presence of a signal peptide sequence, characteristic of proteins that are translocated across membranes. The NH_2-terminal hydrophobic amino acids are flanked by a Gly, characteristic of a signal peptide (Fig. 6-12). The absence of the signal peptide in mature UDPGTs was shown by microsequence analysis of the purified PNP-GT, which suggests that the NH_2-terminal hydrophobic amino acids predicted from the cDNA sequence were removed from purified protein by proteolysis.[164] In addition, transcription of the UDPGT$_{r3}$ cDNA in vitro, followed by translation of its RNA in vitro, resulted in the appearance of polypeptides with molecular weights of 52 and 44 kDA.[169] When the same RNA was translated in the presence of dog pancreatic microsomes, the proteins migrated at molecular weight values estimated at 50 and 42 kDa. The generation of the faster migrating polypeptides, resulting from the action of the signal peptidase of dog pancreatic microsomes, is indicative of signal peptide cleavage.[169]

Another feature of the UDPGTs is the presence of a conserved hydrophobic segment

```
GT-IA1   MACLLPAARLPAGFLFLVL---WGSVLGDKLLVVPQDGSHWLSMKEIVEHLSERGHDIVV
GT-IIB1  MS-----MKQTSVFLLIQLICYFRPGACGKVLVWPTEYSHWINIKIILNELAQRGHEVTV
GT-IIA2  MP-----GKWISALLLLQISCCFQSGNCGKVLVWPMEFSHWMNIKTILDELVQRGHEVTV
         *.      .  ..*.. .       *.** * . ***...* *...* .***...*

GT-IA1   LVPEVNLLLGESKYYRRK--SFPVPYNLEELRTRY-------RSFGNNHFAASSPLMAP
GT-IIB1  LVSSASILIEPTKESSINFEIYSVPLSKSDLEYSFAKWIDEWTRDFETLSIWTYYSKMQK
GT-IIA2  LKPSAYYVLDPKKSPDLKFETFPTSVSKDELENYFIKLVDVWTYELQRDTCLSYSPLLQN
         *  ...   ...  .*        .    ...    ...*

GT-IA1   L-REYRNNMIVIDMCFFSCQSLLKDSATLSFLRENQFDALFTDPAMPCGVILAEYLKLPS
GT-IIB1  VFNEYSDVVENL------CKALIWNKSLMKKLQGSQFDVILADAVGPCGELLAELLKTPL
GT-IIA2  MIDGFSDYYLSL------CKDTVSNKQLMAKLQESKFDVLLSDPVAACGELIAEVLHIPF
         . ....    .     *.. .   . *....**....*.. .** ..** *. *

GT-IA1   IYLFR---GFPCSLEHIGQSPSPVSYVPRFYTKFSDHMTFPQRLANFIANILENYLYHCL
GT-IIB1  VYSLRFCPGYRCE-KFSGGLPLPPSYVPVVLSELSDRMTFVERVKNMLQMLYFDFWFQPF
GT-IIA2  LYSLRFSPGYKIE-KSSGRFILPPSYVPVILSGMGGPMTFIDRVKNMICTLYFDFWFHMF
         .* .*  *.  . .  *    * ****  . ....***.*. *...

GT-IA1   YSK-YEILASDLLKRDVSLPA-LHQNSLWLLRYDFVFEYPRPVMPNMIFIGGTNCKKKGN
GT-IIB1  KEKSWSQFYSDVLGRPTTLTEMMGKADIWLIRTFWDLEFPHPFLPNFDFVGGLHCKPAKP
GT-IIA2  NAKKWDPFYSEILGRPTTLAETMGKAEMWLIRSYWDLEFPHPTLPNVDYIGGLQCRPPKP
          .* .. ..*..* ..**.. ....**.* .  .*.*.* .**  ..** .*.

GT-IA1   LSQEFEAYVNASGEHGIVVFSLGSMVSEIPEKKAMEIAEALGRIPQTLLWRYTGTRPSNL
GT-IIB1  LPREMEEFVQSSGEHGVVVFSLGSMVKNLTEEKANVVASALAQIPQKVVWRFDGKKPDTL
GT-IIA2  LPKDMEDFVQSSGEHGVVVFSLGSMVSSMTEEKANAIAWALAQIPQKVLWKFDGKTPATL
         *....*..*..***** .********....*.** .* **..***...*...*. *..*

GT-IA1   AKNTILVKWLPQNDLLGHPKARAFITHSGSHGIYEGICNGVPMVMMPLFGDQMDNAKRME
GT-IIB1  GSNTRLYKWIPQNDLLGHPKTKAFVAHGGTNGIYEAIYHGIPIVGIPLFADQPDNINHMV
GT-IIA2  GPNTRVYKWLPQNDLLGHPKTKAFVTHSGANGVYEAIYHGIPMVGIPMFGEQHDNIAHMV
         . ** . **.**********..**..*.*..*.**.*..*.*.* .*.*..* ** .*

GT-IA1   TRGAGVTLNVLEMTADDLENALKTVINNKSYKENIMRLSSLHKDRPIEPLDLAVFWVEYV
GT-IIB1  AKGAAVRVDFSILSTTGLLTALKIVMNDPSYKENAMRLSRIHHDQPVKPLDRAVFWIEYV
GT-IIA2  AKGAAVTLNIRTMSKSDLFNALKEIINNPFYKKNAVWLSTIHHDQPMKPLDKAVFWIEFV
         ..**.* ..   ...* .*** ..*. **.* ..** .*.*.*..*** ****.*.*

GT-IA1   MRHKGAPHLRPAAHDLTWYQYHSLDVIGFLLAIVLTVVFIVYKSCAYGCRKCFGGKGRVK
GT-IIB1  MRHKGAKHLRSTLHDLSWFQYHSLDVIGFLLLCVVGVVFIITKFCLFCCRK-----TAN
GT-IIA2  MRHKGAKHLRPLGHDLPWYQYHSLDVIGFLLTCSAVIAVLTVKCFLFIYRL-----FVK
         ****** ***. ***.*.************   ... * ..*

GT-IA1   KSHKSKTH
GT-IIB1  MGKK-KKE
GT-IIA2  KEKKMKNE
         ...* *..
```

Fig. 6-12. Alignment of UDP-glucuronosyltransferase sequences. The UDP-glucuronosyltransferase sequences GT-IA1, GT-IIB1, and GT-IIA2 (Table 6-8) were aligned to each other. The boxed area on the 5′ portion of the sequences delineates the signal sequences. The asterisks at the bottom of the rows indicate perfect matches with all three sequences, while the dots represent conserved amino acid substitutions at those positions. Note the large degree of similarity in the COOH-terminal portions of the sequences. This area contains the halt-transfer sequences that secure the protein to the membrane and also may contain the portions of the enzymes that bind UDPGA, which is a cofactor for all the UDP-glucuronosyltransferases.

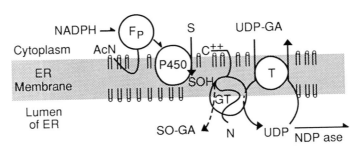

Fig. 6-13. The vectorial transport model for drug biotransformation catalyzed by both the cytochrome P450 system and UDP-glucuronosyltransferase in the membrane of the endoplasmic reticulum. The model indicates that a drug substrate is hydroxylated by the cytochrome P450 system (phase I reaction) and the hydroxylated product (SOH) is glucuronidated by UDPGT (phase II reaction), which is hypothesized to be located on the luminal side of the endoplasmic reticulum membrane. The postulated translocation protein (T) catalyzes translocation of UDPGA from the cytoplasmic compartment to the lumen, possibly by a coupled exchange with UDP. Alternatively, free UDP generated by the action of UDP-glucuronosyltransferase may be hydrolyzed by nucleoside diphosphatase. The charged segment at the COOH-terminal of the GT is marked with C + + . (Fp = NADPH-cytochrome P450 reductase; GT = glucuronosyltransferase; T = translocation protein for UDPGA; S = drug substrate; SOH = hydroxylated product; SO-GA, glucuronide conjugate of SOH; NDPase = nucleoside diphosphatase; ER = endoplasmic reticulum). (From Iyanagi et al.,[164] with permission.)

located in the COOH-terminal end of the proteins. The COOH-terminal transmembrane region is highly conserved among UDPGTs. In addition, this region is flanked by positively charged segments, reminiscent of halt-transfer signals (e.g., this region may function to secure the molecule to the membrane).

With the NH₂ terminus serving as a signal sequence for translocation, it is predicted that the remainder of the protein is translocated across the membrane to the luminal surface as it is synthesized. The protein is secured to the membrane by the hydrophobic COOH terminal, which terminates with the highly charged amino acid region, which remains on the cytoplasmic surface.

A model for the functioning of UDPGTs in the membrane has been presented by Iyanagi et al.[164] and is shown in Figure 6-13. It is based on studies showing that when reagents such as detergents and chaotropic compounds disrupt the integrity of the endoplasmic reticulum, they activate the UDPGTs. This disruption may increase the accessibility of UDPGA and other aglycones to the enzymes. It has been proposed that the active sites of UDPGTs are positioned on the luminal side of the membrane.

With the UDPGTs on the luminal surface and the cytochrome P450 enzymes on the cytoplasmic surface, drug metabolism may be considered as a vectorial process. The model in Figure 6-13 suggests that hydroxylated substrates formed at the cytoplasmic surface pass through the membrane into the lumen of the endoplasmic reticulum, where the UDPGTs transform them to glucuronidated products. It is also assumed, but it has not been demonstrated, that UDPGA reaches the luminal surface through some sort of transport process.

REFERENCES

1. Johnson EF, Zounes MC, Muller-Eberhard U: Characterization of three forms of rabbit microsomal cytochrome P-450 by peptide mapping utilizing limited proteolysis in sodium dodecyl sulfate and analysis by gel electrophoresis. Arch Biochem Biophys 192:282, 1979

2. Botelho LH, Ryan DE, Levin W: Amino acid compositions and partial amino acid sequences of three highly purified forms of liver microsomal cytochrome P-450 from rats treated with polychlorinated biphenyls, phenobarbital, or 3-methylcholanthrene. J Biol Chem 254:5635, 1979

3. Nebert DW, Nelson DR, Adesnik M, et al: The P450 superfamily: Updated listing of all genes and recommended nomenclature of the chromosomal loci. DNA 8:1, 1989

4. Gonzalez FJ: The molecular biology of cytochrome P450s. Pharmacol Rev 40:243, 1988

5. Schwab GE, Johnson EF: Enzymology of rabbit cytochrome P-450. p. 55. In Guengerich FP (ed): Mammalian Cytochromes P-450. CRC Press, Boca Raton, FL, 1987

6. Guengerich FP: Enzymology of rat liver cytochromes P-450. p. 1. In Guengerich FP (ed): Mammalian Cytochromes P-450. Vol. 1. CRC Press, Boca Raton, FL, 1987

7. Nebert DW, Adesnik M, Coon MJ, et al: The P450 Gene Superfamily. Recommended Nomenclature. DNA 6:1, 1987

8. Guengerich FP (ed): Mammalian Cytochromes P-450. CRC Press, Boca Raton, FL, 1987

9. Pelkonen O, Nebert DW: Metabolism of polycyclic aromatic hydrocarbons: Etiologic role in carcinogenesis. Pharmacol Rev 34:189, 1982

10. Sundheimer DW, Caveness MB, Goldstein JA: Differential metabolism of acetanilide versus ethoxycoumarin and benzo(a)pyrene by two 3-methylcholanthrene-inducible forms of rat liver cytochrome P-450. Arch Biochem Biophys 226:548, 1983

11. Ryan DE, Thomas PE, Levin W: Hepatic microsomal cytochrome P-450 from rats treated with isosafrole. J Biol Chem 255:7941, 1980

12. Johnson EF, Muller-Eberhard U: Multiple forms of cytochrome P-450: Resolution and purification of rabbit liver aryl hydrocarbon hydroxylase. Biochem Biophys Res Commun 76:644, 1977

13. Liem HH, Muller-Eberhard U, Johnson EF: Differential induction by 2,3,7,8-tetrachlorodibenzo-p-dioxin of multiple forms of rabbit microsomal cytochrome P-450: Evidence for tissue specificity. Mol Pharmacol 18:565, 1980

14. Goldstein JA, Linko P: Differential induction of two 2,3,7,8-tetrachlorodibenzo-p-dioxin-inducible forms of cytochrome P-450 in extrahepatic versus hepatic tissues. Mol Pharmacol 25:185, 1984

15. Domin BA, Philpot RM: The effect of substrate on the expression of activity catalyzed by cytochrome P-450: Metabolism mediated by rabbit isozyme 6 in pulmonary microsomal and reconstituted monooxygenase systems. Arch Biochem Biophys 246:128, 1986

16. Thomas PE, Reik LM, Ryan DE, Levin W: Regulation of three forms of cytochrome P-450 and epoxide hydrolase in rat liver microsomes. J Biol Chem 256:1044, 1981

17. Levin W, Thomas PE, Ryan DE, Wood AW: Isozyme specificity of testosterone 7α-hydroxylation in rat hepatic microsomes: Is cytochrome P-450a the sole catalyst? Arch Biochem Biophys 258:630, 1987

18. Matsunaga T, Nagata K, Holsztynska EJ, et al: Gene conversion and differential regulation in the rat P-450 IIA gene subfamily. J Biol Chem 263:17995, 1988

19. Harada N, Negishi M: Substrate specificities of cytochrome P-450, C-P-$450_{16\alpha}$ and P-$450_{15\alpha}$, and contribution to steroid hydroxylase activities in mouse liver microsomes. Biochem Pharmacol 37:4778, 1988

20. Lang MA, Juvonen R, Jarvinen P, et al: Mouse liver P450Coh: Genetic regulation of the pyrazole-inducible enzyme and comparison with other P450 isoenzymes. Arch Biochem Biophys 271:139, 1989

21. Serabjit-Singh CJ, Albro PW, Robertson IGC, Philpot RM: Interactions between xenobiotics that increase or decrease the levels of cytochrome P-450 isozymes in rabbit lung and liver. J Biol Chem 258:12827, 1983

22. Domin BA, Serabjit-Singh CJ, Vanderslice RR, et al: Tissue and cellular differences in the expression of cytochrome P-450 enzymes. p. 219. In Paton W, Mitchell J, Turner P (eds): 9th IUPHAR International Congress of Pharmacology, Proceedings, MacMillan Press, London 1984

23. Guengerich FP: Characterization of human microsomal cytochrome P-450 enzymes. Annu Rev Pharmacol Toxicol 29:241, 1989
24. Ryan DE, Iida S, Wood AW, et al: Characterization of three highly purified cytochromes P-450 from hepatic microsomes of adult male rats. J Biol Chem 259:1239, 1984
25. Kimura H, Yoshioka H, Sogawa K, et al: Complementary DNA cloning of cytochrome P-450s related to P-450(M-1) from the complementary DNA library of female rat livers. J Biol Chem 263:701, 1988
26. Zaphiropoulos PG, Mode A, Strom A, et al: cDNA cloning, sequence, and regulation of a major female-specific and growth hormone-inducible rat liver cytochrome P-450 active in 15-beta-hydroxylation of steroid sulfates. Proc Natl Acad Sci USA 85:4214, 1988
27. Dieter HH, Johnson EF: Functional and structural polymorphism of rabbit microsomal cytochrome P-450 form 3b. J Biol Chem 257:9315, 1982
28. Johnson EF, Griffin KJ: Variations in hepatic progesterone 21-hydroxylase activity reflect differences in the microsomal concentration of rabbit cytochrome P-450 1. Arch Biochem Biophys 237:55, 1985
29. Raucy JL, Johnson EF: Variations among untreated rabbits in benzo[a]pyrene metabolism and its modulation by 7,8-benzoflavone. Mol Pharmacol 27:296, 1985
30. Waxman DJ, Walsh C: Cytochrome P-450 isozyme 1 from phenobarbital-induced rat liver: Purification, characterization and interactions with metyrapone and cytochrome b5. Biochemistry 22:4846, 1983
31. Leighton JK, Kemper B: Differential induction and tissue-specific expression of closely related members of the phenobarbital-inducible rabbit cytochrome P-450 gene family. J Biol Chem 259:11165, 1984
32. Finlayson MJ, Kemper B, Browne N, Johnson EF: Evidence that rabbit cytochrome P-450 K is encoded by the plasmid pP-450 PBc2. Biochem Biophys Res Commun 141:728, 1986
33. Finlayson MJ, Dees JH, Masters BSS, Johnson EF: Differential expression of cytochrome P-450 1 and related forms in rabbit liver and kidney. Arch Biochem Biophys 252:113, 1986
34. Imai Y: Characterization of rabbit liver cytochrome P-450 (laurate ω-1 hydroxylase) synthesized in transformed yeast cells. J Biochem 103:143, 1988
35. Tukey RH, Okino ST, Barnes HJ, et al: Multiple gene-like sequences related to the rabbit hepatic progesterone 21-hydroxylase cytochrome P-450 1. J Biol Chem 260:13347, 1985
36. Idle JR, Smith RL: Polymorphisms of oxidation at carbon centers of drugs and their clinical significance. Drug Metab Rev 9:301, 1979
37. Gonzalez FJ, Matsunaga T, Nagata K, et al: Debrisoquine 4-hydroxylase: Characterization of a new P450 gene subfamily, regulation, chromosomal mapping and molecular analysis of the DA rat polymorphism. DNA 6:149, 1987
38. Gonzalez FJ, Skoda RC, Kimura S, et al: Characterization of the common genetic defect in humans deficient in debrisoquine metabolism. Nature 331:442, 1988
39. Ishida N, Tawaragi Y, Inuzuka C, et al: Four species of cDNAs for cytochrome P450 isozymes immunorelated to P450c-M/F encode for members of P450IID subfamily, increasing the number of members within the subfamily. Biochem Biophys Res Commun 156:681, 1988
40. Wong G, Itakura T, Kawajiri K, et al: Gene family of male-specific testosterone 16α-hydroxylase (C-P-450$_{16\alpha}$) in mice. Organization, differential regulation, and chromosome localization. J Biol Chem 264:2920, 1989
41. Koop DR, Coon MJ: Purification of liver microsomal cytochrome P-450 isozymes 3a and 6 from imidazole-treated rabbits. Mol Pharmacol 25:494, 1984
42. Ingelman-Sundberg M, Jornvall H: Induction of the ethanol-inducible form of rabbit liver microsomal cytochrome P-450 by inhibitors of alcohol dehydrogenase. Biochem Biophys Res Commun 124:375, 1984
43. Ryan DE, Ramanathan L, Iida S, et al: Characterization of a major form of rat hepatic microsomal cytochrome P-450 induced by isoniazid. J Biol Chem 260:6385, 1985
44. Ryan DE, Koop DR, Thomas PE, et al: Evidence that isoniazid and ethanol induce the same

microsomal cytochrome P-450 in rat liver, an isozyme homologous to rabbit liver cytochrome P-450 isozyme 3a. Arch Biochem Biophys 246:633, 1986

45. Johansson I, Ekstrom G, Scholte B, et al: Ethanol-, fasting-, and acetone-inducible cytochromes P-450 in rat liver: Regulation and characteristics of enzymes belonging to the IIB and IIE gene subfamilies. Biochemistry 27:1925, 1988

46. Song B-J, Veech RL, Park SS, et al: Induction of rat hepatic N-nitrosodimethylamine demethylase by acetone is due to protein stabilization. J Biol Chem 264:3568, 1989

47. Yang CS, Koop DR, Wang T, Coon MJ: Immunochemical studies on the metabolism of nitrosamines by ethanol-inducible cytochrome P-450. Biochem Biophys Res Commun 128:1007, 1985

48. Tu YY, Yang CS: Demethylation and denitrosation of nitrosamines by cytochrome P-450 isozymes. Arch Biochem Biophys 242:32, 1985

49. Levin W, Thomas PE, Oldfield N, Ryan DE: N-Demethylation of N-nitrosodimethylamine catalyzed by purified rat hepatic microsomal cytochrome P-450: Isozyme specificity and role of cytochrome b5. Arch Biochem Biophys 248:158, 1986

50. Nef P, Heldman J, Lazard D, et al: Olfatory-specific cytochrome P-450. cDNA cloning of a novel neuroepithelial enzyme possibly involved in chemoreception. J Biol Chem 264:6780, 1989

51. Ding X, Coon MJ: Purification and characterization of two unique forms of cytochrome P-450 from rabbit nasal microsomes. Biochemistry 27:8330, 1988

52. Wrighton SA, Schuetz EG, Watkins PB, et al: Demonstration in multiple species of inducible hepatic cytochromes P-450 and their mRNAs related to the glucocorticoid-inducible cytochrome P-450 of the rat. Mol Pharmacol 28:312, 1985

53. Combalbert J, Fabre I, Fabre G, et al: Metabolism of cyclosporin A. IV. Purification and identification of the rifampicin-inducible human liver cytochrome P-450 (cyclosporin A oxidase) as a product of P450IIIA gene subfamily. Drug Metab Dispos 17:197, 1989

54. Larrey D, Funck-Brentano C, Breil P, et al: Effects of erythromycin on hepatic drug-metabolizing enzymes in humans. Biochem Pharmacol 32:1063, 1983

55. Wrighton SA, Maurel P, Schuetz EG, et al: Identification of the cytochrome P-450 induced by macrolide antibiotics in rat liver as the glucocorticoid responsive cytochrome P-450 P. Biochemistry 24:2171, 1985

56. Bork RW, Muto T, Beaune PH, et al: Characterization of mRNA species related to human liver cytochrome P-450 nifedipine oxidase and the regulation of catalytic activity. J Biol Chem 264:910, 1989

57. Komori M, Nishio K, Ohi H, et al: Molecular cloning and sequence analysis of cDNA containing the entire coding region for human fetal liver cytochrome P-450. J Biochem (Tokyo) 105:161, 1989

58. Hardwick JP, Song B-J, Huberman E, Gonzalez FJ: Isolation, complementary DNA sequence, and regulation of rat hepatic lauric acid ω-hydroxylase (cytochrome P-450LAω). J Biol Chem 262:801, 1987

59. Earnshaw D, Dale JW, Goldfarb PS, Gibson GG: Differential splicing in the 3′ noncoding region of rat cytochrome P-452 (P450 IVA1) mRNA. FEBS Lett 236:357, 1988

60. Williams DE, Hale SE, Okita RT, Masters BSS: A prostaglandin ω-hydroxylase cytochrome P-450 (P-450 PG-ω) purified from lungs of pregnant rabbits. J Biol Chem 259:14600, 1984

61. Matsubara S, Yamamoto S, Sogawa K, et al: cDNA cloning and inducible expression during pregnancy of the mRNA for rabbit pulmonary prostaglandin ω-hydroxylase (cytochrome P-450p-2). J Biol Chem 262:13366, 1987

62. Robertson IGC, Serabjit-Singh C, Croft JE, Philpot RM: The relationship between increases in the hepatic content of cytochrome P-450, form 5, and in the metabolism of aromatic amines to mutagenic products following treatment of rabbits with phenobarbital. Mol Pharmacol 24:156, 1983

63. Vanderslice RR, Domin BA, Carver GT, Philpot RM: Species-dependent expression and in-

duction of homologues of rabbit cytochrome P-450 isozyme 5 in liver and lung. Mol Pharmacol 31:320, 1987

64. Nelson DR, Strobel HW: Evolution of cytochrome P-450 proteins. Mol Biol Evol 4:572, 1987
65. Adesnik M, Atchison M: Genes for cytochrome P-450 and their regulation, CRC Crit Rev Biochem 19:247, 1985
66. Dawson JH: Probing structure-function relations in heme-containing oxygenases and peroxidases. Science 240:433, 1988
67. Gotoh O, Tagashira Y, Iizuka T, Fujii-Kuriyama Y: Structural characteristics of cytochrome P-450. Possible location of the heme-binding cysteine in determined amino-acid sequences. J Biochem 93:807, 1983
68. Raag R, Poulos TL: The structural basis for substrate-induced changes in redox potential and spin equilibrium in cytochrome P-450$_{CAM}$. Biochemistry 28:917, 1989
69. White RE, Coon MJ: Oxygen activation by cytochrome P-450. Annu Rev Biochem 49:315, 1980
70. Poulos TL, Finzel BC, Howard AJ: High-resolution crystal structure of cytochrome P450$_{CAM}$. J Mol Biol 195:687, 1987
71. Atkins WM, Sligar SG: The roles of active site hydrogen bonding in cytochrome P-450$_{CAM}$ as revealed by site-directed mutagenesis. J Biol Chem 263:18842, 1988
72. Haugen DA, Armes LG, Yasunobu KT, Coon MJ: Amino-terminal sequence of phenobarbital-inducible cytochrome P-450 from rabbit liver microsomes: Similarity to hydrophobic amino-terminal segments of preproteins. Biochem Biophys Res Commun 77:967, 1977
73. Sakaguchi M, Katsuyoshi M, Sato R: Signal recognition particle is required for cotranslational insertion of cytochrome P-450 into microsomal membranes. Proc Natl Acad Sci USA 81:3361, 1984
74. Monier S, Van Luc P, Kreibich G, et al: Signals for the incorporation and orientation of cytochrome P450 in the endoplasmic reticulum membrane. J Cell Biol 107:457, 1988
75. Sakaguchi M, Mihara K, Sato R: A short amino-terminal segment of microsomal cytochrome P-450 functions both as an insertion signal and as a stop-transfer sequence. EMBO J 6:2425, 1987
76. Szczesna-Skorupa E, Browne N, Mead D, Kemper B: Positive charges at the NH_2 terminus convert the membrane-anchor signal peptide of cytochrome P-450 to a secretory signal peptide. Proc Natl Acad Sci USA 85:738, 1988
77. Szczesna-Skorupa E, Kemper B: NH_2-terminal substitutions of basic amino acids induce translocation across the microsomal membrane and glycosylation of rabbit cytochrome P450IIC2. J Cell Biol 108:1237, 1989
78. DuBois RN, Simpson ER, Tuckey J, et al: Evidence for a higher molecular weight precursor of cholesterol side-chain-cleavage cytochrome P-450 and induction of mitochondrial and cytosolic proteins by corticotropin in adult bovine adrenal cells. Proc Natl Acad Sci USA 78:1028, 1981
79. Brown CA, Black SD: Membrane topology of mammalian cytochromes P-450 from liver endoplasmic reticulum. Determination by trypsinolysis of phenobarbital-treated microsomes. J Biol Chem 264:4442, 1989
80. Nelson DR, Strobel HW: On the membrane topology of vertebrate cytochrome P-450 proteins. J Biol Chem 263:6038, 1988
81. Black SD, Coon MJ: Structural features of liver microsomal NADPH-cytochrome P-450 reductase. Hydrophobic domain, hydrophilic domain, and connecting region. J Biol Chem 257:5929, 1982
82. Potenza CL, Pendurthi UR, Strom DK, et al: Regulation of the rabbit cytochrome P450 3c: Age-dependent expression and transcriptional activation by rifampicin. J Biol Chem 264:16222, 1989
83. Yamamoto S, Kusunose E, Kaku M, et al: Effect of peroxisomal proliferators on microsomal prostaglandin A omega-hydroxylase. J Biochem 100:1449, 1986

84. Yamamoto S, Kusunose E, Ogita K, et al: Isolation of cytochrome P-450 highly active in prostaglandin ω-hydroxylation from lung microsomes of rabbits treated with progesterone. J Biochem 96:593, 1984

85. Schimke RT, Doyle D: Control of enzyme levels in animal tissues. Annu Rev Biochem 39:929, 1970

86. Shiraki H, Guengerich FP: Turnover of membrane protein: Kinetics of induction and degradation of seven forms of rat liver microsomal cytochrome P-450, NADPH-cytochrome P-450 reductase, and epoxide hydrolase. Arch Biochem Biophys 235:86, 1984

87. Watkins PB, Wrighton SA, Schuetz EG, et al: Macrolide antibiotics inhibit the degradation of the glucocorticoid-responsive cytochrome P-450p in rat hepatocytes in vivo and in primary monolayer culture. J Biol Chem 261:6264, 1986

88. Watkins PB, Bond JS, Guzelian PS: Degradation of the hepatic cytochromes P-450. p. 173. In Guengerich FP (ed): Mammalian Cytochromes P-450. Vol. 2. CRC Press, Boca Raton, FL. 1987

89. Okino ST, Quattrochi LC, Barnes HJ, et al: Cloning and characterization of cDNAs encoding 2,3,7,8-tetrachlorodibenzo-p-dioxin-inducible rabbit mRNAs for cytochrome P-450 isozymes 4 and 6. Proc Natl Acad Sci USA 82:5310, 1985

90. Giachelli CM, Omiecinski CJ: Regulation of cytochrome P-450b and P-450e mRNA expression in the developing rat. Hybridization to synthetic oligodeoxyribonucleotide probes. J Biol Chem 261:1359, 1986

91. Omiecinski CJ: Tissue-specific expression of rat mRNAs homologous to cytochromes P-450b and P-450e. Nucleic Acids Res 14:1525, 1986

92. Song B-J, Gelboin HV, Park S-S, et al: Complementary DNA and protein sequences of ethanol-inducible rat and human cytochrome P-450s. J Biol Chem 261:16689, 1986

93. Atchison M, Adesnik M: A cytochrome P-450 multigene family. Characterization of a gene activated by phenobarbital administration. J Biol Chem 258:11285, 1983

94. Simmons DL, McQuiddy P, Kasper CB: Induction of the hepatic mixed-function oxidase system by synthetic glucocorticoids. J Biol Chem 262:326, 1987

95. Gonzalez FJ, Song B-J, Hardwick JP: Pregnenolone 16α-carbonitrile-inducible P-450 gene family: Gene conversion and differential regulation. Mol Cell Biol 6:2969, 1986

96. Pasco DS, Boyum KW, Merchant SN, et al: Transcriptional and post-transcriptional regulation of the genes encoding cytochromes P-450c and P-450d in vivo and in primary hepatocyte cultures. J Biol Chem 263:8671, 1988

97. Silver G, Krauter KS: Expression of cytochromes P-450c and P-450d mRNAs in cultured rat hepatocytes. J Biol Chem 263:11802, 1988

98. Poland A, Glover E: Chlorinated dibenzo-p-dioxins: Potent inducers of delta-aminolevulinic acid synthetase and aryl hydrocarbon hydroxylase. Mol Pharmacol 9:736, 1973

99. Thomas PE, Kouri RE, Hutton JJ: The genetics of aryl hydrocarbon hydroxylase induction in mice: A single gene difference between C57BL/6J and DBA/2J. Biochem Genet 6:157, 1972

100. Poland AP, Glover E, Robinson JR, Nebert DW: Genetic expression of aryl hydrocarbon hydroxylase activity. Induction of monooxygenase activities and cytochrome P_1-450 formation by 2,3,7,8-tetrachlorodibenzo-p-dioxin in mice genetically "nonresponsive" to other aromatic hydrocarbons. J Biol Chem 249:5599, 1974

101. Poland A, Glover E, Kende AS: Stereospecific, high affinity binding of 2,3,7,8-tetrachloro-dibenzo-p-dioxin by hepatic cytosol. Evidence that the binding species is a receptor for induction of aryl hydrocarbon hydroxylase. J Biol Chem 251:4936, 1976

102. Greenlee WF, Poland A: Nuclear uptake of 2,3,7,8-tetrachlorodibenzo-p-dioxin in C57BL/6J and DBA/2J mice. J Biol Chem 254:9814, 1979

103. Legraverend C, Hannah RR, Eisen HJ, et al: Regulatory gene product of the Ah locus: Characterization of receptor mutants among mouse hepatoma clones. J Biol Chem 257:6402, 1982

104. Miller AG, Israel D, Whitlock JP Jr: Biochemical and genetic analysis of variant mouse hepatoma cells defective in the induction of benzo(a)pyrene-metabolizing enzyme activity. J Biol Chem 258:3523, 1983

105. Hankinson O: Dominant and recessive aryl hydrocarbon hydroxylase-deficient mutants of mouse hepatoma line, Hepa-1, and assignment of recessive mutants to three complementation groups. Somatic Cell Genet 9:497, 1983

106. Gudas JM, Hankinson O: Regulation of cytochrome P-450c in differentiated and dedifferentiated rat hepatoma cells: Role of the Ah receptor. Somatic Cell Genet 13:513, 1987

107. Okey AB, Bondy GP, Mason ME, et al: Regulatory gene product of the Ah locus. Characterization of the cytosolic inducer-receptor complex and evidence for its nuclear translocation. J Biol Chem 254:11636, 1979

108. Gustafsson J-A, Carlstedt-Duke J, Poellinger L, et al: Biochemistry, molecular biology, and physiology of the glucocorticoid receptor. Endocrinol Rev 8:185, 1987

109. Wilhelmsson A, Wikstrom A-C, Poellinger L: Polyanionic-binding properties of the receptor for 2,3,7,8-tetrachlorodibenzo-p-dioxin. A comparison with the glucocorticoid receptor. J Biol Chem 261:13456, 1986

110. Cuthill S, Poellinger L: DNA binding properties of dioxin receptors in wild-type and mutant mouse hepatoma cells. Biochemistry 27:2978, 1988

111. Denis M, Cuthill S, Wikström A-C, et al: Association of the dioxin receptor with the M_r 90,000 heat shock protein: A structural kinship with the glucocorticoid receptor. Biochem Biophys Res Commun 155:801, 1988

112. Perdew GH: Association of the Ah receptor with the 90-kDa heat shock protein. J Biol Chem 263:13802, 1988

113. Evans RM: The steroid and thyroid hormone receptor superfamily. Science 240:889, 1988

114. Schultz G: Control of gene expression by steroid hormones. Hoppe Seylers Z Biol Chem 369:77, 1988

115. Jones PBC, Durrin LK, Fisher JM, Whitlock JP Jr: Control of gene expression by 2,3,7,8-tetrachlorodibenzo-p-dioxin: Multiple dioxin-responsive domains 5'-ward of the cytochrome P_1-450 gene. J Biol Chem 261:6647, 1986

116. Fujisawa-Sehara A, Sogawa K, Yamane M, Fujii-Kuriyama Y: Characterization of xenobiotic responsive elements upstream from the drug-metabolizing cytochrome P-450c gene: A similarity to glucocorticoid regulatory elements. Nucleic Acids Res 15:4179, 1987

117. Sogawa K, Fujisawa-Sehara A, Yamane M, Fujii-Kuriyama Y: Location of regulatory elements responsible for drug induction in the rat cytochrome P-450c gene. Proc Natl Acad Sci USA 83:8044, 1986

118. Gonzalez FJ, Nebert DW: Autoregulation plus upstream positive and negative control regions associated with transcriptional activation of the mouse P_1-450 gene. Nucleic Acids Res 13:7269, 1985

119. Fujisawa-Sehara A, Yamane M, Fujii-Kuriyama Y: A DNA-binding factor specific for xenobiotic responsive elements of P-450c gene exists as a cryptic form in cytoplasm: Its possible translocation to nucleus. Proc Natl Acad Sci USA 85:5859, 1988

120. Denison MS, Fisher JM, Whitlock JP Jr: Inducible, receptor-dependent protein-DNA interactions at a dioxin-responsive transcriptional enhancer. Proc Natl Acad Sci USA 85:2528, 1988

121. Denison MS, Fisher JM, Whitlock JP Jr: The DNA recognition site for the dioxin-ah receptor complex. J Biol Chem 263:17221, 1988

122. Hapgood J, Cuthill S, Denis M, et al: Specific protein-DNA interactions at a xenobiotic-responsive element: Copurification of dioxin receptor and DNA-binding activity. Proc Natl Acad Sci USA 86:60, 1989

123. Negishi M, Nebert DW: Structural gene products of the Ah locus. Genetic and immunochemical evidence for two forms of mouse liver cytochrome P-450 induced by 3-methylcholanthrene. J Biol Chem 254:11015, 1979

124. Quattrochi LQ, Tukey RH: Human cytochrome P450IA2 gene contains regulatory elements responsive to 3-methylcholanthrene. Mol Pharmacol 36:66, 1989

125. Bass NM, Kirsch RE, Tuff SA, Saunders SJ: Ligandin heterogeneity: Evidence that the two non-identical subunits are the monomers of two distinct proteins. Biochim Biophys Acta 492:163, 1977

126. Jakoby WB, Ketterer B, Mannervik B: Glutathione transferases: Nomenclature. Biochem Pharmacol 33:2539, 1984

127. Danielson UH, Mannervik B: Kinetic independence of the subunits of cytosolic glutathione transferase from the rat. Biochem J 231:263, 1985

128. Mannervik B, Alin P, Guthenberg C, et al: Identification of three classes of cytosolic glutathione transferase common to several mammalian species: Correlation between structural data and enzymatic properties. Proc Natl Acad Sci USA 82:7202, 1985

129. Beale D, Ketterer B, Carne T, et al: Evidence that the Ya and Yc subunits of glutathione transferase B (ligandin) are the products of separate genes. Eur J Biochem 126:459, 1982

130. Alin P, Mannervik B, Jornvall H: Structural evidence for three different types of glutathione transferase in human tissues. FEBS Lett 182:319, 1985

131. Telakowski-Hopkins CA, Rodkey JA, Bennett CD, Lu AYH: Rat glutathione S-transferases. J Biol Chem 260:5820, 1985

132. Ding GJ-F, Lu AYH, Pickett CB: Rat liver glutathione S-transferases. Nucleotide sequence analysis of a Yb1 cDNA clone and prediction of the complete amino acid sequence of the Yb1 subunit. J Biol Chem 260:13268, 1985

133. Alin P, Mannervik B, Jornvall H: Cytosolic rat liver glutathione transferase 4-4. Primary structure of the protein reveals extensive differences between homologous glutathione transferases of classes alpha and mu. Eur J Biochem 156:343, 1986

134. Ding GJ-F, Ding VD-H, Rodkey JA, et al: Rat liver glutathione S-transferases: DNA sequence analysis of a Yb2 cDNA clone and regulation of the Yb1 and Yb2 mRNAs by phenobarbital. J Biol Chem 261:7952, 1986

135. Tu C-PD, Qian B: Human liver glutathione S-transferases: Complete primary sequence of an Ha subunit cDNA. Biochem Biophys Res Commun 141:229, 1986

136. DeJong JL, Chang C-M, Whang-Peng J, et al: The human liver glutathione S-transferase gene superfamily: Expression and chromosome mapping of an Hb subunit cDNA. Nucleic Acids Res 16:8541, 1988

137. Kano T, Sakai M, Muramatsu M: Structure and expression of a human class π glutathione S-transferase messenger RNA. Cancer Res 47:5626, 1987

138. Rothkopf GS, Telakowski-Hopkins CA, Stotish RL, Pickett CB: Multiplicity of glutathione S-transferase genes in the rat and association with a type 2 Alu repetitive element. Biochemistry 25:993, 1986

139. Tu C-PD, Weiss MJ, Li N-Q, Reddy CC: Tissue-specific expression of the rat glutathione S-transferase. J Biol Chem 258:4659, 1983

140. Pickett CB, Telakowski-Hopkins CA, Ding GJ-F, et al: Rat liver glutathione S-transferases: Complete nucleotide sequence of a glutathione S-transferase mRNA and the regulation of the Ya, Yb, and Yc mRNAs by 3-methylcholanthrene and phenobarbital. J Biol Chem 259:5182, 1984

141. Rhoads DM, Zarlengo RP, Tu C-PD: The basic glutathione S-transferases from human livers are products of separate genes. Biochem Biophys Res Commun 145:474, 1987

142. Lai H-CJ, Qian B, Grove G, Tu C-PD: Gene expression of rat glutathione S-transferases. J Biol Chem 163:11389, 1988

143. Telakowski-Hopkins CA, Rothkopf GS, Pickett CB: Structural analysis of a rat liver glutathione S-transferase Ya gene. Proc Natl Acad Sci USA 83:9393, 1986

144. Okuda A, Sakai M, Muramatsu M: The structure of the rat glutathione S-transferase P gene and related pseudogenes. J Biol Chem 262:3858, 1987

145. Cowell IG, Dixon KH, Pemble SE, et al: The structure of the human glutathione S-transferase π gene. Biochem J 255:79, 1988

146. Lai H-CJ, Grove G, Tu C-PD: Cloning and sequence analysis of a cDNA for a rat liver glutathione S-transferase Yb subunit. Nucleic Acids Res 14:6101, 1986

147. Chow N-WI, Whang-Peng J, Kao-Shan C-S, et al: Human glutathione S-transferases. J Biol Chem 263:12797, 1988

148. Ding VD-H, Pickett CB: Transcriptional regulation of rat liver glutathione S-transferase genes by phenobarbital and 3-methylcholanthrene. Arch Biochem Biophys 240:553, 1985

149. Prochaska HJ, DeLong MJ, Talalay P: On the mechanisms of induction of cancer-protective enzymes: A unifying proposal. Proc Natl Acad Sci USA 82:8232, 1985

150. Telakowski-Hopkins CA, King RG, Pickett CB: Glutathione S-transferase Ya subunit gene: Identification of regulatory elements required for basal level and inducible expression. Proc Natl Acad Sci USA 85:1000, 1988

151. Gorski JP, Kasper CB: UDP-glucuronosyltransferase: Phospholipid dependence and properties of the reconstituted apoenzyme. Biochemistry 17:4600, 1978

152. Erickson RH, Zakim D, Vessey DA: Preparation and properties of a phospholipid-free form of microsomal UDP-glucuronyltransferase. Biochemistry 17:3706, 1978

153. Tukey RH, Billings RE, Autor AP, Tephly TR: Phospholipid-dependence of oestrone UDP-glucuronyltransferase and p-nitrophenol UDP-glucuronyltransferase. Biochem J 179:59, 1979

154. Irshaid YM, Tephly TR: Isolation and purification of two human liver UDP-glucuronosyl-transferases. Mol Pharmacol 31:27, 1987

155. Gorski JP, Kasper CB: Purification and properties of microsomal UDP-glucuronosyltransferase from rat liver. J Biol Chem 252:1336, 1977

156. Burchell B: Substrate specificity and properties of uridine diphosphate glucuronyltransferase purified to apparent homogeneity from phenobarbital-treated rat liver. Biochem J 173:749, 1978

157. Falany CN, Tephly TR: Separation, purification and characterization of three isoenzymes of UDP-glucuronyltransferase from rat liver microsomes. Arch Biochem Biophys 227:248, 1983

158. Puig JF, Tephly TR: Isolation and purification of rat liver morphine UDP-glucuronosyltrans-ferase. Mol Pharmacol 30:558, 1986

159. Von Meyerinck L, Coffman BL, Green MD, et al: Separation, purification, and characterization of digitoxigenin-monodigitoxoside UDP-glucuronosyltransferase activity. Drug Metab Dispos 13:700, 1985

160. Coughtrie MWH, Burchell B, Bend JR: Purification and properties of rat kidney UDP-glucuronosyltransferase. Biochem Pharmacol 36:245, 1987

161. Mackenzie PI, Gonzalez FJ, Owens IS: Cloning and characterization of DNA complementary to rat liver UDP-glucuronosyltransferase mRNA. J Biol Chem 259:12153, 1984

162. Tukey RH, Tephly TR: Purification and properties of rabbit liver estrone and p-nitrophenol UDP-glucuronyltransferases. Arch Biochem Biophys 209:565, 1981

163. Falany CN, Green MD, Tephly TR: The enzymatic mechanism of glucuronidation catalyzed by two purified rat liver steroid UDP-glucuronosyltransferases. J Biol Chem 262:1218, 1987

164. Iyanagi T, Haniu M, Sogawa K, et al: Cloning and characterization of cDNA encoding 3-methylcholanthrene inducible rat mRNA for UDP-glucuronosyltransferase. J Biol Chem 261:15607, 1986

165. Jackson MR, Burchell B: The full length coding sequence of rat liver androsterone UDP-glucuronyltransferase cDNA and comparison with other members of this gene family. Nucleic Acids Res 14:779, 1986

166. Kimura T, Owens IS: Mouse UDP glucuronosyltransferase. cDNA and complete amino acid sequence and regulation. Eur J Biochem 168:515, 1987

167. Harding D, Fournel-Gigleux S, Jackson MR, Burchell B: Cloning and substrate specificity of a human phenol UDP-glucuronosyltransferase expressed in COS-7 cells. Proc Natl Acad Sci USA 85:8381, 1988

168. Jackson MR, McCarthy LR, Harding D, et al: Cloning of a human liver microsomal UDP-glucuronosyltransferase cDNA. Biochem J 242:581, 1987

169. Mackenzie PI: Rat liver UDP-glucuronosyltransferase. Identification of cDNAs encoding two enzymes which glucuronidate testosterone, dihydrotestosterone, and β-estradiol. J Biol Chem 262:9744, 1987

170. Harding D, Wilson SM, Jackson MR, et al: Nucleotide and deduced amino acid sequence of rat liver 17β-hydroxysteroid UDP-glucuronosyltransferase. Nucleic Acids Res 15:3936, 1987

171. Mackenzie PI: Rat liver UDP-glucuronosyltransferase. cDNA sequence and expression of a form glucuronidating 3-hydroxyandrogens. J Biol Chem 261:14112, 1986
172. Mackenzie PI: Rat liver UDP-glucuronosyltransferase. Sequence and expression of a cDNA encoding a phenobarbital-inducible form. J Biol Chem 261:6119, 1986
173. Harding D, Wilson SM, Jackson MR, et al: Nucleotide and deduced amino acid sequence of rat liver 17β-hydroxysteroid UDP-glucuronosyltransferase. Nucleic Acids Res 15:3936, 1987
174. Matchio M, Hakozaki M: Discontinuous variation in hepatic uridine diphosphate glucuronyltransferase toward androsterone in wistar rats. A regulatory factor for in vivo metabolism of androsterone. Biochem Pharmacol 28:411, 1979
175. Green MD, Falany CN, Kirkpatrick RB, Tephly TR: Strain differences in purified rat hepatic 3alpha-hydroxysteroid UDP-glucuronosyltransferase. Biochem J 230:403, 1985
176. Ketterer B, Geyer DJ, Clark AG: Soluble glutathione isozymes. p. 73. In Sies H, Ketterer B (eds). Glutathione Conjugation: Mechanisms and Biological Significance. Academic Press, San Diego, CA, 1988

7

Pharmacogenetics

Daniel W. Nebert
Wendell W. Weber

Pharmacogenetics is a field concerned with unusual (*idiosyncratic*) drug responses that have a *hereditary* basis.[1] An idiosyncratic drug response should be distinguished from unanticipated reactions such as accidental overdosage or allergic phenomena. The term *drugs* is meant here to include numerous foreign chemicals and other substances, in addition to the hundreds of clinically prescribed agents. The total number of compounds to which the body is exposed may amount to more than 1 million. For example, more than 400 chemicals have been isolated from red wine and structurally characterized. A lighted cigarette produces more than 1,000 chemicals, many of which have been identified. Each year farmland in the United States receives more than 75,000 agricultural chemicals in the form of pesticides, herbicides, and fertilizing agents. In any given day and quite independently of industrial hazards, we are routinely exposed to thousands of chemicals in the food and drink we ingest, the air we breathe, and the soaps, perfumes, deodorants, and other substances that we apply to our skin.

When any drug or other chemical is presented to a population, there will be differences in response. The response may be favorable in some patients (e.g., efficient seizure control, relief from pain) and unfavorable in others (e.g., rash, diarrhea, increased risk of cancer). The response will always be modulated by the genetic predisposition of the patient. This observation ultimately implies that genes encoding enzymes or proteins that play a role in the drug response differ in some respect from one individual to the next.

Much of an individual's pharmacogenetic response reflects genetic difference in foreign chemical metabolism (Ch. 5). That is, a drug may be either detoxified more rapidly or converted to reactive (toxic) intermediates more efficiently than in the majority of individuals. For some drugs, there is a delicate balance in each tissue between enzymes that form toxic intermediates and those that detoxify these highly reactive intermediates. Other factors contributing to an individual's susceptibility to drug toxicity include age, concurrent disease, nutritional status, hormone levels, diurnal variations in drug disposition or sensitivity, environmental factors that induce or inhibit drug metabolism, efficiency of

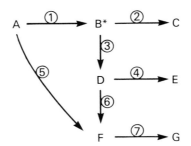

Fig. 7-1. Schematic representation of cascading pathways by which drugs may be metabolized. A is the parent drug; B* through G are various metabolites; circled numbers depict enzymes. (From Thorgeirsson et al.,[2] with permission.)

repair mechanisms (both protein replacement and DNA repair), and immunologic competence.

Most drugs are metabolized by a number of pathways (Fig. 7-1).[2] Given this complexity of interacting pathways, one might expect that pharmacogenetic differences in drug metabolism leading to toxicity would be typified by polygenic multifactorial traits in much the same way as one's stature, intelligence quotient, or blood pressure are influenced by multiple genetic loci. This hypothesis has often been shown *not* to be the case. Why not? If, for example (Fig. 7-1), compound A causes toxicity, any factor decreasing enzyme *1* or *5* would increase the steady-state level of compound A, thereby enhancing its duration of action and toxic effects. On the other hand, if compound A requires metabolism to convert it to the toxic intermediate B*, any factor decreasing enzyme *2*, *3*, or *5* or increasing enzyme *1* would enhance the steady-state level of the reactive intermediate, thereby causing greater toxicity. Moreover, if any of the other, more distant enzymes such as *4*, *6*, or *7* were rate-limiting for the overall pathway, any factor changing the level of such an enzyme could be most important in affecting the steady-state level of compound A or B*. If the enzyme responsible for the rate-limiting step can vary by a large amount, allelic differences in the gene encoding that enzyme would predominate over any subtle changes in the remainder of the enzymes involved. Thus, the finding is not unexpected that a genetic variation affecting just one enzyme in an interacting set of metabolizing enzymes can alter in a substantial way the toxic response to a drug.

GENETICS IN PHARMACOLOGY

Pharmacogenetic disorders are inherited in the same ways that "inborn errors of metabolism" are inherited. The important difference between pharmacogenetic disorders and inherited metabolic diseases lies in the fact that individuals affected with a pharmacogenetic alteration may live their entire lives without ever being challenged with the

Fig. 7-2. Classical examples of modes of inheritance. In the first three cases the *a* allele is the mutant allele. Under "Additive" inheritance, *stippling* denotes an intermediate effect, and *hatching* indicates an afflicted individual. *Circles* always denote females, *squares* indicate males. Sex-linked, or X-linked, inheritance is one in which the defective allele (X^a) on the X chromosome denotes phenotypic expression of a disorder when paired with a Y chromosome but not when paired with a "normal" allele (X^b) on an X chromosome.

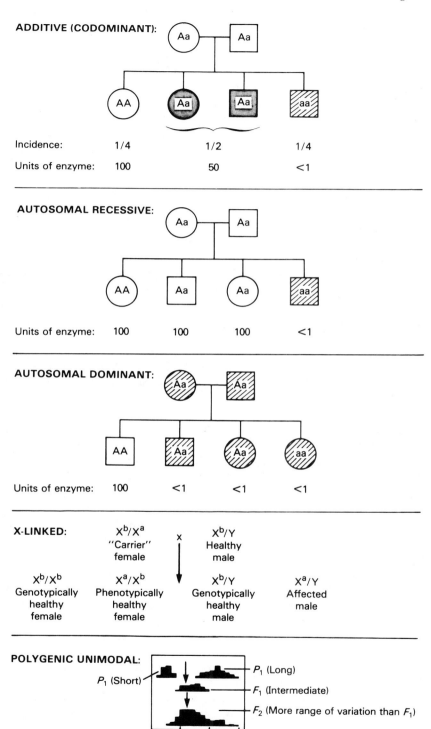

ADDITIVE (CODOMINANT):

Incidence:	1/4	1/2	1/4
Units of enzyme:	100	50	<1

AUTOSOMAL RECESSIVE:

Units of enzyme:	100	100	100	<1

AUTOSOMAL DOMINANT:

Units of enzyme:	100	<1	<1	<1

X-LINKED:

X^b/X^a x X^b/Y
"Carrier" female   Healthy male

X^b/X^b X^a/X^b X^b/Y X^a/Y
Genotypically healthy female   Phenotypically healthy female   Genotypically healthy male   Affected male

POLYGENIC UNIMODAL:

P_1 (Short) P_1 (Long)
F_1 (Intermediate)
F_2 (More range of variation than F_1)

3   9   15   21
LENGTH (cm)

particular drug (or class of drugs) that will precipitate the idiosyncratic response. Hence, pharmacogenetic disorders may be regarded as "silent" until the phenotype is expressed following exposure to the environmental stimulus.

To familiarize the reader with genetic terminology as used in this chapter, the five most common modes of inheritance are illustrated in Fig. 7-2. A gene, or a genetic locus, represents two *alleles* at a particular chromosomal site—one allele on each member of a chromosomal pair in diploid organisms (eukaryotes). All chromosomes other than the sex chromosomal pair are called *autosomes*. The term *phenotype* describes an observed genetic trait (e.g., blue eyes) or clinical finding (e.g., hypercholesterolemia), whereas the term *genotype* describes the trait specifically at the gene level (e.g., the hemoglobin *S* allele responsible for sickle cell anemia).

If one allele does not predominate over the other, these traits are called *additive* (also codominant, midparent, and gene-dose). The majority of enzymes (or other proteins) in eukaryotes are inherited additively. Figure 7-2 (at top) shows the *A/A* individual having 100 units of enzyme, the *A/a* heterozygote 50 units, and the *a/a* individual less than 1 unit. This gene-dose effect is called *autosomal autonomous*. According to strict mendelian terminology, this condition would be called autosomal dominant if the heterozygote is clinically affected. However, the term *autonomous* provides a useful distinction for situations in which the severity of phenotypic response can be predicted on the basis of whether the individual is heterozygous or homozygous for the variant gene.

If the normal allele predominates over the mutant allele, the disorder is inherited as an *autosomal recessive* trait, and if the mutant allele predominates over the normal allele, the trait is inherited as an *autosomal dominant* trait (Fig. 7-2). Slow acetylation of isoniazid is an example of autosomal recessive inheritance. Hepatic porphyrias are examples of autosomal dominant traits.

Some pharmacogenetic traits are transmitted in a sex-linked manner. The allele X^a in Fig. 7-2, for example, represents a mutant allele located on the X chromosome. If an apparently healthy "carrier" female mates with a healthy male, the expected distribution of offspring is one-fourth genotypically healthy females, one-fourth phenotypically healthy females (i.e., carrier females), one-fourth genotypically healthy males, and one-fourth afflicted males. Half of all males born to a carrier female will thus express the X-linked trait under consideration. Hypoxanthine-guanine phosphoribosyltransferase-deficient gout and glucose-6-phosphate-deficient hemolysis are examples of *X-linked inheritance*. Furthermore, the trait is designated *sex-linked dominant* if the female carrier (X/X^a) is affected, and *sex-linked recessive* if expression requires a double dose of the variant gene (e.g., X^a/X^a).

Two or more genes expressed concomitantly and contributing to the same phenotypic response represent *polygenic unimodal* inheritance (e.g., the ear length in corn shown in Fig. 7-2 at bottom). Such multifactorial inheritance is generally unimodal (no distinct groupings), being either distributed in gaussian fashion or skewed to the left or right. A trait might also be expressed with partial (or incomplete) penetrance. This means that modifier genes or other unknown factors most likely contribute to the phenotypic expression in a manner not yet fully understood.

The Hardy-Weinberg distribution of alleles p and q follows the binomial expansion described by the equation $(p + q)^2 = p^2 + 2pq + q^2$, where p is usually the more common allele and q is the less common allele. Several examples using the Hardy-Weinberg law will be given later in the chapter.

INVESTIGATIVE APPROACHES TO PHARMACOGENETICS

It seems reasonable that genetic variation in any of the subcellular steps involved in pharmacokinetics could lead to idiosyncratic drug responses: (1) transport (absorption, plasma protein binding); (2) transducer mechanisms (receptors, enzyme induction, or inhibition); (3) biotransformation; and (4) excretory mechanisms (renal and biliary transport). Genetic differences in drug transport are very rare. There exist significant, (i.e., two- to threefold) interindividual differences in the displacing effect of drugs such as sulfisoxazole, salicylic acid, and salicyluric acid on bilirubin plasma binding.[3] Genetically inherited structural differences in the albumin molecule (one binding site versus two binding sites) may affect the transport of drugs such as warfarin.[4] Examples of transducer mechanisms and alterations in biotransformation will be discussed later in this chapter. As yet, there have been no reports of genetic differences involving drug excretion (certain syndromes with anatomic anomalies such as biliary or renal atresia are excluded here).

There are two ways in which identification of pharmacogenetic subgroups becomes possible. First, if one specific aspect of drug disposition assumes paramount importance in the overall host response to that drug, genetic variation in that process may be identified as a discontinuous response in the population. An example is atypical pseudocholinesterase, which was first detected as a prolonged apneic response to succinylcholine. When the patient who has received succinylcholine does not breathe for a long while, this can be dramatic. Second, one can assay a drug concentration or an enzyme activity, rather than looking for an atypical clinical drug response. Examples include clinical surveys for polymorphisms of dopamine β-hydroxylase activity,[5] catechol *O*-methyltransferase activity,[6] and barbiturate metabolites in the urine.[7] The drug acetylation polymorphism[8] was uncovered following documentation that genetic variability exists in the rate of isoniazid metabolism in humans.[9,10]

Four general investigative approaches have long been used to uncover new atypical drug responses that have a genetic basis: clinical observations, family or twin studies, protein polymorphisms, and animal model systems. Two new investigative approaches are being used to predict individual risk of drug toxicity: restriction fragment length polymorphisms and gene expression assays. These two newer approaches will be described later in this chapter.

Clinical Observations

The approach of clinical investigation is often hampered by the frequent occurrence of multifactorial variation. However, a prolonged apneic response to succinylcholine, a temperature of more than 40°C during general anesthesia, allopurinol-induced gouty arthritis, and unusual sensitivity to the anticoagulant dicumarol are examples of dramatic clinical presentations that have led to the detailed characterization of a pharmacogenetic disorder. In many instances, the abnormal drug response has been ascribed to allelic variants at a single genetic locus.

Family or Twin Studies

By use of twins several investigators have established that interindividual differences in drug metabolism are largely under genetic control. Examples of drugs thus studied

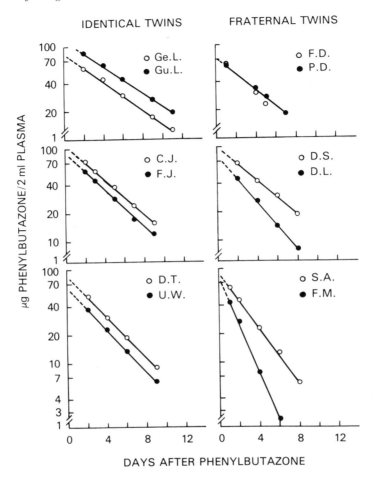

Fig. 7-3. Decline of phenylbutazone in the plasma of three sets of identical twins (*left*) and of three sets of fraternal twins (*right*) following a single oral dose of the drug (6 mg/kg). Note the similar slope of the decay curves within each set of identical twins as against the different slopes within each set of fraternal twins. (From Vesell,[18] with permission.)

include isoniazid,[9] phenylbutazone, antipyrine, dicumarol.[11] nortryptyline,[12] ethanol,[13] halothane,[14] phenytoin,[15] salicylate,[16] and amobarbital.[17] Figure 7-3 illustrates an example in which the drug response is compared in pairs of identical (homozygous) and fraternal (heterozygous) twins.[18] Twin zygosity was confirmed by means of typing for about 30 blood groups. Fraternal twins typically showed wide variations in plasma half-lives, as commonly seen in human populations or among siblings, whereas each pair of identical twins showed remarkably similar half-lives. For the most ideal clinical study the two members of a pair should live apart, so that environmental factors will be equally diverse among all subjects. The subjects were all adults who had not taken drugs for at least 1 month. Almost all lived in different households, had different diets, and presumably were exposed in varying degrees to environmental chemicals that might influence the liver's drug-metabolizing systems.[11]

The contribution of heredity to the large individual variations in plasma half-life can be estimated quantitatively as a *heredity coefficient h* from the formula

$$h^2 = \frac{V_d - V_m}{V_d}$$

where V_d is the variance within pairs of dizygotic (fraternal) twins and V_m is the variance within pairs of monozygotic (identical) twins.[9] Values can theoretically range from zero, indicating little or no genetic contribution to the variance seen in the twin pairs, to $+1.0$, indicating complete genetic influence. For dicumarol, antipyrine, phenylbutazone, ethanol, halothane, and nortriptyline,[11–14] the values range between $+0.88$ and 0.98.

Rates of metabolism of certain drugs often appear to vary together. For the case of bishydroxycoumarin and phenylbutazone, individuals who metabolize one drug slowly are likely also to metabolize the other slowly. Similar correlations have been found for desmethylimipramine, nortriptyline, and oxyphenylbutazone.[19] This is not a general rule, however, as a person may metabolize one drug unusually slowly and another at a normal rate, or even unusually rapidly. Thus, it appears that the relatively specific metabolism of certain drugs is the result of quite independent genetic control. As will be discussed later in this chapter, a defect in one P450 gene in the midst of other normal P450 genes can account for very specific metabolic differences between individuals.

Twin studies have also provided information about the genetic control of phenobarbital-induced increases in drug metabolism. For example, the reduction in plasma half-life of antipyrine in response to phenobarbital yielded a heredity coefficient of 0.99. In this study, there were no marked differences in phenobarbital blood levels, but there was a direct relationship between the initial antipyrine half-life and the extent to which the half-life was shortened by phenobarbital.[20] Thus, subjects who metabolize antipyrine slowly show the greatest increase in metabolism due to phenobarbital.

Family studies have suggested that metabolism is under polygenic control for dicumarol,[21] phenylbutazone,[22] and nortriptyline.[23] Differences in response to inducers of drug metabolism, such as phenobarbital, are genetically controlled.[24] For certain drugs, determination of plasma half-life, steady-state plasma concentration, or rates of urinary metabolite excretion can provide quite specific estimates of metabolism. In instances in which drug response is easily measured and shown directly to reflect tissue levels (e.g., in the initiation and maintenance of anesthesia), clinical observation may allow estimation of the rate of drug metabolism. It is anticipated that as more is understood about genetic variability of specific drug-metabolizing enzymes, new polymorphisms will be discovered.

Protein Polymorphisms

Investigation of protein polymorphisms of potential pharmacologic significance represents another approach. It has been estimated that 30 percent of randomly selected gene products may exhibit polymorphic variation (i.e., frequency greater than 0.01) for variant alleles.[25] Many such structural variants are functionally normal in vitro (i.e., with respect to enzymatic activities or, in the case of hemoglobin variants, oxygen-carrying capacities). It is quite possible, however, that such *isoallelic* variants may be responsible for significant functional derangements in vivo. A suitable qualitative test, such as an electrophoretic or isoelectric focusing pattern, is often required to detect enzyme variants with appreciable differences in activity, especially in heterozygotes of autosomal traits. Several examples will be described later.

Animal Models

Animal systems may provide examples of mutants that are likely to be stable in mammalian gene pools. Several pharmacologically important genetic models have been described, including warfarin resistance in rats,[26] susceptibility to chemical carcinogenesis in mice,[27] polymorphic acetylation in rabbits, mice, and hamsters,[28] and thiopurine methyltransferase activity in mice.[29] The obvious advantages of animal studies are that a pharmacogenetic disorder can be explored in great detail in numerous species, strains, and tissues in animals of known phenotype. Sophisticated predictions can then be made for the human, based on detailed understanding of the disorder in other mammals. Any pharmacogenetic disorder characterized in an animal model system is not likely to be identical to that found in the human, although laboratory animals and humans may exhibit striking similarities. For example, the caffeine-sensitive type of human malignant hyperthermia may reflect two or more genes,[30] and the same phenomenon is probably also true in the pig.[31] Also, "low" catechol *O*-methyltransferase activity is inherited as an autosomal recessive trait both in the rat and in the human.[32]

Both the well-known human pharmacogenetic disorders and some polymorphisms of potential pharmacogenetic interest are summarized in Table 7-1. In the remainder of this chapter the well-defined pharmacogenetic disorders will be discussed in the order in which they appear in the table.

LESS ENZYME OR DEFECTIVE PROTEIN

Succinylcholine Apnea

Succinylcholine is a depolarizing type of neuromuscular blocking agent, widely used to produce muscular relaxation during surgical procedures. The deserved popularity of succinylcholine rests upon its capacity to cause skeletal muscle relaxation of short duration because of its very rapid metabolic degradation by the cholinesterases of plasma and liver (acylcholine acyl hydrolase, sometimes called pseudocholinesterase or butyrylcholinesterase). The plasma concentration, established quickly and maintained readily by intravenous infusion, drops rapidly within a few minutes after drug administration is discontinued. The degradative reaction is a simple hydrolysis to the pharmacologically inert succinylmonocholine.

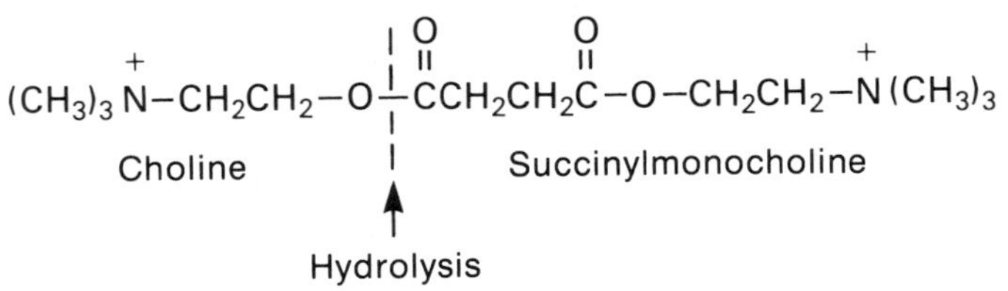

$$(CH_3)_3 \overset{+}{N} - CH_2CH_2 - O - \overset{O}{\overset{\|}{C}}CH_2CH_2\overset{O}{\overset{\|}{C}} - O - CH_2CH_2 - \overset{+}{N}(CH_3)_3$$

Choline   ↑   Succinylmonocholine

Hydrolysis

Succinylcholine (succinyldicholine)

Occasionally, a patient will manifest a bizarre response to succinylcholine, namely, prolonged muscular relaxation and apnea lasting as long as several hours after discontinuation

Table 7-1. Classification of Human Pharmacogenetic Disorders

Less enzyme or defective protein
    Succinylcholine apnea
    Acetylation polymorphism
        Isoniazid-induced neurotoxicity
        Drug-induced lupus erythematosus
        Phenytoin-isoniazid interaction
        Isoniazid-induced hepatitis
        Arylamine-induced bladder cancer
    Increased susceptibility to drug-induced hemolysis
        Glucose-6-phosphate dehydrogenase deficiency
        Other defects in glutathione formation or use
        Hemoglobinopathies
    Hereditary methemoglobinemia
    Hypoxanthine-guanine phosphoribosyltransferase (HPRT)-deficient gout
    P450 monooxygenase polymorphisms
        Debrisoquine 4-hydroxylase deficiency
        Vitamin D–dependent rickets type I
        C21-Hydroxylase polymorphism
    Enzymes of methyl conjugation
    Hyperbilirubinemia
        Crigler-Najjar syndrome type II
        Gilbert's disease
    Fish-Odor syndrome

Increased resistance to drugs
    Inability to taste phenylthiourea
    Coumarin resistance
    Possibility of (or proven) defective receptor
        Steroid hormone resistance
        Cystic fibrosis
        Trisomy 21
        Dysautonomia
        Leprechaunism
    Defective absorption
        Juvenile pernicious anemia
        Folate absorption-conversion
    Increased metabolism
        Succinylcholine resistance
        Atypical liver alcohol dehydrogenase
        Atypical aldehyde dehydrogenase

Change in drug response due to enzyme induction
    The porphyrias
    The *Ah* locus

Abnormal drug distribution
    Thyroxine (hyperthyroidism or hypothyroidism)
    Iron (hemochromatosis)
    Copper (Wilson's disease)

Disorders of unknown etiology
    Corticosteroid-induced glaucoma
    Malignant hyperthermia associated with general anesthesia
    Halothane-induced hepatitis
    Chloramphenicol-induced aplastic anemia
    Phenytoin-induced gingival hyperplasia
    Thromboembolic complications caused by anovulatory agents

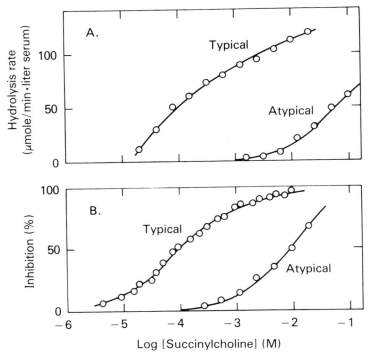

Fig. 7-4. Interactions of succinylcholine with plasma cholinesterase. (Adapted from Kalow,[1] with permission.)

of the infusion. Investigation has revealed that these individuals usually have atypical plasma cholinesterase.

The atypical cholinesterase hydrolyzes various substrates at considerably reduced rates. This decrease alone might suggest merely that the amount of enzyme is reduced. However, the entire pattern of affinities for substrates and inhibitors differs from the normal. The affinity of the atypical enzyme for succinylcholine can be decreased more than 100-fold compared with the normal (Fig. 7-4). The concentrations of succinylcholine that are used clinically to produce neuromuscular paralysis during anesthesia are well below those required to saturate the normal enzyme. Consequently, the decreased affinity of the abnormal enzyme for succinylcholine is sufficient to cause the abnormally prolonged duration of drug action in patients with atypical cholinesterase.

It has proved convenient to use dibucaine, a local anesthetic that is completely stable in the presence of cholinesterase, to characterize the serum enzyme in vitro. The inhibitory effect of dibucaine on the normal cholinesterase is about 20 times its effect on the atypical enzyme. Under arbitrarily standardized conditions, with benzoylcholine as substrate and dibucaine at 10^{-5} M, the rate of hydrolysis of benzoylcholine by the normal enzyme is inhibited by about 80 percent, but the atypical cholinesterase is little affected. The percentage inhibition by dibucaine under these conditions is called the *dibucaine number*. Most of the subjects cluster in a roughly normal distribution around dibucaine number 78 (Fig. 7-5A), with a remarkably small coefficient of variation (about 4 percent). A small group has intermediate dibucaine numbers in the range 40 to 70; there is no overlap with

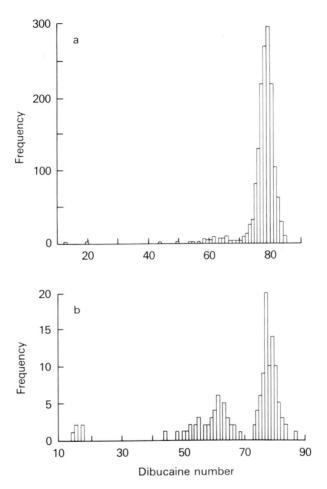

Fig. 7-5. Frequency distribution of dibucaine numbers. Dibucaine numbers represent percentage inhibition of plasma cholinesterase activity by dibucaine at a fixed concentration in a standardized test with benzoylcholine as substrate. **(A)** Distribution of dibucaine numbers in a large number of randomly selected people; **(B)** distribution of dibucaine numbers among families of subjects with low or intermediate dibucaine numbers. (From Kalow,[1] with permission.)

the normal range. Two subjects have very low dibucaine numbers (less than 20). In investigations on an even larger scale, it has been found that the incidence of very low dibucaine numbers is about 1 in 3,000; these people invariably respond to succinylcholine by prolonged paralysis.

Family studies leave no doubt that the presence of atypical cholinesterase is a genetically determined characteristic. Very low dibucaine numbers correspond to the homozygous condition. Intermediate values apparently arise from plasma containing a mixture of normal (usual) and atypical enzyme (Fig. 7-6). The behavior of the "intermediate" plasma is what would be expected of a mixture; inhibition is first manifested at the very low inhibitor concentration to which the normal plasma responds, but complete inhibition is approached only at the very high concentrations required by the atypical enzyme. Studies

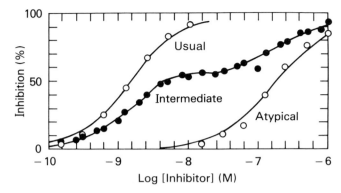

Fig. 7-6. Inhibition of plasma cholinesterase by a neostigmine analog. The inhibitor used was an analog of neostigmine known by the code name Ro2-0683. The substrate was benzoylcholine. The percent inhibition of enzyme activity is shown for three kinds of plasma. (*Left*) usual plasma; (*right*) atypical plasma; (*middle curve*) plasma with intermediate dibucaine number. (Modified from Kalow,[1] with permission.)

of families of subjects with low or intermediate dibucaine numbers have been carried out. The frequencies of low and intermediate dibucaine numbers in such families are much greater than those in the population as a whole (Fig. 7-5B). All the data are compatible with the existence of two alleles at a single genetic locus. Thus, the defect occurs in and is transmitted by both sexes. Homozygous normals produce a given quantity of the normal enzyme; individuals homozygous for the abnormal gene produce only atypical cholinesterase. Heterozygotes produce a mixture of the enzymes.

The gene for atypical cholinesterase has a widespread distribution throughout the world. Application of the Hardy-Weinberg law to the frequencies of the phenotypes has led to estimates of the gene frequency of about 2 percent in British, Greek, Portuguese, North African, Jewish, and some Asiatic ethnic groups.[33] The allele is nondetectable in Japanese, Eskimos, and South American Indians and very rare in blacks, Australian aborigines, Filipinos, and Orientals other than Japanese.[34]

In addition to succinylcholine, diacetylmorphine (heroin) and substance P have been shown to be substrates for serum cholinesterase.[35,36] Since cocaine hydrolysis is mediated by a human plasma cholinesterase,[37] it would be of interest to see if differences in response to this drug are also related to the cholinesterase polymorphism.

Human serum cholinesterase is known to be a tetramer of relative molecular weight (M_r) 340,000.[38] The human enzyme has been sequenced,[39] and this has allowed its allelic variants to be isolated and sequenced.[40]

Other variants of the plasma cholinesterase have been discovered. The atypical cholinesterase already discussed is relatively insensitive to inhibitors other than dibucaine; one of these is the fluoride ion. In family studies it was found that some individuals have an enzyme with normal sensitivity to dibucaine but resistance to fluoride inhibition. The fluoride resistance was found to be determined by a different allele of the same gene. Only the homozygote for fluoride resistance exhibits prolonged apnea when exposed to succinylcholine, just as is true of the dibucaine-resistant atypical enzyme variant.

Another variant discovered through family studies is the so-called silent allele, whose gene product is qualitatively altered so as to lack enzyme activity.[41] More sensitive assay techniques have revealed a complex heterogeneous mixture of defective enzymes in these cases, some with very low but measurable enzyme activity and most with abnormal immunologic properties.

Four bands (designated C1 to C4) are ordinarily found after electrophoresis of human serum cholinesterase. It is now clear that these four bands represent one, two, three, and four subunits of the M_r 340,000 tetramer. Rarely, a patient's serum is found to yield an additional band (C5) in electrophoresis. The cholinesterase activity in such cases is about 30 percent higher than normal; the sensitivity to inhibition by dibucaine or fluoride is not decreased. Since normal cholinesterase is present along with the additional activity represented by the unusual electrophoretic band, these individuals would not be expected to show any unusual response to succinylcholine; an increase of this magnitude in the rate of destruction of succinylcholine would in all likelihood escape detection in view of its already rapid metabolism. Family studies indicated that the abnormality is transmitted as an autosomal autonomous trait. About 5 percent of healthy British subjects have this variant.[42]

The role of various genotypes in determining the idiosyncratic response to succinylcholine has been studied in 78 patients who displayed prolonged apnea after receiving the drug.[43] Enzyme activity was measured with acetylcholine as substrate; dibucaine and fluoride numbers were also determined. The genotypes were deduced from the results of these determinations and confirmed in family studies in about one-fourth of the cases. Atypical homozygotes accounted for 38 percent of the patient group, whereas the frequency of this genotype in the population as a whole is about 1 in 3,000. Curiously, one-third of all the patients who experienced prolonged apnea were of normal genotype with normal plasma cholinesterase activity.[43]

Finally, a variant has been found to have enzyme activity that is two to three times higher than normal and is associated with *resistance* to succinylcholine.[44] This so-called Cynthiana variant will be discussed later.

Acetylation Polymorphism

Acetylation is one of several conjugation reactions that determine the fate of drugs and other environmental chemicals in humans and animals. The chemicals that undergo biologic acetylation are for the most part either aromatic amines or hydrazines. Acetylation occurs primarily in liver and gut mucosa but also in other tissues. This reaction is catalyzed by N-acetyltransferases and involves the transfer of the acetyl group from acetyl coenzyme A to the acceptor amines, resulting in the formation of amides.

The N-acetylating capacity of individuals is genetically determined and is essentially constant over the life span of an individual, but acetylating capacity can vary remarkably from one person to another. These hereditary differences are attributable to differences in the activity of cytosolic N-acetyltransferases located in liver and in intestinal gut mucosa. Studies in animal genetic models make it clear that the hereditary difference between rapid and slow acetylators is due not to a quantitative difference in the amount of liver acetylating enzyme but rather to a qualitative difference associated with isozymic variants of the liver enzyme. Biochemical and immunologic studies indicate that livers of rapid and slow acetylating individuals possess a single isozymic variant of N-acetyltransferase.[45] This trait was initially called the *isoniazid acetylation polymorphism* because it was first recognized in tuberculosis patients treated with isoniazid. Isoniazid is metabolized principally by N-acetylation, but a small amount of the drug is hydrolyzed to a pyridine carboxylic acid (isonicotinic acid).

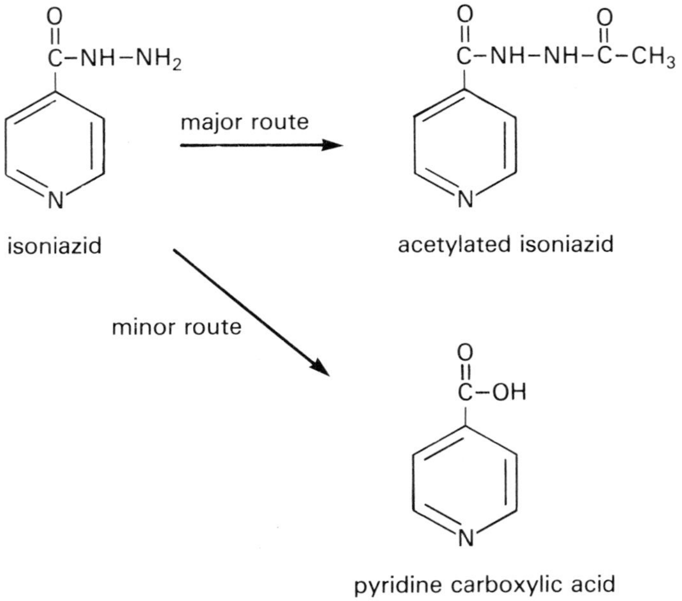

isoniazid   major route →   acetylated isoniazid

minor route → pyridine carboxylic acid

This trait is now usually referred to as the *acetylation polymorphism* since it affects the metabolic fate of many drugs and environmental chemicals.[28]

By determining the plasma concentration of a test drug such as isoniazid at a specified time after administration of a fixed dose, individuals can be identified as rapid or slow acetylators. Human family studies have shown that rapid and slow acetylators differ by a single autosomal gene: phenotypic slow acetylators are homozygous for a slow allele (r/r) while rapid acetylators are either homozygous (R/R) or heterozygous (R/r) for the rapid allele.[10] *N*-Acetylating capacity is thus bimodally (or trimodally) distributed in human and animal populations expressing this trait (Fig. 7-7). Extensive studies in different races and different countries have shown that acetylator gene frequencies vary greatly. For example, the slow gene frequency varies from approximately 0.10 in Japanese populations to nearly 0.90 in some Middle Eastern peoples; in the United States[46] the slow gene frequency is approximately 0.72.

Evans and co-workers[10] found that 152 out of 291 unrelated persons exhibited the slow isoniazid acetylation phenotype ($\overline{S}$). They postulated that slow acetylators are homozygous for a recessive slow inactivator allele r. Thus, the proportion of $\overline{S}$ inactivators (r/r) is $152/291 = 0.52$. According to the Hardy-Weinberg Law, $(p + q)^2 = 1$, or in this case, $(R + r)^2 = R^2 + 2Rr + r^2 = 1$. The proportion of $\overline{S}$ inactivators, 0.52, is equal to r^2. Therefore, the frequency of the slow allele r in the population under study is $\sqrt{0.52} = 0.72$, and the frequency of the rapid allele R in this population is $1 - r = 0.28$. This allelic distribution is shown graphically in Figure 7-8. Matings of the slow ($\overline{S}$) phenotype with the slow phenotype should give only slow (r/r) offspring, and as shown in Table 7-2, this is what was found.

Matings involving the rapid ($\overline{R}$) phenotype are more complicated. From the box diagram we can estimate the frequency of the $\overline{R}$ phenotype as $0.08 + 0.20 + 0.20 = 0.48$. The only time that an $\overline{S}$ phenotype child can result from an $\overline{R} \times \overline{S}$ mating is when the $\overline{R}$ parent is R/r. The fraction of $\overline{R}$ phenotype that are actually R/r heterozygotes is $0.40/0.48 = 0.83$. Hence, for $\overline{R} \times \overline{S}$ matings, the expected fraction of r/r children $= 0.40/0.48 \times \frac{1}{2}$

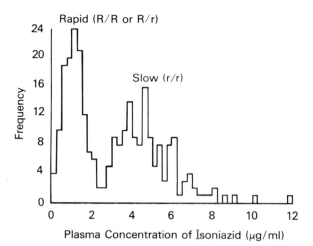

Fig. 7-7. Plasma isoniazid concentrations 6 hours after drug ingestion. Results were obtained in 267 members of 53 complete family units. All subjects received approximately 9.8 mg of isoniazid per kilogram of body weight. (From Evans et al.,[10] with permission.)

= 0.42. The reason for the factor ½ is that $R/r \times r/r$ matings will lead to a ratio of half r/r ($\overline{S}$) phenotype children and half R/r ($\overline{R}$) children. Among the 70 children from $\overline{R} \times \overline{S}$ matings (Table 7-2), the expected number of r/r children is therefore $70 \times 0.42 = 29.4$, and the observed number is 28.

The only time that an $\overline{S}$ phenotype child can result from an $\overline{R} \times \overline{R}$ mating is when both parents are R/r. For $\overline{R} \times \overline{R}$ matings the expected fraction of r/r offspring = 0.40/0.48 × 0.40/0.48 × ¼ = 0.174. The reason for the factor ¼ is that $R/r \times R/r$ matings will produce r/r children at a frequency of 1 in 4. Among the 38 offspring from $\overline{R} \times \overline{R}$ matings (Table 7-2), the expected number of r/r children is $38 \times 0.174 = 6.6$, and the observed number is 7. The data therefore confirm the hypothesis that the allele r represents an autosomal recessive trait exhibited phenotypically as slow isoniazid acetylation ($\overline{S}$).

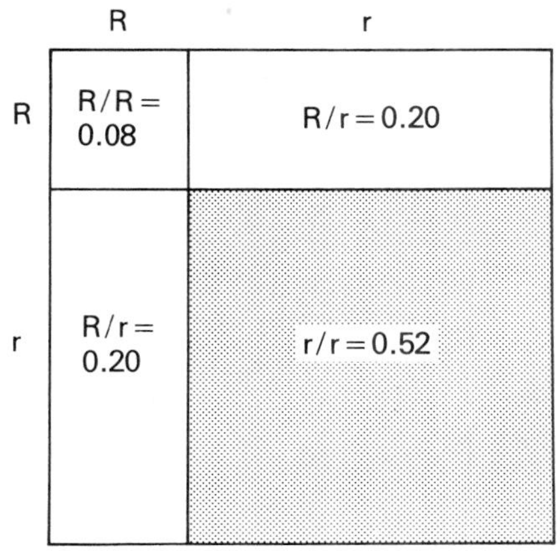

Fig. 7-8. Distribution of slow inactivator (r) and rapid inactivator (R) alleles for isoniazid inactivation in the population studied by Evans and co-workers.[10]

Table 7-2. Rates of Isoniazid Metabolism in Parents and Children

| Parental Phenotypes | No. of Matings | No. of Children | No. of Children of Each Phenotype[a] | | | |
| | | | Rapid | | Slow | |
			Expected	Observed	Expected	Observed
Slow × slow	16	51	0	0	51	51
Rapid × slow	24	70	40.6	42	29.4	28
Rapid × rapid	13	38	31.3	31	6.6	7
Total	53	159		73		86

[a] Numbers in the expected categories are computed on the basis of the hypothesis that slow metabolism of isoniazid is due to a recessive allele, as described in the text.
(From Evans et al.,[10] with permission.)

Acetylator status has remarkable effects on the metabolic fate of drugs such as isoniazid, hydralazine, procainamide, aminoglutethimide, dapsone, and various sulfonamides. The acetylation phenotype also modulates the metabolism of carcinogenic aromatic amines such as benzidine and β-naphthylamine. In addition, the acetylator status influences the fate of drugs that do not originally have a free amine group but may have one introduced metabolically; caffeine, sulfasalazine, nitrazepam, and clonazepam are examples.

Differences in the capacity of individuals to N-acetylate arylamines and hydrazines are frequently reflected in their pharmacologic and toxicologic profiles. Therein lies the significance of the acetylation polymorphism to the clinical sciences. The neurotoxicities from isoniazid, the lupus erythematosus from hydralazine and procainamide, the hemolytic anemia from sulfasalazine, and the phenytoin toxicity accompanying the combined use of phenytoin and isoniazid are examples of adverse drug effects based on the N-acetylation polymorphism. In these conditions, genetically slow acetylators usually have higher serum concentrations of the drug than rapid acetylators at any time after drug ingestion. As would be anticipated, these toxicities are dose-dependent and are usually more common and more severe in slow acetylators.

For some other disorders associated with prolonged intake of arylamine and hydrazine drugs or with occupational exposure to these chemicals, relationships to acetylator status are just emerging, as is the case for urinary bladder cancer resulting from exposure to benzidine. For others, such as isoniazid-induced hepatitis, phenelzine toxicity, and spontaneous (i.e., idiopathic) lupus erythematosus, the precise relationship, if any, to acetylator status is not clear. In certain spontaneous disorders in which there is no obvious rationale for a dependence on the acetylator polymorphism, studies alluding to this trait as a predisposing host factor have been reported. These studies suggest an association between rapid acetylation and diabetes, a possible association between rapid acetylation and both breast cancer and colorectal cancer, a greatly increased prevalence of slow acetylation in Gilbert's disease (mild chronic unconjugated hyperbilirubinemia), an earlier age of onset of thyrotoxicosis (Grave's disease) in slow acetylators than in rapid acetylators, and a possible association of slow acetylation with the severity of leprosy symptoms in Chinese patients. Several of these toxicities are further discussed below because they illustrate the manifold ways in which the clinical outcome may be modified by pharmacogenetic traits. A more complete account of these relationships is provided in reviews by Weber and Hein[28] and by Evans.[47]

Isoniazid-Induced Neurotoxicity

Isoniazid-induced peripheral polyneuropathy was the first recognized instance of drug toxicity associated with slow acetylation. The occurrence and severity of this disorder is related to the total dose of isoniazid ingested by slow acetylators treated chronically with the drug. This clinical manifestation of isoniazid toxicity is unusual now, but it still may be seen occasionally and is more pronounced in patients who suffer from severe malnutrition. The neurotoxicity is due to isoniazid-induced vitamin B_6 (pyridoxine) deficiency.

Isoniazid is also a potent irritant of the central nervous system. No human studies of the relationship between acetylator status and acute central nervous system toxicity from isoniazid have been reported, but several animal studies suggest that such a relationship might exist. The possible significance of the acetylation polymorphism to this disorder is best illustrated by the pronounced differences in survival times exhibited by rapid and slow acetylator rabbits receiving isoniazid.[48] Thus, all rapid acetylator rabbits receiving injections of the drug, (30 mg/kg) once a day, survived an experiment for 12 weeks, whereas all slow acetylator rabbits died in an average of 3.4 weeks of seizures and respiratory arrest. As in humans, pyridoxine was found to be a useful antagonist of isoniazid-induced seizures in the rabbit model.

Drug-Induced Lupus Erythematosus

Lupus erythematosus has been linked to at least 35 drugs, many of which contain a primary amine group. The most important of these are the aromatic amines such as procainamide and the hydrazines such as hydralazine. Hydralazine was introduced as an antihypertensive drug in 1952, and the first case of hydralazine-induced lupus was reported soon thereafter. Subsequently, cases associated with procainamide and isoniazid were reported. Since the mid-1970s procainamide has been ranked as the commonest cause of drug-induced lupus in adults. It was not until 1967 that the connection between hydralazine-induced lupus and slow drug acetylation was documented,[49] stimulating a spate of investigations that confirmed the prevalence of slow acetylators among both hydralazine- and procainamide-induced lupus patients.

Hydralazine and procainamide are the only drugs that produce the lupus syndrome often enough to permit assessment of the relationship of this disorder to acetylator status. In general, the clinical features and laboratory manifestations of drug-induced lupus are similar to those of lupus erythematosus and must fulfill at least 4 of 11 internationally accepted criteria for spontaneous (idiopathic) lupus. In addition, the patient must have received the drug before onset of the syndrome, and the signs and symptoms should abate promptly when the drug is discontinued. About 1 year of drug ingestion is required before onset, but this varies greatly with the drug used, the dose selected, and the acetylator status of the patient.[50] The development of antinuclear antibodies, a characteristic of lupus that always precedes the onset of symptoms of hydralazine- or procainamide-induced lupus, affords a valuable means of monitoring the onset and course of this disorder.

Acetylator status has effects on individual response that are qualitatively similar for hydralazine- and procainamide-induced disease, but quantitatively these effects are more pronounced for procainamide. For example, in a prospective study of procainamide therapy in a series of patients, the incidence of lupus was 29 percent, but with longer-term therapy this incidence increased.[51] The duration of therapy required to induce antinuclear antibodies in 50 percent of slow and rapid acetylators was 2.9 and 7.3 months, respectively. Also, the median total procainamide dose at the time that antibodies were detected was 1.5 and 6.1 g/kg body weight in slow acetylators and rapid acetylators, respectively. Retrospective evaluation[52] of the relationship between acetylator status and the rate of lupus development yielded a mean duration of therapy at onset of 12 ± 5 months for slow acetylators and 48 ± 22 months for rapid acetylators ($P < 0.002$). Antinuclear antibodies and clinical manifestations of lupus erythematosus thus develop preferentially in slow acetylators at lower cumulative doses of procainamide and after shorter periods of procainamide therapy.

The protective effect exerted by rapid acetylation against the development of antinuclear antibodies and of lupus affords somewhat greater protection against hydralazine-induced than against procainamide-induced disease. This observation appears to be accounted for by differences in the pharmacokinetics and metabolism of procainamide and hydralazine. The high first-pass metabolism of ingested hydralazine, owing to the acetylation of this drug in the gut wall and liver, contributes much more to hydralazine elimination than to procainamide elimination; procainamide depends more on renal excretion than does hydralazine.[52]

The prevalence of slow acetylators in patient populations at risk of developing lupus erythematosus is obviously much greater than the prevalence of the disease. For instance, only 1 to 3 percent of populations of which at least 50 percent are slow acetylators develop hydralazine-induced lupus.[53] This discrepancy may be largely explained by the fact that additional genetic traits are important in predisposing individuals to lupus. For example, in a study of 26 patients with hydralazine-induced lupus, 25 were slow acetylators, and there was a 4:1 ratio of women to men among them.[54] In addition, the frequency of HLA-DR4 antigen was 73 percent in lupus patients compared with 32.7 percent in healthy controls. All slow acetylator, DR4-positive women to whom hydralazine was administered developed lupus, but only the men who were DR4-positive and had received a high dose of hydralazine (200 mg or more daily) were affected. These observations strongly suggest that most cases of hydralazine-induced lupus might be avoided by withholding the drug from females who are both slow acetylators and HLA-DR4-positive.

Phenytoin-Isoniazid Interaction

Attention was drawn to the phenytoin-isoniazid interaction in 1962 when a trial of isoniazid therapy in a group of epileptic patients who had received phenytoin for years led to an unexpected outbreak of phenytoin toxicity.[55] Central nervous system side effects observed with administration of both drugs were qualitatively similar to those in patients receiving phenytoin alone but were several times more frequent than, and distinctly different from, those of isoniazid. It was found that there was a highly significant association between slow acetylation and susceptibility to phenytoin toxicity.[56] Toxicity was accompanied by elevations of phenytoin concentration in blood, the greatest elevations occurring in the slowest of the slow acetylators. Further studies demonstrated that isoniazid acts as a noncompetitive inhibitor of phenytoin hydroxylation, thereby retarding its renal excretion and enhancing its accumulation. It is thought that decreases in the activity of certain P450 enzymes that are specifically inhibited by isoniazid may account for the interaction between these two drugs.[57]

Isoniazid-Induced Hepatitis

Initial data on acetylator status from epidemiologic studies suggested that isoniazid might be more hepatotoxic for rapid than for slow acetylators.[58] It was reasoned that rapid acetylators ingesting isoniazid would produce monoacetylhydrazine (a metabolite of isoniazid) more effectively than slow acetylators. This metabolite would then be converted, in greater amounts in rapid than in slow acetylators, to potent reactive electrophiles, which would bind covalently to hepatic tissue, thereby initiating necrosis. This hypothesis was questioned on the grounds that monoacetylhydrazine, like isoniazid, is polymorphically acetylated.[59] Rapid acetylators transform this metabolite further to the relatively nontoxic diacetylhydrazine metabolite at least four times as fast as do slow acetylators. Thus, it was argued that rapid acetylators should not be more susceptible to isoniazid-induced liver damage because exposure to the toxic metabolite generated was similar between the two phenotypes.[59] These observations received additional support from both human studies[60] and biochemical studies in the rabbit genetic model for the human acetylation polymorphism.[48]

There are now more than a dozen epidemiologic studies of the relationship between acetylator status and isoniazid-induced hepatitis, and the findings are conflicting.[61] Recently, a 20-year experience with the incidence of hepatitis with jaundice was summarized for 1,757 slow and 1,238 rapid acetylators treated with isoniazid alone or in combination with other antituberculosis drugs. The overall incidence of liver damage measured in this way was 1.9 percent in slow and 1.2 percent in rapid acetylators. This difference is statistically insignificant, and it was concluded that the incidence of clinical hepatotoxicity with jaundice is unrelated to acetylator status.[62] Part of the difficulty in determining a genetic basis for individual susceptibility to isoniazid-induced liver damage relates to whether one uses clinical or biochemical evidence of hepatitis. It is well established that isoniazid treatment is associated with hepatotoxicity more frequently in older individuals (over 35 years of age) than in younger patients. In a prospective study using biochemical criteria for hepatic damage it was observed: (1) that slow acetylators older than 35 years have a high risk (37 percent), compared with a moderate risk (13 percent) for rapid acetylators; (2) that slow acetylators younger than 35 also have a moderate risk (13 percent); and (3) that rapid acetylators younger than 35 have a relatively low risk (4 percent) of developing significant liver abnormality.[63] In another study, liver damage measured in terms of transaminase elevations was found to be significantly greater among slow acetylators (46.6 percent) than among rapid acetylators (13.3 percent), and the most severe signs of damage were confined to slow acetylators.[64]

These observations indicate that rapid acetylators are not predisposed to isoniazid-induced liver disease; indeed, the opposite appears to be true. In addition, they indicate that the significance of the acetylator difference as a predictor of susceptibility to this disorder depends on the criterion chosen to measure injury. That is, if clinical jaundice is the criterion, "liver damage" is unrelated to acetylator status, but if a biochemical index such as transaminase levels is chosen, there is a relationship. Clearly, failure to define adequately the disease entity can lead to loss of valuable information, if not invalidate any conclusions.

Arylamine-Induced Bladder Cancer

Occupational exposure to arylamines constitutes a grave bladder cancer hazard. The unusual occurrence of such malignancies among fuchsin dye workers was first reported in 1895, but it was not until 50 years later that the risk of contracting bladder cancer was shown to be approximately 30 times greater for exposed dyestuff workers than for the general population.[65] This classic study greatly advanced our knowledge of the epidemiology of this disorder. On the basis of both human investigations[66,67] and investigations in animal models of acetylation polymorphism,[68,69] it now seems that acetylator status is a determinant of arylamine-induced bladder cancer.

Analysis of data from five controlled studies giving information on the acetylator pheno-

Table 7-3. Acetylator Phenotypes and Industrial Bladder Cancer

Acetylator Type	Chemical Workers[a]	Never Chemical Workers[a]	Cancer Invasiveness Low[b]	Cancer Invasiveness High[b,c]
Slow	22 (96%)	52 (59%)	59	14
Rapid	1	36	33	3
Total	23	88		

[a] Chi-square value for slow vs. rapid = 12.2 ($P < 0.00005$).
[b] Chi-square value for high vs. low = 2.77 ($P < 0.096$).
[c] Chi-square value for high vs. controls = 4.60 ($P < 0.032$).
(Data from Cartwright et al.[66])

types of bladder cancer patients demonstrates a statistically significant association between the occurrence of this disorder and slow acetylation.[67] The slow phenotype is present in about 39 percent excess compared to the rapid acetylator phenotype. In one of the studies[66] a striking excess of slow acetylators was observed in a group of chemical workers employed in the dye industry in Yorkshire (Table 7-3). This group, which was exposed to benzidine, showed a 40 percent excess of slow acetylators ($P < 0.00005$) as compared with controls from a nearby village. A high proportion of these slow acetylators developed generalized bladder disease with both carcinoma in situ and deeper invasion of the bladder wall.

It is possible that the association observed between slow acetylation and bladder cancer signifies that rapid acetylators are protected because of their greater capability to render aromatic amines noncarcinogenic by acetylation. It is also possible that slow acetylators survive longer than rapid acetylators with bladder cancer. These hypotheses require further investigation.

Increased Susceptibility to Drug-Induced Hemolysis

Glucose-6-Phosphate Dehydrogenase Deficiency

The antimalarial drug primaquine causes acute hemolysis in approximately 10 percent of black Americans. The finding that reduced glutathione (GSH) concentration is diminished in primaquine-sensitive erythrocytes led to the discovery of red cell glucose-6-phosphate dehydrogenase (G6PD) deficiency in affected individuals.[70] This enzyme, which is part of the hexose monophosphate shunt, is one of the principal sources of NADPH in the normal red cell (Fig. 7-9).[71] NADPH is, in turn, the cofactor for glutathione reductase, which reduces the dimeric oxidized glutathione (GS-SG). More than 280 G6PD protein variants have been described, and at least 200 million individuals are affected worldwide.[72,73] The two principal variants occur in black Americans (A- type) and in Mediterranean populations. Hemolysis associated with the A- type enzyme is usually mild and self-limited, affecting mainly the older erythrocytes. In the Mediterranean type, however, red-cell G6PD is generally lower in younger cells, and this condition is associated with more severe hemolysis.[74]

Numerous drugs (Table 7-4) are known to precipitate hemolytic crises in G6PD-deficient subjects.[75] The precise mechanism whereby G6PD deficiency leads to hemolysis is not fully understood. It is commonly felt that oxidation of GSH plays a central role, since GSH is essential for maintaining protein sulfhydryl groups in the reduced state, thereby preventing denaturation of enzymes and hemoglobin (i.e., Heinz body formation) and perhaps even preserving the integrity of the erythrocyte membrane. Perturbations of intracellular thiol and calcium ion homeostasis may be important early events in the de-

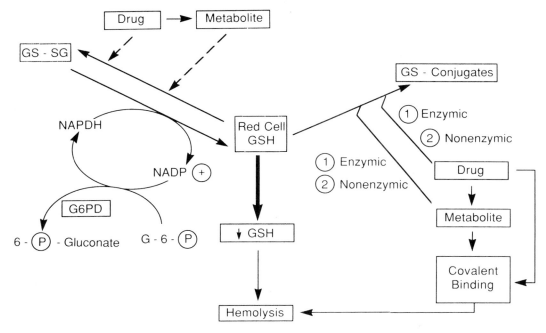

Fig. 7-9. Mechanisms by which erythrocyte glutathione may become depleted. A drug or metabolite may, because of differences in redox potential, oxidize reduced glutathione (GSH) to the dimer GS-SG or may become conjugated enzymatically or nonenzymatically with GSH to form GS conjugates. Regeneration of GSH from GS-SG requires glucose-6-phosphate dehydrogenase (G6PD). Depletion of GSH and covalent binding of drug or metabolite, perhaps to the cell membrane, causes hemolysis. (From Atlas et al.,[71] with permission.)

velopment of toxicity in cells of many types. Many of the substances listed in Table 7-4 require metabolic activation before they can produce hemolysis.[76] It is therefore quite likely that toxic intermediates of such agents directly cause red cell damage.

Primaquine, phenylhydrazine, and ascorbic acid greatly increase the metabolic rate of the hexose monophosphate shunt in normal erythrocytes in vitro (Fig. 7-9) by enhancing the rate of oxidation of GSH to GS-SG. This increased oxidation is probably due to the generation of peroxides.[77] The availability of GS-SG as substrate for the glutathione reductase reaction results in formation of NADP. As NADPH levels are lowered and NADP levels are increased, the inhibition of G6PD is relieved and glucose-6-phosphate is oxidized at a higher rate.

The first demonstration that intrinsic erythrocytic factors are critical in the pathogenesis of hemolysis in G6PD deficiency came from studies on the fate of ^{51}Cr-labeled red cells

Table 7-4. Drugs and Chemicals That Have Clearly Been Shown to Cause Clinically Significant Hemolytic Anemia in G6PD Deficiency

Acetanilide	Nitrofurantoin	Primaquine	Sulfapyridine
Methylene blue	Pamaquine	Sulfacetamide	Thiazolesulfone
Nalidixic acid	Pentaquine	Sulfamethoxazole	Toluidine blue
Naphthalene	Phenylhydrazine	Sulfanilamide	Trinitrotoluene
Niridazole			

(From Beutler,[75] with permission.)

in normal recipients treated with hemolytic agents.[78] Six of eight aniline derivatives studied produced significant hemolysis of transfused enzyme-deficient cells but not of transfused normal cells. However, it is also clear that extraerythrocytic factors, including hepatic drug metabolism, are important for hemolysis in vivo.

Although high concentrations of primaquine may cause lysis of G6PD-deficient erythrocytes in vitro, normal cells are equally susceptible.[78] Sequestration of deformed cells by the reticuloendothelial system (the spleen) in vivo is probably essential for the observed hemolytic effect; however, absence of metabolic potentiation of primaquine in the in vitro system may also account for this discrepancy. Metabolites of several hemolyzing agents (including primaquine) are more effective than the parent compounds in causing increased mechanical fragility of erythrocytes in vitro. This finding was correlated in some cases with a decrease in red cell GSH content. It was postulated[76] that metabolites possessing a higher redox potential might be converted in the red cell to an oxidant capable of damaging the erythrocyte membrane, which is somewhat analogous to the model proposed for methemoglobin formation by aromatic amines.[79]

Many of the agents capable of inducing hemolysis and their metabolites (Table 7-4) are substrates for the mammalian drug-metabolizing enzyme systems, in particular P450 enzymes and N-acetyltransferases. Acetylation reactions may be important in some species in which P450-dependent N-hydroxylation of certain aromatic amines appears to be facilitated by prior N-acetylation.[79] The O-demethylation and 5-hydroxylation of 8-aminoquinolines such as pentaquine or primaquine lead to the formation of quinonimines,[80] which are far more potent in vitro than the parent compounds in causing increased mechanical fragility and methemoglobin formation in G6PD-deficient red cells.[76] Finally, microsomal (non-P450) amine oxidase catalyzes N-oxide formation from aliphatic and aromatic tertiary amines.[81] Several N-oxides are able to produce methemoglobinemia.[79] Potential substrates for the amine oxidase, such as N-substituted aniline derivatives, quinoline derivatives, and heterocycle-containing sulfonamides might, via their N-oxide derivatives, also play a role in hemolysis because N-oxides are known to be nonenzymically reduced to tertiary amines by GSH.[81]

Active metabolites produced principally in the liver must be sufficiently stable to reach the erythrocyte before the red cell can be injured. However, additional *intraerythrocyte* catalytic activities probably play a role in the pathogenesis of hemolysis. Several hemolytic drugs can interact with hemoglobin to generate low levels of hydrogen peroxide, which, like organic hydroperoxides, may result in oxidation of GSH via erythrocyte glutathione peroxidase. The glutathione transferases are a potentially important group of enzymes, which has hitherto not been suspected of playing a role in G6PD-deficient hemolysis. At least one of these cytosolic activities is known to exist in human red cells. The reactions result either in depletion of intracellular GSH (via thioether or mixed disulfide formation) or in net oxidation to GS-SG. The best studied of these is thioether formation,[82] resulting from nucleophilic attack by GSH at electrophilic sites on the substrate; the resulting GSH conjugates are subsequently metabolically degraded to mercapturic acids, which are excreted in the urine. Finally, quinones may lead to both oxidation and depletion of GSH, independently of possible epoxide formation. For example, menadione reacts with glutathione to yield equal amounts of thioether conjugates and hydroquinone; the latter may be reoxidized to the quinone, liberating stoichiometric amounts of hydrogen peroxide, which can oxidize GSH via glutathione peroxidase.[83]

G6PD deficiency is inherited as an autonomous X-linked defect. Because males carry the defect on their single X chromosome (they are hemizygous), it is expressed phenotypically; this is the primaquine-sensitive group, with very low GSH values in the in vitro test. Female heterozygotes have intermediate values because the normal gene on one X chromosome and the defective allele on the other are both expressed. Heterozygous females will pass the defect to half of their sons (Fig. 7-2). Affected males will have normal sons because they pass only their Y chromosome to them, and they will have heterozygous daughters because they pass the defective X chromosome to all of them. If there were really complete phenotypic expression without dominance, heterozygotes should fall into a well-defined intermediate group, and the frequency of the intermediates would be mathematically determined by the known gene frequency. This does not seem to occur. In the population studied, more women were found with normal values in the GSH test than would be expected from the frequency of affected males (which, for a sex-linked trait, is the same as the gene frequency). This finding and the wide dispersion of values suggest that there is variable expression (variable penetrance). Thus, in some instances the gene can be carried without causing a detectable disorder in the red cell. In other words, some other factors influence the degree to which the trait is expressed in identical genotypes.

Subsequent studies have shown that G6PD deficiency is not a simple absence of the enzyme but rather a very heterogeneous trait. At least 12 dozen distinct variants of the enzyme have been identified, with different levels of activity, affinities for G6PD or NADP, pH optima, thermal stability, and electrophoretic mobility. A few examples from different ethnic groups are shown in Table 7-5.[84] Severe deficiency of enzyme activity is generally correlated with sensitivity to drug-induced hemolysis provided that in vitro measurements are made at the same concentrations of substrates and cofactors that would occur in vivo.

The G6PD abnormality itself is usually without demonstrable adverse effect unless the erythrocytes are challenged by certain drugs; however, there is some evidence of decreased life expectancy among affected males.[85] From the point of view of genetic theory, high incidence of an abnormal gene in a given ethnic group implies some significant survival value for the heterozygous carrier females. Analogous reasoning with respect to carriers of the sickling trait led to the discovery that such heterozygotes are more resistant to serious forms of malaria than is the normal population. Prepubertal (especially infant) mortality from malaria is considerably lower in those individuals. Reactors to primaquine and fava beans are also found predominantly among groups that live in, or trace their ancestry to, malaria-hyperendemic areas.

The postulated resistance to malaria infection of G6PD-deficient erythrocytes has been confirmed. One of the X chromosomes in every cell of a female is known to be inactivated during its maturation, apparently on a random basis. Thus, females are mosaics with respect to traits controlled by the X chromosome. A female heterozygous for G6PD deficiency was shown to contain two kinds of erythrocytes. During acute *Plasmodium falciparum* infection, the normal erythrocytes were much more heavily infested with parasites than were the deficient ones.[86]

A curious by-product of the primaquine studies was the finding that all newborn infants are susceptible to drug-induced hemolytic anemia. This phenomenon is due to a low or absent G6PD in the newborn, presumably on a developmental immaturity basis. Among the eliciting drugs are menadione and other vitamin K analogs, which are naphthoquinone derivatives. These drugs are used to prevent neonatal hemorrhage, but they can also cause hemolysis. Even though low GSH levels are found, there is apparently no true G6PD defect in the erythrocytes of normal infants, because this abnormality persists for only 1 or 2 weeks.

The molecular weight of G6PD is about 110,000, representing a dimer of two polypep-

Table 7-5. Ethnic Differences in the Incidence
of G6PD Deficiency

Group	Incidence (%)
Ashkenazic Jews (males)	0.4
Sephardic Jews (males)	
Kurds	53
Iraq	24
Persia	15
Cochin	10
Yemen	5
North Africa	<1–4
Arabs	4
Iranians	8
Sardinians (males)	4–30
Greeks (including Cyprus and Crete)	0.7–3
Blacks	
American	13
Nigerians	10
Bantu	20
Leopoldville	18–23
Bashi	14
Pygmies	4
Watusi	1–2
Asiatics	
Chinese	2
Filipinos	13
Indians-Parsees	16
Javanese	3
Micronesians	0–1
American Indians	
Oyana (males)	16
Carib (males)	2
Peruvian (males)	0
Eskimos	0

(From Marks et al.,[84] with permission.)

tides. The amino acid composition suggests about 18 sulfhydryl groups per dimer and probably no disulfide bridges. A histidine residue may be important in the catalytic activity of G6PD. The G6PD gene has been cloned and localized to the X chromosome. It encodes a 2.3-kb mRNA, which leads to 531 amino acids in the protein.[87] Several diverse point mutations may account for a large amount of the phenotypic heterogeneity of G6PD deficiency.[88,89] Many of the allelic variants should soon be characterized by restriction fragment length polymorphism (RFLP) patterns or through interesting differences in regulation of the G6PD gene(s).

Other Defects in Gluathione Formation or Use

Inherited deficiencies in several other enzymes related to GSH production and utilization have been associated with both spontaneous and drug-induced hemolysis. These polymorphic enzymes and their modes of inheritance are summarized in Table 7-6.

Hemoglobinopathies

In several abnormal hemoglobins, amino acid substitutions occur at or near the histidine residues that serve as the sixth ligand for heme iron (residue 58 in the α chain and residue 63 in the β chain), the site for reversible oxygen binding. Such hemoglobins are "unstable"

Table 7-6. Other Enzyme Deficiencies Possibly Associated with Increased Susceptibility to Drug-Induced Hemolysis

Enzyme	Inheritance	Hemolysis
Defects in GSH[a] synthesis		
γ-Glutamylcysteine synthetase	[?] Two cases	Yes
GSH synthetase		
With 5-oxoprolinuria	Autosomal recessive	Yes
Without 5-oxoprolinuria	Autosomal recessive	Yes
Defects in maintenance of reduced GSH		
GSH reductase	[?] Autosomal dominant	Yes
6-Phosphogluconate dehydrogenase	Autosomal autonomous	[?]
6-Phosphogluconolactonase	Autosomal dominant	Yes
Defects in GSH utilization		
GSH peroxidase	Autosomal autonomous	Yes

[a] GSH = glutathione
(Table compiled from information in Beutler,[75] Flohe et al.,[82] Wellner et al.,[90] Spielberg et al.,[91] and Beutler et al.[92])

and are easily denatured to form Heinz bodies.[74] Of the five known α chain substitutions and the 22 known β chain substitutions, three variant hemoglobins are documented to be associated with drug-induced hemolysis: Torino [$^{43}\alpha^{Phe \to Val}$], Zürich [$^{63}\beta^{His \to Arg}$] and Shepherds Bush [$^{74}\beta^{Gly \to Asp}$].[93] Phenotypically, all three are inherited as autosomal dominant traits and are associated with susceptibility to sulfonamide-induced hemolysis. In addition, hemolysis due to primaquine and other quinoline derivatives has been reported in individuals with hemoglobin Zürich.[74]

Hereditary Methemoglobinemia

It is difficult to separate entirely the discussions of drug-induced hemolysis and drug-induced methemoglobinemia, since many of the same considerations discussed in the preceding section that apply to metabolic activation of causative agents also apply to methemoglobin formation. Nitrites, chlorates, and quinones can produce methemoglobin in vitro, which suggests that direct chemical oxidation rather than metabolic potentiation is involved.[94] Nitrates are converted to nitrites by intestinal bacteria before they become effective. There is considerable evidence that metabolism of aromatic amines (e.g., aniline derivatives) is necessary before such agents may cause methemoglobinemia.[79] N-Hydroxylation appears to be the most important activation step, although formation of aminophenols and N-oxides may also play a role. Nitrobenzenes may be activated by reduction to the corresponding arylhydroxylamine.

Figure 7-10 compares the effect of a single dose of sodium nitrite in a patient with hereditary methemoglobinemia and in a normal person.[95] The amount of methemoglobin formed initially is about the same in both subjects, but the methemoglobin almost disappears within 6 hours in the normal person whereas there is no conversion of methemoglobin to hemoglobin in the patient with methemoglobinemia.

Table 7-7 presents several drugs that may be responsible for causing methemoglobinemia. These agents should be avoided if at all possible in people with hereditary methemoglobinemia. Methylene blue and oxygen are the agents of choice in the therapeutic management of methemoglobinemia.

Several genetic lesions can lead to methemoglobinemia, including deficiencies in the activity of NADH-methemoglobin reductase, cytochrome b_5, and phenacetin O-deethy-

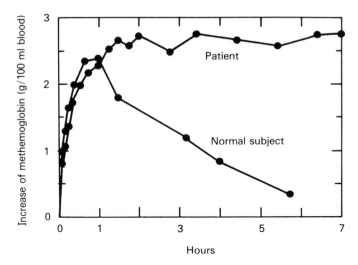

Fig. 7-10. Effect of nitrite on a patient with hereditary methemoglobinemia. At zero time, 0.5 g sodium nitrite was injected intravenously into a normal subject and into a patient with this pharmacogenetic disorder. Increase in blood methemoglobin content is shown on the vertical axis. (From Eder et al.,[95] with permission.)

lase. In the red cell, NADH-methemoglobin reductase is the most important oxidoreductase involved in the reduction of ferric heme iron. The complete absence of this diaphorase from erythrocytes is inherited as an autosomal recessive trait[96] and is associated with congenital cyanosis as well as with drug-induced exacerbations. Genetically determined alterations in the structure of hemoglobin itself can also be responsible for drug-induced methemoglobinemia. In several abnormal hemoglobins, collectively known as hemoglobin M (for "methemoglobinemia"), at least two of the four heme irons are especially prone to oxidation by drugs. These amino acid substitutions occur near the heme binding sites on the α and β chains.[93] Inheritance is autosomal dominant. Hemoglobin H, a β tetramer found in certain patients with recessively inherited α-thalassemia, is also associated with drug-induced methemoglobinemia.

Table 7-7. Drugs That Can Cause Methemoglobinemia

Direct oxidants (effective in vitro and in vivo)
  Nitrites
  Nitrates (reduced to nitrite by bacteria in gut)
  Chlorates
  Quinones
  Methylene blue (high doses)

Indirect oxidants (not usually effective in vitro but effective in vivo)
  Arylamino and arylnitro compounds
  Aniline
  Acetanilide
  Acetophenetidin
  Nitrobenzenes
  Nitrotoluenes
  Sulfonamides

(Adapted from Prankerd,[94] with permission.)

Hypoxanthine-Guanine Phosphoribosyltransferase–Deficient Gout

Complete deficiency of hypoxanthine-guanine phosphoribosyltransferase (HPRT) is responsible for the Lesch-Nyhan syndrome, an X-linked inborn error of metabolism in which neurologic abnormalities, mental retardation, and compulsive self-mutilation are associated with marked hyperuricemia.[97] A less severe deficiency is found in certain patients with gout who possess about 1 percent of normal HPRT activity. This disorder is also inherited as an X-linked recessive trait. Phosphoribosyltransferase is the enzyme of principal importance in the purine salvage pathway (Fig. 7-11), and when it is deficient, conversion of guanine and hypoxanthine to their respective nucleotides is diminished. Since these nucleotides are feedback inhibitors of the rate-limiting initial step in de novo purine biosynthesis, a decrease in the steady-state concentration of guanine and hypoxanthine nucleotides results in an increased (unregulated) rate of purine synthesis and is therefore the major cause of hyperuricemia in affected individuals. At least five different variant forms of the enzyme have been characterized.[98]

Because purine base analogues used in cancer chemotherapy and immunosuppression must be converted to their respective nucleotides by the transferase in order to inhibit purine biosynthesis, the antimetabolites shown in Fig. 7-11 would be expected to be in-

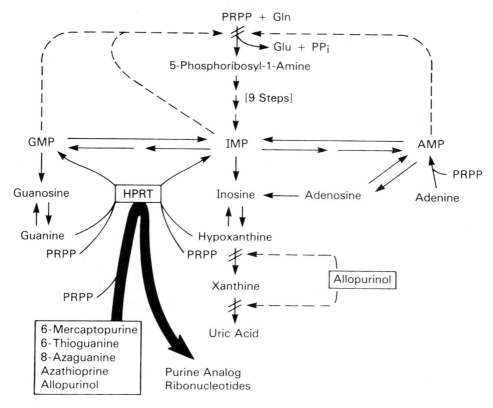

Fig. 7-11. Purine biosynthetic, salvage, and oxidative pathways. PRPP is phosphoribosyl pyrophosphate; PP_i is inorganic pyrophosphate. The dashed lines denote feedback inhibition. (From Atlas et al.,[71] with permission.)

effective in patients with a deficiency of the enzyme. This possibility has been documented for both 6-mercaptopurine and the immunosuppressive agent azathioprine.

As discussed in Chapter 5, allopurinol, one of the major drugs used in the treatment of gout, inhibits uric acid production principally by blocking xanthine oxidase. In normal individuals the resulting accumulation of hypoxanthine leads, via HPRT, to increased levels of the nucleotide inosine monophosphate (IMP) and thus to feedback inhibition of purine biosynthesis. In addition, allopurinol is a substrate for the phosphoribosyltransferase and in the ribonucleotide form it inhibits de novo purine synthesis. These latter two effects of allopurinol are absent in patients with HPRT-deficient gout, thereby accounting for a somewhat atypical drug response. Normal individuals taking allopurinol exhibit a decrease in both uric acid and total purine urinary excretion; HPRT-deficient patients taking allopurinol show a decrease in uric acid excretion only. Total purine urinary output, accounted for primarily by the oxypurines hypoxanthine and xanthine, is unchanged or slightly increased. Although allopurinol may still be effective in treating gout and in preventing formation of urinary calculi composed of uric acid in HPRT-deficient individuals, such patients may develop xanthine stones while taking allopurinol.

At least three genetic variants of phosphoribosyl pyrophosphate (PRPP) synthetase (also X-linked) have been shown[97] to increase production of PRPP and therefore to enhance the rate of purine biosynthesis de novo, leading to hyperuricemia. This enzyme defect in purine metabolism will respond to allopurinol therapy in the usual manner, however, with urinary decreases in both uric acid and total purine.

The HPRT gene has been cloned, sequenced, and expressed in cell culture. In one study the majority of lymphoblast cell lines from 24 unrelated HPRT-deficient patients showed normal levels of mRNA but undetectable quantities of enzyme.[99] These molecular biology studies have already provided insight into the heterogeneous collection of genetic lesions in the Lesch-Nyhan syndrome. Moreover, the HPRT gene is high on the list for gene therapy. When transfected with a transmissible retroviral vector, the gene provides partial correction of human HPRT-deficient lymphoblasts, and the human gene has been expressed in the central nervous system of transgenic mice.

P450 Monooxygenase Polymorphisms

Debrisoquine 4-Hydroxylase Deficiency

Debrisoquine is an adrenergic blocking agent used as an antihypertensive. The drug was introduced in the United Kingdom in 1966 and has been used on a limited basis since that time. Marked variations in optimal dose requirements (20 to 400 mg daily) for control of hypertension[100] and variations in recoveries of the nonmetabolized parent drug in the urine (8 to 70 percent) suggested striking interindividual differences. Moreover, variations in recovery of the unchanged drug were shown not to be due to variations in oral absorption or in renal clearance. It was also clear from these studies that there was a significant correlation between excretion of the unchanged drug (i.e., impaired metabolism) and increased sensitivity to the drug's effect (exaggerated hypotension).

Debrisoquine is known to be metabolized principally by ring hydroxylation, with a minor pathway of ring opening (Fig. 7-12).[101] A comparative metabolic study of the ^{14}C-labeled drug was carried out in four volunteers, one of whom was characterized by the excretion of large amounts of the drug (Table 7-8). For three of the subjects the major urinary metabolite is clearly the 4-hydroxy derivative; small amounts of the 5-, 6-, 7-, and 8-hydroxy metabolites are also excreted. The metabolic picture of subject no. 4, however,

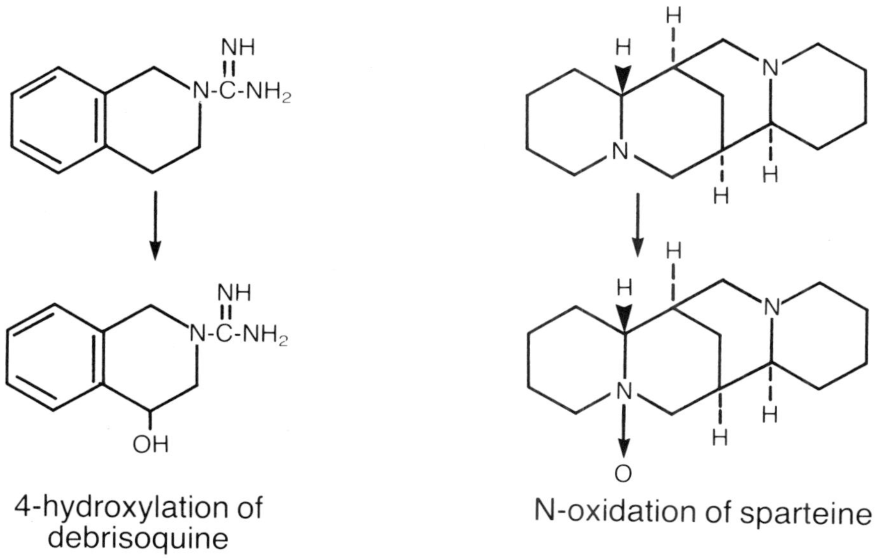

4-hydroxylation of
debrisoquine

N-oxidation of sparteine

Fig. 7-12. 4-Hydroxylation of debrisoquine and *N*-oxidation of sparteine.

is very different; most of the radioactivity in the urine represents the unchanged drug, together with only small amounts of 4-hydroxydebrisoquine and the other four phenols. Hence, the metabolic ratio was calculated as the percentage of the dose excreted as unchanged debrisoquine divided by the percentage excreted as 4-hydroxydebrisoquine. For the three extensive metabolizers ($\overline{\text{EM}}$) in Table 7-8, the metabolic ratio ranges between 0.69 and 1.5 while for subject no. 4, regarded as a poor metabolizer ($\overline{\text{PM}}$), the metabolic ratio is 20.

Subsequent population studies (Fig. 7-13) in which the $\log_{10}$ of the metabolic ratio was plotted as a function of frequency in the population under study indicated that two distinct phenotypes emerge.[102,103] Extensive metabolizers exhibit metabolic ratios between 0.01 and 10, whereas poor metabolizers display metabolic ratios between 20 and 200. There is no overlap. It is worth noting that there is a range of metabolic ratios from 0.01 to 200,

Table 7-8. Identification of an "Aberrant" Metabolizer
of Debrisoquine

	[a] *Percent of Dose Eliminated in Urine by Four Subjects*			
Metabolite	*1*	*2*	*3*	*4*
Debrisoquine	45	28	27	40
4-Hydroxydebrisoquine	30	37	39	2
5-Hydroxydebrisoquine	0.5	1.3	2.3	0.2
6-Hydroxydebrisoquine	0.7	1.0	3.6	0.9
7-Hydroxydebrisoquine	1.2	1.9	6.3	4.0
8-Hydroxydebrisoquine	0.3	0.6	1.5	0.2

[a] Four volunteers took an oral dose (40 mg, 10 μCi) of ^{14}C-labeled debrisoquine, and the urine samples were collected for 0 to 24 hours and assayed for debrisoquine and its hydroxylated metabolites by gas chromatography.

(From Idle et al.,[102] with permission.)

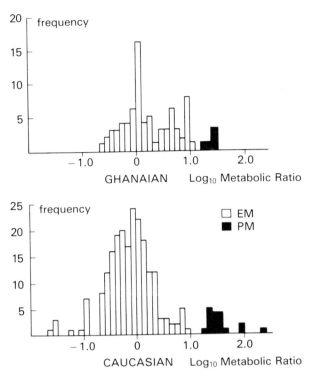

Fig. 7-13. Semilog frequency distribution histograms of debrisoquine 4-hydroxylation (metabolic ratio) in Ghanaians and Caucasians. (From Woolhouse et al.,[103] with permission.)

with 1 in 12 patients being a poor metabolizer. Use of a metabolic ratio between drug and metabolite makes good theoretical sense only if the metabolism of the drug is rate-limiting. Usually, the metabolic ratio will vary, depending upon pharmacokinetic parameters, such as the renal clearance of unchanged drug. The metabolic ratio, therefore, is useful as a screening mechanism to separate phenotypes but it is not necessarily closely related to variations in clinical response to the drug.[104]

Family studies of the kind described in detail for acetylation polymorphism have been carried out for debrisoquine metabolism. Debrisoquine 4-hydroxylase deficiency was determined to be an autosomal recessive trait,[102] the phenotype occurring in about 8 percent of British whites. This means that the frequency of the debrisoquine poor metabolizer allele (D^{PM}) = 0.28 and of the debrisoquine extensive metabolizer allele (D^{EM}) = 0.72. This represents the same type of analysis detailed for acetylation polymorphism.

Ethnic variations in debrisoquine 4-hydroxylation have been observed in numerous ethnogeographic populations.[105] About 1.5 percent of the population have the $\overline{PM}$ phenotype in Egypt, about 12 percent in Ghana, about 15 percent in Nigeria, and about 3 percent in Sweden. No $\overline{PM}$ phenotypes were found in 100 Japanese patients.[106]

There is a growing list of other drugs that also are metabolized poorly in patients who are poor debrisoquine metabolizers. This point is particularly important because, although debrisoquine has not been introduced on the U.S. drug market, many of these other drugs are used in the United States and worldwide. Guanoxan is an antihypertensive drug chemically and pharmacologically related to debrisoquine and guanethidine. In studies using volunteers of known debrisoquine metabolizer status, guanoxan 6- and 7-hydroxylation was found to be deficient in subjects having defective debrisoquine 4-hydroxylation and high in subjects having extensive debrisoquine 4-hydroxylation. Similar conclusions have been drawn for: the *N*-oxidation of sparteine; the *O*-deethylation of phenacetin; the *S*-oxidation of metiamide; the *O*-demethylation of 4-methoxyamphetamine and dextromethorphan; the aromatic 4-hydroxylation of phenytoin; the *E*- but not the *Z*-10-hydroxylation of nortriptyline; the 4-hydroxylation of phenformin; metoprolol metabolism; and the 1'-hydroxylation of bufuralol.[102,103,107–109] This genetic defect in P450 metabolism does have some specificity since, for example, antipyrine metabolite formation is the same in poor metabolizers and extensive metabolizers of debrisoquine.

The debrisoquine polymorphism appears to be associated with cancer risk. The metabolic ratio was examined in a group of 59 Nigerian patients with cancer of the liver and gastrointestinal tract and compared with that for a group of noncancer patients.[110] (Fig. 7-14). The cancer group contained a disproportionately greater number of individuals who were extensive metabolizers of debrisoquine, which suggests that the extensive metabolizers may be more prone to liver and gastrointestinal cancer than poor metabolizers. The latter observation, if true, would most likely be an example of enhanced metabolism of some dietary procarcinogen(s) to an active carcinogen by the same enzyme system involved in debrisoquine metabolism.

In a study of 245 patients with bronchogenic carcinoma, the cancer patients also represented a preponderance of debrisoquine extensive metabolizers relative to 234 smokers without evidence of carcinoma.[111] On the other hand, no relationship between debriso-

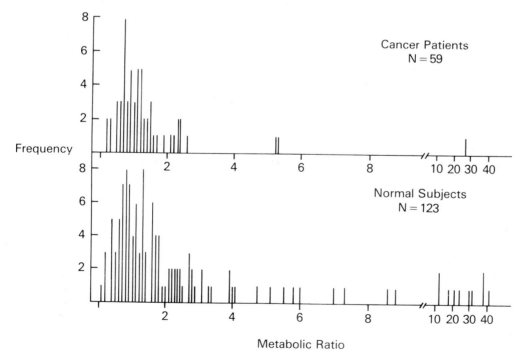

Fig. 7-14. Metabolic (oxidation) ratio frequency distribution for 59 Nigerian cancer patients and 123 healthy volunteers ($P < 0.005$). (From Idle et al.,[110] with permission.)

quine metabolic phenotype and cancer was found among 122 patients with bladder cancer.[112] These findings suggest that genetic polymorphisms of P450 oxidation may contribute to risk of cancer caused by environmental agents and might be specific for the route of entry of the procarcinogens and the ultimate tissue in which the malignancy develops.

A possible relationship between debrisoquine polymorphism and Parkinson's disease has also been proposed.[113] It has been postulated that many potentially toxic substances might be metabolized more slowly by defective P450 enzymes, leading to the chronic degenerative condition of Parkinson's disease, which is believed to be caused by a combination of environmental and genetic factors. Significantly more patients with Parkinson's disease exhibited the $\overline{PM}$ phenotype than controls; the poor metabolizers also tended to experience an earlier onset of the disease.[113] The data base of information concerning the potential relationships between debrisoquine hydroxylation polymorphism and the human disorders mentioned above is very limited. Virtually all these claims are drawn from retrospective studies that may contain unknown biases. Hence, until these results are confirmed (preferably by prospective studies), one must reserve final judgment as to their validity.

The molecular basis for debrisoquine polymorphism is now being defined. Studies of human liver biopsies have demonstrated that the clinically poor metabolizers of debrisoquine have a deficiency or absence of hepatic (P450) enzymatic activity and that this form of P450 protein displays a relatively well defined substrate specificity.[114] The DA inbred rat is a useful animal model of debrisoquine 4-hydroxylase deficiency. Defective substrate binding for debrisoquine, sparteine, and five other drugs in DA rat liver microsomes suggests that the defect might reflect an abnormal substrate binding site on the enzyme. The P450 responsible for DA rat liver debrisoquine 4-hydroxylase has been purified, and the antibody to the rat enzyme has been found to cross-react to some extent with the human debrisoquine 4-hydroxylase.[115]

Four P450 proteins involved in the 4-hydroxylation of debrisoquine have been purified from human liver[116] and designated P450db, P450pa, P450mp-1, and P450mp-2. Each form represents only a small fraction of total P450 content in human liver microsomes. P450db has relatively high catalytic activity toward debrisoquine, sparteine, bufuralol, encainide, and propranolol and appears to be the enzyme involved in the debrisoquine 4-hydroxylase polymorphism. On the basis of immunochemical inhibition and reconstitution studies involving more than a dozen catalytic activities, it would appear that the four P450 polymorphisms all involve different P450 enzymes.[116] One possibility is that the debrisoquine metabolic polymorphism represents defects in more than one form of P450; this would suggest that a regulatory gene mutation is involved rather than a structural gene mutation (i.e., a defect in only the P450db protein itself).

Five rat P450db cDNA genes have been cloned, sequenced, and consequently assigned to one of the subfamilies of the P450II gene family.[117] The cloning and sequencing of cDNAs from livers of humans with the $\overline{PM}$ phenotype has led to the identification of three variant messenger RNAs that are products of mutant genes producing incorrectly spliced P450db1 pre-mRNA.[118] Extension of these studies should enable one to identify $\overline{PM}$ and $\overline{EM}$ individuals on the basis of restriction fragment length polymorphism (RFLP) patterns, and/or expression vector assays, rather than having to phenotype patients by administering a radioactive drug and collecting urine samples.

Vitamin D-Dependent Rickets Type I

Several forms of vitamin D–refractory syndromes exist and have in common a partial or complete inability to respond to pharmacologic doses of the vitamin. The basic and clinical aspects of vitamin D, including the prohormone, and the mechanism of action of $1\alpha,25$-dihydroxy-D_3, which is regarded as the active hormone (Fig. 7-15), have been extensively reviewed.[119] Vitamin D_3 (cholecalciferol) is hydroxylated in the 25-position by a microsomal enzyme located predominantly in the liver of mammals. This enzyme is inhibited by its product, 25-hydroxyvitamin D_3 (25-OH-D_3). Vitamin D_3 may also be hydroxylated by a liver mitochondrial enzyme responsible mainly for the 25-hydroxylation of cholesterol; this alternate pathway is not subject to product inhibition, which explains how pharmacologic doses of vitamin D may bypass the normal regulatory step. 25-OH-D_3 is subsequently hydroxylated to $1\alpha,25$-dihydroxy-vitamin D_3 ($1\alpha,25$-diOH-D_3) by a kidney mitochondrial enzyme similar to some of the adrenal P450-mediated steroid hydroxylases. The $1\alpha,25$-diOH-D_3 promotes intestinal calcium absorption and, together with parathormone, enhances bone recalcification. The $1\alpha,25$-diOH-D_3 is the active form of vitamin D.

In patients with vitamin D–dependent rickets type I, the defect is inherited as an autosomal recessive trait. This disorder represents either a complete absence of the renal 1α-hydroxylase or a congenital defect in its regulation.[120] Patients with vitamin D–dependent rickets thus respond normally to physiologic doses of $1\alpha,25$-diOH-D_3, whereas abnormally large doses of vitamin D and 25-OH-D_3 are required to maintain normocalcemia.

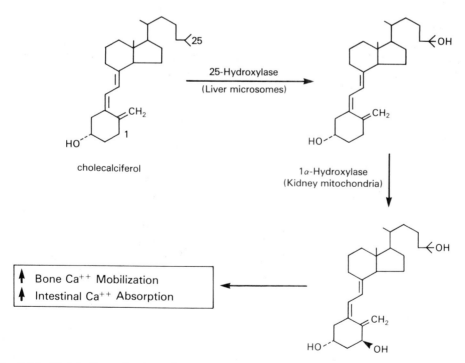

Fig. 7-15. Metabolic activation of cholecalciferol. (From Atlas et al.,[71] with permission.)

In contrast to patients with vitamin D–dependent rickets type I, patients with hypophosphatemic vitamin D–resistant rickets do not respond favorably to $1\alpha,25$-diOH-D_3; there is some increase in intestinal calcium absorption but no improvement in their profound hypophosphatemia. These disorders, which are inherited in both X-linked and autosomal dominant forms, are generally due to a primary defect in renal tubular reabsorption of phosphorus.

Vitamin D-dependent rickets type II represents end organ refractoriness to $1\alpha,25$-diOH-D_3 because high levels of the circulating hormone are found. These patients have normal binding of $1\alpha,25$-diOH-D_3 to its receptor,[121] which suggests that the lesion lies at the level of the transcription-regulating function of the receptor or with some other protein required for receptor activity. This defect will be mentioned later in connection with steroid hormone resistance.

C21-Hydroxylase Polymorphism

Many of the enzyme defects in congenital adrenal hyperplasia include mutant forms of P450 genes, which are currently under intensive investigation. These are regarded as pharmacogenetic disorders because the P450-mediated metabolite formation of both endogenous and synthetic steroids is markedly affected in individuals with these defects. Although the cholesterol side-chain cleavage, 11β-hydroxylase and 17α-hydroxylase deficiencies are being studied, the C21-hydroxylase deficiency disorder is best understood.

The most common form of congenital adrenal hyperplasia is due to decreased or totally absent C21-hydroxylase activity, resulting in diminished cortisol synthesis (Fig. 7-16). The defect occurs in about 1 in 5,000 births, represents an autosomal recessive trait, and is tightly linked to the HLA complex.[122] In 95 percent of cases, 21-hydroxylation is impaired in the zona fasciculata of the adrenal cortex, so that 17-hydroxyprogesterone is not converted to 11-deoxycortisol (Fig. 7-16). Because of decreased cortisol synthesis, corticotropin levels increase, resulting in overproduction and accumulation of cortisol precursors (particularly 17-hydroxyprogesterone) proximal to the block. This causes excessive production of androgens, resulting in virilization of varying degrees—usually more striking in females. In about half the cases there is an additional defect in aldosterone synthesis (converison of progesterone to 11-deoxycorticosterone) in the zona glomerulosa. If untreated, this latter disorder ("salt-wasting" form) can lead to shock or death in the neonatal period from inability to conserve urinary sodium.

The C21-hydroxylase gene has been cloned and sequenced, and shown to be within the *HLA-Bw47* region in the human[123] and within the S region of the mouse *H-2* locus.[124] Of interest, the C21 and C4 (complement) genes in the human and the mouse equivalent [C21, C4, and Slp (sex-limited protein)] had duplicated more than 100 million years ago, resulting in C21A and C21B genes. Restriction fragment length polymorphism (RFLP) studies[125] indicate that the human C21B gene is active but the C21A gene is not. Termination codons in the second exon explain the mechanism for the inactive human C21A gene. Cortico-

---

$\longrightarrow$

Fig. 7-16. Steroid pathways in the adrenal cortex cell. The pathway shown in the bottom half takes place in the mitochondrion, and the one in the top half occurs in the endoplasmic reticulum. The four participating P450 proteins are labeled 1 through 4; P450scc is the form that catalyzes the side-chain cleavage of cholesterol. The other three enzymes catalyze 17α-, 21-, and 11β-hydroxylation, respectively.

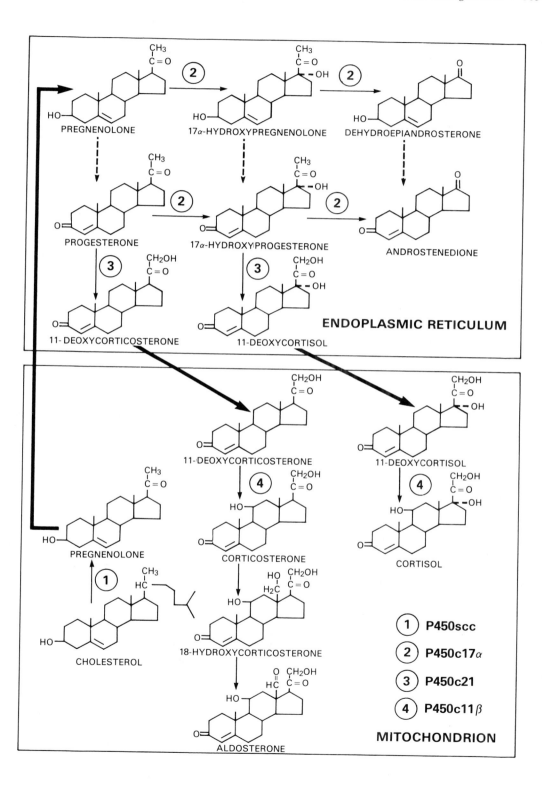

tropin-stimulated adrenal-specific expression of the mouse C21-hydroxylase gene activity has been demonstrated in mouse cell culture, and the situation in the mouse is the reverse of that in the human: the C21A gene is active while the C21B gene is not. Further molecular study of this system should provide a better understanding of this pharmacogenetic disorder, as well as important insight into P450 gene regulation.[117] Important RFLP patterns in the *HLA-Bw47* region may also aid in diagnosis, prediction of clinical severity of disease, and genetic counseling.

Enzymes of Methyl Conjugation

Catechol *O*-methyltransferase catalyzes the *O*-methylation of endogenous catecholamines and such catechol drugs as isoproterenol (Fig. 7-17). Data from family studies are compatible with an allele for low human erythrocyte catechol *O*-methyltransferase, which is inherited in an autosomal recessive fashion. Gene frequencies for the high and low alleles are about equal in white populations of northern European origin. The genetically controlled expression of the *O*-methyltransferase parallels the level of enzyme activity in other tissues and is significantly correlated with individual variations in the methyl conjugation of catechol drugs such as L-dopa and methyldopa. The significance of this polymorphism is not known, since the regulation of the enzyme in experimental animals is known to vary from tissue to tissue.[126]

In addition to catechol *O*-methyltransferase, thiopurine methyltransferase and thiol methyltransferase are important in the methyl conjugation of drugs and environmental chemicals. Thiopurine methyltransferase is controlled by two alleles at a single locus; incidence of the high-activity allele was 0.94 and incidence of the low-activity allele was 0.06 in a white U.S. population sample.[127] This methyltransferase catalyzes the *S*-methylation of thiopurines and thiopyrimidines. The red cell activity parallels the methyltransferase in other tissues such as the kidney and lymphocyte. The thiol methyltransferase catalyzes the S-methylation of drugs such as captopril and D-penicillamine. On the basis

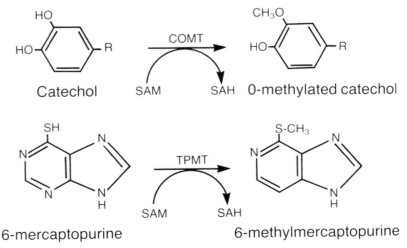

Fig. 7-17. Reactions catalyzed by catechol *O*-methyltransferase (COMT) and thiopurine methyltransferase (TPMT). SAM, *S*-adenosyl-L-methionine; SAH, *S*-adenosyl-L-homocysteine.

of family studies, the heritability index of the red cell thiol methyltransferase activity is approximately 0.98.

These pharmacogenetic defects in methyl conjugation may have clinical significance. For example, an association between cephalosporin-induced hypoprothrombinemia and thiol methylase deficiency has been reported,[128] and hereditary thiopurine methyltransferase deficiency has been correlated with 6-mercaptopurine toxicity in patients with acute lymphoblastic leukemia.[129]

Defects in Uridine Diphosphate Glucuronosyltransferase

There are two inborn errors of metabolism that present as hyperbilirubinemia but can also be responsible for idiosyncratic drug responses; these are Crigler-Najjar syndrome type II and Gilbert's disease. Both diseases are generally benign, and improvement will occur (i.e., serum bilirubin will be lowered) following treatment with phenobarbital. The phenobarbital therapy is believed to induce the defective uridine diphosphate glucuronosyltransferase and/or improve the hepatic canalicular excretion of bilirubin.

Crigler-Najjar syndrome type II is inherited as an autosomal recessive trait.[130] In liver samples from patients with this condition, formation of glucuronide conjugates in vitro is normal with *p*-nitrophenol, markedly decreased with 4-methylumbelliferone and *o*-aminophenol, and totally undetectable with bilirubin as substrate.[130] Impairment of the capacity for glucuronidation of acetaminophen, tetrahydrocortisol, chloral hydrate, menthol trichloroethanol, and salicylate has been described in affected individuals.[130]

Gilbert's disease is believed to be inherited as an autosomal dominant trait. As with Crigler-Najjar syndrome type II, hepatic biopsies of patients with Gilbert's syndrome have shown abnormal responses to menthol and bromsulphalein in vitro.[131] Although no cases of dramatic drug sensitivities have been reported for either syndrome, these individuals would be expected to exhibit a greater susceptibility to adverse reactions from drugs that are conjugated appreciably by the particular glucuronosyltransferase that is defective.

Fish-Odor Syndrome

The extent to which trimethylamine undergoes N-oxidation appears to be polymorphic in a British white population.[132] The trait of impaired N-oxidation is inherited as an autosomal recessive and leads to a very rancid odor of the afflicted person's urine and perspiration. The frequency of the gene is not yet known but appears to be less than 2 percent. The defect most likely lies in a deficient flavin adenine dinucleotide-containing (non-P450) monooxygenase.

INCREASED RESISTANCE TO DRUGS

Inability to Taste Phenylthiourea

Receptors with a high degree of stereospecificity for chemical agents mediate the senses of taste and olfaction, somehow acting as transducers between the chemical stimuli and the specific sensory signals that are transmitted to the brain. Hereditary abnormalities of sensory receptors are known for both taste and smell. The inability to taste phenylthiourea (also called phenylthiocarbamide) is the best characterized of these defects.

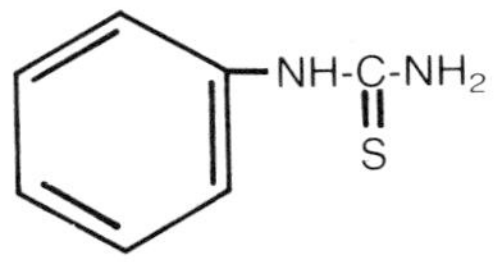

phenylthiourea

Phenylthiourea is perceived by most subjects as a very bitter substance at concentrations of less than 0.15 mM, but a minority note no bitterness at all until much higher concentrations (sometimes 100 times higher) are reached. With a dilution series test in which each concentration differs by a factor of 2 from the one before, a fairly reproducible taste threshold can be established for each subject.[133] A bimodal distribution was found with phenylthiourea but not with quinine.[134] This finding indicates that all bitter tastes do not activate the same chemoreceptors and that people who are deficient in their ability to taste phenylthiourea may nevertheless taste quinine quite normally. Subjects who taste phenylthiourea only at very high concentrations are categorized as the *nontaster* ($\overline{NT}$) phenotype.

The question of whether the trait is dominant or recessive can be answered either by means of mating analysis and application of the Hardy-Weinberg law, as was illustrated for isoniazid metabolism, or by a second method of calculation, which is offered here. In Table 7-9 we see that taster × taster ($\overline{T}$ × $\overline{T}$) matings yield both tasters and nontasters in large numbers, whereas $\overline{NT}$ × $\overline{NT}$ matings yield almost entirely nontaster offspring (the few exceptions in a study such as this could be due to misclassification and/or illegitimacy). This finding strongly suggests that the $\overline{NT}$ trait is recessive, the $\overline{T}$ trait dominant. Quantitative agreement with this hypothesis can be assessed as outlined earlier, with use of the frequency of nontasters in the whole population (0.30, based on more than 3,000 persons tested)[133] to estimate the gene frequencies. Thus, if $q^2 = 0.30$, then $q = 0.55$, where q is the frequency of the nontaster allele. The expected frequency of nontasters derived from $\overline{T}$ × $\overline{T}$ matings would be

$$\left(\frac{q}{p + 2q}\right)^2 = \left(\frac{0.55}{1.55}\right)^2 = 0.127$$

and that from $\overline{T}$ × $\overline{NT}$ matings would be

$$1\frac{q}{p + 2q} = \frac{0.55}{1.55} = 0.357.$$

The results shown in Table 7-9 agree very well with the observed data, indicating that the postulated recessive mode of inheritance can be accepted. Moreover, because of random occurrence of the trait among both sexes,[134] the trait is autosomal recessive.

Among the white U.S. population tested, 30 percent exhibits the $\overline{NT}$ phenotype. The

Table 7-9. Inheritance of the Inability to Taste Phenylthiourea

Parents	No. of Families	Offspring Taster[a]	Offspring Nontasters[a]	Fraction of Nontasters Observed	Fraction of Nontasters Expected
Taster × taster	425	929	130	0.123	0.127
Taster × nontaster	289	483	278	0.366	0.357
Nontaster × nontaster	86	5	218	0.978	1.000

[a] The expected fraction of nontasters was computed from the Hardy-Weinberg law on the assumption that it is a recessive trait, as described in the text.
(From Snyder,[133] with permission.)

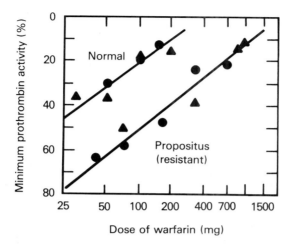

Fig. 7-18. Dose-response relationship for warfarin in a normal and a resistant subject. Response is expressed as the minimum level of prothrombin complex activity attained after a single dose, in terms of percent of normal activity. Circles are oral doses, triangles are intravenous doses (From O'Reilly et al.,[136] with permission.)

frequency of nontasters was found to be only 2 percent among American Indians, 3 percent among Africans, 16 percent among Chinese, and 37 percent among Arabs.[135] As with other pharmacogenetic ethnic differences, the long-term selective pressures for this recessive allele among several different geographic environments are not known. It is also possible that this gene is tightly linked to another (more important) gene that has undergone the selective pressures from particular ethnic and geographic influences.

Coumarin Resistance

The coumarin anticoagulants inhibit blood clotting by blocking the synthesis of four proteins essential to the clotting process: factors II (prothrombin), VII (proconvertin), IX (plasma thromboplastin component), and X (Stuart-Prower factor). Vitamin K is required for the synthesis of these specific proteins in the liver, and the coumarins are similar in chemical structure to vitamin K.

A report of a patient who was found to require 20 times the average daily dose of warfarin to maintain the desired prolongation of prothrombin clotting time[136] led to the discovery of a genetic trait that confers resistance to all the coumarins. In Figure 7-18, the responses to warfarin are compared in this patient (the propositus) and a normal subject. The minimum level of prothrombin activity achieved after each dose is plotted against the logarithm of the dose. The striking insensitivity of the propositus is apparent. Since oral and intravenous doses produced equivalent responses in the normal subject and in the propositus, it was concluded that defective absorption is not the cause of the warfarin resistance. Moreover, the rate of disappearance of warfarin, as judged by the return of prothrombin activity to normal levels after discontinuance of the drug, was found to be exactly the same in the propositus and in the normal subject. This finding suggests that increased metabolism of warfarin does not account for this 20-fold increase in resistance. Also, the extent of serum protein binding of warfarin was not unusual in the propositus.

Two large kinships with coumarin resistance have been studied.[136,137] It was found that the trait: (1) is expressed in successive generations; (2) appears in both sexes; (3) is transmitted by both sexes; and (4) is only sometimes transmitted in matings between affected and normal individuals. The trait appears to be exceedingly rare. Many thousands of people have been given coumarin anticoagulants, and most of them have been under rigorous laboratory control of their prothrombin clotting times; yet only two kindreds with coumarin resistance have been found. A rare trait with this demonstrated pattern of inheritance must be autosomal dominant, and the affected individuals are most likely heterozygotes.

Vitamin K appears to act in the carboxylation of glutamyl residues of precursor proteins of the four clotting factors. Coumarin anticoagulants do not affect the synthesis of these proteins directly, but they may alter the metabolism of vitamin K to promote accumulation of the inactive vitamin K epoxide at the expense of vitamin K itself, perhaps by inhibiting the reduction of epoxide continuously formed in the liver.[138] The molecular basis of coumarin resistance is not yet known, but the shape of the normal and abnormal response curve to warfarin (Fig. 7-18) is consistent with an altered epoxide reductase.[136–138] The aberrant enzyme can reduce vitamin K epoxide but is not as sensitive to inhibition by coumarin as the normal enzyme.

Warfarin has been used as a rodenticide for half a century. Warfarin resistance has been observed among wild rats in several regions of Europe and North America.[139] As in humans, the resistance in rats appears to be due to an alteration in the vitamin K epoxide reductase gene; however, the resistant rat has a higher than normal requirement for vitamin K. As with insect resistance to insecticides and bacterial resistance to antibiotics, if an agent is lethal to most of a population and if genes conferring resistance are at all present, such strong selective pressure will lead to replacement of the original sensitive alleles in the population by the resistant allele.

Other Disorders of Increased Drug Resistance Possibly Due to Defective Receptor

Steroid Hormone Resistance

Hormone resistance is defined as a lack of response to both endogenous and exogenously administered hormones, including synthetic analogs.[140] Vitamin D-dependent rickets type II is an example. As discussed above, both forms of this syndrome appear to represent an end-organ refractoriness to the hormone $1\alpha,25$-dihydroxycholecalciferol, possibly in combination with impaired parathyroid hormone secretion. Among the classical steroid hormones, primary resistance to androgen is the only clearly defined pharmacogenetic syndrome.

The actions of hormones are complex, as exemplified by the effects of androgen; not only may different testosterone metabolites display diametrically opposite effects, but the steroid has different actions at different stages of life, from embryogenesis to old age. According to molecular, genetic, anatomic, and endocrine parameters, at least six androgen-resistant syndromes have been described: 5α-reductase deficiency, complete testicular feminization, incomplete testicular feminization, Reifenstein syndrome, infertility in men, and male pseudohermaphroditism.[141] Except for 5α-reductase deficiency, which occurs as an autosomal recessive trait in females,[142] the syndromes are X-linked recessive and represent receptor disorders. Since the gene for the androgen receptor is on the X chromosome,[143] defects in the androgen receptor become clinically manifest in the hemizygous (XY) state. If the gene were autosomal, most mutations would probably become manifest only in the homozygous state.

Other Syndromes with Possibly Defective Receptors

Cystic fibrosis patients have abnormal responses to α-adrenergic, β-adrenergic, and cholinergic agents, which indicates that the disease is associated with a lesion at or, more likely, beyond the level of the autonomic receptors.[144] Channels for cations or anions are clear candidates. Down's syndrome (trisomy 21) includes an increased sensitivity to atropine and β-adrenergic hyperresponsiveness.[145] The Riley-Day syndrome (dysautonomia) is an autosomal recessive trait associated with norepinephrine hypersensitivity and absence of the usual flare in response to intradermal histamine.[146] A primary insulin receptor defect in an infant with leprechaunism has been characterized.[147]

Defective Absorption

Juvenile Pernicious Anemia

Patients with juvenile pernicious anemia are resistant to massive oral doses of vitamin B_{12} because of defective ileal absorption of the drug. Several causes of the disorder have been described, including congenital absence of intrinsic factor[148] and secretion of a functionally defective intrinsic factor with normal immunologic properties.[149] Although the mode of transmission is not clear, genetic control seems likely from the high incidence of the condition among siblings.[148] The disease can be effectively treated by administration of vitamin B_{12} intramuscularly.

Folate Absorption

Congenital defects in folic acid absorption and its conversion to one-carbon carrier forms include dihydrofolate reductase deficiency,[150] formiminotransferase deficiency syndromes,[151] methylene tetrahydrofolate reductase deficiency,[152] and tetrahydrofolate methyltransferase deficiency.[152] Folates, cobalamin, and analogs of chemically similar structure (e.g., methotrexate) may produce atypical drug responses in these patients.

Increased Metabolism

Succinylcholine Resistance

Just as there are variant alleles that encode a defective serum pseudocholinesterase leading to increased succinylcholine sensitivity, as described earlier, there are also genetic variants that lead to a three- to fourfold increase in enzyme activity and result in a greater resistance to succinylcholine and other acylcholines. The Cynthiana variant was described in one American family. This defect appears to represent an increased number of enzyme molecules rather than any structural change in the enzyme.[44] A second variant has been described in members of two German families.[153] In contrast to the Cynthiana variant, this atypical pseudocholinesterase exhibits a different electrophoretic pattern from the normal enzyme.

Atypical Alcohol Dehydrogenase

An atypical alcohol dehydrogenase was found with frequencies of 20 percent in 59 liver samples from Switzerland and 4 percent in 50 liver biopsies from England.[154] This atypical cytosolic enzyme displays a five- to sixfold increase in the rate of ethanol oxidation in vitro, while ethanol metabolism in these patients appears to be increased only 40 to 50 percent. Increased ethanol metabolism can increase blood acetaldehyde levels, which are known to be elevated in alcoholics and in patients whose primary relatives suffer from chronic alcoholism. The incidence of atypical alcohol dehydrogenase has been studied in several populations and is particularly high in Japan.[155]

Human liver alcohol dehydrogenase is able to oxidize the 3β-hydroxy moiety of digitoxigenin, digoxigenin, and gitoxigenin, the pharmacologically active principles of the corresponding cardiac glycosides. The Michaelis-Menten V_{max} and K_m values toward these digitalis derivatives are similar to those toward the substrate ethanol.[156] In view of the large polymorphism of alcohol dehydrogenase isozymes,[157] the potential relationship between digitalis metabolism and atypical alcohol dehydrogenase will require further study.

Atypical Aldehyde Dehydrogenase

High and low metabolizers of alcohol and chlorpropamide have been determined in members of a dozen families.[158] Ingestion of these drugs is accompanied by facial flushing related to poor metabolism, whereas high metabolizers are resistant to these effects. There are pharmacoethnic differences in this polymorphism—the high-affinity form of aldehyde dehydrogenase is absent in nearly half the Oriental and American Indian population.[159] In these subjects, therefore, acetaldehyde tends to accumulate and cause the same unpleasant consequences that individuals with the normal form of aldehyde dehydrogenase can experience by ingesting alcohol after taking disulfuram (see Chapter 5).[160]

ENZYME INDUCTION

The Porphyrias

The hepatic and erythropoietic porphyrias include both inherited and acquired disorders characterized by defects in specific enzymes of the heme biosynthesis pathway. Consequently, there is increased accumulation and excretion of those intermediates preceding the genetic block in the heme pathway, wherever it may lie (Fig. 7-19). For reasons that are not entirely clear, clinical symptoms include neurologic abnormalities and cutaneous photosensitivity. Depending on the site of expression of the gene defect in each disorder, the porphyrias are classified as either hepatic or erythroid. In all inherited forms of the disease, *environmental factors*—steroid hormones, drugs, alcohol, environmental chemicals, changes in menstrual cycle, surgery, infections and other types of stress, and even low-calorie diets—play a major role in determining the extent of clinical expression of the gene defect.

The idiosyncratic drug response in porphyria patients is caused by enzyme induction. Because many drugs, environmental agents, alcohol, and some steroids induce P450, the endogenous heme pool becomes depleted as the heme is used up during the formation of the active P450 hemoprotein (Fig. 7-19). Consequently, δ-aminolevulinic acid. (δALA) synthetase activity increases (through the synthesis of new enzyme), and the entire heme biosynthetic pathway is stimulated. In porphyric patients, an enzyme defect "downstream" from δALA synthetase results in accumulation of various heme precursors. How the buildup of these metabolites causes the clinical manifestations in porphyria patients is unclear. The porphyrias therefore represent an important model system for studying the host-environment interaction in the pathogenesis of human disease.

All hereditary porphyrias are autosomal dominant, except for congenital erythropoietic

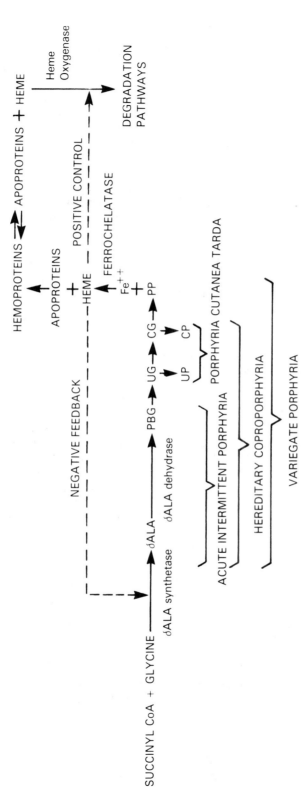

Fig. 7-19. Biochemical defects in the hepatic porphyrias. Heme biosynthesis is shown, as well as the intermediates excreted in excessive amounts in the several types of porphyria. (δALA = δ-aminolevulinic acid; PBG = porphobilinogen; UG = uroporphyrinogen; UP = uroporphyrin; CG = coproporphyrinogen; CP = coproporphyrin; PP = protoporphyrin.)

porphyria, which is autosomal recessive. Erythropoietic protoporphyria (ferrochelatase deficiency) and the extremely rare congenital erythropoietic porphyria (uroporphyrinogen III cosynthase deficiency) are not markedly affected by drugs and environmental pollutants and will not be considered further.

Acute intermittent porphyria is characterized by approximately 50 percent of normal porphobilinogen (PBG) deaminase activity (Fig. 7-19) in every tissue that has been examined.[161] Porphyrin overproduction is not so striking, and thus photosensitivity is minor. The disease is latent before puberty and highly variable during and after puberty, although PBG deaminase deficiency remains about the same at all ages. About 90 percent of all patients with the PBG deaminase defect actually remain clinically latent throughout adult life. Among the 10 percent with clinical symptoms, the majority are female, and subtle endocrine disorders (e.g., hepatic steroid 5α-reductase deficiency) seem to contribute to the increased susceptibility to active porphyria. The steroid 5α-reductase defect is not present in the 90 percent who remain clinically silent throughout adult life.

Hereditary coproporphyria is generally milder than acute intermittent porphyria and is associated with overproduction of coproporphyrinogen III, PBG, and δALA (Fig. 7-19) during acute crises of the disease. The underlying enzyme defect in hereditary coproporphyria is a 50 percent decrease in coproporphyrinogen III oxidase; coproporphyrinogen III therefore accumulates in the liver and skin, somehow causing the neurovisceral symptoms and photosensitivity.[162]

Variegate porphyria is most common in South African whites and reflects a defect in either protoporphyrinogen oxidase[163] or ferrochelatase (Fig. 7-19). As with the two disorders discussed above, a clinical attack is brought on by drugs, alcohol, hormones, and diet, and the defect is inherited as an autosomal dominant trait.

Porphyria cutanea tarda is the most common porphyria. It usually is first expressed in middle or late adult life, and it is more common in males.[164] The defect appears to represent hepatic uroporphyrinogen (UG) decarboxylase deficiency (Fig. 7-19), but it is still not established that this enzyme is defective in all cases of porphyria cutanea tarda. In some instances this enzyme has been reported as defective in red cells as well as liver, and in other cases as defective in liver but not in red cells. The UG decarboxylase cDNA has been cloned and sequenced, and the replacement of a glycine by a glutamic acid residue at position 281 in the mutant enzyme is believed to enhance markedly the rate of degradation of UG decarboxylase.[165] Hexachlorobenzene, 2,3,7,8-tetrachlorodibenzo-*p*-dioxin (TCDD)

hexachlorobenzene   tetrachlorodibenzo-*p*-dioxin

and other halogenated hydrocarbons can inhibit UG decarboxylase in the liver and produce a syndrome very similar to porphyria cutanea tarda without affecting the activity of the red cell enzyme.

A growing list of drugs that are unsafe (category I), potentially unsafe (category II), probably safe (category III), and safe (category IV) is available for patients with known or suspected porphyria. Although few drugs are known definitely to induce δALA synthetase in human liver (phenobarbital, phenytoin, and alcohol), the presumed mechanism by which each unsafe and potentially unsafe drug is porphyrinogenic is believed to be correlated with the drug's potency as an inducer of P450. It is also possible that "suicide substrates" that destroy P450, thereby commanding δALA synthetase induction with resultant synthesis of new P450, would be porphyrinogenic drugs. No correlation has been found, however, between levels of metabolites or covalent binding of metabolites and the hepatic porphyrogenic effects of hexachlorobenzene.[166] In order to provide guidance in the treatment of porphyria patients, there is clearly a need to screen drugs for their capacity to induce δALA synthetase and P450 and for their capacity to destroy P450.

Some of the chemicals that are most dangerous to victims of hereditary porphyria are also capable of causing porphyria in normal people as well as in experimental animals or even in cultured hepatic cells. Such toxic porphyrias have been well documented in human populations. A large-scale epidemic occurred in Turkey in 1956 after widespread consumption of wheat that had been treated with the fungicide hexachlorobenzene. Another massive outbreak occurred in 1964 among workers in a factory producing the herbicide 2,4,5,-triphenoxytricloroacetic acid (2,4,5-T); the responsible agent was identified as TCDD, present as a contaminant.[167] Porphyria patients are merely more sensitive than normal individuals to compounds that are intrinsically capable of disturbing heme synthesis.

The *Ah* Locus

The *Ah* locus is a genetic system that was first named for an observation in which a certain P450-mediated activity, that of aryl hydrocarbon hydroxylase (AHH) (benzo[a]pyrene being the hydrocarbon in this case), was markedly induced in some inbred mouse strains but not others.[168] AHH catalyzes the oxygenation of polycyclic aromatic hydrocarbons such as benzo[a]pyrene to phenolic products and epoxides (Fig. 7-20), some of which are toxic, mutagenic, and carcinogenic. The lack of AHH induction behaved as an autosomal recessive trait between C57BL/6 and DBA/2 mice, and the first inducing chemicals to be characterized were aromatic hydrocarbons (e.g., 3-methylcholanthrene and benzo[a]anthracene), whence the name *Ah* locus. A receptor defect, inherited as an additive trait, was subsequently found to be responsible for the lack of induction in DBA/2 mice.[169] The Ah receptor has been characterized in detail through the use of the very potent inducer TCDD, the porphyrinogenic environmental pollutant described earlier.[169,170]

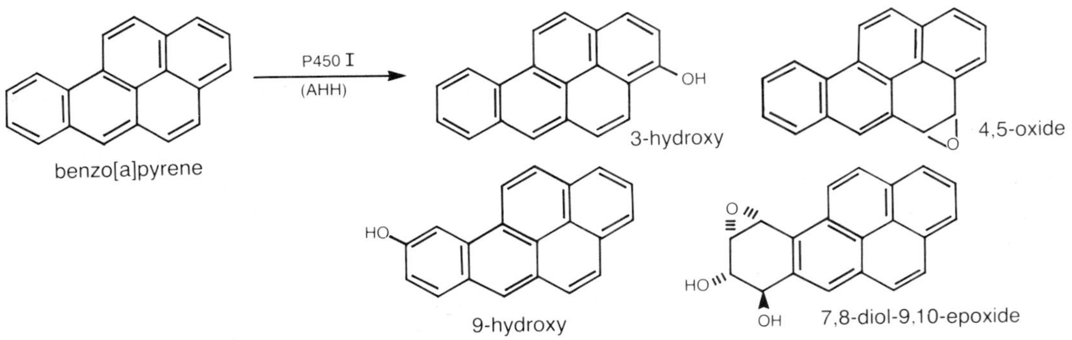

Fig. 7-20. AHH-catalyzed oxidation of benzo[a]pyrene to phenol and epoxide products.

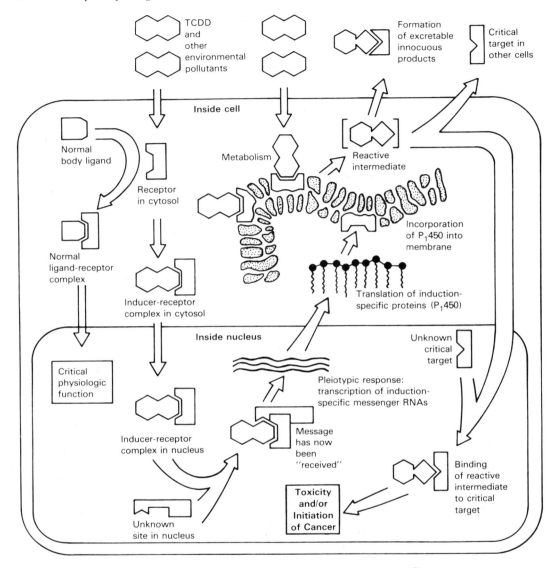

Fig. 7-21. Diagram of the *Ah* locus in a cell. (Adapted from Nebert,[172] with permission.)

Many molecular details of this gene system have been elucidated in the inbred mouse and via somatic cell genetics.[168,171] Procarcinogens formed as combustion products (e.g., benzo[a]pyrene and more than a dozen other polycyclic hydrocarbons) bind to the cytosolic Ah receptor (Fig. 7-21) with an apparent dissociation constant of less than 1.0 nM. The endogenous ligand is not known, but it appears that these foreign chemicals have appropriated the Ah receptor for stimulating their own metabolism.[172]

As we have discussed in chapter 6, following translocation of the TCDD-receptor complex to the nucleus, the expression of several genes is augmented. Included among the six or more TCDD-inducible genes are $P_1 450$ and $P_3 450$ (the equivalent genes in the rat and rabbit have been called P450c and P450d and forms 6 and 4, respectively). The $P_1 450$ and $P_3 450$ genes are known to be transcriptionally activated,[173] and induced concentrations

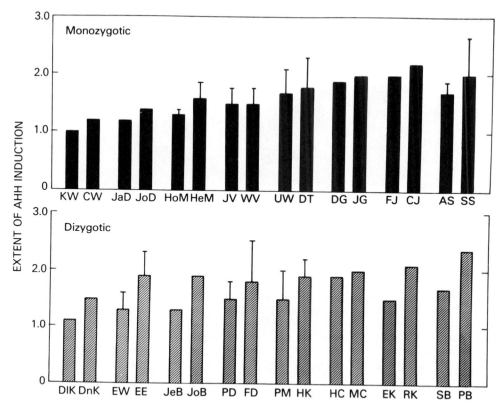

Fig. 7-22. Variance in the extent of AHH induction in cultured mitogen-activated lymphocytes from identical and fraternal twins. In the presence of mitogen, the cultures were treated with the inducer 3-methylcholanthrene and assayed for AHH activity after 72 or 96 hours in culture. (From Atlas et al.,[179] with permission.)

of the mRNAs lead to increased levels of the P_1450 and P_3450 proteins in the endoplasmic reticulum[174] and corresponding rises in benzo[a]pyrene and acetanilid metabolism, respectively.[175] Although detoxification is generally regarded to be an important function of the P450 family of proteins, P_1450 and P_3450 (the two genes in the P450I gene family[117]) are responsible for AHH activity (i.e., the conversion of combustion products and a variety of other procarcinogens to reactive intermediates that are carcinogenic, mutagenic, teratogenic, and toxic).[176,177] Higher amounts of P450I proteins and/or a more efficiently functioning Ah receptor may therefore lead to an increased risk of chemically produced cancer or to toxicity.

Genetic differences in human AHH (*CYP1A1*) inducibility have been demonstrated.[178] If one compares the variance between pairs of identical twins in Figure 7-22 with the variance between pairs of fraternal twins, the heritability index (described earlier in this chapter) is 0.80 for the 16 pairs of twins, all of whom were tested two to five times.[179] This value is consistent with a single gene, or a very small number of genes, being responsible for human AHH inducibility.

Figure 7-23 shows a significant correlation between high AHH inducibility and enhanced risk of bronchogenic carcinoma in cigarette smokers.[180] The original report of a relation-

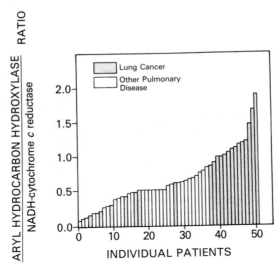

Fig. 7-23. Correlation of cigarette-induced bronchogenic carcinoma with high AHH inducibility. Lymphocytes from 51 patients were cultured for 4 days in the presence of mitogen and the AHH inducer 3-methylcholanthrene and then assayed for AHH and NADH-cytochrome *c* reductase activities. It can be seen that most lung cancer patients have the high AHH inducibility phenotype. (From Kouri et al.,[180] with permission.)

ship between cigarette-induced lung cancer and high AHH inducibility[181] could not be substantiated for several years in many laboratories. A modified assay for AHH inducibility,[180] however, expresses the enzyme activity per unit of NADH-cytochrome *c* reductase, a marker for the proliferating endoplasmic reticulum during mitogen activation of cultured lymphocytes. This assay is substantially improved over, and much more reproducible than, previous assays. The correlation between the high AHH inducibility phenotype and increased risk of polycyclic hydrocarbon–induced cancer in the human (Fig. 7-23) has also been demonstrated in numerous studies with inbred mice.[27]

The low AHH inducibility phenotype is associated with increased risk of polycyclic hydrocarbon–induced aplastic anemia and leukemia in the mouse.[182] A similar relationship between the low AHH inducibility phenotype and spontaneous leukemia has been reported in the human,[183] but this conclusion has been disputed.[184]

Three pharmacogenetic disorders described in this chapter show an association with malignancy. Chemical dye workers who are slow isoniazid acetylators have an increased risk of bladder cancer[66]; extensive metabolizers of debrisoquine have a disproportionately higher risk of liver and gastrointestinal tract cancer[110] and if they are cigarette smokers, of lung cancer[111]; and individuals of high AHH inducibility exhibit an increased risk of cigarette-induced bronchogenic carcinoma.[180] These examples point out several pharmacogenetic principles: (1) the phenotype most likely to exhibit an acute aberrant drug response need not be the same as that most likely to develop the chronic drug response; (2) malignancy is included among the chronic drug responses correlated with pharmacogenetics; and (3) the same response, such as enhanced risk of lung cancer, can exist in two or more quite unrelated pharmacogenetic polymorphisms (e.g., the debrisoquine polymorphism is associated with aberrant mRNA splicing in the P450IID gene subfamily, and the *Ah* locus is associated with inducibility of the P450I gene family[117]).

The human P_1450 gene has been cloned and sequenced,[185] and RFLP patterns do not correlate with AHH inducibility.[185,186] It is quite likely that differences in the P450I regulatory genes [i.e., the Ah receptor gene(s)] will be correlated with AHH inducibility rather than differences in the P450I structural genes. However, Ah receptor levels are—curiously—extremely low, virtually undetectable, in a number of human cell lines displaying high AHH inducibility,[187] which suggests that the properties of the human receptor might differ from those of the mouse or rat receptor.

The P450I gene family is located on human chromosome 15q22-qter,[186,188] and the P450IID gene subfamily exists on human chromosome 22q11.2-qter.[189] Further molecular biologic studies of these genes should provide important insight into the clinical diagnosis and the mechanisms of gene regulation.[117]

ABNORMAL DRUG DISTRIBUTION

Thyroxine (Hyperthyroidism or Hypothyroidism)

A genetic abnormality in the binding of a drug to a plasma protein involves thyroxine. This hormone is carried in the plasma bound in approximately equal amounts to three kinds of plasma protein: (1) albumin; (2) a prealbumin, which migrates more rapidly toward the anode on electrophoresis than does albumin; and (3) thyroxine-binding globulin. Thyroxine-binding globulin also binds triiodothyronine. The affinity of thyroxine-binding globulin is much greater for thyroxine than for triiodothyronine, less than 0.1 percent of total plasma thyroxine being present in the free form, and this probably explains why triiodothyronine is distributed so much more readily into the tissues. A kinship with greatly elevated serum protein-bound iodine has been studied, and the pattern of inheritance found to be consistent with an autosomal dominant trait.[190] A deficiency of thyroxine-binding globulin capacity has also been found[191]; family studies indicate that this defect is genetically determined and sex-linked.[192] Proof of the X chromosome linkage of the trait was provided by the discovery of a female with Turner's syndrome (XO), who must have inherited the trait from her mother, since her father had normal thyroxine-binding globulin.[193]

Iron (Hemochromatosis)

Genetically determined abnormal distribution of iron characterizes the diseases known as primary idiopathic hemochromatosis, in which there is a progressive accumulation of iron in the tissues. The body of a normal young adult contains about 1 g of iron, and this amount remains fairly constant throughout life. In the patient with hemochromatosis, the steady state is somehow disturbed, and there is a daily excess of iron absorption over iron excretion in the amount of about 2 mg. The disease is rarely seen until middle age, presumably because a certain number of years are required for the iron content of tissues to reach damaging levels. One distinguishing feature of primary hemochromatosis is an elevation of the plasma iron concentration, which results in an abnormally high occupation of binding sites on transferrin, the plasma iron-binding protein. Transferrin is capable of binding essentially all plasma iron up to concentrations of about 350 μg/ml. In the normal adult, the plasma iron concentration is approximately 120 μg/ml, representing a transferrin occupancy of 35 percent. In the patient with hemochromatosis, the plasma iron and the transferrin occupancy are both twice the normal levels. The total plasma transferrin is not increased, and there is no evidence of change in its affinity for iron.

Hereditary hemochromatosis (HC) is inherited as an autosomal recessive trait. The *HC* gene is believed to lie telomeric to the *HLA-A* locus on chromosome 6, meaning that the trait is usually inherited with the HLA-A allele and the HLA-A, B, DR haplotype within families (L. W. Powell, personal communication).

Copper (Wilson's Disease)

Wilson's disease, or hepatolenticular degeneration, is a genetically determined abnormality of copper metabolism, resulting in copper deposition in tissues. A specific copper-containing protein, the α_2-globulin called *ceruloplasmin*, is deficient or absent from the plasma. The disease is inherited as an autosomal recessive trait. It is exceedingly rare; there are probably only a few cases per million population. The accumulation and deposition of copper occurs in all tissues but is especially marked in the liver and brain. Ceruloplasmin is evidently the only copper protein that is deficient in this disease; others, such as tyrosinase and erythrocuprein, are present in normal amounts. Ceruloplasmin normally contains about 98 percent of the plasma copper; the copper is not reversibly bound but is incorporated into the protein structure at the time of synthesis. The specific drug for treatment or prevention is penicillamine, which chelates copper and eliminates it from the body. Because penicillamine is highly effective, it is all the more important to detect ceruloplasmin deficiency early in life. Routine screening of all infants might not be considered practical in view of the rarity of the condition, but certainly all relatives of patients in whom the diagnosis has been made should be investigated thoroughly and treated when evidence of the abnormality is found. The ceruloplasmin gene has been cloned, and marked decreases in the rate of ceruloplasmin gene transcription have been found in four patients with Wilson's disease.[194]

DISORDERS OF UNKNOWN ETIOLOGY

Several other pharmacogenetic disorders result in an increased sensitivity to drugs, but there is no basis as yet to classify them under decreased metabolism or defective receptor. These disorders do have either proven or suspected modes of inheritance and are therefore briefly covered here.

Corticosteroid-Induced Glaucoma

Glaucoma induced by corticosteroids is particularly worthy of mention because about 5 percent of the U.S. population is homozygous for the autosomal recessive allele.[195] The afflicted individual is prone to develop glaucoma from the use of corticosteroid-containing ophthalmic agents. The mechanism of the pathogenesis is not known.

Malignant Hyperthermia Associated with General Anesthesia

Malignant hyperthermia is a syndrome initiated by a hypermetabolic state of skeletal muscle. The first episode was described in a patient with a fear of anesthesia that had been prompted by the death of 10 of 24 relatives who had received general anesthesia. The anesthesia-induced disorder is characterized by tachycardia, arrhythmias, very high fever, and muscular rigidity. The body temperature may reach 43°C, and the rate at which the temperature rises can be 1°C every 5 minutes.

The incidence of malignant hyperthermia is one in 15,000 anesthetic administrations in children and one in 50,000 to 100,000 in adults.[196] These statistics do not reflect the true incidence of susceptible persons undergoing anesthesia, since 50 percent of the patients in whom the syndrome develops have had prior anesthesia without recognized malignant hyperthermia. The disorder appears to be inherited as an autosomal dominant trait,[197] but it may be multifactorial.[198]

The underlying defect appears to be an idiopathic increase in sarcoplasmic calcium ion.[199] During general anesthesia there is a two- to threefold increase in total body oxygen consumption in patients with the disorder.[200] Development of symptoms can vary from insidious to fulminant. The fulminant form is usually associated with the concurrent administration of halogenated inhalation anesthetics plus succinylcholine.

The only reliable diagnostic test at present requires a sample of viable muscle for in vitro studies of contracture. Skeletal muscle from susceptible persons shows abnormal contracture in response to caffeine or halothane. In the muscle of patients with malignant hyperthermia, contracture occurs at lower caffeine doses. Halothane, when bubbled through a muscle bath, produces an increase in the electrically evoked twitch tension of normal muscle and sometimes a small contracture response; in muscle from malignant hyperthermia patients, however, the reaction to halothane is a large, abnormal contracture.[201] A similar, if not identical, syndrome has been characterized in pigs.[200]

Halothane-Induced Hepatitis

The anesthetic halothane causes both a *dose-dependent* and a rare *dose-independent* hepatitis, which occurs at an incidence of probably less than 1 in 10,000 courses of administration.[202] The dose-independent halothane hepatitis syndrome seems to be genetically controlled.[203,204] Halothane appears to be anaerobically reduced by P450,[205] and it is the phenobarbital-induced rather than the 3-methylcholanthrene-induced P450 that preferentially catalyzes this reaction,[206] which indicates that the P450II gene family and not the P450I family is primarily involved in the toxicity. The postulated P450-mediated pathway is $CF_3CHClBr \rightarrow CF_3CHCl \rightarrow CF_3COX$ (where X denotes covalently bound P450 protein), with the last oxidative metabolite being so reactive that it becomes a "suicide substrate," which covalently binds to, and consequently destroys, the P450 protein catalyzing the reaction.[207]

When lymphocytes from normal subjects are incubated with phenytoin in a system containing phase II inhibitors to maximize P450 metabolism, as outlined in Figure 7-24, genetic differences in phenytoin toxicity have been demonstrated.[208] When lymphocytes from 11 patients with halothane hepatotoxicity were studied in this type of assay, they exhibited about an eightfold greater sensitivity to phenytoin toxicity as compared with 39 control individuals (including 15 persons with other forms of acute liver disease).[204] This *phenytoin toxicity susceptibility factor* was also demonstrated among members of four families of the patients with halothane hepatitis.[204] Further studies will be necessary to characterize this interesting pharmacogenetic disorder in more detail.

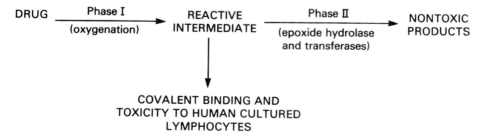

Fig. 7-24. Hypothetical scheme whereby a test drug can be evaluated for possible covalent binding and toxicity to human cultured lymphocytes. Mammalian liver microsomal P450 can be added to augment the formation of reactive intermediates. Inhibitors of phase II enzymes can be added to the cells in order to enhance the interaction of reactive metabolites with the cultured lymphocytes. Increased toxicity under these conditions is consistent with P450-mediated conversion to a toxic species.

Chloramphenicol-Induced Aplastic Anemia

Chloramphenicol remains the leading *known* cause of drug-induced aplastic anemia. As is the case with halothane-induced liver toxicity, chloramphenicol produces two distinct forms of bone marrow toxicity: (1) the common *dose-dependent* reversible marrow suppression involving primarily the erythroid series; and (2) a rare bone marrow aplasia, which is *dose-independent*. This latter form is regarded as a pharmacogenetic disorder. Whereas concentrations of chloramphenicol greater than 100 μg per milliliter of growth medium are necessary to inhibit gross DNA or RNA synthesis in cultures of marrow taken from normal subjects, inhibition has been demonstrated at significantly lower concentrations of chloramphenicol in marrow cells taken from patients who have recovered from chloramphenicol-induced aplastic anemia.[209] It has been suggested that the single oxamyl chloride intermediate is responsible for the drug's covalent binding to protein, mediated by a P450 enzyme(s).[210] The mode of inheritance of this pharmacogenetic disorder is not known.

Other Disorders of Unknown Etiology

Phenytoin-induced gingival hyperplasia occurs at an increased incidence in families of affected individuals. Although the mechanisms are not known, phenytoin induces a greater amount of protein synthesis and collagen production in cultured fibroblasts from afflicted individuals than in cultured control fibroblasts.[211]

There is an increased incidence of thromboembolic complications caused by anovulatory drugs among persons of the A, B, and AB blood groups.[212]

FUTURE DIRECTIONS

The information presented in this chapter can be classified into three fundamentally different areas: (1) the influence of existing genetic variability on *acute* responses to drugs; (2) the influence of underlying genetic predisposition on *chronic* responses (e.g., neurotoxicity, lupus syndrome, or malignancy) to drugs and other foreign chemicals; and (3) the natural selection of various genes by altered environments. These areas of study have been referred to as *pharmacogenetics*,[213] *ecogenetics*,[214] and *pharmacoanthropology*.[215]

Pharmacogenetics

Pharmacogenetic disorders have been detected and subsequently examined by initial clinical observations, family or twin studies, protein polymorphism characterizations, and animal model studies. To these four investigative approaches we can now add a fifth—DNA polymorphism characterizations.

Restriction fragment length polymorphism (RFLP) patterns of allelic variants have been described for dozens of inborn errors of metabolism, and this technique is now utilized widely.[216] The use of RFLPs for identification of the glucose-6-phosphate dehydrogenase, hypoxanthine-guanine phosphoribosyltransferase, steroid 21-hydroxylase, and human P450I genes has been considered in this chapter. A variety of other new techniques are becoming popular for detecting a single nucleotide difference in a mutant allele.[217] Transfection of genes linked to expression vectors into appropriate cell cultures, followed by studies of gene expression, has also become commonplace. These types of studies have been carried out with the human genes encoding hypoxanthine-guanine phosphoribosyltransferase, steroid 21-hydroxylase, and numerous P450 genes. These genetic detection methods should be particularly valuable to the field of pharmacogenetics because drug administration would not be required to identify susceptible individuals. Presently, the most common method of evaluation involves administration of the test drug followed by measurement of the drug (or metabolites) in the blood or urine. Often low levels of radioactivity must be used, and the possibilities of unanticipated idiosyncratic drug responses must always be guarded against. Modern advances in analytical methods are leading to the detection of a parent drug and its metabolites in increasingly smaller amounts. Owing to pharmacokinetic differences between large and small drug doses, however, it might be undesirable to study certain pharmacogenetic polymorphisms with very small doses of drugs.

Ecogenetics

Ecogenetics refers to differences in the effect of the environment on individuals due to underlying genetic variability.[214] Environment is broadly defined here and it includes physical, chemical, infectious, atmospheric, and climatic agents, as well as foodstuffs. Examples of ecogenetic disorders in this chapter include the associations of malignancy with the acetylation, debrisoquine, and *Ah* locus, polymorphisms; of neurotoxicity with the acetylation and debrisoquine polymorphisms; and of lupus erythematosus and hemolytic anemia with the acetylation polymorphism. Whereas the bladder cancer/acetylation polymorphism studies were carried out in chemical workers and the cancers are therefore presumed to be caused by industrial chemicals, the other malignancies and toxicities described are presumably caused by cigarette smoking, food substances, and other, unknown environmental factors.

In 1938, Haldane proposed the possibility of screening susceptible workers in an attempt to prevent certain environmental diseases.[218] As more is known about ecogenetics-related genes and as tests such as the RFLP patterns mentioned above become simpler, less expensive, and more sensitive, it is anticipated that the genetic screening of individuals in hazardous industrial settings will become more and more routine. Such screening programs may be financially more feasible than attempting to lower the concentration of an industrial chemical in the air by a factor of, say, 10.

Pharmacoanthropology

Anthropology is the study of populations. The term *pharmacoanthropology* has been proposed as the study of the causes of quantitative differences in drug metabolism between populations; this definition thereby emphasizes the medical and biologic (rather than social or economic) nature of the enquiry.[215] Another suggested term has been *ethnopharmacology*. Genetic variation can probably be expected for polymorphic loci regulating drug disposition among racial and ethnic groups. The interaction between diet and genetic constitution lies within the concern of pharmacoanthropology. The subject matter is therefore more of a statistical than a clinical nature.

Well known are the classical cases of balanced polymorphisms, such as sickle cell anemia. It is clear that the heterozygote for hemoglobin S has an adaptational advantage in mosquito-infested regions of Africa owing to protection of this individual against malaria. However, for the acetylation polymorphism, why is the population of the slow acetylation phenotype about 10 percent in Japanese and almost 90 percent in Middle Eastern populations? For the glucose-6-phosphate dehydrogenase polymorphism, why is the frequency more than 50 percent in certain Jewish groups, yet less than 1 percent in others? For the phenylthiourea taster polymorphism, why are Arabs 37 percent nontasters while American Indians are 2 percent nontasters? These ethnic differences may reflect natural evolutionary selection pressures, or "balanced" polymorphisms, similar to those occurring with sickle cell anemia. Alternatively, these differences may be incidental associations of drug response due to chromosomal linkage of these pharmacogenetic genes with other genes actually exposed to the selective pressures.

As with the pharmacogenetic and ecogenetic studies described above, methods that have been developed for the study of individuals are not necessarily the best methods for studying large populations. Hence, the use of simple, inexpensive, and highly sensitive methodology will be needed for large-scale studies of pharmacogenetics-related genes within human populations. Use of DNA polymorphisms (RFLP patterns) and perhaps of simplified gene expression assays again appears more reasonable than many of the current cumbersome drug-dosing clinical tests or equivocal assays of enzyme activity in various tissues. Knowledge gained from pharmacoanthropologic research should provide insight into human evolution and ethnic origins, as well as a better understanding of the medical and biologic aspects of many human diseases.

REFERENCES

1. Kalow W: Pharmacogenetics: Heredity and the Response to Drugs. WB Saunders, Philadelphia, 1962
2. Thorgeirsson SS, Nebert DW: The *Ah* locus and the metabolism of chemical carcinogens and other foreign compounds. Adv Cancer Res 25:149, 1977
3. Oie S, Levy G: Interindividual differences in the effect of drugs on bilirubin plasma binding in newborn infants and in adults. Clin Pharmacol Ther 21:627, 1977
4. Wilding G, Paigen B, Vesell ES: Genetic control of interindividual variations in racemic warfarin binding to plasma and albumin of twins. Clin Pharmacol Ther 22:831, 1977
5. Weinshilboum RM: Serum dopamine β-hydroxylase. Pharmacol Rev 30:133, 1979
6. Weinshilboum RM, Raymond FA: Inheritance of low erythrocyte catechol *O*-methyltransferase activity in man. Am J Hum Genet 29:125, 1977
7. Tang BK, Kalow W, Grey AA: Amobarbital metabolism in man: *N*-Glucoside formation. Res Commun Chem Pathol Pharmacol 21:45, 1978
8. Evans DAP, White TA: Human acetylation polymorphism. J Lab Clin Med 63:394, 1964
9. Bönicke R, Lisboa BP: Über die Erbbedingtheit der intraindividuellen Konstanz der Isoniazidausscheidung beim Menschen. Naturwissenschaften 44:314, 1957
10. Evans DAP, Manley K, McKusick VA: Genetic control of isoniazid metabolism in man. Br Med J 2:485, 1960
11. Vesell ES: Advances in pharmacogenetics. Prog Med Genet 9:291, 1973
12. Alexanderson B, Evans DAP, Sjöqvist F: Steady state plasma levels of nortriptyline in twins: Influence of genetic factors and drug therapy. Br Med J 4:764, 1969
13. Vesell ES, Page JG, Passananti GT: Genetic and environmental factors affecting ethanol metabolism in man. Clin Pharmacol Ther 12:192, 1971
14. Cascorbi HF, Vesell ES, Blake DA, Hebrich M: Genetic and environmental influence on halothane metabolism in twins. Clin Pharmacol Ther 12:50, 1971
15. Andreasen PB, Froland A, Skovsted L, et al: Diphenylhydantoin half-life in man and its inhibition by phenylbutazone: The role of genetic factors. Acta Med Scand 193:561, 1973
16. Furst ED, Gupta N, Paulus HE: Salicylate metabolism in twins. Evidence suggesting a genetic influence and induction of salicylurate formation. J Clin Invest 60:35, 1977
17. Endrenyi L, Inaba T, Kalow W: Genetic study of amobarbital elimination based on its kinetics in twins. Clin Pharmacol Ther 20:701, 1977

18. Vesell ES: Drug therapy, pharmacogenetics. N Engl J Med 287:904, 1972
19. Hammer W, Martens S, Sjöqvist F: A comparative study of the metabolism of desmethylimipramine, nortriptyline, and oxyphenylbutazone in man. Clin Pharmacol Ther 10:44, 1969
20. Vesell ES, Page JG: Genetic control of phenobarbital-induced shortening of plasma antipyrine half-lives in man. J Clin Invest 48:2202, 1969
21. Motulsky AG: Pharmacogenetics. Prog Med Genet 3:49, 1964
22. Whittaker JA, Evans DAP: Genetic control of phenylbutazone metabolism in man. Br Med J 4:323, 1970
23. Åsberg M, Evans DAP, Sjöqvist F: Genetic control of nortriptyline kinetics in man: A study of relatives of propositi with high plasma concentrations. J Med Genet 8:129, 1971
24. Vesell ES: Genetic and environmental factors affecting drug response in man. Fed Proc 31:1253, 1972
25. Harris H: The Principles of Human Biochemical Genetics. Elsevier/North-Holland Biomedical Press, New York, 1975
26. Greaves JH, Ayres P: Heritable resistance to warfarin in rats. Nature 215:877, 1967
27. Kouri RE, Nebert DW: Genetic regulation of susceptibility to polycyclic hydrocarbon-induced tumors in the mouse. In Hiatt HH, Watson JD, Winsten JA (eds): Origins of Human Cancer. Cold Spring Harbor Laboratory, Cold Spring Harbor, NY, 1977, p. 811
28. Weber WW, Hein DW: N-Acetylation pharmacogenetics. Pharmacol Rev 37:25, 1985
29. Otterness DM, Keith RA, Weinshilboum RM: Thiopurine methyltransferase: Mouse kidney and liver assay conditions, biochemical properties and strain variation. Biochem Pharmacol 34:3823, 1985
30. Kalow W, Britt BA, Richter A: Individuality in human skeletal muscle, as revealed by studies of malignant hyperthermia. Can J Genet Cytol 18:565, 1976
31. Britt BA, Kalow W, Endrenyi L: Malignant hyperthermia—pattern of inheritance in swine. In Aldrete JA, Britt BA (eds): Malignant Hyperthermia. Grune & Stratton, Orlando, FL, 1978, p. 195
32. Scanlon PD, Raymond FA, Weinshilboum RM: Catechol O-methyltransferase: Thermolabile enzyme in erythrocytes of subjects homozygous for allele for low activity. Science 203:63, 1979
33. Lehmann H, Liddell J: Genetical variants of human serum pseudocholinesterase. Prog Med Genet 3:75, 1964
34. Lubin AH, Garry PJ, Owen GM: Sex and population differences in the incidence of a plasma cholinesterase variant. Science 173:161, 1971
35. Lockridge O, Mottershaw-Jackson N, Eckerson HW, La Du BN: Hydrolysis of diacetylmorphine (heroin) by human serum cholinesterase. J Pharmacol Exp Ther 215:1, 1980
36. Lockridge O: Substance P hydrolysis by human serum cholinesterase. J Neurochem 39:106, 1982
37. Stewart DJ, Inaba T, Tang BK, Kalow W: Hydrolysis of cocaine in human plasma by cholinesterase. Life Sci 20:1557, 1977
38. Lockridge O, Eckerson HW, La Du BN: Interchain disulfide bonds and subunit organization in human serum cholinesterase. J Biol Chem 254:8324, 1979
39. Lockridge O, Bartels CF, Vaughan TA, et al: Complete amino acid sequence of human serum cholinesterase. J Biol Chem 262:549, 1987
40. McGuire MC, Nogueira CP, Bartels CF, et al: Identification of the structural mutation responsible for the dibucaine-resistant (atypical) variant form of human serum cholinesterase. Proc Natl Acad Sci USA 86:953, 1989
41. Altland K, Goedde HW: Heterogeneity in the silent gene phenotype of pseudocholinesterase of human serum. Biochem Genet 4:321, 1970
42. Harris H, Hopkinson DA, Robson EB, Whittaker M: Genetical studies on a new variant of serum cholinesterase detected by electrophoresis. Ann Hum Genet 26:359, 1963
43. Thompson JC, Whittaker M: A study of the pseudocholinesterase in 78 cases of apnoea following suxamethonium. Acta Genet Statist Med 16:209, 1966

44. Yoshida A, Motulsky AG: A pseudocholinesterase variant (E Cythiana) associated with elevated plasma enzyme activity. Am J Hum Genet 21:486, 1969
45. Patterson E, Radtke HE, Weber WW: Immunochemical studies of rabbit *N*-acetyltransferases. Mol Pharmacol 17:367, 1980
46. Karim AKMB, Elfellah MS, Evans DAP: Human acetylator polymorphism: Estimate of allele frequency in Libya and details of global distribution. J Med Genet 18:325, 1981
47. Evans DAP: Survey of the human acetylator polymorphism in spontaneous disorders. J Med Genet 21:243, 1984
48. Hein DW, Weber WW: Polymorphic *N*-acetylation of phenelzine and monoacetylhydrazine by highly purified rabbit liver isoniazid *N*-acetyltransferase. Drug Metab Dispos 10:225, 1982
49. Perry HM, Tan EM, Carmody S, Sakamoto A: Relationship of acetyl transferase activity to antinuclear antibodies and toxic symptoms in hypertensive patients treated with hydralazine. J Lab Clin Med 76:114, 1970
50. Uetrecht JP, Woosley RL: Acetylator phenotype and lupus erythematosus. Clin Pharmacokinet 6:118, 1981
51. Henningsen NC, Cederberg A, Hanson A, Johansson BW: Effects of long-term treatment with procainamide. Acta Med Scand 198:475, 1975
52. Woosley RL, Drayer DE, Reidenberg MM, et al: Effect of acetylator phenotype on the rate at which procainamide induces antinuclear antibodies and the lupus syndrome. N Engl J Med 298:1157, 1978
53. Mansilla-Tinoco R, Harland SJ, Ryan PJ, et al: Hydralazine, antinuclear antibodies, and the lupus syndrome. Br Med J 284:936, 1982
54. Batchelor JR, Welsh KI, Mansilla-Tinoco R, et al: Hydralazine-induced systemic lupus erythematosus: Influence of HLA-DR and sex on susceptibility. Lancet 1:1107, 1980
55. Murray FJ: Outbreak of unexpected reactions among epileptics taking isoniazid. Am Rev Respir Dis 86:729, 1962
56. Brennan RW, Dehejia B, Kutt H, et al: Diphenylhydrantoin intoxication attendant to slow inactivation of isoniazid. Neurology 20:687, 1970
57. Muakassah SF, Bidlack WR, Yang CT: Mechanism of the inhibitory action of isoniazid on microsomal drug metabolism. Biochem Pharmacol 30:1651, 1981
58. Mitchell JR, Zimmerman HJ, Ishak KG, et al: Isoniazid liver injury: Clinical spectrum, pathology and probable pathogenesis. Ann Intern Med 84:181, 1976
59. Ellard GA, Gammon PT: Pharmacokinetics of isoniazid metabolism in man. J Pharmacokinet Biopharm 4:83, 1976
60. Timbrell JA, Wright JM, Baillie TA: Monoacetylhydrazine as a metabolite of isoniazid in man. Clin Pharmacol Ther 22:602, 1977
61. Weber WW, Hein DW, Litwin A, Lower GM: Relationship of acetylator status to isoniazid toxicity, lupus erythematosus, and bladder cancer. Fed Proc 42:3086, 1983
62. Gurumurthy P, Krisnamurthy MS, Nazareth R, et al: Lack of relationship between hepatic toxicity and acetylator phenotype in three thousand South Indian patients during treatment with isoniazid for tuberculosis. Am Rev Respir Dis 129:58, 1984
63. Dickinson DS, Bailey WC, Hirschowitz BI, et al: Risk factors for isoniazid (INH)-induced liver dysfunction. J Clin Gastroenterol 3:271, 1981
64. Musch E, Eichelbaum M, Wang JK, et al: Die Häufigkeit hepatoxischer Nebenwirkungen der tuberkulostätischen Kombinationstherapie (INH, RMP, EMB) in Abhängigkeit vom Acetylierphänotyp. Klin Wochenschr 60:513, 1982
65. Case RAM, Hosker ME, McDonald DB, Pearson JT: Tumours of the urinary bladder in workmen engaged in the manufacture and use of certain dyestuff intermediates in the British chemical industry. Br J Ind Med 11:75, 1954
66. Cartwright RA, Glashan RW, Rogers HJ, et al: The role of *N*-acetyltransferase phenotypes in bladder carcinogenesis: A pharmacogenetics epidemiological approach to bladder cancer. Lancet 2:842, 1982

67. Evans DAP, Eze LC, Whitley EJ: The association of the slow acetylator phenotype with bladder cancer. J Med Genet 20:330, 1983

68. Glowinski IB, Radtke HE, Weber WW: Genetic variation in *N*-acetylation of carcinogenic arylamines by human and rabbit liver. Mol Pharmacol 14:940, 1978

69. Weber WW: Acetylation pharmacogenetics: Experimental models for human toxicity. Fed Proc 43:2332, 1984

70. Carson PE, Flanagan CL, Ickes CE, Alving AS: Enzymatic deficiency in primaquine sensitive erythrocytes. Science 124:484, 1956

71. Atlas SA, Nebert DW: Pharmacogenetics and human disease. In Parke DV, Smith RL (eds): Drug Metabolism from Microbe to Man. Taylor & Francis, London, 1977, p. 393

72. Yoshida A, Beutler E: G-6-PD variants: Another up-date. Ann Hum Genet 47:25, 1983

73. Vergnes HA, Bonnet LG, Grozdea JD: Genetic variants of human erythrocyte glucose-6-phosphate dehydrogenase: New characterization data obtained by multivariate analysis. Ann Hum Genet 49:1, 1985

74. Beutler E: Disorders due to enzyme defects in the red blood cell. Adv Metab Disord 6:131, 1972

75. Beutler E: Hemolytic Anemia in Disorders of Red Cell Metabolism. Plenum, New York, 1978

76. Fraser IM, Vesell ES: Effects of drugs and drug metabolites on erythrocytes from normal and glucose-6-phosphate dehydrogenase–deficient individuals. Ann NY Acad Sci 151:777, 1968

77. Orrenius S, Moldeus P: The multiple roles of glutathione in drug metabolism. Trends Pharmacol Sci 5:432, 1984

78. Dern RJ, Beutler E, Alving S: The hemolytic effect of primaquine. V. Primaquine sensitivity as a manifestation of a multiple drug sensitivity. J Lab Clin Med 45:30, 1955

79. Kiese M: The biochemical production of ferrihemoglobin-forming derivatives from aromatic amines, and mechanisms of ferrihemoglobin formation. Pharmacol Rev 18:1091, 1966

80. Strother A, Allahyari R, Buchholz J, et al: In vitro metabolism of the antimalarial agent primaquine by mouse liver enzymes and identification of a methemoglobin-forming metabolite. Drug Metab Dispos 12:35, 1984

81. Bickel MH: The pharmacology and biochemistry of *N*-oxides. Pharmacol Rev 21:325, 1969

82. Flohe L, Benöhr HC, Sies H, et al. Glutathione. Academic Press, Orlando, FL, 1974

83. Nickerson WJ, Falcone G, Strauss G: Studies on quinone-thioethers. I. Mechanism of formation and properties of thiodione. Biochemistry 2:537, 1963

84. Marks PA, Banks J: Drug-induced hemolytic anemias associated with glucose-6-phosphate dehydrogenase deficiency: A genetically heterogeneous trait. Ann NY Acad Sci 123:198, 1965

85. Petrakis NL, Wiesenfeld SL, Sams BJ, et al: Prevalence of sickle-cell trait and glucose-6-phosphate dehydrogenase deficiency. Decline with age in the frequency of G-6-PD-deficient Negro males. N Engl J Med 282:767, 1970

86. Luzzatto L, Usanga EA, Reddy S: Glucose-6-phosphate dehydrogenase deficient red cells: Resistance to infection by malarial parasites. Science 164:839, 1969

87. Takizawa T, Huang I-Y, Ikuta T, Yoshida A: Human glucose-6-phosphate dehydrogenase: Primary structure and cDNA cloning. Proc Natl Acad Sci USA 83:4157, 1986

88. Hirono A, Beutler E: Molecular cloning and nucleotide sequences of cDNA for human glucose-6-phosphate dehydrogenase variant A(−). Proc Natl Acad Sci USA 85:3951, 1988

89. Vulliamy TJ, D'Urso M, Battistuzzi G et al: Diverse point mutations in the human glucose-6-phosphate dehydrogenase gene cause enzyme deficiency and mild or severe hemolytic anemia. Proc Natl Acad Sci USA 85:5171, 1988

90. Wellner VP, Sekura R, Meister A, Larsson A: Glutathione synthetase deficiency, an inborn error of metabolism involving the γ-glutamyl cycle in patients with 5-oxoprolinuria (pyroglutamic aciduria). Proc Natl Acad Sci USA 71:2505, 1974

91. Spielberg SP, Garrick MD, Corash LM, et al: Biochemical heterogeneity in glutathione synthetase deficiency. J Clin Invest 61:1417, 1978

92. Beutler E, Kuhl W, Gelbart T: 6-Phosphogluconolactonase deficiency, a hereditary eryth-

rocyte enzyme deficiency: Possible interaction with glucose-6-phosphate dehydrogenase deficiency. Proc Natl Acad Sci USA 82:3876, 1985

93. Comings DE: Hemoglobinopathies associated with unstable hemoglobin. In Williams WJ, Beutler E, Erslev AJ, Rundles RW (eds): Hematology. McGraw-Hill, New York, 1972
94. Prankerd TAJ: The Red Cell. Charles C Thomas, Springfield, IL, 1961
95. Eder HA, Finch C, McKee RW: Congenital methemoglobinemia. A clinical and biochemical study of a case. J Clin Invest 28:265, 1949
96. Scott EM: The relation of diaphorase of human erythrocytes to inheritance of methemoglobinemia. J Clin Invest 39:1176, 1960
97. Boss GR, Seegmiller JE: Hyperuricemia and gout. Classification, complications and management. N Engl J Med 300:1459, 1979
98. Wilson JM, Young AB, Kelly WN: The molecular basis of the clinical syndromes. N Engl J Med 309:900, 1983
99. Wilson JM, Stout JT, Palella TD, et al: A molecular survey of hypoxanthine-guanine phosphoribosyltransferase deficiency in man. J Clin Invest 77:188, 1986
100. Athanassiadis D, Cranston WI, Juel-Jensen BE, Oliver DO: Clinical observations on the effects of debrisoquine sulphate in patients with high blood-pressure. Br Med J 2:732, 1966
101. Allen JG, East PB, Francis RJ, Haigh JL: Metabolism of debrisoquine sulfate. Identification of some urinary metabolites in rat and man. Drug Metab Dispos 3:332, 1975
102. Idle JR, Smith RL: Polymorphisms of oxidation of carbon centers of drugs and their clinical significance. Drug Metab Rev 9:301, 1979
103. Woolhouse NM, Andoh B, Mahgoub A, et al: Debrisoquine hydroxylation polymorphism among Ghanaians and Caucasians. Clin Pharmacol Ther 26:584, 1979
104. Inaba T, Otton SV, Kalow W: Debrisoquine hydroxylation capacity: Problems of assessment in two populations. Clin Pharmacol Ther 29:218, 1981
105. Kalow W: Ethnic differences in drug metabolism. Clin Pharmacokinet 7:373, 1982
106. Nakamura K, Goto F, Ray WA, et al: Interethnic differences in genetic polymorphism of hydroxylation between Japanese and Caucasian populations. Clin Pharmacol Ther 38:402, 1985
107. Inaba T, Otton SV, Kalow W: Deficient metabolism of debrisoquine and sparteine. Clin Pharmacol Ther 27:547, 1980
108. Schmid B, Bircher J, Preisig R, Küpfer A: Polymorphic dextromethorphan metabolism: Cosegregation of oxidative O-demethylation with debrisoquin hydroxylation. Clin Pharmacol Ther 38:618, 1985
109. Boobis AB, Murray S, Hampden CE, Davies DS: Genetic polymorphism in drug oxidation: In vitro studies of human debrisoquine 4-hydroxylase and bufuralol 1'-hydroxylase activities. Biochem Pharmacol 34:65, 1985
110. Idle JR, Mahgoub A, Sloan TP, et al: Some observations on the oxidation phenotype status of Nigerian patients presenting with cancer. Cancer Lett 11:331, 1981
111. Ayesh R, Idle JR, Ritchie JC, et al: Metabolic oxidation phenotypes as markers for susceptibility of lung cancer. Nature 312:169, 1984
112. Cartwright RA, Philip PA, Rogers HJ, Glashan RW: Genetically determined debrisoquine oxidation capacity in bladder cancer. Carcinog Compr Surv 5:1191, 1984
113. Barbeau A, Cloutier T, Roy M, et al: Ecogenetics of Parkinson's disease: 4-Hydroxylation of debrisoquine. Lancet 1:1213, 1985
114. Boobis AR, Murray S, Kahn GC, et al: Substrate specificity of the form of cytochrome P-450 catalyzing the 4-hydroxylation of debrisoquine in man. Mol Pharmacol 23:474, 1983
115. Distlerath LM, Guengerich FP: Characterization of a human liver cytochrome P-450 involved in the oxidation of debrisoquine and other drugs by using antibodies raised to the analogous rat enzyme. Proc Natl Acad Sci USA 81:7348, 1984
116. Shimada T, Misono KS, Guengerich FP: Human liver microsomal cytochrome P-450 mephenytoin 4-hydroxylase, a prototype of genetic polymorphism in oxidative drug metabolism. Purification and characterization of two similar forms involved in the reaction. J Biol Chem 261:909, 1986

117. Nebert DW, Gonzalez FJ: P450 genes. Their structure, evolution and regulation. Annu Rev Biochem 56:945, 1987

118. Gonzalez FJ, Skoda RC, Kimura S, et al: Characterization of the common genetic defect in humans deficient in debrisoquin metabolism. Nature 331:442, 1988

119. DeLuca HF: Vitamin D metabolism and function. In Gross F, Labhart A, Mann T, Zander J (eds): Monographs on Endocrinology. Springer-Verlag, Berlin, 1979, p. 1

120. DeLuca HF: Vitamin D metabolism and function. Arch Intern Med 138:836, 1978

121. Griffin JE, Zerwekh JE: Impaired stimulation of 25-hydroxyvitamin D-24-hydroxylase in fibroblasts from a patient with vitamin D-dependent rickets, type II. J Clin Invest 72:1190, 1983

122. Dupont B, Oberfield SE, Smithwick EM, et al: Close genetic linkage between HLA and congenital adrenal hyperplasia (21-hydroxylase deficiency). Lancet 2:1309, 1977

123. White PC, New MI, Dupont B: HLA-linked congenital adrenal hyperplasia results from a defective gene encoding a cytochrome P-450 specific for steroid 21-hydroxylation. Proc Natl Acad Sci USA 81:7505, 1984

124. White PC, Chaplin DD, Weis JH, et al: Two steroid 21-hydroxylase genes are located in the murine S region. Nature 312:465, 1984

125. White PC, Grossberger D, Onufer BJ, et al: Two genes encoding steroid 21-hydroxylase are located near the genes encoding the fourth component of complement in man. Proc Natl Acad Sci USA 82:1089, 1985

126. Weinshilboum RM: Catecholamine biochemical genetics in human populations. In Breakefield XO (ed): Neurogenetics: Genetic Approaches to the Nervous System. Elsevier/North-Holland Biomedical Press, New York, 1979, p. 257

127. Weinshilboum RM, Sladek SL: Mercaptopurine pharmacogenetics: Monogenic inheritance of erythrocyte thiopurine methyltransferase activity. Am J Hum Genet 32:651, 1980

128. Kerremans AL, Lipsky JJ, Van Loon J, et al: Cephalosporin-induced hypoprothrombinemia: Possible role for thiol methylation of 1-methyltetrazone-5-thiol and 2-methyl-1,3,4-thiadizole-5-thiol. J Pharmacol Exp Ther 235:382, 1985

129. Lennard L, van Loon JA, Lilleyman JS, Weinshilboum RM: Thiopurine pharmacogenetics in leukemia: Correlation of erythrocyte thiopurine methyltransferase activity and 6-thioguanine nucleotide concentrations. Clin Pharmacol Ther 41:18, 1987

130. Arias IM, Gartner LM, Cohen M, et al: Chronic nonhemolytic unconjugated hyperbilirubinemia with glucuronyl transferase deficiency; clinical, biochemical, pharmacologic and genetic evidence for heterogeneity. Am J Med 47:395, 1969

131. Berk PD, Jones EA, Howe RB, Berlin NI: Disorders of bilirubin metabolism. In Bondy PK, Rosenberg LE (eds): Metabolic Control and Disease. 8th Ed. WB Saunders Philadelphia 1980, p 1009

132. Al-Waiz M, Ayesh R, Mitchell SC, et al: A genetic polymorphism of the N-oxidation of trimethylamine in humans. Clin Pharmacol Ther 42:588, 1987

133. Snyder LH: Studies in human inheritance. IX. The inheritance of taste deficiency in man. Ohio J Sci 32:436, 1932

134. Leguebe A: Génétique et anthropologie de la sensibilité à la phenylthiocarbamide. I. Fréquence du gène dans la population belge. Bull Inst R Sci Nat Belg 36:article 27, 1960

135. Barnicot NA: Taste deficiency for phenylthiourea in African negroes and Chinese. Ann Eugenics 15:248, 1950–51

136. O'Reilly RA, Aggeler PM, Hoag MS, et al: Hereditary transmission of exceptional resistance to coumarin anticoagulant drugs. The first reported kindred. N Engl J Med 271:809, 1964

137. O'Reilly RA: The second reported kindred with hereditary resistance to oral anticoagulant drugs. N Engl J Med 282:1448, 1970

138. Whitlon DS, Sadowski JA, Suttie JW: Mechanisms of coumarin action: Significance of vitamin K epoxide reductase inhibition. Biochemistry 17:1371, 1978

139. Jackson WB, Kaukeinen D: Resistance of wild Norway rats in North Carolina to warfarin rodenticide. Science 176:1343, 1972

140. Verhoeven GFM, Wilson JD: The syndromes of primary hormone resistance. Metabolism 28:253, 1979

141. Griffin JE, Wilson JD: The syndromes of androgen resistance. N Engl J Med 302:198, 1980

142. Imperato-McGinley J, Gautier T: Inherited 5α-reductase deficiency in man. Trends Genet 2:130, 1986

143. Meyer WJ III, Migeon BR, Migeon CJ: Locus on human X chromosome for dehydrotestosterone receptor and androgen insensitivity. Proc Natl Acad Sci USA 72:1469, 1975

144. Davis PB, Shelhamer JR, Kaliner M: Abnormal adrenergic and cholinergic sensitivity in cystic fibrosis. N Engl J Med 302:1453, 1980

145. McSwigan JD, Hanson DR, Lubiniecki A, et al: Down syndrome fibroblasts are hyperresponsive to β-adrenergic stimulation. Proc Natl Acad Sci USA 78:7670, 1981

146. Ziegler MG, Lake CR, Kopin IJ: Deficient sympathetic nervous response in familial dysautonomia. N Engl J Med 294:630, 1976

147. Schilling EE, Rechler MM, Grunfeld C, Rosenberg AM: Primary defect of insulin receptors in skin fibroblasts cultured from an infant with leprechaunism and insulin resistance. Proc Natl Acad Sci USA 76:5877, 1979

148. McIntyre OR, Sullivan LW, Jeffries GH, Silver RH: Pernicious anemia in childhood. N Engl J Med 272:981, 1965

149. Katz M, Lee SK, Cooper BA: Vitamin B_{12} malabsorption due to a biologically inert intrinsic factor. N Engl J Med 287:425, 1972

150. Tauro GP, Danks DM, Rowe PB, et al: Dihydrofolate reductase deficiency causing megaloblastic anemia in two families. N Engl J Med 294:466, 1976

151. Russell A, Statter M, Abzug-Horowitz S: Methionine dependent glutamic acid formiminotransferase deficiency. In Sperling O, de Vries H (eds): Inborn Errors of Metabolism in Man. S. Karger, Basel, 1978, p. 65

152. Erbe RW: Genetic aspects of folate metabolism. In Harris H, Hirschorn K (eds): Advances in Human Genetics. Vol. 9. Plenum, New York, 1979, p. 293

153. Delbrück A, Henkel E: A rare genetically determined variant of pseudocholinesterase in two German families with high plasma enzyme activity. Eur J Biochem 99:65, 1979

154. Von Wartburg JP, Schürch PM: Atypical human liver alcohol dehydrogenase. Ann NY Acad Sci 151:936, 1968

155. Stamatoyannopoulos G, Chen SH, Fukui M: Liver alcohol dehydrogenase in Japanese: High population frequency of atypical form and its possible role in alcohol sensitivity. Am J Hum Genet 27:789, 1975

156. Frey WA, Vallee BL: Digitalis metabolism and human liver alcohol dehydrogenase. Proc Natl Acad Sci USA 77:924, 1980

157. Bosron WF, Li T-K, Vallee BL: New molecular forms of human liver alcohol dehydrogenase: Isolation and characterization of $ADH_{Indianapolis}$. Proc Natl Acad Sci USA 77:5784, 1980

158. Ohlin H, Jerntop P, Bergstrom B, Almer L-O: Chlorpropamide-alcohol flushing, aldehyde dehydrogenase activity, and diabetic complications. Br Med J 285:838, 1982

159. Impraim C, Wang G, Yoshida A: Structural mutation in a major human aldehyde dehydrogenase gene results in loss of enzyme activity. Am J Hum Genet 34:837, 1982

160. Harada S, Agarwal DP, Goedde HW, et al: Possible protective role against alcoholism for aldehyde dehydrogenase isozyme deficiency in Japan. Lancet 2:827, 1982

161. Meyer UA: Intermittent acute porphyria: Clinical and biochemical studies of disordered heme biosynthesis. Enzyme 16:334, 1973

162. Nordmann Y, Grandchamp B: Hereditary coproporphyria: Demonstration of a genetic defect in coproporphyrinogen metabolism. Monogr Hum Genet 10:217, 1978

163. Brenner DA, Bloomer JR: The enzymatic defect in variegate porphyria. Studies with human cultured skin fibroblasts. N Engl J Med 302:765, 1980

164. De Verneuil H, Aitken G, Nordmann Y: Familial and sporadic porphyria cutanea: Two different diseases. Hum Genet 44:145, 1978

165. De Verneuil H, Grandchamp B, Beaumont C, et al: Uroporphyrinogen decarboxylase structural mutant ($Gly^{281} \rightarrow$ Glu) in a case of porphyria. Science 234:732, 1986

166. Stewart FP, Smith AG: Metabolism of the "mixed" cytochrome P-450 inducer hexachlorobenzene by rat liver microsomes. Biochem Pharmacol 35:2163, 1986

167. Poland A, Glover E: 2,3,7,8-Tetrachlorodibenzo-*p*-dioxin: a potent inducer of σ-aminolevulinic acid synthetase. Science 179:476, 1973

168. Eisen HJ, Hannah RR, Legraverend C, et al: The *Ah* receptor: Controlling factor in the induction of drug-metabolizing enzymes by certain chemical carcinogens and other environmental pollutants. In Litwack G (ed): Biochemical Actions of Hormones. Vol. 10. Academic Press, Orlando, FL, 1983, p. 227

169. Poland AP, Glover E, Kende AS: Stereospecific, high affinity binding of 2,3,7,8-tetrachlorodibenzo-*p*-dioxin by hepatic cytosol. Evidence that the binding species is the receptor for the induction of aryl hydrocarbon hydroxylase. J Biol Chem 251:4936, 1976

170. Hannah RR, Nebert DW, Eisen HJ: Regulatory gene product of the *Ah* complex. Comparison of 2,3,7,8-tetrachlorodibenzo-*p*-dioxin and 3-methylcholanthrene binding to several moieties in mouse liver cytosol. J Biol Chem 256:4584, 1981

171. Nebert DW, Jones JE: Regulation of the mammalian cytochrome P_1450 (*CYP1A1*) gene. Int J Biochem 21:243, 1989

172. Nebert DW: Multiple forms of inducible drug-metabolizing enzymes. A reasonable mechanism by which any organism can cope with adversity. Mol Cell Biochem 27:27, 1979

173. Gonzalez FJ, Tukey RH, Nebert DW: Structural gene products of the *Ah* locus. Transcriptional regulation of cytochrome P_1-450 and P_3-450 mRNA levels by 3-methylcholanthrene. Mol Pharmacol 26:117, 1984

174. Negishi M, Jensen NM, Garcia CS, Nebert DW: Structural gene products of the murine *Ah* locus. Differences in ontogenesis, membrane location, and glucosamine incorporation between liver microsomal cytochromes P_1-450 and P-448 induced by polycyclic aromatic compounds. Eur J Biochem 115:585, 1981

175. Negishi M, Nebert DW: Structural gene products of the *Ah* locus. Genetic and immunochemical evidence for two forms of mouse liver cytochrome P-450 induced by 3-methylcholanthrene. J Biol Chem 254:11015, 1979

176. Pelkonen O, Nebert DW: Metabolism of polycyclic aromatic hydrocarbons: Etiologic role in carcinogenesis. Pharmacol Rev 34:189, 1982

177. Kouri RE, McLemore T, Jaiswal AK, Nebert DW: Current cellular assays for measuring clinical drug metabolizing capacity—Impact of new molecular biologic techniques. In Goedde HW, Kalow W (eds): Ethnic Differences in Adverse Reactions to Drugs and Other Xenobiotics. Alan R Liss, New York, 1986, p. 453

178. Kellermann G, Luyten-Kellermann M, Shaw CR: Genetic variation of aryl hydrocarbon hydroxylase in human lymphocytes. Am J Hum Genet 25:327, 1973

179. Atlas SA, Vesell ES, Nebert DW: Genetic control of interindividual variations in the inducibility of aryl hydrocarbon hydroxylase in cultured human lymphocytes. Cancer Res 36:4619, 1976

180. Kouri RE, McKinney CE, Slomiany DJ, et al: Positive correlation between high aryl hydrocarbon hydroxylase activity and primary lung cancer as analyzed in cryopreserved lymphocytes. Cancer Res 42:5030, 1982

181. Kellermann G, Shaw CR, Luyten-Kellermann M: Aryl hydrocarbon hydroxylase inducibility and bronchogenic carcinoma. N Engl J Med 289:934, 1973

182. Legraverend C, Harrison DE, Ruscetti FW, Nebert DW: Bone marrow toxicity induced by oral benzo[a]pyrene: Protection residues at the level of the intestine and liver. Toxicol Appl Pharmacol 70:390, 1983

183. Blumer JL, Dunn R, Esterhay MD, et al: Lymphocyte aromatic hydrocarbon responsiveness in acute leukemia of childhood. Blood 58:1081, 1981

184. Levine AS, McKinney CE, Echelberger CK, et al: Aryl hydrocarbon hydroxylase inducibility among primary relatives of children with leukemia or solid tumors. Cancer Res 44:358, 1984

185. Jaiswal AK, Gonzalez FJ, Nebert DW: Human P_1-*450* gene sequence and correlation of mRNA with genetic differences in benzo[a]pyrene metabolism. Nucl Acids Res 13:4503, 1985

186. Jaiswal AK, Nebert DW: Two RFLPs associated with the human $P_1$450 gene near the MPI locus on chromosome 15. Nucleic Acids Res 14:4376, 1986

187. Jaiswal AK, Nebert DW, Eisen HJ: Comparison of aryl hydrocarbon hydroxylase and acetanilide 4-hydroxylase induction by polycyclic aromatic compounds in human and mouse cell lines. Biochem Pharmacol 34:2721, 1985

188. Hildebrand CE, Gonzalez FJ, McBride OW, Nebert DW: Assignment of the human 2,3,7,8-tetrachlorodibenzo-p-dioxin-inducible cytochrome P_1-450 gene to chromosome 15. Nucleic Acids Res 13:2009, 1985

189. Gonzalez FJ, Vilbois F, Hardwick JP, et al: Human debrisoquine 4-hydroxylase (P450IID1): cDNA and deduced amino acid sequence and assignment of the *CYP2D* locus to chromosome 22. Genomics 2:174, 1988

190. Beierwaltes WH, Carr EA Jr, Hunter RL: Hereditary increase in the thyroxine-binding sites in the serum alpha globulin. Trans Assoc Am Physicians 74:170, 1961

191. Ingbar SH: Clinical and physiological observations in a patient with an idiopathic decrease in the thyroxine-binding globulin of plasma. J Clin Invest 40:2053, 1961

192. Marshall JS, Levy RP, Steinberg AG: Human thyroxine-binding globulin deficiency. A genetic study. N Engl J Med 274:1469, 1966

193. Refetoff S, Selenkow HA: Familial thyroxine-binding globulin deficiency in a patient with Turner's syndrome (XO). Genetic study of a kindred. N Engl J Med 278:1081, 1968

194. Czaja MJ, Weiner FR, Schwarzenberg SJ, et al: Molecular studies of ceruloplasmin deficiency in Wilson's disease. J Clin Invest 80:1200, 1987

195. Armaly MF: Genetic factors related to glaucoma. Ann NY Acad Sci 151:861, 1968

196. Britt BA, Kalow W: Malignant hyperthermia: A statistical review. Can Anaesth Soc J 17:293, 1970

197. Kalow W, Britt BA, Chan F: Epidemiology and inheritance of malignant hyperthermia. Int Anesthesiol Clin 17:119, 1979

198. Ellis FR, Cain PA, Harriman DGF: Multifactorial inheritance of malignant hyperthermia susceptibility. In Aldrete JA, Britt BA (eds): Proc 2nd Int Symp Malignant Hyperthermia. Grune & Stratton, Orlando, FL, 1978, p. 329

199. Gronert GA: Malignant hyperthermia. Anesthesiology 53:395, 1980

200. Gronert GA, Theye RA: Halothane-induced porcine malignant hyperthermia: Metabolic and hemodynamic changes. Anesthesiology 44:36, 1976

201. Moulds RFW, Denborough MA: Identification of susceptibility to malignant hyperpyrexia. Br Med J 2:245, 1974

202. Cousins MJ, Sharp JH, Gourlay GK, et al: Hepatotoxicity and halothane metabolism in an animal model with application for human toxicity. Anaesth Intensive Care 7:9, 1979

203. Hoft RH, Bunker JP, Goodman HI, Gregory PB: Halothane hepatitis in three pairs of closely related women. N Engl J Med 304:1023, 1981

204. Farrell G, Prendergast D, Murray M: Halothane hepatitis. Detection of a constitutional susceptibility factor. N Engl J Med 313:1310, 1985

205. Trudell JR, Bösterling B, Trevor AJ: Reductive metabolism of halothane by human and rabbit cytochrome P-450. Binding of 1-chloro-2,2,2-trifluoroethyl radical to phospholipids. Mol Pharmacol 21:710, 1982

206. Krieter PA, Van Dyke RA: Cytochrome P-450 and halothane metabolism. Decrease in rat liver microsomal P-450 in vitro. Chem Biol Interact 44:219, 1983

207. Satoh H, Gillette JR, Davies HW, et al: Immunochemical evidence of trifluoroacetylated cytochrome P-450 in the liver of halothane-treated rats. Mol Pharmacol 28:468, 1985

208. Spielberg P, Gordon GB, Blake DA, et al: Predisposition to phenytoin hepatotoxicity assessed in vitro. N Engl J Med 305:722, 1981

209. Yunis AA: Chloramphenicol-induced bone marrow suppression. Semin Hematol 10:225, 1973

210. Miller NE, Halpert J: Analogues of chloramphenicol as mechanism-based inactivators of rat liver cytochrome P-450: Modifications of the propanediol side chain, the *p*-nitro group, and the dichloromethyl moiety. Mol Pharmacol 29:391, 1986
211. Hassell TM, Page RC, Narayanan AS, Cooper CG: Diphenylhydantoin (Dilantin) gingival hyperplasia: Drug-induced abnormality of connective tissue. Proc Natl Acad Sci USA 73:2909, 1976
212. Lewis GP, Jick H, Slone D, Shapiro S: The role of genetic factors and serum protein binding in determining drug response as revealed by comprehensive drug surveillance. Ann NY Acad Sci 179:729, 1971
213. Motulsky AG: Drug reactions, enzymes and biochemical genetics. JAMA 165:835, 1957
214. Omenn GS, Motulsky AG: "Eco-genetics": Genetic variations in susceptibility to environmental agents. In Cohen B, Lilienfeld AM, Huang PC (eds): Genetic Issues in Public Health and Medicine. Charles C Thomas, Springfield, IL, 1978, p. 83
215. Kalow W: Pharmacoanthropology: Outline, problems, and the nature of case histories. Fed Proc 43:2314, 1984
216. Botstein D, White R, Skolnick M, Davis RW: Construction of a genetic linkage map in man using restriction fragment length polymorphisms. Am J Human Genet 32:314, 1980
217. Landegren U, Kaiser R, Caskey CT, Hood L: DNA diagnostics—Molecular techniques and automation. Science 242:229, 1988
218. Haldane JBS: Heredity and Politics. WW Norton, New York, 1938

GENERAL REFERENCES

Boobis AR, Caldwell J, DeMatteis F, Elcombe CF: Microsomes and Drug Oxidations. Taylor & Francis, London, 1985
Brown SS, Kalow W, Pilz W, et al: The plasma cholinesterases: A new perspective. Adv Clin Chem 22:1, 1981
Evans DAP: Survey of the human acetylator polymorphism in spontaneous disorders. J Med Genet 21:243, 1984
François J: Corticosteroid glaucoma. Ophthalmalogica 188:76, 1984
Jakoby WB: Enzymatic Basis of Detoxication. Vol. 1. Academic Press, Orlando, FL, 1980
Kalow W: Contribution of hereditary factors to the response to drugs. Fed Proc 24:1259, 1965
Lieber CS: Medical disorders of alcoholism. Pathogenesis and treatment. Major Prob Intern Med 22:589, 1982
Nebert DW: Genetic differences in susceptibility to chemically induced myelotoxicity and leukemia. Environ Health Perspect 39:11, 1981
Nebert DW, Nelson DR, Adesnik M, et al: The P450 superfamily: Updated listing of all genes and recommended nomenclature for the chromosomal loci. DNA 8:1, 1989
New MI: Congenital Adrenal Hyperplasia. The New York Hospital–Cornell Medical Center, New York, 1985
Omenn GS, Gelboin HV: Genetic Variability in Responses to Chemical Exposure, Banbury Report 16. Cold Spring Harbor Laboratory, Cold Spring Harbor, NY, 1984
Pratt WB, Fekety R: The Antimicrobial Drugs. Oxford University Press, New York, 1986
Stanbury JB, Wyngaarden JB, Fredrickson DS, et al: The Metabolic Basis of Inherited Disease. 5th Ed. McGraw-Hill, New York, 1983
Stern C: Principles of Human Genetics. 3rd Ed. WH Freeman, San Francisco, 1973
Vesell ES: On the significance of host factors that affect drug disposition. Clin Pharmacol Ther 31:1, 1982
Weber WW: The Acetylator Genes and Drug Response. Oxford University Press, New York, 1987
Weinshilboum RM: ASPET Symposium on "Human Pharmacogenetics." Fed Proc 43:2295, 1984

8

Drug Allergy

William B. Pratt

Drug allergy is an adverse reaction to a drug resulting from previous sensitization to that same drug or a closely related one. The term *hypersensitivity* has often been used to describe the allergic state. This word is inappropriate as applied to drug allergy because its literal meaning invites confusion with other kinds of adverse drug reaction. One could properly describe as hypersensitive the normal therapeutic responses of the people at the lower end of the frequency distribution in a quantal log dose-response curve (i.e., those individuals who are sensitive to a very low dose of a drug). One could also reasonably describe as hypersensitivity an idiosyncratic response at a low dosage level to the therapeutic or toxic effects of a drug in a genetically predisposed person. There has been a lack of precision in the diagnosis of drug allergies and often a failure to apply clear-cut criteria to their classification. Ambiguous terminology adds to the confusion. We shall avoid the term hypersensitivity and describe as drug allergy those drug reactions that have an obvious (or inferred) immunologic basis.[1–7]

In order for a drug to produce an allergic reaction, a prior *sensitizing* contact is required, either with the same drug or with one closely related chemically. A period of time is required—usually about 7 to 14 days—for the synthesis of significant amounts of drug-specific antibodies. Then exposure to the drug (the *eliciting* contact) results in an antigen-antibody interaction, which provokes the typical manifestations of allergy. However, there need be no drug-free interval between the sensitizing contact and the eliciting contact; thus, allergic sensitization could occur early and allergic response later during the same course of treatment. The manifestations of allergy are numerous. They involve various organ systems, and they range in severity from minor skin lesions to fatal anaphylactic shock. The pattern of allergic response differs in different species. In humans, involvement of the skin is most common, whereas in the guinea pig, for example, bronchiolar constriction leading to asphyxia is typical. The pattern of response is somewhat conditioned by the route of sensitization and the route of subsequent administration and by the particular drug employed. A certain drug may preferentially elicit one or several responses from among the whole pattern of possible responses. Sulfonamide allergy, for example, is usually manifested by dermatitis, conjunctivitis, or fever; penicillin, on the other hand, most frequently elicits urticaria ("hives") and generalized itching. Unrelated drugs, once they have sensitized, may also elicit the same allergic response, such as dermatitis, anaphylaxis, or angioedema. Thus, the allergic response is a consequence of the antigen-antibody interaction and has nothing directly to do with the chemical structure of the eliciting drug.

Drug allergy may be compared and contrasted with drug toxicity and drug idiosyncrasy, as follows:

1. *Occurrence*. This is not necessarily a distinguishing criterion, since all three kinds of adverse drug reactions may be common or rare, depending upon the drug. Most idiosyncrasies are rare because any given abnormal genotype is likely to be rare, but if a genetic polymorphism (such as inability to taste phenylthiocarbamide [PTC]) is related to a drug idiosyncrasy, the frequency may be quite high. Although drug allergy, with most drugs, is seen in no more than a few percent of all who are exposed, some chemicals can cause allergic sensitization in nearly everyone exposed to them. Genetic predisposition to allergy may play a role in that atopic persons (i.e., persons with allergies in general) appear to have an increased susceptibility to immediate allergic reactions of the anaphylactic type.[3] Other types of allergic drug reactions occur at about the same frequency in atopic individuals as in the general population. In contrast, individuals experiencing an idiosyncratic drug reaction have a clear genetic predisposition to an unusual reaction to a particular drug or class of drugs.
2. *Dose relationship*. Toxic side effects are clearly dose-related, as are idiosyncratic responses in susceptible individuals. In both cases the usual dose-effect principles apply, since the responses are mediated directly by specific drug-receptor interactions. In contrast, allergic responses have an erratic relationship to dosage. Extremely small doses (e.g., traces of antibiotics in foodstuffs) suffice to sensitize in some cases. It is also clear that minute doses can elicit allergic responses in previously sensitized individuals, and the magnitude of the response has little to do with the size of the eliciting dose. Sometimes a mere trace of drug (e.g., a fraction of a microgram contaminating a syringe) elicits life-threatening manifestations of allergy; sometimes full therapeutic doses evoke only mild allergic effects. It appears that the magnitude of an allergic response is determined primarily by immunologic factors in the individual and that the drug (at whatever dose) may serve chiefly to "trigger" the reaction.
3. *Prior contact with drug*. Although prior exposure to a drug is not necessary for toxic side effects or idiosyncratic responses, it is essential for allergic reactions. However, sensitization may occur covertly by environmental or dietary exposure (e.g., penicillin in cow's milk or in moldy foods) so that allergic responses may occur without known prior exposure.
4. *Chemical specificity*. Toxic side effects and drug idiosyncrasies are directly and specifically determined by the chemical structure of the drug, and typical structure-activity relationships can be established. In drug allergy, the responses are determined by antigen-antibody reactions, and they are largely independent of which drug molecule elicits them. Here the structure-activity relationships concern the chemical structures of the sensitizing drugs and of the eliciting drugs. Some are more effective than others in sensitizing. If a particular drug does sensitize, then only this drug or closely related congeners will elicit the allergic response. Thus, the interactions

leading to the allergic state as well as those producing allergic responses may show a high degree of specificity related to chemical structure, as discussed later in this chapter.

5. *Mechanisms.* In drug allergy, the immunologic basis can often be established by demonstrating circulating antibodies in serum or altered immunologic responses in tissues. The antibodies are specific for the sensitizing drug and closely related compounds, but as already indicated, the manifestations of drug allergy are unrelated to any particular drug. In contrast, the nature of a toxic or idiosyncratic reaction to a drug is determined by that drug. A corollary is that toxic or idiosyncratic reactions are overcome or prevented by antagonists that are specific for the drug that precipitated the reaction. In drug allergy, on the other hand, specific drug antagonists are useless, but antihistamines, epinephrine, and hydrocortisone, whose actions are directed toward the general manifestations of the allergic response, may be effective.

IMMUNOLOGIC BASIS OF DRUG ALLERGY

Vertebrates have evolved a variety of defenses against infection that are collectively referred to as *the immune system.* It was observed in ancient times that prior exposure to an infectious disease afforded protection against subsequent attacks by the infectious organism. To achieve that state of immunity, the immune system has to be able not only to identify the organism or foreign agent but to recognize it as different from itself and then to mount a very specific response to it through the synthesis of antibodies. The immune system possesses another remarkable quality and that is memory, for each time it comes in contact with that organism or agent, it recognizes it and responds by again synthesizing antibody.

There are two arms of the immune system: one is the lymphocytic division, which is associated with cellular immunity, and the other is the plasmacytic division, which is responsible for humoral immunity. Cell-mediated immunity is considered to be that form of immunity that can be transferred by cells rather than serum; in addition to affording protection against pathogens, it is also implicated in graft rejection and in certain delayed allergic drug reactions. Humoral immunity refers to the production of circulating antibodies, and the immunity can be transferred either by serum or by the antibody-producing cells. In humoral immunity the plasma cells are the most important cell type involved in antibody synthesis, with lymphoblasts also responsible for some antibody production. A wide variety of allergic drug reactions are due to humoral antibodies that either are freely circulating or have become fixed to a cell surface (so-called cytotropic or reagenic antibodies).

Immunoglobulins

In 1939 Tiselius and Kabat[8] demonstrated that antibody activity is associated with the γ-globulin fraction of serum. Because of the heterogeneity of the molecules that function as antibodies, they are referred to as *immunoglobulins.* The immunoglobulins can be subdivided into five distinct classes: IgA, IgG, IgM, IgD, and IgE.[9-12] The common feature of the immunoglobulins, shown in Figure 8-1, is a symmetrical structure of heavy and light chains, each with a variable and a constant region. In the constant region of a given immunoglobulin class, the polypeptide chain is composed of an identical or near identical

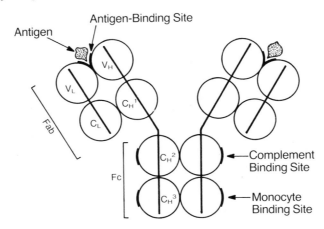

Fig. 8-1. Structure of a typical immunoglobulin molecule. The polypeptide chains are shown as solid lines; NH_2-terminal regions comprise the antigen binding site. V_H = variable region, heavy chain; C_H = constant regions, heavy chain; V_L, C_L = variable and constant regions, light chain. Limited proteolytic attack at the hinge region (the angle in the line defining the heavy chain) cleaves the molecule into Fab and Fc fragments.

amino acid sequence. This homology extends across species and is found even in primitive organisms. In contrast, the variable region is composed of a variety of different amino acid sequences, although the total number of amino acid residues remains the same.

The antigen binding sites are formed by residues contributed by the variable portions of a light and a heavy chain. It is generally accepted that lymphoid cells differentiate in such a way that a given cell retains the capacity to produce only a single immunoglobulin. All the lymphoid cells together, however, produce thousands of different immunoglobulins. According to the clonal theory,[13] if a cell comes into contact with an antigen any part of which happens to "fit" its antigen binding site, that cell is stimulated to divide and increase its production of that particular globulin. Since each region of a given antigen may more or less fit a number of different antigen binding sites, a considerable array is likely to be produced of different antibodies directed toward the several antigenic determinants of the antigen molecule. Some types of antibodies, such as IgG and IgM, are secreted into the plasma, where they comprise the well-known soluble γ-globulins. Others, such as IgE, are found in serum only in very small amounts and are cytotropic—they are carried to cells in the skin and other tissues, where they become fixed to the cell surface.

In normal serum, IgG is the major immunoglobulin class. IgG has a molecular mass of about 150,000 and is the type of immunoglobulin predominantly produced following a secondary antigenic challenge. IgM has a molecular mass of about 900,000 and is synthesized largely during a primary immune response. In fact, IgM immunoglobulins are the first class detected following primary exposure to antigen. The IgA immunoglobulins are present selectively at mucosal surfaces, in saliva, tears, and colostrum and in secretions of the tracheobronchial, gastrointestinal, and genitourinary tracts. The IgD immunoglobulins are located on B lymphocytes, where they appear to regulate activation and suppression of the lymphocyte. After its secretion from plasma cells, IgE becomes bound almost exclusively to mast cells and basophilic leukocytes.

Some of the immunoglobulins contain complement-binding sites. Complement is a system of at least 11 serum proteins that are activated by an antigen-antibody complex of the IgG or IgM class. Formation of the antigen-antibody complex exposes a complement-binding site (Fig. 8-1). A cascade of protein conversions is initiated, much as in the blood coagulation system. The resulting liberation of proteins, with deleterious effects on cell surfaces, may cause cell death or may lead to release of histamine from mast cells and platelets, enhanced phagocytosis by leukocytes, contraction of smooth muscle and release of a variety of mediators such as leukotrienes (SRSA [slow-reacting substance of anaphylaxis]), platelet-aggregating factor, interleukins, and lymphokines.[14]

Classification of Allergic Reactions

Allergic responses may be classified according to the basic mechanism underlying the pathophysiologic response[15,16] (Fig. 8-2).

Type I: Immediate or Anaphylactic Reaction. The type I reaction occurs when drugs cause the production of IgE antibodies that become fixed to the surface of basophils or mast cells. On subsequent exposure, the drug binds to cell-fixed IgE, causing the release of pharmacologically active substances, such as histamine, serotonin, and slow-reacting substance of anaphylaxis (SRSA), which trigger an immune reaction that can be rapid in onset. The effects may be localized to the bronchial tree, as in an asthmatic attack or acute laryngeal edema, or to the skin, as in urticaria or hives, or they may be more generalized and result in hypotension, edema, and shock (anaphylactic shock). Type I reactions are sometimes called *reagin-dependent* reactions, and they cause the local wheal and flare response observed during the skin testing of patients for the presence of drug allergy.

Type II: Antibody-Dependent Cytotoxicity. In a type II reaction, the drug binds to or reacts with surface components of a cell, such as a red cell, causing it to appear to be foreign. This evokes the production of antibodies that can react with the cell-bound drug. The subsequent antigen-antibody reaction may trigger the activation of the complement system or permit attack by mononuclear killer cells. The results may be death of the target cell. In the case of the red cell, for example, drug-induced hemolysis occurs.

Type III: Damage Due to Immune Complexes. A type III reaction occurs when the drug antigen reacts in blood or tissue spaces with soluble antibody. The resulting immune complexes may deposit on the walls of blood vessels, at basement membranes, etc., causing local inflammation or complement activation. Serum sickness, allergic arteritis, granulocytopenia, hemolysis, and some forms of allergic nephritis are examples of type III reactions induced by drugs.

Type IV: Cell-Mediated Reaction. The type IV reaction is also called a *delayed* or *tuberculin-type* reaction because hours or days elapse for the reaction to occur after administration of an eliciting dose of antigen to a sensitized person or animal. In the type IV reaction a cell-mediated immune response is activated, resulting in the infiltration of mononuclear cells. This type of drug reaction occurs mainly in the skin, where the drug combines with the skin proteins, making them appear foreign to the immune system and evoking the cell-mediated immune response. Sensitized T lymphocytes, which produce T cell receptors appropriate for reacting with the protein-bound or membrane-bound drug antigen, recognize it and release lymphokines, which produce local edema and inflammation. In this type of drug reaction the skin is the major route of sensitization and the chief site of allergic response.

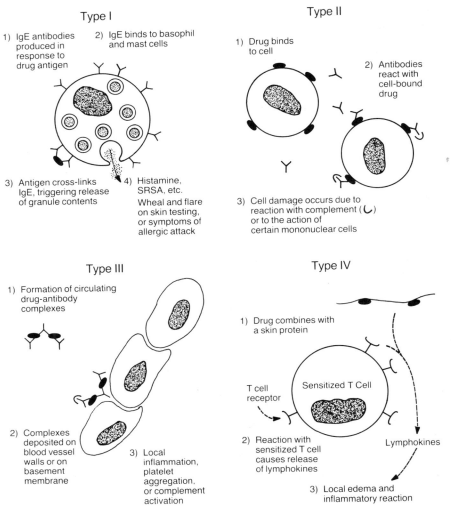

Fig. 8-2. Classification of allergic reactions according to four basic mechanisms. *Type I* includes reactions of the immediate or anaphylactic type; *type II,* antibody-dependent cytotoxicity reactions; *type III,* damage due to antigen-antibody complexes; and *type IV,* cell mediated reactions. This classification according to mechanism underlying the pathophysiologic response is sometimes referred to as the Coombs-Gell classification.[15] See text for details.

Covalently Bonded Drug-Protein Conjugates

Some drugs, such as the hormone insulin or the enzyme L-asparaginase, which is used in the treatment of cancer, are large enough to act as complete antigens and by themselves to elicit the production of antibodies. There is, however, a general limit below which molecules do not have sufficient molecular mass to be immunogenic. It was found with a series of oligo-L-lysine derivatives, for example, that molecules with fewer than seven amino acids, about 1,100 daltons, are not immunogenic, whereas polymers above this limit are immunogenic.[17] Most drugs have molecular masses less than 1,100, and to elicit an immune response they must be covalently bound to larger molecules, usually proteins.

Because of this requirement for coupling to larger molecules, special techniques had to be developed to investigate the immunologic basis of drug allergies. These techniques were worked out in the course of a remarkable series of experiments, largely in the laboratory of Karl Landsteiner (1892–1943) who summarized the methods and results in a classic treatise.[18] Prior to these experiments it was assumed that antigen specificity resided entirely in the protein used as antigen. The basic discovery that upset this idea and opened the way to further progress was the finding that when proteins were acylated they would display altered specificity as antigens. Acylation was carried out with the anhydrides or chlorides of butyric, isobutyric, trichloroacetic, and anisic acids. These groups were coupled chiefly to ε-amino groups of lysine residues. Immune serum prepared against an acylated protein would react more strongly with the acylated protein than with the same protein that had not been acylated. Numerous compounds of low molecular weight could be linked to proteins by acylation or by diazo coupling reactions (to tyrosine, histidine, or lysine residues) to form "artificial conjugated antigens." The simple chemicals thus conjugated to proteins were called *haptens*.

The proof that immunologic specificity could be directed against a hapten was obtained by experiments in which the same hapten was used for immunizing and for testing but was attached to proteins derived from different species (e.g., hapten-horse serum for immunizing a rabbit and hapten-chicken serum for testing the antibodies by a precipitin reaction). In these investigations it was discovered that antibodies to a given hapten also reacted in varying degree with chemically related compounds. Sometimes a particular grouping of atoms could act as an antigenic determinant—e.g., the 2-chlorobenzene portion of a complex azobenzene derivative.[19]

Table 8-1 presents a selection of these experimental results. The high degree of specificity of the immune sera is shown by the reactivity of immune serum prepared against *o*-aminocinnamic acid (A), which did not react with any other hapten, even *o*-aminobenzenesulfonic acid (E). The other data in this table well illustrate the limits of specificity and of cross-reactivity.

A modification of the technique described above permits the use of hapten molecules themselves in the testing procedure. If an immune serum has been prepared against a certain hapten-protein conjugate and the same hapten (unconjugated) is introduced into the incubation mixture at the time of testing, it will compete for antibody and thus inhibit the precipitin reaction. The reason is that the complex of the small hapten molecule with the immunoglobulin remains soluble. This phenomenon is known as *hapten inhibition*. Competition for antigen combining sites is also the basis of immunoassay procedures. Another method permits allergic hemagglutination reactions to be tested and quantitated in vitro. A hapten-erythrocyte conjugate, which can be formed in vitro, is used to sensitize an appropriate animal (usually a rabbit). The antibodies that appear in the rabbit serum will then react in vitro with erythrocytes bearing hapten molecules, causing their agglutination.[20] The usefulness of this technique in studying the basis of allergic drug phenomena is illustrated by investigations on penicillin allergy, discussed later in the chapter.

The principles developed in the pioneering studies cited above were further applied in investigations dealing with skin sensitization in guinea pigs.[21] Picryl chloride (2,4,6-trinitrochlorobenzene), 2,4-dinitrochlorobenzene, and 2,4-dinitrofluorobenzene were used. These compounds form covalent linkages with free amino groups; 2-4-dinitrofluorobenzene is the same reagent first used to establish the primary sequence of proteins by combining with the NH_2 group of the terminal amino acid at each step of a sequential degradation.[22] When such reagents were injected intradermally into guinea pigs, local

Table 8-1. Specificity and Cross-Reactivity of Immune Sera to Azoprotein Antigens

Antigens	Immune Sera[a]			
	(A)	(B)	(C)	(D)
(A)	+ + +	0	0	0
(E)	0	+ + +	0	0
(B)	0	+ + + +	+	+
(C)	0	0	+ + + +	+ + +

(*continued*)

Table 8-1. (*continued*)

Antigens	Immune Sera[a]			

Immune Sera header compounds:

- (A) o-aminocinnamic acid type: NH₂ benzene with CH=CHCOOH
- (B) m-aminobenzenesulfonic acid: NH₂ benzene with SO₃H (meta)
- (C) p-aminobenzenesulfonic acid: NH₂ benzene with SO₃H (para)
- (D) aminotoluenesulfonic acid: NH₂ benzene with CH₃ and SO₃H

Antigen	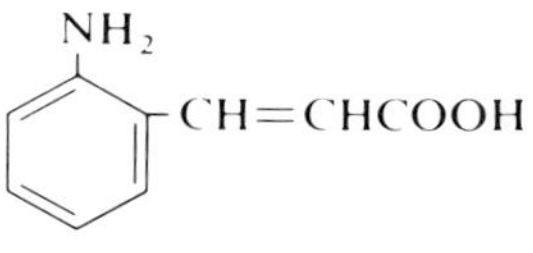 (A)	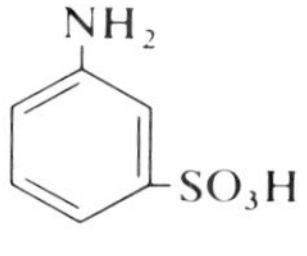 (B)	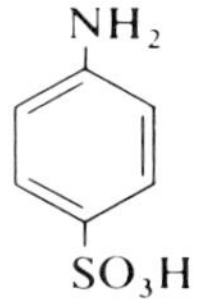 (C)	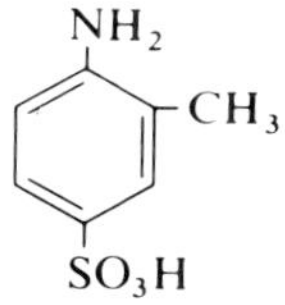 (D)
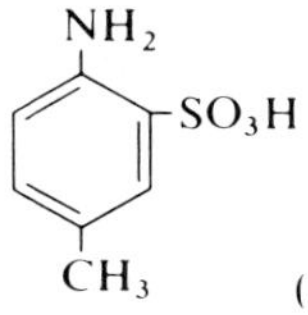 (F) NH₂/SO₃H/CH₃	0	+ +	0	0
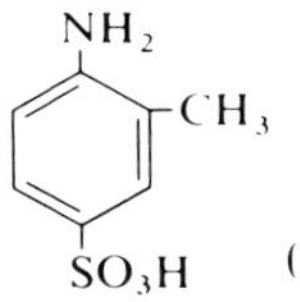 (D) NH₂/CH₃/SO₃H	0	0	+ + +	+ + + +
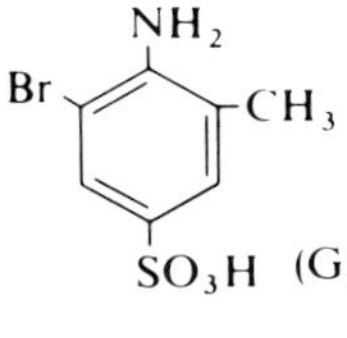 (G) Br, NH₂/CH₃/SO₃H	0	0	0	+ + +
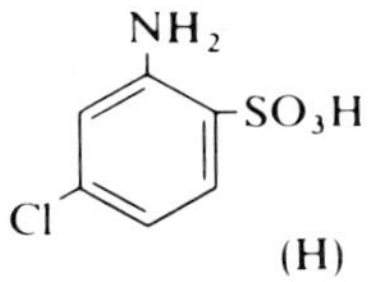 (H) NH₂/SO₃H/Cl	0	+	0	0

[a] The compounds shown at top (A to D) were diazotized and coupled to horse serum proteins. These were used to immunize rabbits, and the rabbit antisera were used in the tests. The same four compounds and four others (A to H) were diazotized and coupled to chicken serum proteins; these were used as antigens in the tests. The testing procedure consisted of adding a few drops of an immune serum to a dilute solution of the hapten-protein antigen and recording the intensity of precipitation (0 to 4 +). (Modified from Landsteiner and Lampl,[19] with permission.)

sensitization resulted, and skin reactions could be elicited subsequently by reapplication of the same reagent. Sensitization of the skin could also be brought about by intraperitoneal injection of the allergenic agent accompanied by killed mycobacteria as adjuvant. (An adjuvant is a substance, usually not antigenic itself, that enhances antibody formation in response to an antigen.) Even better skin sensitization resulted from coupling the reactive chemical to erythrocyte stromata and injecting this artificial conjugate intraperitoneally. Combined injection of the artificial conjugates with mycobacteria in paraffin oil led to sensitization when the intramuscular route was used. The sensitivity to delayed-type contact dermatitis thus induced could be passively transferred to a recipient animal by lymphocytes or by cell exudates from lymphocytes.[23] After injection of such cellular material, the skin of the recipient, which had never been exposed to the allergenic chemical, acquired specific sensitivity within 12 hours to 2 days.

These studies of sensitization of the skin are of interest because they mimic so closely the course of events in human contact dermatitis. Sensitization appears to be most effective by direct application of the allergen to the skin, presumably because conjugates have to be formed with the skin proteins. Subsequently the dermatitis can be elicited either by topical reapplication of the allergen or by its administration via a systemic route. It has been shown[24] that when dinitrochlorobenzene is applied to guinea pig skin, nearly all of it that becomes fixed in the epidermis is bound to lysine groups in the proteins of the malpighian layer at the junction of the epidermis and corium. This binding is thought to be essential for the development of the typical delayed-type skin allergy (type IV in Fig. 8-2). Dinitrochlorobenzene conjugates with homologous (i.e., guinea pig) serum or with heterologous protein (egg albumin) caused sensitization of the immediate type (type I in Fig. 8-2), with circulating antibodies demonstrable but no skin allergy. On the other hand, conjugates of the same hapten with guinea pig skin protein injected into the foot pad of the guinea pig led to a typical delayed-type allergy of the contact dermatitis type (type IV in Fig. 8-2); no circulating antibodies developed, but passive transfer could be achieved with lymphoid cells. Thus, the development of allergic contact dermatitis requires sensitization with a conjugate of hapten and skin protein.

The success of these experimental approaches in producing suitable models of drug allergy raised the question of whether a hapten must necessarily form a covalent linkage to a protein in order to act as an antigen. In one study,[25] a series of reactive chemicals was tested on rabbits to see if there was any correlation between antigenicity and the ability to combine with free amino groups of proteins. The highest antibody titers were found with those compounds that were capable of forming covalent bonds at body pH and at low temperature and were not readily metabolized. A similar and even more dramatic indication of the importance of covalent attachment came from experiments with 2,4-dinitrochlorobenzene.[18] This compound causes an allergic contact dermatitis in factory workers exposed to it, and as indicated above, guinea pigs can also be sensitized to it. There are approximately 90 chloro- and nitro-substituted benzenes. In experiments carried out with 17 of these, it was found that guinea pigs could be sensitized to 10. Not one of the 7 inert compounds would combine with the amino groups of aniline in vitro, but all 10 that sensitized were able to do so. On the other hand, most drugs in therapeutic use, including many that are prone to cause allergic sensitization, are not chemically reactive compounds—at least they are certainly not comparable in reactivity with the diazotizing, acylating, or amine-combining reagents used experimentally. This paradox has led to the concept that allergenic drugs are transformed in vivo to more reactive derivatives. These are the true immunogens that form covalent bonds with body proteins, analogous to the artificial conjugates used to produce experimental allergy.

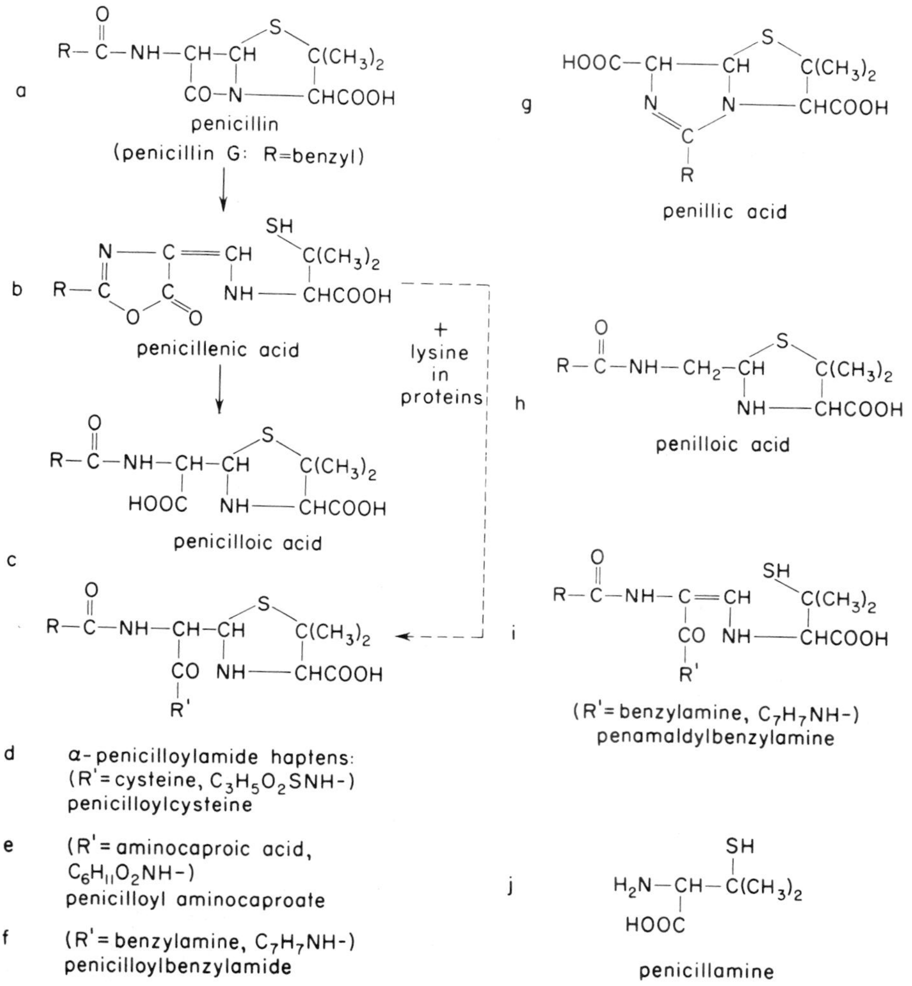

Fig. 8-3. (A–J) Structures of penicillin and derivatives. Arrows indicate spontaneous transformations of the penicillin structure. The derivatives shown here are referred to in Figure 8-4. (Adapted from de Weck,[27] with permission.)

The strongest evidence for covalent binding in hapten-protein interactions in vivo comes from investigations on penicillin allergy.[26–29] It has been shown that both in vitro and in vivo penicillin undergoes slow transformation to much more reactive derivatives. Figure 8-3 shows the initial molecular rearrangement of penicillin to penicillenic acid and the subsequent transformation of this intermediate to penicilloic acid. Penicillenic acid can react with amino groups (e.g., ϵ-amino groups of lysine residues in proteins) prior to molecular rearrangement (as shown by the broken arrow in Figure 8-3) to yield α-amide derivatives of the penicilloic acid structure. A number of lines of investigation have implicated these penicilloic acid–protein conjugates as the most frequent antigenic determinants in penicillin allergy.

Typical evidence is presented in Figure 8-4. The method of hemagglutination was used.

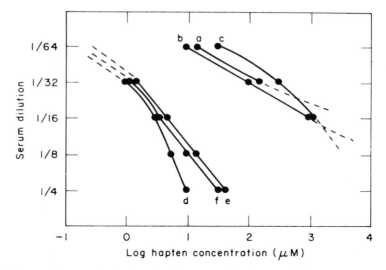

Fig. 8-4. Inhibition of hemagglutination by haptens related to penicillin. The designation of the various haptens refers to Fig. 8-3. A suspension of erythrocytes was preincubated with benzylpenicillin (a, Fig. 8-3) and then added to rabbit benzylpenicillin antiserum. Hemagglutination resulted up to a serum dilution of 1:64. Addition of hapten to the reaction mixture could inhibit hemagglutination by combining with the serum antibody. Each experimental point here represents the hapten concentration needed to achieve complete inhibition of hemagglutination at the given serum dilution. With haptens g, h, i, and j (not shown), no inhibition resulted even at $10^{-3}M$, the highest concentration tested. (Modified from de Weck,[27] with permission.)

Erythrocytes were incubated with penicillin and then added to a reaction mixture containing penicillin antiserum produced by repeated injection of penicillin into a rabbit. The penicillin-treated red blood cells were agglutinated by the antiserum at dilutions up to 1:64. The technique of hapten inhibition was then used to assess the specificity of the antibodies and antigens in the reaction. Addition of the same hapten to which the antibodies were formed inhibits the hemagglutination by occupying the antigen binding site on the antibody molecules. The hapten inhibition was quantitated by finding what hapten concentration was needed to inhibit the agglutination completely at various serum dilutions. The resulting curves in Figure 8-4 are remarkable because they show clearly that the compounds whose structures are illustrated in Figure 8-3 fall into three distinct classes. Penicillin itself, penicillenic acid, and penicilloic acid (a, b, and c) were by no means the most effective inhibitors of the hemagglutination, and four related compounds (g, h, i, and j) were entirely ineffective, but the three α-penicilloylamide haptens tested (d, e, and f) were about 100 times more effective than penicillin itself or its two breakdown products. These results imply very strongly that the penicillin antiserum was really directed against such a penicilloyl derivative and, thus, by inference, that a penicilloyl conjugate was the actual sensitizing agent in vivo.

In summary, the argument that covalently bonded conjugates between a drug and a body protein are necessary for the development of drug allergy rests on two kinds of evidence. First, experimental allergy in animals has been produced readily with reagents capable of forming covalent bonds with proteins, whereas attempts to make animals allergic to drugs that are not particularly reactive have been unsuccessful. Second, the antigenic determinants in penicillin allergy, both in animals and in humans, are penicilloyl or related covalent conjugates with proteins (as described above) rather than the original penicillin molecule itself. In most cases, drugs that elicit allergic responses are enzymatically metabolized to reactive forms that then form covalent conjugates with host proteins. In some cases, drug molecules react with each other in solution to form polymers that are large enough to be antigenic.

DRUG ALLERGY IN HUMANS

In this section we shall consider (1) the various manifestations of drug allergy, (2) the frequency of allergic drug reactions in human populations and the factors that determine this frequency, (3) the methods of predicting allergic sensitivity in individual patients, (4) the methods of desensitizing, and (5) the management of allergic reactions. There is little doubt that penicillin is the leading cause of allergic drug reactions in general and also of serious systemic reactions.[30–32] Consequently, a great deal of the research on drug allergy in humans deals with this drug. And because penicillin has been administered to millions of patients, often under controlled conditions in teaching hospitals and clinics, conclusions from such studies are often soundly based on statistically valid data.

Manifestations of Drug Allergy

Because of pharmacologic, chemical, and immunologic factors, there are differences in the spectra of allergic reactions elicited by different drugs. Virtually all types of allergic response have been elicited by one drug or another, and some immunogenic drugs elicit a wide variety of responses.[5] The reactions caused by penicillins, for example, encompass virtually every sort of allergic manifestation. Their onset may be immediate, accelerated (occurring 1 to 72 hours after administration) or delayed for several days or even weeks (Table 8-2).[33]

Immediate Reactions

Allergic reactions may be localized or widespread. Spasm of smooth muscle, edema of the mucous membranes, and vascular damage characterize the immediate-type response. Target organs are the respiratory and gastrointestinal tracts, blood vessels, and skin. The

Table 8-2. Allergic Reactions to Penicillins

Immediate allergic reactions (occur 2 to 30 minutes after penicillin administration) 　Urticaria 　Flushing 　Diffuse pruritis 　Hypotension or shock 　Laryngeal edema 　Wheezing	Late allergic reactions (occur after more than 72 hours) 　Morbilliform eruptions 　　(occasionally occur as early as 18 hours after initiation of penicillin) 　Urticarial eruptions 　Erythematous eruptions 　Recurrent urticaria and arthralgia 　Local inflammatory reactions
Accelerated reactions (occur after 1 to 72 hours) 　Urticaria or pruritis 　Wheezing or laryngeal edema 　Local inflammatory reactions	Some relatively unusual late reactions 　Immunohemolytic anemia 　Drug fever 　Acute renal insufficiency 　Thrombocytopenia

(Modified from Levine et al.[33] with permission.)

most dangerous immediate allergic reaction is anaphylaxis. Symptoms develop with alarming rapidity after an eliciting dose, which may be extremely small. Anxiety and a sensation of generalized warmth are followed by complaints of substernal pressure, difficulty in breathing, collapse of blood pressure, and anoxia. Death can occur within a few minutes. This potentially fatal syndrome has occurred after the sting of a single bee and after the administration of a test dose of less than 1 μg of penicillin. Obstructive edema of the upper respiratory tract, laryngospasm, and bronchospasm are the usual causes of death in such instances. Cytotropic antibodies of the IgE type are implicated in anaphylactic reactions (type I in Fig. 8-2). IgG molecules have a high affinity for surface receptors on mast cells; attachment of allergen to the combining site of a fixed IgE molecule leads to massive release of histamine, prostaglandins, serotonin, pharmacologically active peptides, and leukotrienes (SRSA). A generalized release of these mediators, which act on smooth muscles and vascular tissue, causes the symptoms of shock. The incidence of anaphylaxis with the penicillins is in the order of 0.04 percent,[32] and treatment consists of administration of epinephrine, together with intravenous fluids to restore plasma volume, administration of oxygen, and provision of an adequate airway.[34]

Other manifestations of the immediate type are conjunctivitis and rhinitis (as in hay fever), bronchospasm (wheezing), acute laryngeal edema, generalized urticaria, and angioedema of various tissues. Angioedema (also called angioneurotic edema) consists of swellings of the face, hands, feet, genitalia, and other regions. The syndrome is caused by dilatation and altered permeability of small blood vessels, chiefly in the subcutaneous tissues.

Skin Reactions

The most common allergic drug reactions occur in the skin. In a survey of 464 patients suffering from drug eruptions treated by a Finnish dermatology service, exanthematous (maculopapular, morbilliform, and erythematous) rashes accounted for 46 percent of allergic reactions.[35] Urticaria accounted for 23 percent, followed by fixed eruptions in 10 percent, erythema multiforme in 5 percent, exfoliative dermatitis in 4 percent, and photosensitivity in 3 percent. In this study 19 patients experienced Stevens-Johnson syndrome, a severe form of erythema multiforme associated with widespread bullous lesions of mucous membranes, often accompanied by systemic manifestations of fever, malaise, dehydration, and generalized toxemia.[36] Stevens-Johnson syndrome is a relatively rare reaction, but the incidence was thought to be especially high with long-acting sulfonamides, which were withdrawn from the U.S. market for this reason.[37]

Allergic reactions in the skin are most often delayed in onset and reactions to systemic drug administration vary from localized fixed eruptions to widespread exfoliative dermatitis. Fixed eruptions are remarkable in that they occur in precisely the same cutaneous areas, sometimes no bigger than a fingertip, whenever the eliciting drug is administered.[38] Contact dermatitis is the allergic response of skin to direct application of an eliciting drug. Lymphocytes infiltrate the cutis underlying the area of contact, and there is vascular dilatation manifested by erythema. The role of histamine in allergic skin reactions is well established. Histamine is certainly released from skin as a consequence of the antigen-antibody reaction, and injection of histamine into the skin produces the "triple response" of erythema, flare, and wheal formation, symptoms that also characterize the response observed on skin testing for drug allergy in sensitized individuals.[39,40] Moreover, prior administration of antihistaminic drugs is effective in antagonizing these phenomena when they occur as part of an allergic syndrome.

Hematologic Reactions

Many drugs have been held responsible for allergic disorders of the blood and the blood-forming tissues, such as hemolytic anemia,[41] granulocytopenia[42] (reduced number of circulating granulocytic leukocytes), and thrombocytopenia[43] (reduced number of platelets). Often there is a mere coincidence in time between administration of the drug and onset of the disease, without rigorous proof of an allergic basis, and sometimes the disorder is actually an idiosyncratic one, as, for example, the hemolytic anemia due to primaquine and other oxidizing drugs in patients with glucose-6-phosphate dehydrogenase deficiency (see Ch. 7). In many instances, however, it has been possible to demonstrate that drug allergy underlies the pathologic changes by demonstrating the presence of an antibody that reacts specifically with the suspected drug in a manner that can account for the destruction of blood cells.

Two general mechanisms for allergic drug reactions involving formed blood elements have been defined.[44] Most reactions appear to be due to the formation of immune complexes that become adsorbed on the surface of the red cell, leukocyte, or platelet (type III in Fig. 8-2).[41–43] The blood cell is destroyed, either because the immune complex-coated cells are eliminated from the circulation by the reticuloendothelial system or because the complement system is activated, leading to cell lysis. For the complement system to become activated, the first circulating plasma protein component, C1q, must bind to the complement binding site on the Fc portion of IgG or IgM (see Fig. 8-1). Fc aggregation appears to be a prerequisite for interaction of the immunoglobulin with C1q. This interaction does not proceed easily with soluble immune complexes but initiation of the complement cascade is enhanced when the immune complex is bound to a cell and the cell membrane is in the vicinity of the reaction. A second mechanism of drug-induced allergic injury to blood cells follows the type II mechanism shown in Figure 8-2. This mechanism is not common but it has been clearly demonstrated with penicillins, cephalosporins, and some other drugs.[41–42] In this case the drug reacts with a red cell, for example, forming a penicilloyl–red cell conjugate, which in turn reacts with antibody. Cell agglutination may then occur with subsequent removal of the affected cells by the reticuloendothelial system, or alternatively, the complement system may be activated leading to cell lysis.

Serum Sickness, Drug Fever, Vasculitis, and Lupus Erythematosus

Several generalized delayed reactions may be manifestations of drug allergy. The serum sickness syndrome was first recognized as a response to antitoxin preparations containing horse serum, but a similar syndrome can be elicited by drugs. Most patients develop urticaria, angioedema, arthralgias with periarticular edema, and low-grade fever. The syndrome may occur within a few hours, but more often it starts several days to 2 weeks after the drug is first given. Serum sickness is an example of an immune-complex disease (type III reaction). Drug fever may have an allergic basis, occasionally appearing as the only indication of drug allergy and otherwise as a manifestation of serum sickness, allergic vasculitis, drug-induced lupus erythematosus, or other allergic phenomena.[5] The fever is presumably due to the release of immune mediators, which act as pyrogens. Several drugs induce allergic vasculitis or a syndrome similar to systemic lupus erythematosus.

The drug-induced lupus syndrome is of special interest because it serves as an experimental model of the disease, and the eventual definition of the mechanism may provide considerable insight into the pathophysiologic mechanisms underlying idiopathic lupus erythematosus. The most frequent symptoms of the lupus-like syndrome are malaise, fever, arthralgias, arthritis, and pleuritic pain; unlike the idiopathic condition, rash and renal involvement are unusual. Patients commonly have a positive lupus erythematosus cell reaction and a positive test for antinuclear antibody. The antihypertensive drug hydralazine was reported in early studies to produce a lupus-like reaction in about 12 percent of patients treated for prolonged periods, with induction of antinuclear antibodies in at least 27 percent of patients.[45] With current hydralazine therapy the incidence of clinical lupus is probably 1 to 3 percent.[46] The mechanism of the drug-induced allergic lupus syndrome is not known.[47] Patients with the drug-induced syndrome develop antibodies against the protein components of nucleoprotein (primarily against histones), but they do not develop anti-DNA antibodies, as do patients with idiopathic systemic lupus erythematosus.[48,49] The patients also have antibodies against hydralazine, but the antibodies do not cross-react with the antideoxyribonucleoprotein antibodies.[48] In contrast to humans with hydralazine-induced lupus, it is interesting that rabbits immunized with protein-hydralazine conjugates develop antihydralazine antibodies that cross-react with both native and single-stranded DNA.[50] It has been shown that hydralazine reacts with thymidine and deoxycytidine in a manner that is enhanced by ultraviolet light,[51] and if such modification of DNA takes place in the body, it might be responsible for initiating the drug-induced lupus syndrome.

An interesting relationship exists between hydralazine-induced allergic lupus erythematosus and the human *N*-acetyltransferase polymorphism involved in drug metabolism. Individuals who are ''slow acetylators'' (i.e., have low levels of *N*-acetyltransferase activity) develop antinuclear antibodies and symptomatic disease earlier and after lower total drug intake than ''rapid acetylators.''[47,52] The same relationship has been shown in patients receiving procainamide, which also induces an allergic lupus syndrome. The relationship between the *N*-acetyltransferase polymorphism and drug-induced lupus is discussed in detail in Chapter 7; it is mentioned here only to point out that genetically determined differences in drug metabolism may predispose some individuals to the development of certain allergic drug reactions when the reactive hapten is a drug metabolite.

Renal and Hepatic Reactions

Because of their role in drug metabolism and excretion, the liver and kidney are exposed to very high levels of drug metabolites and are of special interest as potential sites of allergic reactions. Most drug-induced renal damage results from dose-related toxicity, but occasionally allergic reactions occur. Patients with systemic allergic reactions, such as vasculitis or, less commonly, serum sickness or drug-induced lupus erythematosus, may experience associated renal involvement. Immune complexes circulating in the blood can become deposited at the glomerular basement membrane, causing a reversible decrease in renal function.

Several drugs, most notably penicillins, cephalosporins, and sulfonamides, rarely cause interstitial nephritis.[53] Patients with interstitial nephritis experience fever, rash, eosinophilia, hematuria, and proteinuria.[54] The syndrome is reversible on withdrawal of the drug. Both tubular damage and interstitial infiltration by mononuclear cells and eosinophils are seen in renal biopsy specimens, but there are no glomerular abnormalities nor is there evidence of arteritis.[55] Penicillins are excreted via tubular secretion, and high concentrations of drug are achieved in tubular cells. IgG, the C3 component of the complement system and penicilin haptenic groups were demonstrated at the tubular basement membrane (but not at the glomerular basement membrane) in renal biopsies from two affected patients.[56,57] The patients were shown to have antibodies that react with tubular (but not with glomerular) basement membrane and are likely involved in the pathogenesis of the condition.[56,57] One mechanism suggested by these findings is that the drug may have reacted with tubular basement membrane to form an antigen that can elicit the production of antitubular basement membrane antibodies by a type II mechanism. These antibodies would then react with the basement membrane (either normal membrane or membrane derivatized with drug) to produce the pathology. Another possibility that must be considered is that the drug caused tubular injury by another mechanism and that the resulting release of tubular antigens led to antibody development.

A variety of drugs produce hepatocellular injury and many of the reactions are thought to be allergic in nature, although in most cases there is no direct immunologic evidence of allergy.[5] The hepatic damage caused by erythromycin estolate is of particular interest with regard to understanding how the interaction of basic pharmacologic mechanisms can lead to clinically important effects. Erythromycin estolate can cause a cholestatic hepatitis that is characterized by fever, abdominal pain, eosinophilia, and elevated serum bilirubin and transaminase.[58] Other forms of erythromycin, such as erythromycin base or other esters, do not produce hepatic reactions. The first reaction usually occurs 10 to 20 days after initiation of erythromycin estolate therapy. In a patient who has had a previous reaction, the reaction occurs rapidly, within hours of drug administration. As there is no direct evidence for an immunologic mechanism in patients,[59] some investigators have suggested that the reaction reflects an intrinsic toxicity to the liver coupled with a drug allergy.[60]

In the normal process of excreting the erythromycin, the liver concentrates the drug manyfold in the bile. Thus, liver cells are exposed to very high concentrations of whatever erythromycin preparation is administered. Erythromycin estolate is the lauryl sulfate salt of erythromycin propionate. Erythromycin propionate is clearly toxic to liver cells in suspension at concentrations at which other forms of the drug have no effect.[61,62] The nature of this toxic effect is not known, but the toxicity of the propionyl derivative may explain why cholestatic hepatitis is seen only with this form. The toxicity may reflect a reaction with cell components. The rapid recurrence of symptoms when patients are rechallenged with the propionyl compound must be explained on an immunologic basis. One could postulate a type II mechanism similar to that proposed above for interstitial nephritis. In this case the liver is the site of toxicity because it concentrates the drug in the process of excretion. The propionyl derivative is more reactive than the other forms of erythromycin, and enough drug reacts with the cells of the canaliculi of the biliary system to elicit an immune response specific for this derivative. Thus, rechallenge triggers an immune reaction, which leads to cell damage and the symptoms of cholestatic hepatitis. One can see from this example how pharmacologic factors of drug disposition and elimination and the intrinsic toxicity of a drug derivative may interact to determine an organ-specific drug allergy.

Frequency of Allergic Reactions to Drugs

The frequency of drug allergy in humans is dependent upon the nature of the drug, the route of administration, the genetic predisposition of those who receive the drug, and the extent of prior exposure to and of cross-reactivity with the same or related drugs. There

550 • *Principles of Drug Action*

is really no way at present to arrive at a valid estimate of the frequency of allergic reactions to all drugs. In many cases, toxic or idiosyncratic reactions are considered allergic, while some allergic reactions are attributed to other causes. Even were there no diagnostic difficulty, however, the pertinent statistical questions could not be answered. One would like to know what fraction of all patients treated with a given drug develop symptoms of allergy. One would like to know which of two drugs is less likely to cause allergy. Retrospective fact gathering and haphazard reporting of reactions lead to distorted impressions. The only useful sort of investigation includes all patients who receive a drug, and all have to be followed to determine who has an allergic reaction and, equally important, who does not. As matters now stand, the mild allergic reactions, which are much more common than the severe ones, are usually not even reported; they are treated by physicians everywhere, and the information is nowhere pooled or analyzed. Severe allergic reactions often result in hospitalization; hence, they are more likely to come to general attention. But knowing how many severe allergic reactions are attributable to a given drug does not help one assess the relative risk of using that drug unless one also knows how frequently the drug is administered. The number of allergic drug reactions, as an isolated statistic, is about as informative as the number of Fords, Chevrolets, and Alfa Romeos involved in automobile accidents in a year without knowledge of the number or kinds of cars on the highways or the miles driven per car. It now appears from large-scale surveillance studies that allergic responses account for less than 10 percent of all adverse drug reactions.[63]

Drug allergy may be induced by any route of administration but not with equal efficiency. The oral route is associated with a lower incidence of allergic sensitization than any other, whereas topical application of drugs to the skin is especially prone to sensitize. Industrial exposure to chemicals often results in the development of contact dermatitis among production workers. In one survey of more than 3,000 cases of dermatitis due to occupational exposure, approximately one-sixth could be attributed to allergenic substances.[64] The number of compounds that are capable of causing contact dermatitis is extremely large and continually increases as new chemicals are synthesized. Contact dermatitis in workers engaged in the production of a new drug may serve as an omen of the probable later development of drug allergy in patients after the drug is introduced for therapeutic use.

We have already seen that prior exposure to a drug is essential for the sensitization that must precede an allergic response. The allergic patient, however, may be unaware of any prior exposure. It has been found, for example, that antibodies against penicillin are detectable in most patients who have been treated with the drug in the past and that they are also present in many people who have never knowingly been exposed to these drugs.[65] In the case of the penicillins, people may become sensitized from drinking milk or eating meat from farm animals that have been treated with these antibiotics, even though they have never themselves been treated with these drugs. It should be borne in mind that mere absence of a recorded history of previous exposure by no means rules out the possibility of allergy, since histories of this kind are notoriously unreliable. Patients are commonly unaware of what medication they receive, multiple irrational drug mixtures abound, and memories tend to be much less persistent than antibody-forming capacity. Moreover, enough is known about cross-sensitization to make it apparent that the initial exposure may have been to a different but related drug or environmental chemical.

In the mid-1940s an investigation was conducted on the effect of prior exposure to sulfonamides upon the incidence of allergy.[66,67] The allergic responses considered were

Table 8-3. Frequencies of Several Allergic Responses to Sulfonamides During First and Second Courses of Drug Treatment

Reaction to First Course	Sulfonamides Administered During Second Course	Total No. of Patients	Patients Developing Allergic Reactions During Second Course	
			Number	Percent
No	Different drug	169	6	3.6
No	Same drug	144	16	11.1
Yes	Different drug	30	5	16.7
Yes	Same drug	48	33	68.8
	Control series of persons receiving one course only	737	37	5.0

The allergic responses considered here were drug fever, dermatitis, and conjunctivitis.
(From Dowling et al.,[67] with permission.)

those characteristic of the sulfonamide compounds—drug fever, dermatitis, and conjunctivitis. Three sulfonamides were used: sulfathiazole, sulfapyridine, and sulfadiazine. Before starting a course of therapy, a careful history was taken to see if the patient had previously been exposed to any sulfonamide and, if so, to which one, and also to ascertain if the previous exposure had resulted in an allergic reaction. The results are summarized in Table 8-3. In a very large series of patients receiving a sulfonamide for the first time (control series), the incidence of allergic reactions developing during the course of therapy was 5.0 percent. In most of these, presumably, the drug was administered for weeks, long enough for sensitization and subsequent elicitation of the reaction to occur. Patients who had had previous treatment with a different drug and had not reacted to it were no more likely to develop an allergic reaction during their second course of treatment (incidence 3.6 percent) than if they were receiving the drug for the first time. But if the second course involved administration of the same drug as during the first course, even though there had been no reaction during the first course, the incidence of allergy was increased (to 11.1 percent). If there had been a reaction to the first course, then the incidence of reaction during the second course was still higher (16.7 percent), even when a different drug was used. Most significant, if the same drug that had caused an allergic reaction during the first course was administered again at a second course, the incidence of allergy jumped to 68.8 percent. The evidence is therefore clear that in the sulfonamide series there is both specificity and cross-reactivity. Patients sensitized to one drug are more likely to react to a second drug than if they had never been sensitized at all, but they are less likely to react to the second drug than to the one that sensitized them.

Both because they are allergenic and because they are frequently used in therapy, the penicillins are responsible for more allergic reactions than any other class of drugs. Within the penicillin series, as with the sulfonamides, there is both specificity of allergic sensitization and cross-reactivity. From the clinical point of view, however, sensitization to penicillin in general is more important than sensitization to a specific penicillin. Although there are cases in which patients have been shown to be allergic to one penicillin and not to others,[68,69] these are largely of academic interest, and a physician treating a penicillin-allergic patient should assume cross-reactivity with all the penicillins.

About 5 percent of patients in the United States and Canada will claim sensitivity to penicillin when questioned,[32,70] but the actual incidence of reaction in the random population is less. In a very large study of reaction frequencies in patients treated in venereal disease clinics, 155 of 24,906 patients with a negative history experienced a penicillin

• *Principles of Drug Action*

Table 8-4. Immediate and Delayed Reactions in
Penicillin Allergy

Reaction	Number of Cases[a]
Immediate	7
Delayed	
Less than 24 hours	24
1 to 7 days	33
8 to 14 days	14
Over 14 days	3
Period not specified	10
Total	91

Based on survey of 6,832 patients receiving penicillin.
(From Research Committee of the New South Wales Faculty,[71] with permission.)

reaction, yielding a reaction frequency of 6.2 reactions per 1,000 patients treated.[32] Of 78 patients with positive histories who were treated, 10 experienced a reaction, a reaction frequency of 128 per 1,000. Penicillin reactions occur most commonly 1 to 7 days after initiation of therapy (Table 8-4), and the most frequent reaction is urticaria (Table 8-5).[32,71]

Because systemic anaphylactic reactions are potentially fatal, the frequency of their occurrence is of special interest. Out of 94,655 courses of penicillin therapy monitored in venereal disease clinics, 52 patients had anaphylactic reactions, which yields a frequency of 0.55 per 1,000 patients treated. About half of these reactions were considered mild, which yields an occurrence of severe anaphylaxis of about 0.025 percent.[32] This rate is consistent with other large studies, which suggest rates of severe anaphylactic reaction in the range of 0.04 percent.[31] The risk of death is probably less than 1 in 50,000 (0.002 percent) for ambulatory patients.[31] Even though this risk is very low, it is not acceptable if treatment was inappropriate.

Although the rate of anaphylaxis is much higher with drugs that are large proteins[34] (e.g., L-asparaginase), penicillins are administered much more frequently, and in terms

Table 8-5. Symptoms and Signs in Penicillin Allergy

Clinical Features	Number of Cases[a]
Fever	9
Arthralgia	20
Skin signs	
Bullae	4
Erythema	46
Purpuric spots	1
Urticaria	64
Subsequent desquamation	11
Mouth signs	
Dryness	3
Oral bullae	1
Respiratory signs	
Laryngeal obstruction	2
Bronchospasm	2
General collapse (coldness, sweating, etc.)	9
Paresthesias	2

[a] Based on survey of 6,832 patients receiving penicillin.
(From Research Committee of the New South Wales Faculty,[71] with permission.)

of the absolute number of reactions they predominate over all other drugs. Of 43 deaths due to anaphylaxis recorded by the U.S. Armed Forces Institute of Pathology up to 1972, for example, 32 were due to penicillins.[72] A nationwide survey,[73] covering 29 percent of all general hospital beds in the country over a 3-year period, revealed 1,070 cases of life-threatening drug reactions, of which 901 (84 percent) were caused by penicillin. Of these 901 patients, 83 died, corresponding to a fatality rate of nearly 10 percent. Since the survey covered about one-third of all hospital beds in the country but included data for 3 years, it would appear that there were somewhat less than 100 fatalities per year in the country as a whole. The frequencies of anaphylaxis and of other reagenic, type I responses are increased in atopic individuals,[3] and they increase with repeated courses of therapy.[74] Anaphylaxis occurs less frequently after oral than after parenteral drug administration,[73,75] presumably because of the slower entry of the drug into the circulation.

Both age and disease state influence the frequency of allergic reaction. Allergic reactions to drugs appear to be less common in children than adults.[76] Part of the reason for this may be that children have had less exposure and therefore less opportunity to become sensitized. Although no documentation is available, it is reasonable to assume that immune suppression caused either by disease or by the effects of other drugs might alter the incidence of allergic drug reaction.

In patients with impaired renal function, there is an increased risk of hemolysis occurring by a type II mechanism. When large doses of penicillin are given for a prolonged period (typically at least 10 million units daily for a week or more), hemolysis may occur because penicillin becomes bound to red cell membranes and antibodies of the IgG class react with the cell-bound drug.[77] Complement is not usually involved in this reaction, and intravascular hemolysis rarely occurs. As penicillins are excreted by the kidney, patients with impaired renal function have a higher probability of having prolonged high levels of drug in the body and are thus at increased risk of this complication.

The incidence of rashes is higher with ampicillin than with other penicillins,[78] but the rash peculiar to ampicillin is later in onset and somewhat different in character than rashes occurring with penicillins in general.[79] About 90 percent of patients with mononucleosis who are treated with ampicillin will experience a maculopapular eruption.[80] Mononucleosis patients have been shown to have IgM and IgG antibodies that react with ampicillin.[81] Patients with hyperuricemia,[82] chronic renal disease, or lymphocytic leukemia[7] also have a maculopapular rash with ampicillin therapy at a frequency higher than occurs in the general population. This is thought to reflect a delayed hypersensitivity to ampicillin polymers,[7] but the mechanism has not really been not defined.

Testing for Drug Allergy

In view of the potential seriousness of drug allergies, it would obviously be valuable to have a reliable and safe method of testing for allergic sensitivity before administering a drug. For many years, skin and conjunctival tests were in vogue in which a very small amount of the drug solution was injected intradermally or dropped into the conjunctival sac. Local erythema or conjunctival inflammation was taken as sign of allergic sensitivity. These tests fell into disrepute for two reasons. First, they were unreliable in a capricious way. Patients with positive tests who were nevertheless given the drug therapeutically because of serious need often did not have allergic reactions, whereas patients with negative tests might have reactions of life-threatening severity. Second, the test itself could precipitate a full-blown anaphylactic response in some patients; indeed, deaths have been recorded as a result of skin testing, even though the amount used was only a minute fraction of the usual therapeutic dose.

Although skin testing with most drugs is unreliable, very useful information may be obtained in skin testing for the potential of allergic reaction to penicillins. As a result of competition studies with penicilloylamide haptens like that shown in Figure 8-4 but using serum from penicillin-allergic patients,[83] it was realized that allergic patients commonly possess antibodies directed against the penicilloyl-lysyl structure. Thus, a penicilloyl derivative of lysine was developed as a test substance. Penicilloyl-polylysine (PPL) is a multivalent antibody composed of approximately 20 lysine residues with 12 to 15 penicilloyl groups per unit.[84] A small amount of PPL solution is administered intradermally, and after 20 minutes the injected area is examined for evidence of a wheal and erythema response. The reaction is graded negative, 2 +, or 4 + depending upon the magnitude of the response. Because of its molecular size, penicilloyl-polylysine diffuses more slowly from the site of injection than penicillin, and systemic reaction is rare. Nevertheless, some danger still persists. For example, 4 of 16,239 patients tested developed generalized skin reactions after the test, and 1 had bronchospasm.

The predictive value of the PPL test can be assessed in the data presented in Table 8-6 and Figure 8-5. If history of prior contact with penicillin is ignored, then a strong correlation between skin test result and subsequent allergic reaction is seen (Table 8-6). Among those with negative skin tests, only 0.5 percent experienced any reaction. The percent experiencing an allergic reaction increased with increasing positivity of the skin test, to 10.2 percent among the group that had reacted most strongly. However, even in this strongly positive group, 9 out of 10 patients given penicillin therapeutically did not react adversely.

Figure 8-5 shows that the predictive value was even greater when previous history was taken into account. Of the patients with a history of penicillin sensitivity as well as a positive skin test, more than one in four experienced an allergic reaction; in the remaining categories, the response frequency was graded in an orderly manner. A meaningful way of summarizing these studies is to say that if a person without any history of penicillin allergy reacts positively to the skin test, the probability is greatly increased that that person will experience an allergic reaction to therapeutically administered penicillin, as compared with one whose skin test is negative.

Because most penicillin-allergic patients have antibodies directed against the penicilloyl

Table 8-6. Relationship Between Skin Test Result and Subsequent Reaction to Penicillin

Skin Test Response[a]	No. of Patients Given Penicillin Therapeutically	Percent of Patients Reacting Allergically to Therapeutic Course
—	13,530	0.5
±	782	1.3
2 +	212	4.2
4 +	206	10.2

[a] The skin test with penicilloyl-polylysine was scored according to size of wheal and erythema (−, negative response; ±, ambiguous response, wheal less than 12 mm in diameter; 2 +, positive, wheal 12–20 mm in diameter; 4 +, strongly positive, wheal more than 20 mm in diameter). Patients with 2 + or 4 + skin tests were given penicillin therapeutically only when it was felt that the need outweighed the risk.
(Data from Brown et al.[84])

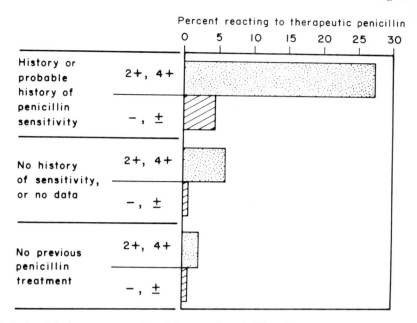

Fig. 8-5. Relationship between previous history of penicillin allergy, skin test response, and subsequent allergic reaction to penicillin. The percent of patients reacting to a therapeutic course of penicillin is shown as a function of previous history of allergic reaction to penicillin and of reaction to the penicilloyl-polylysine skin test. These results are those of the patients analyzed in Table 8-6, and the meaning of skin test categories is the same as given there. (From Brown et al.,[84] with permission.)

structure, this has been called the "major determinant" of penicillin allergy. Testing with PPL will detect patients allergic to the penicilloyl group, but the physician cannot rely on this test alone for predicting a patient's reaction to subsequent penicillin therapy. Patients may have developed antibodies to minor determinants that do not recognize the penicilloyl group. The use of the word *minor* to describe these determinants is unfortunate, since people who are allergic to the minor determinants are more likely than those with penicilloyl-specific antibodies to experience an immediate immune reaction upon therapeutic administration of the drug. Thus, it is important to test patients with minor determinants as well as with PPL. The best way to do this may be to use a minor determinant mixture (MDM), which usually contains crystalline benzylpenicillin, sodium benzylpenicilloate, and α-benzylpenicilloyl-amine. If this mixture is not available from the hospital pharmacy, one can test the PPL-negative patient with benzylpenicillin alone.

The predictive value of skin testing with both PPL and MDM is indicated by the data in Table 8-7. Skin tests with PPL and MDM were performed on 217 patients with a history of allergic reaction to penicillins. Of 185 patients in whom both skin tests were negative, only one accelerated reaction occurred when penicillin was given therapeutically; 32 patients (15 percent) had positive skin tests with PPL, MDM, or both. Seven patients who were negative on testing with PPL and who might have been considered at low risk if judged on the basis of that test alone, were positive on testing with MDM. These and other similar data indicate that negative skin tests to PPL and MDM virtually exclude the possibility that the patient will experience an immediate and possibly life-threatening

556 • *Principles of Drug Action*

Table 8-7. Relation of Immediate Skin Tests with PPL and MDM to Immediate and Accelerated Allergic Reactions to Penicillin[a]

Patients with History of Penicillin Allergy	Skin Tests		Immediate or Accelerated Reaction to Penicillin Therapy
	PPL	MDM	
185	−	−	One had a mild accelerated urticarial reaction
9	+	−	Not treated with penicillins
4	−	+	Not treated with penicillins
8	+	+	Not treated with penicillins
8	+	−	Five of eight had accelerated urticarial reactions
3	−	+	Two had accelerated reactions (urticarial or diffuse flush); one had an immediate urticarial reaction

[a] In skin test–positive patients, penicillin therapy was started by gradual administration. In skin test–negative patients, penicillin therapy was initiated without an attempt at desensitization.
(From Levine and Zolov,[85] with permission.)

allergic reaction to penicillin.[85,86] A negative response also markedly reduces the probability of an accelerated reaction. It has been shown that the testing procedure can be applied by medical service residents in a hospital ward setting in a useful and safe manner.[87] PPL testing can be initiated with intradermal injection, and if this is negative, one may proceed to MDM (or benzylpenicillin) scratch testing and then intradermal testing. No one should be tested for a drug sensitivity without trained personnel, syringes, epinephrine, and appropriate airway support immediately available.

It would be advantageous to have a method of reliably testing for drug allergy without exposing the patient to the risk of reaction. The radioallergosorbent test (RAST) method has been employed to detect penicilloyl-specific IgE antibodies. In this test the drug is coupled to an insoluble matrix, which is then incubated with the patient's serum. The matrix is then washed, and the presence of antibody is detected by using radiolabeled antiserum to human immunoglobulins. There appears to be a good correlation between the RAST results and those obtained by skin testing with PPL.[88]

A disadvantage of the RAST technique is that it only demonstrates IgE. An enzyme-linked immunosorbent assay (ELISA) has been developed for detecting antipenicillin antibodies of several immunoglobulin classes.[89] In this assay human transferrin is conjugated with penicilloyl groups and the resulting hapten-carrier conjugate is coated onto the inside of polystyrene tubes. The antigen-coated tubes are then incubated first with the patient's serum and then with rabbit anti-human IgG, IgA, IgM, or IgE. One now has the immobilized drug hapten, which is bound by antibody present in the patient's serum, and this in turn is bound by a rabbit antibody against the appropriate immunoglobulin class. After washing the tubes thoroughly to remove unbound antibody, sheep anti-rabbit IgG that is conjugated to horseradish peroxidase is added to detect the presence of rabbit antibody, which is only present if a portion has bound to antipenicilloyl antibody of the patient. The peroxidase enzyme permits detection of the complex by a rapid colorimetric assay. Although ELISA is more sensitive at detecting penicillin-allergic individuals than RAST or the older hemagglutination test, all the tests fail to detect many penicillin-allergic individuals who react positively on skin testing.[89]

ELISA, RAST, and the hemagglutination test detect only humoral antibodies present in serum. As cell-mediated allergy is suspected in many drug reactions, another interesting test called the *lymphocyte transformation test* has been developed.[16] When circulating lymphocytes of allergic individuals are cultured in vitro in the presence of the specific antigen (but not otherwise), the cells undergo a transformation; they become larger, develop a basophilic cytoplasm, show increased RNA and DNA synthesis, and may even

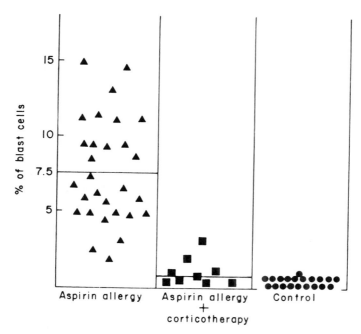

Fig. 8-6. Lymphocyte transformation test for drug allergy. Each point represents a result from one test on one patient's lymphocytes. Patients known to be allergic to aspirin are shown at left, controls at extreme right. Center panel shows results in allergic patients treated with an anti-inflammatory corticosteroid. (From Halpern,[16] with permission.)

develop mitotic figures over a period of about 4 days. These blast cells are readily counted. When cells were cultured without antigen or with an antigen unrelated to the allergenic drug to which patients were sensitized, fewer than 1 percent of the lymphocytes were transformed. Cells from patients allergic to penicillin, when cultured in the presence of penicillin, showed transformation in 4 to 45 percent. In cells from patients who had received penicillin without allergic manifestations, the frequency of transformation rarely exceeded 1 percent. Figure 8-6 shows similar results in aspirin allergy. The greatest advantage of the test is that it is conducted in vitro, with no possible risk to the patient. Its major disadvantage is that 4 days are required to obtain the result.

Administration of Drug to a Patient with a History of Drug Allergy

In technically advanced nations, there are so many drugs available that the physician can almost always treat a patient with a history of drug allergy with an appropriate drug from a different class. This problem of choosing an appropriate drug in the presence of an allergic history occurs most often with local anesthetics and penicillins. Although only about 1 percent of reactions to local anesthetics are allergic, the physician or dentist commonly encounters patients who maintain they are allergic to "cains," meaning such drugs as procaine, tetracaine, and benzocaine. The benzoic acid ester group of local anesthetics does not cross-react with amides, such as lidocaine and dibucaine, or other nonester drugs that are appropriate alternatives.[90] Only in rare cases is skin testing for allergy to local anesthetics necessary, although this is the only group of drugs other than the β-lactams for which the results of skin tests are reliable.[5,90]

In the case of a patient with a history of allergic reaction to a penicillin, one minimizes the risk of an allergic reaction by choosing an antibiotic that is not a member of the β-lactam group. A physician should never substitute one penicillin for another in the treatment of the allergic patient. Because of the toxicity associated with some of the alternative antibiotics, physicians will often treat the patient with a history of penicillin allergy with a cephalosporin. Although they are in many ways structurally different from the penicillins, the cephalosporins are β-lactam antibiotics, and some cross-reactivity with the penicillins exists. In a large clinical trial that included 15,708 patients, 701 (4.5 percent) had a history of allergy to penicillin, and 57 (8.1 percent) of these had an allergic reaction on administration of a cephalosporin.[70] Of the 15,007 patients treated with a cephalosporin who did not have a history of penicillin allergy, 285 (1.9 percent) had an allergic reaction. Thus, a patient with a history of penicillin allergy is about four times as likely to have an allergic reaction to a cephalosporin as a patient without a history of penicillin allergy. The physician should be aware that there have been several reports of anaphylaxis following administration of a cephalosporin to patients who were allergic to penicillins.[53]

Several precautions should be taken to minimize risk in a patient who gives a history of a drug reaction:

1. In most cases the patient should be treated with a drug from a different structural class.
2. In the case of the penicillins, skin testing with PPL and MDM (or penicillin G) can be very helpful, particularly in identifying those patients who have a high risk of an immediate reaction. There is risk to skin testing for penicillin allergy, and at least three deaths from penicillin skin tests have been recorded in the literature.[91]
3. When skin testing for drug allergy, one should always have a syringe containing epinephrine (1:1,000) and appropriate airway support on hand.
4. A slow-release injectable form of drug, such as procaine penicillin, should never be given to a patient with a history of allergic reaction.
5. A cephalosporin should not be administered to a patient with a history of an immediate reaction to penicillins.
6. Cephalosporins are often appropriate alternative drugs in patients with a history of a delayed penicillin reaction. The risk of a reaction to a cephalosporin in such a patient is about 8 percent, which is four times the risk in a patient without a history of penicillin reaction.

Desensitization

In very rare instances in which appropriate alternatives are not available, it may be necessary to administer a drug such as a penicillin to an allergic patient. In such a case desensitization may be attempted. Desensitization with a penicillin generally begins with the intradermal administration of very small amounts of drug (about 5 units of penicillin G). In the absence of reaction, this is followed by increasing doses administered by intradermal, subcutaneous, and finally intramuscular injection according to a prudent desensitization schedule.[92] Because the incidence of allergic reaction, particularly fatal reaction, is much less after oral than parenteral administration, desensitization protocols with penicillin may begin with somewhat higher initial doses given orally, followed at the end by subcutaneous and then intramuscular injection of therapeutic doses.[93] Desensitization is a dangerous procedure, which should be carried out only in a hospital by a physician. An intravenous infusion line should be established prior to the procedure, and epinephrine and theophylline prepared for injection, as well as other emergency medications and equipment, should be at the bedside. After successful desensitization and establishment of routine drug administration, there should be no lapses in therapy that might permit resensitization.

The scientific basis of desensitization is evidently complex. If a large amount of the allergen can be introduced without triggering the allergic reaction, the allergic state is inhibited. In animals some striking examples have been demonstrated. When guinea pigs were fed 2,4-dinitrochlorobenzene for several weeks and then given a typical sensitizing course intracutaneously, there was a dramatic inhibition of the expected development of allergic sensitivity.[94] The protection was manifest even 6 months later. The protective effect of prefeeding was highly specific for the particular antigen; another hapten, *o*-chlorobenzoyl chloride, sensitized as usual even when it was given at the same time as the ineffective 2,4-dinitrochlorobenzene. Similar experiments with neoarsphenamine had been conducted many years before, with essentially the same result.[95] In all such cases, the protective feeding of hapten has to precede the attempted sensitization; the allergic responses cannot be modified once sensitization has occurred. Quite clearly, some form of acquired unresponsiveness develops during the desensitization procedure that is maintained during full-dose parenteral therapy. The response of the patient to skin testing may change from positive to negative during therapy. A number of factors may contribute to the desensitized state, including mediator depletion, some type of antigen-specific cellular unresponsiveness to IgE-mediated signals, hapten binding by IgG and IgM blocking antibodies, or hapten inhibition like that observed in Figure 8-4.[93]

Another approach to treatment of the penicillin-allergic patient has utilized the principle of hapten inhibition shown in Figure 8-4. In this case a small, stable, univalent penicilloyl hapten is administered to compete for antigen binding sites on IgE antibodies.[6] It has been shown that the synthetic hapten benzylpenicilloylformyllysine (BPO-FLYS) inhibits systemic anaphylaxis caused by penicillin in sensitized guinea pigs and inhibits skin reactions to PPL in humans.[96] BPO-FLYS has been administered to patients who had previously experienced acute allergic reactions to penicillin, and the patients were then able to receive penicillin therapy without experiencing allergic symptoms under cover of the hapten.[97] In animal models it has been shown that the univalent haptens do not themselves elicit the production of benzoylpenicilloyl-specific IgE antibodies.[98] This approach is obviously very limited, as it could be applied only to a subgroup of the penicillin-allergic population (i.e., those who are allergic only to penicilloyl groups by virtue of IgE-mediated reactions). It is, however, an interesting demonstration of how basic molecular principles may be translated into a method of treating an allergic patient.

Management of Drug Allergies

In the mild types of allergic reaction, the signs and symptoms subside when the drug is withdrawn. Antihistamines are helpful in relieving urticaria and itching. Anti-inflammatory steroids are effective in suppressing annoying skin reactions and hasten remission in more seriously affected patients with some systemic reactions such as drug fever, lupus erythematosus, and thrombocytopenia.

Life-threatening allergic manifestations develop very quickly and require immediate treatment. Initial treatment is directed to maintenance of an airway and of the circulatory system. This is best accomplished by subcutaneous injection of aqueous epinephrine

1:1,000 (0.3 to 0.5 ml in an adult). If the airway is obstructed, then an airway must be established by intubation or tracheotomy, and oxygen should be administered. If the drug causing the reaction has been injected into an extremity, a tourniquet may be applied above the injection site to slow entry of the drug into the general circulation. Epinephrine may be injected locally to cause vasoconstriction and slow drug absorption. An intravenous infusion should be established to permit administration of fluids to restore plasma volume and of aminophylline, which may aid in reducing airway obstruction. Cardiac arrhythmias may develop during anaphylaxis, and patients should be monitored. It is not clear that H_1 antihistamines are useful in anaphylaxis and they are usually not administered. Corticosteroids do not produce any effect during the critical first hour of treatment, but they should be administered to reduce the possibility of late recurrence of symptoms (after 6 to 8 hours) following initial successful management with sympathomimetic amines.

Although subcutaneous administration of epinephrine is the best treatment for anaphylaxis, there is bound to be some delay, even when a physician is at hand; the procedure is often impractical in the absence of a physician. An excellent first-aid treatment is inhalation of an epinephrine aerosol. A stable suspension of epinephrine microcrystals, 3- to 5-μm particle size (cf. Ch. 3), is available in an automatic aerosol dispenser. Each dose of the inhalant delivers 0.16 mg of epinephrine to the respiratory tract, where it can act on the laryngeal tissues to prevent edema and on the bronchial tree to prevent smooth muscle contraction. At the same time the systemic absorption of the epinephrine is rather limited; thus, even five or more inhalations may produce only slight cardiovascular effects. Such an epinephrine aerosol device should obviously be included in any emergency kit and should also be carried by people known to be prone to anaphylactic reactions from drugs, foods, and bee stings. Those persons should also carry with them a syringe and epinephrine prepared for injection.

REFERENCES

1. de Weck AL, Bundgaard H (eds): Allergic Reactions to Drugs. Springer-Verlag, Berlin, 1983
2. Dash CH, Jones HEH (eds): Mechanisms in Drug Allergy. Williams & Wilkins, Baltimore, 1972
3. Parker CW: Drug allergy. Parts 1, 2, and 3. N Engl J Med 292:511, 732, 957, 1975
4. Whittingham S, Mackay IR: Adverse reactions to drugs: Relationship to immunopathic disease. Med J Aust 1:486, 1976
5. Van Arsdel PP Jr: Adverse drug reactions. Ch. 63. In Middleton E, Reed CE, Ellis EF (eds): Allergy: Principles and Practice. CV Mosby, St. Louis, 1983
6. de Weck AL: Low molecular weight antigens. Ch. 3. In Sela M (ed): The Antigens. Vol. 2. Academic Press, Orlando, FL, 1974
7. Dewdney JM: Immunology of the antibiotics. p. 77. In Sela M (ed): The Antigens. Vol. 4. Academic Press, Orlando, FL, 1977
8. Tiselius A, Kabat EA: An electrophoretic study of immune sera and purified antibody preparations. J Exp Med 69:119, 1939
9. Paul WE (ed): Fundamental Immunology. Raven Press, New York, 1984
10. Roitt IM: Essential Immunology. 5th Ed. Blackwell Scientific Publications, Oxford, 1984
11. Middleton E, Reed CE, Ellis EF (eds): Allergy: Principles and Practice. 2nd Ed. CV Mosby, St. Louis, 1983
12. Lachmann PJ, Peters DK (eds): Clinical Aspects of Immunology. 4th Ed. Blackwell Scientific Publications, Oxford, 1982
13. Burnet FM: The Clonal Selection Theory of Acquired Immunity. Vanderbilt University Press, Nashville, 1959

14. Ruddy S, Gigli I, Austen KF: The complement system of man. N Engl J Med 287:489, 545, 592, 642, 1972
15. Coombs RRA, Gell PGH: Classification of allergic reactions responsible for clinical hypersensitivity and disease. p. 575. In Gell PGH, Coombs RRA (eds): Clinical Aspects of Immunology. 2nd Ed. Blackwell Scientific Publications, Oxford, 1968
16. Halpern BN: Antibodies produced by drugs and methods for their detection. In International Encyclopedia of Pharmacology and Therapeutics. Vol. 1, Sec. 75: Hypersensitivity to drugs. Pergamon Press, Oxford and New York, 1972
17. Stupp Y, Paul WE, Benacerraf B: Structural control of immunogenicity. II. Antibody synthesis and cellular immunity in response to immunization with mono-ε-oligo-L-lysines. Immunology 21:583, 1971
18. Landsteiner K: The Specificity of Serological Reactions. Harvard University Press, Cambridge, 1945
19. Landsteiner K, Lampl H: Uber die Abhängigkeit der serologischen Spezifizität von der chemischen Struktur. (Darstellung von Antigenen mit bekannter chemischer Konstitution der spezifischen Gruppen). XII. Mitteilung über Antigene. Biochem Z 86:343, 1918
20. Bullock WE, Kantor FS: Hemagglutination reactions of human erythrocytes conjugated covalently with dinitrophenyl groups. J Immunol 94:317, 1965
21. Chase MW: Experimental sensitization with particular reference to picryl chloride. Int Arch Allergy Appl Immunol 5:163, 1954
22. Sanger F, Tuppy H: The amino-acid sequence in the phenylalanyl chain of insulin. I. The identification of lower peptides from partial hydrolysates. Biochem J 49:463, 1951
23. Chase MW, Dameshek W, Haberman S, et al: A symposium on the role of the formed elements of the blood in allergy and hypersensitivity. J Allergy Clin Immunol 26:219, 1955
24. Salvin SB: Contact hypersensitivity, circulating antibody, and immunologic unresponsiveness. Fed Proc 24:40, 1965
25. Gell PGH, Harrington CR, Rivers RP: The antigenic function of simple chemical compounds: Production of precipitins in rabbits. Br J Exp Pathol 27:267, 1946
26. Parker CW: Immunochemical mechanisms in penicillin allergy. Fed Proc 24:51, 1965
27. De Weck AL: Studies on penicillin hypersensitivity. I. The specificity of rabbit "anti-penicillin" antibodies. Int Arch Allergy Appl Immunol 21:20, 1962
28. De Weck AL: Studies on penicillin hypersensitivity. II. The role of the side chain in penicillin antigenicity. Int Arch Allergy Appl Immunol 21:38, 1962
29. Levine BB: Immunochemical mechanisms involved in penicillin hypersensitivity in experimental animals and in human beings. Fed Proc 24:45, 1965
30. Arndt KA, Jick H: Rates of cutaneous reactions to drugs. A report from the Boston Collaborative Drug Surveillance Program. JAMA 235:918, 1976
31. Idsoe O, Guthe T, Wilcox RR, De Weck AL: Nature and extent of penicillin side-reactions with particular reference to fatalities from anaphylactic shock. Bull WHO 38:159, 1968
32. Rudolph AH, Price EV: Penicillin reactions among patients in venereal disease clinics. A national survey. JAMA 223:499, 1973
33. Levine BB, Redmond AP, Voss HE, Zolov DM: Prediction of penicillin allergy by immunological tests. Ann NY Acad Sci 145:298, 1967
34. Boston Collaborative Drug Surveillance Program: Drug-induced anaphylaxis. JAMA 224:613, 1973
35. Kuokkanen L: Drug eruptions: A series of 464 cases in the Department of Dermatology, University of Turku, Finland, during 1966–1970. Acta Allergol 27:407, 1972
36. Bianchine JR, Macaraeg PFJ, Lasagna L, et al: Drugs as etiologic factors in the Stevens-Johnson syndrome. Am J Med 44:390, 1968
37. Carroll OM, Bryan PA, Robinson RJ: Stevens-Johnson syndrome associated with long-acting sulfonamides. JAMA 195:179, 1966
38. Derbes VJ: The fixed eruption. JAMA 190:765, 1964

39. Dale HH, Laidlaw PP: The physiological action of β-iminazolylethylamine. J Physiol 41:318, 1910
40. Lewis T: The Blood Vessels of the Human Skin and Their Responses. Shaw & Sons, London, 1927
41. Worlledge SM: Immune hemolytic anemia. Semin Hematol 10:327, 1973
42. Pisciotta AV: Immune and toxic mechanisms in drug-induced agranulocytosis. Semin Hematol 10:279, 1973
43. Miescher PA: Drug-induced thrombocytopenia. Semin Hematol 10:311, 1973
44. Kerr RO, Cardamone J, Dalmasso AP, Kaplan ME: Two mechanisms of erythrocyte destruction in penicillin-induced hemolytic anemia. N Engl J Med 287:1322, 1972
45. Perry HM: Late toxicity to hydralazine resembling systemic lupus erythematosus or rheumatoid arthritis. Am J Med 54:58, 1973
46. Mansilla-Tinoco R, Harland SJ, Ryan PJ, et al: Hydralazine, antinuclear antibodies, and the lupus syndrome. Br Med J 284:936, 1982
47. Reidenberg MM, Drayer DE: Genetic regulation of drug metabolism and systemic lupus erythematosus. p. 857. In Lahita RG (ed): Systemic Lupus Erythematus. Churchill Livingstone, New York, 1987
48. Carpenter JR, McDuffie FC, Sheps SG, et al: Prospective study of immune response to hydralazine and development of antideoxyribonucleoprotein in patients receiving hydralazine. Am J Med 69:395, 1980
49. Fritzler MJ, Tan EM: Antibodies to histones in drug-induced and idiopathic lupus erythematosus. J Clin Invest 62:560, 1978
50. Yamauchi Y, Litwin A, Adams L, et al: Induction of antibodies to nuclear antigens in rabbits by immunization with hydralazine–human serum albumin conjugates. J Clin Invest 56:958, 1975
51. Dubroff LM, Reid RJ: Hydralazine-pyrimidine interactions may explain hydralazine-induced lupus erythematosus. Science 208:404, 1980
52. Perry HM Jr, Tan EM, Carmody S, Sakamoto A: Relationship of acetyl transferase activity to the antinuclear antibodies and toxic symptoms in hypertensive patients treated with hydralazine. J Lab Clin Med 176:114, 1970
53. Pratt WB, Fekety FR: The Antimicrobial Drugs. Oxford University Press, New York, 1986
54. Galpin JE, Shinaberger JH, Stanley TM, et al: Acute interstitial nephritis due to methicillin. Am J Med 65:756, 1978
55. Baldwin DS, Levine BB, McCluskey RT, Gallo GR: Renal failure and interstitial nephritis due to penicillin and methicillin. N Engl J Med 279:1245, 1968
56. Border WA, Lehman DH, Egan JD, et al: Antitubular basement-membrane antibodies in methicillin-associated interstitial nephritis. N Engl J Med 291:381, 1974
57. Bergstein J, Litman N: Interstitial nephritis with anti-tubular-basement-membrane antibody. N Engl J Med 292:875, 1975
58. Braun P: Hepatotoxicity of erythromycin. J Infect Dis 119:300, 1969
59. Tolman KG, Sannella JJ, Freston JW: Chemical structure of erythromycin and hepatotoxicity. Ann Intern Med 81:58, 1974
60. Kendler J, Anuras S, Laborda O, Zimmerman HJ: Perfusion of the isolated rat liver with erythromycin estolate and other derivatives. Proc Soc Exp Biol Med 139:1272, 1972
61. Dujovne CA, Shoeman D, Biachine J, Lasagna L: Experimental bases for the different hepatotoxicity of erythromycin derivatives in man. J Lab Clin Med 79:832, 1980
62. Dujovne CA, Salhab AS: Erythromycin estolate vs. erythromycin base, surface excess properties and surface scanning changes in isolated liver cell systems. Pharmacology 20:285, 1980
63. Borda IT, Slone D, Jick H: Assessment of adverse reactions within a drug surveillance program. JAMA 205:645, 1968
64. Klauder JV: Actual causes of certain occupational dermatoses. Arch Dermatol 85:441, 1962
65. Klaus MV, Fellner MJ: Penicilloyl-specific serum antibodies in man. Analysis in 592 individuals from the newborn to old age. J Gerontol 28:312, 1973

66. Dowling HF, Lepper MH: "Drug fever" accompanying second courses of sulfathiazole, sulfadiazine and sulfapyridine. Am J Med Sci 207:349, 1944
67. Dowling HF, Hirsh HL, Lepper MH: Toxic reactions accompanying second courses of sulfonamides in patients developing toxic reactions during a previous course. Ann Intern Med 24:629, 1946
68. Warrington RJ, Simons FER, Ho HW, Gorski BA: Diagnosis of penicillin allergy by skin testing: The Manitoba experience. Can Med Assoc J 118:787, 1978
69. Van Dellen RG, Walsh WE, Peters GA, Gleich GJ: Differing patterns of wheal and flare skin reactivity in patients allergic to the penicillins. J Allergy 47:230, 1971
70. Petz LD: Immunologic cross-reactivity between penicillins and cephalosporins: A review. J Infect Dis suppl, 137:S74, 1978
71. Research Committee of the New South Wales Faculty of the Australian College of General Practitioners: Report on a survey of allergic reactions to penicillin. Med J Aust 1:827, 1959
72. Delage C, Irey NS: Anaphylactic deaths: A clinicopathologic study of 43 cases. J Forensic Sci 17:525, 1972
73. Welch H, Lewis CN, Weinstein HI, Boeckman BB: Severe reactions to antibiotics. A nationwide survey. Antibiot Med 4:800, 1957
74. Girard JP, Cuevas M: Clinical and immunological analysis of 1047 allergic reactions to penicillin. Schweiz Med Wochenschr 105:953, 1975
75. Simmonds J, Hodges S, Nicol F, Barnett D: Anaphylaxis after oral penicillin. Br Med J 2:1404, 1978
76. Bierman CW, Van Arsdel PP Jr: Penicillin allergy in children. J Allergy 43:267, 1969
77. Garraty G, Petz LD: Drug-induced immune hemolytic anemia. Am J Med 58:398, 1975
78. Shapiro S, Slone D, Siskind V: Drug rash with ampicillin and other penicillins. Lancet 2:969, 1969
79. Bierman CW, Pierson WE, Zeitz SJ, et al: Reactions associated with ampicillin therapy. JAMA 220:1098, 1972
80. Pullen H, Wright N, Murdoch JM: Hypersensitivity reactions to antibacterial drugs in infectious mononucleosis. Lancet 2:1176, 1967
81. McKenzie H, Parratt D, White RG: IgM and IgG antibody levels to ampicillin in patients with infectious mononucleosis. Clin Exp Immunol 26:214, 1976
82. Boston Collaborative Drug Surveillance Program: Excess of ampicillin rashes associated with allopurinal or hyperuricemia. N Engl J Med 286:505, 1972
83. Levine BB, Ovary Z: Studies on the mechanism of the formation of the penicillin antigen. J Exp Med 114:875, 1961
84. Brown BC, Price EV, Moore MB Jr: Penicilloyl-polylysine as an intradermal test of penicillin sensitivity. JAMA 189:599, 1964
85. Levine BB, Zolov D: Prediction of penicillin allergy by immunological tests. J Allergy Clin Immunol 43:231, 1969
86. Sullivan TJ, Wedner HJ, Shatz GS, et al: Skin testing to detect penicillin allergy. J Allergy Clin Immunol 68:171, 1981
87. Adkinson NF, Thomson WL, Maddrey WC, Lichtenstein LM: Routine use of penicillin skin testing on an inpatient service. N Engl J Med 285:22, 1971
88. Kraft D, Wide L: Clinical patterns and results of radioallergosorbent test (RAST) and skin tests in penicillin allergy. Br J Dermatol 94:593, 1976
89. De Haan P, Boorsma DM, Kalsbeek GL: Penicillin hypersensitivity. Determination and classification of anti-penicillin antibodies by the enzyme-linked immunosorbent assay. Allergy 34:111, 1979
90. De Shazo RD, Nelson HS: An approach to the patient with a history of local anesthetic hypersensitivity. Experience with 90 patients. J Allergy Clin Immunol 63:387, 1979
91. Van Dellen RG: Skin testing for penicillin allergy. J Allergy Clin Immunol 68:169, 1981
92. Fellner MJ, Van Hecke E, Rozan M, Baer RL: Mechanisms of clinical desensitization in urticarial hypersensitivity to penicillin. J Allergy 45:55, 1970

93. Sullivan TJ, Yecies LD, Shatz GS, et al: Desensitization of patients allergic to penicillin using orally administered β-lactam antibiotics. J Allergy Clin Immunol 69:275, 1982
94. Chase MW: Inhibition of experimental drug allergy by prior feeding of the sensitizing agent. Proc Soc Exp Biol Med 61:257, 1946
95. Sulzberger MB: Hypersensitiveness to arspenamine in guinea pigs. I. Experiments in prevention and in desensitization. Arch Dermatol 20:669, 1929
96. De Weck AL, Schneider CH: Specific inhibition of allergic reactions to penicillin in man by a monovalent hapten. I. Experimental immunological and toxicologic studies. Int Arch Allergy Appl Immunol 42:782, 1972
97. De Weck AL, Girard JP: Specific inhibition of allergic reactions to penicillin in man by a monovalent hapten. II. Clinical studies. Int Arch Allergy Appl Immunol 42:798, 1972
98. Nakagawa T, Otz U, De Weck AL, Schneider CH: Induction of immunological tolerance to the penicilloyl antigenic determinant. III. Suppression of benzylpenicilloyl-specific IgE antibody formation by cleavable penicilloylated dextran. Int Arch Allergy Appl Immunol 64:210, 1981

9

Drug Resistance

William B. Pratt

ORIGIN OF ACQUIRED DRUG RESISTANCE

Drug resistance is a state of insensitivity or of decreased sensitivity to drugs that ordinarily cause growth inhibition or cell death.[1,2] The term is customarily used in reference to microorganisms or to populations of neoplastic cells (cancer cells) that are undergoing continuous growth in higher organisms. We are concerned here primarily with *acquired* resistance (i.e., with populations initially sensitive that undergo a change in the direction of insensitivity).[3-5]

Resistance—A Heritable Change in Drug Response

The typical course of events in the development of drug resistance is that a strain of microorganisms exposed to a growth-inhibitory or lethal drug responds normally at first. The growth rate is reduced or the population size is diminished. Eventually, however, although the drug is still present, growth resumes. The organisms that display this renewed growth are no longer susceptible to the same drug concentration. If the organism is a pathogen and the resistance has developed in a patient under treatment, the patient relapses and the infection becomes refractory to the old drug regimen. This phenomenon has been recognized since the latter part of the nineteenth century in microorganisms, and more recently, in mammalian cells in vitro and in cancer cells in vivo. Acquired drug resistance is an important limitation to the use of antibiotics and many other antimicrobial and anticancer agents.

Microorganisms are said to be *susceptible* to a drug if cells are killed or their growth is inhibited at drug concentrations in the blood or in another body compartment, such as urine or a body fluid, that are lower than the concentration achieved during therapy. In some cases a population of cells may be susceptible to a drug, but many cells within the population are not killed because the conditions of their environment permit them to *escape* the consequences of the drug blockade. This is sometimes seen, for example, in the treatment of purulent infections with sulfonamides.[1] Sulfonamides inhibit the growth of microorganisms by blocking the synthesis of folic acid, which is required as a cofactor in a variety of one-carbon transfer reactions that occur in the synthesis of thymidine, purines, and the amino acids methionine and serine. In an abscess, pus may contain substantial concentrations of these substances because of tissue necrosis and the resulting hydrolysis of nucleic acids and proteins. In a purulent infection, even though the sulfonamide may be inhibiting the appropriate reaction in a sensitive bacterium, the organism may be able to utilize products of the blocked reaction sequence that are present in the growth environment and thereby escape the consequences of the drug blockade. Thus, although the drug is acting in an appropriate manner, the microorganism is not susceptible to the drug because of its growth conditions.

A similar effect of environment on the response to therapy occurs in the chemotherapy of solid tumors, in which cells may respond very differently to treatment with an anticancer drug depending upon their location within the tumor. The cells on the periphery of a solid tumor are closer to the blood supply, where the concentrations of nutrients and oxygen are optimal for growth. These cells proliferate rapidly, whereas those cells located at the relatively anoxic core of the tumor, where growth conditions are unfavorable, are more likely to be dormant. In general, cells that are dividing rapidly are more susceptible to the cytotoxic effects of anticancer drugs than "resting" cells (the so-called G_o cells), which are not dividing.[2] When the patient is treated with an effective anticancer drug, the cells on the periphery will be killed and the tumor may shrink, but the dormant cells towards the core are the most likely to survive a course of chemotherapy and subsequently proliferate, regenerating the tumor.

In these examples, some of the cells in a drug-sensitive population have escaped the consequences of the drug effect. Because of the failure to obtain an expected response to drug therapy, physicians may sometimes refer to these cells as being resistant. The cells, however, are not resistant. They are sensitive and, if they were present in a different environment, they would have responded to therapy. To satisfy the definition of acquired drug resistance the cells must undergo a *heritable change* that decreases its sensitivity, or renders it insensitive, to the drug. This change in the genetic composition of the cell may occur by three different mechanisms:

1. The DNA in the sensitive cell may undergo a *mutation* such that a protein that is normally produced by the cell is altered in its ability to interact with the drug or to perform a function required for the drug effect.

2. The sensitive cell may acquire drug-resistance genes from another microorganism via *gene transfer*. This is the most common mechanism responsible for the drug resistance that is observed clinically in patients with bacterial infections. The transfer of resistance genes among microorganisms is responsible for the rapid spread of drug resistance among pathogenic bacteria that has occurred on a worldwide basis since the introduction of antibiotics into human and veterinary medicine.

3. The sensitive cell may undergo *gene amplification*. In this case the gene determining the production of a normal cell product becomes multiplied. Cells that contain more copies of the gene synthesize more of the gene product and are able to survive at drug concentrations that would normally be lethal. This mechanism is responsible for drug resistance in both bacteria and higher organisms. It now seems likely that gene amplification is a major mechanism by which cancer cells become resistant during chemotherapy.

Acquired Resistance Versus Intrinsic Resistance

A microorganism that is inherently insensitive to a drug is said to be *intrinsically resistant*. If, for example, a wild-type microorganism lacks the receptor for a drug or if a drug cannot enter a cell and reach its site of action in the interior, then the cell is intrinsically resistant. The difference between intrinsic and acquired resistance can be appreciated from the different ways in which organisms respond to the polyene family of antibiotics. These drugs (e.g., amphotericin B, nystatin) kill fungi by binding very tightly to sterols in the fungal cell membrane and altering membrane permeability.[1] The presence of sterol is absolutely required for the drug action, and since bacteria do not contain sterols in their cell membranes, they are intrinsically resistant.

There are some microorganisms that are either sensitive or intrinsically resistant to polyenes, depending upon their growth conditions. *Acholeplasma laidlawii*, for example, does not synthesize sterols and when grown in sterol-free medium, it is insensitive to polyene antibiotics.[6,7] As shown in Table 9-1, however, when the organism is grown in a cholesterol-containing medium, the sterol is incorporated into the cell membrane, and the cell is readily killed by the drug.[6] Similarly, when the organism is again grown in a sterol-free medium, it becomes intrinsically resistant to the drug. This change from a drug-sensitive to a drug-insensitive state is not an acquired drug resistance because no heritable change has taken place.

Although acquired resistance to the polyene antibiotics is uncommon, occasionally, resistant fungi (defined by growth at or above an amphotericin B concentration of 2 μg/ml) have been recovered from patients who have undergone long-term therapy with these drugs. These resistant isolates, like polyene-resistant fungi that have been selected in the

Table 9-1. Interconversion of *Acholeplasma laidlawii* Between Sensitivity and Intrinsic Resistance to the Polyene Antibiotic Amphotericin B

Cell Type[a]	Survivors after a 2-Hour Exposure to Amphotericin B (%)
Cholesterol-grown cells (S cells)	2
Cholesterol-free cells (R cells)	200
S cells incubated in cholesterol-free medium for 2 hours at	
37°C	150
4°C	5
R cells incubated in cholesterol-containing medium for 2 hours at	
37°C	3
4°C	180

[a] *Acholeplasma laidlawii* were grown in medium with (sensitive, S cells) and without (resistant, R cells) 20 μg/ml cholesterol. Cells were harvested, washed, suspended in cholesterol-free medium, and assayed for viability with and without 25 μg/ml of amphotericin B. Cholesterol was then added to the R cells, each parent culture was divided in half for further incubation at either 4 or 37°C, and viability tests were performed as before. *A. laidlawii* has a generation time of about 2 hours. Therefore, if the drug had no effect on cell growth during the 2-hour incubation in the presence of amphotericin B, the number of cells would be expected to double and approach 200 percent of the initial viability assay. If the drug had a killing effect, then the percentage of survivors would be less than 100 percent (i.e., less than the initial viability assay carried out before exposure to the drug). Growing the R cells at 37°C in cholesterol medium makes them drug-sensitive, whereas the S cells are made drug-insensitive by growth at 37°C without cholesterol.
(From Feingold,[6] with permission.)

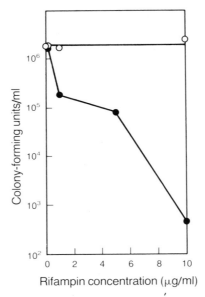

Fig. 9-1. Effect of amphotericin B on the sensitivity of fungal cells to rifampin. Aliquots of a suspension of *Saccharomyces cerevisiae* cells were inoculated into growth medium or medium containing 30 ng/ml of amphotericin B, and the cultures were incubated for 7 days in the presence of various concentrations of rifampin. After 7 days viability was measured by the colony-forming capacity of the cells. ●, with amphotericin B; ○, without amphotericin B. (From Medoff et al.,[10] with permission.)

laboratory, have decreased amounts of or are completely lacking in ergosterol, which is the principal sterol in fungal cell membranes.[8,9] The organisms with acquired resistance appear to have undergone mutations that impair enzymatic functions required for ergosterol synthesis.

Often, microorganisms contain the drug receptor, but the cell membrane or structures external to the cell membrane prevent passage of the drug into the cell. This is the case with the antibiotic rifampin, which is not able to enter and is not particularly effective against fungi. As shown in Figure 9-1, however, when fungi are exposed to rifampin in the presence of a low concentration of a polyene antibiotic that does not by itself affect cell growth, rifampin kills the fungal cells.[10,11] The effect of the drug combination is due to increased entry of rifampin into the cell where it binds to RNA polymerase and inhibits RNA synthesis.[11] The exact mechanism by which the polyene antibiotic amphotericin B increases the entry of rifampin into the cells is unknown. Amphotericin B also enhances the entry of 5-fluorocytosine into fungi, and the two drugs administered together have been shown to produce synergism in vitro.[10] These two drugs have been used together successfully to treat patients with fungal meningitis.[12] In these examples of combined drug effects, the role of amphotericin B is to reduce the threshold of intrinsic resistance to rifampin or 5-fluorocytosine, rendering the organism susceptible to the second drug.

RESISTANCE TO THE β-LACTAM ANTIBIOTICS

A variety of intrinsic and acquired factors interact to determine whether a microorganism is susceptible or resistant to an antimicrobial drug. The factors that determine the response of a bacterium to the β-lactam antibiotics (e.g., the penicillins and cephalosporins) are particularly well understood, and they serve as a good example of how multiple properties determine a drug's spectrum of antimicrobial action. The major factors are: (1) the ability of the β-lactam drugs to penetrate to their receptors, which are cell wall–synthesizing enzymes located at the external surface of the cell membrane; (2) the ability of the drugs to interact with these enzymes and inhibit their action; and (3) the ability of the drugs to be substrates for β-lactamase enzymes, which cleave the β-lactam structure. It is the interplay of all three of these factors that determines whether a bacterium will be susceptible or resistant to a penicillin or a cephalosporin.

Mechanism of β-Lactam Action

The penicillins and cephalosporins all possess a four-membered β-lactam ring structure (Fig. 9-2), which is essential for their biological action. These antibiotics are structural analogs of D-alanyl-D-alanine, a dipeptide contained in the basic repeating units that are

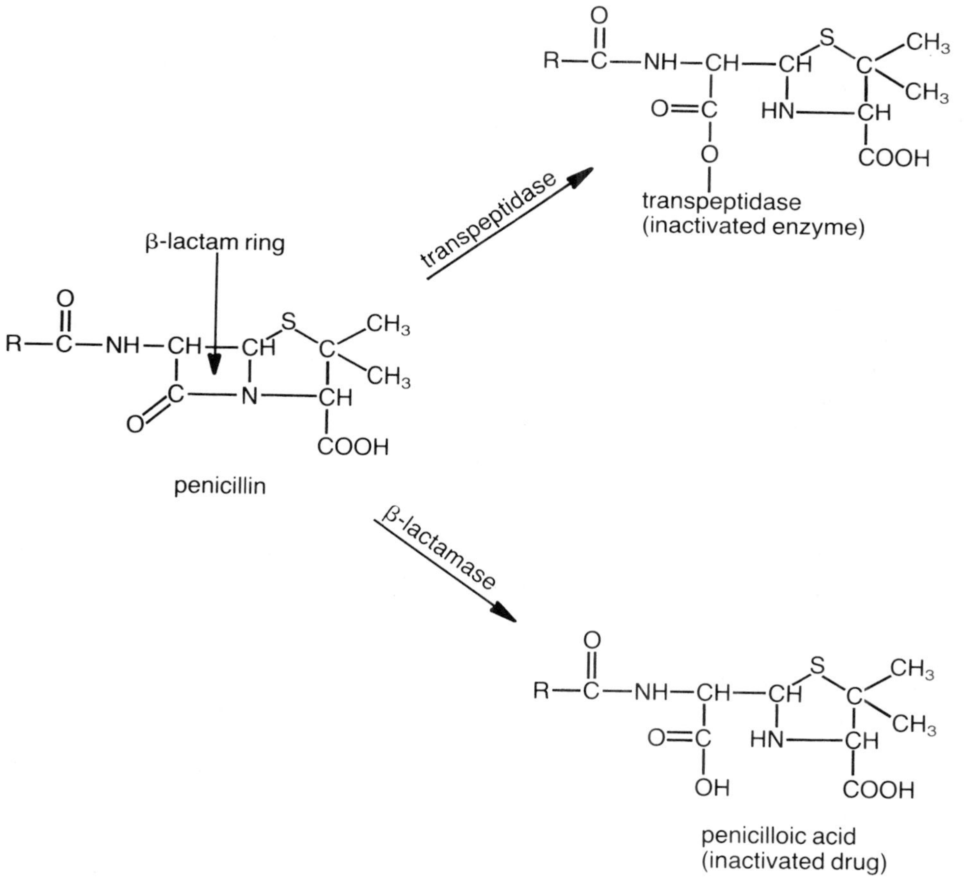

Fig. 9-2. Reaction of penicillin with a transpeptidase or with a β-lactamase. When penicillins interact with cell wall modifying enzymes such as the transpeptidases, the β-lactam ring in the drug is cleaved, and a stable penicillin-enzyme product is formed. When penicillins interact with β-lactamases, the β-lactam ring is hydrolyzed, and the drug is inactivated.

polymerized and cross-linked to form bacterial cell walls.[1] Under most circumstances, inhibition of cell wall synthesis leads to cell death. The terminal reactions in cell wall synthesis are directed by a variety of enzymes, which cross-link and modify the cell wall. Some of the cross-linking enzymes are transpeptidases involved in wall synthesis during cell elongation, whereas other enzymes are required for functions such as determining the shape of the bacterium or forming the septum when the newly formed bacterial cells separate. Many of these cell wall-modifying enzymes act specifically on the D-alanyl-D-alanine portion of the wall precursor units. Thus, these enzymes have substrate sites that recognize either the D-alanyl-D-alanine structure in the cell wall or the analogous β-lactam ring structure in the penicillins and cephalosporins. When the enzymes react with the cell wall, the peptide bond between the two D-alanyl moieties is cleaved, the terminal D-alanine is eliminated, and a second peptide bond is formed, linking the remaining D-alanine in the repeating unit with another polymer in the cell wall structure. When the substrate site on the enzyme is occupied by a penicillin or a cephalosporin, the C—N bond in the β-lactam ring structure is attacked by the enzyme in the same manner as the C—N peptide bond between the two D-alanines, but a stable, covalent complex is formed between the drug and a serine moiety in the active site of the enzyme (Fig. 9-2). The β-lactam antibiotic-enzyme complex can be regarded as an analog of the covalent transition state complex between the normal substrate and the enzyme. Thus, the cell wall-modifying enzymes are inactivated. Collectively, these enzymes are called *penicillin-binding proteins*, and they are the receptors for the β-lactam antibiotics.

Resistance Due to Binding Protein Mutations

The β-lactam antibiotics vary with regard to their relative affinities for the critical binding proteins of different bacteria. Mecillinam, for example, is an amidinopenicillin that readily fits into the substrate site of a cell wall, modifying enzyme that is required for maintaining the rod shape of gram-negative enterobacteria. The drug does not, however, interact with appreciable affinity with other penicillin-binding proteins. Although mecillinam has remarkably high activity against *Escherichia coli* and other enterobacteria, its activity against gram-positive cocci, which do not possess the high-affinity binding protein, is very poor.[13] This difference in the binding proteins determines a very narrow spectrum of action for mecillinam which is limited to the enterobacteria. The gram-positive cocci may be regarded as intrinsically resistant to mecillinam because they do not possess the most sensitive target for the drug's action.

Clearly, acquired resistance to the β-lactam antibiotics can develop as a result of mutations that alter the binding proteins. For example, mutants of *Bacillus subtilis* that are resistant to cloxacillin (a penicillinase-resistant penicillin) have been selected in the laboratory and shown to have a binding protein with altered affinity for cloxacillin but normal affinity for penicillin G.[14] The mutation apparently has altered the configuration of the substrate binding site on the enzyme in a subtle way so that it no longer accepts the cloxacillin structure but retains its ability to accept penicillin G, to which it remains sensitive. Mutations resulting in altered binding may be responsible for the highly penicillin-resistant strains of pneumococci and gonococci that have been isolated from patients.[15,16] These strains do not produce β-lactamases and they have been called intrinsically resistant. The mutations that lead to the production of these resistant strains are very rare events, but in the case of the gonococci, the therapeutic and social consequences of infections by strains bearing this type of resistance have been quite profound in some regions of the world.

Resistance Due to Porin Mutations

Before they can react with their binding proteins at the external surface of the cell membrane, the β-lactam antibiotics must first pass through the outer envelope of the cell. The gram-positive bacterial cell envelope does not present a significant barrier to drug diffusion, but the gram-negative envelope contains an outer membrane that must be traversed if the antibiotic is to arrive at its site of action. The relationship between the cell membrane, the cell wall, and the outer membrane in a gram-negative bacterium is shown in Figure 9-3. In order for small hydrophilic drug molecules, such as those of the β-lactam antibiotics, to traverse the outer membrane they must pass through pores that are formed by proteins called *porins*.[17,18]

The β-lactam antibiotics vary with regard to their relative abilities to pass through pores in the outer membrane. It has been shown that the more hydrophilic β-lactam antibiotics pass through the pores more readily than do the more hydrophobic ones.[18] Indeed, among the penicillins the broad-spectrum drugs (e.g., ampicillin and carbenicillin) are those that readily pass through the outer membrane pores, whereas the narrow-spectrum penicillins (e.g., penicillin G and the penicillinase-resistant penicillins) are the more hydrophobic compounds that pass through the pores very poorly. Thus, some gram-negative bacteria are intrinsically resistant to the narrow-spectrum penicillins because the drugs cannot pass through the outer membrane barrier. Mutations that affect the porin system can produce acquired resistance to broad-spectrum penicillins and to cephalosporins.[19,20] β-Lactam-resistant bacteria with markedly decreased amounts of or altered porin proteins can be selected from drug-sensitive, wild-type populations in the laboratory. Several strains of bacteria with resistance due to decreased drug permeability have been isolated from patients undergoing antibiotic treatment,[21] but it is not yet clear how commonly this type of resistance occurs in clinical specimens.[22]

The gram-negative bacterium *Pseudomonas aeruginosa* is a clinically important pathogen intrinsically resistant to a large number of antibiotics that are otherwise active against a broad spectrum of bacteria.[23] Some of this resistance is accounted for by very poor drug penetration of the outer membrane barrier. Mutants of *P. aeruginosa* with unusually high sensitivity to β-lactam antibiotics have been selected and shown to have altered permeability properties permitting easy access of the drugs to their target proteins on the cell membrane.[24]

Resistance Due to β-Lactamases

Many different types of bacteria have the ability to synthesize β-lactamase enzymes, which inactivate the β-lactam antibiotics by cleaving the C—N bond in the β-lactam ring (see Fig. 9-2). Production of β-lactamases is by far the most common mechanism of acquired resistance to these drugs. It is ironic that the genes that determine the production of β-lactamase were probably derived originally from the genes that code for the cell wall–modifying enzymes that are the targets of the drug action.[1] There are many different β-lactamases, and they can be distinguished from each other on the basis of their substrate and inhibitor specificities, physical properties (e.g., pH optima, isoelectric points) and immunologic differences.[25] The β-lactamases vary considerably with respect to their ability to inactivate the β-lactam antibiotics. Some of the enzymes hydrolyze primarily pen-

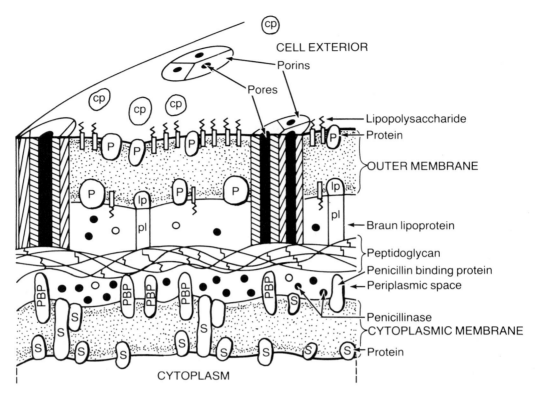

Fig. 9-3. Structure of the gram-negative cell envelope. The three-layered envelope of gram-negative bacteria consists of two membranes separated by the periplasmic space containing the cell wall composed of peptidoglycan. Hydrophobic regions are stippled. Each membrane has protein as well as phospholipid and lipopolysaccharide components; s and p designate the protein components of these membranes. There are also extramembrane proteins. Some of these are capsular proteins (cp), and others are located in the periplasmic zone. Gram-negative bacilli that produce β-lactamase retain most of the enzyme in the periplasmic space. The outer membrane is attached to the peptidoglycan by bridges of Braun lipoprotein; pl and lp refer to the protein and lipid portions, respectively, of these bridging units. The penicillin-binding proteins (PBP), which are the targets of β-lactam antibiotic action, are attached to the cytoplasmic membrane and extend into the periplasmic space. The antibiotics pass through the outer membrane by diffusing through pores formed by porins, which extend from the outside of the cell to the peptidoglycan. In *E. coli* and some other enterobacteria, the porins are arranged as trimers, each monomeric unit contributing a channel. (Adapted from Costerton et al.,[17] and Nikaido et al.,[18] with permission.)

icillins, some hydrolyze primarily cephalosporins, and others hydrolyze a wide variety of β-lactam antibiotics. Many bacteria produce a low level of β-lactamase, which may be induced to higher levels by the presence of β-lactam antibiotics. The genes for β-lactamases may be located either on plasmids or on the bacterial chromosome. Table 9-2 presents a useful classification of the β-lactamases according to substrate specificity, location of the gene, and inducibility.[25]

In general, the gram-positive bacteria produce β-lactamases that act on penicillins but not cephalosporins (penicillinases), the synthesis of the enzyme is usually inducible, and

Table 9-2. Classification of β-Lactamases

Type[a]	Substrate Characteristics	Gene Location	Inducibility
Gram-positive	Primarily penicillinases	r plasmid	Most are inducible
Gram-negative			
I	Primarily cephalosporinases	Chromosome	Many are inducible
II	Primarily penicillinases	Chromosome	Constitutive
III	Broad-spectrum β-lactamases	R plasmid	Constitutive
IV	Broad-spectrum β-lactamases	Chromosome	Constitutive
V	β-Lactamases that hydrolyze methicillin and isoxazolyl β-lactam substrates	R plasmid	Constitutive

[a] The β-lactamases of gram-negative bacteria are classified here according to criteria published by Sykes and Mathew.[25] R plasmid refers to plasmids that are transferred by conjugation and r plasmid to those transferred by transduction. Group III includes the TEM enzymes. Isoxazolyl penicillins include oxacillin, cloxacillin, and dicloxacillin. Methicillin and the isoxazolyl penicillins are called penicillinase-resistant penicillins because they are not substrates for gram-positive or types I to IV gram-negative β-lactamases.

large amounts of enzyme are released into the surrounding medium. The gram-positive β-lactamases have substrate affinities that are usually much higher than those of the enzymes synthesized by gram-negative bacteria. The β-lactamase produced by a gram-positive bacterium is diluted extensively when it is released into the surrounding medium; thus, the ability to produce large amounts of enzyme with high substrate affinity is important for protecting the gram-positive organism against the antibiotic.[1] Gram-positive bacteria, such as many strains of *Staphylococcus aureus*, when fully induced, may generate an impressive drug-destroying activity in their environment. Occasionally, physicians have noted, for example, that streptococcal infections of the respiratory tract do not respond appropriately to treatment with penicillin even though the pathogen cultured from the infection site is very sensitive to the drug when tested in vitro.[26] In this case sufficient numbers of the drug-sensitive pathogenic bacteria are protected from the effect of the drug by a penicillinase secreted into the local environment by small numbers of β-lactamase-producing drug-resistant organisms (such as staphylococci), so that the clinical infection may return even though the patient was treated with very high doses of drug.

In contrast to the gram-positive bacteria, β-lactamase-producing gram-negative bacteria can attain a high level of resistance to the penicillins with the production of a relatively small amount of enzyme. Much of the enzyme produced by gram-negative bacteria is retained in the periplasmic space between the cytoplasmic and outer membranes (see Fig. 9-3). This cell-bound β-lactamase may have a very high level drug-inactivating effect in the periplasmic space. Thus, in the gram-negative organism, a penicillin or cephalosporin must first pass through the outer membrane barrier and then traverse the β-lactamase-containing environment of the periplasmic space before reaching the cell wall-modifying enzymes with which it interacts. The effectiveness of a β-lactam antibiotic against a gram-negative bacterium is therefore a function of both its ability to pass through the pores in the outer membrane and its sensitivity to hydrolysis by the periplasmic β-lactamases.

This interplay of permeability and enzymatic barriers in a gram-negative bacterium is illustrated by the way in which strains of *E. coli* that produce the TEM β-lactamase may respond to ampicillin or cephaloridine.[27] The TEM β-lactamase (type III in Table 9-2) is a common, broad-spectrum enzyme produced by gram-negative bacteria, and it hydrolyzes ampicillin and cephaloridine at similar rates.[28] Cephaloridine, however, passes through the outer membrane pores of *E. coli* much better than does ampicillin.[18,29] *E. coli* strains that produce the TEM β-lactamase are almost always resistant to ampicillin, but some of those organisms may still be killed by cephaloridine.[27] This is because large amounts of cephaloridine pass into the periplasmic space, and the β-lactamase activity may not be sufficient to hydrolyze all of the drug, even though the same amount of β-lactamase activity may be adequate to protect the cell from the smaller amounts of ampicillin that arrive in the periplasmic space. In contrast to ampicillin, the penicillinase-resistant penicillins methicillin and cloxacillin are not hydrolyzed by the TEM enzyme at all, yet *E. coli* are not susceptible to these drugs, solely because they do not pass through the pores in the outer membrane.

The Development of New β-Lactam Antibiotics

In an effort to overcome the intrinsic and acquired factors that limit β-lactam action, the pharmaceutical industry has developed several β-lactamase-resistant penicillins as well as a number of penicillins with enhanced permeation properties that have a relatively broad spectrum of action against gram-negative bacteria. There are no penicillins that are both β-lactamase-resistant and broad-spectrum in action. Some of the cephalosporins, however, possess both excellent permeation properties and a high degree of β-lactam resistance. Although all clinically useful cephalosporins permeate fairly well, the individual cephalosporins do differ from one another with regard to their abilities to pass through the porin system. However, the primary factor that determines the spectrum of action of a cephalosporin is the ability of the drug to serve as a substrate for hydrolysis by gram-negative β-lactamases. The cephalosporins that first came into clinical use, the so-called first generation of cephalosporins, are more readily inactivated by gram-negative β-lactamases than the second generation cephalosporins, which are effective against a broader variety of gram-negative bacteria. Table 9-3 shows the relative rates of hydrolysis of several of the first- and second-generation drugs by four gram-negative β-lactamases.[30] The newest cephalosporins of the third generation are inactivated by very few β-lactamases and have an even broader spectrum of action against gram-negative bacteria.

Another advance in the development of β-lactam antibiotics has come with the development of drugs that destroy β-lactamase enzymes. Several naturally occurring β-lactamase inhibitors and inactivators have been isolated. Clavulanic acid, a β-lactam compound isolated from *Streptomyces clavuligerus*, interacts poorly with penicillin-binding

Table 9-3. Relative Rates of Hydrolysis of First- and Second-Generation Cephalosporins by Several Gram-Negative β-Lactamases

Antibiotic	Rate of Hydrolysis			
	Ia	Id	IIIa	IVc[a]
First generation				
Cephaloridine	100	100	100	100
Cephalothin	100	60	25	68
Cefazolin	45	110	15	75
Second generation				
Cefamandole	0.1	0	20	60
Cefoxitin	0	0.1	0	0
Cefuroxime	0	0	0.1	1.3

[a] Enzymes Ia and Id are cephalosporinases from *Enterobacter cloacae* and *Pseudomonas aeruginosa*; IIIa is the major broad-spectrum TEM enzyme produced by a wide range of gram-negative bacteria; IVc is a broad-spectrum β-lactamase from *Klebsiella aerogenes*. Rates are expressed relative to an arbitrary value of 100 for cephaloridine.
(From Richmond et al.,[30] with permission.)

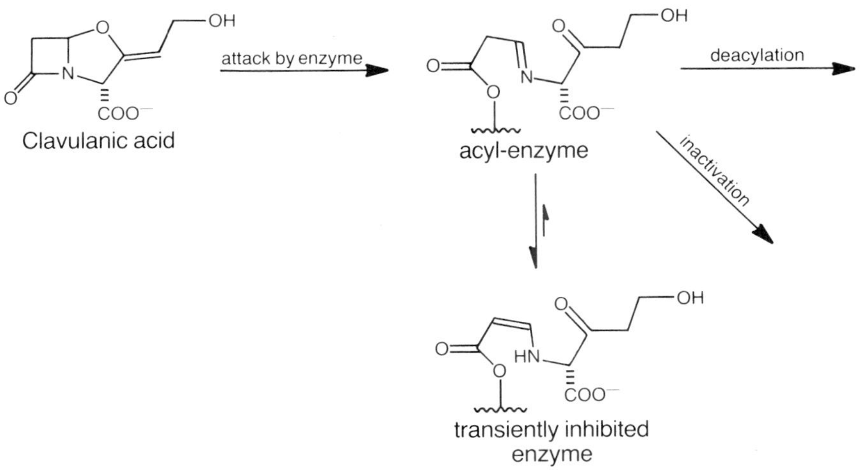

Fig. 9-4. Reaction of clavulanic acid with β-lactamase. Clavulanic acid first acylates the enzyme, after which the acyl-enzyme has three possible fates: the enzyme can be transiently inhibited, a variety of irreversibly inactivated enzyme species may be formed, or deacylation may occur. (Reaction scheme proposed by Charnas et al.[31])

proteins and has only a weak antibacterial activity, but it is a potent and progressive inhibitor of β-lactamases. As diagrammed in Figure 9-4, clavulanic acid first interacts with β-lactamase to form an acyl-enzyme intermediate. This complex can undergo a rearrangement to form a transiently inhibited enzyme, or the drug can act as a mechanism-based inactivator and leave the enzyme permanently inactivated.[31] It is not surprising that the combination of a β-lactamase inhibitor and a β-lactamase-sensitive penicillin may act synergistically against β-lactamase-producing bacteria. Table 9-4 shows the synergism that can be obtained against some β-lactamase-producing strains of bacteria with the combination of clavulanic acid and ampicillin.[32]

The discovery of clavulanic acid has stimulated a great deal of interest in the synthesis of β-lactam drugs that are mechanism-based inhibitors with a broad spectrum of anti-β-lactamase action combined with a greater intrinsic antibacterial potency that is obtained through both improved permeation and high-affinity interaction with the penicillin-binding proteins. It is clear that the extensive effort to understand the intrinsic and acquired factors that determine bacterial response to β-lactam antibiotics has provided an impressive foundation for new drug development. The antimicrobial activities of some of the new β-lactam drugs, like the penems and carbapenems, suggest that the goals of high-affinity

Table 9-4. Antimicrobial Activity of Ampicillin Alone and In the Presence of Clavulanic Acid Against β-Lactamase-Producing Strains of *Staphylococcus aureus*, *Proteus mirabilis*, and *Escherichia coli*.

Antibiotic	Minimum Inhibitory Concentration (μg/ml)		
	S. aureus	*P. mirabilis*	*E. coli*
Clavulanic acid alone	15	62–125	31
Ampicillin alone	500	>2,000	>2,000
Ampicillin in the presence of 5 μg/ml of clavulanic acid	0.02	8	4

(From Reading et al.,[32] with permission.)

interaction with penicillin-binding proteins and potent β-lactamase inhibition will be incorporated together in developing new generations of highly effective β-lactam antibiotics.

ANTIBIOTIC USE AND THE PREVALANCE OF RESISTANCE

Once an organism is altered such that it is partially or completely resistant to a drug, there is a selective advantage for its survival in a drug-containing environment where the drug-sensitive organisms are killed. This process of enrichment for resistant cells in a population is called *selection* and the presence of the drug is said to exert a *selective pressure* in favor of the resistant microorganisms. The selective pressure exerted by antibiotic use on the relative abundance of resistant organisms may be observed both within the hospital environment and in the community at large.

Antibiotic Use and Resistance in Staphylococci

When penicillin was first introduced into clinical medicine in the early 1940s, very few organisms were resistant to the drug. Of 120 strains of *S. aureus* isolated from patients at the Boston City Hospital prior to 1946, 82 percent were susceptible in vitro to 0.04 μg/ml of penicillin G.[33,34] The rest responded to increasing concentrations of drug, but all organisms were susceptible to 25 μg/ml or less. By 1947 only 25 percent of the staphylococci at this hospital were sensitive to 0.04 μg/ml, and 32 percent were resistant to 25 μg/ml; by 1951 resistance to 25 μg/ml had increased to 73 percent of *S. aureus*. For several years the incidence of resistance was higher among strains acquired in the hospital than among strains acquired in the community, where there is a less intensive use of antibiotics. By 1967, however, the incidence of penicillin resistance in *S. aureus* strains recovered at the Boston City Hospital from both inpatients and outpatients was in the range of 80 to 85 percent, and in 1978 it was still in this range.[33] Virtually all these strains acquired the ability to produce penicillinase enzymes. Penicillinases clearly existed before the introduction of penicillin into therapy, but few strains of bacteria produced them. With the selection pressure caused by widespread antibiotic use, however, penicillinase-producing strains became more prevalent.

Several factors determine the ease with which drug resistance makes its appearance and then spreads in a human or animal population. One factor is the intensity of endemic or epidemic infection in that population, and another is the extent of drug use. If the total number of parasites harbored in the host population is high and the drug is widely used, opportunity is provided for the transfer of resistance as well as for selection of the resistant genotype so that it becomes dominant. This principle frequently operates in shifts from sensitivity to resistance among numerous pathogenic microorganisms.

An example studied particularly carefully[35,36] is summarized in Figure 9-5. In preparation for the introduction of the then new antibiotic erythromycin at a contagious disease hospital in Chicago, nose and throat cultures were obtained from all patients and from all personnel concerned with patient care. Whenever staphylococci were found, their sensitivity to erythromycin was determined in vitro. On September 28, 1952, the use of erythromycin was begun. Nose and throat cultures were made periodically. In February the use of erythromycin was discontinued. Figure 9-5 shows that at the outset, the incidence of erythromycin resistance was negligible. It rose quickly, so that by January 60 percent of the staphylococci cultured from hospital personnel were resistant. The incidence among patients on discharge exactly paralleled this trend. For the first several months, no resistant organisms were harbored by patients at the time of their admission

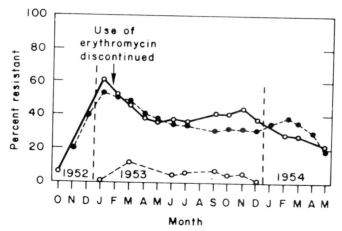

Fig. 9-5. Erythromycin resistance among strains of *S. aureus* in a hospital population. Nose and throat culture data were collected periodically at a hospital for contagious diseases. Resistance of staphylococci to a high concentration (100 μg/ml) of erythromycin was determined. (Sensitive strains responded to 1 μg/ml.) Erythromycin was introduced at the end of September 1952 and discontinued in February 1953. The vertical axis shows the percentage of all strains isolated that were resistant to the drug; the horizontal axis shows month and year. The solid curve represents hospital personnel, the upper broken curve patients at time of discharge from hospital, and the lower broken curve patients on admission to hospital. (From Dowling et al.,[36] with permission.)

to the hospital. By March 1953, however, this was no longer true, presumably because of the widespread use of the antibiotic in the community by that time. The data show clearly that the resistant strains were being transmitted from hospital personnel to the patients, and that the bacterial flora in the carriers became resistant to erythromycin coincident with its introduction into use in the hospital. The conclusions about transmission of the resistant strains were confirmed by detailed analyses of the serologic types of the organisms. Following discontinuance of erythromycin, there was a gradual decline in the frequency of resistant strains. Similar observations on the rise and decline of bacterial resistance associated with intensity of therapeutic use have been made with other antibiotics.[34]

The Evidence for the Association Between Antibiotic Use and Resistance

Although it is widely accepted that the increasing use of antimicrobials is a critical factor accounting for the increase in frequency of drug-resistant bacteria, it has been difficult to prove the cause and effect relationship. The evidence supporting the relationship can be summarized as follows[37]:

1. Antimicrobial resistance is more prevalent in bacterial strains that cause infection in the hospital (nosocomial infection), where there is more intensive use of antibiotics, than in organisms recovered from patients who acquired their infection in the community.
2. During outbreaks of bacterial infections, patients with resistant strains are more likely to have received prior antimicrobial therapy than are patients infected with drug-susceptible strains of the same organism.

3. Changes in antimicrobial drug usage are paralleled by changes in the prevalence of resistance.
4. Areas within the hospital that have the highest antimicrobial usage (e.g., intensive care units, burn units, special care units for newborns) have the highest incidence of antibiotic-resistant bacteria.
5. The likelihood of a patient being colonized by or infected by resistant organisms increases with increasing duration of exposure to antibiotics in the hospital.

The overwhelming weight of correlative evidence supports the hypothesis that the prevalence of antimicrobial resistance among microorganisms is directly related to the extent of antimicrobial drug use. Virtually all experts in infectious disease agree that the two most important approaches that can be used to control resistant bacteria in the hospital environment are: (1) careful and discriminating use of antimicrobial drugs to reduce the selective pressure for drug resistance, and (2) appropriate isolation and containment procedures to block transmission of resistant organisms or of the plasmids that determine the drug resistance.[37,38]

Drug Resistance in Malaria

One of the most dramatic and certainly global examples of the association of antimicrobial drug use with pathogen resistance occurred when many strains of the plasmodium that causes falciparum malaria became resistant to chloroquine. Malaria is the major infectious disease killer of humans, and the social and economic impact of the disease on the societies of Africa, Asia, and South America is severe.[39] During the 1950s and 1960s chloroquine was used for suppressive prophylaxis in programs of mass drug administration, in which every person in an endemic area was treated. Mass drug administration was carried out in conjunction with a program to control the mosquito vector in the attempt to eliminate the disease in a local area. It is widely accepted that such eradication programs accelerated the selection of resistant parasites.[40]

Chloroquine-resistant strains of *Plasmodium falciparum* were first reported in South America in 1961. Within a few years resistance became widespread throughout both South America and Southeast Asia, and more recently it has been reported in East Africa.[41] In Africa most malaria cases are caused by *P. falciparum*, and epidemiologists have dreaded the day when chloroquine resistance would emerge on that continent. There is a marked correlation between the development of drug resistance in *P. falciparum* and the extent to which a drug has been used in a particular area.[40,42] In some areas where there has now been long-standing chloroquine resistance, strains of *P. falciparum* have also developed resistance to *Fansidar*, a fixed-ratio combination of pyrimethamine and sulfadoxine, which is the major alternative to chloroquine for suppressive prophylaxis of the disease.[43] The presence of such multiple drug resistance makes therapy considerably more difficult.

Much has been learned from the experience with drug resistance in malaria, and major efforts are being made to reduce the incidence of resistance by reducing chloroquine use. For example, it is now considered inappropriate to continuously treat every resident in an endemic malarial area. In some malarial control programs, a single dose of chloroquine is administered weekly only to those in the population who are at highest risk of morbidity and mortality, such as children and pregnant women. In other areas the potential selective pressure is reduced even further by administering the drug in a program of presumptive treatment.[44] In this case, instead of administration of chloroquine on a regular prophylactic basis, a single dose of the drug is administered to children only when they have a fever. All fevers are presumed to be due to malaria, and the dose of chloroquine is large enough to completely cure the patient.

The experience with chloroquine and pyrimethamine resistance has led to extreme caution in the way the new and highly effective antimalarial drug mefloquine is employed. For several years, the distribution of mefloquine was under the rigorous control of the World Health Organization (WHO), and the drug was made available only for limited use with certain high risk groups in regions where drug-resistant (particularly multidrug-resistant) *P. falciparum* poses a serious problem.[45] Like chloroquine, mefloquine is not active against the sexual forms of the malarial parasite, which are the forms that transfer resistance from the human host to the mosquito vector in the normal life cycle of the organism. To reduce even further the risk of transmitting any mefloquine resistance that might develop, it has been recommended that a dose of primaquine be given with mefloquine therapy, as primaquine kills the sexual forms of the parasite. This is a unique example of the use of one drug specifically for the purpose of preventing the spread of resistance to another drug.

RESISTANCE VIA MUTATION AND SELECTION

At one time it was assumed that resistance arose because the drug played some directive role in causing a biochemical adaptation. It has become clear that this view is incorrect for resistance arising via mutation or gene transfer. Instead, the genetic composition of the cell undergoes alteration spontaneously by mutation or gene transfer, and the resulting resistant cells survive and give rise to a wholly new, drug-resistant population. The only role played by the drug is to provide a strong selective pressure in favor of the resistant cell by preventing the growth of all the wild-type sensitive cells. Thus, in acquired drug resistance the bulk of the initial population usually does not become resistant. It responds to the drug in the expected way, and it is then replaced by cells of a different kind, which are less sensitive to the drug action.[46,47] Occasionally a growth-inhibitory drug may have mutagenic properties and thus nonspecifically increase the probabilities of many kinds of mutation; no example is known of a drug that selectively increases the mutation rate at the particular gene locus concerned with sensitivity and resistance to itself.

Evidence for the Mutational Origins of Drug Resistance

The question of whether or not exposure to a drug is instrumental in causing development of resistance to that drug remained controversial for a long time. The difficulty arose from the fact that the drug necessarily had to be present in order to demonstrate resistance. How, then, could one tell if it had played a part in causing the altered cell response? Was drug resistance an adaptation to the drug or a spontaneous change having survival value? The first solution to this problem was reached by means of an ingenious statistical approach known as a *fluctuation test*.[48] In its original form, this test was used to prove that acquired resistance of bacteria to bacteriophage arose spontaneously, before contact with the phage. Later, the same procedure was applied to determine the origin of bacterial resistance to a number of antibacterial drugs.

The design of the fluctuation test is illustrated in Figure 9-6. It was applied as follows to streptomycin resistance.[49] A drug-sensitive culture was diluted so that very small inocula (50 to 300 cells) could be placed in each of a series of culture tubes. By plating an appropriate portion of the original culture on an agar test plate containing a lethal con-

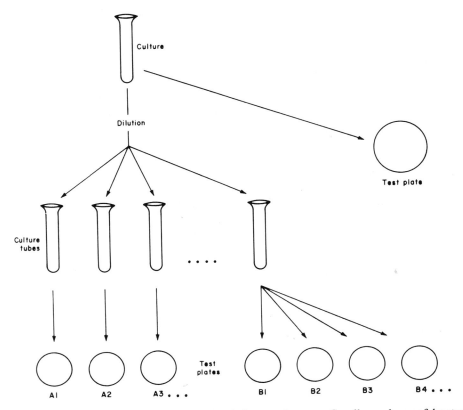

Fig. 9-6. Fluctuation test to determine origin of drug resistance. Small numbers of bacteria are inoculated into culture tubes and after growing out are plated onto test plates. Only the test plates contain drug. The numbers of drug-resistant colonies on the plates of series A are compared with those of series B. (Modified from Luria et al.,[48] with permission.)

centration of streptomycin, the frequency of drug-resistant cells in the original culture was estimated; each resistant cell would give rise to a resistant colony on the test plate, whereas no other cells would grow. It could then be asserted with confidence that none of the small inocula contained any cells already resistant to streptomycin; for example, if the frequencey of resistant cells was 10^{-5}, then there would be only one chance in 1,000 that a given inoculum of 100 cells contained a resistant cell. The culture tubes were incubated to permit multiplication of the small inocula to full-grown cultures (10^8 to 10^9 cells). Then came the critical step in the test. A sample from each culture tube was plated on a single test plate containing drug; about 20 culture tubes were thus plated (series A). From the twenty-first tube, identical platings were made onto 15 more test plates containing drug (series B). Now the plates of both series were incubated, and the numbers of resistant colonies were counted.

Let us suppose that drug resistance arises only after contact of bacteria with drug. Then in this experimental design, drug resistance would arise on the test plates. Since all test plates received equal inocula, the numbers of resistant colonies should be approximately the same on them all. On the other hand, if the drug resistance arose prior to contact with drug (i.e., in the culture tubes), then there might well be differences in the numbers of drug-resistant cells in the different tubes. If a spontaneous event leading to drug resistance occurred early in the growth of a culture, then by the time of plating onto the test plates, a sizable clone of resistant cells would have developed. If the spontaneous event occurred late, then only a few resistant cells would be present in that tube when it was plated. The variation between plates in series B affords a measure of the random fluctuations to be expected from the experimental technique itself, when all platings are made from the same culture.

The question, then, is whether the variation in series A is substantially greater than the variation in series B. The answer was unambiguous. The mean number of resistant colonies was very similar in both series; however, the variation was much greater in series A. In series A, the mean was 106 colonies per plate, the variance was 2,914, and the range was 48 to 291. In series B the mean was 131, but the variance was only 151, and the range was 110 to 155. When numbers of items or events are counted, the random variation in repeated counts is expected to be such that the variance will be equal to the mean. This was approximately true in series B, but the variance in series A was much greater than could reasonably have come about by chance ($P < 0.001$). In other words, events in the tubes, but not in the plates, determined the numbers of drug-resistant cells obtained. Thus, it was concluded that phage resistance, streptomycin resistance, and so on, owed their origins to spontaneous random events occurring during growth of a culture of microorganisms. Several variants of the fluctuation test, some much simpler to perform, all led to the same conclusions.[50] An interesting application of the same concept to mice with transplantable leukemia yielded a similar indication about the origin of drug resistance of the leukemic cells to a cancer chemotherapeutic agent.[51]

A more direct and perhaps more convincing way of showing that resistant variants are present prior to contact with a drug is by means of the *replica plate technique*.[52] A culture of bacteria is spread uniformly over the surface of an ordinary nutrient agar plate and incubated until confluent heavy growth is present. This master plate is then pressed onto a sterile velvet surface, so that many cells from every part of the plate are transferred to the pile of the fabric. Fresh agar plates are then pressed, in succession, onto the same velvet surface; a few cells from every part of the velvet are thus transferred onto the surface of each "replica" plate. The replica plates (but not the master plate) contain the growth-inhibitory drug or antibacterial agent, so that only resistant cells will be able to grow. Figure 9-7 shows the outcome of such an experiment in which the antibacterial agent was phage. Eleven resistant colonies grew on one replica plate, eight on the other. Of these colonies, five pairs occupied identical locations on the two plates. Obviously, in these same positions on the master plate (which contained no phage) small clones of resistant cells must have been already present. It was concluded, therefore, that phage resistance arose spontaneously prior to contact with the selective antibacterial agent. Similar results have been obtained with streptomycin, penicillin, and other antibacterial drugs.

An extension of the replica plate procedure permitted the isolation of a pure strain of streptomycin-resistant *E. coli* that had never been exposed to streptomycin at any stage of the procedure. Replica plating was used to locate a position on the master plate corresponding to that of a resistant colony on a replica plate. A bacteriologic loop was used to transfer cells from this position into a culture tube containing broth. After incubation, this culture was used to prepare a fresh master plate, and the entire procedure of replica plating was repeated. A large number of resistant colonies was now obtained on the replica plates. Again, cells were taken from a position on the new master plate corresponding to

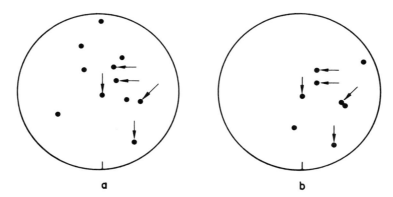

Fig. 9-7. Replica plate demonstration of origin of resistance. Plates a and b were spread with phage. By means of velvet, as described in the text, a master plate with confluent growth of a phase-sensitive bacterial population was replicated onto plates a and b. All phage-resistant colonies are shown; arrows indicate those in congruent positions in both plates. (From Lederberg,[52] with permission.)

a resistant colony on the replica plate, and the whole procedure was repeated. Eventually, a pure culture of a streptomycin-resistant strain was obtained in this way, despite the fact that the cells had never been in contact with streptomycin. The drug was contained only in the replica plates; the cultures, progressively enriched for resistant cells, were grown only on master plates and in broth tubes containing no drug.

In the mutational development of the chromosomal type of drug resistance, two distinct patterns are seen: the *multiple-step* ("penicillin type") and the facultative *large-step* ("streptomycin type") patterns. In the multiple-step pattern,[53] each isolation of resistant organisms in the laboratory leads only to a small increase in the degree of resistance. If a culture is placed in contact with a very high concentration of drug, all cells are affected and none will grow. At a suitable low concentration, while most of the population is held in check, a few resistant mutants will grow. These mutants are still sensitive to the drug at a somewhat higher concentration. Evidently no possible mutation can confer a high degree of resistance. On the other hand, if the population of mutants having a low level of resistance is grown in the presence of a somewhat higher drug concentration, one can select for another mutation superimposed on the first, which will confer a higher degree of resistance. In this way, step by step, quite high levels of resistance can be achieved. It was formerly thought that this pattern necessarily implied a multigenic determination of resistance (i.e., that each mutation affected one gene and many such genes were concerned in the action of the drug) so that the effects of successive mutations would be more or less additive. It is now known that a single gene can be involved but that mutations at different sites within this gene can lead to corresponding alterations at different positions on the gene product. Consider an enzyme the target of the drug action. The configuration of the combining site will be subject to modification by amino acid substitutions throughout the protein, and the configurational change might be expected to show additive effects when several substitutions are introduced. Each small change could reduce the affinity for the drug by a small amount, and these affinity decrements could be additive.

The *facultative large-step pattern* in mutational development of drug resistance is seen typically with streptomycin. If a sensitive culture is plated on a low concentration of the antibiotic, resistant colonies of different kinds can be obtained. Some are resistant to a low concentration of drug, others to a higher concentration; a few are completely insensitive to streptomycin at any concentration. It has been shown by recombination techniques that the various kinds of resistant genotypes represent alleles of the same gene locus. Evidently, mutational substitution at certain sites leads to much greater change in drug sensitivity than at others. The gene locus that determines streptomycin resistance is the *strA* locus, and the gene product is the S12 protein, which is a component of the 30S subunit of the bacterial ribosome.[54,55] The S12 protein is required for streptomycin to bind to its receptor site on the 30S ribosome subunit and inhibit protein synthesis. Analysis of S12 proteins purified from several highly streptomycin-resistant (*strA*) mutant bacteria demonstrated that resistance results from mutations that determine a single amino acid replacement at one of two positions in the molecule.[56]

Combination Chemotherapy

A principle of chemotherapy that emerges from the multiple-step pattern of resistance is that administration of low doses of antibiotics that produce subinhibitory concentrations of drug at the infection site promotes the selection of resistant subpopulations. This has been noted, for example, with nosocomial strains of *P. aeruginosa* where several investigators have correlated the emergence of resistance with inadequate dosing of aminoglycoside antibiotics.[57] The resistance in this case appears to reflect the selection of strains that are deficient in drug uptake.[1] It is a principle of chemotherapy that one should adminster enough antibiotic to obtain clear killing or growth-inhibitory levels at the infection site. This is obviously necessary if one is to obtain the optimal therapeutic effect, but it also reduces the probability of selecting organisms with sequential mutations that confer low-level resistance. This principle was epitomized by Ehrlich in the early days of chemotherapy by the injunction "Frapper fort et frapper vite!"[58]

In the large-step pattern of resistance, an infectious disease may escape from therapeutic control abruptly. This may occur because of a mutation occuring during treatment or, more commonly, because the drug selects for resistant cells that existed as a minor component of the infection prior to the initiation of treatment. The probability of selecting cells that are resistant to therapy is decreased if two drugs with different mechanisms of action and different biochemical pathways of resistance are administered together in combination chemotherapy. The basis of combined chemotherapy is the complete independence of the mutational events leading to resistance to different drugs provided that the drugs are not simply congeners acting by the same mechanism. Suppose two drugs, X and Y, which inhibit growth of a pathogen, and a spontaneous mutation rate 10^{-6} for resistance to each of these. If 10^6 cells divide once, there will arise, on the average, one resistant to X and one mutant resistant to Y. But because the mutational events are independent, the probability is vanishingly small (10^{-12}) that a cell resistant to both drugs will arise. Thus, X-resistant mutants will be killed by Y, Y-resistant mutants will be killed by X, and the disease will be kept under control.

The first application of combination therapy for suppression of drug resistance was in the treatment of tuberculosis. In 1959 it was shown that administration of both streptomycin and isoniazid to tuberculosis patients markedly reduced the emergence of drug-resistant strains of the tubercle bacillus.[59] Both for this reason and because the use of more than one drug can yield a greater killing effect, the initial intensive therapy of tuberculosis is always carried out with two and sometimes with three drugs. The tubercle bacillus is different from most other bacteria in that the only mechanism by which antibiotic resistance arises is mutation. Although combination therapy is an effective approach to preventing the emergence of resistance in tuberculosis, it is probably not effective in most bacterial infections in which resistance is due to transfer of multiple drug resistance genes rather than to mutation of chromosomal genes.

Drug combinations are also used in cancer treatment with the goals of obtaining a greater killing effect and preventing resistance to treatment. The potential suppression of resistance was, historically, probably the most important factor that prompted studies of the effects of drug combinations in cancer treatment.[60] It should be noted, however, that although drug resistance through mutation and selection has been demonstrated for human tumor cells growing in vitro, it is very difficult to obtain convincing evidence for mutational drug resistance in cancer patients undergoing treatment. Nevertheless, there is a sound theoretical basis for the use of drug combinations, and combination chemotherapy has had a profound impact on the treatment of many cancers.

The initial attempts at treatment of acute lymphocytic leukemia in childhood, for example, involved treatment with a single cytotoxic drug. Although remissions in the disease were often induced, subsequent courses of therapy with the same drug were progressively less successful, and the median survival was about 6 months. It was then demonstrated that the use of certain drug combinations resulted in a marked increase in the response rate. Although there was a clear therapeutic advantage to such combined drug treatment, subsequent courses of therapy with the same drugs were progressively less successful. There are clearly many factors besides resistance that account for this therapeutic failure. For example, a few cancer cells may have invaded compartments such as the intrathecal space, where they are protected from the great majority of the anticancer drugs, which do not pass through the choroid plexus. Another possibility is that cells resistant to both drugs in the combination may have been selected during multiple courses of therapy over a prolonged period.

To circumvent these problems, elaborate combined drug protocols have been developed to treat these patients.[2] A combination of drugs (e.g., vincristine and prednisone) is administered on a short-term basis to induce remission of the disease, and this initial treatment is followed by continuous therapy designed to maintain the remission. This second, so-called maintenance phase of therapy consists of continuous treatment with two other drugs (e.g., methotrexate and mercaptopurine) with mechanisms of action and resistance that are different from each other and from the drugs used to induce remission. Simlutaneously, the patient receives a course of prophylactic therapy with intrathecal methotrexate and/or a course of radiotherapy to the head in order to eliminate leukemia cells that may already have invaded the central nervous system. Because different drugs are used for maintaining the disease remission, there should be no selective advantage for cells that may be resistant to the drugs used to induce remission. Thus, the inducing drug combination may be useful in obtaining subsequent remissions if there is a renewal of the disease. In the case of acute lymphocytic leukemia in children, combination therapy has been so effective that a significant percentage of patients may now expect to achieve a normal life span.

RESISTANCE VIA GENE TRANSFER

Although bacteria may develop resistance to antibiotics through the process of mutation and selection, it is clear that in the great majority of cases drug resistance encountered clinically among pathogenic bacteria is due to transfer of drug resistance genes from one bacterial strain to another. Often, several genes are transferred simultaneously into the drug-susceptible population, determining resistance to several antibiotics with entirely different mechanisms of action. In this case treatment with any of the drugs selects for strains that are resistant not only to that drug but to other drugs to which the bacterial population has not been exposed. This method of drug resistance acquisition is known as *infectious* or *transmissible multiple drug resistance*.[61]

The Original Observations

At the end of the Second World War, the sulfonamides were introduced into Japan for treating outbreaks of bacillary (*Shigella*) dysentery. The treatment was initially successful, and the incidence of the disease decreased. By 1952, however, the incidence of the disease had increased again despite the extensive use of sulfonamides, and more than 80 percent of the *Shigella* isolates were highly resistant to sulfonamides. The antibiotics streptomycin, chloramphenicol, and tetracycline were introduced to Japan in 1950 and were widely used to treat the sulfonamide-resistant shigellae. After 1952 Japanese health officials isolated a *Shigella* strain from each dysentery epidemic and tested it for resistance to these three antibiotics.[62] It can be seen from the data in Table 9-5 that, initially, strains were resistant to either streptomycin or tetracycline alone, but by 1957 many of the strains were simultaneously resistant to two or three of these antibiotics.

The rapid emergence of the multiple drug resistance observed in *Shigella* isolates obtained in 1957 could not be explained solely on the basis of mutation and selection, as the probability of a single strain mutating to resistance to all three antibiotics would be vanishingly small. In fact, the incidence of multiple drug resistance after 1957 was higher than that of resistance to only one or two drugs (Table 9-5). It was found that *Shigella* strains isolated from some patients were completely sensitive, whereas serologically identical strains isolated from other patients in the same epidemic were resistant to multiple drugs. On occasion, stool cultures from a single patient contained both sensitive and multiple drug-resistant strains of the same serotype. Importantly, it was observed that administration of only one antibiotic to patients infected with sensitive *Shigella* could be followed by the appearance of organisms that were resistant to several drugs. These observations were tied together when the Japanese investigators proposed that multiple drug resistance could be transferred from multiple drug-resistant *E. coli* to drug-sensitive *Shigella* in the patient's intestine.[61] When multiple drug-resistant *E. coli* were cultured in vitro with drug-sensitive *Shigella*, it was found that the multiple drug resistance could be transferred to *Shigella* without the simultaneous transfer of a number of genetic markers that are part of the *E. coli* genome.[63] Subsequently, it was shown that the genes for transmissible drug resistance are located on circular pieces of extrachromosomal DNA called *plasmids*.

Table 9-5. Antibiotic Resistance in *Shigella* Strains Isolated from Epidemics of Dysentery in Japan

Year	*Number of Strains Tested*	*[a]Number of Strains Resistant to:*						
		Sm	Tc	Cm	Sm, Cm	Sm, Tc	Cm, Tc	Sm, Cm, Tc
1953	4,900	5	2	0	0	0	0	0
1956	4,399	8	4	0	0	0	1	0
1958	6,563	18	20	0	7	2	0	193
1960	3,396	29	36	0	61	9	7	308

[a] One strain of *Shigella* was isolated from each dysentery epidemic and tested for sensitivity to streptomycin (Sm), tetracycline (Tc), and chloramphenicol (Cm).
(From Watanabe,[62] with permission.)

Mechanisms of Resistance Transfer

There are three mechanisms by which genes are transferred from one bacterium to another—transformation, transduction, and conjugation. In *transformation*, small pieces of DNA containing the genes for drug resistance are taken up from the environment by a drug-sensitive bacterium and incorporated into the bacterial chromosome. This mechanism of resistance transfer is not of great clinical importance. In *transduction*, antibiotic resistance genes are transferred from one bacterium to another by a bacteriophage[64] (Fig. 9-8). This mechanism is of considerable clinical importance, particularly among the gram-positive bacteria. The great majority of the pencillin-resistant staphylococci, for example, acquired the genes for β-lactamase via phage-mediated transduction.[65] In *conjugation*, drug resistance genes contained in a plasmid are passed from one cell to another through a direct connection formed by a sex pilus. Such conjugative transfer (Fig. 9-8) occurs primarily among the gram-negative bacilli and it is the principal mechanism by which resistance is transferred among enterobacteria such as *Shigella* and *E. coli*.

If a drug resistance plasmid is self-transmissible through conjugation, it is called an R

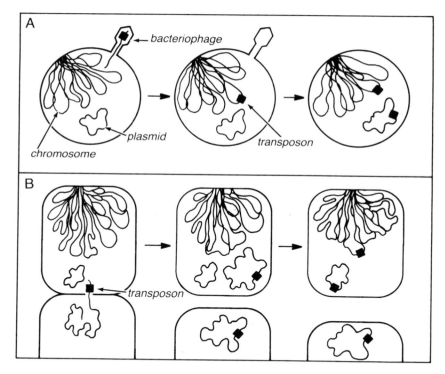

Fig. 9-8. Transfer of antibiotic resistance genes. Resistance genes are being transferred into a bacterial host via transduction with bacteriophage (**A**) or through self-transmission via conjugation (**B**). If the resistance genes are on transposons (solid squares), they can be transferred from the entering plasmid or phage DNA to the host cell chromosome or to preexisting resident plasmids. In the case of plasmid transfer, the replicating plasmid donates one copy to the recipient cell while the donor cell retains its own copy (Fig. B, first and second diagrams). Even if the incoming plasmid is unstable, the drug resistance transposon can become stabilized in the new host by insertion into its chromosome or into a resident plasmid (Fig. B, diagram 3). (From Levy,[64] with permission.)

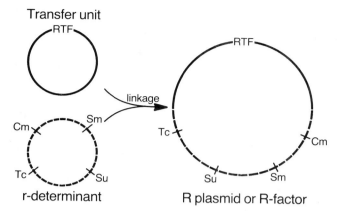

Transfer unit

r-determinant   R plasmid or R-factor

Fig. 9-9. Diagram of the units contained in an R plasmid. The genetic determinants for antibiotic resistance (r determinants) and the genetic determinants for transfer of the whole plasmid during bacterial conjugation (resistance transfer factors [RTF]) can exist as independent closed circles of DNA or they may exist combined as a self-transmissible, conjugative R plasmid (R factor). The plasmid contains genes determining resistance to tetracycline (Tc), sulfonamide (Su), streptomycin (Sm), and chloramphenicol (Cm). (From Pratt, et al.,[2] with permission.)

plasmid, and if it is not self-transmissible (nonconjugative), it is called an r plasmid. The r plasmids are smaller than the R plasmids because they do not contain the genes for conjugative transfer. The r plasmids are found in a wide variety of bacteria, but they are particularly important in staphylococci and other gram-positive bacteria, in which they are responsible for most or all of the plasmid-mediated drug resistance. The r plasmids usually encode for resistance to a single antibiotic and, infrequently, for resistance to two antibiotics. Clinical isolates of staphylococci may be resistant to multiple drugs because they contain several r plasmids, each of which exists in multiple copies in the cell.

The conjugative (R) resistance plasmids usually encode for resistance to several antibiotics, and they consist of two components, the genes encoding for drug resistance (r determinants) and the genes that mediate the transfer of the plasmids during bacterial conjugation (resistance transfer factor [RTF]). As shown in Figure 9-9, the two units can exist as separate closed circles of extrachromosomal DNA or can be combined in the form of an R plasmid (R factor). Each of these units (r determinants, RTF, or the composite R plasmid) is a plasmid containing its own genes for replication and it replicates autonomously; that is, its replication is not linked to replication of the chromosomal DNA. The composite R plasmid has at least two origins at which replication can be initiated, and under certain conditions the r determinant component can undergo extensive gene amplification and recombination to form R plasmids composed of one RTF and multiple tandem copies of r determinants.[66] Bacteria that contain R plasmids with an amplified r determinant may be resistant to very high concentrations of antibiotic.

Like other plasmids, drug resistance plasmids are classified according to incompatibility groups. Plasmids of the same incompatibility group possess considerable DNA homology, but they cannot stably coexist with each other in the same bacterial cell. They can, however, cohabit with plasmids of any other incompatibility set, and a bacterium may contain several plasmids as long as they belong to different incompatibility groups.

Transposons and the Spread of Drug Resistance

Some drug resistance genes (e.g., the TEM β-lactamase) have been found in both plasmid and chromosomal locations in a wide variety of bacteria. For a number of years it was not clear how specific drug resistance genes could have spread so rapidly throughout the bacterial kingdom. Although plasmids and bacteriophages are vectors for resistance transfer, their existence in and of themselves could not explain how different bacterial genera could have acquired virtually the same gene for resistance to a specific drug. It is now clear that this dissemination of resistance genes is due to the existence of transposable genetic elements (transposons); these are discrete, movable DNA elements that can integrate into numerous nonhomologous sequences of DNA, and they are able to "jump" (transpose) from one plasmid to another, from a plasmid to the bacterial chromosome, and from the chromosome to a plasmid in a manner that does not require the recombination functions of the bacterium.[67] The ability to transpose drug resistance genes from one site to another depends in part upon the presence of insertion sequences (IS), which are discrete DNA sequences that range in length from 800 to 1,800 base pairs. A span of one or more genes with an IS at each end is called a *transposon*. A transposon may encode for resistance to one drug or to multiple drugs.

Figure 9-10 presents a genetic map of the IS segments of R_{100}, a well studied R plasmid originally found in enterobacteria.[68] This R plasmid contains two drug resistance transposons. One transposon (Tn2571) encodes for resistance to chloramphenicol, streptomycin, and sulfonamide and contains IS1 elements at each end. The plasmid also contains transposon Tn10 for tetracycline resistance, which is bordered on each end by the insertion sequence IS10. The IS10 elements exist as inverted repeated sequences of DNA, which can anneal to each other to form a stem-loop structure containing the tetracycline resistance determinant. The transposon also contains genes encoding for proteins required to direct the translocation process. As diagramed in the bottom half of Figure 9-10, the transposon can be excised from the plasmid and integrate into another plasmid or into the bacterial chromosome at certain favored "hot spots" for insertion.[67] The mechanisms by which transposable elements move from one genetic site to another are not yet completely defined, but the result is the transfer of the complete resistance gene from one locus to another.

Transposition permits the spread of drug resistance genes to an even wider range of bacteria than can be reached by the plasmid vectors alone. Plasmid DNA can be introduced into bacteria in which the plasmid cannot replicate, but if the plasmid contains a transposon for drug resistance, the drug resistance genes can be rescued by transposition into the bacterial chromosome or into a resident plasmid (see panel B of Fig. 9-8). The transposed DNA can replicate even though the plasmid that donated the drug resistance is lost. In this way drug resistance genes (such as TEM β-lactamase genes) from plasmids of enterobacteria may be acquired by species of *Hemophilus* and other genera. Thus, the existence of both transposons and plasmids, some of which have very wide host ranges and can be conjugated to many different bacterial species, accounts for the fact that identical mechanisms of drug resistance determined by nearly homologous resistance determinants are found in widely different bacteria. When these forms of resistance gene transfer are combined with the selective pressure of widespread antibiotic use, one can account for the rapid spread of drug resistance that has occurred since the introduction of antibiotics.

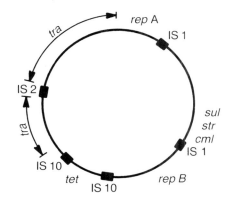

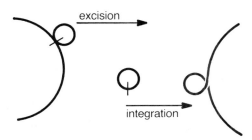

Fig. 9-10. Genetic map of the resistance plasmid R100 and diagram of the transposition process. The determinants for tetracycline resistance, *tet*, are located in the 9.3 kilobase tetracycline resistance transposon, Tn10, which contains an IS10 insertion sequence at each end.[67] The determinants governing conjugal transferability, *tra,* are split by another insertion sequence, IS2. The genes governing replication of R plasmids are *rep*A and *rep*B, and *sul, str,* and *cml* are resistance determinants for sulfanilamide, streptomycin, and chloramphenicol, respectively. The scheme at the bottom of the figure illustrates the excision and subsequent integration of the transposon into another plasmid or into bacterial chromosomal DNA. (From Mitsuhashi,[68] with permission.)

Antibiotic Use and Resistance Transfer

The transfer of drug resistance from one strain of bacterium to another has resulted in some major changes in the therapy of specific infections. Some of these changes are so prominent that they are appreciated by the general public outside of the health care field. One such example is the spread of penicillin resistance among *S. aureus* strains during the 1950s, which was discussed previously in this chapter. This resistance in staphylococci was due almost entirely to the selection of r plasmids encoding for β-lactamases. A similar spread of β-lactamase genes among strains of *Neisseria gonorrhoeae* led to the worldwide spread of penicillin-resistant gonorrhea.

In some cases the transfer of drug resistance genes necessitates rather sudden changes in the recommendations for optimal therapy of a particular disease. This occurred during the 1970s, for example, with the treatment of severe infections due to *Hemophilus influenzae*. *H. influenzae* is the most common cause of bacterial meningitis in children under 2 years of age. For approximately 10 years ampicillin, a broad-spectrum penicillin, was the drug of first choice for treating *H. influenzae* meningitis. In 1974, however, ampicillin-resistant *H. influenzae* isolates were reported in North America. For this reason it became necessary to initiate treatment with another antibiotic, chloramphenicol. The sudden change in the recommendations for optimal therapy was necessitated by the transfer of genes encoding for TEM-type β-lactamases. DNA hybridization studies have shown a high degree of sequence homology between some β-lactamase genes on *H. influenzae* plasmids and a family of transposons called TnA (transposon for ampicillin resistance), which are commonly found in enteric gram-negative bacilli, such as *E. coli* and *Shigella*.[69] Several of the small plasmids of *H. influenzae* and *N. gonorrhoeae* have also been found to share a considerable DNA sequence homology related to the Tn2 transposon for ampicillin resistance. These examples point out the important role of transposons in facilitating the spread of drug resistance among clinically important pathogens. The mobilization of transposons from one bacterium to another via plasmid and phage vectors makes virtually all organisms vulnerable to drug resistance gene transfer.

One fact that is not widely appreciated by physicians is that nonpathogenic bacteria resident in the intestinal tract (coliform bacteria) serve as a reservoir of plasmid-mediated resistance that can be transmitted to pathogens. For example, resistance to the broad-spectrum penicillin carbenicillin in *P. aeruginosa* strains that were infecting patients in a hospital burn unit was shown to be due to R plasmids derived from bacteria of other genera residing in the intestinal tract.[70] The clinical problem that resulted in the burn unit may have been considered by the medical personnel to be an epidemic of a drug-resistant bacterium, but from the point of view of the microbiologist it is really an epidemic of a plasmid. Treatment of a patient with an antibiotic is followed by the rapid conversion of the gut flora to the appropriate resistance pattern. Sometimes as many as 90 percent of all strains isolated from the intestinal tract are resistant within a few days of the initiation of antibiotic treatment.[70] Since the resistance determinants are usually multiple, one can enrich for coliform resistance to penicillins and aminoglycosides, for example, while treating a patient with a tetracycline. When antibiotic treatment is ended, the percentage of resistant flora usually declines.

The prevalence of resistance plasmids in a community reflects the selective pressure exerted by antibiotic use. Table 9-6 shows the incidence of antibiotic resistance among coliform organisms isolated from areas of high antibiotic use compared with adjacent residential areas.[71] In this study the investigators sampled the effluent of sewers draining two general hospitals, a mental hospital, and adjacent residential areas.[71] Coliform bacteria were cultured, and antibiotic sensitivity was determined on each strain. It is clear that

Table 9-6. Antibiotic Resistance of Coliform Bacteria Cultured from Sewers Emanating from Areas of High and Low Exposure to Antibiotics

Area	Premises	Number of Samples	[a]*Percentage of Coliform Bacilli Resistant to:*		
			Streptomycin	*Chloramphenicol*	*Tetracycline*
A	General hospital	3	48.8	0.4	24.3
	Residential area	3	0.6	0.007	0.1
B	General hospital	3	34.7	0.7	32.0
BC	Residential area	3	6.5	0.02	1.3
C	Mental hospital	2	9.5	0.03	0.4

[a] Coliform organisms were cultured from effluent of sewers serving restricted premises, such as hospitals or adjacent residential areas. The coliform bacilli were then tested for antibiotic sensitivity by the disc diffusion (Kirby-Bauer) method.
(From Linton et al.,[71] with permission.)

there was a high incidence of resistance in coliform organisms cultured from the sewage of general hospitals as compared with that of residential areas or the mental hospital. It was documented in this study that a wider variety of antibiotics and many more courses of treatments were administered in the general hospitals than in the mental hospital. It was also shown that the coliform bacilli cultured from the sewage of the general hospitals contained more R plasmids and a greater proportion of R plasmids carrying multiple drug resistance than sewage bacteria from residential and other sources. Despite the fact that the concentration of R plasmid-carrying bacteria was much higher in sewage from hospitals, it was calculated that less than 5 percent of the R plasmids discharged into the sewage of this English city were derived from hospital patients.

As the normal population seems to be the greatest source of R plasmids, one must ask what accounts for this reservoir of drug resistance. The answer to this question has not been defined, but one factor that may contribute to the pool of resistance plasmids is the selective pressure created by the widespread use of antibiotics in animal feeds. The addition of some antibiotics to feeds promotes animal growth. Although the basis for the effect is not well understood, the economic advantage of the practice has been clearly demonstrated.[72] About half of the antibiotics produced in the United States are used in animal feeds,[73] and there has been widespread discussion, both in the scientific community and in the popular press, regarding the effect of this selective pressure on the pool of transmissible drug resistance determinants and their transmission to humans. It is clear that the use of antibiotics in animal feeds selects for multiple-drug resistance plasmids that are shared between animal and human bacteria,[74] but it has not been possible to provide a quantitative estimate of the extent to which the use of these drugs as feed additives has contributed to the reservoir of antibiotic resistance in humans who are not farm personnel.

Although antibiotics are added to animal feeds in amounts that are subtherapeutic, there is, nevertheless, a rapid selection for drug-resistant strains among the bacteria of the intestinal tract.[75,76] There is clear evidence that the multiple-drug resistance that develops in animals emerges in the intestinal flora of farm personnel as a result of the sharing of resistance plasmids.[76,77] In the case of *Salmonella*, there is evidence that multiple drug resistance selected by the use of subtherapeutic amounts of tetracycline to promote growth in animals has been transferred to humans who are not farm workers or meat processors. The major reservoir of salmonellosis in humans is *Salmonella* in food-producing animals and their products.[73] Surveys performed during the 1960s and 1970s revealed a steady increase in antibiotic resistance among *Salmonella* isolates obtained from humans in the United States.[78] The case fatality rate for patients infected with multiple drug-resistant *Salmonella* was found to be 4.2 percent, which is 21 times higher than the case fatality rate associated with antibiotic-susceptible *Salmonella*.[79] When *Salmonella* resistance plasmids were submitted to "fingerprinting" analysis by digestion with restriction endonuclease, identity or near identity between plasmids from several human and animal isolates was demonstrated, indicating extensive resistance gene transfer between the animal and human bacteria.[74]

In one study of a salmonella outbreak, it was shown that multiple drug-resistant *Salmonella* derived from animals fed subtherapeutic amounts of chlortetracycline caused serious illness in humans who had consumed processed meat sold in widely separated areas.[80] The infecting organism was a strain of *Salmonella* that was resistant to ampicillin and tetracycline, and transmission was confirmed by endonuclease digestion of the resistance plasmids recovered from patient isolates and from a dairy herd located next to the fattening pens that were the source of the contaminated meat. Of the 18 persons who were infected, 12 had taken a penicillin for medical problems other than diarrhea in the 12 to 24 hours before the onset of salmonellosis. The rapid onset of gastrointestinal illness in these patients after taking an antibiotic suggested that most of the patients had an asymptomatic infection, and that the use of antimicrobials to which the *Salmonella* was resistant constituted a selective pressure that allowed the growth of the organisms. Thus, although the degree to which the use of antibiotics as feed additives contributes to the reservoir of antibiotic resistance in humans is not known, it is known that antimicrobial-resistant bacteria of animal origin can cause serious human disease, especially in persons taking antimicrobials. One may conclude in the case of this outbreak of salmonellosis that the emergence and selection of such R plasmid-containing, antibiotic-resistant organisms are complications of subtherapeutic antimicrobial use.

RESISTANCE VIA GENE AMPLIFICATION

In some cases a population of cells exposed to selective conditions may survive because individual cells undergo spontaneous amplification of a gene coding for an essential function required for cell survival. Amplification of both chromosomal and plasmid drug-resistance genes can be readily demonstrated in bacteria,[81] and it is clear that resistance via amplification occurs under in vitro selection conditions in protozoa[82] and in mammalian cells.[83] Resistance to anticancer drugs arises via gene amplification in cancer patients undergoing treatment,[84] and it may very well be that gene amplification and selection will be found to be as common a mechanism for clinical resistance to cancer chemotherapeutic agents as mutation and selection.

Resistance to several clinically useful anticancer drugs has been demonstrated in cultured cell lines that overproduce the target enzymes for drug action. The example that has been examined in the greatest detail is resistance to methotrexate, a folate analog, which selects for cells that overproduce dihydrofolate reductase.[83,84] 5-Fluorouracil is an inhibitor of thymidylate synthetase, and in cells in which that inhibition is responsible for the killing effect, resistance can arise due to amplification of the gene for thymidylate synthetase.[85,86] The antileukemia drug hydroxyurea inhibits ribonucelotide reductase and cells may become resistant as a result of overproduction of that enzyme.[87] N-(Phosphonacetyl)-L-aspartate (PALA) is a transition state analog inhibitor of aspartate transcarbamylase, and resistance may result from amplification of the gene for CAD (carbamyl-P synthetase, aspartate transcarbamylase, and dihydroorotase),[88] a multifunctional enzyme that catalyzes the first three reactions of de novo uridine monophosphate biosynthesis.

Methotrexate Resistance and Amplification of the Dihydrofolate Reductase Gene

Methotrexate is an anticancer drug that is a structural analog of folic acid:

	R_1	R_2
Folic acid	OH	H
Methotrexate	NH_2	CH_3

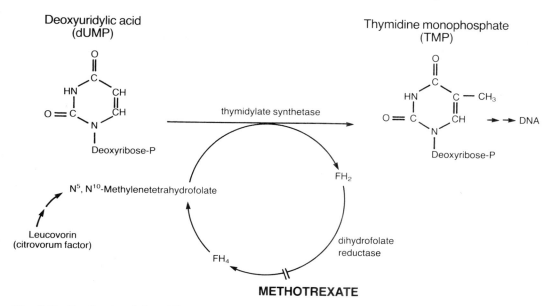

**Deoxyuridylic acid
(dUMP)**

**Thymidine monophosphate
(TMP)**

thymidylate synthetase

DNA

N^5, N^{10}-Methylenetetrahydrofolate

FH_2

Leucovorin
(citrovorum factor)

dihydrofolate
reductase

FH_4

METHOTREXATE

Fig. 9-11. Synthesis of thymidine monophosphate from deoxyuridine monophosphate. In this reaction a one-carbon fragment is transferred from the tetrahydrofolate cofactor to deoxyuridylic acid (dUMP) with the formation of thymidine monophosphate (TMP) and dihydrofolate (FH_2). Tetrahydrofolate (FH_4) must then be regenerated by reduction of FH_2, the reaction blocked by methotrexate. (From Pratt et al.,[2] with permission.)

It acts by competitively inhibiting dihydrofolate reductase (DHFR), the enzyme that reduces dihydrofolate to tetrahydrofolate in the presence of NADPH.[2] Since tetrahydrofolate is converted to a variety of coenzymes that are necessary for one-carbon transfer reactions involved in the synthesis of thymidylate, purines, methionine, and glycine, inhibition of dihydrofolate reductase leads to inhibition of DNA, RNA, and protein synthesis. In many cells the critical effect leading to death after exposure to methotrexate is the inhibition of thymidylate synthesis. As shown in Figure 9-11, thymidine monophosphate is synthesized by transfer of a one-carbon unit from N^5, N^{10}-methylenetetrahydrofolate to deoxyuridine monophosphate under the direction of the enzyme thymidylate synthetase. In this reaction the coenzyme is oxidized and dihydrofolate is formed. To keep the system running, dihydrofolate must be reduced to tetrahydrofolate by the reductase. Stoichiometric amounts of the tetrahydrofolate cofactor are required for thymidine monophosphate synthesis, and when the DHFR activity is inhibited by methotrexate, the folate cofactors are rapidly depleted, with the folate being trapped in the inactive dihydrofolate form.

Cultured cells can become resistant to methotrexate by at least three biochemical mechanisms: (1) by altered transport of methotrexate into the cell[89]; (2) by mutation in DHFR leading to a reduced affinity for methotrexate[90]; and (3) by overproduction of DHFR.[91,92] The mechanism encountered most frequently has been overproduction of DHFR, and in all cases studied the overproduction of DHFR is due to a proportional amplification in the DHFR gene.[84,93] The resistant cells accumulate sufficiently high DHFR levels to maintain some free enzyme in the presence of drug.[94]

The relationship between the degree of methotrexate resistance and the number of DHFR gene copies was first demonstrated in murine sarcoma 180 (S-180) cells. Many years ago it was shown that cultured S-180 cells selected for resistance to methotrexate had levels of DHFR activity that were increased in proportion to the degree of resistance.[94] Schimke and his coworkers subsequently demonstrated that the methotrexate-resistant AT-3000 line of S-180 cells contained high levels of immunologically reactive DHFR protein.[91] The DHFR from resistant cells had the same physical, kinetic, and immunochemical properties as the sensitive cell enzyme, and the increased amount of enzyme protein was due entirely to an increased rate of synthesis of DHFR in the resistant cells relative to the sensitive cells.[91]

It was shown by immunoprecipitation that DHFR comprises as much as 7 to 8 percent of the continuously labled, soluble protein in the resistant cells. As this abundance of DHFR protein reflected an increased amount of mRNA for the enzyme, the mRNA could be readily purified and used to synthesize a tritium-labeled cDNA via a viral reverse transcriptase. The dihydrofolate reductase–specific [^{3}H]cDNA was used as a probe in hybridization experiments to quantitate the relative number of DHFR mRNA sequences and gene copies in the methotrexate-resistant subline (AT-3000) and in the drug-sensitive wild type S-180 cells (S-3).[93] As shown in Table 9-7, the specific activity of DHFR in the resistant subline is 250 times higher than that of the drug-sensitive cells, and this increase is accounted for by a 220-fold increase in mRNA sequences and a 180-fold increase in DHFR gene copies.

An interesting characteristic of the AT-3000 cell line is that high levels of resistance are lost when these cells are grown in the absence of methotrexate.[94] A partially revertant line called Rev-400 was established by growing the resistant S-180 cells in the absence of methotrexate for 400 cell doublings. The level of DHFR in the Rev-400 line has declined to a value that is approximately 10 times as great as that of the sensitive cells. As shown in Table 9-7, this decrease in the relative synthesis of DHFR is accompanied by comparable decreases in the level of reductase-specific mRNA sequences and the relative number of DHFR gene copies.[93] Thus, in this case the overproduction of DHFR is due to the selection of cells with an increased number of genes coding for the production of a normal enzyme, and the degree of resistance reflects the gene dosage. Although the resistant cells usually produce a normal enzyme, resistance can also arise from the selection of amplified sequences that code for an altered enzyme with reduced affinity for the drug.[95]

Table 9-7. Relative Level of Dihydrofolate Reductase Activity, mRNA, and Gene Copies in Methotrexate-Sensitive and Resistant Murine Sarcoma 180 Cell Lines

| Line | *Relative DHFR* | | |
	Specific Activity	mRNA Sequences	Gene Copies
S-180			
S-3	1	1	1
AT-3000	250	220	180
Rev-400	10	7	10

[a] The specific activity of DHFR was determined by an immunologic procedure, and the number of DHFR-specific mRNA sequences and gene copies were determined by hybridization with a DHFR-specific [^{3}H]cDNA probe. The S-3 cells are methotrexate-sensitive, the AT-3000 line is highly methotrexate-resistant, and the Rev-400 line is a partial revertant obtained by growing AT-3000 cells in the absence of methotrexate for 400 cell duplications. Each value is expressed relative to that obtained in the drug-sensitive S-3 cells.

(From Alt et al.,[93] with permission.)

Mechanism of Gene Amplification

Cells with amplified DHFR genes are selected by a multiple, small-step selection process, and resistant lines with 100 to 1,000 gene copies may be obtained by gradually increasing the concentration of methotrexate in the medium by stepwise increments.[84] There is good experimental evidence in support of the proposal that amplifications occur in small steps and that it may not be possible to achieve a high degree of methotrexate resistance via gene amplification with a single, large-step selection protocol.[96]

When resistant cells containing amplified genes are grown in the absence of drug, the cells may retain a stable resistance phenotype, or the amplified genes and the resistance phenotype may be unstable, with a decline in resistance occurring over multiple cell generations. The stable genes are located on chromosomes, often in regions that are expanded in length and lack the characteristic banding patterns observed on chromosome staining by the trypsin-Giemsa technique.[97] In the case of methotrexate resistance, these *homogeneously staining regions*, known as *HSRs*, have been shown by in situ hybridization with radiolabled cDNA probes to contain multiple DHFR genes.[98] In the unstably amplified state, the DHFR genes are located on extrachromosomal elements that often exist in pairs and are called *double minute chromosomes or DMs*.[98] The DMs are self-replicating but they differ from normal chromosomes in that they lack centromeres and tend to be spontaneously eliminated during mitosis under nonselective conditions.[98] Cultured mammalian cells or protozoa that contain unstably amplified (extrachromosomal) DHFR genes when they are initially selected for methotrexate resistance may convert to a population of cells containing stably amplified (chromosomal) genes if they are maintained under selection conditions in the presence of drug.[82,83]

A fluorescence-activated cell sorting procedure has been used to demonstrate that gene amplification occurs spontaneously in the absence of drug selection.[99] To perform the experiments, cells were grown in medium containing glycine, hypoxanthine, and thymidine, which shunt around the methotrexate-blocked functions and permit cell growth in the presence of drug. Cells were exposed to a fluorescein derivative of methotrexate, which binds very tightly to DHFR, permitting individual cells with a high content of DHFR to be identified by their high fluorescence and separated from the general cell population by fluorescence-activated cell sorting. In this manner, 10 successive rounds of growth and sorting under nonselective conditions yielded a population of cells that showed a 50-fold increase in fluorescence intensity, was highly resistant to methotrexate, and was amplified 40-fold in DHFR gene content.[99] The spontaneous frequency of a twofold increase in gene copy number was estimated to be about 10^{-3} per cell per generation in methotrexate-sensitive Chinese hamster ovary cells in the absence of selection pressure. Cells that already have amplified genes (i.e., some resistance), however, undergo increases or decreases in gene copy number at an even more rapid rate (as high as 3×10^{-2} amplification events per cell division).[99]

As we have discussed in a previous section, it was shown by fluctuation testing and replica plating approaches that mutation to resistance occurs in the absence of drug and that the sole role of the drug is to select for the resistant cell population. For years, it has been a principle in the field of drug resistance that the presence of drug does not alter the frequency at which the events that determine drug resistance occur. In the case of gene amplification, however, the presence of drug can increase the frequency at which drug resistance events occur.[100] Indeed, it has been found that a variety of agents (e.g., tumor promoters,[101] anticancer drugs,[102] ultraviolet rays,[103]) that alter DNA replication or DNA structure facilitate amplification of DHFR genes and emergence of methotrexate resistance. It has been proposed that a variety of treatments, including exposure to the cytotoxic drugs themselves, can result in a "misfiring" during cell replication such that "illegitimate" extra rounds of replication occur in segments of DNA, leading to amplification.[104] The exact mechanism for such disproportionate replication is not known; however, according to one attractive model based on the observation that the replicating DNA of eukaryotic cells can exist as loop structures moving through fixed sites of replication,[105] one can envision how secondary rounds of replication and recombination could generate extrachromosomal circular structures in the form of double minute chromosomes. Two models of disproportionate replication[105,106] involving more than a single initiation of replication in a portion of a chromosome within a single DNA synthesis phase (S phase) of the cell cycle are diagrammed in Figure 9-12.

It has been shown that the DHFR gene in Chinese hamster ovary cells is replicated during the first 2 hours of S phase, a time when only about 10 percent of the total genome has been replicated. If DNA synthesis is inhibited by the anticancer drug hydroxyurea for 6 hours, beginning 2 hours after the initiation of S phase, the frequency with which cells become resistant to a 100-fold increment in methotrexate is markedly increased.[102] When DNA synthesis resumes following removal of hydroxyurea, essentially all the DNA that was replicated in the first 2 hours prior to the hydroxyurea inhibition is replicated a second time, including the gene for DHFR. This ability of one anticancer drug (hydroxyurea) to promote resistance to another drug (methotrexate) via gene amplification is another factor of potential significance to be considered when designing multidrug treatment protocols for cancer chemotherapy.

Gene Amplification and Clinical Resistance to Anticancer Drugs

Although it is not yet possible to predict the relative frequency at which gene amplification versus gene mutation is responsible for clinical resistance to anticancer drugs, from single case studies it is clear that gene amplification occurs in tumor cells of patients undergoing chemotherapy. Lymphoblasts obtained from myeloid leukemia patients prior to and during treatment with methotrexate, for example, were assayed for DHFR gene copy number by hybridization with cDNA probes. The patients became clinically resistant to methotrexate, and tumor cells obtained after repeated courses of therapy with methotrexate showed both elevated DHFR activity and a three- to six-fold increase in DHFR gene copies when compared with pretreatment controls.[107,108] The amplification phenomenon is not restricted to myeloid cells, as increased DHFR gene copies have been observed by in situ hybridization in tumor cells obtained from a patient with ovarian adenocarcinoma.[109] Although this patient had not received methotrexate for treatment of the tumor, she had received low-dose methotrexate twice weekly for 3 years for treatment of psoriasis. As noted above, cells with amplified DHFR genes are selected by a multiple, small-step selection process, and prolonged exposure to a low dosage of a cytotoxic drug such as methotrexate would provide optimal conditions for the emergence of resistance via gene amplification.

There is a good reason to anticipate that the principles of resistance via gene amplification that have been defined in cultured cell systems apply to human tumor cells exposed to anticancer drugs during treatment. When gene amplification first occurs in cultured cells, for example, it is often unstable and associated with the existence of minichromosomes. Figure 9-13 shows a metaphase chromosome plate of tumor cell cultured from

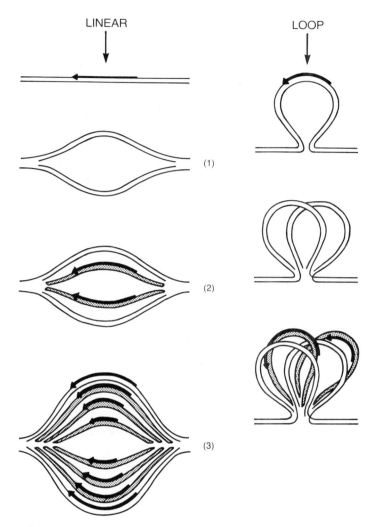

Fig. 9-12. Two models of gene amplification by disproportionate replication. During the S phase of the eukaryotic cell cycle, the DNA is normally replicated once. When conditions exist that alter DNA replication or DNA structure, more than one initiation of replication may occur on a portion of a chromosome within a single S phase of the cell cycle, leading to gene amplification via disproportionate replication. In the linear model on the left, additional rounds of replication (stippled strands) produce the so-called onion skin replication bubble,[106] in which replication complexes are moving on fixed DNA. In the loop model on the right, replicating DNA is moving through fixed sites of replication with the generation of loop structures.[105] One can envision how, through various patterns of ligation and recombination, the amplified genes may exist as extrachromosomal structures (double minutes) or as repeating units that are incorporated into the chromosome in the form of multiple head-to-tail or head-to-head copies of drug resistance genes. The reader is referred to Schimke[83] for detailed discussion of the basis for the models. Another general mechanism that produces gene amplification involves the unequal crossing over of sister chromatids (not shown). (From Schimke,[84] with permission.)

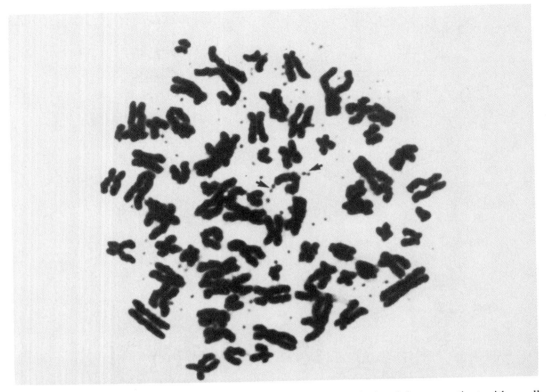

Fig. 9-13. Metaphase plate of methotrexate-resistant tumor cell isolated from a patient with small cell carcinoma of the lung. The presence of double minute chromosomes is indicated by the arrows. As shown in Table 9-8, tumor cells cultured from this patient were shown to have a high level of DHFR activity and an increased number of DHFR genes. As described in the text, both the amplified DHFR genes and the minichromosomes were lost as the tumor cells underwent serial passage under nonselective conditions. (From Curt et al.,[110] with permission.)

a patient with small cell lung cancer who was treated with methotrexate.[110] When the cells were initially cultured from the patient, they had a high level of DHFR activity and contained the double minute chromosomes indicated by the arrows in the figure. As the cell line underwent serial pasage in tissue culture, however, the cells reverted from methotrexate resistance to sensitivity, and both the DHFR activity and the amount of DHFR protein (as indicated by methotrexate binding activity) declined (Table 9-8). The loss of DHFR activity was accompanied by a loss of double minute chromosomes and a return of DHFR gene copy number to levels existing in a methotrexate-sensitive small cell lung tumor cell line isolated from a patient with newly diagnosed disease who had not received prior methotrexate therapy.[110]

Taken together, the case studies strongly suggest that amplification of the DHFR gene is responsible for clinical methotrexate resistance due to elevated DHFR activity. As indicated in the beginning of this section, resistance to other commonly used anticancer drugs, such as fluorouracil, has been shown to arise in cultured cells via amplification of a gene that codes for an enzyme target, and it is reasonable to predict that similar resistance

Table 9-8. Unstable Methotrexate Resistance in Human Small Cell Carcinoma Associated with Double Minute Chromosomes and DHFR Gene Amplification

[a]*Tumor Cell Line*	*Relative DHFR Activity*	*Relative Methotrexate Binding Capacity (Amount of DHFR Protein)*	*Relative DHFR Gene Copy Number*
NCI-H187	1	1	1
NCI-H249P			
Initial tumor line	11.7	11.2	2.4
After 6 mo in culture	0.8	1.3	1

[a] Tumor cells were isolated from a patient who was treated with high-dose methotrexate but no longer responded to the drug, and a cell culture (NCI-H249P) was established. Cells were assayed for DHFR activity by a spectrophotometric assay, for amount of DHFR protein by high-affinity binding of methotrexate, and for number of DHFR gene copies by filter hybridization using the ^{32}P-labeled mouse DHFR gene as the probe. Assays were performed immediately and after 6 months of serial passage in the absence of drug. Similar assays were performed on a continuous tumor cell line isolated from a patient with small cell lung cancer who had not been treated with methotrexate (NCI-H187), and the results of the assays were expressed relative to the value obtained in this sensitive cell line as 1. After 6 months in culture, the NCI-H249P cells had lost their double minute chromosomes and had reverted from resistance to sensitivity to methotrexate, as determined by a soft agar cytotoxicity assay. (From Curt et al.[110] with permission.)

via gene amplification will be established as the cause of clinical resistance to other anticancer drugs. The amplified gene product need not be an enzyme that is the target for the drug effect. In a subsequent section of this chapter concerned with multidrug resistance, we will review a type of resistance occurring in tumor cells in vitro in which a cross-resistance develops to several drugs with very different mechanisms of action. This multidrug resistance phenotype results from increased transport of the anticancer drugs out of the cell, and it is associated with the amplification of several tumor cell genes. It is likely that such multidrug resistance also arises in cancer patients during treatment, and an understanding of the mechanisms may allow modifications in therapy that will improve the drug treatment of cancer.

Schimke[84] has noted several principles of chemotherapy that may emerge from the study of drug resistance via gene amplification in cultured tumor cells. One principle that obtains regardless of whether resistance arises via gene mutation or amplification is that multiple drugs that are not incompatible should be used together to decrease the probability of selection of cells resistant to the therapeutic regimen. As transient inhibition of replication favors gene amplification, one should ensure that an effective concentration of the anticancer drug is delivered to the tumor for sufficient time to produce cell death. As gene amplification is often initially unstable and becomes stable only when cells are maintained under selective conditions for a long time, prolonged exposure to a single treatment regimen should perhaps be avoided. Resistance arising from brief exposure to one treatment regimen may decrease during treatment with a second treatment regimen and thus permit drugs in the initial regimen to be used again. Because conditions that damage DNA may facilitate gene amplification, it may be that DNA-damaging drugs, such as the alkylating agents, have the ability to promote drug resistance when they are used to treat tumors in which a major portion of the cells are actively replicating. If this consideration proves to be of clinical importance, it may be that alkylating agents would be most effective when used against tumors containing largely noncycling cells.

As one proceeds down the evolutionary ladder from the mammals to more rapidly growing eukaryotic organisms, one encounters instances in which resistance via gene amplification may have broad societal consequences. The demonstration of methotrexate resistance via DHFR gene amplification in *Leishmania*[82] suggests that gene amplification could be responsible for drug resistance in other protozoa, such as the plasmodia that cause malaria. It is also possible that gene amplification contributes to the extraordinary rapidity at which insect populations can become resistant to insecticides. In prokaryotes all three mechanisms for undergoing a change in gene composition may operate together to determine a resistant pheontype. That is, genes that have undergone mutation and selection for decreased drug response may be picked up by plasmids, in which they are amplified and subsequently transferred to drug-sensitive microbes, thus conferring a high degree of drug resistance.

BIOCHEMICAL MECHANISMS OF DRUG RESISTANCE

Microorganisms and eukaryotic cells in culture can become resistant to most cytotoxic drugs through mutation, acquisition, or amplification of genes determining cell functions required for the drug effect or of genes determining functions that in some way depress or overcome the drug effect. Thus, a wide variety of biochemical mechanisms that determine drug resistance have been defined.[1-5] The mechanisms fall within several general classifications, and in this section we will review some examples in each class. The examples are chosen either because of their clinical importance or because they illustrate some of the extraordinarily clever ways by which cells become resistant to drugs.

The study of biochemical mechanisms underlying drug resistance has contributed immensely to our understanding of how antimicrobial and anticancer drugs work at the cellular and molecular level. The study of resistance mechanisms has also led to improvements in therapy. In some cases (as discussed above for clavulanic acid and penicillinase), it has been possible to block the resistance mechanism and utilize combined drug regimens that are effective against the resistant organism. In other cases (e.g., with the animoglycoside antibiotics and the new β-lactams), modification of old drugs to prevent attack by resistance enzymes has led to the creation of new, potent drugs that are effective against resistant organisms. There are also a few instances in which delineation of a resistance mechanism has led to unique applications of established therapy in order to obtain a selective effect against the resistant cell (e.g., the use of high-dose methotrexate therapy followed by thymidine rescue in certain fluorouracil-resistant tumor cell populations).

From the outset the reader should realize that although only one resistance mechanism may be discussed below for a particular drug, several biochemical mechanisms of resistance have been defined for most of the common classes of antimicrobial and anticancer drugs.[1,2] Similarly, one should realize that if the biochemical pathway affected by a genetic alteration is one that is shared by several drugs, then cells that are selected for resistance to one of the drugs may display cross-resistance to the others. When resistance arises to drugs with different chemical structures and mechanisms of action, it is called *multidrug resistance* or *pleiotropic resistance*. In bacteria, resistance to multiple drugs is most often due to the acquisition of plasmids containing multiple resistant genes, each one of which determines a different drug resistance mechanism. In cancer cells, however, multidrug resistance is due to either gene mutation or gene amplification. It has been thought that multidrug resistance is uncommon in the clinical treatment of the cancer patient, but it is now clear that it occurs clinically[111] and it may be relatively common. The concept of cross-resistance is important from a therapeutic standpoint, as an awareness of cross-resistance patterns may permit design of specific second-line therapies for relapsing cancer patients that avoid drugs unlikely to be useful. Several biochemical mechanisms defining resistance to multiple drugs will be presented in the following sections.

Mechanism 1. Decreased Intracellular Drug Level

If an antimicrobial or anticancer drug is to be effective, adequate cytotoxic levels of the drug must be achieved at the site of drug action at the cell membrane or in the cell interior. Resistance based on a decreased intracellular level of drug is one of the most common types of resistance encountered clinically in the treatment of both infectious diseases and cancer. A variety of factors determine the intracellular concentration of a drug. Drugs enter cells by processes of passive diffusion, facilitated diffusion, and active transport, and once inside the cell, they may be transported out again, they may be bound to cellular constituents, or they may be chemically modified in such a manner that rapid efflux does not occur. Resistance may develop as a consequence of decreased drug entry or increased drug efflux, and alterations in each of the factors that determine intracellular drug levels have been associated with drug resistance.

As discussed previously in this chapter, in order for hydrophilic antibiotics such as the penicillins and cephalosporins to be active against gram-negative bacteria, they must first diffuse through pores in the outer membrane that are formed by proteins called *porins*. Gram-negative bacteria can develop a high level of drug resistance as a result of mutations that determine altered porin proteins and thus decreased passive drug diffusion.[18] A reduction in the rate of facilitated diffusion or active transport is frequently responsible for resistance to sulfonamides,[112] to the antifungal drug flucytosine,[113] and to several classes of anticancer drugs.[2] In some cases bacteria may become resistant to antimicrobial drugs by acquiring genes that determine an active efflux system. Tetracycline resistance is the best described example of this mechanism.

Tetracycline

In a study of 433 isolates of Enterobacteriaciae stored between 1917 and 1954, only 9 tetracycline-resistant strains were identified.[114] As a result of widespread selection and resistance transfer, however, tetracycline resistance is now the most common resistance determinant among all species of bacteria.[115] A large proportion of the tetracycline resistance determinants in both gram-negative and gram-positive bacteria are located on transposons, such as the Tn10 resistance transposon shown in the map of the R100 plasmid in Figure 9-10. In most bacteria with plasmid-determined tetracycline resistance, the property is inducible. That is, the level of resistance increases in response to the presence of subinhibitory concentrations of the drug.[116] In the great majority of clinical isolates, tetracycline resistance is associated with a decreased ability to accumulate the antibiotics. The biochemical basis for the resistance has been studied most extensively in *E. coli*.

The tetracyclines are cytotoxic by virtue of their ability to inhibit bacterial protein synthesis.[1] In a gram-negative bacillus such as *E. coli*, the drug enters the cell by diffusing through pores in the outer membrane (see Fig. 9-3) and then passing through the inner membrane, utilizing an active uptake system that is driven by the electrochemical gradient (proton-motive force). Thus, the drug utilizes processes of both passive diffusion and active uptake to reach its site of action in the cell interior. The mechanism of active uptake across the inner membrane is not well defined, as it has not yet been possible to demonstrate a saturable tetracycline carrier protein for this process. Drug-sensitive *E. coli* also contain an active efflux system that transports tetracycline from the inside of the cell

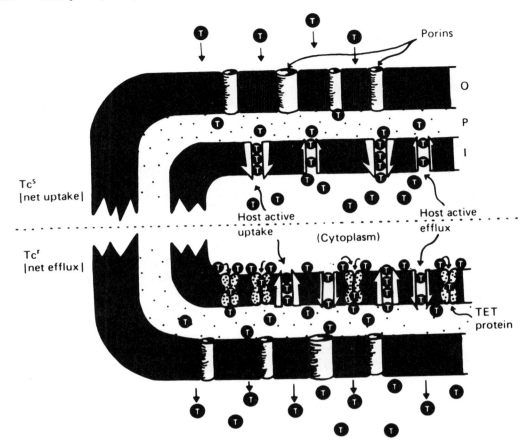

Fig. 9-14. Diagram of the components involved in tetracycline accumulation in sensitive (Tc^s, *top*) and resistant (Tc^r, *bottom*) cells. Sensitive cells show a net active uptake of tetracycline whereas resistant cells show a net active efflux. Tetracycline (T) passes through the outer membrane (O) of *E. coli* via pores formed by porin IA and diffuses across the periplasmic space (P) to the inner membrane (I), which it traverses via an active uptake system (probably carrier-mediated), which is driven by the electrochemical gradient (proton-motive force) across the membrane. A weaker active efflux system exists in the inner membrane, and the net active uptake of drug is determined by all three processes. Both the host uptake and efflux systems appear to operate normally in resistant cells, but there is in addition a higher-affinity efflux system provided by the plasmid-encoded, tetracycline-resistance protein TET. The TET protein appears to bind tetracycline and transport it from the inside surface of the inner membrane back into the periplasmic space. (From Levy,[115] with permission.)

back into the periplasmic space between the inner and outer membranes.[117] The entire system is diagrammed in Figure 9-14. The relative rate of tetracycline uptake and the intracellular drug level depends on the rate of drug entry through the outer cell membrane and the subsequent rates of relative uptake or efflux at the inner membrane. In the drug-sensitive bacterium the rate of efflux is relatively slow, and cytotoxic levels of drug rapidly accumulate in the cell.

There are several biochemical mechanisms that determine decreased drug accumulation in tetracycline-resistant strains of *E. coli.* Some tetracycline-resistant mutants have been shown to be deficient in porin IA, which permits tetracycline penetration of the outer membrane.[18] These porin mutants are often cross-resistant to the antibiotic chloramphenicol, which diffuses through the same pores.[18] The great majority of tetracycline-resistant bacterial strains encountered clinically have low intracellular levels of tetracycline because they have acquired plasmids that determine an energy-dependent system that actively transports the antibiotic out of the cell.[118] Four genetic classes of tetracycline resistance determinants residing on plasmids have been identified in *E. coli*, and each has been associated with an energy-dependent decrease in antibiotic accumulation in whole cells.

As shown in Figure 9-15, both tetracycline-sensitive *E. coli* and a strain infected with a resistance plasmid accumulate tetracycline at a similar rate in the absence of energy (+DNP), but when energy production is normal, the sensitive cells accumulate higher levels of drug, and the resistant cells accumulate much lower levels.[118] This observation suggests that the resistant cells are either actively preventing entry of tetracycline or actively effluxing the drug. The question was resolved by preparing everted inner membrane vesicles from resistant cells and examining drug uptake. In the everted vesicle the inside surface of the bacterial inner membrane is located on the outside of the vesicle, so that the efflux system now carries the drug to the vesicle interior. As shown in Figure 9-16, everted vesicles prepared from the inner membrane of *E. coli* bearing a resistance plasmid actively concentrate tetracycline when adenosine triphosphate (ATP) or lactate is present as an energy source, but the drug is lost from the vesicle when an energy inhibitor (CCCP) is added to the external solution.[115] The plasmid-determined drug efflux system does not affect the host-determined drug uptake system, which is completely functional in resistant cells. This was demonstrated with cells containing resistance plasmids bearing Tn10 mutants that showed temperature-sensitive drug efflux: at the non-permissive temperature an active uptake system typical of drug-sensitive cells was seen, but at the lower temperature there was drug efflux.[115]

The tetracycline resistance determinants have been shown to code for production of a

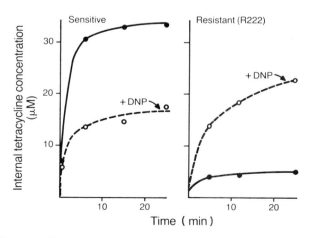

Fig. 9-15. Uptake of tetracycline by sensitive *E. coli* and by an induced resistant strain containing the R222 plasmid. Tetracycline uptake was assayed in the presence (○) or absence (●) of the energy inhibitor 2,4-dinitrophenol (DNP). (From McMurry et al.,[118] with permission.)

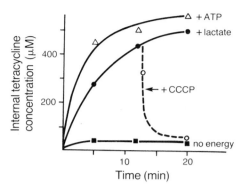

Fig. 9-16. Energy-dependent accumulation of tetracycline into everted inner membrane vesicles prepared from tetracycline-resistant *E. coli.* Everted vesicles were prepared from *E. coli* containing the resistance plasmid R222, and the uptake of tetracycline was determined in the absence of substrate (■) or in the presence of ATP (△) or lactate (●) as an energy source. At 12 minutes, the energy inhibitor carbonyl cyanide-*m*-chlorophenylhydrazone (CCCP) was added to vesicles in lactate (○), and sampling was continued. Energy inhibition caused loss of accumulated drug. (From Levy,[115] with permission.)

hydrophobic membrane protein called TET. The TET protein is a 34,000- to 43,000-dalton inner membrane protein,which is needed for drug efflux and presumably binds tetracycline. As indicated in the diagram of Figure 9-14, the TET protein is thought to span the membrane. Small amounts of TET protein are produced in uninduced resistant cells, but in the presence of inducer (i.e., tetracycline) the TET gene is derepressed and the synthesis of TET is markedly increased. An organizational map of the tetracycline resistance transposon, Tn10, is shown in Figure 9-17. Two protein products are expressed by the resistance determinant: one is a 23,000- to 25,000-dalton repressor and the other is the TET protein. The repressor and the TET protein sequences are transcribed in opposite directions, and there are two repressor-sensitive operator regions controlling overlapping promoters.[119,120] A similar genetic organization has been shown for all four classes of resistance determinants in *E. coli.*[115]

Although the major form of tetracycline resistance in clinical strains results from plasmid-mediated or transposon-mediated genes, tetracycline resistance in laboratory strains

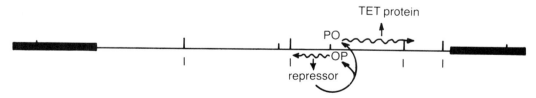

Fig. 9-17. Organizational map of the tetracycline resistance transposon Tn10. Tn10 is bordered on each end by the insertion sequence IS10 arranged as inverted repeated sequences. The genes for the repressor and the TET protein are transcribed in opposite directions. The locations of operators (O) and promoters (P) for the repressor and TET protein are shown. The arrows indicate that the repressor binds to two repressor-sensitive operator regions controlling divergent, overlapping promoters for each gene. I refers to cleavage sites for the HpaI restriction enzyme. (From Wray et al.,[120] with permission.)

can arise by stepwise selection of plasmid-free, wild-type *E. coli* in increasing concentrations of tetracyclines or chloramphenicol.[121] This resistance is due to gene amplification, and the resistance phenotype is not to tetracycline alone but also to chloramphenicol, the penicillins, the cephalosporins, nalidixic acid, and rifampin. The mechanism of resistance for tetracycline involves drug efflux that occurs at the inner membrane and is driven by energy supplied by the proton-motive force. The mechanisms of resistance to the other antibiotics are not yet known, but at least four separate loci on the *E. coli* chromosome are required for this form of amplifiable multidrug resistance.[122] This form of tetracycline resistance occurs only with growth in the presence of antibiotic, and upon removal of the selecting agent the level of resistance quickly declines. The tetracycline resistance gene is usually cryptic in the *E. coli* chromosome, but the drug selects for amplified forms of the gene. There is a striking similarity between this mechanism of tetracyline resistance encoded by the chromosome and the resistance determined by the plasmid-mediated TET protein.[115]

Methotrexate

Lymphoid cells selected for resistance to methotrexate, either in vivo or in vitro, may be resistant as a result of impaired membrane transport.[123,124] As discussed above, methotrexate-resistant cells often have increased DHFR activity, but transport mutants occur relatively frequently, and amplification of DHFR and decrease in methotrexate transport often exist together in the same resistant cell line.[124] A decrease in transport could result from a change in the affinity (K_m) of the transporter for the drug or from a decrease in maximum transport rate (V_{max}). In most cases resistant cells have been found to have a decreased V_{max}.[124,125] A decrease in V_{max} implies a decrease either in the amount of transporter in the cell membrane or in the rate of transport through the cell membrane in the resistant cell line.

Uptake of methotrexate into tumor cells can occur via two pathways. At relatively low drug concentrations (in the micromolar range), the drug is taken up by carrier-mediated, energy-dependent transport, but at high concentrations (in the millimolar range), the drug enters the cell predominantly by passive diffusion.[126] In the case of cells that become transport-resistant or in the case of tumors that are intrinsically resistant to therapy because of poor transport, high concentrations of drug may still be effective. Thus, methotrexate is sometimes administered in high-dose therapy in which serum concentrations of 0.1 millimolar (mM) or higher are achieved and uptake into the tumor is primarily via passive diffusion.[2] Because the high serum levels are toxic to the bone marrow, the epithelial mucosa, and other normal proliferative tissues of the host, leucovorin is administered at a carefully timed interval after administration of high-dose methotrexate in order to "rescue" these normal cells. As the normal cells have a normal transport mechanism, they will concentrate leucovorin, which bypasses the methotrexate block (see Fig. 9-11) and they will survive, whereas the tumor cells will be killed.

A second approach that has been used against transport-resistant tumor cells has been to use antifolate drugs containing lipophilic structures that enter more readily by passive diffusion.[125,127] In some cases resistant cells have not only responded well to such lipophilic compounds but they have demonstrated collateral sensitivity.[125,127,128] The term *collateral sensitivity* describes a poorly understood phenomenon in which a cell population that is resistant to one or more drugs is more sensitive to the cytotoxic effects of another drug or drugs than the wild-type parent cell population.[129] Although it is clear that collateral sensitivity occurs, the molecular bases for it are not known, and the observation of the phenomenon has been a chance event. If systematic patterns of collateral sensitivity could be identified, regimens of selective therapy could be devised for tumors displaying certain drug resistance phenotypes.

Fluorouracil

For many years 5-fluorouracil and its metabolite 5-fluoro-2'-deoxyuridine have been used to treat colon cancer. No other single drug or combination of drugs has been shown to be superior to treatment with fluorouracil. Between 20 and 40 percent of patients with colon carcinoma experience tumor regression with fluorouracil, but complete remission is rare or nonexistent.[2] Remissions, when they are obtained, are short-lived because of the development of drug resistance. Fluorouracil and fluorodeoxyuridine are taken into the cell via a facilitated diffusion system, which accepts a wide variety of purine and pyrimidine nucleosides as well as their analogs.[130] A fluorodeoxyuridine-resistant human colon carcinoma cell line has been isolated in vitro by stepwise selection in the presence of the drug.[131] After selection the cells showed a 700-fold resistance to fluorodeoxyuridine and various degrees of cross-resistance to several purine and pyrimidine analogs. The resistant cells failed to take up fluorodeoxyuridine from the medium.

It is possible that in the future oncologists may be able to selectively inhibit the growth of uptake-deficient cells of this type. Unlike neoplastic cells, the normal stem cell population in the bone marrow and gastrointestinal tract does not become resistant to the fluoropyrimidines. Thus, the stem cells will take up purines and pyrimidines, such as hypoxanthine and thymidine, in a normal manner. Methotrexate is taken up by a different route, and its efficacy should be unchanged in fluorodeoxyuridine-resistant tumor cells. Thus, one might be able to administer high-dose methotrexate to treat the tumor and then rescue the normal stem cells by administering thymidine, which bypasses the methotrexate-blocked reaction. As thymidine enters the cell by the same uptake system that is deficient in the resistant tumor cells, the cells would not be rescued and a selective effect would be obtained. Studies in vitro have shown that administration of thymidine protected the drug-sensitive human colon carcinoma cell line whereas the fluorodeoxyuridine-resistant subline was selectively killed.[132]

The Multidrug Resistance Phenotype

An interesting multidrug resistance is obtained by stepwise selection for resistance to any of several anticancer drugs, such as vincristine or vinblastine, which prevent tubulin polymerization, or actinomycin D or anthracycline antibiotics, which interact directly with DNA.[133,134] The cross-resistance pattern also includes colcemid, another inhibitor of microtubule function, and puromycin, an inhibitor of protein synthesis.[135] This multidrug resistance phenotype has also been called pleiotropic drug resistance because cross-resistance develops to a group of drugs with widely different structures and mechanisms of action. The only common features are that the drugs have a hydrophobic aromatic ring and a tendency to be positively charged at neutral pH.[136] The resistance is due to decreased drug accumulation in the cell. The observation that exposure to metabolic inhibitors increases intracellular drug levels in resistant cells suggested that decreased drug accumulation is due to accelerated drug efflux,[137] much as described above for tetracycline-resistant bacteria. It is now known that the resistant cells have a normal capacity for drug uptake but overproduce a transporter that is responsible for the drug efflux.[138-140]

Examination of membrane proteins in drug-sensitive parent cells and in multidrug-resistant mutants showed that highly resistant cell lines produce large amounts of a 170,000 dalton glycoprotein that is called P170 or P-glycoprotein.[141] P-glycoprotein can represent 3 to 4 percent of the total plasma membrane protein in the multidrug-resistant cells, and it is clearly overproduced as a result of gene amplification.[142] Multidrug resistance has been associated with the presence of both double-minute chromosomes and homogeneously staining regions in the same manner as methotrexate resistance due to DHFR gene amplification. The degree of overproduction of the P-glycoprotein correlates well with the degree of resistance, as shown in cell lines with different levels of resistance during stepwise selection and in revertant lines with reduced drug resistance.[143,144]

cDNAs encoding the 170,000 dalton P-glycoprotein have been cloned from several species, including mouse[145] and human.[146] Several observations provide solid support for the proposal that the P-glycoprotein is the transporter responsible for multidrug resistance: (1) P-glycoprotein has a binding site for drugs that are transported out of multidrug-resistant cells. This has been determined by directly labeling the 170,000 dalton protein with a photoaffinity derivative of vinblastine and demonstrating that the covalent drug binding is inhibited by some other drugs involved in multidrug resistance.[147] (2) Amplification of specific DNA sequences known to contain the P-glycoprotein gene correlates with the development of multidrug resistance, and reversion toward drug sensitivity is accompanied by an appropriate reduction in the number of gene copies.[142] (3) The cDNAs for the human *mdr*1 (*mdr* for *m*ulti*d*rug *r*esistance) and the mouse *mdr*1 genes coding for the P-glycoprotein have been cloned into expression vectors and transfected into drug-sensitive cell lines, with resulting conversion of the cells to the multidrug-resistant phenotype.[148,149]

A model of the multidrug transporter based on the deduced amino acid sequence is shown in Figure 9-18.[139] It can be seen that there is considerable conservation of amino acid sequence between the mouse and human P-glycoproteins, both of which contain

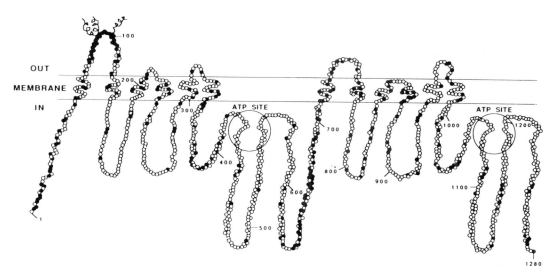

Fig. 9-18. Linear model of P-glycoprotein structure. The amino acids that differ between the mouse and human *mdr*1 sequences are shown as solid circles. Potential *N*-linked sugars are indicated as curly lines, and ATP binding sites are circled. (From Gottesman et al.,[139] with permission.)

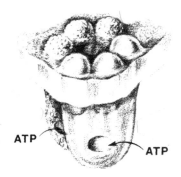

ATP   ATP

Fig. 9-19. Three-dimensional model of P-glycoprotein. The six membrane-spanning loops shown in Figure 9-18 have been arranged to form a central pore in the transporter. The two ATP binding sites lie at the inside surface of the plasma membrane. (Modified from Ames,[150] with permission.)

about 1,280 amino acids and 12 predicted transmembrane domains. The first half of the protein has more than 40 percent identity with the second half, which suggests that the two halves were generated by a gene duplication event. Interestingly, the hydrophilic regions lying at the inside of the cell membrane share strong homology with the ATP binding components of a number of bacterial permeases.[145,146] The bacterial permeases are complex systems containing at least 4 proteins that transport a variety of substrates (sugars, amino acids, ions, and peptides) into bacteria. The homology of the P-glycoprotein with the permease ATP-binding proteins includes the ATP binding site and extends well beyond it, indicating that there is a strongly conserved function. As diagrammed in Figure 9-19,[150] the six membrane-spanning loops of the P-glycoprotein are thought to form a pore, with the ATP binding sites and presumably a substrate binding site located at the inside of the membrane. It is thought that ATP hydrolysis drives a conformational change in the pore that results in efflux of the drug. The process of drug efflux is diagrammed on the left side of Figure 9-20.

Hybridization studies suggest that amplified DNA from multidrug-resistant cells contain a small family of related *mdr* genes, although, as discussed above, a single gene coding for a P-glycoprotein is sufficient to confer multidrug resistance. Nevertheless, other cellular changes have been correlated with multidrug resistance, including the overexpression of a 19,000 to 22,000 dalton acidic cytosolic protein that has been found in several multidrug-resistant cell lines obtained when the anticancer drug vincristine was employed as the selecting agent.[138] Table 9-9[147] illustrates a phenomenon that may be related to the existence of multiple *mdr* genes. When colchicine was used as the selecting drug in the human KB carcinoma cell line, the cells were most resistant to colchicine (1750-fold) and less resistant to vinblastine (254-fold) and doxorubicin (159-fold). Cells submitted to stepwise selection in vinblastine, however, are actually more resistant to doxorubicin than to vinblastine or colchicine. Thus, somewhat different patterns of cross-resistance can be seen when the same cell line is exposed to selection with different drugs. It is difficult to explain the existence of different cross-resistance patterns on the basis of amplification of the gene for a single P-glycoprotein transporter, and these differences may reflect modifying effects of other amplified gene products.

Studies of P-glycoprotein expression in normal tissues show relatively high levels in

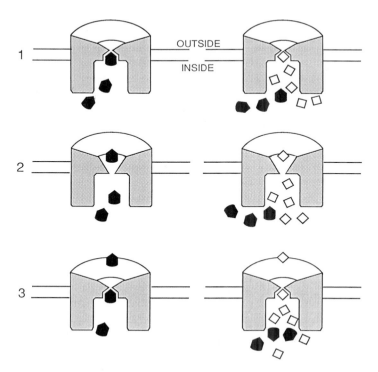

Fig. 9-20. Model of P-glycoprotein mediating drug efflux. The three stages on the left depict the outward transport of a drug in the absence of a competitor and, on the right, in the presence of a competitor, such as verapamil (open squares). (1) Both the drug and the competitor can occupy the transport site. (2) The hydrolysis of ATP then drives a conformational change in the transporter with release of the substrate at the external surface. (3) The transporter returns to the substrate-binding conformation.

kidney, liver, pancreas, small intestine, colon, and adrenal gland, with very low levels being found in most other tissues.[138,139] With the exception of the cells of the adrenal gland, where it is distributed diffusely throughout the plasma membrane, P-glycoprotein is localized to the luminal or apical surface of cells. Thus, it is found in the brush border of renal proximal tubular cells, on hepatocyte surfaces that line the bile canaliculi and bile ductules, at the pancreatic ductules, and on the luminal surface of the villus cells in the intestinal mucosa.[151] This localization suggests that the P-glycoprotein may have a normal physiologic role in secretory processes. Its presence in the liver, kidney, and bowel suggest that it may function normally in the elimination of drugs and other xenobiotics from the body. Thus, the multidrug resistance phenotype in the cancer cell may reflect amplification of genes that are normally responsible for elimination of drugs and other xenobiotics, or, in the case of the adrenal gland, for transport of endogenous metabolites.

Given the fact that the P-glycoprotein transports drugs with widely different structures, it is not surprising that a variety of compounds can compete with anticancer drugs for

Table 9-9. Relative Resistance of Human KB Carcinoma Cells to
Three Anticancer Drugs

	Relative Resistance		
Cell Line[a]	Vinblastine	Colchicine	Doxorubicin
KB-3-1	1	1	1
KB-C4	254	1750	159
KB-C4-R	3	6	4
KB-V1	213	170	458
KB-V1-R	1	1	1

[a] Multidrug-resistant sublines were prepared from drug-sensitive
human KB carcinoma cells (KB-3-1) by stepwise selection with either
colchicine (KB-C4) or vinblastine (KB-V1). KB-C4-R and KB-V1-R are
revertant lines prepared by growing the multidrug-resistant lines under
nonselective conditions. The concentration of each drug required to produce 50 percent inhibition of growth was determined for each cell line
and it is expressed here relative to the concentration required to inhibit
the growth of the drug-sensitive parent KB-3-1 cells.
(Data from Cornwell et al.[147])

the efflux mechanism, as depicted in the diagram on the right side of Figure 9-20. Several noncytotoxic drugs, such as the calcium channel blocker verapamil and the antiarrhythmic agent quinidine, inhibit the efflux of cytotoxic drugs from multidrug-resistant cells. The ability of verapamil to increase the intracellular content of the anticancer drug vinblastine in a multidrug-resistant subline of human cells is shown in Figure 9-21.[152] This effect suggests a form of combined drug therapy in which one drug in the combination is given specifically to compete for drug efflux, thus permitting cytotoxic drugs to achieve killing levels within otherwise resistant cells. It has been suggested that the intrinsic resistance of renal, hepatic, and gastrointestinal adenocarcinomas to a broad variety of anticancer drugs may be due in part to the relatively high normal expression of P-glycoprotein in

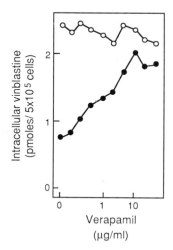

Fig. 9-21. Vinblastine accumulation in multidrug-resistant and sensitive KB cells in the presence of various concentrations of verapamil. Drug-sensitive parent cells (open circles) or a multidrug-resistant subline (closed circles) were incubated for 1 hour with 15 nM [3H]vinblastine and various concentrations of verapamil. At the end of the incubation, cells were washed and the intracellular radioactivity was assayed. (From Fojo et al.,[152] with permission.)

these tissues that was discussed above. If this is the case, combined therapy with cytotoxic drugs and drugs that block their efflux might enhance the efficacy of initial chemotherapy (i.e., prior to any selection for drug resistance) in these tumors, which are traditionally refractory to drug treatment.

Earlier in this chapter, we discussed the widespread emergence of chloroquine resistance in many strains of the plasmodium that causes falciparum malaria. It has been known since the 1960s that resistant strains of *P. falciparum* accumulate less chloroquine than susceptible strains.[1] It now seems clear that this reduced accumulation is due to more rapid efflux of the drug from the resistant parasite. As in the case of the multidrug-resistant cancer cells, verapamil inhibits chloroquine efflux and reverses chloroquine resistance in *P. falciparum* in vitro. Desipramine and some other tricyclic antidepressant drugs have been shown to reverse chloroquine resistance in *P. falciparum* in vitro at concentrations observed in the plasma of human patients treated for depression.[153] In what may constitute a very important therapeutic advance, it was shown that combined chloroquine and desipramine treatment of owl monkeys infected with chloroquine-resistant *P. falciparum* resulted in rapid suppression of parasitemia. As we mentioned earlier in the chapter, *P. falciparum* has the propensity to become resistant to multiple antimalarial drugs, and combined therapy with desipramine and chloroquine was also shown to effectively suppress parasitemia in monkeys infected with such a multidrug-resistant strain.[153]

The logical extension of these observations would be the design of compounds that are themselves pharmacologically inert but that can be used to block cytotoxic drug efflux. Such compounds could be very useful in combination drug therapy of patients with multidrug-resistant tumors, for limited prophylaxis against, as well as treatment of, acute clinical attacks of drug-resistant falciparum malaria, and perhaps for initial treatment of patients with intrinsically resistant cancers, if such cancers are refractory to treatment because of intrinsically high P-glycoprotein expression.

Mechanism 2. Increased Inactivation of Drug

As many of the antibiotics are produced by soil microorganisms, it is perhaps not surprising that bacteria living in the environment of antibiotic-producing organisms might produce enzymes that render antibiotics biologically inert. As the genes determining the inactivating enzymes can be transferred on plasmids and by transposition, the abundance of these genes in the pool of common pathogenic bacteria has increased markedly with the selective pressure of widespread antibiotic use. Resistance due to increased drug inactiviation and resistance due to decreased drug uptake are the two most common biochemical mechanisms accounting for the antibiotic resistance that is encountered in the clinical treatment of bacterial infections.[1] Antibiotics are inactivated either by enzymatic cleavage or by chemical modification such that they no longer interact with the target site or are no longer taken up by the organism. The classic example of drug inactivation via enzymatic cleavage is the inactivation of penicillins and cephalosporins by β-lactamase enzymes, which was reviewed earlier in this chapter. Inactivation by chemical modification is the major mechanism of clinical resistance to the aminoglycoside antibiotics and to chloramphenicol. Perhaps the most far-reaching example of resistance via chemical inactivation is the worldwide development of resistance to insecticides.

Aminoglycoside Antibiotics and Chloramphenicol

The aminoglycoside antibiotics include such commonly used drugs as gentamicin, tobramycin, kanamycin, amikacin, streptomycin, and neomycin. They are all bactericidal drugs by virtue of their ability to bind to the 30S ribosomal subunit and inhibit protein synthesis.[1] Three mechanisms of resistance have been identified in clinical isolates: (1) resistance due to mutations in a protein that forms part of the drug receptor site on the ribosome; (2) resistance due to decreased drug uptake; and (3) resistance due to aminoglycoside-modifying enzymes. More than 20 aminoglycoside-modifying enzymes have been identified, and they fall within three general classes: O-phosphotransferases, O-nucleotidyltransferases (adenylyltransferases), and N-acetyltransferases.[154,155] The enzymes are associated with the bacterial cell membrane, and it is probably at the internal surface of the membrane, where the ATP and coenzyme A cofactors are readily available, that the aminoglycosides are inactivated. When the capacity for drug modification exceeds the rate of drug uptake across the membrane, most or all of the drug that is accumulated is inactivated, and the bacterium is resistant. The genes for the aminoglycoside-modifying enzymes are carried on plasmids and are expressed in a constitutive manner. Each of the aminoglycoside antibiotics can be modified by more than one enzyme, and each enzyme can modify more than one antibiotic. A chemical modification that inactivates one aminoglycoside may not markedly affect the antibacterial activity of another. Thus, different resistance profiles develop, depending upon whether the bacterium harbors one plasmid conferring one enzyme or several plasmids conferring different modifying enzymes.

The clinical usefulness and the spectrum of action of aminoglycosides are inversely related to their ability to serve as substrates for the modifying enzymes. The study of the modifying enzymes has led to the design and synthesis of aminoglycosides that are not substrates for the enzymes and are thereby effective against resistant strains. Amikacin, a semisynthetic derivative of the older drug kanamycin, is one of the more successful of these compounds introduced into clinical use. Figure 9-22 shows the structures of kanamycin A and amikacin. Kanamycin A is a substrate for at least 14 aminoglycoside-modifying enzymes, and because of this resistance to kanamycin is widespread, and the drug is no longer very useful clinically. In contrast, amikacin is a substrate for only three modifying enzymes produced by gram-negative bacteria, and its relative insensitivity to enzymatic modification is reflected in the relatively low incidence of amikacin resistance in clinical isolates.

Chloramphenicol binds to the larger subunit (50S) of the bacterial ribosome and inhibits protein synthesis. Bacteria generally become resistant to chloramphenicol by acquiring plasmids that determine the production of chloramphenicol acetyltransferase.[157] Chloramphenicol has the following structure:

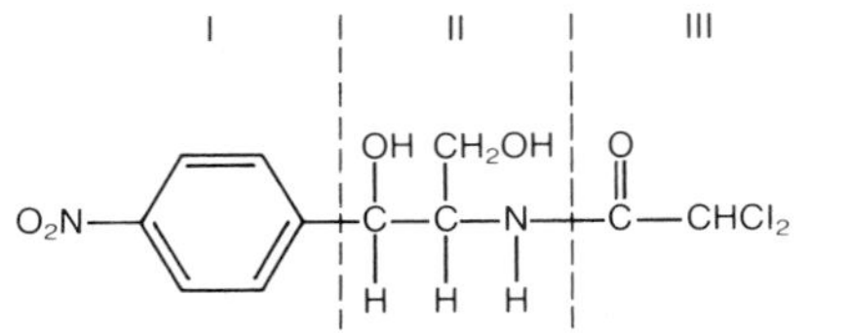

Chloramphenicol

The aromatic ring system (I) and the acetyl side chain (III) of chloramphenicol can be extensively substituted without loss of antibacterial potency, whereas very little substitution is permitted in the propanediol moiety (II).[158] The acetyltransferase acetylates the

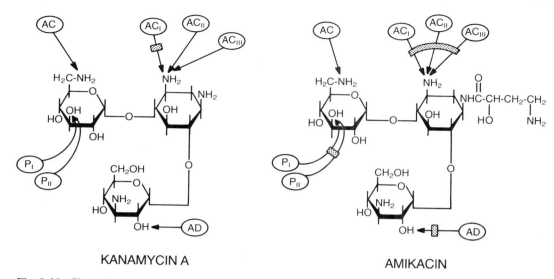

KANAMYCIN A   **AMIKACIN**

Fig. 9-22. Sites where kanamycin A and amikacin are modified by several aminoglycoside-modifying enzymes. The arrows point to sites modified by *N*-acetyltransferases (AC), *O*-phosphotransferases (P) and an *O*-adenylyltransferase (AD). The hatched bars indicate that the enzyme is not able to modify the site. Kanamycin A is attacked by at least 14 different enzymes, of which 6 are shown in the figure. The modification of the kanamycin structure that yielded amikacin rendered the molecule susceptible to attack by only one of the six enzymes. Thus, amikacin is effective against many bacteria that are resistant to kanamycin. (From Moellering,[156] with permission.)

drug at the 3-hydroxy position in the propanediol moiety,[159] and the modified drug is no longer able to bind to its receptor site on the 50S subunit of the bacterial ribosome.[160]

Insecticides

During the 1950s and 1960s the emergence of mutant insect strains that are resistant to the commonly used insecticides became a major worldwide problem.[161,162] By 1970, for example, resistant populations had developed in 224 species, of which 105 species were of public health or veterinary importance. Among the anopheline and culicine mosquitoes, resistance to DDT, dieldrin, and malathion had been observed. Populations of houseflies in California, Florida, and Japan had become resistant to four major insecticide groups–chlorinated hydrocarbons (DDT), cyclodienes (dieldrin), organophosphates, and carbamates.

The typical mechanism of resistance is by production of a drug-metabolizing enzyme.[163,164] For example, houseflies resistant to DDT demonstrated a greatly enhanced capacity to inactivate the toxic compound by dehydrochlorination. Houseflies resistant to carbamate insecticides have been shown to degrade these compounds more rapidly than do the sensitive strains.[165] The most extensive studies in insects have dealt with resistance to organophosphate cholinesterase inhibitors such as malathion. Malathion becomes an active inhibitor only upon its conversion to an oxygen analog known as *malaoxon*. Both malathion and malaoxon can be degraded by a phosphatase and by a carboxyesterase:

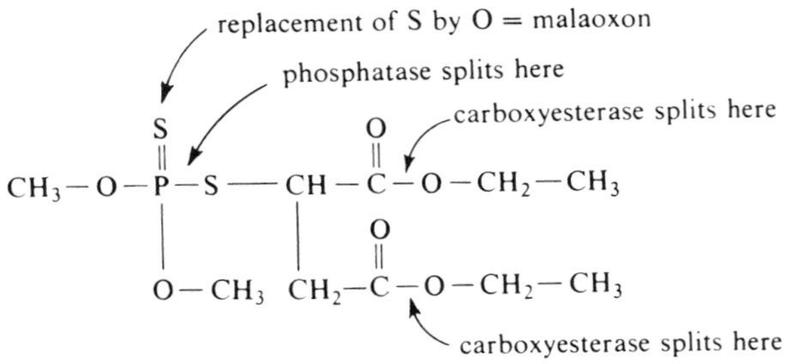

During the widespread use of malathion as a larvicide against mosquitoes, a resistant strain emerged.[166] Larvae of this strain were found to contain greatly increased activity of a mitochondrial carboxyesterase that degraded malathion to the monoester and the succinic acid derivative. Thus, less malathion remained available for conversion to malaoxon. The degradation of malaoxon was also increased in this strain as compared with the sensitive strain. The enhanced esterase activity was thought to be due to an increased amount of the normal enzyme, since no alterations in affinity for malathion were found. However, affinities for other substrates were not studied, nor were pH optima or thermal stability.

Mating experiments showed that the increased carboxyesterase activity was inseparable from the malathion resistance. The data are shown in Table 9-10. The resistant larvae required 42 times higher malathion concentration for a 50 percent kill than did the sensitive strain; under the conditions of the assay, the carboxyesterase activity was 5.5 times higher. There was no difference in phosphatase activity between the two strains. The first-generation hybrid (F_1) showed a resistance level somewhat lower than the resistant strain and a higher carboxyesterase activity. Selection for malathion resistance was carried out among the F_1 hybrids. Survivors of exposure to malathion (1 part per million) were crossed back to the sensitive line to obtain strain B_1. The same procedure was repeated with B_1, survivors being mated with the sensitive strain to obtain B_2. Table 9-10 shows that the high carboxyesterase activity was retained in B_1 and B_2 strains, despite their genomes being 3/4 and 7/8, respectively, derived from the sensitive stock. Thus, selection for mal-

Table 9-10. Carboxyesterase Activity and Malathion Resistance in Mosquito Larvae

Larvae[a]	Malathion LC50 (ppm)	Carboxyesterase products (%)	Phosphatase products (%)
Resistant	1.8	4.4 ± 0.6	4.3 ± 0.8
Sensitive	0.043	0.8 ± 0.3	3.2 ± 0.9
F_1 hybrid	0.80	4.5 ± 1.0	
B_1 back-cross	0.75	4.2 ± 0.4	
B_2 back-cross	0.80	5.4 ± 0.6	

[a] Larvae of *Culex tarsalis* were tested for sensitivity to malathion by determining the LC50 (concentration, in parts per million, killing 50 percent of the larvae). Carboxyesterase and phosphatase products were measured by an in vitro assay using radioactive malathion and identifying products by a chloroform extraction procedure; the data are percent of total radioactivity found in products in 30 minutes at 23°C.

(From Matsumura et al.[166] with permission.)

athion resistance resulted in associated high activity of the particular degradative enzyme. It was concluded that the gene conferring malathion resistance is an allele of the wild-type gene that determines carboxyesterase activity.

A similar investigation[167] of malathion resistance in houseflies showed that although resistance was accompanied by increased esterase activity toward malathion or malaoxon, there was decreased activity toward other ester substrates (e.g., methoxybutyrate). In mating experiments, this decreased activity was inseparable from the increased activity toward malathion or the resistance to malathion. Thus, it seems likely that the enhanced ability to degrade the insecticide resulted from a qualitatively altered enzyme rather than a simple increase in amount of normal enzyme. The increase in esterase activity toward malathion and the concomitant decrease in activity toward methoxybutyrate suggested that the resistant strain might prove to be sensitive to a methyl ester analog of malathion; this was demonstrated to be true.[168] Thus, resistance to one particular insecticide does not necessarily confer cross-resistance, even to closely related congeners.

Most insecticides are oxidatively metabolized, apparently by a system involving NADPH and a cytochrome P450 resembling that found in mammalian liver.[169] Induction of microsomal enzyme activity by insecticides is not usually observed; however, resistance emerges through selection of resistant mutants. Certain compounds, known as synergists, act as inhibitors (actually competitive substrates) of the P450 system, thereby protecting an active insecticide against destruction. An example shown below is piperonyl butoxide, which can saturate the microsomal system, thus enhancing the potency of another compound against resistant strains.[170]

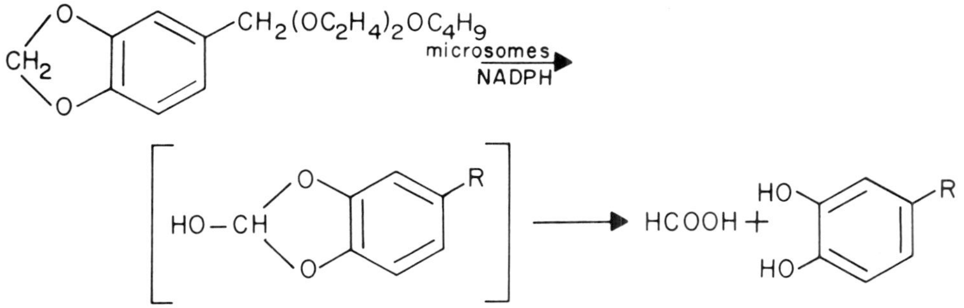

Mechanism 3. Decreased Conversion of Drug to a More Active Compound

If a drug is inactive in the form in which it is administered but is converted to an active inhibitor once it is inside the target cell, then alterations that impair drug conversion will confer resistance. This mechanism of resistance occurs most often with drugs that act as antimetabolites, and it arises via mutation and selection.

Methotrexate

After it is transported into the cell, methotrexate, like natural folate cofactors, is converted to polyglutamate derivatives that contain two to six covalently linked γ-glutamyl residues. The polyglutamate derivatives are selectively retained by cells, probably because of both an increased affinity of binding to target enzymes such as DHFR and a decreased affinity for the outward transport system responsible for methotrexate efflux. Synthesis of polyglutamate derivatives of methotrexate is associated with prolonged inhibition of

DNA synthesis and is positively correlated with cytotoxicity as measured by clonogenic assays.[171] Although resistance of human tumor cells to methotrexate is most commonly due to increased production of DHFR, altered affinity of DHFR, or impaired membrane transport, it can also be due to decreased formation of polyglutamate derivatives.[172,173] In a careful study of a methotrexate-resistant subline of human breast cancer cells, resistance was associated with multiple defects, including a threefold decrease in transport of the drug into the cell, a threefold decrease in the activity of thymidylate synthetase, and a virtual absence of polyglutamate formation.[173] The resistance was not associated with an apparent change in the activity of polyglutamyl synthetase in cell-free extracts or with any alteration in the apparent K_m of the enzyme for methotrexate. This leads to the speculation that the differences between the resistant cells and the parental cell line from which they were derived by stepwise selection may represent an alteration in the intracellular regulation of polyglutamyl synthetase activity.[173] It is interesting that these methotrexate-resistant cells are cross-resistant to antifolate analogs that can be converted to polyglutamate derivatives, yet they remain relatively sensitive to antifolate analogs that cannot be converted to polyglutamate forms.

Purine and Pyrimidine Analogs

Drugs that are purine and pyrimidine analogs must be converted to nucleotides before they become cytotoxic.[2] The anticancer drug 5-fluorouracil (FU), for example, must be converted to 5-fluorouridine 5'-monophosphate (FUMP) before it exerts its cytotoxicity via inhibition of thymidylate synthetase and subsequent inhibition of DNA synthesis or via incorporation into RNA. The relative contribution of the DNA-directed versus the RNA-directed effect to the cytotoxicity varies according to cell type.[174] Two pathways by which the drug is activated are shown in Figure 9-23. In one pathway the drug is first converted to FUMP via a reaction with phosphoribosyl pyrophosphate catalyzed by a pyrimidine phosphoribosyltransferase. The second pathway involves conversion to fluorouridine (FUR), which is then phosphorylated by uridine kinase. Subsequent reactions convert the drug to the nucleotide triphosphate, which is incorporated into RNA, and to 5-fluoro-2'-deoxyuridine 5'-monophosphate (FdUMP), which is the form that inhibits thymidylate synthetase.[2] Depending upon the type of tumor cell, one pathway of FUMP

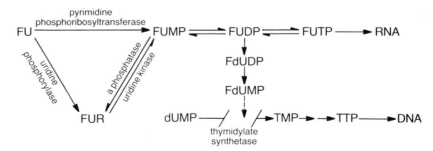

Fig. 9-23. Conversion of fluorouracil (FU) to its active cytotoxic forms. To exert its cytotoxic effect FU has to be converted to either fluorodeoxyuridine monophosphate (FdUMP), which inhibits thymidylate synthetase, or to flurouridine triphosphate (FUTP), which is incorporated into RNA. Resistance to FU in tumor cells has been associated with decreased activity of pyrimidine phosphoribosyltransferase, uridine phosphorylase, and uridine kinase.

formation or the other may predominate. Resistance to FU based on decreased conversion to FUMP has been demonstrated in several animal tumor systems. The resistance mechanisms include decreased activity of pyrimidine phosphoribosyltransferase[175] and uridine kinase,[176] as well as the absence of uridine phosphorylase activity.[177]

In most cases a decrease in or a lack of converting enzyme activity reflects the selection of cells that have undergone mutations in the structural genes for the enzymes. The activities of the converting enzymes are influenced by a variety of factors, however, and resistance to purine and pyrimidine analogs can develop via ingeniously indirect mechanisms. A clone of mouse lymphoma cells, for example, was selected for resistance to the RNA-directed cytotoxic effects of FU by culturing them in the presence of both FU and thymidine. The cells were also less sensitive than the parental cells to the cytotoxic nucelosides fluorouridine (FUR) and arabinosylcytosine. The resistance was found to result from an alteration in the enzyme CTP synthetase, such that it was no longer subject to allosteric regulation by cytidine triphosphate (CTP).[178] CTP synthetase catalyzes the de novo synthesis of CTP from UTP, and it is subject to feedback inhibition by its product. Because the enzyme in resistant cells is refractory to inhibition by CTP, the resistant cells contain elevated levels of cytidylate nucelotides. The elevated levels of CTP inhibit uridine kinase, the enzyme that converts FUR to FUMP (see Fig 9-23). Thus, the resistant cells survive exposure to FU because they cannot convert the drug to its active form. In addition to accounting for FU resistance, the genetic loss of normal allosteric inhibition of CTP synthetase activity also confers a high spontaneous mutator phenotype. Apparently, the alteration in deoxynucelotide pools in these cells leads to errors of nucleotide incorporation during DNA replication and consequently to a higher rate of mutation. Thus, these FU-resistant mutants display elevated rates of spontaneous mutation to resistance to other anticancer drugs, such as dexamethasone or thioguanine, which possess very different mechanisms of action.[179]

In contrast to the pyrimidine analogs, purine analogs are converted to their nucleotides in mammalian cells only via reaction with phosphoribosylpyrophosphate, the so-called "salvage pathway." The enzyme responsible for the activation of the anticancer drug 6-mercaptopurine is hypoxanthine-guanine phosphoribosyltranferase. A number of 6-mercaptopurine-resistant cell lines and experimental tumors are deficient in or have lost their hypoxanthine-guanine phosphoribosyltransferase activity.[180] As this enzyme also activates 6-thioguanine, the tumor cells are cross-resistant to both drugs. 6-Methylmercaptopurine riboside, synthesized with the goal of circumventing this type of resistance, is transported into mammalian cells, where it is phosphorylated by a purine kinase.[181] Some experimental tumor cells that are resistant to 6-mercaptopurine will respond to 6-methylmercaptopurine riboside; however, the drug does not induce remissions in patients with 6-mercaptopurine-resistant acute leukemia.[182]

Mechanism 4. Increased Concentration of Metabolite Antagonizing the Drug Action

If a drug acts as an antimetabolite, then alterations in the cell that lead to an increased production of the normal metabolite will compete for the drug effect and lead to resistance.

One of the earliest investigations of sulfonamide resistance disclosed a striking example of this mechanism.[183] The sulfonamides are structural analogs of the para-aminobenzoic acid component of folic acid, and they inhibit the growth of microorganisms by inhibiting folate synthesis. When the amount of para-aminobenzoic acid in sulfonamide-resistant *staphylococci* was compared with that in the drug-sensitive parent strain, an increase on the order of 100-fold was found in the resistant cells. This increase was sufficient to account for the observed degree of resistance through competitive antagonism of the sulfonamide inhibition. Overproduction of a metabolite implies that there has been mutational loss of control in a pathway that is subject to regulation by end product ("feedback") inhibition or by end product repression of enzymes. It is conceivable, however, that an organism could overproduce a metabolite by acquiring or amplifying genes that determine its production.

Resistance to the antifungal drug flucytosine can also result from overproduction of a metabolite. Flucytosine itself is not cytotoxic; to become cytotoxic, it must be transported into the fungal cell, where it is deaminated to yield FU, which in turn must be converted to the appropriate cytotoxic nucelotides (see Fig. 9-23). Flucytosine is selectively toxic to fungi because most cells in the mammlian host do not possess cytosine deaminase, which is required for conversion to FU. Clinical resistance to flucytosine is extremely common. The resistance may result from a decrease in the activity of the cytosine-specific permease responsible for drug uptake,[184] a loss of cytosine deaminase activity,[185] or a decrease in the activity of uridine monophosphate (UMP) pyrophosphorylase,[184] which converts FU to 5-fluorouracil monophosphate. Mutant organisms created in the laboratory have been shown to be resistant by all of these mechanisms and also by the absence of feedback inhibition of pyrimidine synthesis.[186] Normally, aspartic transcarbamylase, the first enzyme in the pyrimidine biosynthetic pathway, is under feedback inhibitory control by uridine triphosphate (UTP). A mutation that results in a loss of this regulation leads to increased endogenous synthesis of uridine nucleotides, which compete with the fluorine-containing uridine analogs derived from the drug and overcome the antifungal effect.

Mechanism 5. Altered Amount of Target Enzyme or Receptor

Increase in Target Enzyme

If a drug acts by inhibiting an enzyme that is critical for cell growth, then cells that produce greater amounts of the enzyme may be able to produce a sufficient amount of the metabolic product to survive in the presence of the drug concentrations that are usually attained in clinical treatment. When cancer cells are exposed to a stepwise protocol of selection in vitro, cells with an amplified number of gene copies for the target enzyme may be selected. The example of methotrexate resistance arising via amplification of the gene for DHFR has been discussed in detail in a previous section of this chapter. Another well established example of this mechanism is resistance to FU which can arise in certain cells that overproduce thymidylate synthetase, the enzyme that is inhibited by FdUMP. Again the overproduction of this enzyme is clearly due to gene amplification.[85,86] Microorganisms may become resistant to high levels of drug as a result of infection by resistance plasmids containing multiple copies of the genes for the target enzyme. This is seen, for example, in some bacteria that are resistant to the folate analog trimethoprim because they contain plasmids with amplified copies of the DHFR gene. A third mechanism for overproduction of a target enzyme is via a mutation in a regulatory gene that controls the expression of the structural gene for the enzyme. For example, if a gene for a drug target enzyme is under the influence of a repressor, a mutation in the repressor gene that renders the repressor protein inactive would result in constitutive synthesis of the target enzyme and possibly in drug resistance.

Decrease in Receptor

In certain cases in which the receptor for a drug is not an enzyme required for cell growth, resistance can result from decreased production of the receptor or from a mutation that eliminates the ability of the receptor to perform its biologic functions.

The glucocorticoid steroids are used to treat a variety of tumors of lymphatic origin, and resistance often arises during therapy. As these steroids are cytotoxic for some thymus-derived lymphocytes that grow in cell culture, it is easy to select single-step mutants that are glucocorticoid-resistant and to study the resistance mechanism in vitro. Most of these resistant cells contain variant receptors.[187] The specific receptor protein for glucocorticoids exists in cytoplasm, where steroid binding occurs. Once it has bound the drug, the receptor is transformed to a state that has a high affinity for DNA, and it is rapidly transferred into the cell nucleus, where it acts by regulating gene transcription. Two receptor functions, binding of steroid and binding to DNA or nuclei, can be readily assayed in cell-free systems. Three types of receptor defects have been identified in cultured murine thymic lymphocytes selected for resistance to the potent glucocorticoid dexamethasone.[188] Most of the resistant variants are classed as receptor-negative (r⁻). This category includes cells with no steroid binding activity and cells with low levels of binding activity. In some cases it has been shown that the levels of receptor protein are decreased or absent in the r⁻ cells, which shows that the resistance does not simply reflect a mutation in the steroid binding site that renders the receptor unable to bind the drug.

In addition, two types of receptor defects have been identified in which hormone binding is roughly normal but interaction of the steroid-receptor complex with the cell nucleus or DNA is affected. In one class of these mutants, nuclear binding of the receptors is particularly low. These resistant cells are called *nuclear transfer-deficient* (nt⁻). The nt⁻ receptors are the same size as receptors in the wild-type parent cells, but they have undergone mutations that render them unable to bind with high affinity to DNA.[189] The other class of mutants with normal steroid binding is characterized by an increased binding of receptors to nuclei. These resistant cells are called *nuclear transfer-increased* (ntⁱ), and they contain receptors with a molecular weight of 40,000 daltons as compared with 100,000 for the wild-type murine receptor.[189] These ntⁱ mutants contain the steroid-binding domain of the receptor protein and the DNA-binding domain, but they lack the portion of the receptor that is apparently involved in modulating DNA and nuclear binding of the receptor. The 60,000-dalton portion of the receptor that is missing is obviously in some way critical for the hormone effect because the cells are resistant in spite of normal binding of steroid to the receptor and increased binding of the receptor to nuclei.

Mechanism 6. Decreased Affinity of Receptor for Drug

If the gene for a protein that is the target for a drug action undergoes a mutation that changes the conformation of the drug-binding site, resistance may result. Usually, there is a modest decrease in affinity for the drug, and if the organism is exposed to high enough concentrations, the drug will still have a cytotoxic effect. Under conditions of stepwise selection, high levels of resistance may result because additional mutations alter the receptor site in such manner that the affinity for the drug is decreased further with each selection step. On occasion, a single mutation may alter the receptor so much that essentially no affinity for the drug remains. Mutations of this type have been very useful in defining the target sites responsible for the cytotoxic action of a variety of drugs.

It is often the case that a drug inhibits a variety of cellular reactions, and by using solely biochemical approaches, it is difficult to determine which effect is critical for the cytotoxic action. If drug resistance is associated with decreased affinity for binding to a particular site, however, it can be concluded that this site is in some way critical for the drug action. Careful examination of herpes simplex virus strains selected for high-level resistance to the antiviral drugs vidarabine and acyclovir, for example, showed that the resistance mutations mapped to the viral DNA polymerase gene locus.[190] Thus, it could be concluded either that inhibition of the viral DNA polymerase or that incorporation of the drug by the enzyme into viral DNA is critical for the antiviral effect.

In some cases a drug resistance mutation in a target enzyme has led to the identification of a previously undefined enzyme function. The target of the antimicrobial compound nalidixic acid, for example, was identified when it was found that a crude extract from a nalidixic acid-sensitive strain of *E. coli* conferred drug sensitivity on phage DNA replication directed by enzymes from a nalidixic acid-resistant strain (*nal*A^r) of *E. coli*.[191,192] This assay system permitted the purification of the *nal*A gene product, a 105,000-dalton protein, which is a subunit of DNA gyrase and is the target of nalidixic acid action. DNA gyrase is one of a class of enzymes called *topoisomerases*, which control the amount of supercoiling in bacterial DNA and are essential for DNA replication in the intact cell. There are two 105,000-dalton A subunits in each molecule of gyrase in *E. coli*. The A subunits nick and close one strand of DNA during the process of forming negative DNA supercoils. The study of nalidixic acid resistance permitted identification of this nicking-closing function.

Antibiotics That Inhibit Protein Synthesis

Several commonly administered antibiotics act by binding to sites on the bacterial ribosome and inhibiting protein synthesis. Mutations in ribosomal proteins that form the binding sites confer resistance. The so-called ribosomal type of resistance to streptomycin is a well-defined example of this resistance mechanism. As mentioned in a previous section of this chapter, single-step mutation to a high level of streptomycin resistance results from mutations in the *str*A locus, a gene that determines the production of a component of the 30S subunit of the bacterial ribosome called *protein S12*.[54] The experiment presented in Table 9-11 demonstrates that mutations in the S12 protein lead to decreased binding of streptomycin to the ribosome. Bacterial ribosomes are composed of 50S and 30S subunits. In this experiment 30S subunits were isolated from streptomycin-sensitive and resistant *E. coli* and then further fractionated into their 16S RNA and 21 different protein components. Hybrid 30S particles were then constructed in which all of the proteins except protein S12 were derived from one bacterial strain and protein S12 was derived from the other. The binding of radiolabeled dihydrostreptomycin to the reconstructed ribosomal subunits was then assayed by a simple filtration technique. The data show that there is significant binding of dihydrostreptomycin to reconstituted ribosomes only when the S12 protein is derived from sensitive cells. Thus, the S12 protein is a necessary component of the streptomycin receptor site. This high-level streptomycin resistance results from mutations in the *str*A locus that determine a single amino acid replacement at one of two positions in the S12 protein.[56] Streptomycin is an aminoglycoside antibiotic, and the most common mechanism of clinical resistance to this class of drugs in gram-negative bacilli involves increased drug inactivation. Streptomycin is frequently used to treat tuberculosis,

Table 9-11. Binding of Dihydrostreptomycin to 30S Ribosome Subunits Prepared with Proteins from Drug-Sensitive and Resistant Strains of Bacteria

[a]*Origin of Proteins used for Reconstituted 30S Subunits*		
All Proteins but S12	**Protein S12**	*Bound Dihydrostreptomycin (cpm)*
S	S	1198
S	r	65
S	—	83
r	r	31
r	S	691
Control 30S (S)		943
Control 30S (r)		35

[a] 30S ribosomal particles were reconstituted from 16S ribosomal RNA and purified 30S subunit proteins isolated from streptomycin-sensitive or streptomycin-resistant *E. coli*. The reconstituted particles were then incubated at 30°C with radioactive dihydrostreptomycin, and after 20 minutes the bound drug–30S complex was separated from the free drug by filtration. The amount of bound dihydrostreptomycin is expressed as counts per minute (cpm) per 1.5 OD_{260}, units of 30S particles. S, sensitive; r, resistant.

(From Ozaki et al.,[55] with permission.)

however, and among tubercle bacilli, resistance due to an alteration in the ribosomal binding site for streptomycin is quite common.[1]

In contrast to streptomycin, the ribosomal binding sites for the antibiotics erythromycin, chloramphenicol, and the lincomycins lie on the 50S ribosome subunit. These antibiotics are structurally quite different from one another, and they inhibit different steps in the process of protein synthesis.[1] Nevertheless, we know from studies of drug binding that the receptor sites for each of these drugs overlap or interact in some way. For example, the binding of radiolabeled chloramphenicol to ribosomes is inhibited by erythromycin and lincomycin,[193] and the binding of radiolabeled lincomycin is inhibited by erythromycin.[194] The binding of radiolabeled erythromycin is not inhibited by chloramphenicol or lincomycin[195,196]; thus the binding sites are not identical. Laboratory strains of erythromycin-resistant *E. coli* have been selected that do not bind erythromycin because of a single amino acid replacement in the L4 protein of the 50S subunit.[197] One of the L4 protein mutants also binds chloramphenicol with decreased affinity.[198] Another type of mutation also suggests a similarity in the interactions of the three antibiotics with the 50S subunit. A strain of *E. coli* has been selected that is absolutely dependent on the presence of erythromycin for growth.[199] The erythromycin-dependent cells presumably have a mutation in one of the ribosomal proteins such that the ribosomes are not functional in the absence of drug. When erythromycin binds to the altered 50S subunit, it restores the ribosome to a more normal configuration, which is functional in protein synthesis. Lincomycin and chloramphenicol also permit growth of this mutant, although they are less effective than erythromycin.

A unique form of inducible multidrug resistance based on altered ribosomal RNA has been demonstrated in staphylococci.[200] It was shown many years ago that some erythromycin-resistant clinical isolates of bacteria were resistant to other macrolide antibiotics if they were grown in the presence of a very low concentration of erythromycin. Subsequently, it was found that exposure of these organisms to low concentrations of erythromycin results in resistance to high concentrations of erythromycin, other macrolide antibiotics, and lincomycins.[201] After exposure to low erythromycin concentrations, the bacteria contain a unique methylated base (a dimethyladenine) in the 23S RNA component

Table 9-12. Binding of Erythromycin to Ribosomes from Erythromycin-Sensitive and Resistant Strains of *Staphylococcus aureus*

Source of Ribosomes[a]	Amount of Erythromycin Bound (cpm/OD_{260} unit)
Drug-sensitive strain	274
Constitutively resistant strain	15
Inducibly resistant strain	
Noninduced	281
Induced	36

[a] Ribosomes were isolated from different strains of *S. aureus* MS353 and incubated at 27°C for 30 minutes with radiolabeled erythromycin. The bound drug–ribosome complex was separated from unbound drug by passage through a column of Sephadex G-100. The inducible resistant strain of *S. aureus* is resistant only after it has been exposed to a low concentration of erythromycin that is not sufficient to inhibit growth but is sufficient to cause methylation of 16S ribosomal RNA. Ribosomes were prepared from both induced, drug-resistant and non-induced, drug-sensitive states of this inducible strain. Binding of radiolabeled erythromycin is expressed as cpm per OD_{260} unit of ribosomes.
(From Mitsuhashi et al.,[200] with permission.)

of the 50S ribosomal subunit.[202] Hybrid 50S ribosomal subunits have been assembled in which the 23S RNA is derived from drug-sensitive or induced-resistant staphylococci and the other components are derived from *Bacillus stearothermophilus*. These hybrid subunits were used in a protein synthesizing system in which it was shown that lincomycin inhibits synthesis when the ribosomes contain 23S RNA from the drug-sensitive parent but not when they contain the methylated 23S RNA from the induced-resistant cells.[203] Staphylococci with this type of resistance have acquired a plasmid that contains a gene for an inducible RNA methylase.[204] In the presence of small amounts of erythromycin or lincomycin (at concentrations that are too low to inhibit protein synthesis), the enzyme is induced, so that on subsequent exposure to the usual growth-inhibitory concentrations of erythromycin or lincomycin, the drugs are no longer effective. As demonstrated by the data in Table 9-12, the drugs are no longer effective because ribosomes containing the methylated RNA have a markedly decreased affinity for the antibiotic. It is interesting that of 10 streptomycetes tested for resistance to erythromycin and lincomycin, only *Streptomyces erythreus*, the organism used for production of erythromycin, was found to be resistant to both classes of antibiotics and to contain dimethyladenine in the 23S ribosomal RNA.[205] Thus, the organism that produces the antibiotic is protected from the drug effect in the same manner as resistant clinical isolates of staphylococci.

Rifampin

Rifampin is an antibiotic that is used primarily to treat infections by mycobacteria. The drug kills bacteria by interacting directly with RNA polymerase to inhibit RNA synthesis.[1] Rifampin binds tightly to RNA polymerases from sensitive bacteria but not to RNA polymerases from resistant bacteria.[206] Bacerial RNA polymerases are complex enzymes composed of several polypeptide chains. The core enzyme from *E. coli*, for example, contains at least four subunits (two α, one β, and one β'). The enzyme core binds another unit called the δ *factor*, which recognizes the promoter regions of the DNA where tran-

Table 9-13. Sensitivity of RNA Polymerase Components to Rifampin

	[a] *Specific Activity of Enzyme (mU/mg)*		Inhibition by Rifampin (%)
	Minus Rifampin	*Plus Rifampin*	
Original sensitive enzyme	242	1.5	99
Original resistant enzyme	124	120	3
Reconstituted enzyme			
$\alpha + \beta + \beta' + \sigma$	52	1.4	97
$\alpha_r + \beta_r + \beta_r' + \sigma$	27	25.6	5
$\alpha_r + \beta + \beta' + \sigma$	40	0.6	98
$\alpha + \beta_r + \beta' + \sigma$	88	69	22
$\alpha + \beta + \beta_r' + \sigma$	17.5	1.4	92

[a] Purified RNA polymerases from rifampin-sensitive and rifampin-resistant *E. coli* were dissociated, and the α, β, and β' subunits were separated by electrophoresis. The subunits were then mixed in stoichiometric ratio, δ factor was added, and the units were permitted to reassociate. Enzyme activity was then assayed in the presence and absence of rifampin. The subscript *r* refers to subunits derived from the rifampin-resistant polymerase. Enzyme activity is expressed as milliunits per milligram enzyme protein.
(From Heil et al.,[207] with permission.)

scription is initiated. Rifampin inhibits the initiation of RNA synthesis, but it inhibits initiation via an interaction with the β subunit of the core enzyme and not with the δ initiation factor. That the β subunit is the target for the drug effect was shown in crossover experiments with reconstituted hybrid enzymes, such as that presented in Table 9-13.[207] The reconstituted enzymes are only about 20 percent as active as the drug-sensitive and drug-resistant polymerases from which the subunits were derived, but it is clear that the β subunit must be derived from the sensitive polymerase for rifampin to produce substantial inhibition. Rifampin does not bind to the isolated β subunit, but it does bind to the holoenzyme ($\alpha_2\beta\beta'\delta$) or to a partially reconstituted enzyme consisting of $\alpha_2\beta$.[208] Thus, we know that the β subunit is the target site for rifampin, but rifampin is bound tightly only when the β subunit is in the conformation it assumes when it is associated with two α subunits.

Antifolate Drugs

Antifolate drugs are used to treat bacterial and protozoal infections as well as cancer. There are clear differences in the ability of different folate analogs to inhibit DHFRs obtained from bacteria, protozoa, and mammals. For example, 30,000- to 60,000-fold higher concentrations of the drug trimethoprim are required to inhibit human DHFR as are required to inhibit DHFR from *S. aureus* or *E. coli*.[209] Similarly, 3,600- and 5,000-fold higher concentrations of the antimalarial drug pyrimethamine are required to inhibit purified human and *E. coli* DHFR, respectively, as are required to inhibit DHFR purified from the malarial parasite *Plasmodium berghei*.[209] These differences in the sensitivity of DHFR to inhibition by different folate analogs provide the major basis for their use as antibacterial or antiprotozoal drugs.[1] Regardless of whether antifolate drugs are being used to treat cancer, bacterial infections, or malaria, resistance can arise as a result of mutations in the DHFR gene that determine a decreased affinity for the drug.

In the case of tumor cells, amplification of the DHFR gene and decreased drug uptake are the most common mechanisms of resistance, but mutations leading to a decreased affinity of DHFR for methotrexate also occur.[90] The most common mechanism by which bacteria become resistant to trimethoprim is by producing DHFR with reduced affinity for the drug.[210] The trimethoprim-resistant reductases that have been characterized differ from all other DHFRs in molecular weight, subunit structure, and kinetic properties. The production of trimethoprim-resistant DHFR is mediated by either plasmids or chromosomal genes. One can appreciate that particularly high levels of resistance can develop if a bacterium acquires a plasmid containing multiple copies of a gene that codes for a DHFR with decreased affinity for trimethoprim.

Malarial organisms that develop resistance to pyrimethamine may be resistant because they contain increased amounts of DHFR, an altered enzyme with decreased affinity for the drug, or both.[211] The altered enzyme has different physical properties from the wild-type DHFR, and there is evidence that the genes for the variant enzyme can be transferred from one species of plasmodium to another. The evidence is derived from an intriguing experiment in which mice were simultaneously inoculated with pyrimethamine-resistant *Plasmodium vinckei* and pyrimethamine-sensitive *P. berghei*, and both organisms were allowed to multiply.[212,213] After a period of growth in the mice, the plasmodia were transferred to a hamster, which was subsequently treated with high doses of pyrimethamine. Since *P. vinckei* is not able to grow in hamsters, the animal serves as a biologic filter to select for *P. berghei* that have become drug-resistant. Drug-resistant *P. berghei* was recovered from the hamster, and the physical properties of the DHFR purified from these newly resistant plasmodia were intermediate in character between those of the original drug-sensitive *P. berghei* and the drug-resistant *P. vinckei*, which produced an enzyme with a 225-fold lower affinity for pyrimethamine. It is postulated that there was transfer of genetic material from the drug-resistant to the drug-sensitive plasmodium while both species were infecting the same red cell. As the enzyme from the newly resistant *P. berghei* was intermediate in character between the original drug-sensitive and drug-resistant enzymes, it seems likely that only a part of the DHFR gene in the donor strain was transferred to the recipient. Although the design of this experiment was not such that the results prove gene transfer, the observation brings to mind the mechanism of drug resistance transfer via transformation described in an earlier section of this chapter. As mixed plasmodial infections are common in humans in the tropics, such resistance transfer could prove to be of epidemiologic interest.

Mechanism 7. Enchanced Biochemical Mechanisms for Repairing the Drug-Sensitive Reaction

There are only a few examples in which acquired drug resistance is due to an enhanced ability to repair lethal damage caused by the drug. This mechanism is limited to drugs that react with DNA to form chemical adducts with bases (e.g., alkylating agents), to drugs that cross-link DNA strands or form DNA-protein cross-links (e.g., alkylating agents, platinum compounds, mitomycin C), and to drugs that cause DNA strand breakage (e.g., bleomycin, nitrofurans).[214] An example of this form of resistance is the ability of certain bacterial strains to repair damaged DNA resulting from exposure to alkylating agents or x-rays. The β-chlorethylamine alkylating agents (e.g., mechlorethamine, also called nitrogen mustard) react with the N-7 atom of guanine residues of DNA[2] by the mechanism shown in Figure 11-4. The bifunctional alkylating agents crosslink DNA strands, forming diguanin-7-yl derivatives joined by a $-CH_2CH_2-N(CH_3)-CH_2CH_2-$ bridge. With a sulfur mustard, the bridge contains S instead of N. Such crosslinked DNA is incapable of normal strand separation and replication. Mutant strains of *E. coli* resistant to the lethal effects of sulfur mustard were isolated. In these cells the alkylation reactions

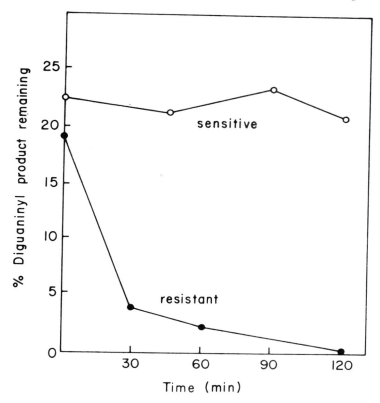

Fig. 9-24. Excision of crosslinks in DNA treated with an alkylating agent. Cultures of a sensitive and a resistant strain of *E. coli* were treated briefly with [^{35}S]mustard gas, a potent bifunctional alkylating agent. The cultures were diluted and aerated to remove the toxic gas, then sampled at various times. DNA was extracted and hydrolyzed to remove purine residues. Diguanyl and guanine residues were separated, and their radioactivity was determined. The graph shows the bifunctionally alkylated guanine as a percentage of total aklylated guanine, representing the degree of crosslinking of the DNA in vivo. *Top curve:* sensitive strain. *Bottom curve:* resistant strain. (From Venitt,[215] with permission.)

proceeded as in sensitive strains, but repair processes were capable of excising the diguanyl residues, replacing the missing purines, and thus restoring functional DNA to the cell.[215] The experiment illustrated in Figure 9-24 shows the enhanced repair activity in a radiation-resistant strain of *E. coli* that is cross-resistant to bifunctional alkylating drugs.

The repair process involves a number of different enzymes. Endonucleases recognize the abnormal base and cut the DNA at the damaged site. Exonucleases then degrade the damaged segment of DNA, and a repair polymerase synthesizes a new segment, utilizing the opposing DNA strand as a template. The end of the newly synthesized segment is then covalently linked to the preexisting strand by a ligase enzyme to reconstitute the original double-stranded DNA. The entire process is called *excision repair*, and the two pathways shown in Figure 9-25 have been identified in mammalian cells.[216] In *short-patch* repair only three or four nucleotides are excised; this pathway repairs damage caused by some alkylating agents and by x-rays. In *long-patch* repair up to 120 nucleotides are

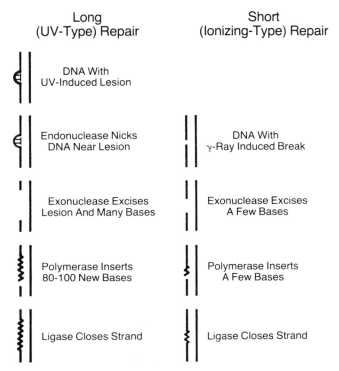

Fig. 9-25. Two pathways of DNA repair in human cells. (From Regan et al.[216] with permission.)

excised; this pathway repairs damage caused by agents that produce bulky substituents in DNA, as when dimers are formed under ultraviolet irradiation.

Mutant bacteria with altered DNA repair systems have in some cases proved to be useful tools for establishing the lethal effect of some drugs. It was known for some years, for example, that nitrofuran compounds, such as the urinary tract antiseptic nitrofurantoin, caused DNA strand breakage. The drug is metabolized by reduction to short-lived metabolites, which cause DNA strand breakage either by direct interaction with DNA or by their ability to generate oxygen free radicals.[1] Important evidence showing that it is the DNA damage that is the primary event leading to bacterial cell killing came from studies comparing the sensitivity of wild-type *E. coli* with that of mutants that are defective in DNA repair. Both *E. coli* mutants that lack the ability to carry out postreplication repair (*recA* mutants) and mutants lacking the excision repair system (*uvr* mutants) are more sensitive to nitrofurantoin than are the parent strains.[217] As the sensitivity of the bacterium varies inversely with its ability to repair drug-induced DNA damage, it is reasonable to propose that DNA damage is the critical event responsible for cytotoxicity.

Mechanism 8. Decreased Activity of an Enzyme Required to Express the Drug Effect

In an earlier section of this chapter we discussed the mechanism of action of the β-lactam antibiotics and several mechanisms by which bacteria become resistant to these drugs. There is an additional mechanism of resistance that is unique to inhibitors of bacterial cell wall synthesis (e.g., penicillins, cephalosporins, bacitracin, vancomycin). These antibiotics are usually bactericidal when added to growing cultures of sensitive cells. Although we have described how the β-lactam antibiotics inhibit cell wall biosynthesis, this does not explain how the drugs cause cell death. Cell death results from cell lysis, which occurs as a result of cell membrane rupture at discrete growth regions on the bacterium. In addition to the cell wall synthetic enzymes, the growth regions contain autolytic enzymes, which degrade the cell wall. The natural biologic role of these auto-lysins (murein hydrolases) is subject to speculation, but it is clear that in many bacteria autolytic enzyme activity is required for cell lysis and death to occur when cell wall synthesis is inhibited by antibiotics.[218] Thus, the autolytic enzyme activity is required to express the killing effect of these drugs. In the absence of autolytic enzyme activity, the antibiotics that inhibit cell wall synthesis inhibit cell growth, but they do not kill the bacterium. Thus, the antibiotic effect is bacteriostatic rather than bactericidal.

The response of an autolysin-deficient mutant strain to penicillin is shown in Figure 9-26.[219] In the autolysin-deficient mutant bacteria, low concentrations of penicillin stop cell growth, but the bacteria remain viable. These mutants have been called *tolerant* organ-

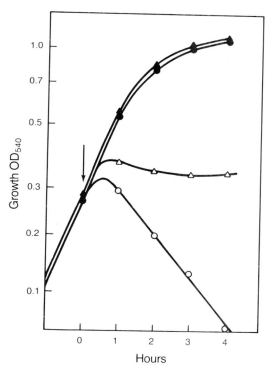

Fig. 9-26. Effect of penicillin on the growth of a parent strain of *Bacillus subtilis* with normal autolytic enzyme activity and an autolysin-deficient mutant. Penicillin was added to cultures of *B. subtilis* in the middle log phase of growth, and growth was assayed by turbidity at 540 nm. The arrow indicates the time of drug addition. ●, parent strain; ○, parent strain plus penicillin; ▲, autolysin-deficient mutant; △, mutant plus penicillin. The parent strain was lysed, whereas the growth of the mutant was halted without lysis. The same phenomenon was observed upon addition of cycloserine, vancomycin, or bacitracin. (From Ayusawa et al.,[219] with permission.)

628 • *Principles of Drug Action*

Table 9–14. Susceptibility of 60 Strains of *Staphylococcus aureus* to Oxacillin

Isolates	[a]MIC (μg/ml)	[a]MBC (μg/ml)
Sensitive group	0.30 (0.1–1.6)	2.2 (0.2–12.5)
Tolerant group	0.33 (0.1–0.8)	> 100 (50–> 100)

[a] The minimum concentration of oxacillin required to inhibit growth (MIC) and the minimum concentration required to kill 99.9 percent of organisms (MBC) were determined for 60 randomly selected clinical isolates of *S. aureus*. The penicillin was bactericidal against 27 strains and only bacteriostatic against the other 33. It should be noted that the "tolerant" organisms will die very slowly if kept in the presence of a high concentration of oxacillin for many hours. The data represent the mean MIC and MBC for each group, with the range of values shown in parenthesis.
(From Mayhall et al.,[220] with permission.)

isms. They differ from other resistant organisms in that they are still susceptible to the growth-inhibiting effect of the antibiotic but they are resistant to the lytic action. The mutant used in the experiment of Figure 9-26 was also resistant to some other antibiotics, such as cycloserine, vancomycin, and bacitracin, which inhibit cell wall synthesis by mechanisms that are different from that of the β-lactams. Thus, mutations resulting in deficient autolytic enzyme activity represent a unique mechanism of multiple drug resistance, which is due to the modification of an enzymatic process that is unaffected by the drug but is necessary for the drug's killing effect.

This tolerance phenomenon is not limited to organisms selected under controlled laboratory conditions. Penicillin-tolerant bacteria have been isolated from patients with persistent or relapsing infections. Because the drugs still inhibit cell growth, the tolerant organisms are characterized by the fact that they have the same MICs (minimum inhibitory concentrations) for β-lactam antibiotics as susceptible strains; however, because they are deficient in lytic activity, their MBCs (minimum bactericidal concentrations) are very high.[218] This difference is demonstrated in Table 9-14 by the response of clinical isolates of *S. aureus* to oxacillin, a penicillinase-resistant penicillin.[220]

REFERENCES

1. Pratt WB, Fekety FR: The Antimicrobial Drugs. Oxford University Press, New York, 1986
2. Pratt WB, Ruddon RW: The Anticancer Drugs. Oxford University Press, New York, 1979
3. Bryan LE (ed): Antimicrobial Drug Resistance. Academic Press, Orlando, FL, 1984
4. Mitsuhashi S (ed): Drug Resistance in Bacteria. Thieme-Stratton, New York, 1982
5. Fox BW, Fox M (eds): Handbook of Experimental Pharmacology. Vol. 72. Antitumor Drug Resistance. Springer-Verlag, New York, 1984
6. Feingold DS: The action of amphotericin B on *Mycoplasma laidlawii*. Biochem Biophys Res Commun 19:261, 1965
7. De Kruijff B, Gerritsen WJ, Oerlemans A, et al: Polyene antibiotic-sterol interactions in membranes of *Acholeplasma laidlawii* cells and lecithin liposomes. I. Specificity of the permeability changes induced by the polyene antibiotics. Biochim Biophys Acta 339:30, 1974
8. Dick JD, Merz WG, Saral R: Incidence of polyene-resistant yeasts recovered from clinical specimens. Antimicrob Agents Chemother 18:158, 1980

9. Pierce AM, Pierce HD, Unrau AM, Oehlschlager AC: Lipid composition and polyene resistance of *Candida albicans* mutants. Can J Biochem 56:135, 1978

10. Medoff G, Kobayashi GS, Kwan CN, et al: Potentiation of rifampicin and 5-fluorocytosine as antifungal antibiotics by amphotericin B. Proc Natl Acad Sci USA 69:196, 1972

11. Kobayashi GS, Cheung SC, Schlessinger D, Medoff G: Effects of rifamycin derivatives, alone and in combination with amphotericin B, against *Histoplasma capsulatum*. Antimicrob Agents Chemother 5:16, 1974

12. Bennett JE, Dismukes WE, Duma RJ, et al: A comparison of amphotericin B alone and combined with flucytosine in the treatment of cryptococcal meningitis. N Engl J Med 301:126, 1979

13. Gotfredsen WO: An introduction to mecillinam. J Antimicrob Chemother 3:suppl.B, 1, 1977

14. Buchanan CE, Strominger JL: Altered penicillin-binding components in penicillin-resistant mutants of *Bacillus subtilis*. Proc Natl Acad Sci USA 73:1816, 1976

15. Williamson R, Zighelboim S, Tomasz A: Penicillin-binding proteins of penicillin-resistant and penicillin-tolerant *Streptococcus pneumoniae*. p. 215. In Salton M, Shockman GM (eds): β-Lactam Antibiotics. Academic Press, Orlando, FL, 1981

16. Dougherty TJ, Koller AE, Tomasz A: Penicillin-binding proteins of penicillin-susceptible and intrinsically resistant *Neisseria gonorrhoeae*. Antimicrob Agents Chemother 18:730, 1980

17. Costerton JW, Cheng K-J: The role of the bacterial cell envelope in antibiotic resistance. J Antimicrob Chemother 1:363, 1975

18. Nikaido H, Nakae T: The outer membrane of gram-negative bacteria. Adv Microb Physiol 20:163, 1979

19. Komatsu Y, Murakami K, Nishikawa T: Penetration of moxalactam into its target proteins in *Escherichia coli* K-12: comparison of a highly moxalactam-resistant mutant with its parent strain. Antimicrob Agents Chemother 20:613, 1981

20. Harder KJ, Nikaido H, Matsuhashi M: Mutants of *Escherichia coli* that are resistant to certain beta-lactam compounds lack the *omp*F porin. Antimicrob Agents Chemother 20:549, 1981

21. Irvin RT, Govan JWR, Fyfe JAM, Costerton JW: Heterogeneity of antibiotic resistance in mucoid isolates of *Pseudomonas aeruginosa* obtained from cystic fibrosis patients: role of outer membrane proteins. Antimicrob Agents Chemother 19:1056, 1981

22. Gutmann L, Williamson R, Collatz E: The possible role of porins in bacterial antibiotic resistance. Ann Intern Med 101:554, 1984

23. Brown MRW (ed): Resistance of *Pseudomonas aeruginosa*. John Wiley & Sons, London, 1974

24. Zimmermann W: Penetration of β-lactam antibiotics into their target enzymes in *Pseudomonas aeruginosa*: Comparison of a highly sensitive mutant with its parent strain. Antimicrob Agents Chemother 18:94, 1980

25. Sykes RB, Mathew M: The β-lactamases of gram-negative bacteria and their role in resistance to β-lactam antibiotics. J Antimicrob Chemother 2:115, 1976

26. Weinstein L, Dalton AC: Host determinants of response to antimicrobial agents. N Engl J Med 279:580, 1968

27. Richmond M: Beta-lactamases and bacterial resistance to beta-lactam antibiotics. p. 261. In Salton M, Shockman G (eds): β-Lactam Antibiotics. Academic Press, Orlando, FL, 1981

28. Mathew M: Plasmid-mediated β-lactamases of gram-negative bacteria: Properties and distribution. J Antimicrob Chemother 5:349, 1979

29. Zimmerman W, Rosselet A: Function of the outer membrane of *Escherichia coli* as a permeability barrier to β-lactam antibiotics. Antimicrob Agents Chemother 12:368, 1977

30. Richmond MH, Wotton S: Comparative study of seven cephalosporins: Susceptibility to beta-lactamases and ability to penetrate the surface layers of *Escherichia coli*. Antimicrob Agents Chemother 10:219, 1976

31. Charnas RL, Knowles JR: Inactivation of RTEM β-lactamase from *Escherichia coli* by clavulinic acid and 9-deoxyclavulinic acid. Biochemistry 20:3214, 1981

32. Reading C, Cole M: Clavulinic acid: A beta-lactamase-inhibiting beta lactam from *Streptomyces clavuligerus*. Antimicrob Agents Chemother 11:852, 1977

33. Murray BE, Moellering RC: Patterns and mechanisms of antibiotic resistance. Med Clin North Am 62:899, 1978

34. Finland M: Emergence of antibiotic resistance in hospitals, 1935–1975. Rev Infect Dis 1:4, 1979

35. Lepper MH, Moulton B, Dowling HF, et al: Epidemiology of erythromycin-resistant staphylococci in a hospital population—effect on therapeutic activity of erythromycin. Antibiot Annu 1953–54, p. 308

36. Dowling HF, Lepper MH, Jackson GG: Clinical significance of antibiotic-resistance bacteria. JAMA 157:327, 1955

37. McGowan JE Jr: Antimicrobial resistance in hospital organisms and its relation to antibiotic use. Rev Infect Dis 5:1033, 1983

38. Weinstein RA, Kabins SA: Strategies for prevention and control of multiple drug-resistant nosocomial infection. Am J Med 70:449, 1981

39. Wernsdorfer WH: The Importance of Malaria in the World. p.1. In Kreier JP (ed): Malaria. Vol.1. Academic Press, Orlando, FL, 1980

40. Wernsdorfer WH, Kouznetsov RL: Drug-resistant malaria—occurrence, control, and surveillance. Bull WHO 58:341, 1980

41. Weniger BG, Blumberg RS, Campbell CC, et al: High level chloroquine resistance of *Plasmodium falciparum* acquired in Kenya. N Engl J Med 307:1561, 1982

42. Thaithong S, Beale GH, Chutmongkonkul M: Susceptibility of *Plasmodium falciparum* to five drugs: An *in vitro* study of isolates mainly from Thailand. Trans Soc Trop Med Hyg 77:228, 1983

43. Centers for Disease Control: *Plasmodium falciparum* malaria contracted in Thailand resistant to chloroquine and sulfonamide-pyrimethamine—Illinois. Morbid Mortal Weekly Rep 29:493, 1980

44. Population Information Program: Community-based health and family planning. Population Reports Series L, No. 3:L-77, 1982

45. Development of mefloquine as an antimalarial drug. Bull WHO 61:169, 1983

46. Bryson V, Demerec M: Bacterial resistance. Am J Med 18:723, 1955

47. Bryson V, Szybalski W: Microbial drug resistance. Adv Genet 7:1, 1955

48. Luria SE, Delbrück M: Mutations of bacteria from virus sensitivity to virus resistance. Genetics 28:491, 1943

49. Demerec M: Origin of bacterial resistance to antibiotics. J Bacteriol 56:63, 1948

50. Newcombe HB, Hawirko R: Spontaneous mutation to streptomycin resistance and dependence in *Escherichia coli*. J Bacteriol 57:565, 1949

51. Law LW: Origin of the resistance of leukaemic cells to folic acid antagonists. Nature 169:628, 1952

52. Lederberg J, Lederberg EM: Replica plating and indirect selection of bacterial mutants. J Bacteriol 63:399, 1952

53. Eagle H: The multiple mechanisms of penicillin resistance. J Bacteriol 68:610, 1954

54. Nomura M, Mizushima S, Ozaki M, et al: Structure and function of ribosomes and their molecular components. Cold Spring Harbor Symp Quant Biol 34:49, 1969

55. Ozaki M, Mizushima S, Nomura M: Identification and functional characterization of the protein controlled by the streptomycin-resistant locus in *E. coli*. Nature 222:333, 1969

56. Funatsu G, Wittman HG: Ribosomal proteins. XXXIII. Location of amino acid replacements in protein S12 isolated from *Escherichia coli* mutants resistant to streptomycin. J Mol Biol 68:547, 1972

57. Weinstein RA, Nathan C, Gruensfelder R, Kabins SA: Endemic aminoglycoside resistance in gram-negative bacilli: Epidemiology and mechanisms. J Infect Dis 141:338, 1980

58. Ehrlich P: Chemotherapeutics: Scientific principles, methods, and results. Lancet 2:445, 1913

59. Conn, ML, Middlebrook G, Russell WF: Combined drug treatment of tuberculosis. I. Prevention of emergence of mutant populations of tubercle bacilli resistant to both streptomycin and isoniazid *in vitro*. J Clin Invest 38:1349, 1959

60. De Vita VT, Young RC, Canellos GP: Combination versus single agent chemotherapy: A review of the basis for selection of drug treatment of cancer. Cancer 35:98, 1975
61. Falkow S: Infectious Multiple Drug Resistance. Pion Ltd., London, 1975
62. Watanabe T: Infective heredity of multiple drug resistance in bacteria. Bacteriol Rev 27:87, 1963
63. Akiba T, Koyama K, Ishiki Y, et al: On the mechanism of the development of multiple-drug-resistant clones of *Shigella*. Jpn J Microbiol 4:219, 1960
64. Levy SB: Microbial resistance to antibiotics: An evolving and persistent problem. Lancet 2:83, 1982
65. Lacey RW: Antibiotic resistance plasmids of *Staphylococcus aureus* and their clinical importance. Bacteriol Rev 39:1, 1975
66. Rownd RH, Womble DD: Molecular nature and replication of R factors. p.161. In Mitsuhashi S (ed): R Factor Drug Resistance Plasmid. University Park Press, Baltimore, 1977
67. Kleckner N: Transposable elements in prokaryotes. Annu Rev Genet 15:341, 1981
68. Mitsuhashi S: Translocatable drug resistance determinants. p.77. In Mitsuhashi S (ed): R Factor Drug Resistance Plasmid. University Park Press, Baltimore, 1977
69. Degraaff J, Elwell LP, Falkow S: Molecular nature of two β-lactamase specifying plasmids isolated from *Haemophilus influenzae* type b. J Bacteriol 126:439, 1976
70. Richmond MH: R Factors in man and his environment. p.27. In Schlessinger D (ed): Microbiology—1974. American Society of Microbiology, Washington, 1975
71. Linton KB, Richmond MH, Bevan R, Gillespie WA: Antibiotic resistance and R factors in coliform bacilli isolated from hospital and domestic sewage. J Med Microbiol 7:91, 1974
72. Visek WJ: The mode of growth promotion by antibiotics. J Anim Sci 46:1447, 1978
73. Bennett JV: Antibiotic use in animals and human salmonellosis. J Infect Dis 142:631, 1980
74. O'Brien TF, Hopkins JD, Gilleece ES, et al: Molecular epidemiology of antibiotic resistance in *Salmonella* from animals and human beings in the United States. N Engl J Med 307:1, 1982
75. Pohl P: Relationship between antibiotic feeding in animals and emergence of bacterial resistance in man. J Antimicrob Chemother 3:suppl.C, 67, 1977
76. Levy SB, Fitzgerald GB, Macone AB: Changes in intestinal flora of farm personnel after introduction of a tetracycline-supplemented feed on a farm. N Engl J Med 295:583, 1976
77. Marsik FJ, Parisi JT, Blenden DC: Transmissible drug resistance of *Escherichia coli* and *Salmonella* from humans, animals, and their rural environments. J Infect Dis 132:296, 1975
78. Ryder RW, Blake PA, Murlin AC, et al: Increase in antibiotic resistance among isolates of *Salmonella* in the United States, 1967–1975. J Infect Dis 142:485, 1980
79. Holmberg SD, Wells JG, Cohen ML: Animal-to-man transmission of antimicrobial-resistant *Salmonella*: Investigations of U.S. outbreaks, 1971–1983. Science 225:833, 1985
80. Holmberg SD, Osterholm MT, Senger KA, Cohen ML: Drug-resistant *Salmonella* from animals fed antimicrobials. N Engl J Med 311:617, 1984
81. Anderson RP, Roth JR: Tandem genetic duplications in phage and bacteria. Annu Rev Microbiol 31:473, 1977
82. Beverley SM, Coderre JA, Santi DV, Schimke RT: Unstable DNA amplifications in methotrexate-resistant *Leishmania* consist of extrachromosomal circles which relocalize during stabilization. Cell 38:431, 1984
83. Schimke RT: Gene amplification in cultured animal cells. Cell 37:705, 1984
84. Schimke RT: Gene amplification, drug resistance, and cancer. Cancer Res 44:1735, 1984
85. Jenh CH, Geyer PK, Baskin F, Johnson LF: Thymidylate synthetase gene amplification in fluorodeoxyuridine-resistant mouse cell lines. Mol Pharmacol 28:80, 1985
86. Berger SH, Jenh CH, Johnson LF, Berger FG: Thymidylate synthetase overproduction and gene amplification in fluorodeoxyuridine-resistant human cells. Mol Pharmacol 28:461, 1985
87. Lewis WH, Kuzin BA, Wright JA: Assay of ribonucleotide reduction in nucleotide-permeable hamster cells. J Cell Physiol 94:287, 1978
88. Wahl GM, Padgett RA, Stark GR: Gene amplification causes overproduction of the first three

enzymes of UMP synthesis in *N*-(phosphonacetyl)-L-aspartate-resistant hamster cells. J Biol Chem 254:8679, 1979

89. Sirotnak FM, Kurita S, Hutchison DJ: On the nature of a transport alteration determining resistance to amethopterin in the L1210 leukemia. Cancer Res 28:75, 1968

90. Flintoff WE, Davidson SV, Siminovitch L: Isolation and partial characterization of three methotrexate-resistant phenotypes from Chinese hamster ovary cells. Somatic Cell Genet 2:245, 1976

91. Alt FW, Kellems RE, Schimke RT: Synthesis and degradation of folate reductase in sensitive and methotrexate-resistant lines of S-180 cells. J Biol Chem 251:3063, 1976

92. Hanggi UJ, Littlefield JW: Altered regulation of the rate of synthesis of dihydrofolate reductase in methotrexate-resistant hamster cells. J Biol Chem 251:3075, 1976

93. Alt FW, Kellems RE, Bertino JR, Schimke RT: Selective multiplication of dihydrofolate reductase genes in methotrexate-resistant variants of cultured murine cells. J Biol Chem 253:1357, 1978

94. Hakala MT, Zakrzewski SF, Nichol CA: Relation of folic acid reductase to amethopterin resistance in cultured mammalian cells. J Biol Chem 236:952, 1961

95. Haber DA, Beverley SM, Kiely ML, Schimke RT: Properties of an altered dihydrofolate reductase encoded by amplified genes in cultured mouse fibroblasts. J Biol Chem 256:9501, 1981

96. Rath H, Tlsty T, Schimke RT: Rapid emergence of methotrexate resistance in cultured mouse cells. Cancer Res 44:3303, 1984

97. Biedler JL, Spengler BA: Metaphase chromosome anomaly: Association with drug resistance and cell-specific products. Science 191:185, 1976

98. Schimke RT, Brown PC, Kaufman RJ, et al: Chromosomal and extrachromosomal localization of amplified dihydrofolate reductase genes in cultured mammalian cells. Cold Spring Harbor Symp Quant Biol 55:785, 1981

99. Johnston RN, Beverley SM, Schimke RT: Rapid spontaneous dihydrofolate reductase gene amplification shown by fluorescence-activated cell sorting. Proc Natl Acad Sci USA 80:3711, 1983

100. Tlsty T, Brown PC, Johnston R, Schimke RT: Enhanced frequency of generation of methotrexate resistance and gene amplification in cultured mouse and hamster cell lines. p.231. In Schimke RT (ed): Gene Amplification. Cold Spring Harbor Laboratory, Cold Spring Harbor, NY, 1982

101. Varshavsky A: Phorbol ester dramatically increases incidence of methotrexate-resistant mouse cells: Possible mechanisms and relevance to tumor promotion. Cell 25:561, 1981

102. Mariani BD, Schimke RT: Gene amplification in a single cell cycle in Chinese hamster ovary cells. J Biol Chem 259:1901, 1984

103. Tlsty TD, Brown PC, Schimke RT: UV irradiation facilitates methotrexate resistance and amplification of the dihydrofolate reductase gene in cultured 3T6 mouse cells. Mol Cell Biol 4:1050, 1984

104. Varshavsky A: On the possibility of metabolic control of replicon "misfiring": Relationship to emergence of malignant phenotypes in mammalian cell lineages. Proc Natl Acad Sci USA 78:3673, 1981

105. Vogelstein B, Pardoll DM, Coffey DS: Supercoiled loop and eukaryotic DNA replication. Cell 22:79, 1980

106. Botchan MW, Topp W, Sambrook J: Studies on SV40 excision from cellular chromosomes. Cold Spring Harbor Symp Quant Biol 43:709, 1979

107. Horns RC, Dower WJ, Schimke RT: Gene amplification in a leukemic patient treated with methotrexate. J Clin Oncol 2:2 1984

108. Carman MC, Schornagel JH, Rivest RS, et al: Resistance to methotrexate due to gene amplification in a patient with acute leukemia. J Clin Oncol 2:16, 1984

109. Trent JM, Buick RN, Olson S, et al: Cytologic evidence for gene amplification in methotrexate-resistant cells obtained from a patient with ovarian adenocarcinoma. J Clin Oncol 2:8, 1984

110. Curt GA, Carney DM, Cowan KH, et al: Unstable methotrexate resistance in human small-cell carcinoma associated with double minute chromosomes. N Engl J Med 308:199, 1983

111. Bell DR, Gerlach JH, Kartner N, et al: Detection of P-glycoprotein in ovarian cancer: A molecular marker associated with multidrug resistance. J Clin Oncol 3:311, 1985

112. Benveniste R, Davies J: Mechanisms of antibiotic resistance in bacteria. Annu Rev Biochem 42:471, 1973

113. Block ER, Jennings AE, Bennett JE: 5-Fluorocytosine resistance in *Cryptococcus neoformans*. Antimicrob Agents Chemother 3:649, 1973

114. Hughes VM, Datta N: Conjugative plasmids in bacteria of the "pre-antibiotic" era. Nature 302:725, 1983

115. Levy SB: Resistance to the tetracyclines. p.191. In Bryan LE (ed): Antimicrobial Drug Resistance. Academic Press, Orlando, FL, 1984

116. Chopra I, Howe TGB, Linton AH, et al: The tetracyclines: Prospects at the beginnings of the 1980s. J Antimicrob Agents Chemother 8:5, 1981

117. McMurry L, Aronson DA, Levy SB: Susceptible *Escherichia coli* cells can actively excrete tetracyclines. Antimicrob Agents Chemother 24:544, 1983

118. McMurry L, Petrucci RE, Levy SB: Active efflux of tetracycline encoded by four genetically different tetracycline resistance determinants in *Escherichia coli*. Proc Natl Acad Sci USA 77:3974, 1980

119. Jorgensen RA, Reznikoff WS: Organization of structural and regulatory genes that mediate tetracycline resistance in transposon Tn10. J Bacteriol 138:705, 1979

120. Wray LV, Jorgensen RA, Reznikoff WS: Identification of the tetracycline resistance promoter and repressor in transposon Tn10. J Bacteriol 147:297, 1981

121. George AM, Levy SB: Amplifiable resistance to tetracycline, chloramphenicol, and other antibiotics in *Escherichia coli*: Involvement of a non-plasmid-determined efflux of tetracycline. J Bacteriol 155:531, 1983

122. George AM, Levy SB: Gene in the major cotransduction gap of the *Escherichia coli* K-12 linkage map required for the expression of chromosomal resistance to tetracycline and other antibiotics. J Bacteriol 155:541, 1983

123. Sirotnak FM, Moccio DM, Kelleher LE, Goutas LJ: Relative frequency and kinetic properties of transport-defective phenotypes among methotrexate-resistant L1210 clonal cell lines derived *in vivo*. Cancer Res 41:4447, 1981

124. Niethammer D, Jackson RC: Changes in molecular properties associated with the development of resistance against methotrexate in human lymphoblastoid cells. Eur J Cancer 11:845, 1975

125. Ohnoshi T, Ohnuma T, Takahashi I, et al: Establishment of methotrexate-resistant human acute lymphoblastic leukemia cells in culture and effects of folate antagonists. Cancer Res 42:1655, 1982

126. Warren RD, Nichols AP, Bender RA: Membrane transport of methotrexate in human lymphoblastoid cells. Cancer Res 38:668, 1978

127. Rosowsky A, Lazarus H, Yuan GC, et al: Effects of methotrexate esters and other lipophilic antifolates on methotrexate-resistant human leukemic lymphoblasts. Biochem Pharmacol 29:648, 1980

128. Diddens H, Niethammer D, Jackson RC: Patterns of cross-resistance to the antifolate drugs trimetrexate, metoprine, homofolate, and CB3717 in human lymphoma and osteosarcoma cells resistant to methotrexate. Cancer Res 43:5286, 1983

129. Hill BT: Collateral sensitivity and cross-resistance. p.673. In Fox BW, Fox M (eds): Antitumor Drug Resistance. Springer-Verlag, New York, 1984

130. Plageman PGW, Wohlhueter RM: Permeation of nucleosides, nucleic acid bases and nucleotides in animal cells. Curr Top Membr Transp 14:225, 1980

131. Sobrero AF, Moir RD, Bertino JR, Handschumacher RE: Defective facilitated diffusion of nucleosides, a primary mechanism of resistance to 5-fluoro-2'-deoxyuridine in the HCT-8 human carcinoma line. Cancer Res 45:3155, 1985

132. Sobrero AF, Handschumacher RE, Bertino JR: Highly selective drug combinations for human colon cancer cells resistant *in vitro* to 5-fluoro-2'-deoxyuridine. Cancer Res 45:3161, 1985

133. Biedler JL, Riehm H, Peterson RHF, Spengler BA: Membrane mediated drug resistance and phenotypic reversion to normal growth behavior of Chinese hamster cells. JNCI 55:671, 1975

134. Kartner N, Shales M, Riordan JR, Ling V: Daunorubicin-resistant Chinese hamster ovary cells expressing multidrug resistance and a cell-surface P-glycoprotein. Cancer Res 43:4413, 1983

135. Debenham PG, Kartner N, Simenovitch L, et al: DNA-mediated transfer of multiple drug resistance and plasma membrane glycoprotein expression. Mol Cell Biol 2:881, 1982

136. Borst P: DNA amplification and multidrug resistance. Nature 309:580, 1984

137. Inaba M, Kobayashi H, Sakurai Y, Johnson RK: Active efflux of daunorubicin and Adriamycin in sensitive and resistant sublines of P388 leukemia. Cancer Res 39:2200, 1979

138. Bradley G, Juranka PF, Ling V: Mechanism of multidrug resistance. Biochim Biophys Acta 948:87, 1988

139. Gottesman MM, Pastan I: The multidrug transporter, a double-edged sword. J Biol Chem 263:12163, 1988

140. Pastan I, Gottesman M: Multiple drug resistance in human cancer. N Engl J Med 316:1388, 1987

141. Riordan JR, Ling V: Purification of P-glycoprotein from plasma membrane vesicles of Chinese hamster ovary cell mutants with reduced colchicine permeability. J Biol Chem 254:12701, 1979

142. Roninson IB, Abelson HT, Housman DE, et al: Amplification of specific DNA sequences correlates with multi-drug resistance in Chinese hamster cells. Nature 309:626, 1984

143. Kartner ND, Evernden-Porelle G, Bradley G, Ling V: Detection of P-glycoprotein in multi-drug-resistant cell lines by monoclonal antibodies. Nature 316:820, 1985

144. Robertson SM, Ling V, Stanners CP: Coamplification of double minute chromosomes, multiple drug resistance and cell surface P-glycoprotein in DNA-mediated transformants of mouse cells. Mol Cell Biol 4:500, 1984

145. Gros P, Croop J, Housman D: Mammalian multidrug resistance gene: complete DNA sequence indicates strong homology to bacterial transport proteins. Cell 47:371, 1986

146. Chen CJ, Chin JE, Ueda K, et al: Internal duplication and homology with bacterial proteins in the mdr1 (P-glycoprotein) gene from multidrug-resistant human cells. Cell 47:381, 1986

147. Cornwell MM, Safa AR, Felsted RL, et al: Membrane vesicles from multidrug-resistant human cancer cells contain a specific 150- to 170-kDa protein detected by photoaffinity labeling. Proc Natl Acad Sci USA 83:3847, 1986

148. Gros P, Ben-Neriah Y, Croop J, Housman DE: Isolation and expression of a cDNA clone that confers multidrug resistance. Nature 323:728, 1986

149. Ueda K, Cardarelli C, Gottesman MM, Pastan I: Expression of a full-length cDNA for the human ''MDR1'' gene confers resistance to colchicine, doxorubicin, and vinblastine. Proc Natl Acad Sci USA 84:3004, 1987

150. Ames GF: The basis of multidrug resistance in mammalian cells: homology with bacterial transport. Cell 47:323, 1986

151. Thiebault F, Tsuruo T, Hamada H, et al: Cellular localization of the multidrug-resistance gene product P-glycoprotein in normal human tissues. Proc Natl Acad Sci USA 84:7735, 1987

152. Fojo A, Akiyama S, Gottesman MM, Pastan I: Reduced drug accumulation in multiply drug-resistant human KB carcinoma cell lines. Cancer Res 45:3002, 1985

153. Bitonti AJ, Sjoerdsma A, McCann PP, et al: Reversal of chloroquine resistance in malaria parasite *Plasmodium falciparum*. Science 242:1301, 1988

154. Shannon K, Phillips I: Mechanisms of resistance to aminoglycosides in clinical isolates. J Antimicrob Chemother 9:91, 1982

155. Bryan LE: Aminoglycoside resistance. p.241. In Bryan LE (ed): Antimicrobial Drug Resistance. Academic Press, Orlando, FL, 1984

156. Moellering RC: Microbiological considerations in the use of tobramycin and related aminoglycosidic aminocyclitol antibiotics. Med J Aust, special suppl. 2:4, 1977

157. Davies J, Smith DI: Plasmid-determined resistance to antimicrobial agents. Annu Rev Microbiol 32:469, 1978

158. Pongs O: Chloramphenicol. p.26. In Hahn FE (ed): Antibiotics. Springer-Verlag, New York, 1979

159. Thibault G, Guitard M, Daigneault R: A study of the enzymatic inactivation of chloramphenicol by highly purified chloramphenicol acetyltransferase. Biochim Biophys Acta 614:339, 1980

160. Piffaretti JC, Froment Y: Binding of chloramphenicol and its acetylated derivatives to *Escherichia coli* ribosomal subunits. Chemotherapy 24:24, 1978

161. Insecticide resistance—the problem and its solution. WHO Chron 25:214, 1971

162. Brown AWA, Pal R: Insecticide resistance in arthropods. WHO Monograph Series No. 38, 2nd Ed., Geneva, 1971

163. Oppenoorth FJ: Resistance in insects: The role of metabolism and the possible use of synergists. Bull WHO 44:195, 1971

164. O'Brien RD, Yamamoto I, (ed): Biochemical Toxicology of Insecticides. Academic Press, Orlando, FL, 1970

165. Georghiou GP, Metcalf RL: The absorption and metabolism of 3-isopropylphenyl *N*-methylcarbamate by susceptible and carbamate-selected strains of house flies. J Econ Entomol 54:231, 1961

166. Matsumura F, Brown AWA: Biochemistry of malathion resistance in *Culex tarsalis*. J Econ Entomol 54:1176, 1961

167. Oppenoorth FJ, van Asperen K: Allelic genes in the housefly producing modified enzymes that cause organophosphate resistance. Science 132:298, 1960

168. Dauterman WC, Matsumura F: Effect of malathion analogs upon resistant and susceptible *Culex tarsalis* mosquitoes. Science 138:694, 1962

169. Casida JE: Insect microsomes and insecticide chemical oxidations. p.517. In Gillette JR, Conney AH, Cosmides GJ, et al (eds): Microsomes and Drug Oxidations. Academic Press, Orlando, FL, 1969

170. Casida JE: Mixed-function oxidase involvement in the biochemistry of insecticide synergists. J Agr Food Chem 18:753, 1970

171. McGuire JJ, Mini E, Hsieh P, Bertino JR: Role of methotrexate polyglutamates in methotrexate- and sequential methotrexate-5-fluorouracil-mediated cell kill. Cancer Res 45:6395, 1985

172. Curt G, Carney D, Jolivet J, et al: Defective methotrexate (MTXG$_1$) polyglutamation: A mechanism of drug resistance in human small cell lung cancer (SCLC). Proc Am Assoc Cancer Res 24:283, 1983

173. Cowan KH, Jolivet J: A methotrexate-resistant human breast cancer cell line with multiple defects, including diminished formation of methotrexate polyglutamates. J Biol Chem 259:10793, 1984

174. Maybaum J, Ullman B, Mandel HG, et al: Regulation of RNA- and DNA-directed actions of 5-fluoropyrimidines in mouse T-lymphoma (S-49) cells. Cancer Res 40:4209, 1980

175. Reyes P, Hall TC: Synthesis of 5-fluorouridine 5-phosphate by a pyrimidine phosphoribosyltransferase of mammalian origin. II. Correlation between the tumor levels of the enzyme and the 5-fluorouracil-promoted increase in survival of tumor-bearing mice. Biochem Pharmacol 18:2587, 1969

176. Sköld O: Studies on resistance against 5-fluorouracil. IV. Evidence for an altered uridine kinase in resistant cells. Biochim Biophys Acta 76:160, 1963

177. Reichard P, Sköld O. Klein G: Possible enzymatic mechanism for the development of resistance against fluorouracil in ascites tumors. Nature 183:939, 1959

178. Aronow B, Watts T, Lassetter J, et al: Biochemical phenotype of 5-fluorouracil-resistant murine T-lymphoblasts with genetically altered CTP synthetase activity. J Biol Chem 259:9035, 1984

179. Weinburg G, Ullman B, Martin DW: Mutator phenotypes in mammalian cell mutants with

distinct biochemical defects and abnormal deoxyribonucleoside triphosphate pools. Proc Natl Acad Sci USA 78:2447, 1981

180. Brockman RW: Resistance to purine antagonists in experimental leukemia systems. Cancer Res 25:1596, 1965

181. Bennett LL, Brockman RW, Schnebli HP, et al: Activity and mechanism of action of 6-methylmercaptopurine ribonucleoside in cancer cells resistant to 6-mercaptopurine. Nature 205:1276, 1965

182. Luce JK, Frenkel EP, Vietti TJ, et al: Clinical studies of 6-methylmercaptopurine riboside (NSC-40774) in acute leukemia. Cancer Chemother Rep 51:535, 1967

183. Landy M, Larkum NW, Oswald EJ, Streightoff F: Increased synthesis of *p*-aminobenzoic acid associated with the development of sulfonamide resistance in *Staphylococcus aureus*. Science 97:265, 1943

184. Block ER, Jennings AE, Bennett JE: 5-Fluorocytosine resistance in *Cryptococcus neoformans*. Antimicrob Agents Chemother 3:649, 1973

185. Hoeprich PD, Ingraham JL, Kleker E, Winship MJ: Development of resistance to 5-fluorocytosine in *Candida parasilosis* during therapy. J Infect Dis 130:112, 1974

186. Jund R, Lacrute F: Genetic and physiological aspects of resistance to 5-fluoropyrimidines in *Saccharomyces cerevisiae*. J Bacteriol 102:607, 1970

187. Ip MM: Steroids. p.633. In Fox BW, Fox M (eds): Antitumor Drug Resistance. Springer-Verlag, New York, 1984

188. Gehring U: Cell genetics of glucocorticoid responsiveness. p.205. In Litwack G (ed): Biochemical Actions of Hormones. Vol. 7. Academic Press, Orlando, FL, 1980

189. Gehring U, Hotz A: Photoaffinity labeling and partial proteolysis of wild-type and variant glucocorticoid receptors. Biochemistry 22:4013, 1983

190. Coen DM, Furman PA, Gelep PT, Schaffer PA: Mutations in the herpes simplex virus DNA polymerase gene can confer resistance to 9-β-D-arabinofuranosyl adenine. J Virol 41:909, 1982

191. Sugino A, Peebles CL, Kreuzer KN, Cozzarelli NR: Mechanism of action of nalidixic acid: Purification of *Escherichia coli nal*A gene product and its relationship to DNA gyrase and a novel nicking-closing enzyme. Proc Natl Acad Sci USA 74:4767, 1977

192. Gellert M, Mizuuchi K, O'Dea MH, et al: Nalidixic acid resistance: A second genetic character involved in DNA gyrase activity. Proc Natl Acad Sci USA 74:4772, 1977

193. Oleinick NL, Wilhelm JM, Corcoran JW: Nonidentity of the site of action of erythromycin A and chloramphenicol on *Bacillus subtilis* ribosomes. Biochim Biophys Acta 114:277, 1966

194. Chang FN, Weisblum B: The specificity of lincomycin binding to ribosomes. Biochemistry 6:826, 1967

195. Tanaka K, Teraoka H, Nagira T, Tamaki M: [^{14}C]Erythromycin-ribosome complex formation and non-enzymatic binding of amino-acyl-transfer RNA to ribosome-messenger RNA complex. Biochim Biophys Acta 123:435, 1966

196. Teraoka H, Tanaka K, Tamaki M: The comparative study on the effects of chloramphenicol, erythromycin and lincomycin on polylysine synthesis in an *Escherichia coli* cell-free system. Biochim Biophys Acta 174:776, 1969

197. Wittmann HG, Stöffler G, Aprion D, et al: Biochemical and genetic studies on two different types of erythromycin resistant mutants of *Escherichia coli* with altered ribosomal proteins. Mol Gen Genet 127:175, 1973

198. Tanaka K, Tamaki M, Takata R, Osawa S: Low affinity for chloramphenicol of erythromycin-resistant *Escherichia coli* ribosomes having an altered protein component. Biochem Biophys Res Commun 46:1979, 1972

199. Sparling PF, Blackman E: Mutation to erythromycin dependence in *Escherichia coli* K-12. J Bacteriol 116:74, 1973

200. Mitsuhashi S, Inoue M: Resistance to macrolides and lincomycins. p.279. In Bryan LE (ed): Antimicrobial Drug Resistance. Academic Press, Orlando, FL, 1984

201. Weisblum B, Siddhikol C, Lai J, Demohn V: Erythromycin-inducible resistance in *Staphylococcus aureus*: Requirements for induction. J Bacteriol 106:835, 1971

202. Lai CJ, Weisblum B: Altered methylation of ribosomal RNA in an erythromycin-resistant strain of *Staphylococcus aureus*. Proc Natl Acad Sci USA 68:856, 1971

203. Lai CJ, Weisblum B, Fahnstock SR, Nomura M: Alteration of 23S ribosomal RNA and erythromycin-induced resistance to lincomycin and spiramycin in *Staphylococcus aureus*. J Mol Biol 74:67, 1973

204. Horinouchi S, Weisblum B: Posttranscriptional modification of mRNA conformation: Mechanism that regulates erythromycin-induced resistance. Proc Natl Acad Sci USA 77:7079, 1980

205. Graham MY, Weisblum B: 23S ribosomal ribonucleic acid of macrolide-producing streptomycetes contains methylated adenine. J Bacteriol 137:1464, 1979

206. Wehrli W, Knüsel F, Schmid K, Staehelin M: Interaction of rifamycin with bacterial RNA polymerase. Proc Natl Acad Sci USA 61:667, 1968

207. Heil A, Zillig W: Reconstitution of bacterial DNA-dependent RNA polymerase from isolated subunits as a tool for the elucidation of the role of the subunits in transcription. FEBS Lett 11:165, 1970

208. Lill UI, Hartmann GR: Formation of a RNA polymerase sub-assembly composed of subunit α from *Escherichia coli* and of subunit β from *Micrococcus luteus*. Hoppe-Seyler's Z Physiol Chem 358:1605, 1977

209. Burchall JJ, Hitchings GH: Inhibitor binding analysis of dihydrofolate-reductases from various species. Mol Pharmacol 1:126, 1965

210. Burchall JJ, Elwell LP, Fling ME: Molecular mechanisms of resistance to trimethoprim. Rev Infect Dis 44:246, 1982

211. Ferone R: Dihydrofolate reductase from pyrimethamine-resistant *Plasmodium berghei*. J Biol Chem 245:850, 1970

212. Yoeli M, Upmanis RS, Most H: Drug-resistance transfer among rodent plasmodia. Parasitology 59:429, 1969

213. Ferone R, O'Shea M, Yoeli M: Altered dihydrofolate reductase associated with drug-resistance transfer between rodent plasmodia. Science 167:1263, 1970

214. Fox M: Drug resistance and DNA repair. p.335. In Fox BW, Fox M (eds): Antitumor Drug Resistance. Springer-Verlag, New York, 1984

215. Venitt S: Interstrand cross-links in the DNA of *Escherichia coli* B/r and B$_{s-1}$ and their removal by the resistant strain. Biochem Biophys Res Commun 31:355, 1968

216. Regan JD, Setlow RB: Two forms of repair in the DNA of human cells damaged by chemical carcinogens and mutagens. Cancer Res 34:3318, 1974

217. McCalla DR: Biological effects of nitrofurans. J Antimicrob Chemother 3:517, 1977

218. Parr TR, Bryan LE: Nonenzymatic resistance to other cell wall synthesis inhibitors. p.81. In Bryan LE (ed): Antimicrobial Drug Resistance, Academic Press, Orlando, FL, 1984

219. Ayusawa D, Yoneda Y, Yamane K, Maruo B: Pleiotropic phenomena in autolytic enzyme(s) content, flagellation, and simultaneous hyperproduction of extracellular α-amylase and protease in a *Bacillus subtilis* mutant. J Bacteriol 124:459, 1975

220. Mayhall CG, Medoff G, Marr JJ: Variation in the susceptibility of strains of *Staphylococcus aureus* to oxacillin, cephalothin, and gentamicin. Antimicrob Agents Chemother 10:707, 1976

10

Drug Tolerance and Physical Dependence

Brian M. Cox

CHARACTERISTICS OF TOLERANCE AND DEPENDENCE

Drug tolerance is a state of decreased responsiveness to the pharmacologic effect of a drug as a result of prior exposure to that drug or to a related drug. When exposure to drug A produces tolerance to it and also to drug B, the organism is said to be *cross-tolerant* to drug B. The degree of tolerance, in general, may vary within very wide limits. Usually in the tolerant organism, although the ordinarily effective dose is less effective or is even entirely ineffective, an increased dosage will again elicit the typical drug response. Thus, as a rule, tolerance is a quantitative change in sensitivity to a drug. Sometimes, however, the drug effect cannot be obtained at any dosage in the tolerant organism. Tolerance to drug effects can develop very rapidly. The term *tachyphylaxis* is sometimes used to describe rapidly developing tolerance to a drug or endogenous substance; the term *acute tolerance* is also used to describe this phenomenon. The mechanisms of tachyphylaxis or acute tolerance are not necessarily different from those contributing to more slowly developing tolerance.

Physical dependence is a state sometimes associated with drug tolerance, especially with drugs whose primary action is exerted in the nervous system. As a consequence of sustained exposure to the drug, adaptive changes occur, leading to the required presence of the drug for normal function. If the dependent state produced by exposure to drug A can be maintained by continued treatment with drug B in the absence of drug A, then the organism is said to be *cross-dependent* on drug B. The state of physical dependence is revealed by withdrawing the drug that induced the dependence or by antagonizing its action. This elicits various pathophysiologic disturbances known collectively as a *withdrawal syndrome* (also "abstinence syndrome"). The features of the withdrawal syndrome are characteristic of the type of drug inducing the dependent state and also of the species or type of organism in which the dependent state was induced. All manifestations of the withdrawal syndrome can be terminated abruptly and dramatically by readministering the drug.

There is evidence that many different processes contribute to drug tolerance and dependence. Tolerance to drug effects and phenomena analogous to a withdrawal syndrome have been observed in isolated cells exposed to drugs in culture. Thus, local adaptive changes at the primary cellular site of drug action may be responsible for tolerance in some cases. In the intact animal, however, additional mechanisms that affect the amount of drug reaching its target site and modified behavioral responses that result from prior drug exposure may also occur as a result of chronic drug treatment. The relative contributions of these mechanisms will vary considerably depending upon the drug, the physiologic system, and the schedule of drug treatment.

The characteristic features of drug tolerance and dependence vary considerably among different drugs as an inevitable consequence of differences in basic pharmacology between drug classes. Several types of drugs elicit tolerance but not physical dependence, while others induce both tolerance and dependence. Some drugs may induce a marked physical dependence at a time when the degree of tolerance appears modest. In considering the mechanisms by which these various phenomena are produced, it is helpful to have a general appreciation of the features of tolerance and dependence. Experimental procedures that may be used in evaluating the induction of tolerance and dependence by drugs have been summarized in a monograph prepared by the National Institute on Drug Abuse.[1] Most of the features of drug tolerance and dependence are exhibited by two classes of drugs, the opiates and the central depressants, although there are major differences in the tolerance and dependence phenomena induced by these agents. We will therefore describe the characteristic consequences of sustained exposure to these types of drugs before considering the mechanisms that may be responsible for these effects.

Opiate Drug Pharmacology

The opiate class of compounds comprises both the natural opium alkaloids, of which morphine is the prototype, and related synthetic and semisynthetic drugs. Sometimes these drugs are known as *narcotics,* a term with legal connotations that is more appropriately used to describe all neuronal depressants. The compounds that have been studied most intensively are morphine, heroin (diacetylmorphine), and the synthetic congeners levorphanol, meperidine, and methadone.

Opiate drugs have complex pharmacologic effects.[1-3] They are exceedingly valuable clinically for alleviating severe pain and for allaying the anxiety related to pain. In addition, they are anesthetic agents, they are effective cough suppressants, and they provide symptomatic relief of diarrhea. The aspect of their psychotropic action that accounts for their abuse by addicts is described as *euphoria.* This is a peculiar state of well-being which seems to defy exact description. After intravenous administration of morphine or heroin, the addict experiences an immediate sensation of physical pleasure akin to sexual orgasm.[4] A feeling of relaxation follows; sometimes accompanied by increased loquaciousness. With higher doses, sedation is a prominent effect and is accompanied by daydreams and fantasies. Libido and aggressiveness are decreased as subjects become increasingly withdrawn and unresponsive to their surroundings, often drifting into sleep. For many years attempts have been made to develop drugs that would be free of addiction liability while retaining the analgesic properties of the opiates. Some drugs such as pentazocine, nalbuphine, and butorphanol,[3,5] which seem to behave as partial agonists at morphine receptors, begin to approach that goal, but the maximum degree of pain relief that can be provided by these drugs is generally less than that observed with the potentially addictive agents such as morphine and methadone. However, intensive research on structure-activity relationships in the opiate drug series has led to two important developments in our understanding of their complex pharmacology.

The discovery that there are specific receptors for opiate drugs[6-8] led to a quest for the physiologic functions of those receptors. Several endogenous peptides were found with the ability to produce many of the pharmacologic actions of opiate drugs,[9-11] and the localization of the peptides in specific neural pathways and endocrine tissues has led to the concept that these endogenous opioid peptides normally function as neurotransmitters, neuromodulators, and hormones. [12-14] The wide range of pharmacologic actions of opiate drugs is presumed to reflect their ability to mimic physiologic actions of the endogenous opioids. Careful comparisons of the pharmacology of endogenous opioid peptides, synthetic peptide congeners, and opiate alkaloids and their derivatives have resulted in the discovery that these agents act through receptors that are heterogeneous.[15,16] Different types of opioid receptors may be defined on the basis of differing affinities for various series of peptide and alkaloid opiates, as measured by estimates of specific radioligand binding,[17] and by differing sensitivities to opiate antagonists, as measured by apparent antagonist affinities determined from shifts induced in the dose-response curves of agonists.[16,18]

Studies of this nature have suggested the existence of at least four major classes of opioid receptors, although unambiguous physical evidence of their separate identities is not yet available. Drugs chemically similar to morphine, as well as some synthetic peptides, are thought to act primarily through a class of receptor designated μ. The naturally occurring peptides [Leu^5]enkephalin and [Met^5] enkephalin have high affinity for the δ type receptors, although they probably also activate μ receptors. The synthetic drug ethylketocyclazocine and endogenous peptides related to dynorphin are thought to act predominantly through κ-type receptors.[16,18] Some synthetic opiates with psychotomimetic properties are postulated to induce these effects through a fourth type of receptor designated σ,[15,19] although it is unlikely that either the major opiate drugs used in therapy or the currently identified endogenous opioid peptides normally act at σ receptors. Some studies suggest that other receptor types may occur, and some investigators propose the existence of subsets within some of the major opioid receptor classes.[20] The structural relationships and possible interactions between the various receptor forms have not yet been worked out.

The major opiate drugs that are used therapeutically, as well as those opiate drugs most subject to abuse, seem to produce most of their actions through interactions with μ-type receptors.[16,21] There are similarities in the actions of these compounds in different species, although the predominant effects may vary. In humans, monkeys, dogs, rabbits, and rats, sedative actions usually predominate in drug-naïve animals. In horses, cats, and mice, the predominant effects are excitatory. However, in all species both depressant and excitatory actions can be observed. Several studies suggest that inhibition of neurotransmitter release may underly many opiate actions, including pain relief,[22] modulation of hormonal secretion,[23] and inhibition of motility and secretion in the gastrointestinal tract.[24,25] It is possible that the apparent excitatory effects observed in some species or physiologic systems may also arise from opiate-induced inhibition of inhibitory pathways.[26] Respiratory depression occurs in all mammals; it is the cause of death from opiate overdose in humans and most species, including species such as mice in which excitation is the major effect observed at lower doses.

Tolerance to Opiate Drugs

Tolerance to opiates can be readily induced in laboratory animals by repeated injections of the drug, by infusion of the drug through an indwelling catheter, or by release of the drug from an implanted drug reservoir. Tolerance is usually manifested as a shift to the right of the dose-response curve, although in some circumstances the maximum attainable response may be depressed. Most investigations of tolerance to opiates in animals have used analgesia (antinociceptive action) as the pharmacologic end point. In such investigations animals are subjected to a standardized noxious stimulus. Their reaction is then recorded, either as a latency (time) to respond to the standard stimulus or in terms of the minimal stimulus intensity (threshold) required to induce a predetermined behavioral response. Analgesia is defined as the increase in reaction latency or the increase in stimulus threshold induced by a drug. Tolerance after prior drug exposure is indicated by a return toward initial response latency or threshold sensitivity. Tolerance may be overcome by increasing the drug dosage to re-establish the initial drug response. Thus, tolerance may be quantified as the increase in drug dosage required to induce the same response in drug-treated animals that was observed with the initial dose in untreated animals. Figure 10-1A shows the effects of repeated administration over a period of 20 days on the dose-response curves for morphine in two different measures of antinociceptive response in mice.[27] Analgesia was measured by the hot-plate test, in which the response latency of mice placed on a metal surface at 58°C was recorded. The acetic acid writing test, in which the number of abdominal stretches in response to intraperitoneal injection of a small amount of acetic acid was recorded in control, acutely morphine-treated, and chronically morphine-treated animals, was also used to measure analgesia. Morphine reduces the frequency of the abdominal stretch response. This test is a more sensitive measure of the antinociceptive action of morphine than the hot-plate test, as indicated by the lower morphine EC50 in the acetic acid test. Nevertheless, both tests show that morphine pretreatment produced comparable parallel rightward shifts in the morphine dose-response curves. Substantial analgesic responses could still be obtained upon increasing the dose of the drug.

With a more intensive drug exposure to ensure that a pharmacologically active concentration of morphine is maintained in tissues throughout each 24-hour period, it may become impossible to induce the same degree of analgesia observed in previously un-

Fig. 10-1 Effects of morphine pretreatments on the dose-response curves for morphine in five different tests in mice. (A) Analgesic tests: (a) hot plate test in which the reaction time (in seconds) of mice placed on a hot plate at 58°C is plotted on the ordinate; (b) acetic acid test in which the number of abdominal stretches produced over a 10-minute period in response to an intraperitoneal injection of dilute acetic acid is plotted on the ordinate (note the inverted scale). (B) Other actions of morphine: (a) hypothermia test in which reduction in colonic temperature (in °C) is plotted on the ordinate; (b) motor activity test in which increase in motor activity is reported as the number of cage crossings made in 10 minutes by groups of five mice; (c) lethality test in which the percentage mortality in groups of 10 mice is recorded 24 hours after administration of various morphine doses. Morphine pretreatments: ● no pretreatment; △ 64 mg/kg/day for 20 days; ■ 128 mg/kg twice daily for 20 days. Morphine dosage was calculated as the hydrochloride salt, and the drug was injected subcutaneously. Except in the lethality study each data point represents the mean results from at least 15 animals and in most cases 20 to 30 animals. Male mice of the NMRI strain were used. (Redrawn from Fernandes et al.,[27] with permission.)

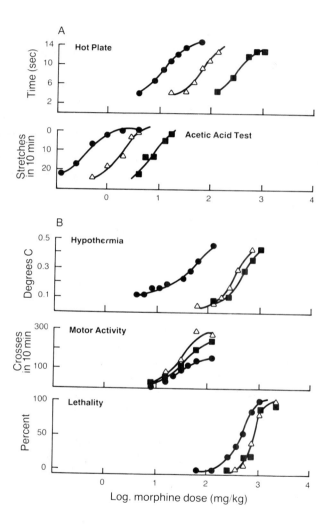

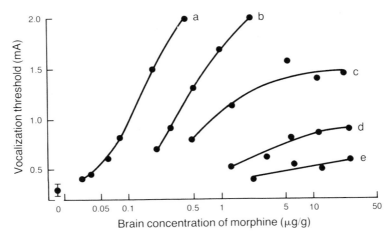

Fig. 10-2. Dose-response curves for morphine-induced analgesia in untreated rats and in rats previously treated with differing amounts of morphine. Analgesia was measured as the increase in vocalization threshold, determined as the minimum current (in milliamperes) applied to the root of the tail required to induce a vocalization response in Sprague-Dawley rats after various doses of morphine. The vocalization threshold has been plotted against estimated levels of morphine (in micrograms per gram wet weight) in brain produced by various morphine doses given subcutaneously, a procedure that takes into account the presence of residual morphine from the tolerance-inducing treatments. Mean results from groups of 12 or more animals are plotted. Tolerance was induced by the subcutaneous implantation of pellets (containing 75 mg morphine base), which slowly released the drug. Morphine pretreatments: (a) No pretreatment; (b) One pellet over a 4-day period; (c) Six pellets over a 10-day period; (d) 13 pellets over a 10-day period; (e) 24 pellets over a 10-day period. (Redrawn from Blasig et al.,[28] with permission.)

treated animals. Figure 10-2 shows an experiment in which tolerance was induced in rats by the subcutaneous implantation of pellets containing morphine. Because the drug was the less soluble free base, morphine was released slowly into the circulation, resulting in maintenance of a constant concentration of morphine in the tissues over a long period of time. The amount of morphine in the brain after each drug treatment was also measured. The minimum electrical stimulus applied to the tail that was required to induce a vocalization response is plotted against the estimated concentration of morphine in the brain after each treatment. With one morphine pellet, the analgesic dose-response curve for morphine was shifted to the right in a roughly parallel fashion. When several pellets were implanted over a period of more than 1 week, however, it became impossible to induce a significant analgesic response with increased amounts of morphine. The maximum response to the drug was depressed. Both the rightward shift in the dose-response curve and the reduction in maximum response can be prevented if the antagonist, naloxone, is administered together with the opiate drug during pretreatment.[29,30]

Interpretation of these results is in part complicated by the complexity of the analgesic response. There are many potential ways in which a drug might modify the latency or threshold of behavioral responses to the application of a noxious stimulus, not all of which are related to analgesia. For example, the drug may paralyze the motor response without affecting sensitivity to pain. Furthermore, there are several potential sites at which opiate drugs might act to modify behavioral responses induced by noxious stimuli. It is now well established that opiates act at the level of the dorsal horn of the spinal cord, in the nucleus raphe magnocellularis of the brain stem, and in the periaqueductal gray region of the midbrain to attentuate responses to a peripheral noxious stimulus.[31] This suggests that analgesia is the result of a composite of opiate actions at different sites.[32] Measures of analgesic tolerance often involve repeated testing of behavioral responses in the same animal, raising the possibility that learned behaviors might influence the outcome of such tests. However, similar tolerance characteristics have been observed to other actions of opiate drugs in which interactions between multiple sites of action or potential modification of test responses by learned behaviors are not likely to be involved.[33,34] Despite the complexity implicit in the measurement of antinociceptive actions, such studies have been very useful in the characterization both of the chemical features necessary to produce analgesia of the opiate type and of the development of tolerance to this action.

Tolerance to opiate drugs can be observed in isolated tissues and in cells maintained in culture. Thus, the phenomenon is not restricted to complex behavioral actions of opiates in intact animals. For example, opiates inhibit the activity of the enzyme adenylate cyclase in cultured neuroblastoma X glioma hybrid (NG 108-15) cells. Chronic exposure of these cells to opiates results in a reduced ability of the drugs to inhibit enzyme activity.[33] There is no evidence suggesting that the development of tolerance to this action of opiates requires interactions between individual cells in the culture. It must therefore be concluded that tolerance can occur in a single cell. Opiate tolerance has also been observed in other simple systems. Morphine reduces the frequency of movement of the developing chick embryo; the effectiveness of morphine is reduced if the embryo is exposed to morphine for a few days.[35] Tolerance has also been observed in vitro in primary cultures of fetal mouse dorsal root ganglia and spinal cord,[36] and in guinea pig ileum myenteric plexus neurons incubated with opiates in vitro.[34]

The development of tolerance in intact animals is not dependent on the access of the opiate drug to a single critical region of the nervous system. While most studies of analgesic tolerance have used systemic drug administration to expose the drug to the entire neuroaxis, repeated discrete localized injections of an opiate to a single site of opiate action in either the spinal cord or midbrain periaqueductal gray region can also induce tolerance to opiate analgesia.[32] Localized injections at other sites may induce tolerance to other actions of opiates while failing to induce analgesic tolerance. Tolerance can be achieved in most physiologic systems in which opiate drugs act.

However, tolerance to all actions of a drug does not develop to the same extent. By quantitating the individual actions of opiates, the extent of tolerance development to each action can be examined in the same study. Figure 10-1B shows the effects of the same morphine pretreatments that produced parallel rightward shifts of the analgesic dose response curves in mice for morphine-induced hypothermia, motor activity, and lethality.[27] A parallel rightward shift was observed in the hypothermia dose-response curve, although a more intensive pretreatment induced little more tolerance than a moderate pretreatment. The rightward shift in the lethality dose-response curve was much less marked, however, and the same pretreatments may have actually sensitized these mice to the motor stimulant actions of morphine. (It should be noted, as will be discussed below, that with different conditions and a different strain of mice, it is possible to demonstrate significant tolerance to opiate-induced increases in motor activity). Thus, it is apparent that the magnitude of the tolerance induced by opiates is dependent not only on the intensity of the pretreatment but also on the nature of the response being measured. When a greater degree of tolerance develops to a desired pharmacologic effect than to the lethal effects of a drug, the margin of safety in the use of that drug becomes much smaller, and the probability of inadvertent drug overdosage is increased.

The rate of tolerance development is related to the frequency and intensity of drug treatment. An illustrative example is provided in studies on locomotor stimulation in mice. This action of an opiate drug can be easily quantified with simple equipment that permits automatic recording of the drug effect. For example, mice were housed in cages fitted with light beams directed across each cage.[37] Each time a mouse interrupted the beam by moving across the cage, a response was recorded by a photocell counter. After the initial exploratory behavior subsided, the animals spent most of the time huddled together in a corner of the cage, so that background activity was very low. Removal from the cage, injection with saline, and replacement in the cage produced very little increase in recorded activity. In contrast, administration of the opiate drug levorphanol produced a great increase in the movement of the mice about the cage. Movement continued at an almost constant rate for about 2 hours and then gradually diminished. When the same dose was injected at regular intervals (e.g., every 8 hours) less "running" activity was produced after each successive dose. At any time during this process, a substantial increase of the drug dose could reinstate the full running activity seen after the initial injection. Thus, the capacity of the mice to move rapidly about the cage was not impaired; only the sensitivity to opiate had decreased. In these mice, tolerance to the locomotor stimulant actions of the opiate was reliably observed, in contrast to the results shown in Figure 10-1B. The difference may relate to the use of a different strain of mice, measurement of activity over a longer time after each drug dose, use of a different opiate drug, or different treatment and test schedules. In all species, opiates produce both stimulant and depressant effects, and the observed effect in intact animals is often dependent on the balance between these functionally opposing actions. It is possible that in the experiments shown in Figure 10-1, tolerance developed more rapidly to the depressant effect of morphine than to its stimulant action, thus exposing an apparent sensitization to morphine-induced stimulation after the drug pretreatment.

The locomotor stimulation experiments shown in Figure 10-3 were carried out with levorphanol at a fixed dose, which caused maximal running activity in a mouse receiving its first injection. As shown in the figure, each decrease in the interval of drug administration led to a different rate of tolerance development and also to a different level of maintained tolerance, as indicated by the plateaus in the curves relating percent of initial drug activity to the number of days of treatment. Injection intervals of 4 or 8 hours resulted in very rapid rates of tolerance development and a high level of tolerance. An interval of 24 hours resulted in slower onset of tolerance and a milder sustained level, while little tolerance developed when levorphanol injections were spaced at 48 hour intervals. Thus, it appears that the processes responsible for tolerance development had completely decayed by 48 hours after each injection.

The best interpretation of these findings is that a single effective dose of an opiate initiates a certain biochemical change, with its own intrinsic time course of onset and decay, which is responsible for the occurrence of tolerance. If the next dose of drug is given before the tolerance-inducing effect produced by the previous dose has decayed, the level of observed tolerance will increase, as in the process of cumulative toxicity. The process of tolerance appears to be completely reversible; complete recovery of sensitivity to the locomotor effects of levorphanol was observed in this study within 48 hours, and when further injections of the drug were given, the rate of tolerance development was the same as before.[37]

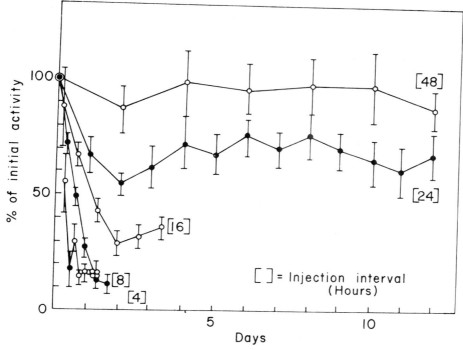

Fig. 10-3. Effects of multiple doses of a narcotic on tolerance in mice. Levorphanol (20 mg kg^{-1}) was injected intraperitoneally on various interval schedules. Running activity was measured initially and after each injection. Points represent running activity as percent of initial running activity for each group of mice. Numbers in brackets represent the injection interval for each curve, 4, 8, 16, 24, and 48 hours. (From Goldstein et al.,[37] with permission.)

These results suggest that tolerance to the locomotor stimulant actions of opiates may be the result of a relatively simple process. More complex events appear to be involved in tolerance to the analgesic actions of opiates. In a study in rats in which the morphine-induced increase in the minimal pressure stimulus applied to the tail in order to induce tail withdrawal was recorded, tolerance was shown to develop rapidly during the course of an intravenous infusion of morphine; within 6 to 8 hours of infusion of a standard concentration of morphine, the stimulus threshold had returned to the level observed prior to the start of the drug infusion.[38] Examination of the rate of recovery of morphine sensitivity after termination of the infusion showed that recovery required more than 2 weeks. This suggested that the mechanisms of analgesic tolerance in rats were more complex than those responsible for tolerance to the motor stimulant actions of morphine in mice. However, interpretation is complicated by the possibility that each dose of opiate used to measure the level of tolerance during the recovery phase of the experiment might itself have reinitiated the tolerance mechanisms and thereby artifactually prolonged the apparent recovery time (even though the level of tolerance was measured in different groups of rats at each time).

The observation that tolerance development can be inhibited by the simultaneous administration of inhibitors of protein synthesis, such as cycloheximide,[38] pointed to a procedure by which the potential tolerance-inducing effects of test doses of drug might be

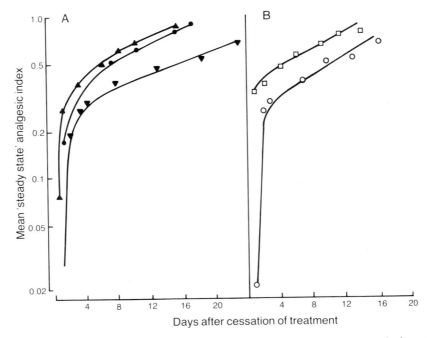

Fig. 10-4. Rates of recovery of responsiveness to morphine infused intravenously in rats that had been rendered tolerant to morphine by different pretreatments. Mean "steady-state" analgesic index was calculated from the morphine-induced increase in minimum pressure on the upper surface of a hind foot that was required to provoke foot withdrawal. This value is plotted against the number of days after cessation of pretreatment with opiate drug. Test doses of morphine were administered by intravenous infusion of morphine hydrochloride at a rate of 5 mg/kg/hr, together with cyclo-heximide (200 μg/g/hr) to prevent tolerance development during the test procedure (see text). The steady-state increase in pressure threshold was measured 4 to 6 hours after start of the test infusions. Since an arbitrary maximum pressure stimulus was employed to prevent foot damage, the observed increase in pressure threshold was expressed as a fraction of the possible increase between the baseline (predrug) threshold and the arbitrary maximum. Results are means from groups of four to six rats. (A) Morphine pretreatments: ▲ twice daily morphine doses increasing to 20 mg/kg over 3 days; ● twice daily morphine doses increasing to 40 mg/kg over 6 days; ▼ twice daily morphine doses increasing to 100 mg/kg over 7 days. (B) Methadone pretreatment □, twice daily methadone doses increasing to 12.5 mg/kg over 4 days; heroin (diacetylmorphine) pretreatment ○, twice daily heroin doses increasing to 20 mg/kg over 4 days. (From Cox et al.,[39] with permission.)

circumvented. By testing tolerance recovery with doses of morphine administered to-gether with cycloheximide, the observed rate of recovery of morphine sensitivity should not be influenced by the rapid reinitiation of tolerance by the test dose. The results of such an experiment are shown in Figure 10-4. This study confirms that the recovery period from tolerance to this analgesic action of morphine in rats is biphasic, consisting of a rapid recovery phase with a half-time of less than 24 hours and a slow phase with a half-time of 10 to 14 days.[39] More than one process may be implicated in tolerance to the analgesic actions of opiates, in contrast to the apparently simpler mechanisms responsible for tolerance to the motor stimulant effects in mice. It is unlikely that any single mechanism will be adequate to explain all the features of opiate tolerance.

Physical Dependence on Opiates

Opiate-tolerant addicts or experimental animals evidently function well as long as they continue to receive the drug. When a high degree of tolerance has been attained, even very high doses of drug may no longer produce euphoria, but drug intake must be maintained in order to avoid withdrawal symptoms. If drug administration is stopped, profound derangements ensue. In humans, opiate withdrawal is characterized initially by restlessness and intense craving for the drug. Yawning, running nose, lacrimation, and perspiration follow, with chills, fever, vomiting, panting respiration, loss of appetite, insomnia, hypertension, aches and pains, and loss of weight occurring in most individuals. The pupils become dilated, and there are associated signs of hyperactivity of the sympathetic nervous system. Pilomotor stimulation producing gooseflesh accounts for the vernacular description of withdrawal as "cold turkey." In animals similar disturbances occur during the withdrawal period, although the predominant symptoms vary among species.[40–43]

The invention of a procedure for quantitating the intensity of the withdrawal syndrome in humans[40] has contributed much to our understanding of its nature and to assessment of the addiction potential of newly developed analgesic drugs. Subjects presently or previously addicted to opiates are stabilized on a dosage regimen of 240 to 340 mg morphine daily or on an equivalent regimen of another opiate. Careful measurements of respiratory rate, blood pressure, body temperature, hours of sleep, caloric intake, and body weight are then made on a regular schedule. The presence of certain signs that are not subject to quantitative measurement, such as yawning, lacrimation, and vomiting, is simultaneously noted. For each observed symptom, a score based on an arbitrary point scale is assigned, with a maximum limit set on some symptom scores, so that the combined score represents a balanced assessment of the intensity of the whole withdrawal syndrome. Evaluations are usually carried out daily, but can be made more frequently for drugs that produce a withdrawal syndrome with rapid onset and decay. Figure 10-5 shows the results of an early study in which 65 addicts were followed with this assessment procedure. The curves show the course of the physiologic variables measured after withdrawal of morphine. The bottom curve illustrates the total point score computed on a daily basis, including all the items listed above. Peak intensity occurs at 2 days, followed by a slow decline over a period of more than 1 week. The total intensity of the withdrawal syndrome is sometimes expressed as the area under such a curve.

The method has proved extremely useful for comparing different drugs. The course of withdrawal is almost the same for morphine and heroin but is very different for methadone, and this has some practical application in the clinical management of withdrawal. Figure 10-6 shows an experiment in which subjects were stabilized on morphine or methadone and then withdrawn.[44] The subsequent withdrawal effects developed more slowly after methadone withdrawal than after morphine withdrawal, and did not reach as great an intensity. However, the total withdrawal period was longer after methadone. Because of the occurrence of cross-tolerance and cross-dependence between opiates, it is possible to use methadone to replace whatever opiate addicts have been taking to maintain their dependence without precipitating withdrawal symptoms. The methadone can then be withdrawn on a predetermined schedule, with a less severe overall intensity of withdrawal symptoms than occurs during morphine or heroin withdrawal.

The relationship between dosage administered during the period of dependence development and the intensity of the subsequent withdrawal syndrome has been studied in a large number of addicts who were stabilized on doses of morphine from 40 to 400 mg

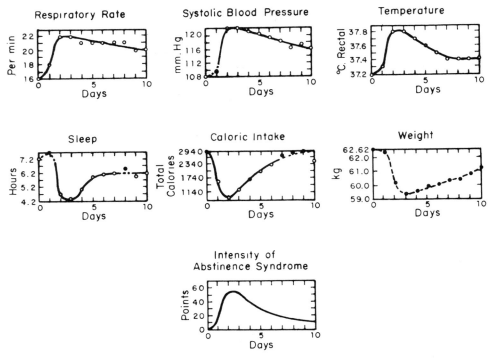

Fig. 10-5. Quantitation of the withdrawal syndrome. Sixty-five addicts were stabilized on a dosage of 240 to 340 mg of morphine daily, then withdrawn abruptly at day zero. Careful observations and measurements were made for 10 days. A representative sampling is shown in the upper two rows. The summation of scores (see text) for all the signs of withdrawal yielded the curve at bottom. (Adapted from Kolb et al.,[40] with permission.)

daily.[45] For each group the total score for intensity of the withdrawal syndrome was summed over 7 days (Fig. 10-7). Clearly, the higher the dosage, the more intense was the subsequent withdrawal syndrome. The shape of the curve is interesting because it suggests that a maximum degree of physical dependence is reached at morphine dosages of about 400 mg day^{-1}. However, this flattening of the curve may be an artifact of the scoring system used to quantify the withdrawal syndrome, since certain scores are not permitted to exceed arbitrary maximum values.

Development of dependence can be prevented if opiate antagonists are administered together with the opiate agonist used to induce dependence.[46,47] As in the case of tolerance development, it appears that activation of opiate receptors to induce a pharmacologic effect is a necessary condition for dependence to develop. In dependent subjects, withdrawal symptoms can usually be prevented by administration of an opiate agonist in sufficient doses.[48] Other types of drugs, such as the α-receptor agonist clonidine,[49] cholinergic antagonists, ganglion blocking agents,[50] and tranquilizers and hypnotic drugs,[51] can modify some of the withdrawal symptoms. These drugs act by altering the function of specific effector systems responsible for the expression of some withdrawal symptoms without affecting the underlying dependence process. Withdrawal symptoms can be induced in opiate-dependent animals and in humans by administration of an opiate receptor antagonist such as naloxone or naltrexone. This action of antagonists is sometimes de-

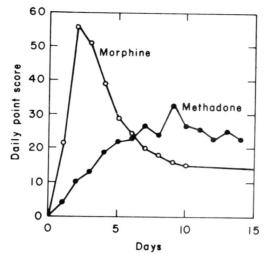

Fig. 10-6. Course of withdrawal syndrome after morphine and after methadone. Morphine and methadone were withdrawn (on day zero) after several months of administration. Intensity of the withdrawal syndrome was scored daily thereafter, as described in the text. Morphine data are average point scores of 65 subjects; methadone data are for five subjects. (From Isbell,[44] with permission.)

scribed as "precipitated withdrawal"; the symptoms are qualitatively similar to withdrawal induced by failure to continue drug administration, but the onset is more rapid and the intensity of symptoms may be more severe.[52] The predominant features of the opiate withdrawal syndrome vary between species. In small laboratory animals, escape reactions, irritability, body shakes, defecation, and weight loss are often the major symptoms observed. Some of these effects lend themselves to quantitative assessment. Thus, in rats and mice escape responses manifested as jumping from an elevated platform can easily be counted by an observer, allowing a quantitative measurement of the intensity of the withdrawal syndrome in these species.[43] Hyperalgesia and changes in body weight have also proved to be quantitatively reliable indicators of withdrawal intensity.[53]

Naloxone-precipitated escape jumping in mice has been used to determine the factors that affect the level of dependence induced by opiate pretreatments. The severity of withdrawal symptoms precipitated by the antagonist is dependent on the dose of naloxone. A convenient measure of sensitivity is therefore the naloxone ED50, computed in the case of escape jumping responses as the naloxone dose required to induce escape jumping in 50 percent of a group of opiate-dependent mice treated with the antagonist. This value is estimated by giving selected groups of mice various naloxone doses around the assumed ED50 dose. Previously untreated nondependent mice seldom jump out of a jar or off an elevated platform, and naloxone does not cause jumping in such mice in doses up to those that induce convulsions and death. However, even a single large dose of an opiate drug can induce a state in which naloxone can induce escape jumping. Figure 10-8 shows that within 2 hours of administration of a 20 mg kg^{-1} dose of levorphanol to mice naloxone-induced escape jumping was apparent, reaching maximum sensitivity after about 8 hours and decaying within 24 hours.[54] This time course was unrelated to that of levorphanol in plasma, which had a measured half-life of less than 1 hour; however, persistent drug at

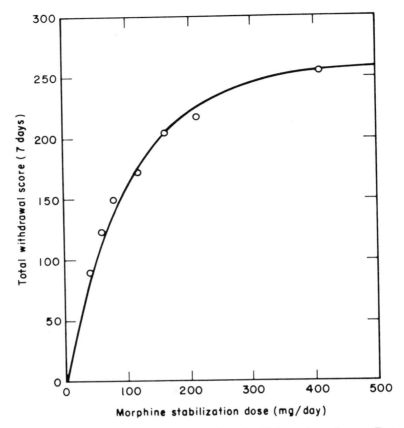

Fig. 10-7. Relationship between dosage and intensity of withdrawal syndrome. Data for intensity of withdrawal syndrome in 127 addicts who had been stabilized on various dosages from 40 to 400 mg of morphine daily before abrupt withdrawal. Total scores for 7 days of withdrawal are plotted against the stabilization dose prior to withdrawal. (Modified from Andrews et al.,[45] with permission.)

tight-binding sites in the central nervous system could not be ruled out. (Precipitated withdrawal after very short exposure to opiate drugs has also been observed in dogs.[41])

After more intensive pretreatment (higher doses, shorter intervals, longer duration of treatment) and simultaneously with the development of higher and higher degrees of tolerance, escape jumping of mice could be elicited with lower and lower doses of naloxone. A similar enhancement of sensitivity to naloxone with increasing intensity of morphine pretreatment of rats was observed when the naloxone-induced loss of body weight was used as an index of withdrawal severity.[53] While it cannot be assumed that there is a linear correspondence between the naloxone ED50 and the degree of the disturbance underlying physical dependence, such studies confirm that the severity of the dependent state increases with the intensity of the opiate treatment.

The time course of onset and disappearance of physical dependence after one dose of levorphanol led to a prediction: that repeated injection of the same dose at 4-hour intervals would lead to intense physical dependence (very low naloxone ED50), whereas injection of the same dose at 16 hour intervals would lead to a measurable but low degree of dependence at the steady state. These predictions were borne out in experiments with

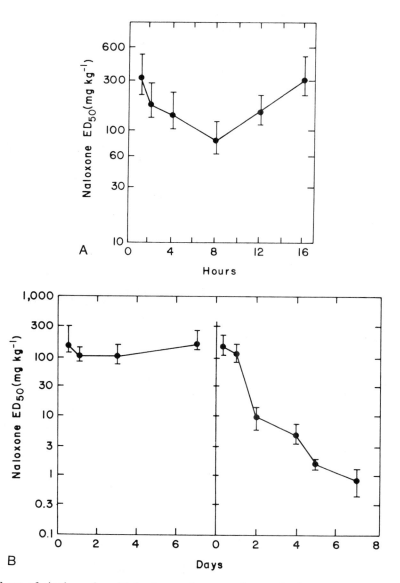

Fig 10-8. Effects of single and multiple doses of a narcotic on physical dependence in mice. Levorphanol (20 mg kg^{-1}) was injected intraperitoneally. Withdrawal was precipitated in groups of mice by naloxone. Points represent naloxone ED50 with standard errors. In untreated animals no dose of naloxone produces jumping. (**A**) Effect of a single dose of levorphanol given at time zero. (**B**) Effect of levorphanol on the steady state degree of dependence when given at 12-hour interval (left) or at 4-hour interval (right). (From Cheney et al.,[54] with permission.)

mice, as shown in Figure 10-8. When measurement of naloxone-precipitated escape jumping is used as an index of the dependent state, the dependence process appears to be completely reversed within 1 to 2 days of termination of opiate drug treatment.[39,54] Thus, the recovery time course is similar to that of tolerance to opiate-induced motor stimulation in mice.[37] However, there are some indications that underlying disturbances persist for a longer time. It was shown, for example, that administration of a single dose of morphine to rats for up to 2 to 3 weeks during the period of recovery from the dependent state exposed an underlying hypersensitivity to naloxone-induced jumping, even though the single dose of morphine used was, by itself, insufficient to produce any substantial degree of dependence in previously untreated animals.[55] Similarly, it has been noted that in morphine-dependent mice, the next dose of opiate in a sequence of opiate injections does not reduce the sensitivity of the animal to naloxone-precipitated withdrawal,[56] as might have been anticipated as a consequence of a competitive interaction between the agonist and antagonist. It appears that in opiate-dependent animals, the ability of an opiate agonist to induce a state characterized by increased sensitivity to antagonists may actually be enhanced. Following the last dose of opiate used to maintain the dependent state, the ability of morphine to reinitiate sensitivity to naloxone-induced escape jumping in mice decays in a biphasic manner, with an initial rapid recovery phase followed by a slow phase with a half-time of 2 to 3 weeks.[55] The rate of recovery is very similar to the rate of recovery from tolerance to opiate-induced analgesia in rats.[39] These kinetics suggest that identical or similar processes might underly the two functions.

Clinical studies suggest that the time courses of recovery from the various components of the dependent state are not identical. As indicated previously, many of the major physical symptoms of opiate withdrawal decline to negligible levels within 6 to 7 days after withdrawal of the opiate (Fig. 10-5). Administration of naloxone during this period initially provokes a more extreme withdrawal reaction, but the overall time course for many of these physical symptoms is shortened by antagonist treatment.[57] Since the severity of some withdrawal symptoms can be alleviated by drugs such as clonidine,[58] some addicts may choose to achieve a rapid detoxification from the dependent state by precipitating withdrawal with an opiate antagonist while using other agents to provide some symptomatic relief.[57] Despite this relatively rapid recovery from many of the features of dependence, however, other symptoms, such as sleep disturbances, show a much longer time course for recovery. Craving for opiate drugs may persist for many months.[59–61] It is not known if the mechanisms underlying these symptoms are sensitized to reactivation by opiate agonists during recovery from dependence. If they were, it would suggest that occasional exposure to an opiate during withdrawal might significantly extend the period of withdrawal distress and drug craving.

Tolerance and Dependence Induced by Central Depressant Drugs

A significant degree of tolerance and dependence is associated with chronic exposure to drugs that produce depression of neuronal function in the central nervous system (CNS), including alcohol, barbiturates, and related drugs. Tolerance and dependence are also observed after repeated or sustained treatment with antianxiety agents of the benzodiazepine type. Although there are qualitative differences among individual classes of depressant drugs in the pharmacologic actions that show tolerance, in the characteristic features of the induced withdrawal syndromes, and in the time courses of dependence development and decay, there are also many similarities, which suggests that common mechanisms may underly the long-term effects of treatment by each type of depressant. There are, however, several differences from opiate tolerance and withdrawal. The degree of tolerance observed with the central depressant drugs is much less marked than with the opiates: the dose of depressant drug required to produce depression is seldom increased as much as 10-fold by chronic drug treatment, in contrast to the 100-fold or greater tolerance that can be induced with opiate drugs. The major features of the withdrawal syndrome also differ substantially.

Alcohol

Tolerance develops to the central depressant effects of alcohol. Most studies have used ethanol, but other alcohols produce similar pharmacologic effects, and cross-tolerance between alcohols occurs. The pharmacologic actions of ethanol are less readily quantified than the motor stimulant or analgesic actions of opiate drugs. In order to demonstrate tolerance, several studies have measured the blood alcohol concentrations at which animal or human subjects show unmistakable symptoms of intoxication, often measured on a drunkenness symptom scale. In an early experiment of this type, it was shown that administration of ethanol to dogs twice daily in their drinking water over a 3-month period resulted in an increase in the concentration of blood alcohol needed to produce a given degree of intoxication.[62] Similar results have been obtained in human subjects.[63,64] In each of these studies the observed degree of tolerance was relatively modest, the required blood concentration of ethanol increasing less than twofold. The ethanol exposure periods of several months after which tolerance development in dogs or human subjects was measured are presumed similar to those for the development of alcohol tolerance in humans. However, studies in dogs and rats have indicated that an acute tolerance to ethanol can arise in periods as short as 1 or 2 hours.[65,66]

Withdrawal of ethanol after a period of chronic intoxication leads to occurrence of a withdrawal syndrome. In alcoholic patients, a characteristic pattern of symptoms emerges on discontinuation of alcohol consumption.[67] A well controlled study at the Addiction Research Center in Lexington showed that the seizures and hallucinatory symptoms (delirium tremens) of alcoholics are associated not with the state of chronic intoxication but with withdrawal from ethanol.[68] Ten former morphine addicts were given enough ethanol to maintain a severe degree of intoxication for up to 13 weeks, followed by abrupt and complete withdrawal. The average daily dose was around ¼ to ½ L of 95 percent ethanol. To avoid any complications due to malnutrition, the subjects were kept on a high-calorie diet supplemented with vitamins. (These studies were performed in the mid 1950s; it is unlikely such studies would be permitted under the stricter current view of ethical human experimentation.)

The "degree of intoxication" was evaluated by trained observers using an arbitrary scale from 0 to 4. There was fairly good agreement between blood levels and the estimated degree of intoxication. Initially, as the daily intake was being increased very cautiously, there was no evidence of intoxication. Then, as the blood concentration rose past 1 mg ml^{-1} the subjects became boisterous, noisy, and silly. During the third week a curious fall in the blood alcohol concentrations occurred without any change in the daily intake. Its cause was not investigated, but it might reflect the appearance of increased activity of the liver enzymes that metabolize ethanol (see below). As the blood ethanol concentration declined at this time, sobriety returned. When the daily dose was increased, the blood level rose again, and the state of intoxication returned. Subsequently, the blood alcohol concentration continued to rise as the daily intake was adjusted upward, but the degree of intoxication lagged behind. Tolerance was demonstrable on electroencephalographic records as well as by gross evaluations. An increase in slow-wave activity occurred initially at the higher blood concentrations, but this effect became less marked as the experiment proceeded despite the rising blood concentration in the final weeks.

During their state of chronic intoxication, none of the subjects developed any hallucinatory or convulsive behavior. The onset of withdrawal symptoms upon discontinuation of alcohol administration was quite rapid. About 8 hours after their last drink, the subjects became nervous, apprehensive, and very weak. Some suffered retching and vomiting. All six of the subjects who had been drinking for 48 days or more manifested tremor, weakness, perspiration, nausea, vomiting, diarrhea, elevated blood pressure, and insomnia. Delirium and hallucinations occurred in four of the subjects, and grand mal seizures developed in two. All the symptoms waned after a few days, and 3 months later the subjects appeared normal in all respects. Three subjects who withdrew from the experiment within the first month developed only slight tremor and anorexia.

It is clear from this and similar experiments[69] that delirium tremens is a typical withdrawal syndrome manifested after prolonged intake of ethanol, that a severe degree of physical dependence may occur, and that the intensity of the withdrawal syndrome depends upon the duration of exposure to ethanol and on the dosage schedule.

Animal models have been developed for the study of ethanol tolerance and dependence. Most laboratory animals will not drink ethanol voluntarily to the point of intoxication, so special techniques of administration are required. Procedures have been employed in which rats or other animals have to consume ethanol in order to satisfy their thirst or hunger by including ethanol in the drinking water or in a liquid diet. While it is clear that dependence on ethanol can be developed by such methods, interpretation of the results may be complicated by fluctuating blood levels of alcohol due to the tendency of rats to satisfy their water and caloric needs by consumption almost exclusively during a few hours at night. To overcome this difficulty, mice were exposed to a fixed concentration of ethanol by housing them in a chamber containing ethanol vapor.[70,71] By administering daily injections of pyrazole, liver alcohol dehydrogenase could be inhibited. With alcohol metabolism thus largely blocked, a near equilibrium could be established across the alveoli so that the ethanol level in blood was linearly related to its concentration in the inspired air, as described for volatile anesthetics in Chapter 4. While in the vapor chamber, the mice were more or less intoxicated, depending on the ethanol concentration. On removing the mice from the chamber, various characteristic withdrawal signs were observed (including convulsions and death), and these could be scored according to their severity. As Figure 10-9A shows, the withdrawal reaction reached its peak intensity at about 10 hours, then subsided completely in about 30 hours. The degree of dependence (intensity of withdrawal reaction) proved to be linearly related to the total exposure to ethanol (i.e., the blood concentration times the duration of exposure), as shown in Figure 10-10. It was found that even a single injection of ethanol produced a very slight but measurable degree of dependence. This technique has also proved useful for studying the effects of various drugs on the progression of the withdrawal reaction. Injections of ethanol abolished all the withdrawal signs immediately, but they returned as the ethanol was eliminated.

Barbiturates

Treatment with barbiturates and related drugs leads to tolerance and dependence with features similar to those described for ethanol. While it is sometimes difficult to demonstrate cross-tolerance between ethanol and barbiturates (because of the difficulty in

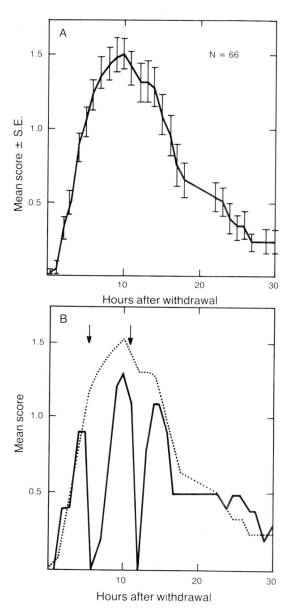

Fig 10-9. Withdrawal reaction of mice removed from vapor chamber. (**A**) Course of the withdrawal reaction in mice exposed for 3 days to a blood alcohol level of 1.8 to 2.3 mg ml^{-1}, then removed from the vapor chamber and left untreated. (**B**) Modification of withdrawal syndrome by pentobarbital injections, 60 mg kg^{-1} at arrows. Dotted curve is that for the untreated mice, as above. (Modified from Goldstein,[71] with permission.)

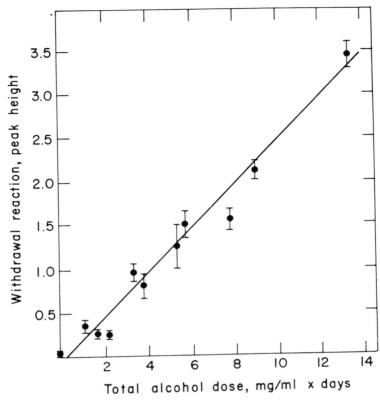

Fig. 10-10. Relationship of withdrawal reaction to alcohol exposure. Each point represents the mean peak withdrawal score for a group of mice. Vertical lines give standard errors. The *x* axis is total alcohol exposure, measured as the product of the constant blood level times the duration in days. (From Goldstein,[70] with permission.)

quantifying relatively low degrees of tolerance in measurements of animal behavior), suppression of ethanol withdrawal symptoms by barbiturates occurs in laboratory animals (Fig. 10-9B) and in humans.[68] In contrast, chlorpromazine, which is not clinically useful in treating alcohol withdrawal, exacerbates the ethanol withdrawal syndrome in mice.[71]

The initial studies of barbiturate tolerance in laboratory animals suggested that tolerance develops more readily to the long-acting drugs phenobarbital and barbital than to shorter-acting drugs such as pentobarbital. In many of these studies, however, drugs were administered in a single daily dose. A series of studies in cats have employed dosage regimens for barbital and pentobarbital in which equivalent degrees of intoxication were induced by progressively increasing doses of each drug given twice daily.[72–74] Under these conditions a greater degree of tolerance was obtained with pentobarbital than with barbital. However, when allowance was made for the accelerated metabolism of pentobarbital as a result of enzyme induction (see below), both the rate of onset of tolerance and the degree of tolerance were comparable for the two drugs.[74] In these studies CNS depression was measured by a rating scale in which symptoms of depression, including ataxia, loss of righting reflex, the rate and mode of respiration (normal or diaphragmatic), and corneal

Table 10-1. Lowering of Seizure Threshold during Barbiturate Withdrawal in Cats

No. of Animals	Duration of Barbiturate Treatment	Threshold for Pentylenetetrazol-Induced Seizures (% of Pretreatment Threshold)	
		20 hr after Terminating Barbiturate	*90 hr after Terminating Barbiturate*
8	26 hr	82	101
7	56 hr	72	107
7	5 days	46	103
4	3 weeks	31	59

Cats were given pentobarbital intravenously three to four times daily, in doses sufficient to cause deep anesthesia. Prior to the injections, seizure threshold was determined in each cat by infusing pentylenetetrazol intravenously and measuring how much was required to produce tonic muscular contractions. Then, after various durations of barbiturate intoxication, seizure threshold was again determined 20 and 90 hours after pentobarbital was discontinued. The data are average thresholds, as percents of initial threshold for each animal group. All the depressed thresholds differ significantly ($P < 0.05$) from the pretreatment value.
(From Jaffe et al.,[75] with permission.)

and skin twitch reflexes, were scored by observers unaware of the treatments administered.

Physical dependence on barbiturates can be produced in laboratory animals. It has been shown, for example, that administration of pentobarbital to cats three or four times a day results in progressively shorter periods of anesthesia.[75] On cessation of drug administration, the cats showed hyperexcitability, tremors, exaggerated startle responses, and myoclonic jerks, even after treatments as short as 3 days. In one cat receiving a longer treatment, withdrawal of the drug induced spontaneous seizures. A convenient indication of the severity of the dependent state was obtained by measuring the threshold dose of pentylenetetrazol (administered by IV infusion) required to induce tonic seizures. The results, given in Table 10-1, show that after treatment with pentobarbital for only 26 hours, the seizure threshold was lowered as compared with the initial threshold measured before treatment. Barbiturate withdrawal in rats induces a similar profile of symptoms.[76,77]

Experiments in human subjects have shown that abrupt withdrawal from chronic treatment with barbiturate precipitates a severe withdrawal syndrome characterized by weakness, tremor, insomnia, anxiety, vomiting, weight loss, increased pulse and respiration rates, increased blood pressure, grand mal seizures, and a psychosis resembling alcoholic delirium tremens.[78,79] The severity of the withdrawal syndrome makes it unwise to withdraw patients abruptly after prolonged treatment with barbiturates. Controlled dosage reduction over a few weeks reduces the severity of the symptoms. The ability of pentobarbital to suppress the symptoms of ethanol withdrawal has already been noted (Fig. 10-9B), and the similarity in symptoms following withdrawal of alcohol and barbiturates suggests that common factors may underly these syndromes.

Benzodiazepines

Because of the widespread use of benzodiazepines, interest has focused on their potential for inducing tolerance and dependence. After treatment of hospitalized patients with 100 to 600 mg of chlordiazepoxide daily for 1 to 7 months, abrupt withdrawal resulted in a series of symptoms, including depression, worsening of psychosis, insomnia, agitation, decreased appetite, and seizures in some patients.[80] Similar symptoms have been reported following the withdrawal of other benzodiazepines, including diazepam, nitrazepam, oxazepam, and temazepam.[81,82]

Careful study of the pharmacologic effects induced by benzodiazepines also indicates that a modest level of tolerance develops during chronic drug administration in anticonvulsant therapy.[83] The overall impression is that most patients receiving benzodiazepines as antianxiety agents on a daily basis do not progressively increase their dose,[82] but significant tolerance may occur when antiepileptic doses are given. In laboratory animals chronic benzodiazepine treatment has been shown to induce tolerance.[84] However, even after animals were maintained on a chlordiazepoxide dosage regimen designed to induce the same degree of CNS depression at each injection, the required dosage only increased four- to fivefold over a 38-day period.[84] Thus, as with other CNS depressant drugs, the degree of tolerance induced by benzodiazepines is relatively low.

Chronic administration of diazepam or chlordiazepoxide to rats results in drug dependence.[85,86] When administration of the drug is stopped, a withdrawal syndrome develops slowly, becoming apparent 10 to 20 hours after the last dose of benzodiazepine and persisting for at least 60 hours. The symptoms of withdrawal include tail erection, explosive awakenings, jerks, tremors, "wet dog shakes," hostility, decreased food and water consumption, and weight loss. There is a general similarity between these symptoms and the symptoms of a mild barbiturate or ethanol withdrawal syndrome. However, frank convulsions are not a feature of benzodiazepine withdrawal. This difference might reflect the different mode of action of benzodiazepines, but it could also reflect a different time course of withdrawal. Since benzodiazepines are metabolized in part to active metabolites with relatively long half-lives, the milder symptoms may simply result from the prolongation of withdrawal by the slow elimination of active metabolites. Benzodiazepine withdrawal symptoms are completely suppressed by diazepam administration. Pentobarbital is fairly effective at suppression, but it does not completely suppress all the symptoms. As might be predicted, diazepam is only partially effective in suppressing symptoms resulting from pentobarbital withdrawal.[85]

In benzodiazepine-dependent rats, the benzodiazepine antagonist Ro15-1788 induces a mild withdrawal syndrome.[87,88] In some ways this withdrawal is analogous to the naloxone-precipitated withdrawal syndrome in opiate-dependent animals; however, there are some significant differences. Ro15-1788, for example, induces a syndrome that, despite its more rapid onset, is noticeably less intense than that produced by drug discontinuation, and increasing the dosage of the antagonist does not induce symptoms of greater severity. This contrasts with naloxone-precipitated opiate withdrawal. The reasons for the differences are not clear. The differences might be related to the fact that Ro15-1788 is a partial agonist, although the opiate partial agonist nalorphine is very effective in precipitating an intense withdrawal syndrome in opiate-dependent animals.[89] Alternatively, it is possible that Ro15-1788 has very low antagonist activity at a subset of benzodiazepine receptors that is essential to the generation and maintenance of the tolerant state. This would stand in contrast to the high affinity of nalorphine at the μ class of opioid receptors through which morphine induces independence. Finally, it must be noted that the degree of tolerance to benzodiazepines is much less than the degree of tolerance that arises to opiates during the induction of the dependent state. Differences in the severity of the withdrawal syndrome precipitated by antagonists might therefore be related to differences in the magnitude of the adaptive changes associated with dependence on benzodiazepines and opiates.

Tolerance and Dependence Induced by Other Centrally Acting Drugs

Tolerance develops following chronic exposure to a number of centrally acting drugs in addition to the opiates and CNS depressant agents. These include nicotine, caffeine, amphetamines, cocaine, marijuana, and LSD. In general, physical dependence is less obvious with these drugs, although clinical experience suggests that a mild degree of physical dependence may develop in humans with some of these agents. Perhaps because of the often subtle effects of these drugs on very selective aspects of CNS function, craving for some of these drugs (nicotine, amphetamine, cocaine), and resulting compulsive use may become severe.

Nicotine produces mild and selective stimulant and depressant effects in humans and laboratory animals. It stimulates the secretion of catecholamines,[90] has both stimulant and depressant effects on motor activity,[91,92] and depresses muscle tone and some reflexes.[93] Nicotine elicits intravenous self-administration behavior in laboratory animals,[94,95] and appears to be very addictive, as judged by its chronic use by a substantial fraction of the adult population and the difficulty experienced by many individuals in giving up cigarette smoking.[96] After repeated administration, tolerance develops to many of the direct actions of nicotine,[90,97] although tolerance is generally less marked to the motor stimulant than to the depressant effects.[92] Some tolerance is detectable after a single dose of drug.[98] The presence of a nicotine withdrawal syndrome after chronic treatment of laboratory animals has not been demonstrated; however, termination of nicotine use in humans is thought to induce a mild withdrawal syndrome.[99]

Repeated administration of amphetamines and cocaine leads to tolerance to the anorectic effect, and there is cross-tolerance between amphetamine and cocaine.[100] However, the ability of amphetamine to stimulate motor activity may actually be enhanced by prior amphetamine or methamphetamine administration.[101] Neurochemical effects of amphetamine, such as impaired synthesis of dopamine and serotonin or elevation of striatal substance P, show tolerance after chronic treatment.[102] Chronic exposure to large doses of amphetamine or cocaine in humans leads to the onset of a state characterized by stereotypic behavior and a toxic psychosis in which paranoid delusions and hallucinations are common. This syndrome, which is often difficult to distinguish from an acute schizophrenic reaction, is clearly associated with the chronic dependent state and is not a withdrawal syndrome.[103] Psychotic behavior ceases when drug administration is discontinued. Within 12 hours of withdrawal, subjects who have received chronic amphetamine treatment become sleepy, depressed, and irritable for about 48 hours. Thus, the withdrawal symptoms following amphetamine use are relatively mild. As with depressant drugs, the withdrawal symptoms are generally the converse of the acute effects of the drug.

Repeated use of marijuana or of hallucinogens such as LSD also induces a degree of tolerance to the subjective effects of the drugs.[104,105] Generally, less tolerance develops to the autonomic effects. There is little cross-tolerance between LSD and marijuana or between these drugs and stimulants such as the amphetamines. These observations suggest that there are significant differences in the processes underlying tolerance to the three drug types. Withdrawal of marijuana in chronically exposed subjects results in a mild withdrawal syndrome characterized by irritability, decreased appetite, weight loss, and insomnia. Withdrawal of LSD is not associated with any consistent pattern of symptoms.

Tolerance to Peripherally Acting Drugs

Tolerance is not restricted to drugs acting on the CNS. Reduced effectiveness of drugs or hormones following repeated administration is a well documented phenomenon in many peripheral systems. Often, the term *tachyphylaxis* is used instead of tolerance in connection with peripherally acting drugs, since some degree of response reduction is apparent when a second dose of drug is given soon after the first. Among peripherally acting drugs, acute tolerance may be particularly rapid and apparent for the indirectly acting sympathomimetic amines and histamine-releasing agents. However, reduced responsiveness on repeated treatment to the direct actions of drugs or endogenous substances on peripheral nerves (e.g., neurotensin), on smooth muscle (e.g., histamine and serotonin), or on vascular tissue (e.g., nitrites and nitrates) may also be observed. Selective tolerance following administration of high doses of smooth muscle stimulants or inhibitors has been used to differentiate the mechanisms by which various agents affect contractile activity.[106]

TOLERANCE BY INDIRECT MECHANISMS

An animal may become tolerant to a drug even though sensitivity at the cellular (or subcellular) site(s) of drug action does not change. The concentration of free drug in contact with the relevant receptors may remain within initial limits despite an increase in the total drug dose that is given to the animal. This could occur by reduced drug absorption into the body, by increased rate of drug metabolism or elimination, by diminution in the passage of drug across biologic membranes that separate the sites of action from the plasma water, or by an increased extent of binding of the drug in an inert complex. It should be noted that such indirect mechanisms may provide an explanation of drug tolerance but they do not explain physical dependence.

Metabolic Tolerance

Metabolic tolerance develops toward any drug that induces synthesis or reduces degradation of enzymes responsible for its own metabolism. Enzyme induction is considered in detail in Chapters 5 and 6. Here, we will simply consider the importance of this phenomenon in drug tolerance. Tolerance resulting from induction of hepatic microsomal drug-metabolizing enzymes has a unique characteristic—its magnitude is strongly dependent upon the route of drug administration and upon the drug effect criteria selected for examination. Suppose such a drug is given intravenously to a normal animal and to one pretreated with the drug for a time sufficient to induce metabolic tolerance. The maximum intensity of drug effect should be the same in both animals, but the effect should be terminated more quickly in the pretreated animal. This should be so because the dose distributes into the same volume of distribution and produces the same immediate drug concentration in the body fluids of both animals, but the increased rate of metabolism in the pretreated animal will cause the concentration to fall faster. If acute lethality were the measure of drug action, we should probably not find very much difference in the LD50 between pretreated and normal animals, but if the total area under the effect-duration curve were the criterion, then the animal that degrades the drug faster will seem to have become tolerant. The situation is different when the drug is given by a route of slow absorption, for then the peak level attained after a single dose is determined by the balance between absorption rate and elimination rate. As the rate of drug metabolism increases, therefore, the peak intensity of drug effect will be reduced, and larger doses will be required to attain the same peak effect.

Among the major groups of drugs in which tolerance occurs, metabolic mechanisms are most significant for those barbiturates, such as pentobarbital, whose duration of action is largely determined by their rate of metabolism. Studies in rats have indicated that the plasma half-life of pentobarbital may be reduced to about one-third of control values by prior chronic treatment with the drug.[107] Sleeping time induced by a standard dose of the drug was much reduced, but the plasma concentration at the time of awakening was similar in the two groups of animals, which suggests that the basis of the tolerance was almost entirely metabolic in this experiment. In contrast, when pentobarbital was given to cats by twice daily injection in a dosage regimen designed to result in a constant degree of CNS depression (to surgical-stage anesthesia with moderate respiratory depression), both metabolic and functional tolerance processes appear to be implicated.

In the example shown in Figure 10-11, tolerance to pentobarbital and to barbital were compared.[74] The daily dose of each drug necessary to maintain the target level of CNS depression increased progressively throughout the 36-day treatment period. However, the pentobarbital dose increased over twofold, while the barbital dose only increased by 35 percent. The plasma half-life for pentobarbital fell from 11 hours to about 6 hours over a period of 12 to 15 days and then remained constant, despite the continuing need for more drug to maintain the CNS depression. When barbital was used to induce the same level of CNS depression, however, the plasma half-life of about 30 hours did not change significantly during the 36-day period of treatment. Thus, increased metabolism appears to contribute significantly to pentobarbital tolerance, but this is not a major factor in tolerance to barbital. The reason for the difference is that the elimination half-life of barbital is determined largely by the rate of its excretion by the kidney, a rate that is unaffected by prior treatment. The tolerance that develops to barbital results from a change in the sensitivity of the CNS to the drug. The elimination half-life of pentobarbital, however, is determined largely by its rate of metabolism by inducible enzymes in the liver, and increased activity of these enzymes results in a reduced concentration of drug in plasma.

Chronic ethanol treatment also induces a significant degree of metabolic tolerance by induction of oxidative enzymes of the hepatic endoplasmic reticulum. In the absence of prior exposure to ethanol or other inducers of drug-metabolizing enzymes, ethanol is largely metabolized by alcohol dehydrogenase to generate acetaldehyde and ultimately CO_2 (see Chapter 5 for discussion of ethanol metabolism). This enzyme requires NAD as a cofactor, and the availability of NAD rapidly becomes the rate-limiting step in ethanol metabolism following the ingestion of a single pharmacologically active dose, which in the case of ethanol is many grams.[108,109]

Microsomal enzymes in the liver also metabolize ethanol to acetaldehyde. This process, which requires molecular oxygen and the cofactor NADPH, is similar to other cytochrome P450-catalyzed oxidation reactions. Because the enzyme is located in the microsomal fraction of liver homogenates, it is sometimes known as the microsomal ethanol oxidizing system (MEOS). Like similar enzymes, MEOS is subject to induction by prior exposure not only to inducers such as phenobarbital but also to ethanol itself.[110] Ethanol treatment

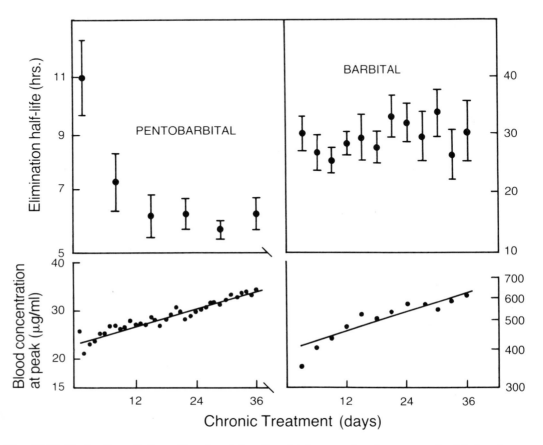

Fig. 10-11 Evaluation of dispositional and functional tolerance development to barbital and pentobarbital. Upper panels: half-lives for elimination of pentobarbital and barbital from blood during chronic treatment. The abscissa represents time of chronic treatment in days, and the ordinate gives the elimination half-life in hours. Half-lives were calculated for each animal by a least squares exponential regression of blood barbiturate concentrations against time. Each point and vertical bar represent mean and standard error estimates. Lower panels: estimates of blood barbiturate concentration at time of equieffective peak effect during chronic treatment. Average pentobarbital concentration was sampled 1 to 1.25 hours after the morning dose of pentobarbital, and the average barbital concentration was sampled 6 to 6.5 hours after each barbital dose. Each point in the figure represents the mean of 15 observations for pentobarbital and 12 observations for barbital. (From Boisse et al.,[74] with permission.)

not only increases the activity of MEOS but behaves like other inducers in increasing levels of cytochrome P450 protein in the liver and in inducing morphologic changes in the endoplasmic reticulum. It is difficult to determine exactly the contribution of the MEOS to the overall metabolism of ethanol after administration of pharmacologically effective doses, but it is generally assumed to play only a minor role in animals not previously treated with agents that induce the drug-metabolizing enzymes. However, the contribution of MEOS appears to become significant after chronic ethanol treatment.

Increased metabolism of ethanol induced by prior exposure has been observed in human subjects. Six men addicted to alcohol were studied under carefully controlled conditions on a hospital ward. Their nutrition was adequate during the course of the experiment, and they received vitamin supplements daily. After a 4-day predrinking period, they were given a small test dose of ethanol by mouth, and 30 minutes later, an intravenous injection of 10 μCi of ethanol-1-^{14}C. Blood ethanol concentrations were assayed, as was the specific activity of carbon dioxide in the expired air, which served as a measure of the rate of oxidation of ethanol.[111] The subjects were then given alcohol in large amounts regularly for 7 days. At the end of that time another test dose was given. The data for one subject are shown in Figure 10-12. In Figure 10-12A it can be seen that the blood level established by the test dose declined much faster after the 7-day period of drinking than before. In Figure 10-12B the specific radioactivity of carbon dioxide in the first 2 hours after the test dose is seen to be much higher after prior ethanol exposure than before. It seems probable that the increased rate of ethanol metabolism is related, at least in part, to an increase in metabolism by the MEOS. However, since the availability of NAD is the rate-limiting factor in the extent of ethanol metabolism by alcohol dehydrogenase, it is possible that enhanced regeneration of NAD might also contribute to the increase in ethanol metabolism. Although an increased rate of metabolism of ethanol contributes to the degree of tolerance observed with this drug, functional and behavioral factors also play a major role. Metabolic tolerance may arise with any drug that is both metabolized by microsomal drug-metabolizing enzymes at a rate sufficient to affect its rate of elimination and is capable of causing induction of these enzymes. Tolerance of this type does not appear to occur to any significant extent for morphine (which is not an effective enzyme inducer), but hepatic enzyme induction may contribute to tolerance to some of the synthetic opiates, such as methadone,[112] and possibly also benzodiazepines.[113]

CELLULAR OR FUNCTIONAL TOLERANCE AND DEPENDENCE MECHANISMS

In many situations tolerance appears to arise from changes in the function of the cell or tissue on which the primary action of the drug or hormone is exerted.[114] Such tolerance might be considered to be a homeostatic adjustment by the tissue (i.e., the tissue attempts to restore the level of activity of the system to that maintained prior to the sustained exposure to drug or hormone). Evidence is accumulating that suggests that there are several mechanisms by which modified tissue responsiveness might be induced, and in

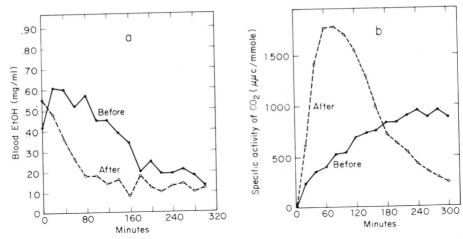

Fig. 10-12 Increased metabolism of ethanol during tolerance. Data from one subject, before and after a 7-day period of alcohol ingestion, during which the subject received 3.2 g of ethanol per kg per day in divided doses. A test dose of ethanol was given by mouth, and ½ hour later 10 μc of ethanol-1-^{14}C was given intravenously. At 20-minute intervals blood samples were removed for ethanol determination, and samples of expired air were collected for CO_2 assay and radioactivity determination. (A) blood ethanol concentrations; (B) specific radioactivity of CO_2. Solid lines, test before the 7-day period of drinking; broken lines, test after 7-day period of drinking. (Modified from Mendelson et al.,[111] with permission.)

the best studied cases it seems likely that several or all of these adaptive processes contribute to the overall level of tolerance observed.

Several general hypotheses have been advanced to account for tolerance and dependence, most of which attempt to explain both features in a unitary theory, since tolerance and dependence often show a close temporal relationship, as though they were reflections of the same biologic change. To explain the phenomena adequately, the theory should also account for the different time courses of acute and chronic effects of the drug. Drug action is immediate (i.e., as soon as the drug can enter the CNS and reach its receptors). Development of the tolerant-dependent state is slower. Presumably more is involved than merely activation of existing neural circuits to oppose the drug action for such events could occur very quickly. The slower time course suggests instead that biochemical changes are involved, such as changes in the quantity of an enzyme, the storage and release of a neurotransmitter, the production and release of a hormone, the pattern of synaptic contacts, or some other process involving biosynthesis and turnover of biochemical components. Support for the view that the time course of the development of tolerance and dependence reflects a process of macromolecular synthesis comes from experiments with inhibitors of RNA and protein synthesis. Actinomycin D, puromycin, and cycloheximide have all been reported to block the development of tolerance and dependence to opiates.[115-117]

Two general theories have been advanced to explain functional tolerance. One postulates a continuous and unchanged interaction between the drug and its receptors, the effects of which are antagonized or compensated for by changes elsewhere in other biochemical pathways or in other neuronal systems. The other attributes tolerance to a change in the drug receptors themselves, either in number or in properties, that makes them less sensitive to the drug. The first theory can be formulated in a very general way[118,119]: the drug action is seen as disturbing homeostasis, and primary drug effects are compensated for by the activation of pathways that produce opposite effects, thus restoring homeostasis in the presence of the drug. By analogy to the way the body deals with other disturbances of homeostasis, it is supposed that neural and hormonal mechanisms that counteract the drug effects may be involved. As a result of such adaptations, a higher drug dose would now be required to produce the original effect. The system would also demonstrate dependency since removing the drug would permit the counteracting mechanism to perturb homeostasis in the opposite direction. The immediate response to removal of the drug would correspond to the withdrawal syndrome, which would then wane as the initial state was gradually restored in the absence of drug. In the specific model proposed by Collier,[114] postsynaptic receptors for an endogenous neurotransmitter become supersensitive, the processes involved being analogous to the well known phenomenon of denervation supersensitivity.[75] As we shall see later, accumulating evidence suggests that chronic drug administration can indeed induce changes in neurotransmitter receptor levels and in neuronal sensitivity to some transmitters. Thus, such changes probably contribute significantly to the tolerant and dependent state.

An alternative type of homeostatic mechanism applies concepts derived from end product regulation of enzyme activity to regulation of the primary target system on which drugs inducing the tolerant and dependent state act.[120,121] Suppose, for example, that the drug X inhibits an enzyme responsible for synaptic transmission or other neuronal function and that the enzyme is subject to product repression. This common biochemical arrangement would account for all the main features of tolerance and dependence. Let C be a product of the enzyme E, which is inhibited by the drug; assume that the function of C is excitatory at the particular synapses where it is released.

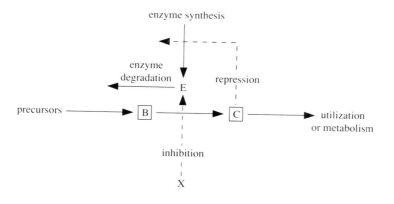

Then the normal steady-state concentration of E and the normal utilization of C determine the concentration of C and the normal state of excitation. The steady-state concentration of E is determined by its rates of synthesis and degradation, according to the plateau principle (Ch. 4).

This model predicts two results, with different time courses. The inhibition of E by the drug X will cause an immediate decline in the concentration or availability of C; if C was mediating an excitatory function, the effect will be depressant on that function. The decrease in C will increase the synthesis of E, and the enzyme concentration will rise. This will be a *delayed* effect, with a time course commensurate with the rate of protein turnover. The increased concentration of E will now produce C from the intermediate B at the initial rate despite its partial inhibition by X, and the concentration of X will have to be raised in order to reduce the concentration of C again in the face of the higher enzyme concentration. Thus, tolerance will develop.

Withdrawal of drug will cause two effects. The *immediate* effect, as soon as drug concentration declines sufficiently, is to disinhibit the large excess of enzyme that is present. An overproduction of C results, with effects (in this instance excitatory) opposite to those of the primary drug effect. This is the withdrawal syndrome. The *delayed* effect, requiring perhaps days, will be a restoration of the original state of affairs. The excess of C represses the new synthesis of E; as the concentration of E declines, the concentration of C also falls. Thus, physical dependence and tolerance develop and disappear together. An even simpler form of this theory requires no end product repression of the rate of enzyme synthesis.[122] It is assumed that the enzyme undergoes continual synthesis and degradation and that the inhibitory interaction of drug with enzyme stabilizes the enzyme. As a consequence, the total amount of enzyme would increase, and tolerance would develop as above. No change in the rate of enzyme synthesis would be required.

This type of hypothesis can be generalized further by supposing that E, the enzyme whose activity is modified by the drug in the example above, might alternatively be the receptor at which the drug exerts its primary action or an enzyme or transport system that is indirectly regulated by activated drug receptors. In the sections following, the evidence that specific components of the receptor-effector system are modified as a result of chronic drug or hormone exposure will be considered.

Receptor Function in Tolerance and Dependence

The receptors through which a drug acts to induce its primary pharmacologic actions may also be implicated in the processes underlying tolerance and perhaps dependence. The case is best argued with respect to opiate drugs. First, it is clear that tolerance and dependence do not develop following treatment with doses of opiate that are too low to induce a pharmacologic effect, and thus it may be presumed that a certain level of receptor occupation is required. Second, although chronic antagonist treatment does not induce tolerance to agonists, concurrent administration of antagonist with an opiate agonist prevents development of these states. This observation indicates that receptor occupation alone is insufficient; a significant fraction of the receptors must be activated for tolerance development. Third, withdrawal can be provoked in dependent animals or in some isolated tissues chronically exposed to opiates by administration of an antagonist. Fourth, the dose of antagonist required to precipitate the withdrawal syndrome decreases with increasing intensity or duration of pretreatment (see Fig. 10-8).

Further evidence of receptor-specific mechanisms in tolerance development arises from studies of the heterogeneity of opiate receptors in isolated tissues such as the mouse vas deferens. In this tissue, μ, δ, and κ opiate receptors all appear to regulate the release of norepinephrine from sympathetic nerve endings.[16,123] After chronic treatment of the mouse with an agonist, such as D-Ala^2-D-Leu^5 enkephalin (DADLE), which in this tissue acts predominantly at δ receptors, significant tolerance to DADLE and cross-tolerance to other δ-selective agonists is observed, although there is little or no cross-tolerance to agonists acting preferentially through μ or κ receptors.[123,124] Similarly, chronic treatment with selective μ agonists (e.g., morphine or sufentanyl) induces μ-specific tolerance with little cross-tolerance to δ or κ agonists.[124,125] The intracellular mechanisms by which each opiate receptor type regulates norepinephrine release in mouse vas deferens are not known, although evidence from other tissues suggests that μ and δ receptors both act by opening potassium channels, while κ receptors reduce transmitter release by a reduction of depolarization-induced calcium entry.[126,127] Since μ and δ receptors probably share a common postreceptor mode of action in regulating norepinephrine release in the mouse vas deferens, the lack of cross-tolerance between these two types of opiate appears to be linked specifically to a change in the function of the receptors initially activated by the drugs.

Direct measures of opiate receptor affinity by radioligand binding in brain membrane preparations (see below) and indirect measures of opiate agonist affinity in isolated guinea pig ileum (measurement of shifts in dose-response relationships induced by treatment with irreversible receptor antagonists) have not shown any change in receptor affinity for agonists after chronic opiate treatment.[128,129] However, the greater sensitivity of opiate-tolerant and opiate-dependent ileum preparations to irreversible antagonists (as indicated by the smaller maximum opiate effect following irreversible antagonist treatment) suggests that induction of the tolerant and dependent state is associated with a reduction in the number of spare receptors.[128,129] Thus, a number of experimental approaches all suggest that a modification in the function or number of the receptors through which opiate drugs act is a likely mechanism for tolerance development and might be associated with the dependence process as well.

Receptor Down Regulation

The apparent reduction in the number of spare receptors in opiate tolerance would be consistent with a loss of functional opiate receptors. In other systems, chronic exposure of receptors to agonists is in many cases known to result in decreased numbers of functional receptors present at the plasma membrane surface, a phenomenon known as receptor down regulation (see Ch. 2). In isolated cell preparations, agonist-induced down regulation of receptors is associated with a significant reduction in agonist effect. This is normally manifest as a reduction in maximum response to the agonist, but when spare receptors are initially present, a parallel shift to the right in the agonist dose-response curve will be observed with low concentrations of irreversible antagonist.

Direct measurements of opiate receptor binding in tissues from morphine-tolerant animals initially failed to reveal any significant differences in either receptor affinity or in number of opiate receptors, either in tissue homogenates[130,131] or in brain in vivo.[132] However, these studies used radioligands that bind to several types of opiate receptors. Changes in one type of receptor may not have been detected if other types were unaffected by the treatment. Altered distribution of receptors between plasma membrane and intracellular membrane compartments may also not be detected in these studies. When binding of radioligands to opiate receptors in intact cells was measured,[133] or when binding specifically to μ type receptors in cortex was estimated,[134] a reduction in μ receptor number by about 30 to 40 percent was noted following the development of tolerance to morphine in rats or guinea pigs. Chronic intracerebral administration to rats of the opiate peptide agonist, which occupies δ receptors with higher affinity than μ receptors, induces a reduction in the number of δ receptors with much less effect on the numbers of μ receptors.[135]

More information regarding receptor down regulation has been obtained from studies of opiate drug exposure in cell lines carrying only one type of opiate receptor. Cultured neuroblastoma X glioma hybrid NG108-15 cells have only the δ type of opiate receptor, which in these cells mediates inhibition of adenylate cyclase.[33] Exposure of these cells to morphine for several hours or longer reduces the ability of opiates to inhibit adenylate cyclase.[136] Several processes appear to contribute to this effect; here I will limit discussion to consideration of receptor down regulation. Incubation of NG108-15 or related neuroblastoma cells with enkephalins or with other opiates that have high affinity for δ receptors (e.g., etorphine) significantly reduces the number of δ binding sites without affecting the affinity of the residual sites.[137,138] Typical results of such an experiment are shown in Figure 10-13, from which it is clear that down-regulation of binding sites was dependent on the concentration of agonist present during the initial incubation and that a substantial reduction in the number of binding sites occurred within 1 hour. The process was temperature-dependent, being much slower at 25°C than at 37°C. When a large series of opiate drugs and opioid peptides was tested, a close correlation was found between their intrinsic activities, defined in terms of their relative abilities to inhibit adenylate cyclase activity in NG108-15 cell membranes, and their ability to induce down regulation of δ receptors.[139]

The mechanisms involved in δ opiate receptor down regulation are probably similar to those implicated in the down regulation of other receptor types (see Chapter 2). Studies in which receptors were visualized on the NG108-15 cell membrane by using a fluorescent enkephalin derivative have shown that agonist occupation induces a clustering of receptors on the cell surface.[140] No internalization of receptors was observed. However, these experiments were conducted at 25°C, a temperature at which down regulation is much reduced. When tritium-labeled DADLE was incubated with NG108-15 cells for 1 hour or longer at 37°C in the presence of chloroquine and the cells were subsequently lysed and fractionated, significant amounts of the labeled DADLE were recovered in fractions enriched in lysosomal membranes.[141] In the absence of chloroquine, no lysosomal accumulation of DADLE was seen. It appears that chloroquine elevates lysosomal pH and therefore prevents the degradation of the receptors by lysosomal enzymes. Internalized receptor-ligand complexes can then accumulate.

The mechanism by which agonist-occupied δ receptor complexes move from the cell surface to lysosomal vesicles is not known. For other types of receptors, it has been shown that, following clustering of the receptors on the cell surface, the membrane invaginates in regions where the internal surface of the plasma membrane is coated with the protein clathrin (see discussion of receptor-mediated endocytosis in Chapter 3). The resulting clathrin-coated vesicles then move into the cell and fuse with lysosomal vesicles. Opiate binding has been observed in purified preparations of clathrin-coated vesicles from bovine brain,[142] which suggests that opiate receptors become internalized by this route even in the absence of pretreatment with drug.

Cells of the prolactin-secreting rat pituitary tumor 7315c carry μ opiate receptors but do not appear to have receptors of the δ or κ type. In these cells, μ receptor activation causes inhibition of adenylate cyclase. Treatment of cultures of these cells with morphine for periods of 24 hours or more results in a significant reduction in the number of μ receptors and loss of the ability of opiate agonists to inhibit adenylate cyclase.[143] Thus, chronic agonist exposure in isolated cells can also induce down regulation of μ opiate

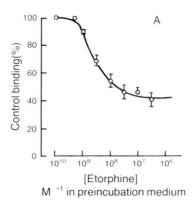

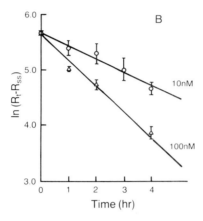

Fig. 10-13 Concentration- and time-dependent decreases in tritiated diprenorphine binding to NG108-15 cells after preincubation with etorphine. NG108-15 hybrid cells were treated **(A)** with various concentrations of etorphine for 24 hours or **(B)** with 10 nM (○) or 100 nM (△) etorphine for various time periods. After removal of excess etorphine, specific ^{3}H-diprenorphine binding to intact cells was measured by a rapid filtration assay. The amount of specific binding to control cells in Fig. A was 449 ± 22 fmol per milligram protein ($n = 13$). In Fig. B, R_t denotes receptor concentration at time t, and R_{ss} denotes receptor concentration at the steady-state level which was 195 ± 18 fmol per milligram of protein ($n = 8$). (From Law et al.,[138] with permission.)

receptors, although a longer period of drug exposure is required to induce a reduction of μ receptors in 7315c cells than of δ receptors in NG108-15 cells.

The studies discussed above indicate that in isolated cells in culture and in brain tissue preparations from morphine-treated rats prolonged exposure to opiate agonists is followed by a down regulation of opiate receptors. This must play some role in opiate tolerance. However, as I shall discuss further below, in cells in culture, the loss of the ability of opiate agonists to inhibit adenylate cyclase occurs before any reduction in the number of opiate receptors on the cell surface is measurable. Thus, it remains unclear how important the down regulation phenomenon is in opiate tolerance. Down regulation is not the only mechanism contributing to the reduced response to opiate agonists, and it may not be the most important mechanism. Down regulation does not provide any explanation for the occurrence of physical dependence. Prolonged exposure of cells to many hormones and neurotransmitters results in receptor down regulation. Such systems exhibit tolerance to the agonist whose receptors have been down-regulated and cross-tolerance to other agents capable of activating the same receptor. However, withdrawal of the agonist does not usually lead to disturbances in cell physiology akin to a withdrawal syndrome. Thus, receptor down regulation may play a part in tolerance development, but it does not provide a full explanation of tolerance and physical dependence.

In contrast to the chronic effects of agonists, treatment of laboratory animals with opiate antagonists for several days is reported to induce an increase in the number of opiate binding sites in brain tissues,[144] a process described as "up regulation" of receptors. Again, the mechanisms are not entirely clear. It is possible that under normal physiologic conditions, sufficient endogenous opioid is present to hold the number of brain opioid receptors at a partially down-regulated level. Chronic naltrexone treatment, by antagonizing the endogenous opioid, would alter the normal rate of receptor turnover. Thus, the number of opioid receptors may be subject to either up or down regulation, depending upon the nature of the ligand that is occupying the receptor.

In the case of the central depressant agents, the role of receptor down regulation is even less certain than with the opiates. Ethanol and the barbiturates may have multiple cellular targets. It does not seem likely that ethanol acts through a specific ethanol receptor, although disturbances of cellular membrane properties induced by ethanol[145] may well perturb or modify the functions of specific receptors for other substances. For example, there is evidence that ethanol at relatively low concentrations inhibits the cation current induced by activation of the N-methyl-D-aspartate type of glutamate receptor.[146] Ethanol also potentiates Y-aminobutyric acid (GABA) receptor-mediated transport of chloride ions by interacting with a multireceptor-chloride ion channel complex containing regulatory sites where barbiturates and benzodiazepines can also serve a regulatory role[147] (cf. Chapter 2). Thus, at least one common site of action has been proposed for these three groups of drugs that produce tolerance and dependence with somewhat similar characteristics. Furthermore, the induction of a withdrawal syndrome in diazepam-dependent animals by the benzodiazepine antagonist Ro15-1788 implicates the benzodiazepine receptor-chloride ion channel complex in the dependence process.[87,88] The increased sensitivity of animals dependent on barbiturates to convulsants such as picrotoxin and pentylenetetrazol, which behave as antagonists at the barbiturate binding site, might also be interpreted as antagonist-precipitated withdrawal. These results suggest that specific receptor-mediated processes are involved in the tolerant and dependent states induced by chronic treatment with barbiturates and benzodiazepines. In studies of benzodiazepine binding after chronic treatment there are conflicting results; some groups have failed to observe a reduction in binding, whereas others have noted significant reductions in the number of benzodiazepine binding sites in brain tissues.[148] A transient increase in the number of benzodiazepine binding sites has been reported two days after withdrawal of benzodiazepines in functionally tolerant animals.[149]

Other studies point to changes in different functional components of the GABA receptor chloride channel complex following chronic barbiturate or benzodiazepine treatment. Mice treated chronically with barbiturates show both reduced sensitivity to GABA-mimetic agents and a lower affinity of GABA for neuronal membrane binding sites.[150] A reduced ability of GABA to enhance benzodiazepine binding has been noted after chronic treatment of rats with diazepam.[151]

Treatment of primary cultures of neurons from young mice or embryonic rat brain with benzodiazepines did not result in significant reductions in the number of benzodiazepine binding sites.[152,153] However, treatment with high concentrations of GABA or muscimol for 48 hours resulted in a reduced number of binding sites for both benzodiazepines and GABA, and a reduced number of chloride channels as measured by the binding of the channel ligand [^{35}S]t-butylbicyclophosphorothionate.[153] Binding to muscarinic, opiate, and α_2-adrenergic receptors was not affected by these treatments. These results suggest a selective effect of high levels of GABA receptor occupancy on the membrane concentrations of several of the regulatory sites associated with the GABA-regulated chloride ion channel. It remains to be determined if these effects contribute to tolerance to central depressants in vivo.

Receptor Desensitization

In some situations following drug or hormone treatment, the effectiveness of agonists may be reduced even though direct measurements of receptor number indicate that the receptors are still present and capable of binding ligands. The occupied receptors appear to becomes less efficient in activating subsequent steps in the chain of events linking receptor occupation to the observed functional event. This phenomenon is described as *desensitization* (mechanisms that might be responsible for it have been discussed in Chapter 2). Obviously, tolerance results when exposure to agonists induces desensitization. In some cases cross-tolerance may be limited to other agonists acting through the same receptor type; this is *homologous desensitization*. In other cases cross-tolerance to other agonists acting on the same cell through different receptors may be observed; this is *heterologous desensitization*. Mechanisms involving changed conformational states of the receptor[154] or covalent modification (e.g., methylation, phosphorylation) have been proposed,[155,156] but much still remains to be learned.

Desensitization seems to be an important component of tolerance to drugs acting on both peripheral tissues and the CNS. Studies of agonist action in tissues maintained in vitro indicate that desensitization is a very common consequence of exposure to agonist. In excitable tissues it may be a usual concomitant of nicotinic receptor activation.[157] Desensitization contributes to the reduced ability of β-adrenoreceptor agonists to activate adenylate cyclase after prolonged exposure to β-agonists,[158] and it may also be responsible for the tolerance to the nitrate-induced increase in cyclic guanosine monophosphate (cGMP) that occurs in vascular tissues.[159]

Desensitization of δ opiate receptors has been observed in NG108-15 cells. A reduced ability of δ-receptor agonists to inhibit adenylate cyclase occurs within a few minutes of exposure of the cells to a potent opiate, and prior to any detectable reduction in receptor number.[136] Exposure of μ opiate receptors in 7315c pituitary tumor cells to morphine results in a loss of μ agonist-mediated inhibition of adenylate cyclase, again before any changes in receptor number are observed.[143] In these cells, the loss of agonist activity is associated with a reduction in agonist affinity for μ receptors and a reduced ability of GTP and its analogs to affect agonist affinity at μ receptors. A loss of guanine nucleotide regulation of agonist affinity has also been observed at μ receptors in brain membranes from animals showing tolerance to morphine.[134] These results suggest that desensitization at μ and δ opiate receptors may follow from a functional uncoupling of the receptors from the G proteins that normally mediate the agonist-induced effects. It is not yet clear if a physical separation of receptor and G protein occurs, or if they remain physically associated despite the inability of agonist-occupied receptors to activate associated G proteins.

Since agonist activity can be completely lost before any change in receptor number is detectable, desensitization of μ or δ receptors may be a primary mechanism in opiate drug tolerance. The role of desensitization mechanisms in tolerance to central depressant drugs and benzodiazepines remains to be established.

Receptor desensitization processes have not been implicated directly in causation of drug withdrawal reactions. While desensitization is a very common concomitant of agonist action, major withdrawal reactions following agonist removal are observed after treatment with only a limited number of drug types. Since the mechanisms responsible for desensitization of opioid receptors are not known, we cannot rule out their possible contributions to opiate dependence.

Postreceptor Adaptive Mechanisms

Postreceptor adaptations to chronic drug or hormone exposure may occur at all steps between the receptor and the ultimate tissue response. Since intervening transduction processes are often unknown, the mechanisms by which they adapt to prolonged activation or inhibition are also uncertain. However, as knowledge of the role of specific second messenger systems accumulates, their adaptive capabilities are also becoming more readily understood. Here, discussion is limited to a few systems for which there is some understanding of the processes underlying postreceptor modulation of a tissue's response to drug or hormone.

Adenylate Cyclase-Mediated Systems

There is evidence that the activity of the enzyme adenylate cyclase is modified following chronic treatment with agents that inhibit this enzyme.[136,160] The potential role of enhanced adenylate cyclase activity in tolerance to inhibitory drugs or hormones was first suggested in relation to opiate-induced inhibition of the enzyme in NG108-15 neuroblastoma X glioma hybrid cells (Fig. 10-14). Treatment of NG108-15 cells with high concentrations of morphine inhibited both basal and hormone-stimulated adenylate cyclase activity and lowered the concentration of cyclic adenosine monophosphate (cAMP) in the cells. When the cells were grown for several days in the presence of morphine or other opiate drugs, however, inhibition of enzyme activity declined. Removal of morphine (or its antagonism by addition of the opiate antagonist naloxone) resulted in an increase in hormone-stimulated adenylate cyclase activity above initial levels. A similar tolerance to inhibition of adenylate cyclase activity in NG108-15 cells has been observed following sustained exposure of the cells to agents that inhibit the enzyme through α_2-adrenergic receptors.[161] Tolerance also occurs in adipocytes following sustained inhibition of adenylate cyclase by adenosine and related agents acting through adenosine A_1 receptors.[162] The adaptive increase in adenylate cyclase activity is apparent only after a few days of treatment with the inhibitory agents. Thus, the time scale of tolerance development is very different from the rapid occurrence of down regulation and receptor desensitization. The mechanisms remain unknown. The increased enzyme activity does not seem to be directly dependent on a change in the properties of the drug or hormone receptor, since effects of stimulatory agents acting through different receptors and of forskolin, a direct activator of the catalytic component adenylate cyclase, are also increased at this time.[33,136,162]

The critical transduction role of guanine nucleotide–binding (G) proteins in receptor-

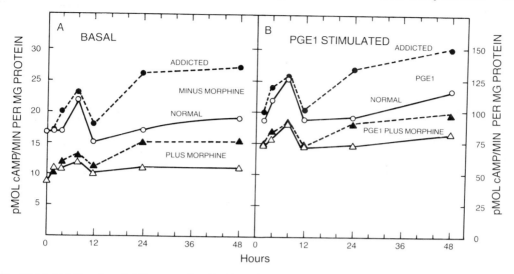

Fig. 10-14 (**A**) Basal and (**B**) prostaglandin E₁ (PGE₁)-stimulated adenylate cyclase activity of homogenates of NG108-15 cells cultured and assayed in the presence or absence of 10 μM morphine and/or PGE₁. Cells at 90 percent, confluence in 100-mm petri dishes were cultured in the presence or absence of morphine for the times indicated and then harvested and washed, and adenylate cyclase activity was assayed immediately. Protein values ranged from 8.2 to 9.2 mg per dish. Filled symbols, cells pre-exposed to morphine (10 μM) for the time indicated: open symbols, no prior morphine exposure; triangles, assayed in the presence of morphine; circles, assayed in the absence of morphine. (From Sharma et al.,[33] with permission.)

effector transduction was first identified in hormonal stimulation of adenylate cyclase (Chapter 2). Proteins of this family have now been shown to be implicated in other transduction systems involving inhibition of adenylate cyclase, phosphatidyl inositol turnover, and ion channel function. Because of their intermediary role between receptors and effector systems, G proteins provide likely sites at which modulation of drug or hormone activity following sustained treatment might occur. The enhanced activity of adenylate cyclase following chronic treatment with inhibitory agents might be related to changes in the relative amounts and/or properties of the various inhibitory and stimulatory G proteins. Changes in the relative amounts of G_s and G_i may be responsible for some examples of heterologous desensitization.[163]

Increased activity of adenylate cyclase activity following long-term treatment with opiate drugs may provide a partial explanation of dependence on opiates. Rapid withdrawal of the opiate or administration of the antagonist naloxone results in an increase in hormone-stimulated enzyme activity above the levels observed in normal cells not exposed to drug.[33,136,160] Thus, the response of the adenylate cyclase system to stimulant agents is enhanced following drug withdrawal. Cyclic AMP-dependent protein phosphorylation is one of the many systems regulating neurotransmitter release.[164] Comparable increases in enzyme capacity in specific systems in an intact animal during drug withdrawal might well result in altered patterns of transmitter release, ultimately manifested as a withdrawal syndrome.

Reduced Availability of Response Mediators

Many drugs and hormones act by stimulating the release of mediators that are stored in some way within the cell. The released mediator may activate other processes within the cell, or it may be released from the cell to induce effects in other cells. Since the stored mediator may be released more rapidly than the store can be replenished, systems of this type are sensitive to the effects of prior agonist exposure.

A classic example is that of the indirectly acting sympathomimetic agents. Drugs such as tyramine and amphetamine induce a rise in blood pressure, which is largely caused by the liberation of norepinephrine from sympathetic nerve terminals. Reserpine treatment, which depletes releasable neuronal stores of norepinephrine by liberating it intracellularly for degradation by monoamine oxidase, abolishes the sympathomimetic action of tyramine and related drugs.[165,166] Tyramine was shown experimentally to release norepinephrine from the nerve ending into the extracellular fluid.[167] With repeated administration of tyramine, the amount of released norepinephrine declined progressively as the releasable stores of norepinephrine were depleted. Depletion of monoamine neurotransmitter stores in the CNS may also contribute to tolerance to the behavioral effects of drugs such as amphetamine. Alternative mechanisms have been proposed in which amphetamine is accumulated in norepinephrine- or dopamine-containing secretory vesicles in CNS neurons and becomes a substrate for enzymes that are normally involved in the biosynthesis of dopamine and norepinephrine. Such an action would lead to the production and accumulation of "false neurotransmitters" at the expense of the more functionally active dopamine or norepinephrine. These hypotheses have been critically reviewed.[168] Neurotransmitter biosynthesis and receptor turnover may also be modified as a result of chronic amphetamine treatment.[102]

Another example of a reduced effect of agonist resulting from prior drug exposure leading to altered availability of cellular mediator is provided by a study of the mobilization of intracellular calcium by norepinephrine and histamine.[169] The system used was a muscle cell line in which calcium mobilization could be activated by norepinephrine (acting through α_1-adrenergic receptors) or histamine (acting through H1 receptors). The investigators were able to show that tolerance to the stimulant effects of norepinephrine was largely dependent on an altered disposition of agonist-sensitive intracellular calcium stores at a point common to the actions of both norepinephrine and histamine. In contrast, tolerance to histamine in the same cells occurred much more rapidly and appeared to be largely caused by H1 receptor desensitization.

Reduced availability of cellular response mediators may account for tolerance but does not necessarily lead to the development of dependence on the stimulating agent. However, depletion of a mediator that is normally secreted as a transmitter regulating the activity of an adjacent cell often leads to adaptive changes in the sensitivity of this cell to this and other transmitters, and this process may contribute to the development of dependence.

Altered Responsivity To Neurotransmitters

As originally predicted by Collier,[114] chronic treatment with morphine alters the responsiveness of peripheral tissues to some neurotransmitters. In isolated longitudinal muscle–myenteric plexus preparations from morphine-pretreated guinea pigs, an enhanced sensitivity was found to many stimulatory agents, including serotonin,[170] nicotine, and potassium chloride, as well as to electrical stimulation.[171] Vas deferens preparations from morphine-treated mice are reported to be supersensitive to norepinephrine.[172] Such changes are not limited to tissues in which morphine exerts a direct, acute action. Rat colon and vas deferens preparations, which are not directly inhibited by morphine, show enhanced sensitivity to serotonin and muscarinic agonists,[173] and guinea pig vas deferens is supersensitive to electrical stimulation.[171]

The mechanisms underlying these effects are not completely understood. Since the supersensitivity is often not limited to one stimulatory agent, it seems more likely that post-receptor mechanisms that affect smooth muscle contraction may be altered. It has been proposed, for example, that chronic morphine treatment induces a reduction in the muscle membrane potential, thus rendering it more sensitive to excitatory agents.[171] A corollary of this hypothesis is that the tissues should be less sensitive to all inhibitory agents, and, at least in the case of guinea pig ileum, reduced sensitivity to inhibition by α_2-adrenoreceptor and adenosine receptor agonists has been shown to accompany the development of opiate tolerance.[174] However, other adaptations in the steps between stimulation and contraction may also occur.

In the CNS there is also evidence that the sensitivity of neurons to other transmitters is altered by chronic opiate treatment. Thus, rat cortical neurons are reported to show supersensitivity to acetylcholine and glutamate following morphine treatment.[175] During opiate withdrawal, rats show considerably enhanced behavioral and motor responsiveness to dopamine, norepinephrine, and serotonin.[176] The motor responses measured in this study, however, were those characteristically associated with opiate withdrawal in rats. An enhanced effect of the neurotransmitters on these behaviors does not necessarily reflect any specific morphine-induced increase in sensitivity of the receptor systems for these agents; rather, it might result from the initial partial activation of the particular motor pathways responsible for these motor effects.

Measurements of radioligand binding have shown that chronic opiate treatment can induce alterations in the number of receptors for certain neurotransmitters. For example, the number of binding sites for the β-adrenergic antagonist dihydroalprenolol is reported to be increased by about 20 to 30 percent in the cortex and brain stems of rats chronically treated with morphine,[177,178] and this increase in binding is accompanied by a comparable increase in norepinephrine stimulation of adenylate cyclase in the cortex.[177] The number of α_2-adrenergic receptors in rat cortex and brain is increased by 30 to 50 percent following chronic morphine treatment, although the number of α_1-adrenergic receptors is unaffected.[178] It has also been shown that the number of binding sites for the adenosine agonists phenylisopropyladenosine and diethylphenylxanthine is increased by 50 to 150 percent in mouse brain tissue 72 hours after implantation of a morphine pellet to induce tolerance and physical dependence.[179] The increase in adenosine binding sites occurs without any change in ligand affinity.

These results indicate that changes in the neurotransmitter binding capacity in brain tissue may be commonplace following the disturbances of neuronal function induced by chronic opiate treatment. It is possible that these effects occur on neurons directly inhibited by opiate drugs. However, they may also occur in other neurons that are not directly sensitive to opiates but whose activity is affected as a result of opiate-induced modulation of the secretion of transmitters to which they are sensitive. It is likely that these changes contribute to the overall modification of neuronal function in tolerance and dependence. The initial increase in receptor number may occur as an adaptive response that reduces the effect of sustained opiate receptor activation, thus leading to tolerance to the opiate.

Comparable changes in neurotransmitter receptors and neuronal sensitivity may occur as a result of long-term exposure to central depressants,[180] although this treatment has been less extensively studied. In view of the widespread effects of central depressants on neuronal activity, it would be surprising if alterations in responses to some neurotransmitters at specific sites in the CNS did not contribute to both tolerance to and dependence on these agents.

Changes in Membrane Properties

It has been suggested that alcohols modify neuronal function, at least in part, by disordering neuronal membranes.[145] Significant increases in membrane fluidity were induced by relatively low concentrations of ethanol, as indicated by the increased rotational mobility of electron spin resonance probes inserted into the membranes. The chemical composition of cell membranes is known to change when cells are grown at different temperatures. The changes may be important for maintaining cell membrane fluidity within the range observed at the usual growth temperature.[181] Some investigators have considered the possibility that changes in membrane composition might occur during chronic ethanol treatment in compensation for the initial increase in fluidity induced by the drug. Experiments with spin-labeled probes have shown, for example, that synaptosomal plasma membranes from ethanol-treated mice are significantly less sensitive to the disordering effect of ethanol than membranes from untreated mice.[146] In these experiments no consistent reduction in membrane fluidity (increase in ordering) was observed when ethanol was removed from membranes obtained from chronic ethanol-treated animals. However, the length of the spin-labeled probe appears to be critical for detecting an increased ordering effect following chronic ethanol treatment. A reduction in membrane fluidity was observed with probes of sufficient length to allow their location in the center of each lipid layer.[182,183] When shorter or longer probes were used, in which the reporter groups were located near the bilayer surface or close to the region between each lipid layer in the bilayer, no effect of chronic ethanol treatment was observed. Thus, there is evidence that changes in membrane properties can occur following chronic ethanol treatment.

Attempts to identify the membrane components that are changed by ethanol treatment have met with only limited success. An increase in the cholesterol/phospholipid ratio in membranes from ethanol-treated mice has been reported,[184] but is not clear that the change in ratio per se affects the ethanol sensitivity.[185]

The significance of ethanol-related alterations in membrane ordering is still uncertain. It is possible that the major consequence of these fluidity changes is alteration of interactions between membrane proteins and their surrounding lipid molecules. Such changes might be of sufficient magnitude to induce conformational changes or an altered lipid environment for active sites in membrane-bound receptors, enzymes, or transporters.

BEHAVIORAL FACTORS IN DRUG TOLERANCE AND DEPENDENCE

Behavioral factors contribute significantly to drug tolerance, when the phenomenon is examined by measurement of drug-mediated effects on behavior in intact animals. Several studies have shown that the degree of tolerance induced by a drug can be varied by manipulating the experimental conditions and the prior experience of the test animal. It is beyond the scope of this chapter to discuss in detail the mechanisms underlying modulation of drug responses by environmental and experiential factors, but a brief overview of this topic is necessary to transmit to the reader a comprehensive view of tolerance in the intact animal.

A striking example of the importance of the time of drug administration in relation to the test sessions in which drug-mediated behaviors are measured is provided by experiments examining the effects of repeated cocaine administration on the amount of milk consumed by rats during daily 15-minute test sessions (Fig. 10-15). The potency of cocaine in inhibiting milk drinking was measured by administering the drug over a range of doses to different groups of rats at the beginning of the experiment. Thereafter, the rats all received 16 mg/kg daily, a dose that initially inhibited milk drinking by 60 to 70 percent. After 75 days of treatment, the potency of cocaine was again measured. In rats that had received the daily dose of cocaine immediately *prior* to each milk drinking session, the cocaine dose-response curve was shifted to the right, with an approximate doubling of the dose of cocaine needed to produce 50 percent inhibition of milk drinking. Cross-tolerance to *d*-amphetamine was also noted. However, in another group of rats, which received their daily dose of cocaine immediately *after* each milk drinking session, no tolerance to either cocaine or amphetamine was observed. In contrast, the animals appeared to be sensitized to cocaine and amphetamine, since the dose-response curve was shifted to the left relative to the curve that was determined initially. Now about half as much cocaine or amphetamine was required to produce a comparable degree of inhibition of milk drinking. Since all the animals had received the same chronic cocaine treatment, the difference in effect must be related to differences in the relative timing of drug administration and behavioral testing.

This experiment demonstrates several features typical of studies of behavioral tolerance. First, the intervals between chronic drug treatment doses were fairly long relative to the rates of metabolism and excretion of the drug, which thus ensured that the acute effects of the drug were only apparent for a small part of each 24-hour period. Processes initiated by each drug dose that might result in metabolic or cellular tolerance may well have decayed between each drug administration. Second, the daily dose of drug was administered either immediately before or immediately after a behavioral training session in which the rats were exposed to stimuli uniquely associated with that training session; thus, drug administration was associated with a specific experimental environment. The nature of the experimental procedure employed does not appear to be critical. In this experiment the training procedure was brief daily exposure to a novel source of fluid and nutrient. In other experiments behavioral tolerance has developed as a result of repeated measurement of pain threshold or the daily measurement of body temperature.[187] The mechanisms responsible for behavioral tolerance are still in dispute. For more information the reader is directed to a more detailed review.[188] As with cellular tolerance, several processes may contribute to behavioral tolerance, the relative importance of each being dependent on the experimental situation.

Behavioral factors may also contribute to the symptoms induced by drug withdrawal.[189] Behavioral responses to external stimuli that are established before withdrawal may be disrupted during the stress of withdrawal. Such behavioral disruption is often one of the most sensitive indicators of withdrawal, and it has been observed following the withdrawal of many types of drug, including those for which the physical withdrawal syndrome is very mild.[190,191] In animals or human subjects experiencing more than one cycle of dependence and withdrawal (a common feature of illicit drug use in humans), withdrawal symptoms may also become conditioned by association of environmental factors with drug withdrawal itself.[192] For example, in humans both the subjective and physical symp-

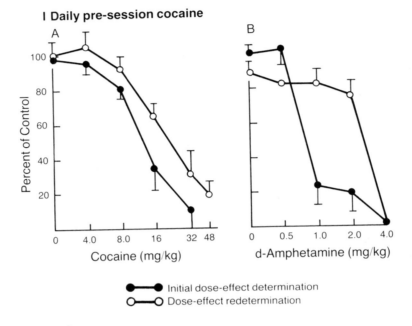

I Daily pre-session cocaine

A

Percent of Control

Cocaine (mg/kg)

B

d-Amphetamine (mg/kg)

●——● Initial dose-effect determination
○——○ Dose-effect redetermination

II Daily post-session cocaine

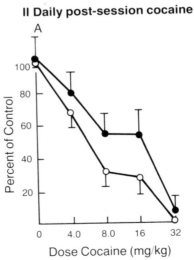

A

Percent of Control

Dose Cocaine (mg/kg)

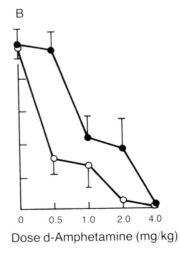

B

Dose d-Amphetamine (mg/kg)

toms of opiate withdrawal can be induced by exposure to an environment in which withdrawal has previously been experienced.[193] Clearly, this phenomenon may contribute to the severity of withdrawal symptoms, and it needs to be considered in the design of studies that require more than one cycle of dependence and withdrawal.

RELATIONSHIP BETWEEN TOLERANCE AND DEPENDENCE

The general hypotheses proposed to account for the components of tolerance and dependence that are not obviously related to drug dispositional factors or to behavioral factors have been based on the assumption that the same fundamental process is responsible for both effects.[114,118,120,121] As more evidence concerning the action of opiate and central depressant drugs has become available, it has become clear that some of the processes that contribute to cellular tolerance (e.g., receptor down regulation and desensitization) do not require the coincident development of dependence. And for many drugs, including LSD, marijuana, amphetamines, cocaine, and nicotine, the development of tolerance is accompanied by little or no physical dependence. (That is not to say that these drugs are not addictive; indeed, craving for some of these drugs may be very intense.) Detailed studies of opiate drug effects on specific tissues have also revealed situations in which tolerance to opiates occurs without any evidence of dependence. This is best documented in the isolated mouse vas deferens preparation, in which considerable degrees of tolerance can be induced by sustained activation of opioid receptors without any concomitant development of dependence.[194] The same result was obtained regardless of whether tolerance was induced selectively through δ or through μ type receptors.

Homeostatic adjustments in postreceptor components of receptor-effector systems have been invoked to explain dependence.[33,114,127,144] Such adjustments include increased activity of enzymes, altered sensitivity or numbers of transmitter receptors, and changes in neuronal membrane composition. These types of mechanisms predict that tolerance and dependence are associated phenomena. It is difficult to test this prediction because it is often much easier to detect the occurrence of withdrawal symptoms than to demonstrate that a quantitative change has occurred in the sensitivity to a drug, especially when quantitative measurements of drug effect are subject to significant experimental error. The available evidence indicates, however, that dependence is associated with the presence of at least a modest degree of tolerance. It seems likely, therefore, that adaptive changes in neural function that are responsible for physical dependence occur at some selective

← —————————————————————————————————————

Fig. 10-15 Effects of cocaine and amphetamine on milk intake in rats after cocaine pretreatments given immediately before or immediately after daily 15-minute milk drinking training sessions. Each panel presents two dose-effect curves, one of which was determined before (●) and the other after (○) a 75-day period of daily injection with 16 mg/kg cocaine. Drug effects on milk intake are expressed as a percentage of nondrug control intake measured prior to the drug treatment. Vertical lines indicate standard errors of the mean values. **I.** Pre-session cocaine: **(A)** the effects of cocaine before and immediately after (redetermination) a period of daily injections of cocaine given 15 minutes before each milk drinking training session: **(B)** the effects of *d*-amphetamine before and during the period of daily injections of cocaine given before each training session. **(II)** Post-session cocaine: **(A)** the effects of cocaine before and after the period of daily injections of cocaine immediately after each milk drinking training session. **(B)** the effects of *d*-amphetamine given before and during the period of daily injections of cocaine immediately after each training session (From Woolverton et al.,[100] with permission.)

sites in the nervous system, while tolerance is manifested both at these sites and at other sites at which the drug acts. Thus, dependence is not an inevitable consequence of drug action, but it requires the presence of specific adaptive machinery in the neural milieu on which the drug acts. This does not necessarily require complex neural circuitry, since evidence of drug dependence has been obtained in cells maintained in culture.[33,160] In the case of opiate drugs, dependence is not specifically associated with one kind of receptor. In intact animals μ receptor–selective opiates are most active as inducers of dependence, but dependence phenomena have also been observed following δ[33,160] and κ[195] receptor activation. The available evidence suggests that if the adaptive response to a primary drug effect leads to the quantitative readjustment of cellular components or to changes in membrane properties and the duration of these changes exceeds the time it takes for the drug to be removed from the system following termination of its administration, then withdrawal symptoms will probably occur.

REFERENCES

1. Brady JV, Lukas SE (eds): Testing drugs for physical dependence potential and abuse liability. Natl Inst Drug Abuse Res Monogr Ser 53: 1984
2. Martin WR: Pharmacology of opioids. Pharmacol Rev 35: 283, 1983
3. Inturrisi CE, Foley KM: Narcotic analgesics in the management of pain. p.257. In Kuhar MJ, Pasternak GW (eds): Analgesics: Neurochemical, Behavioral and Clinical Perspectives. Raven Press, New York, 1984
4. Chessick RD: The "pharmacologic orgasm" in the drug addict. Arch Gen Psychiatry 3:545, 1960
5. Houde RW: Analgesic effectiveness of the narcotic agonist-antagonists. Br J Pharmacol 7:297, 1979
6. Terenius L: Stereospecific interaction between narcotic analgesics and a synaptic plasma membrane fraction of rat cerebral cortex. Acta Pharmacol Toxicol (Copenh) 32:317, 1973
7. Pert CB, Snyder SH: Opiate receptor: Demonstration in nervous tissues. Science 179:1011, 1973
8. Simon EJ, Hiller JM, Edelman I: Stereospecific binding of the potent narcotic analgesic [³H]etorphine to rat brain homogenate. Proc Natl Acad Sci USA 70:1947, 1973
9. Hughes J, Smith TW, Kosterlitz HW, et al: Identification of two related pentapeptides from the brain with potent opiate agonist activity. Nature 258:577, 1957
10. Cox BM, Goldstein A, Li CH: Opioid activity of a peptide, beta-lipotropin-(61-91), derived from beta-lipotropin. Proc Natl Acad Sci USA 73:1821, 1976
11. Goldstein A, Fishli W, Lowney LI, et al: Porcine pituitary dynorphin: Complete amino acid sequence of the biologically active heptadecapeptide. Proc Natl Acad Sci USA 78:7219, 1981
12. Cuello AC: Central distribution of opioid peptides. Br Med Bull 39:11, 1983
13. Vincent SR, Hokfelt T, Christensson I, Terenius L: Dynorphin-immunoreactive neurons in the central nervous system of the rat. Neurosci Lett 33:185, 1982
14. Morley JE, Barabetsky NG, Wingert TD, et al: Endocrine effects of naloxone-induced opiate receptor blockade. J Clin Endocrinol Metab 50:251, 1980
15. Martin WR, Eades CG, Thompson JA, et al: The effects of morphine- and nalorphine-like drugs in the non-dependent and morphine-dependent chronic spinal dog. J Pharmacol Exp Ther 197:517, 1976
16. Lord JAH, Waterfield AA, Hughes J, Kosterlitz HW: Endogenous opioid peptides: Multiple agonists and receptors. Nature 267:495, 1977
17. Gillan MCG, Kosterlitz HW: Spectrum of the mu, delta and kappa-binding sites in homogenates of rat brain. Br J Pharmacol 77:461, 1982

18. Chavkin C, Goldstein A: Specific receptor for the opioid peptide dynorphin: Structure–activity relationships. Proc Natl Acad Sci USA 78:6543, 1981
19. Su TP: Evidence for sigma opioid receptor: Binding of [^{3}H]SKF 10047 to etorphin inaccessible sites in guinea pig brain. J Pharmacol Exp Ther 223:284, 1982
20. Wolozin BL, Pasternak GW: Classification of multiple morphine and enkephalin binding sites in the central nervous system. Proc Natl Acad Sci USA 78:6181, 1981
21. Magnan J, Paterson SJ, Tavani A, Kosterlitz HW: The binding spectrum of narcotic analgesic drugs with different agonist and antagonist properties. Naunyn Schmiedebergs Arch Pharmacol 319:197, 1982
22. Jessell JM, Iversen LL: Opiate analgesics inhibit substance P release from rat trigeminal nucleus. Nature 268:549, 1977
23. Cicero TJ, Badger TM, Wilcox CE, et al: Morphine decreases luteinizing hormone by an action on the hypothalamus. J Pharmacol Exp Ther 203:548, 1977
24. Cox BM, Weinstock M: The effects of analgesic drugs on the release of acetylcholine from electrically stimulated guinea pig ileum. Br J Pharmacol 21:81, 1966
25. Binder HJ, Laurenson JP, Dobbins JW: Role of opiate receptors in regulation of enkephalin stimulation of active sodium and chloride absorption. Am J Physiol 247:G432, 1984
26. Zieglgänsberger W, French ED, Siggins GR, Bloom FE: Opioid peptides may excite hippocampal pyramidal neurons by inhibiting adjacent inhibitory interneurons. Science 205:415, 1985
27. Fernandes M, Kluwe S, Coper H: Quantitative assessment of tolerance to and dependence on morphine in mice. Naunyn Schmiedebergs Arch Pharmacol 297:53, 1977
28. Blasig J, Meyer G, Hollt V, et al: Non-competitive nature of the antagonistic mechanism responsible for tolerance development to opiate-induced analgesia. Neuropharmacology 18:473, 1979
29. Mushin BE, Cochin J: Tolerance to morphine in rat: Its prevention by naloxone. Life Sci 18:797, 1976
30. Mucha RF, Kalant H: Naloxone prevention of morphine LDR curve flattening associated with high dose tolerance. Psychopharmacology (Berlin) 75:132, 1981
31. Basbaum AI, Clanton CH, Fields HL: Opiate and stimulus produced analgesia: Functional anatomy of a medullospinal pathway. Proc Natl Acad Sci USA 73:4685, 1976
32. Yaksh TL: Spinal opiate analgesia: characteristics and principles of action. Pain 11:293, 1981
33. Sharma SK, Klee WA, Nirenberg M: Dual regulation of adenylate cyclase accounts for narcotic dependence and tolerance. Proc Natl Acad Sci USA 72:3092, 1975
34. Karras PJ, North RA: Acute and chronic effects of opiates in single neurons of the myenteric plexus. J Pharmacol Exp Ther 217:70, 1981
35. Newby-Schmidt MB, Norton S: Development of opiate tolerance in the chick embryo. Pharmacol Biochem Behav 15:773, 1981
36. Crain SM, Crain B, Finnigan T, Simon EJ: Development of tolerance to opiates and opioid peptides in organotypic cultures of mouse spinal cord. Life Sci 25:1797, 1979
37. Goldstein A, Sheehan P: Tolerance to opioid narcotics. I. Tolerance to the "running fit" caused by levorphanol in the mouse. J Pharmacol Exp Ther 169:175, 1969
38. Cox BM, Ginsburg M, Osman OH: Acute tolerance to narcotic analgesic drugs in rats. Br J Pharmacol 33:245, 1968
39. Cox BM, Ginburg M, Willis J: The offset of morphine tolerance in rats and mice. Br J Pharmacol 53:385, 1975
40. Kolb L, Himmelsbach CK: Clinical studies of drug addiction. III. A critical review of the withdrawal treatments with method of evaluating abstinence syndromes. Am J Psychiatry 94:759, 1938
41. Martin WR, Eades CG: A comparison between acute and chronic physical dependence in the chronic spinal dog. J Pharmacol Exp Ther 146:385, 1964
42. Cicero TJ, Meyer ER: Morphine pellet implantation in rats: Quantitative assessment of tolerance and dependence. J Pharmacol Exp Ther 184:404, 1973

43. Way EL, Loh HH, Shen F: Simultaneous quantitative assessment of tolerance and physical dependence. J Pharmacol Exp Ther 167:1, 1969
44. Isbell H: Methods and results of studying experimental human addiction to the newer synthetic analgesics. Ann NY Acad Sci 51:108, 1948
45. Andrews HL, Himmelsbach CK: Relation of the intensity of the morphine abstinence syndrome to dosage. J Pharmacol Exp Ther 81:288, 1944
46. Seevers MH, Deneau GA: A critique of the "dual action" hypothesis of morphine physical dependence. Arch Int Pharmacodyn Ther 140:514, 1962
47. Yano I, Takemori AE: Inhibition by naloxone of tolerance and dependence in mice treated acutely and chronically with morphine. Res Commun Chem Pathol Pharmacol 16:721, 1977
48. Dole VP, Nyswander M: A medical treatment for diacetylmorphine (heroin) addiction. A clinical chemical trial with methadone hydrochloride. JAMA 193:646, 1965
49. Fielding S, Wilker J, Haynes M, et al: A comparison of clonidine with morphine for antinociceptive and antiwithdrawal actions. J Pharmacol Exp Ther 207:899, 1978
50. Collier HOJ, Francis DL, Schneider C: Modification of morphine withdrawal by drugs interacting with humoral mechanisms: some contradictions and their interpretation. Nature 327:220, 1972
51. Himmelsbach CK, Andrews HL: Studies on modification of the morphine abstinence syndrome by drugs. J Pharmacol Exp Ther 77:17, 1943
52. Linseman MA: Naloxone-precipitated withdrawal as a function of the morphine-naloxone interval. Psychopharmacology (Berlin) 54:159, 1977
53. Tilson HA, Rech RH, Stolman S: Hyperalgesia during withdrawal as a means of measuring the degree of dependence in morphine dependent rats. Psychopharmacology (Berlin) 28:287, 1973
54. Cheney DL, Goldstein A: Tolerance to opioid narcotics. III. Time course and reversibility of physical dependence in mice. Nature 232:477, 1971
55. Brase DA, Iwamoto ET, Loh HH, Way EL: Re-initiation of sensitivity to naloxone by a single narcotic injection in post-addicted mice. J Pharmacol Exp Ther 197:317, 1976
56. Cheney DL, Judson BA, Goldstein A: Failure of an opiate to protect mice against naloxone precipitated withdrawal. J Pharmacol Exp Ther 182:189, 1972
57. Resnick RB, Kentenbaum RS, Washton A, Poole D: Naloxone-precipitated withdrawal: A method for rapid induction onto naltrexone. Clin Pharmacol Ther 21:409, 1977
58. Gold MS, Redmond DE Jr, Kleber HD: Clonidine blocks acute opiate withdrawal symptoms. Lancet 2:599, 1978
59. Himmelsbach CK: Clinical studies of drug addiction: Physical dependence, withdrawal and recovery. Arch Intern Med 69:766, 1942
60. Martin WR, Jasinski DR: Physical parameters of morphine dependence in man—tolerance, early abstinence, protracted abstinence. J Psychiatr Res 7:9, 1969
61. Wilker, A: Dynamics of drug dependence. Arch Gen Psychiatry 28:611, 1973
62. Newman HW, Lehman AJ: Nature of acquired tolerance to alcohol. J Pharmacol Exp Ther 62:301, 1938
63. Mirsky IA, Piker P, Rosenbaum M, Lederer H: "Adaptation" of the central nervous system to varying concentrations of alcohol in the blood. Q J Stud Alcohol 2:35, 1941
64. Goldberg L: Quantitative studies on alcohol tolerance in man. Acta Physiol Scand 5, suppl. 16:1, 1943
65. Maynert EW, Klingman GI: Acute tolerance to intravenous anesthetics in dogs. J Pharmacol Exp Ther 128:192, 1960
66. Le Blanc AE, Kalant H, Gibbons RJ: Acute tolerance to ethanol in the rat. Psychopharmacology (Berlin) 41:43, 1975
67. Victor M, Adams RD: The effect of alcohol on the nervous system. Res Publ Assoc Res Nerv Ment Dis 32:526, 1953
68. Isbell H, Fraser HF, Wikler A, et al: An experimental study of the etiology of "rum fits" and delirium tremens. Q J Stud Alcohol 16:1, 1955

69. Mendelson JH (ed): Experimentally induced chronic intoxication and withdrawal in alcoholics. Q J Stud Alcohol 25: suppl., 1964

70. Goldstein DB: Relationship of alcohol dose to intensity of withdrawal signs in mice. J Pharmacol Exp Ther 180:203, 1972

71. Goldstein DB: An animal model for testing effects of drugs on alcohol withdrawal reactions. J Pharmacol Exp Ther 183:14, 1972

72. Rosenberg HC, Okamoto M: Eectrophysiology of barbiturate withdrawal in the spinal cord. J Pharmacol Exp Ther 199:189, 1976

73. Boisse NR, Okamoto M: Physical dependence to barbital compared to pentobarbital. I. "Chronically equivalent" dosing method. J Pharmacol Exp Ther 204:497, 1978

74. Boisse NR, Okamoto M: Physical dependence to barbital compared to pentobarbital. II. Tolerance characteristics. J Pharmacol Exp Ther 204:507, 1978

75. Jaffe JH, Sharpless SK: The rapid development of physical dependence on barbiturates. J Pharmacol Exp Ther 150:140, 1965

76. Flint BA, Ho IK: Continuous administration of barbital by pellet implantation. J Pharmacol Methods 4:127, 1980

77. Yutrzenka GJ, Patrick GA, Rosenberger W: Continuous intraperitoneal infusion of pentobarbital: A model of barbiturate dependence in the rat. J Pharmacol Exp Ther 232:111, 1985

78. Isbell H, Altschul S, Kornetsky CH, et al: Chronic barbiturate intoxication: An experimental study. Arch Neurol Psychiatry 64:1, 1950

79. Fraser HF, Isbell H, Eisenman AJ, et al: Chronic barbiturate intoxication: Further studies. Arch Intern Med 94:34, 1954

80. Hollister LE, Motzenberger FP, Degan RO: Withdrawal reactions from chlordiazepoxide. Psychopharmacology (Berlin) 2:63, 1961

81. Mackinnon GL, Parker WA: Benzodiazepine withdrawal syndrome: A literature review and evaluation. Am J Drug Alcohol Abuse 9:19, 1982

82. Owen RT, Tyrer P: Benzodiazepine dependence: A review of the evidence. Drugs 25:385, 1983

83. Lader M, Petersson H: Long-term effects of benzodiazepines. Neuropharmacology 22:527, 1983

84. Ryan GP, Boisse NR: Benzodiazepine tolerance, physical dependence and withdrawal: Electrophysiological study of spinal reflex function. J Pharmacol Exp Ther 231:464, 1984

85. Martin WR, McNicholas LF, Cherian S: Diazepam and pentobarbital dependence in the rat. Life Sci 31:72, 1982

86. Ryan GP, Boisse NR: Experimental induction of benzodiazepine tolerance and physical dependence. J Pharmacol Exp Ther 226:100, 1983

87. Rosenberg HC, Chiu TH: An antagonist-induced benzodiazepine abstinence syndrome. Eur J Pharmacol 81:153, 1982

88. McNicholas LF, Martin WR: The effect of a benzodiazepine antagonist, Ro15-1788, in diazepam dependent rats. Life Sci 31:731, 1982

89. Wikler A, Carter RL: Effect of single doses of *N*-allylnormorphine on hindlimb reflexes of chronic spinal dogs during cycles of morphine addiction. J Pharmacol Exp Ther 109:92, 1953

90. Westfall TC, Brase DA: Studies on the mechanism of tolerance to nicotine-induced elevations of urinary catecholamines. Biochem Pharmacol 20:1627, 1971

91. Morrison CF, Stephenson JA: The occurrence of tolerance to a central depressant effect of nicotine. Br J Pharmacol 45:151, 1972

92. Clarke PBS, Kumar R: The effects of nicotine on locomotor activity in non-tolerant and tolerant rats. Br J Pharmacol 78:329, 1983

93. Domino EF: Neuropharmacology of nicotine and tobacco smoking. p.5. In Dunn WL (ed): Smoking Behavior: Motives and Incentives, Winston & Sons, Washington, 1973

94. Spealman RD, Goldberg SR: Maintenance of schedule-controlled behavior by intravenous injection of nicotine in squirrel monkeys. J Pharmacol Exp Ther 223:402, 1982

95. Cox BM, Goldstein A, Nelson WT: Nicotine self-administration in rats. Br J Pharmacol 83:49, 1984

96. Jaffe JH, Kanzler M: Smoking as an addictive disorder. p.4. In Krasnegor NA (ed): Cigarette Smoking as a Dependence Process. Natl Inst Drug Abuse Res Monogr Ser. 29:4, 1979

97. Stolerman IP, Fink R, Jarvik ME: Acute and chronic tolerance to nicotine measured by activity in rats. Psychopharmacology (Berlin) 30:329, 1973

98. Stolerman IP, Bunker P, Jarvik ME: Nicotine tolerance in rats; role of dose and dose interval. Psychopharmacology (Berlin) 34:317, 1974

99. Shiffman SM, Jarvik ME: Smoking withdrawal symptoms in two weeks of abstinence. Psychopharmacology (Berlin) 50:35, 1976

100. Woolverton WL, Kandel D, Schuster CR: Tolerance and cross-tolerance to cocaine and *d*-amphetamine. J Pharmacol Exp Ther 205:525, 1978

101. Rebec GV, Segal DS: Enhanced responsiveness to intraventricular infusion of amphetamine following its repeated systemic administration. Psychopharmacology (Berlin) 62:101, 1979

102. Schmidt CJ, Gehlert DR, Peat MA, et al: Studies on the mechanisms of tolerance to meth-amphetamine. Brain Res 343:305, 1985

103. Griffith JD, Cavanaugh J, Held J, Oakes JA: Dextroamphetamine: Evaluation of psychomimetic properties in man. Arch Gen Psychiatry 26:97, 1972

104. Rosenberg DE, Wolbach AB, Miner EJ, Isbell H: Observations on direct and cross tolerance of LSD and *d*-amphetamine in man. Psychopharmacology (Berlin) 5:1, 1963

105. Jones RT, Benowitz N, Bachman J: Clinical studies of cannabis tolerance and dependence. Ann NY Acad Sci 282:221, 1976

106. Huidobro-Toro JP, Yoshimura K: Pharmacological characterization of the inhibitory effects of neurotensin on the rabbit ileum myenteric plexus preparation. Br J Pharmacol 80:645, 1983

107. Remmer H: Drugs as activators of drug enzymes. p. 235. In Brodie BB, Erdos EG (eds): Metabolic Factors Controlling Duration of Drug Action, Proc 1st Int Pharmacol Meeting. Vol 6. Macmillan, New York, 1962

108. Theorell H, McKinley-McGee JS: Liver alcohol dehydrogenase. I. Kinetics and equilibria without inhibitors. Acta Chem Scand 15:1797, 1961

109. Khanna JM, Israel Y: Ethanol metabolism. Int Rev Physiol. 21:275, 1980

110. Lieber CS, De Carli LM: Hepatic microsomal ethanol-oxidizing system. In vitro characteristics and adaptive properties in vivo. J Biol Chem 245:2505, 1970

111. Mendelson JH, Stein S, Mello NK: Effects of experimentally induced intoxication on metabolism of ethanol-1-C^{14} in alcoholic subjects. Metabolism 14:1255, 1965

112. Maasten LW, Paterson GR, Burkhalter A, Way EL: Tolerance to methadone lethality and microsomal enzyme induction in mice tolerant to and dependent on morphine. Drug and Alcohol Depend 5:27, 1980

113. Hoogland DR, Miva TS, Bousquet WF: Metabolism and tolerance studies with chlordiazepoxide-2-^{14}C in the rat. Toxicol Appl Pharmacol 9:116, 1966

114. Collier HO: Tolerance, physical dependence and receptors. Adv Drug Res 3:171, 1966

115. Cox BM, Osman OH: The role of protein synthesis inhibition in the prevention of morphine tolerance. Br J Pharmacol 38:157, 1970

116. Way EL, Loh HH, Shen F-H: Morphine tolerance, physical dependence, and synthesis of brain 5-hydroxytryptamine. Science 162:1290, 1968

117. Cohen M, Keats AS, Krivoy W, Ungar G: Effect of actinomycin D on morphine tolerance. Proc Soc Exp Biol Med 119:381, 1965

118. Seevers MH, Deneau GA: Physiological aspects of tolerance and physical dependence. p. 565. In Root WS, Hoffman FG (eds): Physiological Pharmacology: A Comprehensive Treatise. Vol. 1. Academic Press, San Diego, CA, 1963

119. Martin WR, Eisenman AJ: Interactions between nalorphine and morphine in the decerebrate cat. J Pharmacol Exp Ther 138:113, 1962

120. Goldstein DB, Goldstein A: Possible role of enzyme inhibition and repression in drug tolerance and addiction. Biochem Pharmacol 8:48, 1961

121. Shuster L: Repression and de-repression of enzyme synthesis as a possible explanation of some aspects of drug action. Nature 189:314, 1961

122. Goldstein A, Goldstein DB: Enzyme expansion theory of drug tolerance and physical dependence. Res Publ Assoc Res Nerv Ment Dis 46:265, 1968

123. Cox BM, Chavkin C: Comparison of dynorphin-selective kappa receptors in mouse vas deferens and guinea pig ileum. Spare receptor fraction as a determinant of potency. Mol Pharmacol 23:36, 1983

124. Wuster M, Krenss H, Herz A: Lack of cross tolerance on multiple opiate receptors in the mouse vas deferens. Mol Pharmacol 18:395, 1980

125. Schulz R, Wuster M: Are there subtypes (isoreceptors) of multiple opiate receptors in the mouse vas deferens? Eur J Pharmacol 76:61, 1981

126. Cherubini E, North RA: Mu and kappa opioids inhibit transmitter release by different mechanisms. Proc Natl Acad Sci USA 82:1860, 1985

127. Mihara S, North RA: Opioids increase potassium conductance in submucous neurons of guinea pig caecum by activating delta-receptors. Br J Pharmacol 88:315, 1986

128. Forreca F, Burks TF: Affinity of normorphine for its pharmacologic receptor in the naïve and morphine-tolerant guinea pig ileum. J Pharmacol Exp Ther 225:688, 1983

129. Chavkin C, Goldstein A: Opioid receptor reserve in normal and morphine tolerant guinea pig ileum myenteric plexus. Proc Natl Acad Sci USA 81:7253, 1984

130. Klee WA, Streaty RA: Narcotic receptor sites in morphine dependent rats. Nature 248:61, 1974

131. Cox BM, Padhya R: Opiate binding and effect in ileum preparations from normal and morphine pretreated guinea pigs. Br J Pharmacol 61:271, 1977

132. Dum J, Meyer G, Hollt V, Herz A: In vivo opiate binding unchanged in tolerant/dependent mice. Eur J Pharmacol 58:453, 1979

133. Rogers NF, Fakahany EE: Morphine-induced opioid receptor down regulation detected in intact adult rat brain cells. Eur J Pharmacol 124:221, 1986

134. Werling LL, McMahon PN, Cox BM: Selective changes in μ receptor properties induced by chronic morphine exposure. Proc Natl Acad Sci USA 86:6393, 1989

135. Tao P-L, Chang L-R, Law PY, Loh HH: Decrease in δ-opioid receptor density in rat brain after chronic [D-Ala2,D-Leu5]enkephalin treatment. Brain Res 462:313, 1988

136. Sharma SK, Klee WA, Nirenberg M: Opiate-dependent modulation of adenylate cyclase. Proc Natl Acad Sci USA 74:3365, 1977

137. Chang K-J, Eckel RW, Blanchard SG: Opioid peptides induce reduction of enkephalin receptors in cultured neuroblastoma cells. Nature 296:446, 1982

138. Law PY, Hom DS, Loh HH: Opiate receptor down-regulation and desensitization in neuroblastoma X glioma NG 108-15 hybrid cells are two separate cellular adaptation processes. Mol Pharmacol 24:413, 1983

139. Law PY, Hom DS, Loh HH: Opiate regulation of adenosine 3', 5'-cyclic monophosphate level in neuroblastoma X glioma NG 108-15 hybrid cells. Mol Pharmacol 23:26, 1983

140. Hazum E, Chang K-J, Cuatrecasas P: Opiate (enkephalin) receptors of neuroblastoma cells: Occurrence in clusters on the cell surface. Science 206:1077, 1979

141. Law PY, Hom DS, Loh HH: Down regulation of opiate receptor in neuroblastoma X glioma NG 108-15 hybrid cells. Chloroquine promotes accumulation of tritiated enkephalin in the lysosomes. J Biol Chem 259:4096, 1984

142. Bennett DB, Spain JW, Laskowski MB, et al: Stereospecific opiate binding sites occur in coated vesicles. J Neurosci 5:3010, 1985

143. Puttfarcken PS, Werling LL, Cox BM: Effects of chronic morphine exposure on opioid inhibition of adenylyl cyclase in 7315c cell membranes: A useful model for the study of tolerance at μ opioid receptors. Mol Pharmacol 33:520, 1988

144. Zukin RS, Sugarman JR, Fitz-Syage ML, et al: Naltrexone-induced opiate receptor supersensitivity. Brain Res 245:285, 1982

145. Chin JH, Goldstein DB: Drug tolerance in biomembranes: A spin label study of the effects of ethanol. Science 196:684, 1977
146. Lovinger DM, White G, Weight FF: Ethanol inhibits NMDA-activated ion current in hippocampal neurons. Science 243:1721, 1989
147. Suzdak PD, Schwartz RD, Skolnick P, Paul SM: Ethanol stimulates gamma-aminobutyric acid receptor mediated chloride transport in rat brain synaptosomes. Proc Natl Acad Sci USA 83:4071, 1986
148. Crawley JN, Marangos PJ, Stivers J, Goodwin FK: Chronic clonazepam administration induces benzodiazepine receptor subsensitivity. Neuropharmacology 21:85, 1982
149. Miller LG, Greenblatt DJ, Roy RB, et al: Chronic benzodiazepine administration. II. Discontinuation syndrome is associated with upregulation of γ-aminobutyric acid$_A$ receptor complex binding and function. J Pharmacol Exp Ther 246:177, 1988
150. Gray PL, Taberner PV: Evidence for GABA tolerance in barbiturate dependent and withdrawn mice. Neuropharmacology 24:437, 1985
151. Gallagher DW, Lakowski JM, Gonsalves SF, Rauch SL: Chronic benzodiazepine treatment decreases post-synaptic GABA sensitivity. Nature 308:74, 1984
152. Sher PK: Long-term exposure of cortical cell cultures to clonazepam reduces benzodiazepine receptor binding. Exp Neurol 92:360, 1986
153. Maloteaux J-M, Octave J-N, Gossuin A, et al: GABA induces down-regulation of the benzodiazepine-GABA receptor complex in the rat cultured neurons. Eur J Pharmacol 144:173, 1987
154. Katz B, Thesleff S: A study of the 'desensitization' produced by acetylcholine at the motor end-plate. J Physiol 138:63, 1957
155. Goldbeter A, Koshland DE: Simple molecular model for sensing and adaptation based on receptor modification with application to bacterial chemotaxis. Mol Biol 161:395, 1982
156. Sibley DR, Strasser RH, Caron MG, Lefkowitz RJ: Homologous desensitization of adenylate cyclase is associated with phosphorylation of the beta-adrenergic receptor. J Biol Chem 260:3883, 1985
157. Heidmann T, Changeux J-P: Structural and functional properties of the acetylcholine receptor protein in its purified and membrane-bound states. Ann Rev Biochem 47:317, 1978
158. Strulovici B, Cerione RA, Kilpatrick BF, et al: Direct demonstration of impaired functionality of a purified desensitized beta-adrenergic receptor in a reconstituted system. Science 225:837, 1984
159. Murad F: Cyclic guanosine monophosphate as a mediator of vasodilation. J Clin Invest 78:1, 1986
160. Musacchio JM, Greenspan DL: The adenylate cyclase rebound response to naloxone in the NG 108-15 cells. Effects of etorphine and other opiates. Neuropharmacology 25:833, 1986
161. Sabol SL, Nirenberg M: Regulation of adenylate cyclase of neuroblastoma X glioma hybrid cells by alpha-adrenergic receptors. II. Long-lived increase of adenylate cyclase activity mediated by alpha-receptors. J Biol Chem 254:1921, 1979
162. Hoffman BB, Cheng H, Dall'Aglio E, Reavan GM: Desensitization of adenosine receptor-mediated inhibition of lipolysis. The mechanism involves the development of enhanced cyclic adenosine monophosphate accumulation in tolerant adipocytes. J Clin Invest 78:185, 1986
163. Sibley DR, Lefkowitz RJ: Molecular mechanisms of receptor desensitization using the beta-adrenegic receptor coupled adenylate cyclase as a model. Nature 317:124, 1985
164. Cooper JR, Meyer ER: Possible mechanisms involved in the release and modulation of release of neuroactive agents. Neurochem Int 6:419, 1984
165. Burn JH, Rand MJ: The action of sympathomimetic amines in animals treated with reserpine. J Physiol 144:314, 1958
166. Trendelenburg U, Muskus A, Fleming WW, de la Sierra BGA: Modification by reserpine of the action of sympathomimetic amines in spinal cats: a classification of sympathomimetic amines. J Pharmacol Exp Ther 138:176, 1962

167. Axelrod J, Gordon E, Herrting G, et al: On the mechanism of tachyphylaxis to tyramine in the isolated rat heart. Br J Pharmacol 19:56, 1962
168. Demellweek C, Goudie AJ: Behavioral tolerance to amphetamine and other psychostimulants: The case for considering behavioral mechanisms. Psychopharmacology (Berlin) 80:287, 1983
169. Brown RD, Prendiville P, Cain C: Alpha$_1$-adrenergic and H1-histaminergic receptor control of intracellular Ca^{++} in a muscle cell line: The influence of prior agonist exposure on receptor responsiveness. Mol Pharmacol 29:531, 1986
170. Schulz R, Goldstein A: Morphine tolerance and supersensitivity to 5-hydroxytryptamine in the myenteric plexus of the guinea pig. Nature 244:168, 1973
171. Johnson SM, Westfall DP, Howard SA, Fleming WW: Sensitivities of the isolated ileal longitudinal smooth muscle-myenteric plexus and hypogastric nerve–vas deferens of the guinea pig after chronic morphine pellet implantation. J Pharmacol Exp Ther 204:54, 1978
172. Rae GA, Neto JP, de Morae S: Noradrenergic supersensitivity of the mouse vas deferens after long-term treatment with morphine. J Pharm Pharmacol 29:310, 1977
173. Pollock D, Muir TC, MacDonald A, Henderson G: Morphine-induced changes in the sensitivity of the isolated colon and vas deferens of the rat. Eur J Pharmacol 20:321, 1972
174. Taylor DA, Leedham JA, Doak N, Fleming WW: Morphine tolerance and nonspecific subsensitivity of the longitudinal muscle myenteric plexus preparation of the guinea-pig to inhibitory agonists. Naunyn-Schmiedeberg's Arch Pharmacol 338:553, 1988
175. Satoh M, Zieglgänsberger W, Herz A: Supersensitivity of cortical neurons of the rat to acetylcholine and *l*-glutamate following chronic morphine treatment. Naunyn Schmiedeberg's Arch Pharmacol 293:101, 1976
176. Schulz R, Herz A: Naloxone-precipitated withdrawal reveals sensitization to neurotransmitters in morphine tolerant/dependent rats. Naunyn Schmiedeberg's Arch Pharmacol 299:95, 1977
177. Llorens C, Martres MP, Baudry M, Schwartz JC: Hypersensitivity to noradrenaline in cortex after chronic morphine: Relevance to tolerance and dependence. Nature 274:603, 1978
178. Hamburg M, Tallman JF: Chronic morphine administration increases the apparent number of alpha$_2$-adrenergic receptors in rat brain. Nature 291:493, 1981
179. Ahlijanian MK, Takemori AF: Changes in adenosine receptor sensitivity in morphine-tolerant and -dependent mice. J Pharmacol Exp Ther 236:615, 1986
180. Rabin RA, Wolfe BB, Dibner MD, et al: Effects of ethanol administration and withdrawal on neurotransmitter systems in C57 mice. J Pharmacol Exp Ther 213:491, 1980
181. Sinensky M: Homeoviscous adaptation—a homeostatic process that regulates the viscosity of membrane lipids in Escherichia coli. Proc Natl Acad Sci USA 71:522, 1974
182. Lyon RC, Goldstein DB: Changes in synaptic membrane order associated with chronic ethanol treatment in mice. Mol Pharmacol 23:86, 1983
183. Harris RA, Baxter DM, Mitchell MA, Hitzeman RJ: Physical properties and lipid composition of brain membranes from ethanol tolerant-dependent mice. Mol Pharmacol 25:401, 1984
184. Chin JH, Parsons LM, Goldstein DB: Increased cholesterol content of erythrocyte and brain membranes in ethanol tolerant mice. Biochim Biophys Acta 513:358, 1978
185. Johnson DA, Lee NM, Cooke R, Loh HH: Ethanol-induced fluidization of brain lipid bilayers: Required presence of cholesterol in membranes for expression of tolerance. Mol Pharmacol 15:739, 1979
186. Seigel S: Evidence from rats that morphine tolerance is a learned response. J Comp Physiol Psychol 89:498, 1975
187. Seigel S: Tolerance to the hyperthermic effects of morphine in the rat is a learned response. J Comp Physiol Psychol 92:1137, 1978
188. Baker TB, Tiffany ST: Morphine tolerance as habituation. Psychol Rev 92:78, 1985
189. Balster RL: Behavioral studies of tolerance and dependence. p. 403. In Seiden LS, Balster RL (eds): Behavioral Pharmacology: The Current Status. Alan R Liss, New York, 1985
190. Branch MN, Dearing ME, Dee DM: Acute and chronic effects of tetrahydrocannabinol on complex behavior of squirrel monkeys. Psychopharmacology (Berlin) 71:247, 1980

191. Slifer BL, Balster RL, Woolverton WL: Behavioral dependence produced by continuous phencyclidine infusion in rhesus monkeys. J Pharmacol Exp Ther 230:399, 1984

192. Wikler A: Dynamics of drug dependence: Implications of conditioning theory for research and treatment. Arch Gen Psychiatr 28:611, 1973

193. O'Brien CP, Testa T, O'Brien TJ, et al: Conditioned narcotic withdrawal in humans. Science 195:1000, 1977

194. Schulz R, Wuster M, Krenss H, Herz A: Selective development of tolerance without dependence in multiple opiate receptors of mouse vas deferens. Nature 285:242, 1980

195. Gmerek DE, Woods JH: Kappa receptor mediated opioid dependence in rhesus monkeys. Life Sci 39:987, 1986

11

Chemical Mutagenesis

Raymond W. Ruddon

Mutation is a fact of life, a biologic phenomenon that we all live with. Without it, evolution would not occur. In the words of Lewis Thomas: "The capacity to blunder slightly is the real marvel of DNA. Without this special attribute, we would still be anaerobic bacteria and there would be no music."[1] Against the "normal" background of spontaneous mutations occurring constantly in nature, the added burden placed on the DNA of living systems by chemical mutagens present in the environment or added by humans must be considered.

First, a few definitions should be given. A *mutation* is a heritable alteration in cellular DNA. Often, the alteration leads to change in cell phenotype. That is, the mutation leads to a change in the attributes that determine a cell's structure and metabolism. A *mutant* organism results from such a genetic alteration in a parent or *wild type* characteristic. For example, the common bacterium *Escherichia coli* can utilize galactose as a carbon source, and its wild-type state is designated Gal$^+$, whereas a mutant cell unable to utilize this sugar is called Gal$^-$. A similar terminology is used to characterize the nutritional requirements of cells for amino acids, for example, the designation Arg$^+$ or His$^+$ indicates that an organism can synthesize its own supply of arginine or histidine and does not need an exogenous supply of the amino acid in the growth medium, as do Arg$^-$ and His$^-$ mutant cell types, which require an exogenous source of the amino acids for growth. The ability of microorganisms to express a mutant phenotype of the nutritional type has become a valuable tool in the assessment of the genetic risk of various chemicals for higher organisms, including humans.

A *mutagen* is a physical or chemical agent that causes mutations to occur. Examples of the former are x-rays and ultraviolet radiation. Examples of the latter are drugs and chemicals that can directly or indirectly affect DNA structure and its function as a template for DNA replication and RNA transcription. *Mutagenesis* is the process involved in the production of a mutation and may be *spontaneous,* which means it occurs at a certain background rate in nature by usually unknown mechanisms, or *induced,* which indicates that some identifiable exogenous agent or agents are involved.

DNA: THE TARGET FOR MUTAGENIC AGENTS

The sum total of the genetic information that specifies the structure, function, and development of each individual of a species is encoded in the DNA.[2,3] The zygote of sexually reproducing organisms contains two copies of this information, one from the sperm, the other from the ovum. All the information contained in all the genes is in the form of a linear code of three-letter "words," the letters of which are the nucleotide bases adenine (A), guanine (G), cytosine (C), and thymine (T). Thus, the word CGG specifies one piece of information, CAG another, and so forth. The orderly replication of the genetic information is ensured by the mechanism of base pairing by hydrogen bond formation in the double-stranded DNA helix. Since a given base on one strand uniquely specifies its partner on the complementary strand, the letters of the coding alphabet are really the four possible base pairs, A:T, T:A, G:C, and C:G. The obligatory pairing of purine against pyrimidine is ensured by the distance between the phosphate deoxyribose backbones of the two helices; pyrimidine against pyrimidine would leave a gap between, and purine against purine would not fit the available space. The hydrogen bonding relationships are optimal for the matching of adenine to thymine and guanine to cytosine (Fig. 11-1). The process whereby the double helix unwinds during replication, each strand acting as template for the synthesis of a new complementary strand—the semiconservative replication

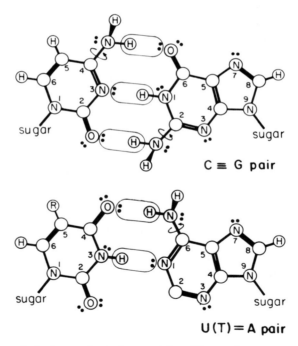

Fig. 11-1. Participation of electron pairs in base pairing. The ovals represent hydrogen bonds in a Watson-Crick structure. Solid pairs of dots represent electron pairs. Electron pairs inside ovals, when involved in hydrogen bonding, are unreactive. Others may react when in double-stranded structures if physically accessible. Note that the oxygens all have a free electron pair that is reactive both in single- and double-stranded polymers. The three exocyclic amino groups may rotate, as indicated by arrows, so that the two hydrogens are equivalent. A substituent may therefore interfere with normal hydrogen bonding if rotated into the base pairing side. (From Singer,[8] with permission.)

mechanism—guarantees that all of the genetic information will be partitioned equally to daughter cells at every cell division and thus be transmitted accurately from generation to generation.[4-7]

It is generally assumed that the target for chemical mutagenesis is DNA itself. This provides the simplest, most direct way to explain the base sequence changes that occur with many mutagens and the heritability of the genetic changes induced by such agents. Indeed, there is substantial evidence indicating that chemical mutagens or their activated metabolites can react directly with DNA to form adducts that would be expected to produce one or more possible aberrations: (1) mispairing of bases during DNA replication; (2) production of "apurinic" sites, causing "holes" in DNA, which could be filled with the wrong base; (3) stacking defects in DNA, which throw the reading frame off in such a way that during DNA replication a "frameshift" occurs by adding an extra base.

In this chapter we will examine these reactions and their possible biologic effects. We will also consider some cellular mechanisms that are involved in the maintenance of the correct sequence of bases, namely, the DNA repair enzymes that continually "edit" the cell's complement of DNA to guard against errors in the genome. A point to keep in mind is that the spontaneous mutation rate is in the range of 10^{-7} to 10^{-9} for prokaryotes and 10^{-10} to 10^{-12} for eukaryotes, meaning that mistakes in DNA replication occur so rarely that there is a 1 in 10 million or less chance that a gene will mutate when a cell divides. Thus, DNA replication in cells must be a highly accurate process under normal background conditions. A mutagen may increase the spontaneous rate by a factor of 10 to 1,000, depending on how powerful it is.

Reaction Sites in DNA

In double helical DNA, certain reaction sites appear to be particularly available for reaction with chemical mutagens. Particularly favored reaction targets appear to be guanine bases in DNA, which are attacked by a variety of alkylating chemicals (Table 11-1). A large number of mutagens are alkylating agents although they differ widely in their mutagenicity. Alkylating agents generate electrophiles, which can react with available nucleophilic (electron-rich) sites in cells. Such reactions are thought to be the ones that produce mutation. In the stacked bases of double helical DNA, the unshared electrons of the N-7 nitrogen atom in guanine are sterically available and appear to produce the greatest amount of reaction with alkylating mutagens. Other biologically significant adducts include the N-1 and N-3 adducts of adenine, the N-3 and O^6 adducts of guanine, and the diesters formed with the phosphate backbone of DNA. Structures of some of the reaction products of mutagenic alkylating agents are shown in Figure 11-2. It should be pointed out that not all these reactions have the same propensity to cause mutagenic events. Many of these adducts are removed by repair enzymes before harm can be done (see below), and certain adducts may be more easily removed than others. For example, in some cell types N-7 adducts appear to be removed more readily than O^6 adducts, and the latter, though quantitatively a minor reaction product, may be potentially more damaging. Reaction with phosphate groups could cause mutations by destabilizing the DNA backbone and producing strand breakage.

It is interesting that the reactivity of various alkylating mutagens with oxygen atoms in the bases of double-stranded DNA correlates with their mutagenicity (e.g., ethylnitrosourea = ethylnitrosoguanidine > methylnitrosourea = methylnitrosoguanidine > ethyl methanesulfonate > methyl methanesulfonate > diethyl sulfate > dimethyl sulfate).[8]

Table 11-1. Alkylation of Double-Stranded Nucleic Acids in Vitro

Alkylation Site	Percent of Total Alkylation					
	Me_2SO_4	MeMS	MeNU	Et_2SO_4	EtMS	EtNU
Adenine						
N-1	1.9	3.8	1.3	2.0	1.7	0.2
N-3	18.0	10.4	9.0	10.0	4.0	4.0
N-7	1.9	(1.8)	1.7	1.5	1.1	0.3
Guanine						
N-3	11.0	(0.6)	0.8	0.9	0.9	0.6
O^6	0.2	(0.3)	6.3	0.2	2.0	7.8
N-7	74.0	83.0	67.0	67.0	65.0	11.5
Thymine						
O^2			0.11	nd	nd	7.4
N-3			0.3	nd	nd	0.8
O^4			0.4	nd	nd	2.5
Cytosine						
O^2	(nd)	(nd)	0.1	nd	nd	3.5
N-3	(<2)	(<1)	0.6	0.7	0.6	0.2
Phosphodiester bonds		0.8	17.0	16.0	13.0	57.0

Analyses were from experiments using DNA from salmon sperm, calf thymus, salmon testes, rat liver and brain, human fibroblasts, and HeLa cells. Me_2SO_4 is dimethyl sulfate; MeMS is methyl methanesulfonate; MeNU is methylnitrosourea; Et analogs are the equivalent ethyl derivatives; nd = not detectable.
(From Singer,[8] with permission.)

Methylating agents are 15 to 20 times more efficient in reacting with nucleic acids in vitro and in vivo than are ethylating agents under the same reaction conditions, but the mutagenicity of ethylating agents is usually higher.

Among the reactive groups in DNA bases are a number of sites that are involved directly or indirectly with base-base hydrogen bond formation in double-stranded DNA (Fig. 11-1). For example, the O^6 of guanine and the N-1 of adenine are involved in base pairing, and they also have available electrons and are sites of adduct formation with mutagenic agents. Other sites of adduct formation, such as N-7 of guanine and N-3 of guanine and adenine, although not directly involved in hydrogen bond formation, can change the tautomeric equilibrium of the bases and also alter the base pairing patterns of purine-pyrimidine dimers. The polycyclic aromatic hydrocarbons, which have both mutagenic and carcinogenic activity, form adducts with the 2-amino groups of guanine, another site involved in base pairing.

The chemical structures of some mutagenic alkylating agents are shown in Figure 11-3. Among these are several drugs used in cancer chemotherapy, including the nitrogen mustards and certain nitrosourea compounds. The DNA adducts formed by reaction of cells in vitro and in vivo with nitrogen mustard are N-7 of guanine, N-1 of adenine, and N-3 of cytosine.[9] The widely used anticancer drug 1,3-bis-(2-chloroethyl)-1-nitrosourea (BCNU) has been shown to form adducts with the N-3 of cytosine and the 4-amino group of cytosine as well as with the N-7 of guanine.[10] As might be predicted, these agents can be both mutagenic and carcinogenic in humans, and the evidence for their carcinogenicity will be discussed in Chapter 12. Chloroethylene oxide is a highly mutagenic metabolite of vinyl chloride and is a carcinogen in humans,[11] causing hemangiosarcoma, a rare form of liver cancer. As in other epoxides, the ring opens, and the product, chloroacetaldehyde, reacts with polynucleotides to form cyclic etheno derivatives of guanine, adenine, and cytosine.[12]

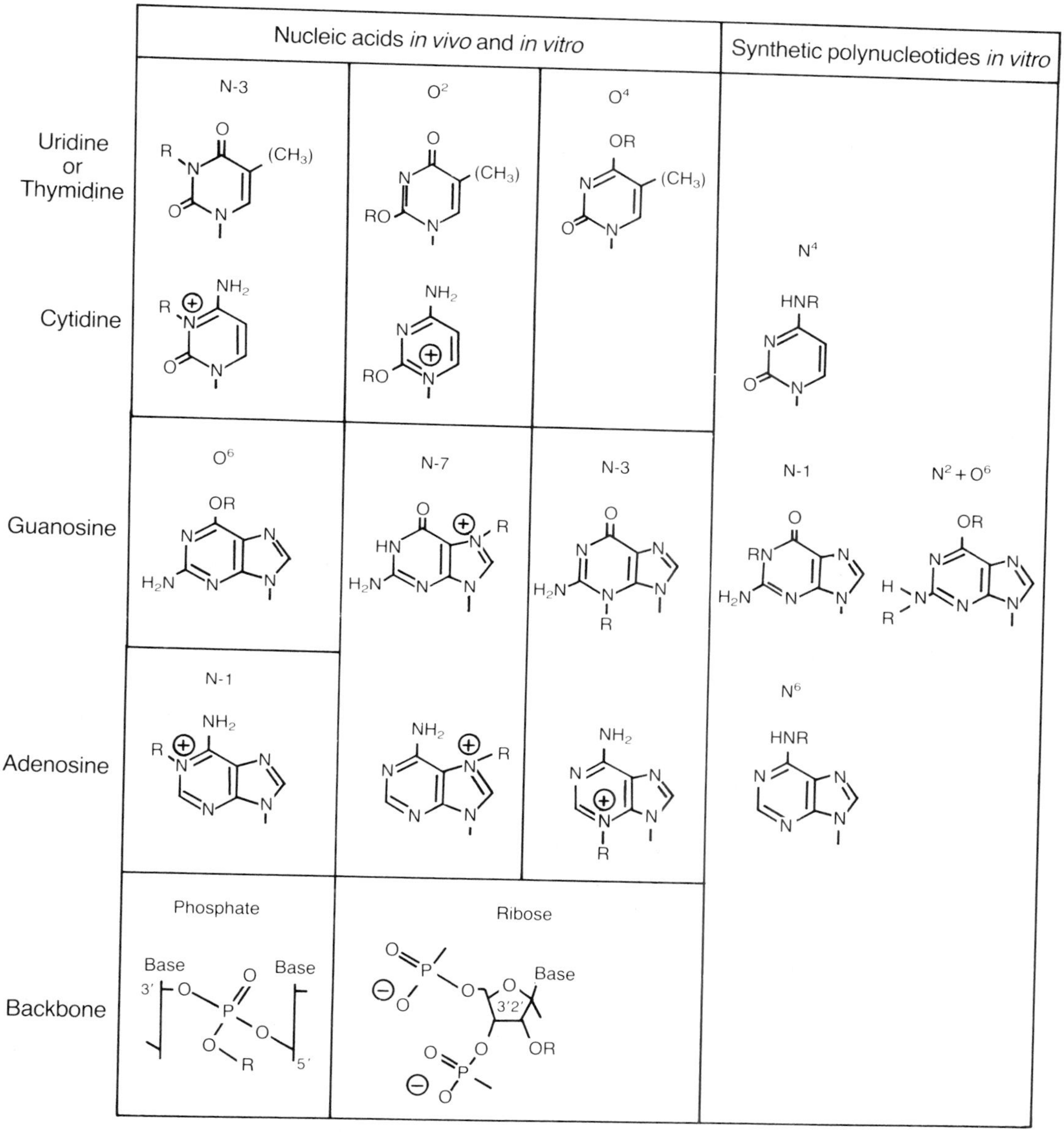

Fig. 11-2. Sites of reaction of mutagenic alkylating agents with nucleic acids or polynucleotides in neutral aqueous solution. All derivatives shown are formed with ethyl and methyl nitrosoureas and nitrosoguanidines. The derivatives on the right side have been found only after reaction with synthetic polynucleotides. (From Singer,[8] with permission.)

Types of Damage to DNA

Several potentially mutagenic alterations of DNA can occur as a result of interaction of living cells with physical or chemical agents.

1. *Alteration of a purine or pyrimidine base by direct adduct formation:* This is perhaps

Alkyl Sulfates

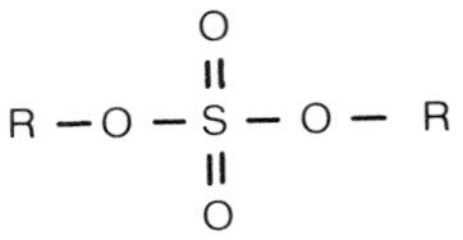

$$R - O - \overset{\overset{O}{\|}}{\underset{\underset{O}{\|}}{S}} - O - R$$

Dialkyl Sulfates (Me_2SO_4, Et_2SO_4)

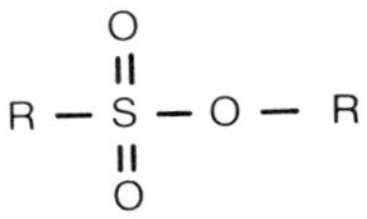

$$R - \overset{\overset{O}{\|}}{\underset{\underset{O}{\|}}{S}} - O - R$$

Alkyl Alkane Sulfonates (MeMS, EtMS, EtES)

N-Nitroso Compounds

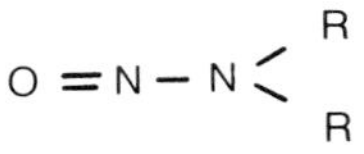

$$O = N - N \underset{R}{\overset{R}{<}}$$

Dialkyl Nitrosamines (DMNA, DENA)

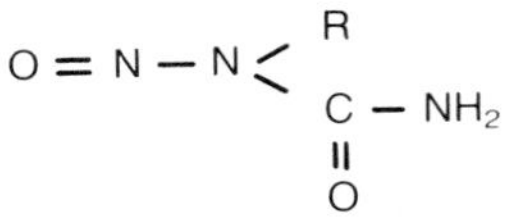

$$O = N - N \overset{R}{\underset{\underset{\underset{O}{\|}}{C - NH_2}}{<}}$$

N-Nitrosoureas (MeNU, EtNU)

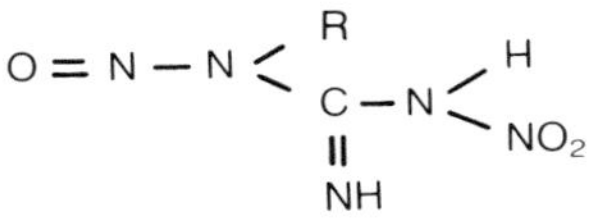

$$O = N - N \overset{R}{\underset{\underset{\underset{NH}{\|}}{C - N \overset{H}{\underset{NO_2}{<}}}}{<}}$$

N-Alkyl-N′-Nitro-N-Nitrosoguanidine (MNNG)

Cyclic Compounds

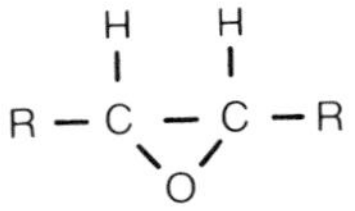

$$R - \overset{H}{\underset{}{C}} \overset{}{\underset{O}{-}} \overset{H}{\underset{}{C}} - R$$

Epoxides (Chloroethylene Oxide, Ethylene Oxide)

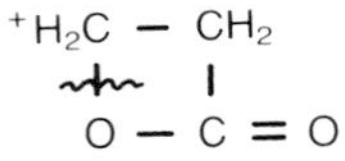

$$^+H_2C - CH_2$$
$$O - C = O$$

Lactones (β-Propiolactone)

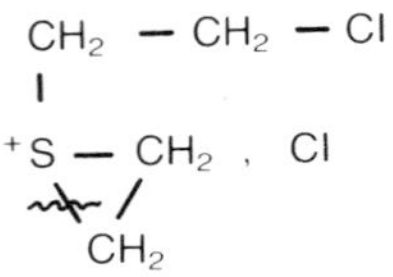

$$CH_2 - CH_2 - Cl$$
$$^+S - CH_2 \quad , \quad Cl$$
$$CH_2$$

S-Mustards (Mustard Gas)

$$CH_2 - CH_2 - Cl$$
$$R - ^+N - CH_2 \quad , \quad Cl$$
$$CH_2$$

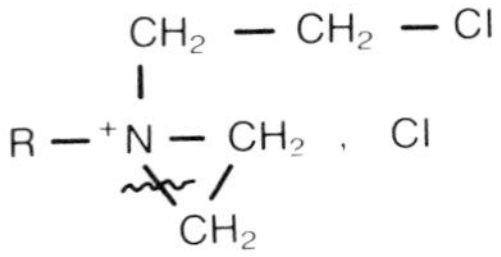

N-Mustards (HN-2)

the most obvious way in which chemical mutagens alter DNA, and we have discussed some of the favored reaction sites above. The biologic consequences of such adduct formation will be discussed below.

2. *Loss of a purine or pyrimidine base:* The loss of bases, particularly purines, from DNA occurs spontaneously at a rather high rate. The rate of spontaneous depurination is approximately 1 purine molecule removed per 300 purine base molecules per day at pH 7 and 37°C, which amounts to about 10^4 purines per day in a mammalian cell.[13] This depurination event results from destabilization and hydrolysis of the *N*-glycosyl bond between deoxyribose and the base. The frequency of base loss can be increased by base modifications similar to those described above. Alkylation of DNA bases weakens the *N*-glycosidic bond and favors hydrolysis. Certain enzymes called DNA glycosylases can also remove modified DNA bases. These *N*-glycosylases occur both in bacteria and in mammalian cells, and they appear to be specific in that each enzyme recognizes a limited range of base modifications.[14]

3. *Deamination:* Spontaneous deamination of cytosine to uracil or of adenine to hypoxanthine occurs in living cells. These events appear to be rather rare, particularly the spontaneous deamination of adenine to hypoxanthine. However, certain agents, such as nitrous acid, increase the frequency of deamination significantly. Nitrous acid converts amino groups in cytosine and adenine to keto groups by oxidative deamination. This modification results in a base alteration that will produce a coding error (see below). For this reason nitrous acid is a powerful mutagen.

4. *Single-strand breaks:* Peroxides and chemicals that can generate oxygen radicals, such as the drug bleomycin, can cause single-strand breaks in the DNA backbone. Ionizing radiation produces DNA strand breaks by intracellular production of free radicals (e.g., hydroxyl radicals) that can attack phosphodiester bonds.

5. *Double-strand breaks:* When DNA strand breakage occurs on opposite strands of DNA within a distance of a few base pairs, a double-strand break can result, the possible consequence of which is the loss of a whole piece of DNA. Double-strand breaks can occur after exposure of cells to highly ionizing radiation such as x-rays or γ-rays.

6. *Cross-linking:* Bifunctional alkylating agents, such as the anticancer drugs nitrogen mustard and the nitrosoureas, can form covalent bonds between a base in one strand of DNA and another base in the same strand (intramolecular) or in the complementary strand (intermolecular)[15] (Fig. 11-4). This cross-linking can prevent strand separation during DNA replication.

DNA Repair

Not all the damage done to DNA in cells or whole organisms exposed to DNA-damaging agents is translated into a biologically destructive event. In fact, most DNA "lesions" or modifications induced by chemical agents are quickly repaired by a variety of editing enzymes called repair enzymes. When the lesions cannot be repaired, as in repair enzyme-

←

Fig. 11-3. Structural formulas and examples of various types of alkylating mutagens. With the exception of dialkyl nitrosamines, all are direct-acting. The lactones and mustard-type agents form unstable cyclic structures (indicated by the wavy line), which open upon reaction with a nucleophile. (Adapted from Singer,[8] with permission.)

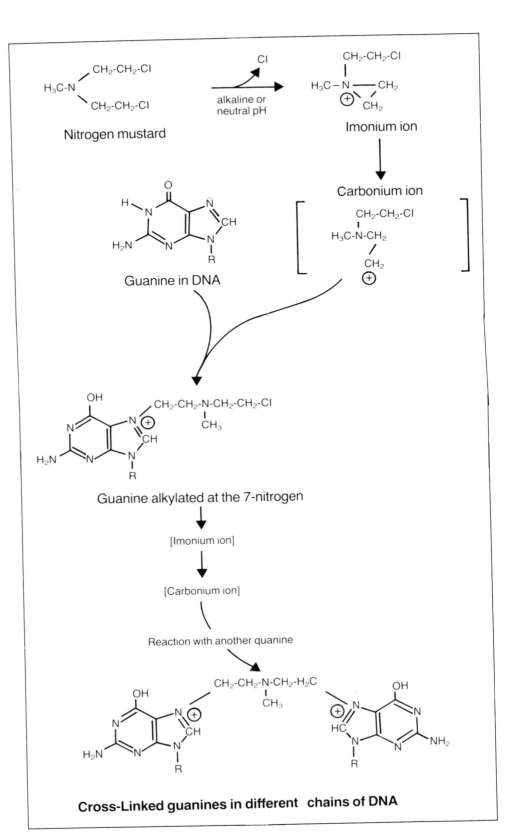

Nitrogen mustard

alkaline or neutral pH

Imonium ion

Carbonium ion

Guanine in DNA

Guanine alkylated at the 7-nitrogen

[Imonium ion]

[Carbonium ion]

Reaction with another quanine

Cross-Linked guanines in different chains of DNA

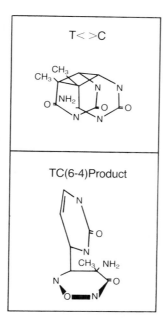

Fig. 11-5. Cyclobutane pyrimidine dimer and (6-4) thymidine-cytosine (TC), photoproducts. (From Haseltine,[19] with permission.)

deficient cells, or when the rate of cell division does not allow time for repair to be completed before DNA replication occurs, there is a much higher chance of mutation.

The existence of a DNA repair system was first observed in *E. coli* that were selected for resistance to the lethal effects of ultraviolet (UV) light.[16–18] Exposure to UV light induces two kinds of lesions in DNA, a cyclobutane pyrimidine dimer and a so-called 6-4 thymidine-cytosine (TC) dimer formed between the 6 position of a 5′-pyrimidine and the 4 position of another pyrimidine located at the 3′ position of the first[19] (Fig. 11-5). Both these reactions produce DNA cross-links that may be repaired in two ways: (1) by exposure of bacterial cells to intense visible light, which results in photoreactivation repair of cyclobutane pyrimidine dimers; and (2) by an enzymatic process called *excision repair,* which can remove the 6-4 TC products as well as cyclobutane dimers. Since strains of *E. coli* lacking excision repair systems are very sensitive to the mutagenic effects of UV light, it is clear that the excision repair system is important for removal of these pre-mutagenic lesions in DNA.[19] It is now known that DNA structural defects other than pyrimidine dimers, such as alkylated bases, can also be repaired by excision repair systems in *E. coli,* as well as in cells from higher organisms, including humans, that possess similar repair systems. Cells taken from individuals with genetically determined defects in their

←

Fig. 11-4. The mechanism by which nitrogen mustard becomes covalently bonded to the N-7 atoms of two guanines. In solution, the drug forms a reactive cyclic intermediate, which reacts with the N-7 of a guanine residue in DNA to form a covalent linkage. The second arm can then cyclize and react with nucleophilic groups such as a second guanine moiety in an opposite DNA strand or in the same strand. (From Pratt et al.,[15] with permission.)

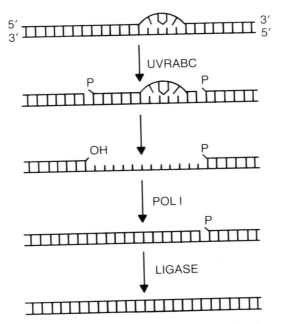

Fig. 11-6. Mechanism of incision at DNA damage sites by *uvr*ABC endonucleases of *E. coli*. (From Haseltine,[19] with permission.)

DNA repair systems lack the ability to excise premutagenic lesions from their DNA, and these individuals have a high incidence of neoplastic diseases (see Ch. 12).

The mechanisms of excision repair are somewhat more complicated than originally envisaged, and a schematic model is presented in Figure 11-6. Much of the evidence for this is based on studies of the *uvr*A, *uvr*B, and *uvr*C nuclease activities in *E. coli*.[20] Incision via a specific endonuclease occurs on both sides of the damaged site in DNA, seven nucleotides toward the 5′ end from the lesion and three nucleotides toward the 3′ end from the damage site (in this example, a dimer). A fragment of 12 nucleotides containing the damaged site is removed. A DNA polymerase (Pol 1) then fills in the gap left by the excised nucleotides, and a DNA ligase completes the resealing by forming the final phosphodiester bond. As discussed in Chapter 9, two excision repair pathways have been identified in mammalian cells (see Fig. 9-25). Most drug-induced and x-ray-induced damage is repaired by the so-called short patch repair mechanism, which is similar to the repair mechanism in *E. coli*. In mammalian cells UV light-induced dimers are repaired by a "long patch" repair system, in which 100 or more nucleotides are excised.

Unfortunately, not all DNA repair is error-free (i.e., reproduces the original DNA base sequence). If DNA is modified by interaction with very bulky chemical groups or if lesions are left unrepaired, as may happen in cells undergoing rapid cell division, an error can occur in the base sequence. In bacteria, a so-called SOS repair system is induced by bulky lesions in DNA. This is a "bypass" system, which allows DNA chain growth across damaged segments at the cost of fidelity of replication. Thus, it is an error-prone process in that random base insertion may occur at the site or sites being bypassed. This, of course, would result in a mutation and in a potentially lethal event. Similarly, if cells are rapidly replicating, they may not have time to repair their DNA before replication but may have to repair DNA after replication; this is called *postreplication repair*. The fidelity of the postreplication repair system is less than that of the excision repair system, and the likelihood of introducing genetic error is higher. Maher and McCormick[21] have shown that the ultimate biologic consequences of lesions introduced in DNA by UV light or various chemical agents (e.g., aromatic amines, polycyclic aromatic hydrocarbons, or nitrosoureas) depend on the rate of excision repair and the time available before the onset of DNA replication. They compared the amount of mutagenesis induced in cell cycle phase-synchronized cultures of fibroblasts from patients with xeroderma pigmentosum (XP), who have a defective excision repair process, and in synchronized cultures of normal human diploid fibroblasts. In both cases the cells were exposed to the mutagenic agents at various times before the DNA synthetic phase. It was demonstrated that the number of mutations was severalfold greater in normal fibroblasts when the cells were exposed to UV light or chemical mutagen just prior to the onset of the DNA synthetic phase rather than 18 hours earlier. The frequency of mutations induced in XP cells was the same whether they were treated just before the DNA synthetic (S) phase or 18 hours earlier because these cells have a repair defect that does not allow removal of the damaged regions even if the time for repair is increased. Interestingly, it was also observed that the activity of excision repair processes in cultured normal fibroblasts decreased the frequency of malignant transformation to tumor-producing cells after UV irradiation. Repair-deficient XP cells had a greater propensity to undergo malignant transformation after UV treatment than did normal fibroblasts.

TYPES OF CHEMICAL MUTAGENS AND MECHANISMS OF CHEMICAL MUTAGENESIS

Various types of chemical mutagens and the alterations in DNA base sequence that they produce are shown in Table 11-2. The production of a mutant requires a change in DNA base sequence, and this can occur by a variety of mechanisms.

Table 11-2. Examples of Mutagenic Agents

Type of Mutagen	Mechanism	Examples	Type of Base Changes in DNA
Alkylating agent	Forms covalent bonds with purine and pyrimidine ring nitrogens or hydroxyl groups; creation of apurinic sites	Alkyl alkanesulfonates, nitrosoureas, nitrogen mustard, nitrosoguanidine	GC → AT transitions, GC → CG, and GC → TA transversions
Deaminating agent	Deaminates adenine to hypoxanthine and cytosine to uracil	Nitrous acid	GC → AT and AT → GC transitions
Base analog	Substitutes for a normal purine or pyrimidine during DNA replication	2-Aminopurine	AT → GC transitions
Intercalating agent	Addition or deletion of base pairs	Acridines, anthracyclines	Shift in DNA reading frame
Agents that cause DNA strand breakage	Unequal crossover; chromosome translocations	Ionizing radiation, certain alkylating agents	Single or multiple base changes

Direct Modification of a Base

Examples of the direct modification of a base are (1) deamination of adenine or cytosine by nitrous acid as described above; (2) reactions that cause a shift in the tautomeric equilibrium of a base; and (3) the alkylation of bases. These events can lead to base pair change by incorporation of the wrong base opposite the modified site during DNA replication. A base change that does not alter the purine-pyrimidine orientation in the daughter DNA strands is called a base *transition* [e.g., guanine-cytosine → adenine-thymine (G:C → A:T)]. When base modification produces a change in purine-pyrimidine orientation in the daughter strands [e.g., guanine-cytosine → thymine-adenine (G:C → T:A)], it is called a base *transversion*. Examples of the genetic consequences of direct base modification are given below.

The deaminating action of nitrous acid is illustrated in Figure 11-7. Nitrous acid is a nonspecific deaminating agent; it attacks all the bases except thymine, which has no amino group. Deamination of adenine forms hypoxanthine, which has the base pairing properties of guanine; the end result is, therefore, a transition of the A:T → G:C type. Nitrous acid also deaminates cytosine to uracil, which behaves like thymine, so the result is a transition of the reverse kind, G:C → A:T. Finally, it deaminates guanine to xanthine, but xanthine apparently acts like guanine in base pairing, so no mutation results.

That the mutagenic action of HNO_2 is due almost entirely to the postulated transitions C → T and A → G is indicated by extensive studies with tobacco mosaic virus (TMV),[22] summarized in Table 11-3. Nineteen different amino acid replacements were observed in the TMV protein after mutagenic treatment with HNO_2. Many of these occurred repeatedly, so that altogether 63 occurrences were identified. The table shows that when the codons for the original amino acid and the replacement amino acids are considered, all but a few of the observations are accounted for by C → U or A → G transitions. In only three instances, representing only one or two occurrences each, was it impossible to account for the result by the postulated transitions, and those may well have been spontaneous rather than mutagen-induced events. Significantly, there was not a single instance suggesting the modification of a uracil residue, in agreement with the chemical impossibility of deaminating uracil.

Among other direct base-modifying mutagenic agents are those that cause a tautomeric shift such that a mispairing event is favored. Hydroxylamine, methoxyamine, and hydrazine form reaction products of the 4-amino group of cytosine, producing a shift in the tautomeric equilibrium of the base that causes it to mispair.[8]

Alkylating agents, such as ethyl methanesulfonate (EMS) and the nitrogen mustards, can carry out electrophilic attack on various nucleophilic functional groups (amino, carboxyl, sulfhydryl, phosphate) in proteins and nucleic acids. The mutagenicity of these compounds is largely attributable to alkylation of nucleophilic sites in DNA bases, including the N-7 and O^6 of guanine, the N-1 and N-3 of adenine, and the N-3 of cytosine. It is not clear which of these reactions is the most mutagenic, but it is likely that the relative ability of these adducts to be removed by repair systems is what determines their mutagenic activity in intact cells. There is some evidence that ethylated base derivatives are poorer substrates for repair in some cell types than are methylated bases.[23] Also, O^6 alkylations of guanine are repaired less well than N-7 alkylations of guanine, and O^6 alkylations correlate better with mutagenic and carcinogenic effects.[24]

Addition of an alkyl group to a purine base, for example to the N-7 of guanine, has two effects, both of which result from the formation of a quaternary form of the ring nitrogen.

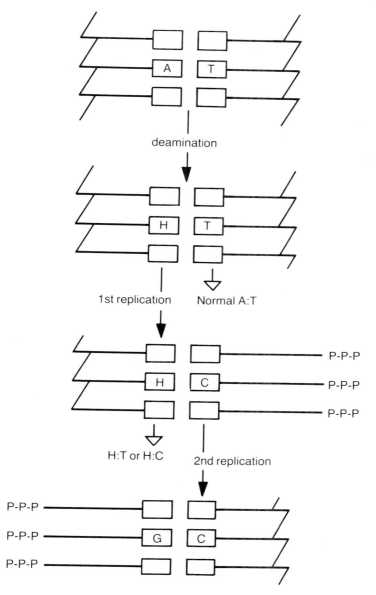

Fig. 11-7. Mechanism of a mutagenic transformation by deamination. Adenine is deaminated to hypoxanthine, which pairs like guanine. The result is a mutagenic transition, A:T → G:C.

In the ionized form the N-7 alkylated guanine can pair with thymine instead of cytosine, producing a C:C → A:T base pair transition[25] (Fig. 11-8). O[6]-Alkylated guanine has also been shown to form a hydrogen bonded mispair with thymine during DNA replication.[26] Interestingly, the amount of 7-methylguanine adducts increase in the livers of rats as they age, suggesting that endogenous methylation of DNA over time could contribute to aging and cancer induction.[27] In addition, aklylated guanine has a labile *N*-glycosidic bond, which hydrolyzes readily to yield a depurinated site. These sites are potentially repairable

Table 11-3. Mutagenic Action of Nitrous Acid on Tobacco Mosaic Virus RNA

Amino Acid Replacement	No. of Occurrences	Probable Codon Alteration	Base Alteration
Thr → Ala	2	AC(x) → GC(x)	A → G
Thr → Ile	10	AC(Py) → AU(Py)	C → U
Thr → Met	3	AC(Pu) → AU(Pu)	C → U
Ser → Phe	8	UC(x) → UU(Py)	C → U
Ser → Leu	2	UC(x) → UU(Pu)	C → U
Asn → Ser	6	AA(Py) → AG(Py)	A → G
Asp → Gly	2	GA(Py) → GG(x)	A → G
Asp → Ala	4	GA(Py) → GC(x)	A → C
Ile → Val	5	AU(Py) → GU(x)	A → G
Ile → Met	1	AU(Py) → AU(Pu)	Py → Pu
Pro → Ser	3	CC(x) → UC(x)	C → U
Pro → Leu	6	CC(x) → CU(x)	C → U
Leu → Phe	1	CU(Py) → UU(Py)	C → U
Gln → Val	2	CA(Pu) → GU(x)	?
Gln → Arg	1	CA(Pu) → CG(x)	A → G
Glu → Gly	2	GA(Pu) → GG(x)	A → G
Arg → Gly	3	AG(Pu) → GG(x)	A → G
Arg → Lys	1	AG(Pu) → AA(x) *or*	G → A *or*
		CG(x) → AA(x)	?
Val → Met	1	GU(x) → AU(Pu)	G → A

The observed amino acid replacements in TMV protein are interpreted in terms of the most probable single-base alterations from the genetic code. The triplet codons are read from 5' at left to 3' at right. Degeneracy in the 3' position is indicated by (x) = any base, (Pu) = ether purine, (Py) = either pyrimidine.
(Modified from Siegel,[22] with permission.)

by an apurinic acid (AP) endonuclease, but replication sometimes precedes this repair. In this case, any base can be converted, after a second round of replication, to an A:T, C:G, or T:A pair, the latter two being base transversions. There appears to be a strong preference for insertion of adenine at apurinic sites in bacteria, and G:C → T:A and A:T → T:A transversions frequently occur at such sites.[28]

N-Methyl-*N'*-nitro-*N*-nitrosoguanidine (MNNG) is a powerful mutagen and one that is often used to produce mutations of experimental interest in bacteria and in mammalian cells in culture. MNNG appears to act by alkylation of DNA bases, such as the amino groups of adenine, and it can be highly mutagenic at a concentration that is not lethal. From an experimental point of view MNNG has the advantage that mutants are easily induced, but one problem with it is that it tends to induce multiple mutations. For example, an MNNG-induced *gal⁻* mutant of *E. coli* may also be *pro⁻*. The mutations tend to be clustered in genes that are close together in the genetic map, possibly because the drug-induced lesions are clustered in the region of DNA that was transversed by the replication fork during exposure to the mutagen.[13] The high mutagenicity of MNNG seems to involve the generation of apurinic sites, since *E. coli* lacking AP endonuclease, the first step in repair of apurinic sites, are more susceptible to the mutagenic effects of MNNG.[29]

Base Analog Incorporation

Certain mutagens can alter the fidelity of DNA replication by becoming incorporated into the base sequence. The thymine analog 5-bromouracil (BU) is a typical example. After being first converted metabolically to the deoxyribose triphosphate, BU is incorporated extensively into DNA in place of thymine by entering the nascent DNA strand opposite adenine on the old strand. The extent of this replacement in some experiments has been quite remarkable, up to about one-half the total number of thymine residues.

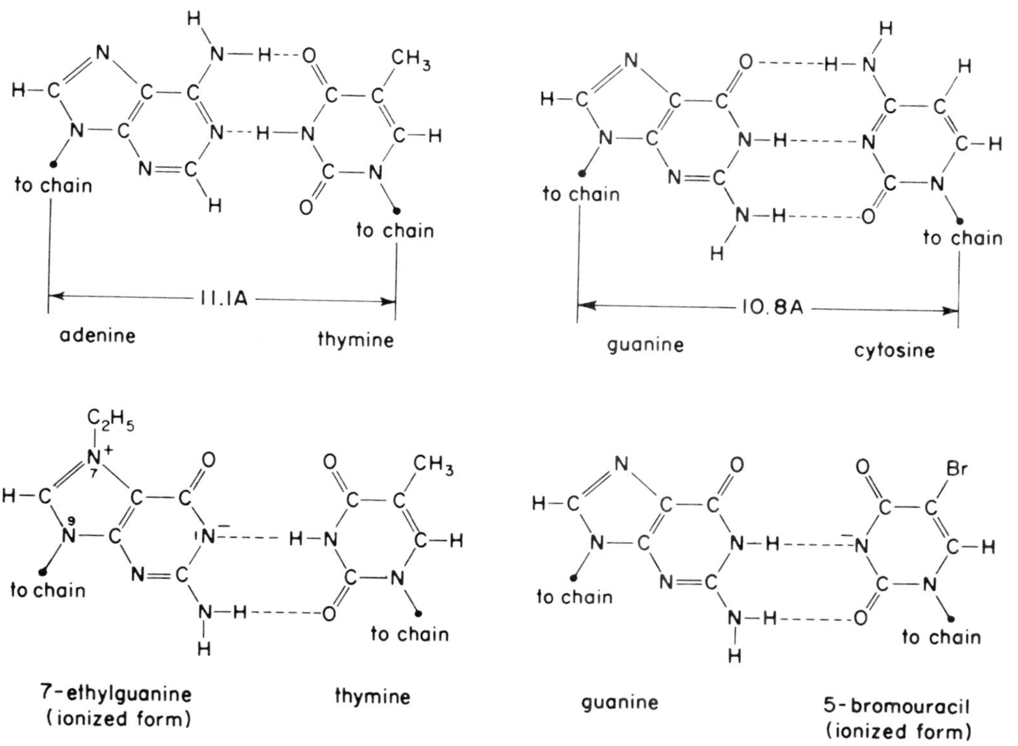

Fig. 11-8. Abnormal base pairing of alkylated guanine and 5-bromouracil. Alkylation of guanine at position 7 permits ionized form to pair with thymine; ionization of 5-bromouracil permits pairing with guanine. All hydrogen bond distances are 2.8 to 3.0 Å. (Modified from Strauss,[25] with permission.)

Obviously, the presence of BU instead of thymine does not seriously affect DNA function—either replication or transcription—since the organisms are viable and continue to grow and divide, either in normal medium or in the continued presence of BU. Thus, the A:BU pair functions like the A:T pair. At replication, BU specifies an incoming adenine on the nascent strand; at transcription, BU specifies adenine on the nascent messenger RNA.

Errors of incorporation or of replication are probably attributable to the ionized form of BU, which undergoes base pairing as though it were cytosine (Fig. 11-8). This results from loss of a proton at N-1, so that a hydrogen bond can be formed with the H atom at N-1 of guanine. When it is being incorporated, BU may occasionally undergo this erroneous base pairing and thus enter opposite guanine, as illustrated in the first replication in Figure 11-9. At subsequent replications this BU might behave "normally," as though it were thymine, and thus the end result would be a G:C → A:T transition. Since it has been shown that BU is more likely to be ionized when it is free (as the deoxynucleoside triphosphate) than after its polymerization into DNA, errors of incorporation (rather than of replication) are probably the principal mechanism of BU mutagenesis.[30] Alternatively, as shown at the third replication in Figure 11-9, a BU molecule incorporated "correctly" in place of thymine, might behave as as though it were cytosine, pairing with an incoming guanine. Then the transition A:T → G:C will be the end result. The patterns of mutation

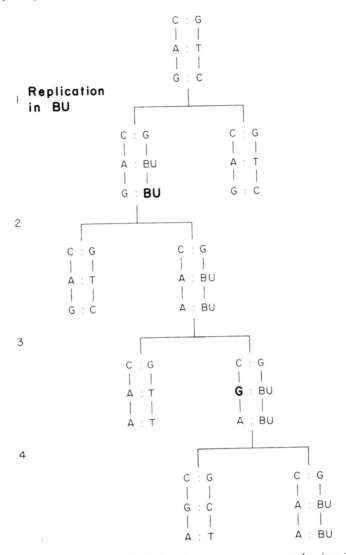

Fig. 11-9. Mutagenesis by 5-bromouracil (BU). The most common mechanism is shown at replication 1; BU enters opposite guanine, and the end result is a G:C → A:T transition. If BU that has already been incorporated pairs with an incoming guanine molecule (as at replication 3), an A:T → G:C transition results.

induction and reversion observed in phage conform to these expectations; transitions of the G:C → A:T type are most frequent, but A:T → G:C transitions also occur.[31] As long as the strand containing BU persists, occasional mutations would be expected to occur at any subsequent replication (i.e., whenever an incoming guanine is paired against BU). This phenomenon has been observed in phage as a peculiar "mottling" of the plaques caused by new mutations that arise after plaque formation has been initiated by phenotypically wild-type phage.

The mechanisms are apparently similar for all the base analogs that can be incorporated.

Purines replace purines and pyrimidines replace pyrimidines, so that transitions always result. The essential requirement is a certain ambiguity of structure with respect to those features that distinguish the normal purines or pyrimidines from each other. Thus, for example, 2-aminopurine resembles guanine at the 2-position but lacks the keto group at the 6-position. It seems to induce transitions in both directions.[4]

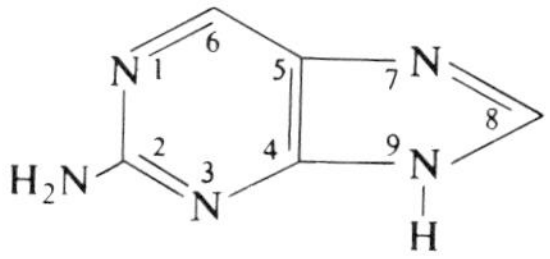

2-Aminopurine 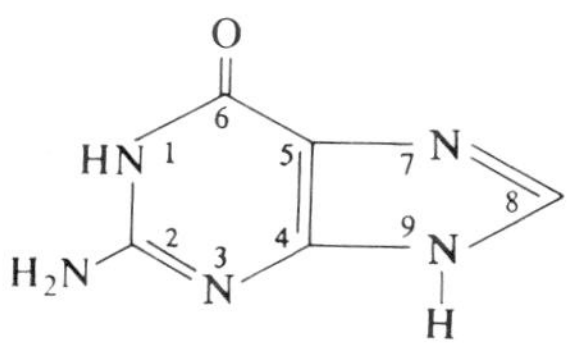   Guanine

A potential base-analog mutagen that may be of some significance in humans is caffeine.[32,33] This is a fully methylated purine. Because it is substituted in the 7-position, it cannot form a stable bond to deoxyribose at the 9-position and is therefore not incorporated into DNA. Because it is known to inhibit some enzymes of purine metabolism, the suggestion has been made that it alters the normal base ratios in the DNA precursor pool, thereby causing errors of base pairing. There is also evidence that caffeine greatly enhances the rate of UV-induced mutation by impairing the operation of the normal repair mechanisms for excising and replacing radiation-damaged segments of DNA.[34]

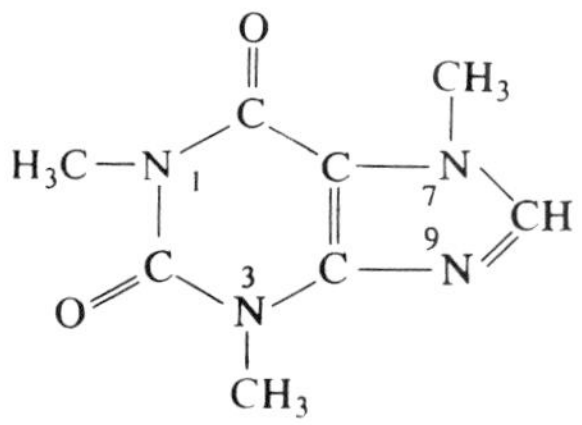

Caffeine (1,3,7-trimethylxanthine)

Many drugs of the base analog type have been employed in cancer chemotherapy in order to produce lethal damage in tumors in which a high percentage of the cells are engaged in DNA synthesis. Some also act as radiation sensitizers, increasing the killing effect of any given x-ray dose.[35] The lethal effect of x-irradiation is dependent upon the G:C content of the DNA. This is in contrast to ultraviolet irradiation, which is most effective upon DNA with high A:T content and which acts by dimerization of adjacent thymine residues. Alkylating agents, which act preferentially upon G:C pairs, have long been recognized to be "radiomimetic" in their actions. Bromouracil and other halogenated uracil compounds that are incorporated into DNA are good x-ray sensitizers.

Intercalation

Agents such as proflavin and acridine yellow are three-ringed planar structures whose dimensions are approximately the same as a purine-pyrimidine base pair. These agents are able to "interdigitate" themselves between the stacked bases in double helical DNA and produce a spatial distortion of the helix. This process is called *intercalation* (Fig. 11-

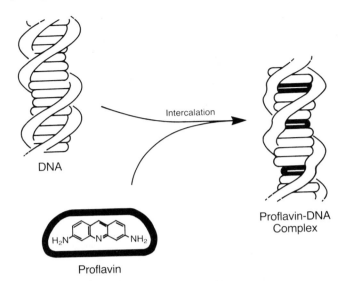

Fig. 11-10. Diagrammatic model of the intercalation of proflavin into double helical DNA. Local distortion of the helix occurs where the stacked base pairs are moved apart by the intercalating agent (dark lines).

10). The intercalation of an acridine-like molecule into DNA causes adjacent base pairs

to move apart by a distance similar to the space occupied by one base pair. When DNA containing an intercalating agent is replicated, additional bases may be inserted into the sequence. Addition of a single base is the usual result although occasionally addition of more than one base may occur. Deletion of bases may also occur, but this is far less common. Addition or deletion of bases alters the whole reading frame of DNA and can induce what are called *frame shift mutations* (see below).

TYPES OF MUTATIONS

Much of the fundamental work that led to our present understanding of the molecular basis of mutagenesis was done with mutants of bacteriophage T4 of *E. coli,* known as rII mutants.[36,37] These are characterized by an abnormal plaque morphology (large plaques with very sharp edges, caused by unusually rapid lysis) and by their inability to grow on bacterial strain K although they grow well on strain B. Thus, mutants are readily recognized by eye from among thousands of wild-type plaques, and wild-type revertants are efficiently selected by growth on bacteria of strain K. The rII mutants arise by a genetic change occurring anywhere within a particular region of the phage genome, designated

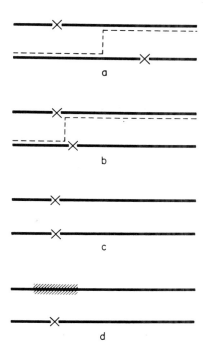

Fig. 11-11. Recombination of mutants defective at different sites. Each diagram represents phage DNA from two strains. Mutant sites are indicated by X. Broken line represents replication or breakage and reunion. Hatched segment is a deletion. (a) Wild-type recombinant is possible because mutations are at different sites. (b) Wild-type recombinant is possible, but will occur less frequently than in a (c & d). Wild-type recombinants impossible because mutations or deletions are at identical sites.

the rII gene. The rII gene directs the synthesis of two proteins. The term *cistron,* in general use to describe the portion of a gene that codes for a single protein, originated in these investigations with rII mutants. It was found that certain pairs of mutants would grow on *E. coli* K if inoculated together but not separately. This phenomenon of complementation obviously depended upon each strain producing a normal gene product that could be used by the other. The test for this property was called a *cis-trans* test, whence the term *cistron.*

The exact location of a given mutation within the gene can be established by the method of recombination. Phage recombination results from breakage and reunion of DNA in two different phage particles. Two mutant strains of phage are inoculated together into a culture of *E. coli* B. The progeny, after lysis of the bacteria, are tested by spreading on strain K. Some wild-type plaques result, and their frequency is determined. If the experiment is done with two mutant strains thought to be different but in fact identical, then very few wild-type plaques representing spontaneous back mutations are found.

As illustrated in Figure 11-11, a wild-type recombinant can arise only if the damaged portions of the genomes do not overlap. If the probability of breakage is constant throughout a gene, the frequency of recombination between two mutant sites is a measure of the linear distance between them. Since the selection of wild-type recombinants on *E. coli* strain K is very efficient, extremely low frequencies of recombination can be detected.

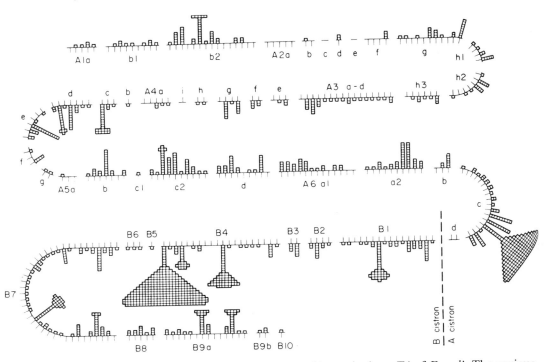

Fig. 11-12. Spontaneous mutation sites in the rII gene of bacteriophage T4 of *E. coli*. The various segments of the A and B cistron are designated by arbitrary numbers and letters. Each small square denotes one independent occurrence of a spontaneous mutation. (From Benzer,[36] with permission.)

Two mutants are presumed to have been altered at the same site if wild-type recombinants cannot be obtained. The resolving power of the method is on the order of a single base pair (i.e., mutants could probably be distinguished if they were mutated at adjacent base pairs). Deletions are recognized by their inability to yield recombinants with a series of mutants already mapped at different sites; deletions of a wide range of sizes have been thus identified.

As detected by this technique, spontaneous mutations and those caused by chemical mutagens were plotted on a map of the rII gene. The sites of a large number of spontaneous mutations are shown in Figure 11-12. They are scattered over the entire gene, but the distribution is far from random; at certain *hot spots* the mutability is many times greater than elsewhere. There are two prominent hot spots for spontaneous mutation, one near the terminus of the A cistron, the other in the middle of the B cistron. The spectrum of mutation sites in the terminal portion of the B cistron after treatment by different chemical mutagens is shown in Figure 11-13. The spontaneous sites for this region are the same as those already depicted in Figure 11-12. These results indicate that the phenomenon of hot spots is not peculiar to spontaneous mutation but is seen with all the mutagens tested. It is also evident that hot spots are mutagen-specific. One of the spontaneous hot spots, for example, has no counterpart in any of the mutagen patterns. The largest hot spot in the 5-bromouracil pattern is not represented even once in the spontaneous pattern. The 2-aminopurine hot spot in segment 8 is represented by only an occasional mutant in any of the other patterns.

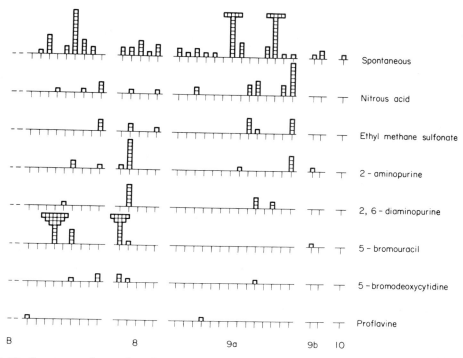

Fig. 11-13. Spectrum of mutation sites for spontaneous mutations and for seven different mutagens. A small part of the rII gene is represented by the terminal portion of the B cistron shown at bottom of Figure 11-12. Each small square denotes one independent occurrence of a mutation. The mutagens are listed next to each row, at the right. Mutation sites are indicated by symbols at bottom. (Modified from Benzer,[36] with permission.)

Hot spots were once taken at face value as representing sites of unusually high mutability. If this were true, a hot spot would have to be imbedded in a special and rather rare sequence of base pairs. The reason for this deduction is simply that the normal base pairs could account, at most, for only four different degrees of mutability, and these would necessarily be associated with numerous sites throughout the gene. To account for exceptionally high mutability at one site, we would have to invoke some influence of neighboring base pairs. Suppose there is one extraordinary hot spot among 1,000 base pairs. Then a special sequence of at least five pairs will be required, since five is the smallest specified sequence that would occur randomly only once in 1,000 base pairs (actual probability $4^{-5} = 1/1024$). However, advances in our understanding of the genetic code and the way it functions render such an explanation unlikely.

First, the very nature of the code makes certain sites more mutable than others. Each of the 20 amino acids is coded in mRNA by more than a single codon, some by as many as six different codons. Most of the degeneracy of the code is attributable to the base in the third (3') position. Every codon has at least one degenerate partner, which differs in the third position but represents the same amino acid; one-half of the codons have three such degenerate partners. Obviously, a transition mutation in the DNA that results in a corresponding change in the third position in the RNA codon (purine for purine, or pyrimidine for pyrimidine) will have no effect whatsoever, (i.e., the "mutation" will be undetectable), and for one-half of the codons even a transversion in the third position would be undetectable. Certain changes in the first position also will have no effect (e.g., AGA → CGA = *Arg*; CUG → UUG = *Leu*).

Second, the apparent mutability of a given site will be determined by the position and nature of the corresponding amino acid in the protein. It is clear that functional proteins tolerate amino acid replacement at some positions but not at others. At certain critical locations any alteration may produce a nonfunctional protein, but often the substitution of chemically similar amino acids (e.g., *Glu → Asp, Gln → Asn, Lys → Arg, Leu → Ile*) has little effect on the protein function. From this point of view, a hot spot could be a site at which the base pair alteration results in a codon specifying an amino acid that is incompatible with protein function when it occupies that particular position in the amino acid sequence. In general, mutations that have large effects upon a phenotypic function will be detected, but mutations at other sites, which lead to tolerated modifications of protein structure, will be overlooked.

Third, the identification of a special role in polypeptide chain termination for the codons UAA and UAG[3,38,39] offers yet another explanation of hot spots. These codons, as well as UGA, specify no amino acid (i.e., "nonsense"). Therefore, codons that can be transformed into these by alteration of a single base pair will seem to be more mutable than codons that cannot because premature chain termination will nearly always produce a complete deficiency of the protein function. Thus, for example, a *Gln* position coded by CAA or CAG could readily be converted to nonsense by the single transition C → U, causing chain termination.

A surprising amount of information about the nature of the base pairs at the various mutant sites in the rII gene can be deduced from observations on induced reversions. A single example will illustrate the method and the argument.[4,28,40,41] As mentioned in a previous section, the base analog 5-bromouracil causes pyrimidine transitions. Most mutations induced by BU are also revertible by BU (see below for definition of genetic reversion). This implies that BU can cause both the transitions C → T and T → C, thereby transforming G:C (or C:G) to A:T (or T:A), and the reverse. Hydroxylamine acts preferentially upon cytosine, causing the transition C:G (or G:C) to T:A (or A:T).[42-45] Most mutants caused by BU cannot be induced to revert by hydroxylamine. From this, it is inferred that most BU mutants have an A:T (or T:A) pair at the mutant site (i.e., that BU itself preferentially induces the transition G:C → A:T or C:G → T:A). This conclusion is further strengthened by the fact that even under conditions that favored the selective modification of guanine residues, most BU mutants could not be made to revert by treatment with an alkylating agent.[46,47] Explicit data about changes induced by chemical mutagens, obtained in studies with tobacco mosaic virus,[22] confirm the earlier conclusions in most respects. Here the virus RNA can be treated directly with a mutagenic agent, then inoculated into the plant host to give a large yield of virus protein. Since the entire amino acid sequence of TMV protein has been determined, the observed changes can be correlated through the genetic code with the actions of the various mutagens. For example, treatment with the known deaminating agent nitrous acid resulted frequently in replacement of a threonine residue by isoleucine. Since the *Thr* codons are ACA, ACG, ACC, and ACU whereas the *Ile* codons are AUC, AUA, and AUU, it is obvious that nitrous acid deaminated cytosine to uracil in the second position of an ACC, ACA, or ACU codon.

There is also evidence for significant variation in mutation rate among regions of the mammalian genome. For example, Wolfe et al.[47] have examined the rates of nucleotide substitution at silent sites for human versus Old World monkeys in a variety of genes. The rates of base substitution differ up to fivefold for some of the genes. For example, the relative rate of substitution for the β-globin gene is 0.039 (a calculation based on the number of substitutions per fourfold degenerate site) and for β-myosin heavy chain is 0.179. The authors show that the rate of silent substitution among mammalian genes is correlated with the base composition of genes and their flanking DNA. They propose that the differences occur because mutation patterns vary with the timing of replication of chromosomal regions in the germline.

Single Base Pair Modifications: Point Mutations

A point mutation is one in which a single base pair of a gene is changed. Most frequently this results from a direct modification of a base or insertion of the wrong base at an apurinic site, leading to a mispairing or base substitution, respectively. Most of the examples given in Figure 11-13 are of this type.

Frame Shift Mutations

Frame shift mutations result from the addition or deletion of a base. This mechanism of mutagenesis was discovered during investigations with acridine dyes such as proflavine and acridine yellow. As discussed above, the mechanism is by intercalation into the stacked bases of double helical DNA. When bacteria infected with phage T4 were treated with an acridine, rII mutants were obtained that differed sharply from those already described in that they could not be reverted by base analogs or by any of the other mutagens that cause transitions. Nor would acridines induce any reversion of transition mutants. On the other hand, many spontaneous mutants that were not revertible by the other mutagens could be reverted by treatment with acridines, and acridine mutants often reverted spontaneously. The elucidation of the mechanism of acridine mutagenesis was accomplished in a series of recombination experiments that also established several fundamental principles of the coding and translation of genetic information.[48] The results of these experiments were interpreted by supposing that acridines caused the insertion or deletion of a base. As a consequence, the reading frame (i.e., the ordered sequence of triplets) would be shifted so that all codons distal to the mutation site would be changed. Clearly, no functional gene product could be synthesized under these circumstances. However, a shift of the reading frame in the opposite direction would restore correct reading, except in the region between the two mutation sites. This is illustrated schematically in Figure 11-14. Each normal codon is represented by a sequence of bases numbered 1-2-3 (line a). The insertion of an extra base (line b) throws all codons to the right out of register (3-1-2 instead of 1-2-3). Finally, deletion of a base (line c) restores the reading frame to the right of the deletion, leaving only the region between the two sites out of register. Presumably, if the original mutation and its suppressor are not too far apart and if they occur in a region of the gene corresponding to a portion of the protein product that will tolerate some amino acid replacements, a partially functional protein can result, and "pseudowild" behavior is seen (i.e., the revertants can grow, form plaques, etc., but they differ in some aspects from true wild-type behavior). Line d of Figure 11-14 shows a similar result when the deletion is to the left of the insertion.

By recombination and appropriate selection procedures it was possible to construct artificial genomes containing any desired combination of (+) or (−) mutations. When two (+) or (−) mutations were combined in the same genome, the result was a typical

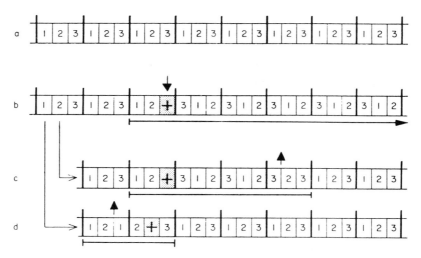

Fig. 11-14. Mechanism of frame shift mutagenesis. Each box represents a base pair. The base pairs in a codon are numbered 1, 2, and 3 in the reading direction from left to right (i.e., $5' \rightarrow 3'$ on the messenger RNA). Original configuration is shown in line a. Addition of a base produces the configuration shown on line b, where all codons to the right of the addition are now missense. On line c deletion of a base restores proper reading frame to the right, leaving a few missense codons between the sites of addition and deletion. On line d the deletion has been made to the left of original addition, with a similar restorative result.

rII mutant; the gene was nonfunctional. Remarkably, however when three (+) or (−) mutations were combined, pseudowild behavior resulted. This constituted strong evidence that the genetic code was indeed a triplet code; for if each codon contained three bases, addition or deletion of that number should restore the reading frame and produce a wild-type protein containing one extra (or one missing) amino acid.

Direct confirmation of the insertion-deletion theory of acridine (and spontaneous) mutagenesis could not be obtained in the rII phage mutants because the gene product was unknown. It was predicted, however, by Crick et al.[48] that if pseudowild double mutants of the (+) and (−) types could be studied in a system in which the protein product of the gene was available, "a string of amino-acids would be altered, covering the region of the polypeptide chain corresponding to the region on the gene between the two mutants." This proof was accomplished with the enzyme lysozyme of phage T4 by amino acid sequence determinations.[49,50] The frame shift predicted by the theory really occurs. An illustration is presented in Figure 11-15. The lysozyme from a pseudowild (+ and −) double mutant was found to differ from the wild-type enzyme with respect to five contiguous amino acids. The codons for all the amino acids in this region are shown. It is clear that the deletion of one base from the -*Thr-Lys-Ser*- codons at the left and the insertion of a guanine or adenine residue in the -*Asn-Ala*- codons at the right would precisely account for the observed amino acid replacements. Because the polarity of each codon is known and it is also known that proteins are assembled from NH_2-terminus to COOH-terminus, this experiment shows conclusively that the genetic message is translated in the direction $5' \rightarrow 3'$ on the mRNA. The reason is that if the mRNA were translated in the direction $3' \rightarrow 5'$, every codon shown in Figure 11-15 would have to be reversed, left to right. If this were so, no set of codons corresponding to the wild-type sequence of amino acids could be converted to the pseudowild sequence by any simple transformation.

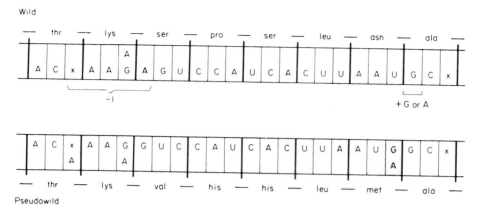

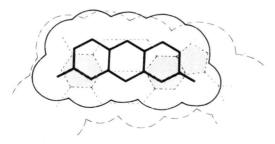

Fig. 11-15. Frame shift mutation in phage T4 lysozyme. Portions of the amino acid sequences for the wild-type protein and for the lysozyme isolated from a pseudowild strain are presented. The pseudowild strain carries two frame shift mutations of opposite sign (i.e., an addition and a deletion). The codons corresponding to each amino acid are shown. The symbol *x* represents any one of the four bases. The polypeptide sequence is written with the NH₂-terminus to the left and the polynucleotide sequence with the 5'-terminus to left. (From Streisinger et al.,[49] with permission.)

Acridine dyes cause the addition or deletion of bases at replication by becoming intercalated between the adjacent base pairs of the DNA.[51] These dyes (and similar compounds) are planar molecules of dimensions similar to those of normal base pairs (Fig. 11-16). Physical measurements of several kinds have given convincing evidence that they do indeed interact with DNA in a manner consistent with intercalation. As indicated in the diagram shown in Figure 11-9, they cause a local spreading of the distance between adjacent base pairs and a localized unwinding of the helix to accommodate this distortion. An elegant proof employed supercoiled circular DNA.[52] Here the local unwinding at the point of intercalation forces a change in the degree of supercoiling, which is readily detectable as an alteration of buoyant density of the DNA.

If spreading apart adjacent base pairs by acridine intercalation permits the insertion of an extra base during replication, how does the same process account for base pair deletions? The similarity of acridine-induced and spontaneous mutations offers a clue. Reciprocal additions and deletions of bases may occur as a result of unequal crossover

Fig. 11-16. Relative sizes of an acridine (proflavin) and a base pair. The purine-pyrimidine base pair is shown shaded, and its three hydrogen bonds are represented by dotted lines. The acridine is superimposed in bold outline. (From Lerman,[51] with permission.)

between homologous chromosomes of diploid organisms at meiosis, or during recombination due to DNA breakage and reunion in bacteria and phage.[5,51,53,54] Unequal crossover produces spontaneous mutation of the frameshift type, and acridines evidently increase the frequency of this event, very likely by interfering with the excision and repair processes.[55,56]

Gene Rearrangements, Deletions, and Duplications

Sometimes gross genetic changes involving hundreds or thousands of bases can occur. This happens spontaneously at a very low rate but it can occur with increased frequency in cells treated with intercalating agents, with agents that induce DNA strand breaks, or with agents that cross-link DNA. When alteration of DNA is severe enough to cause chromatid breakage, abnormal crossover events between sister chromatids can occur.

Crossing over requires either actual breakage and reunion of chromatids or a reciprocal switching of the replication mechanism from one chromatid to another ("copy choice").[57] These possibilities are diagrammed in Figure 11-17. At the top of the figure are shown two homologous chromosomes in synaptic alignment at meiosis. The result, after centromere division, is the emergence of two new chromosomes, the reciprocal recombinants, in addition to the original pair.[58]

Broken ends of chromatids are known to be "sticky" in the sense that they tend to heal together, a process in which the DNA ligases play an important part. An important consequence of this property is that once breakage is produced or repair of broken ends

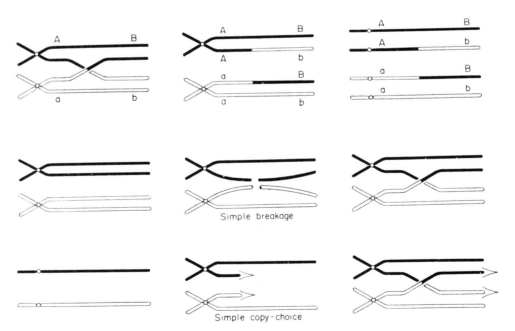

Fig. 11-17. Crossover at meiosis. In the upper line two homologous chromosomes are shown aligned, each consisting of two chromatids. The centromere is the small circle at left. A and B are genes of one chromosome; a and b are the coresponding alleles on the other. Recombination yields two new genomes. The middle and bottom diagrams show alternative theories to account for crossover and recombination. (From Srb et al.,[58] with permission.)

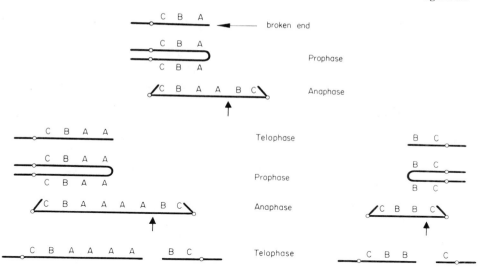

Fig. 11-18. The chromosome breakage-fusion-bridge cycle. A chromosome with a broken end is pictured at top. The open circle represents the centromere and A, B, C are genes. Fusion of broken ends of the two chromatids is shown, yielding a dicentric chromosome. An anaphase bridge results in breakage (shown by arrow), followed by repetition of the cycle. Gene duplications and deletions result, as illustrated. (From McClintock,[60] with permission.)

is inhibited, bizarre alterations of chromosome structure are possible.[59] An illustration of how gene duplications, inversions, and deletions can occur through operation of a cycle of breakage, fusion, and bridge formation is shown in Figure 11-18. At the top of the figure a chromosome from which a terminal segment has been broken is depicted.[60] Such terminal fragments become lost because they are detached from the portion of the chromosome bearing the centromere and therefore cannot move properly at mitosis or meiosis. If such a terminal deletion is compatible with continued life of the cell, the mutant will be defective in those characters controlled by the missing genes. After replication of the chromatid, the sticky broken ends join to form a dicentric chromatid. At the next anaphase the centromeres will be pulled in opposite directions, forming an anaphase bridge, which eventually breaks. The new break heals after replication, and the cycle is repeated. A sequence of genes, A, B, and C, is shown to undergo several possible changes in the course of these events. Sometimes broken ends reunite to form ring chromosomes. Sometimes a whole segment may be transposed elsewhere on the same chromosome or even onto a different chromosome. A photomicrograph showing anaphase bridges, detached terminal fragments, and extensive chromosome breakage is presented in Figure 11-19. Here an alkylating agent was administered to mice bearing a transplantable carcinoma, and the tumor cells were examined 48 hours later.[61]

The precise morphologic classification of the individual chromosomes of a diploid set (the *karyotype*) makes it easy to recognize the kinds of gross chromosome alterations described above. Agreement between deductions from genetic evidence and observed aberrant morphology has been remarkable. Especially in the giant salivary gland chromosomes of *Drosophila* have structural alterations been discernible that were predicted from genetic evidence. In all such cases the modified chromosomes replicate and undergo mitosis normally provided the mutant phenotype is viable. In this way even major chro-

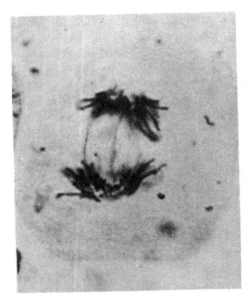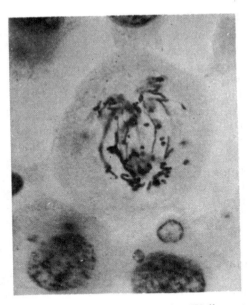

Fig. 11-19. Chromosome abnormalities induced by mechlorethamine. Mice bearing Walker carcinoma 256 were given the nitrogen mustard mechlorethamine, a single dose of 1 mg kg^{-1} intraperitoneally. Photomicrograph at left shows a cell at mitosis 48 hours later. Chromosome bridges (chiasmata) and fragments are evident. Photomicrograph at right shows bridges and more severe fragmentation in a cell at mitosis 56 hours after drug treatment. × 2500. (From Koller,[61] with permission.)

mosome abnormalities can become established in the germ line of the species, and since hereditary defects have been associated with such visible abnormalities, it follows that agents capable of breaking chromosomes are also capable of causing genetic damage.

Alkylating agents are very effective chromosome breakers, mimicking the action of x-irradiation. Chromosome breakage by x-rays requires oxygen, however, whereas that caused by alkylating agents does not. Another difference is that delayed effects are much more commonly encountered with alkylating agents than with x-rays. Crosslinking is evidently not the only mechanism underlying chromosome breakage, since monofunctional alkylating agents are effective, as are many of the chemical mutagens that induce base pair transformations. Bromouracil, for example, is a good chromosome breaker in mammalian cells in vitro.[62,63] Hydroxylamine causes chromatid breaks and also inhibits the repair of breaks caused by x-rays.[64] It seems likely, therefore, that chromosome breakage is related in some fundamental way to other mechanisms of mutagenesis.[65,66] Since breakage and reunion of the genetic material occur normally as part of the cell cycle, inhibition of repair mechanisms may play a central role in the action of chromosome breakers.

Genetic deletions can also occur in many sizes, both spontaneously and consequent to treatment with a mutagen. In bacteriophage T4, deletions were recognized by the fact that they could not be caused to revert to the wild type and that they would not yield wild-type recombinants when crossed with certain point mutants.[37] The extent and position of each deletion was found by crossing it with point mutants whose positions had been mapped; every point mutant with which no wild-type recombinants were obtained must lie within the region of the deletion. The results of such studies led to a simple conclusion. Deletions can occur spontaneously anywhere along the rII gene. Their lengths range from a few base pairs to most of the gene. They can cross the boundary between two adjacent cistrons[67]; when this happens, the region of separation between the two protein products is deleted, and a continuous protein is synthesized with a certain number of amino acids missing where one protein should end and the next should begin. Nitrous acid, it has already been pointed out, causes major deletions in phage DNA, perhaps by interrupting replication at points where guanine has been deaminated to xanthine. Deletions are common results of chromosome breakage in higher organisms because of the loss of terminal segments after single breaks and loss of internal portions of chromatids after double breaks.

Streptonigrin, an antibiotic from a streptomycete, has remarkable effects at extraordinarily low concentration upon chromosomes of cultured human leukocytes.[68] At 2×10^{-9} M this compound produced an average of nearly three breaks per cell in 12 hours; in contrast, bromouracil deoxyriboside at 40,000 times this concentration produced only two breaks per cell after 28 days. The streptonigrin effects involved every kind of abnormality, including chromatid breaks (discontinuity of one chromatid in a pair), isochromatid breaks (discontinuity of both chromatids at the same position), acentric fragments, dicentric chromosomes, translocation cross-configurations, end-to-end association of chromosomes, anaphase bridges, uncoiling, and severe fragmentation.

A wide variety of compounds have been implicated as chromosome breakers.[65] It is true that in most of the experiments plant materials such as bean or onion root tips were used, but whenever human cells have been exposed in vitro to the same mutagens, similar effects have been seen. In most investigations fairly high concentrations of the agents were used in order to produce a large enough number of chromosome abnormalities for ready visualization. It is difficult to say what hazard may be presented by exposure of human cells in vivo to these same agents (some of which are commonly present in the environment) with exposure to low concentrations over a lifetime. This problem is discussed in a wider context in a later section of this chapter.

Gene duplications can also lead to a mutation in the sense that a heritable phenotypic alteration can occur. The best example of this occurs in the development of drug resistance, in the study of which it has been shown that a manyfold replication of a gene coding for an enzyme target or a protein needed for the drug effect can circumvent the lethal action of a drug. The example of amplification of the dihydrofolate reductase gene causing resistance to methotrexate is described in Chapter 9. Methotrexate acts by inhibiting the enzyme dihydrofolate reductase, and resistance to methotrexate can result from overproduction of the enzyme as a consequence of amplification of the gene coding for the enzyme.[69]

BIOLOGIC CONSEQUENCES OF MUTATION

Since the base sequence of DNA in a structural gene ultimately determines the amino acid sequence in a protein, the effects of a DNA-altering event become apparent as a structural or functional change in cells. Depending on where in a protein an amino acid substitution, addition, or deletion occurs, a mutation may be a *missense, nonsense,* or *silent.* A missense mutation occurs when an amino acid substitution produces a partially active protein. This change could be evident as a temperature-sensitive mutation (e.g., a protein that functions at 30°C but not at 40°C). A nonsense mutation results from an alteration producing a base sequence that no longer codes for an amino acid. This often results in formation of an incomplete protein owing to chain termination when the non-coding sequence of the altered mRNA reaches the translation system on the ribosome. A silent mutation is said to occur if a base alteration does not lead to an amino acid change because of redundancy of the genetic code or if a base change produces an amino acid substitution that does not alter function.

The chemical and physical properties of a protein are determined by the amino acid sequence, and a single key amino acid change is capable of inactivating or severely restricting the function of a protein. A classic example is the mutant hemoglobin molecule found in patients with sickle cell anemia, in which a single amino acid substitution (a valine instead of a glutamic acid as the sixth amino acid from the amino terminus of the globin β chain) occurs as a result of a single base change in the triplet code word.[70] How a single amino acid difference can alter a protein so dramatically can be visualized if one considers that the three-dimensional structure can be influenced greatly by disulfide bonds in cystines, electrostatic interactions, hydrophobic forces, and hydrogen bonding. If, for example, an interaction between one positively charged amino acid such as lysine and one negatively charged amino acid such as aspartic acid is crucial, a substitution of a methionine, which is uncharged, for the lysine could completely change the three-dimensional structure and hence the way a protein associates with a cell membrane, reacts with a substrate, recognizes through binding a drug or hormone, and so on. Another example would be a protein conformation stabilized by a cluster of hydrophobic amino acids, in which substitution of a charged amino acid such as glutamic acid for an uncharged one such as leucine would disrupt the surface charge on the protein.

The ultimate biologic consequences of a mutation for a higher organism will vary depending on the nature of the mutation. Obviously, some mutations have been "good" from an evolutionary point of view and have led to traits that we highly value. Most of these mutations have presumably produced proteins of altered but not completely compromised function. Other changes have not been so propitious. Some mutations have produced genetically determined diseases such as hemophilia, sickle cell anemia, and various inborn errors of metabolism. If a mutation is incompatible with life, spontaneous abortion occurs. Congenital malformations may result if the mother is exposed at crucial times during pregnancy to certain mutagens. Most types of cancer, as we shall see in Chapter 12, are probably initiated by a somatic mutation. Thus, the biologic end results of mutations can be either helpful or devastating to the survival of the species, depending on the type of mutation produced.

GENETIC REVERSION

In addition to "forward" mutations from a wild-type or parent phenotype to a mutant phenotype, back mutations or reversions occasionally occur that lead to the regaining of the wild-type phenotype. These reversions can occur in several ways. One obvious way is to restore the parental genotype (i.e. the original base sequence in DNA). This, however, is rare; other mechanisms are more likely. One of these mechanisms is the so-called second-site or suppressor mutation, which occurs at a different site from the original mutation but in the same gene (intragenic reversion) or in a different gene (extragenic reversion). The end result is to restore the original phenotype, and in the case of the intragenic reversion the function, of the original, wild-type protein. There are multiple examples in which it has been shown that the amino acid sequence in a revertant is not the wild-type sequence and that the original amino acid substitution in the mutant is still present in the revertants. A number of ways in which this can occur are demonstrated in Figure 11-20. Revertants are sometimes found to be temperature-sensitive in that a second-site mutation may lead to a protein that has somewhat different thermal stability and may be more easily disrupted by raising the temperature.

Reversions of frameshift mutations almost always are second-site mutations, and, in general, the back mutation must occur at a site in the gene near the original mutation so as to regain the original reading frame register without too much alteration. This is possible when a segment of the mutated polypeptide chain can undergo fairly substantial alteration without major functional change (probably in a segment minimally involved in key interactions with binding sites).

The use of genetic reversion is a powerful tool to detect mutagenic agents. For example, the now classic Ames test (see below) depends on the ability of a potential mutagen to revert a His$^-$ bacterial strain to His$^+$ (i.e., from a strain that requires exogenous histidine for its growth to one that does not). Since frameshift mutagens can revert frameshift mutations but generally do not induce reversion of base-substituting mutagens and vice versa, it is frequently possible to deduce whether a mutagenic agent is of the base substitution or frameshift type by using this simple in vitro test.

USE OF MUTANTS IN PHARMACOLOGY

The use of mutant cells is one of the most powerful tools for examining the molecular mechanisms by which drugs and hormones exert their effects on cells. A few examples below will illustrate this. First, a comment should be made about the potential difficulty of generating such mutants. It is generally much easier to create and select for mutations in bacterial cell populations. Because bacterial cells are haploid and because their replication rate is so rapid, one can much more readily select mutants from within a population. Eukaryotic cells are diploid, have a higher DNA content, have a much slower population doubling time, and generally require a much more complicated growth medium; thus it is more difficult to use nutritional deprivation as a selection technique. Frequently, the use of potent mutagens such as N-methyl-N'-nitro-N-nitrosoguanidine (MNNG) is required to mutagenize cells prior to selection of the desired trait.

The use of drug-resistant mutants has been widely used to determine both the mechanism of action and the mechanisms of resistance to a number of chemotherapeutic agents. For example, the use of bacterial cells resistant to nitrogen mustard revealed that a cell's ability to repair its DNA after drug treatment determines to a large extent its sensitivity to the drug.[71] As discussed above, our understanding of the mechanism of resistance development to the antimetabolite methotrexate was significantly advanced by the discovery of methotrexate-resistant cells that had greatly amplified genes for the enzyme dihydrofolate reductase.[69] A line of S49 mouse lymphoma cells (designated cyc$^-$) that are deficient in G protein, an accessory protein required for adenyl cyclase activation, has been developed by treating the parent line with agents that elevate the intracellular concentration of cyclic adenosine monophosphate (cAMP) to cytotoxic levels and then selecting the resistant clones.[72] The use of these clones has been a tremendous boon to studies designed to discern how adenylate cyclase is coupled to the receptors for various hormones and to identify the individual components of this multicomponent receptor-coupled-adenylate cyclase system.[73]

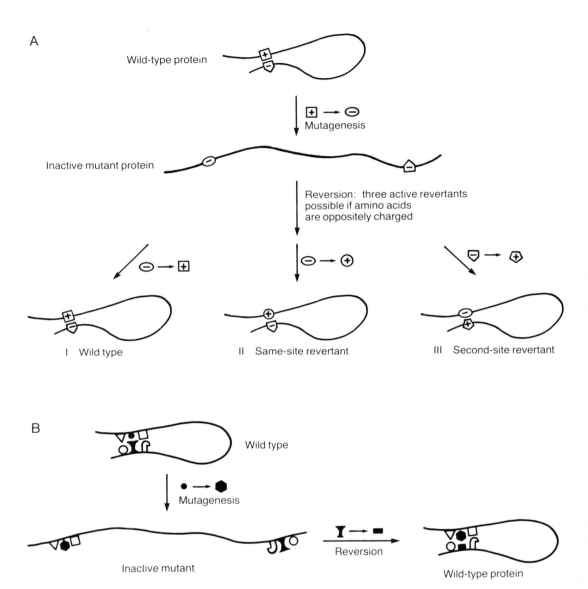

Fig. 11-20. Schematic diagram of several mechanisms of reversion. **(A)** The charge of one amino acid is changed, and the protein loses activity. The activity is returned (I) by restoring the original amino acid; (II) by replacing the (−) amino acid by another (+) amino acid; or (III) by reversing the charge of the original (−) amino acid. In each case the attraction of opposite charges is restored. **(B)** The structure of the protein is determined by interactions between six hydrophobic amino acids. Activity is lost when the small circular amino acid is replaced by the bulky hexagonal one and is regained when complementary hydrophobic ''faces'' are restored by replacing the convex amino acid by the smaller rectangular shaped one. (From Freifelder,[13] with permission.)

CHEMICAL MUTAGENESIS IN ANIMALS AND HUMANS
The Human Germ Line

Inherited defects arise by mutation in the germ line. Each person may be regarded as a differentiated clone of cells derived from the fusion of a paternal and maternal gamete to form a zygote. Mutations can be introduced into the human germ line only during the reproductive life of the individual, a period of about 30 years on the average. If recessive in nature, these mutations may remain concealed for generations until homozygosity makes them manifest.

Primordial germ cells are first distinguishable at about the sixth week of gestation. Development proceeds differently in the two sexes. In the female all the primary oocytes (about 400,000) are produced from undifferentiated oogonia during fetal life. No further cell divisions occur until puberty, when the monthly maturation of a single ovum begins. The maturation process entails two meiotic divisions, followed by the degeneration of three of the four meiotic products as polar bodies.

In the male a population of primary spermatogonia persists in the germinal layer of the seminiferous tubules of the testis. These *stem cells* undergo mitosis about once every 12 days, giving rise to nonequivalent daughter cells. One daughter cell retains the characteristics of a primary spermatogonium, the other migrates toward the lumen of the tubule and becomes a primary spermatocyte, the progenitor of four mature spermatozoa. In this way, stem cell renewal and sperm production continue throughout childhood and reproductive life.[74]

The continuity of the male germ line through one human generation is shown schematically in Figure 11-21. Period 1 contains all the mitotic cycles (about 50 on the average) between the zygote and the population of primordial germ cells; its duration is about 6 weeks. We are not speaking here of the total number of cell divisions, which would be one less than the total cell population at the end of the period under consideration. We are concerned with the number of times the chromosomes of any given cell in the final population have replicated. (In the female another 17 mitotic cycles serve to produce all the primary oocytes in both ovaries.) Period 2 lasts until puberty, about 12 to 14 years; period 3 encompasses the remainder of reproductive life. If the average generation time is taken to be 30 years, then these periods of stem cell renewal (average cycle 12 days) contain about 900 mitotic cycles in the male. (Periods 2 and 3 are absent in the female.) Finally, period 4 comprises the two meiotic divisions by which the male and female gametes are formed. Thus, on the average, a zygote is formed by the union of a sperm whose chromosomes have replicated approximately 950 times since the previous generation, and an ovum whose chromosomes have replicated only about 70 times in the same period.

It will be evident from this account that the occurrence of new mutations might follow a different course in the two sexes. *In the female* mutagens that act only on replicating DNA or on the mitotic process should have effects primarily during fetal life. Mutagens that act on nonreplicating DNA might act throughout the lifetime. Agents that disturb meiosis would act only at the time of conception, when the meiotic divisions occur. This is probably the time when most spontaneous mutations occur. *In the male,* on the other hand, the risk of mutation by agents that act on replicating DNA or on the mitotic process should span the whole reproductive life cycle. The male stem cell line passes through so many more mitotic cycles than does the female that such mutagens should cause the accumulation of many more mutations in sperm than in ova, other factors being equal.

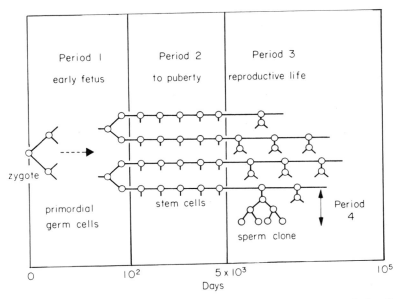

Fig. 11-21. The human germ line. A schematic diagram showing the four periods of possible sensitivity to mutagens in the human male. (In the female, periods 2 and 3 are effectively absent, and period 4 represents the two meiotic divisions at the time of fertilization of the ovum.) (From Goldstein,[75] with permission.)

Agents that only affect meiosis should act in the male during a period of a few weeks prior to the coitus that leads to conception.

It follows that mutations arising in relation to DNA replication and cell division, whatever their cause, should produce genetic defects whose incidence is correlated with paternal age but not with maternal age. Such a correlation is actually observed for two human genetic diseases, hemophilia and chondrodystrophy. Mongolism, on the other hand, is correlated exclusively with maternal age, the implication of which has been discussed. As it remains somewhat uncertain which mutagenic agents act upon what stages of DNA replication or of the mitotic or meiotic cycle, only one practical conclusion can be derived apart from the general injunction to minimize exposure to mutagens. Since by far the greatest number of mitotic cycles in the female germ line occur during the first 2 months of fetal life, it seems wise to avoid unnecessary exposure of pregnant women to any drugs or potentially mutagenic environmental agents from a time just prior to conception through the first trimester of pregnancy. This recommendation relates also to potentially teratogenic agents (cf. Chapter 13).

Large differences in mutagenicity, depending upon the time of treatment with a mutagen, as shown in Table 11-4, are fairly typical. The data reflect differences in sensitivity of the various stages of spermatogenesis.[76] Since spermatogonia in the stem cell line, premeiotic (primary) spermatocytes, postmeiotic (secondary) spermatocytes, spermatids, and spermatozoa are all present simultaneously, they are all necessarily exposed to the mutagen. But if the treatment is brief and matings are conducted on successive days, one can distinguish which stages of germ cell maturation are most sensitive. If the litters conceived shortly after treatment are affected, then the agent must have caused mutations in the mature spermatozoa. The data show, on the contrary, that the most sensitive forms were

Table 11-4. Partial Sterility and Translocations Induced in Mice by an Alkylating Agent

Litter Size in Matings with Treated Males	
Days after Drug	Average Litter Size
1	6.3
2	5.3
3	7.3
10	1.7
11	2.0
12	1.6
13	3.6
Control	8.5

Sterility and Translocations in F_1 Males			
Days after Drug on Which F_1 Males were Conceived	Number Tested	% Sterile or Semisterile	% Showing Translocations
1–3	111	4.5	7.2
10–13	74	14.9	28.4

Triethylenemelamine (0.2 mg kg^{-1}) was administered in a single intraperitoneal injection to male mice. These were mated daily to untreated females 1, 2, and 3 days after injection, and again after 10, 11, 12, and 13 days. F_1 males were tested for partial sterility and examined cytologically for translocations. (Data from Cattanach.[76])

those that required 10 to 13 days to mature after treatment; in mice, these would be the postmeiotic spermatids. In *Drosophila*, too, the spermatids are the germ cells most sensitive to alkylating agents and radiation. The quantitative differences between the stages, in oogenesis as well as in spermatogenesis, may be very great.[77,78]

Risk Assessment

Exposure of human beings to mutagens occurs from chemicals in our diet, water, and air, from products that we use as cosmetics and drugs, and from cigarette smoking. Several mutagenic substances have been identified in cigarette smoke.[79] Mutagens and carcinogens are found among the natural products contained in foods, such as products elaborated by molds (e.g., aflatoxin) or by edible plants that synthesize a variety of toxins, presumably serving to ward off insects, as well as among synthetic chemicals such as pesticides, industrial pollutants, and weed killers.[79,80] We live in a sea of mutagens and carcinogens. Identification of potentially mutagenic substances in our environment is a major public health and political issue. There are a myriad of potential mutagens and carcinogens in our diet, only a few of which have been studied in detail. In addition, over 50,000 synthetic chemicals are produced in the United States, and about 1,000 new chemicals are introduced to the commercial market each year.[79] Only a small number of these were examined for mutagenic and carcinogenic potential before being marketed. Obviously, this is a major epidemiologic problem and one that has major economic impact on private industry as well as on the consumer and taxpayer. What is needed are accurate, rapid, and economically feasible tests to predict the mutagenic and carcinogenic potential of the chemicals in our environment. In practice, however, it has not been possible to develop a "perfect" short-term test. One problem has been that there are inevitably a number of false positive and false negative results with in vitro tests. Since metabolic activation, detoxication, and excretion of compounds are often key to their cytotoxic and mutagenic effects, there is really no perfect substitute for the whole animal. Tests in whole animals involve chronic exposure of large numbers of animals and are, unfortunately, very expensive and time-consuming.

More than 100 short-term tests for mutagenicity and carcinogenicity have been developed. Some of the most widely used are: bacterial mutagenesis (the Ames test); mutagenesis in cell culture systems; direct measurement of damage to DNA or chromosomes in exposed cells; and malignant transformation of cell cultures.[81]

One of the most popular of the short-term tests is the Ames test, developed by Bruce Ames and his colleagues.[82] The basis of this assay is the ability of a chemical agent to induce a genetic reversion in a series of *Salmonella typhimurium* tester strains, which contain either a base substitution or a frameshift mutation, from histidine-requiring (His$^-$) to histidine-nonrequiring (His$^+$). These strains have been specially developed for this assay by selecting clones that have a decreased cell surface barrier to the uptake of chemicals and a decreased excision repair system. Other advantages of the Ames test system are the small genome of the bacterium (4×10^6 base pairs), the large number of cells that can be exposed per culture dish (about 10^9), and the positive selection of the mutated organisms (i.e., only the *mutated* organisms will grow under the test conditions). This system has great sensitivity: only about 1 reversion in 1,000 to 10,000 mutated bacteria is sufficient to give a positive test, and nanogram amounts of a potent mutagen can be detected as a positive.[82] Both base substitution and frameshift mutagens can be detected. By using the appropriate tester strains, the type of mutagen can be deduced, because frameshift mutagens usually only revert tester strains with frameshift mutations and not strains with base substitution mutations, and vice versa. Since many mutagens must be metabolized to be active, a liver homogenate fraction containing microsomes is usually added to the incubation in order to provide the necessary drug-metabolizing enzymes.

The potential of various chemical agents to mutagenize mammalian cells has also been used as a short-term test. Frequently, mutation at the hypoxanthine-guanine phosphoribosyl transferase (HGPRT) locus is used as a marker; the end point of the assay is loss of sensitivity to purine antimetabolites that must be activated by HGPRT in order to be effective, thus leading to the selection of HGPRT$^-$ clones. Cultured fibroblast cell lines such as Chinese hamster V79 or ovary cells (CHO) are frequently used in this way.

Agents that damage DNA can often be detected by examining an index of genotoxicity, such as unscheduled DNA synthesis, sister chromatid exchange, or chromosome breakage in cultured cells exposed to the agents in question.

Carcinogenic potential has been estimated by the ability of chemicals to "transform" smooth, well organized monolayers of normal diploid fibroblasts into cells that grow piled up on one another (transformed foci) or into a cell type that can grow suspended in soft agar (normal fibroblasts do not grow on soft agar). Sometimes, the transformed cells are then injected into immunosuppressed or genetically immunodeficient mice in order to demonstrate that they are malignant. All these estimates of carcinogenic potential are fraught with danger in that a significant number of false negatives or false positives can occur.

No single short-term test is foolproof; however, if definitive evidence of genotoxicity has been obtained in more than one test, a chemical is highly suspect. An agent that is found to be mutagenic, DNA-damaging, and a chromosome breaker is almost certain to be carcinogenic also.[81]

Some Common Methods of Testing Mutagenicity in Animals

Final proof of mutagenicity and carcinogenicity involves the use of in vivo animal model systems. While the short-term in vitro tests have several advantages, a number of important components, such as absorption, pharmacokinetics, tissue distribution, metabolism, age or sex effects, and species specificity cannot be duplicated in vitro. Since direct experiments with chemical mutagens are obviously out of the question in humans, our assessment of the mutagenic hazards associated with exposure to drugs and other agents necessarily rests upon genetic investigations in other animals. One naturally supposes that the sensitivity of the genetic apparatus to mutagens will be almost the same in closely related species. Although much of modern genetics rests upon experiments with *Drosophila*,[83] mice have been used increasingly as a practical mammalian model.[84] Because large-scale breeding is often required, especially to detect low mutation rates, larger mammals are excluded on practical grounds. Induced dominant mutations are readily observed, but detection of induced recessive mutations required the use of specially bred stocks.[85] Since recessive mutations are expressed in the homozygous state, a good test of mutagenesis is to mate an animal treated with a mutagen to an animal that is already heterozygous for certain traits. If the treatment induces a mutation at a corresponding locus, then some of the offspring will be homozygous for the mutant trait. In devising such tests advantage is often taken of the fact that the male is hemizygous for the X chromosome; thus, for example, one-half the male offspring of a treated female with an induced X-chromosome mutation will display the mutant trait.

A good example of the adroit use of sex linkage in a test for mutagenesis is the classical *ClB method* in *Drosophila*.[86] The procedure requires a stock of females heterozygous for two mutant traits carried on the same X chromosome—bar eye (a visible characteristic) and a recessive lethal trait. Males are treated with a mutagen and then mated to the special females. Female F_1 offspring with bar eye are selected for the next round of breeding. These animals will have the maternal X chromosome carrying the bar eye allele and also the recessive lethal gene carried with it. Their other X chromosome is inherited from the treated males. The question is whether any recessive lethal mutations were induced in that X chromosome during the mutagen treatment. We are concerned here with mutations that are not allelic with the recessive lethal already carried by the female. In the occasional instance of induced mutation at the same gene locus, no F_1 offspring would be obtained, since the zygote would be homozygous for the lethal trait. The answer is obtained very simply by breeding these females with ordinary males and examining the sex of F_2 offspring. If a recessive lethal mutation is present in the X chromosome derived from the treated males, there will be no viable male F_2 offspring whatsoever because both maternal X chromosomes would then carry recessive (but nonallelic) lethal mutations and all F_2 males would express one or the other lethal trait. Conversely, if any males are found, then no recessive lethals had been induced.

Dominant lethal mutations are detected by exposing males to a mutagenic treatment, mating them to normal females, and then simply observing the number of viable offspring. This test is frequently employed in mice. To ensure detection of nonviable embryos, the pregnant females are sacrificed just before term in order to count the number of live embryos, the number of dead embryos, and the number of corpora lutea (whence the number of preimplantation deaths can be estimated, since each corpus luteum represents one ovum).[87-89] Dominant lethals are often due to major chromosome abnormalities that are incompatible with development of the zygote.

Chromosome translocations have been observed microscopically in mice after the following selection procedure.[76] The F_1 male offspring of males originally treated with a mutagen were mated with normal females, and their litter size was used as a preliminary screening criterion. Whenever the average litter size derived from a given F_1 male was smaller than normal, a direct cytologic examination of that animal's testis was carried out. If 19 instead of the normal 20 chromosomes were seen consistently in metaphase configurations, a translocation was assumed to be present. Table 11-4 presents data of a typical experiment with an alkylating agent, in which dominant lethals as well as translocations were induced. The size of litters derived from treated males was greatly reduced 10 to 13 days after treatment. The translocation test showed that the male offspring of these same treated males carried translocations and were partially sterile, and again the peak effect was seen in offspring of males mated 10 to 13 days after drug treatment.

Another method, which has yielded important information about radiation mutagenesis in mice, is the *specific locus method*.[90] It depends upon the expression of mutations when they are homozygous; the traits considered here are readily observable, visible abnormalities such as unusual coat color or peculiar shape of the ear. A special stock of mice is bred, heterozygous for seven such traits carried on seven different autosomal genes. Males or females are exposed to the mutagenic treatment and then mated to mice of the opposite sex belonging to the special stock. Then the F_1 offspring are examined. When a mutation has been induced in one of the seven loci in a treated mouse, its offspring will be homozygous for that particular visible trait.

The method can be illustrated by an experiment on radiation mutagenesis. Males were given 600 roentgens of whole-body x-irradiation. They were then allowed to recover from the postirradiation sterility, so that the spermatozoa available for the matings developed from irradiated spermatogonia. These treated males were mated with females of the special stock, and unirradiated control males were also mated. In the control group in which 37,868 offspring were examined, two mutant animals were found. In the irradiated group in which 48,007 offspring were examined, 53 mutants were found. The mean mutation rate induced by x-irradiation was therefore computed to be $2.5 \pm 0.4 \times 10^{-7}$ per roentgen per locus. The disadvantage of this method is evident from the data; enormous numbers of animals have to be bred and examined. And although a good quantitative estimation can be made when mutagenesis is strong, the accuracy of estimate for a weak mutagen (e.g., one that only doubled the spontaneous mutation rate) would be very poor because of the extremely small number of mutations observed. Another problem is that the seven chosen genes differ considerably among themselves in their sensitivities to mutagenic treatments, so that "mean mutation rate" may have no relevance to actual rates at the most sensitive gene loci in humans.

Evaluation of the Hazards of Chemical Mutagens in Humans

The difficulties of arriving at quantitative estimates of mutagenicity for chemical agents in human populations are very great. Even in the case of radiation mutagenesis, which is generally accepted as a fact, most of the evidence comes from animal experimentation. Humans exposed to radiation or to a chemical mutagen are not expected to be affected themselves except at doses large enough to cause sterility. Even the offspring of the exposed person may seem unaffected if the induced mutation is recessive or incompletely expressed. Thus, many induced mutations will only be manifested in future generations through the eventual union of gametes both of which are heterozygous for the same recessive alleles. It follows that much of the data bearing directly upon the human species will have to be epidemiologic rather than experimental. It also follows that a conservative position with respect to mutagenic hazards in humans will be based frequently on common sense judgments rather than on ironclad proofs. By assuming a conservative position we mean that we wish to err, when in doubt, in the direction of overestimating the potential mutagenic hazard.[75,91,92]

A growing number of genetic diseases are being identified in humans. Most estimates show[93] that every sperm or ovum carries several mutant genes accumulated over the past history of the race, and that as many as one person in three carries a new mutation not present in either of his parents. These accumulated and newly altered mutant genes are attributed to past and present "spontaneous" mutation. It is quite clear from what is known about radiation mutagenesis that lifelong exposure to background radiation could not account for more than a small fraction of the total spontaneous mutation rate. Occasionally, a "mutator gene" renders an organism and its progeny subject to very high spontaneous mutation rates, perhaps by production of an endogenous mutagen.[94–98] In addition, the human race is exposed to many chemicals that are known to be mutagenic to lower forms of life. Since no estimates of the "spontaneous" mutation rate in humans have been made in the absence of such exposure, the possibility must be entertained that some part of the apparent spontaneous rate may be due to exogenous chemical mutagens.

In organisms in which chemical mutagenesis has been demonstrated, the concentrations usually employed have been very high compared with those to which humans might be exposed. If extrapolation from such data to humans is to have any validity, a knowledge of the dose-response relationship is essential. This has been worked out for very few mutagens. Especially important is the question of whether the probability of mutation is a simple product of dose (concentration) times duration of exposure. Is prolonged exposure of humans to low doses equivalent in mutagenic efficiency to short exposures at high doses in laboratory experiments? The answer is not clear, and there is debate about whether there is any safe "threshold" dose for exposure of humans to mutagenic and carcinogenic agents. Since all it would take, theoretically, is a single "hit" (e.g., alkylation of a key base pair in an important gene) to produce a mutation, the assumption that there is a "safe" dose of any potent mutagen is tenuous at best. On the other hand, all persons are exposed to a wide variety of these agents during their lifetimes, but not everyone gets cancer, presumably because most of the damage to DNA is repaired. If the repair processes are not functioning well, as in patients with xeroderma pigmentosum, the risk is significantly higher. The risk of damaging mutations may also increase as people age since damage to DNA may accrue over a lifetime of exposure to mutagenic agents and since the efficiency of DNA repair mechanisms appears to decrease with aging.[27]

Clearly, each new chemical introduced into our environment should be examined for its mutagenic and carcinogenic potential. Many types of tests will have to be used to obtain a reasonably high degree of accuracy.

REFERENCES

1. Thomas L: The Medusa and the Snail. Viking Press, New York, 1979
2. Watson JD: Molecular Biology of the Gene. 2nd Ed. Benjamin, Elmsford, NY, 1970
3. The Genetic Code. Cold Spring Harbor Symp Quant Biol 31: 1966
4. Freese E: The difference between spontaneous and base-analog induced mutations of phage T4. Proc Natl Acad Sci USA 45:622, 1959
5. Drake JW: The Molecular Basis of Mutation. Holden-Day, San Francisco, 1970
6. Freese E: Molecular mechanisms of mutations. Ch. 1. In Hollaender A (ed): Chemical Mutagens: Principles and Methods for Their Detection. Plenum, New York, 1971
7. Röhrborn G: Biochemical mechanisms of mutation. Ch. 1. In Vogel F, Röhrborn G (eds): Chemical Mutagenesis in Mammals and Man. Springer-Verlag, New York, 1970
8. Singer B: Mutagenic effects of nucleic acid modification and repair assessed by in vitro transcription. p. 1. In Lawrence W (ed): Induced Mutagenesis. Plenum, New York, 1983

9. Brookes P, Lawley PD: The reaction of mono- and di-functional alkylating agents with nucleic acids. Biochem J 80:496, 1961

10. Ludlum DB, Krame BS, Wang J, Fenselau C: Reaction of 1,3-bis(2-chloroethyl)-1-nitrosourea with synthetic polynucleotides. Biochemistry 14:5480, 1975

11. Barbin A, Bresil H, Croisy A, et al: Liver microsome-mediated formation of alkylating agents from vinyl bromide and vinyl chloride. Biochem Biophys Res Commun 67:596, 1972

12. Green T, Hathway DE: Intereactions of vinyl chloride with rat liver DNA *in vivo*. Chem Biol Interact 22:211, 1978

13. Freifelder D: Molecular Biology: A Comprehensive Introduction to Procaryotes and Eukaryotes. Jones & Bartlett Publishers, Boston, 1983, Ch. 9

14. Lindahl T: DNA repair enzymes. Ann Rev Biochem 51:61, 1982

15. Pratt WB, Ruddon RW: The Anticancer Drugs. Oxford University Press, New York, 1979

16. Setlow RB, Carrier WL: The disappearance of thymine dimers from DNA: An error-correcting mechanism. Proc Natl Acad Sci USA 51:226, 1964

17. Howard-Flanders P, Boyce PR, Simson E, Theriot L: A genetic locus in *E. coli* K12 that controls the reactivation of UV-photoproducts associated with thymine in DNA. Proc Natl Acad Sci USA 48:2109, 1962

18. Pettijohn D, Hanawalt PC: Evidence for repair replication of ultraviolet-damaged DNA in bacteria. J Mol Biol 9:395, 1964

19. Haseltine WA: Ultraviolet light repair and mutagenesis revisited. Cell 33:13, 1983

20. Sancar A, Rupp WD: A novel repair enzyme: *uvr*ABC excision nuclease of *E. coli* cuts a DNA strand on both sides of the damaged region. Cell 33:249, 1983

21. Maher VM, McCormick JJ: Relationship between excision repair and the cytotoxic and mutagenic action of chemicals and UV radiation. p. 271. In Lawrence W (ed): Induced Mutagenesis. Plenum, New York, 1983

22. Siegel A: Artificial production of mutants of tobacco mosaic virus. Adv Virus Res 11:25, 1965

23. Singer B, Brent TP: Human lymphoblasts contain DNA glycosylase activity excising N-3 and N-7 methyl and ethyl purines but not O^6-alkylguanine or 1-alkyladenine. Proc Natl Acad Sci USA 78:856, 1981

24. Bedell MA, Lewis JG, Billings KC, Swenberg JA: Cell specificity in hepatocarcinogenesis: Preferential accumulation of O^6-methylguanine in target cell DNA during continuous exposure of rats to 1,2-dimethylhydrazine. Cancer Res 42:3079, 1982

25. Strauss BS: Chemical mutagens and the genetic code. Prog Med Genet 3:1, 1964

26. Williams LD, Shaw BR: Protonate base pairs explain the ambiguous pairing properties of O^6-methylguanine. Proc Natl Acad Sci USA 84:1779, 1987

27. Park J-W, Ames BN: 7-Methylguanine adducts in DNA are normally present at high levels and increase on aging: Analysis by HPLC with electrochemical detection. Proc Natl Acad Sci USA 85:7467, 1988

28. Kunkel TA: Mutational specificity of depurination. Proc Natl Acad Sci USA 81:1494, 1984

29. Foster PL, Davis EF: Loss of an apurinic/apyrimidinic site endonuclease increases the mutagenicity of *N*-methyl-*N'*-nitro-*N*-nitrosoguanidine to *Escherichia coli*. Proc Natl Acad Sci USA 84:2891, 1987

30. Krieg DR: Specificity of chemical mutagenesis. Prog Nucleic Acid Res Mol Biol 2:125, 1963

31. Howard BD, Tessman I: Identification of the altered bases in mutated single-stranded DNA. II. In vivo mutagenesis by 5-bromodeoxyuridine and 2-aminopurine. J Mol Biol 9:364, 1964

32. Adler ID: The problem of caffeine mutagenicity. Ch. 24. In Vogel F, Röhrborn G (eds): Chemical Mutagens: Principles and Methods for Their Detection. Plenum, New York, 1971

33. Epstein S: The failure of caffeine to induce mutagenic effects or to synergize the effects of known mutagens in mice. Ch. 25. In Vogel F, Röhrborn G (eds): Chemical Mutagens: Principles and Methods for Their Detection. Plenum, New York, 1971

34. Lieb M: Dark repair of UV induction in K12 (λ). Virology 23:381, 1964

35. Kaplan HS, Earle JD, Howsden FL: The role of purine and pyrimidine bases and their analogs in radiation sensitivity. J Cell Physiol 64:suppl 1,69, 1964

36. Benzer S: On the topography of the genetic fine structure. Proc Natl Acad Sci USA 47:403, 1961
37. Benzer S: On the topology of the genetic fine structure. Proc Natl Acad Sci USA 45:1607, 1959
38. Stretton AOW, Brenner S: Molecular consequences of the amber mutation and its suppression. J Mol Biol 12:456, 1965
39. Brenner S, Stretton AOW: The amber mutation. J Cell Physiol 64:suppl 1, 43, 1964
40. Benzer S, Freese E: Induction of specific mutations with 5-bromouracil. Proc Natl Acad Sci USA 44:112, 1958
41. Freese E, Bautz-Freese E, Bautz E: Hydroxylamine as a mutagenic and inactivating agent. J Mol Biol 3:133, 1961
42. Tessman I, Poddar RK, Kumar S: Identification of the altered bases in mutated single-stranded DNA. I. In vitro mutagenesis by hydroxylamine, ethyl methanesulfonate and nitrous acid. J Mol Biol 9:352, 1964
43. Tessman I, Ishiwa H, Kumar S: Mutagenic effects of hydroxylamine in vivo. Science 148:507, 1965
44. Brown DM, Phillips JH: Mechanism of the mutagenic action of hydroxylamine. J Mol Biol 11:663, 1965
45. Freese E, Bautz E, Bautz-Freese E: The chemical and mutagenic specificity of hydroxylamine. Proc Natl Acad Sci USA 47:845, 1961
46. Bautz E, Freese E: On the mutagenic effect of alkylating agents. Proc Natl Acad Sci USA 46:1585, 1960
47. Wolfe KH, Sharp PM, Li W-H: Mutation rates differ among regions of the mammalian genome. Nature 337:283, 1989
48. Crick FHC, Barnett L, Brenner S, Watts-Tobin RJ: General nature of the genetic code for proteins. Nature 192:1227, 1961
49. Streisinger G, Okada Y, Emrich J, et al: Frameshift mutations and the genetic code. Cold Spring Harbor Symp Quant Biol 31:77, 1966
50. Terzaghi E, Okada Y, Streisinger G, et al: Change of a sequence of amino acids in phage T4 lysozyme by acridine-induced mutations. Proc Natl Acad Sci USA 56:500, 1966
51. Lerman LS: Acridine mutagens and DNA structure. J Cell Physiol 64:suppl 1, 1, 1964
52. Gale EF, Cundliffe E, Reynolds PE, et al: Inhibitors of nucleic acid synthesis. Ch. 5. In The Molecular Basis of Antibiotic Action. John Wiley & Sons, New York, 1981
53. Magni GE: Origin and nature of spontaneous mutations in meiotic organisms. J Cell Physiol 64:suppl 1, 165, 1964
54. Magni GE, von Borstel RC, Sora S: Mutagenic action during meiosis and antimutagenic action during mitosis by 5-aminoacridine in yeast. Mutat Res 1:227, 1964
55. Dulbecco R: Summary of 1964 biology research conference. J Cell Physiol 64:suppl 1, 181, 1964
56. Witkin EM: The effect of acriflavine on photoreversal of lethal and mutagenic damage produced in bacteria by ultraviolet light. Proc Natl Acad Sci USA 50:425, 1963
57. Taylor JH: The replication and organization of DNA in chromosomes. Ch. 2. In Taylor JH (ed): Molecular Genetics. Academic Press, New York, 1963
58. Srb AM, Owen RD, Edgar RS: General Genetics. 2nd Ed. WH Freeman, San Francisco, 1965
59. Kihlman BA: Root tips for studying the effects of chemicals on chromosomes. Ch. 18. In Hollaender A (ed): Chemical Mutagens: Principles and Methods for Their Detection. Plenum, New York, 1971
60. McClintock B: The stability of broken ends of chromosomes in Zea mays. Genetics 26:234, 1941
61. Koller PC: Comparative effects of alkylating agents on cellular morphology. Ann NY Acad Sci 68:783, 1958
62. Hsu TC, Somers CE: Effect of 5-bromodeoxyuridine on mammalian chromosomes. Proc Natl Acad Sci USA 47:397, 1961
63. Chu EHY: Effects of ultraviolet radiation on mammalian cells. I. Induction of chromosome aberrations. Mutat Res 2:75, 1965

64. Cohn NS: The effect of hydroxylamine on the rejoining of x-ray-induced chromatid breaks in *Vicia faba*. Mutat Res 1:409, 1964

65. Kihlman BA: Actions of Chemicals on Dividing Cells. Prentice-Hall, Englewood Cliffs, NJ, 1966

66. Kihlman BA: Molecular mechanisms of chromosome breakage and rejoining. In DuPraw EJ (ed): Advances in Cell and Molecular Biology. Academic Press, New York, 1971

67. Benzer S, Champe SP: A change from nonsense to sense in the genetic code. Proc Natl Acad Sci USA 48:1114, 1962

68. Cohen MM, Shaw MW, Craig AP: The effects of streptonigrin on cultured human leukocytes. Proc Natl Acad Sci USA 50:16, 1963

69. Schimke RT: Gene amplification in cultured animal cells. Cell 37:705, 1984

70. Ingram VM: Gene mutations in human haemoglobin: The chemical differences between normal and sickle haemoglobin. Nature 180:326, 1957

71. Yin L, Chun EH, Rutman RJ: A comparison of the effects of alkylation on the DNA of sensitive and resistant Lettre-Ehrlich cells following in vivo exposure to nitrogen mustard. Biochim Biophys Acta 324:472, 1973

72. Bourne HR, Coffino P, Tomkins GM: Selection of a variant lymphoma cell deficient in adenylate cyclase. Science 187:750, 1975

73. Ross EM, Gilman AG: Biochemical properties of hormone-sensitive adenylate cyclase. Ann Rev Biochem 49:533, 1980

74. Leblond CP, Steinberger E, Roosen-Runge EC: Spermatogenesis. Ch. 1. In Hartman CG (ed): Mechanisms Concerned with Conception. Macmillan, New York, 1963

75. Goldstein A: Mutagens currently of potential significance to man and other species. p. 167. In Schull WJ (ed): Mutations. Second Macy Conference on Genetics, University of Michigan Press, Ann Arbor, 1962

76. Cattanach BM: The sensitivity of the mouse testis to the mutagenic action of triethylenemelamine. Z Vererbungs 90:1, 1959

77. Alderson T, Pelecanos M: The mutagenic activity of diethyl sulphate in Drosophila melanogaster. II. The sensitivity of the immature (larval) and the adult testis. Mutat Res 1:182, 1964

78. Pelecanos M, Alderson T: The mutagenic activity of diethyl sulphate in Drosophila melanogaster. III. The sensitivity of the immature (larval) and adult ovary. Mutat Res 1:302, 1964

79. Ames BN: Identifying environmental chemicals causing mutations and cancer. Science 204:587, 1979

80. Ames BN: Dietary carcinogens and anticarcinogens. Science 221:1256, 1983

81. Weisburger JH, Williams GM: Carcinogen testing: Current problems and new approaches. Science 214:401, 1981

82. Ames BN, Durston WE, Yamasaki E, Lee FD: Carcinogens are mutagens: A simple test system combining liver homogenates for activation and bacteria for detection. Proc Natl Acad Sci USA 70:2281, 1973

83. Abrahamson S, Lewis EB: The detection of mutations in Drosophila melanogaster. Ch. 17. In Hollaender A (ed): Chemical Mutagens: Principles and Methods for Their Detection. Plenum, New York, 1971

84. Grahn D: Mammalian radiation genetics. p. 127. In Burdette WJ (ed): Methodology in Mammalian Genetics. Holden-Day, San Francisco, 1963

85. Cattanach BM: Specific locus mutation in mice. Ch. 20. In Hollaender A (ed): Chemical Mutagens: Principles and Methods for Their Detection. Plenum, New York, 1971

86. Muller HJ: The measurement of gene mutation rate in Drosophila, its high variability, and its dependence upon temperature. Genetics 13:279, 1928

87. Partington M, Bateman AJ: Dominant lethal mutations induced in male mice by methyl methanesulphonate. Heredity (Edinburgh) 19:191, 1964

88. Bateman AJ, Epstein SS: Dominant lethal mutations in mammals. Ch. 21. In Hollaender A (ed): Chemical Mutagens: Principles and Methods for Their Detection. Plenum, New York, 1971

89. Epstein SS, Röhrborn G: Recommended procedures for testing genetic hazards from chemicals, based on the induction of dominant lethal mutations in mammals. Nature 230:459, 1971
90. Russell WL: X-ray-induced mutations in mice. Cold Spring Harbor Symp Quant Biol 16:327, 1951
91. Malling HV: Chemical mutagens as a possible genetic hazard in human populations. Am Ind Hyg Assoc J 31:657, 1970
92. Harris M: Mutagenicity of chemicals and drugs. Science 171:51, 1971
93. Stern C. Principles of Human Genetics. 3rd Ed. WH Freeman, San Francisco, 1973
94. Yanofsky C, Cox EC, Horn V: The unusual mutagenic specificity of an *E. coli* mutator gene. Proc Natl Acad Sci USA 55:274, 1966
95. Pierce BLS: The effect of a bacterial gene upon mutation rates in bacteriophage T4. Genetics 54:657, 1966
96. Goldstein A, Smoot JS: A strain of *Escherichia coli* with an unusually high rate of auxotrophic mutation. J Bacteriol 70:588, 1955
97. Treffers HP, Spinelli V, Belser NO: A factor (or mutator gene) influencing mutation rates in Escherichia coli. Proc Natl Acad Sci USA 40:1064, 1954
98. Drake J (ed): The genetic control of mutation. Genetics, suppl., 73: April 1973

12

Chemical Carcinogenesis

Raymond W. Ruddon

Why should a pharmacologist be interested in chemical carcinogenesis? Often this is thought to be the pursuit of the biochemist, cancer biologist, molecular geneticist, and epidemiologist. The magnitude of the cancer problem in the United States and other Western countries, where cancer is the second leading cause of death, is, of course, itself a compelling reason to be interested, but in addition there are several areas that are of experimental interest to pharmacologists. Of primary importance is the fact that a number of drugs, hormones, and food additives are carcinogenic in animals and potentially carcinogenic in humans. Take, for example, the appearance of vaginal adenocarcinomas in young women whose mothers had taken the synthetic estrogen diethylstilbestrol (DES) during pregnancy to prevent spontaneous abortion. This was an accepted treatment in the 1950s and 1960s to maintain pregnancy for women with a high tendency to abort spontaneously, and it was not until 1971 that the carcinogenic effect of this treatment was reported.[1] The continuing controversy over the safety of nonsugar sweeteners for foods and soft drinks highlights another example of the potential carcinogenic effects of compounds consumed as food additives. These chemicals are consumed by the ton, and yet certain of them are suspected of being tumor promoters. A number of anticancer agents have been implicated in the occurrence of secondary acute myelogenous leukemias arising in cancer patients 2 to 10 years after successful treatment.[2] Notable among these compounds are such alkylating agents as melphalan, chlorambucil, and cyclophosphamide, which are known to interact with DNA in a manner similar to some chemical mutagens.

Many carcinogens are detoxified or metabolized to an active carcinogenic moiety by the same enzyme systems (e.g., the P-450 monooxygenases) that metabolize drugs and thus are subject to modulation by agents that induce or inhibit these metabolic pathways. The metabolism of carcinogens is also regulated in genetically determined and species-specific ways. For example, animals and humans that have a slow acetylator as opposed to a fast acetylator phenotype (cf. Ch. 7) are potentially more susceptible to arylamine-induced urinary bladder cancer,[3] possibly because these agents are metabolized more completely in fast acetylators resulting in inactivation of more of the compound before it reaches the urinary bladder, the target tissue. Variation in metabolism between species may also explain why some species are more susceptible than others to certain carcinogens.

Another interesting pharmacologic point is that chemical carcinogens have specific target tissues. Thus, a chemical may cause mainly renal cancers in one species and hepatic tumors in another, for example. Some carcinogens act primarily at the site of their application. If painted on the skin, they produce papillomatous epithelial growths that develop into squamous cell carcinomas. If injected subcutaneously, they produce sarcomas (i.e., malignant growths of the fibroblasts in connective tissues). If given by mouth, they may produce tumors of the gastrointestinal tract. Other carcinogens are principally effective when incorporated into the diet; they act on the liver to produce malignant hepatomas or tumors of the bile ducts. Some carcinogens act at widely dispersed sites throughout the body regardless of the route by which they are taken in. Cutaneous application of such a compound might lead not only to skin cancer at the point of application but also perhaps to cancer of the intestine, lungs, or kidneys. Illustrative of carcinogenesis at a remote site is the effect of the hydrocarbon 3-methylcholanthrene. When this substance was given to rats in the diet, it caused no hepatomas but produced cancer of the mammary glands in all the treated animals.[4] Similarly, administration of naphthylamine by any route leads to cancer of the bladder in susceptible species. The mammary cancers caused by 3-methylcholanthrene, the bladder tumors caused by naphythylamine, and indeed all cancers that develop in tissues remote from the site of carcinogen administration are not metastatic implants. They are primary tumors initiated by the carcinogen itself or by a product of carcinogen metabolism after absorption and distribution have taken place.

Mice have been bred selectively for a high incidence of spontaneous tumors at particular sites. For example, one strain may develop spontaneous mammary gland cancers at a rate of less than 1 percent, whereas the incidence in a specially bred strain may be as high as 90 percent. Sometimes a high susceptibility to spontaneous cancer of a particular tissue is associated with high sensitivity to induced chemical carcinogenesis at the same site, but this is not necessarily so. If a given carcinogen induces sarcomas at the site of subcutaneous injection and also lung carcinomas remote from the injection site, selective breeding may yield one strain in which the carcinogen produces only sarcomas, another in which only lung tumors develop. Azo dyes injected subcutaneously usually cause both sarcomas at the injection site and hepatomas, but some strains of mice develop few tumors of either kind in response to these agents. This pattern of genetic variation in susceptibility to cancer in general, susceptibility to cancer of particular tissues, and susceptibility to individual chemical carcinogens may also apply in the human. It is well known that certain kinds of cancer tend to run in families, and there is also a high concordance rate for the occurrence of specific types of cancer in monozygous twins.

Sex differences in cancer incidence and in responses to carcinogens may be related to hormonal influences.[5,6] A strain of mice that developed mammary cancer at a high rate after administration of a hydrocarbon carcinogen was found to produce unusually large amounts of estrogen. Estrogen administration to other strains was found to increase the yield of mammary tumors caused by the same carcinogen.

Malignant growths of hormone-sensitive organs often remain responsive to the hormones that ordinarily stimulate these organs. For example, prostate cancer can be treated by castration to remove the major source of testosterone or by administration of estrogenic hormones, which antagonize the effects of androgens. Thyroid tumors have been induced by pituitary thyroid-stimulating hormone or thiouracil (which causes increased output of

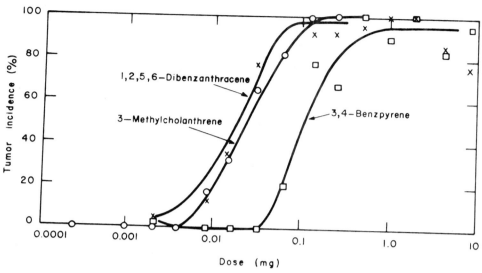

Fig. 12-1. Dose-response relationship for carcinogens. Three hydrocarbon carcinogens were administered subcutaneously, each to a group of 20 mice in a single dose. The incidence of sarcomas at the site of injection was noted. (From Bryan et al.[8])

the pituitary hormone). Pituitary hormones have also been used to produce tumors in the adrenal glands, ovaries, testes, and mammary glands. It is not certain whether the hormones act as carcinogens in their own right or whether they alter the cellular environment in sensitive tissues in a way that makes them more susceptible to endogenous or exogenous carcinogens. Some phenanthrene derivatives having the same carbon ring skeleton as the naturally occurring steroids are potent carcinogens, even on tissues (such as skin) that are not hormone-dependent. No such compounds have been found to arise by metabolism of steroid hormones, but they might possibly be produced from dietary steroids through metabolism by the intestinal flora.[7]

If species, strain, sex, hormonal status, diet, and route of administration are carefully controlled, then reliable dose-response relationships can be found, and the relative potencies of carcinogens can be described quantitatively.[8] Figure 12-1 shows log dose–response curves for three hydrocarbon carcinogens administered to groups of mice by single subcutaneous injections. The eventual incidence of sarcomas at the injection sites was recorded. The curves are approximately parallel, suggesting a similar mechanism of action of the agents. Under these conditions 3,4-benzpyrene was about one-fifth as potent as 1,2,5,6-dibenzanthracene or 3-methylcholanthrene. ED50 values and their confidence limits for carcinogenesis may be found in the same way as for any toxic drug action. At least a 10-fold increase of dose was required to span the range of response from an incidence of a few percent to an incidence of nearly 100 percent. This implies that laboratory experiments may tend to underestimate the likelihood that very small doses of a carcinogen will produce cancer in some animals. The reason is that with a small group of animals (e.g., less than 100) a dosage that causes no tumors at all will be judged ineffective, whereas the same dosage in a large population of the species would cause cancer in some animals. The same argument applies to estimating "safe" dosages of carcinogens in human populations on the basis of experimentation with a limited number of animals.

Perhaps the most interesting pharmacologic question is: What is the mechanism of action of chemical carcinogens? While a number of clues have been found over the years, the answer is not clearly understood. This chapter will attempt to give an overview of the biology of the cancer cell, the epidemiology of cancer, various classes of known and suspected chemical carcinogens, the routes of their metabolic activation, and evidence relating to their mechanism of action.

BIOLOGY OF THE CANCER CELL

Carcinogenic *transformation* occurs in cells that have the capacity to proliferate. The target cells for cancer-causing agents, including chemicals, oncogenic viruses, and radiation are most likely the so-called stem cells of an organ (i.e., those cells that have some capacity to divide when stimulated to do so, for example, after tissue wounding). These are the *renewal cells* of a tissue. It is unlikely that fully differentiated nonproliferating cells are targets for malignant transformation. Thus, cells such as mature neurons and peripheral blood leukocytes are not the cell types that are susceptible to carcinogens. In malignant transformation, the transformed cell becomes blocked during the process of normal differentiation; the genes regulating cell differentiation are shut off or function abnormally while the genes controlling cell proliferation are locked in the "on" position. The exact sequence of changes that the various types of carcinogens produce to bring about these cellular aberrations in gene expression are not clear, but most carcinogens have in common an ability to interact with genomic DNA and thus have the potential to alter the regulatory sequences that control genes coding for the structural proteins and enzymes that modulate cell proliferation and differentiation. It is most likely the control of these regulatory sequences that is altered rather than the structural genes themselves, since changes in the structural genes would probably lead to a nonfunctional or badly damaged gene product, and that could be fatal to the cell. In some cases (as will be described below) the activation of cellular *onc* genes (oncogenes) could lead to increased production of a growth factor or a receptor for a growth factor by the transformed cell.

Several phenotypic changes occur in transformed cells, of which some[9,10] are schematically represented in Figure 12-2. Many of these deviations from the phenotype of normal cells have been observed in cultured cells, and it is not clear for a number of these traits how they relate to the biology of the cancer cell in the living animal or patient. Several alterations, however, that are typical of cancer cells can be listed. In general, cancer tissues, compared with their normal counterpart tissues, contain cells that have larger nuclei, more prominent nucleoli, a decreased differentiation state compared with the mature normal cell of that type, and increased numbers of mitotic cells. This is not to say that cancer cells always proliferate faster than normal cells, because they may not. In the bone marrow, for example, normal stem cells proliferate as rapidly as leukemic cells; the difference between these cell types is in their response to normal regulatory signals that tell them when and how often to divide. It is true, though, that viewed as a population, neoplasms usually have a higher *percentage* of dividing cells than normal surrounding tissue.

Several biochemical changes can be correlated with the increased propensity of cancer cells to proliferate. As might be expected, enzymes involved in nucleic acid synthesis, transport of nutrients, and cell membrane turnover are often increased in cancer cells.[11] In addition, a number of cell surface changes can be observed. There is frequently a change in charge density, probably due to changes in the number and distribution of

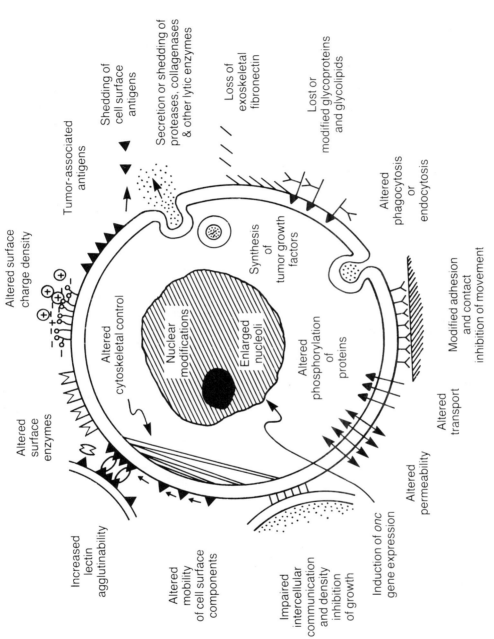

Altered surface charge density

Tumor-associated antigens

Shedding of cell surface antigens

Secretion or shedding of proteases, collagenases & other lytic enzymes

Loss of exoskeletal fibronectin

Lost or modified glycoproteins and glycolipids

Altered phagocytosis or endocytosis

Synthesis of tumor growth factors

Nuclear modifications

Enlarged nucleoli

Altered phosphorylation of proteins

Modified adhesion and contact inhibition of movement

Altered cytoskeletal control

Altered surface enzymes

Altered transport

Altered permeability

Increased lectin agglutinability

Altered mobility of cell surface components

Impaired intercellular communication and density inhibition of growth

Induction of *onc* gene expression

Fig. 12-2. Some cellular alterations observed after neoplastic transformation. (Modified from Nicolson,[10] with permission.)

negatively charged sialic acid molecules on cell surface glycoproteins and glycolipids. Several biochemical alterations in tumor cell surface glycoproteins and glycolipids have been reported. In some cases, there is a ''simplification'' of the oligosaccharide portions of these molecules, reflecting a decrease in the complete processing of the carbohydrate chains to the typical mature, complex chains that predominate in normal cells.[9] Changes in glycoproteins and glycolipids probably also explain to a large extent the altered lectin agglutinability and the modified adhesion properties of cancer cells, as well as the production of tumor-associated antigens. The specific tumor-associated antigens detected by monoclonal antibodies have frequently turned out to be glycoproteins or glycolipids with altered carbohydrate structure.[12] Tumor cells also have an increased propensity to shed lytic enzymes such as glycosidases, proteases, and collagenases, and this may explain, in part, why tumor cells are invasive and have the ability to metastasize to distant organs.

Various intracellular biochemical changes also occur in tumor cells. There may be an altered pattern of protein phosphorylation, perhaps the end result of activation of oncogenes whose products either have or can modulate protein kinase activity.[13,14] Tumor cells may produce their own growth factors, some of which are called TGFs (for transforming growth factors), which stimulate their own proliferation.[15]

CANCER EPIDEMIOLOGY

There are large variations in cancer incidence in various parts of the world[16] (Table 12-1). The variations most likely reflect all the variables in life-style and environment among different populations, including diet and exposure to various chemical agents.[17] In addition to the worldwide variation, there are significant differences within the United States in cancer incidence and mortality rates. The example shown in Figure 12-3 demonstrates the mortality rates for bronchogenic cancer in white males in the United States, by

Table 12-1. Worldwide Variation in the Incidence of Common Cancers. Range of Variation is Expressed for Ages 35 to 64.

Type of Cancer	High-incidence Area	Low-incidence Area	Range of Variation
Skin	Australia (Queensland)	India (Bombay)	>200
Buccal cavity	India	Denmark	>25
Nasopharynx	Singapore[a]	England	40
Bronchus	England	Nigeria	35
Esophagus	Iran	Nigeria	300
Stomach	Japan	Uganda	25
Liver	Mozambique	Norway	70
Colon	U.S.A. (Connecticut)[b]	Nigeria	10
Rectum	Denmark	Nigeria	20
Pancreas	New Zealand[c]	Uganda	5
Breast	U.S.A. (Connecticut)[b]	Uganda	5
Uterine cervix	Colombia	Israel	15
Uterine corpus	U.S.A. (Connecticut)[b]	Japan	10
Ovary	Denmark	Japan	8
Bladder	U.S.A. (Connecticut)[b]	Japan	4
Prostate	U.S.A.[d]	Japan	30
Penis	Uganda	Israel	300

[a] Chinese.
[b] The U.S. data are taken from the Connecticut Tumor Registry because it is the oldest continuous cancer registry based upon a defined population in this country.
[c] Maori.
[d] Blacks.
(Data from Doll.[16])

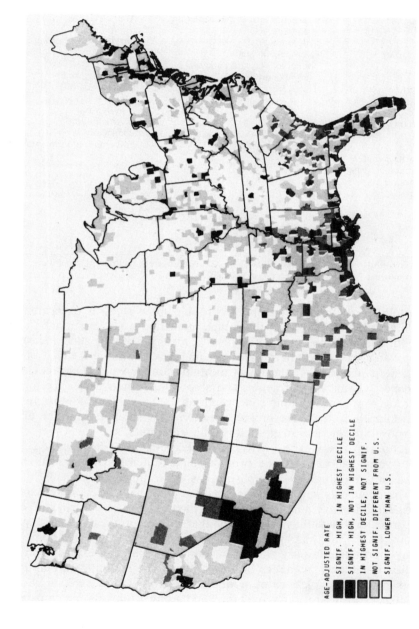

Fig. 12-3. Mortality rates for cancers of the trachea, bronchus, and lung in the United States for white males, by county, 1950 to 1969. (From Blot et al.,[18] with permission.)

AGE-ADJUSTED RATE

SIGNIF. HIGH, IN HIGHEST DECILE

SIGNIF. HIGH, NOT IN HIGHEST DECILE

IN HIGHEST DECILE, NOT SIGNIF.

NOT SIGNIF. DIFFERENT FROM U.S.

SIGNIF. LOWER THAN U.S.

Table 12-2. Chemicals and Industrial Processes Associated with Human Cancer

Carcinogenic for Humans	Probably Carcinogenic for Humans	Possibly Carcinogenic for Humans
4-Aminobiphenyl	Aflatoxins	Acrylonitrile
Arsenic and certain arsenic compounds	Cadmium and certain cadmium compounds[a]	Aminotriazole
Asbestos	Chlorambucil	Auramine
Auramine manufacturing[a]	Cyclophosphamide	Beryllium and certain beryllium
Benzene	Nickel and certain nickel	compounds[a]
Benzidine	compounds[a]	Carbon tetrachloride
N,N-Bis(2-chloroethyl)	Thio TEPA	Dimethyl carbamoyl chloride
-2-naphthylamine		Dimethyl sulfate
Bis(chloromethyl) ether		Ethylene oxide
Chromium and certain chromium		Iron dextran
compounds[a]		Oxymetholone
Diethylstilbestrol		Phenacetin
Underground hematite mining[a]		Polychlorinated biphenyls
Isopropyl alcohol manufacturing by strong acid process[a]		
Melphalan		
Mustard gas		
2-Naphthylamine		
Nickel refining[a]		
Soots, tars, and mineral oils[a]		
Vinyl chloride		

[a] The specific compounds that may be responsible for a carcinogenic effect in humans have not been identified. (Data from International Agency for Research on Cancer.[20])

county.[18] This "clustering" of cancers should provide some clues as to particular environmental and life-style traits found in these high incidence areas, eventually leading, it is hoped, to identification of the immediate causes. Clustering of lung cancer cases occurs in large metropolitan areas, in southern California and Nevada, along the Gulf of Mexico, and along the eastern seaboard. Lung cancer mortality among white males is elevated in counties with paper, chemical, petroleum, and shipbuilding industries. The strong correlation of cigarette smoking with lung cancer mortality[19] most likely contributes heavily to this distribution pattern: there are probably more heavy smokers in urban areas, and they are also exposed to the additional factor of air pollutants.

Although direct occupational exposure to chemical carcinogens is thought to add a small increment to the overall cancer incidence (probably 5 percent or less),[17] there are a number of clear examples in which industrial exposure has led to an increase in the number of cancer cases. The chemicals and industrial processes that have been shown to have or are strongly suspected to have an etiologic role in the development of cancer[20] are listed in Table 12-2. For many years it has been known that workers in the dye industry exposed to aromatic amines such as 2-naphthylamine, 4-aminobiphenyl, and benzidine have an increased risk of contracting urinary bladder cancer.[9] Occupational exposure to asbestos fibers has resulted in a higher incidence of lung cancer.[20] Beginning with Percival Pott's report in 1775 of increased incidence of scrotal cancer in chimney sweeps, it gradually became known that exposure to soot, coal tars, and certain crude oils can cause epithelial cancer in the skin and other organs. We now know that the carcinogenicity of these materials is related to their content of polycyclic aromatic hydrocarbons.

Air and Water Pollutants

Although direct occupational exposure may account for relatively few cancers, many of these same materials find their way into our everyday environment via chemical dump sites, smokestacks, water supplies, and the food chain. It is not clear what carcinogenic effect, if any, chronic long-term exposure to low levels of carcinogens is having on the populace. However, we may be sitting on a time bomb in that it often takes 20 to 25 years for "initiated" cancer cells to be "promoted" and grow to the stage of clinical detection (see below). Since the worldwide pollution of our environment by synthetic chemicals is a relatively recent phenomenon in human history, it may take several more decades before the effects of all these xenobiotics can be ascertained.

An example of the potential problem is the effluents that find their way into drinking water supplies. One study estimated that over 1,000 tons of chlorinated organic compounds are discharged by sewage treatment plants annually into the nation's waterways.[21] Some of these chlorinated compounds are known to be carcinogenic in animals. In another survey about 325 organic chemicals were identified in the drinking water of various cities.[22] Only about 10 percent of these have been carefully studied for carcinogenicity.

Diet

There is strong suggestive evidence that diet is associated with several types of human cancer, including cancers of the stomach, colon, pancreas, breast, ovary, uterine endometrium, and prostate.[23] There is evidence that a high dietary intake of fat, as well as a dietary deficiency of fiber, may play a role in the etiology of colon cancer. The typical U.S. diet, for example, contains 40 to 45 percent of its calories as fat, but in Japan, where the incidence of colon cancer is much lower, only 15 to 20 percent of dietary calories are derived from fat.[23] There is also a correlation between breast cancer mortality in women in various countries and fat consumption[24] (Fig. 12-4). To date, the carcinogenic materials (if any) in dietary fat have not been clearly identified. However, animal fat is a storage depot for many lipid-soluble chemical carcinogens, and they may be passed on via this source to higher species in the food chain. In addition, there is evidence that certain bile acids, secreted into the gastrointestinal tract in response to a high fat diet, can act as tumor promoters.[25]

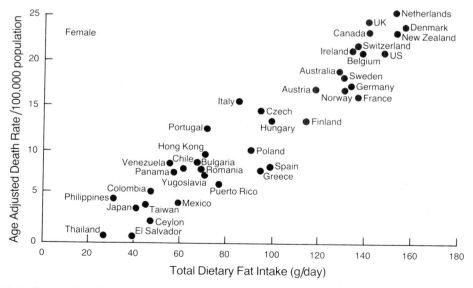

Fig. 12-4. Correlation between breast cancer mortality in various countries and fat consumption. (From Carroll,[24] with permission.)

Certain protective elements in the diet have also been identified. There is evidence that animals fed diets poor in selenium, for example, have a higher tumor incidence when fed carcinogens and that vitamin C can decrease the amount of nitrosamine formed from dietary nitrites and secondary amines.[17] Also, vitamin A-containing foods appear to have some protective effect. Thus, it seems that a well rounded diet, including a reasonable amount of fiber, is a prudent choice. There is no evidence, however, that macrovitamin regimens will protect against cancer, and indeed, such diets may be harmful by causing hypervitaminosis.

A number of naturally occurring toxins with carcinogenic potential are also present in small quantities in the human diet.[26] For example, black pepper contains a small amount of safrole, a carcinogen in rodents. A widely eaten false morel (*Gyromitra esculenta*) contains 11 hydrazine-type compounds, 3 of which are known carcinogens. Pyrrolizidine alkaloids are mutagenic, carcinogenic, and teratogenic and are present in numerous plant species, some of which are ingested by humans in herbs and herbal teas. Gossypol, a major toxin in cottonseed oil and a potent initiator and promoter in the mouse skin carcinogenesis model, may be consumed in appreciable amounts in certain countries such as Egypt, where cottonseed oil is used in cooking. A variety of carcinogens are present in molds that contaminate foods consumed by humans, such as corn, grain, nuts, peanut butter, and fruit. Two of these, sterigmatocystin and aflatoxin, are among the most potent mutagens and carcinogens known.

Clearly, one needs to be cautious in interpreting correlative data. A mere association of a factor with cancer incidence does not prove cause. Since high-fat, high-beef diets tend to be associated with economically well off populations, one could also plot the number of luxury automobiles versus colon cancers and likely find a high correlation coefficient.

Hormones and Drugs

The carcinogenic effect of hormones was demonstrated by Lacassagne in 1932, when he found that mice injected repeatedly with an ovarian extract containing estrogen developed mammary carcinomas. Later, he also showed that the synthetic estrogen diethylstilbestrol (DES) induces mammary tumors in susceptible strains of mice.[27] The discovery of the increased risk of vaginal carcinoma in women whose mothers took DES during early pregnancy, mentioned above, demonstrates that excessive hormone stimulation can also be carcinogenic in humans. A role of hormones in human breast cancer has also been deduced from the known risk factors associated with the disease. These factors relate to prolonged hormonal stimulation, and they include early age of menarche, delayed age of first pregnancy, and delayed menopause.

Exposure to certain drugs has also been implicated in the appearance of some cancers. Anticancer drugs are of particular risk in this regard, but other drugs are also suspected of causing or contributing to the development of cancer in humans. For example, several cases of hepatocellular carcinomas have been reported in patients with blood disorders treated chronically with the androgenic drug oxymetholone.[20] Several studies have indicated that chronic use of analgesic preparations containing phenacetin leads to papillary necrosis of the kidney. It has been suggested that this is related to the subsequent development of transitional cell carcinoma of the renal pelvis in some of these persons.[20]

Cigarette Smoking

There are extensive and compelling data to indicate that cigarette smoking is a major contributing factor to lung cancer and probably to other cancers as well.[19] These data are summarized below.

1. A strong relationship between cigarette smoking and lung cancer mortality in men has been demonstrated in numerous prospective and retrospective studies, with risks for all smokers as a group ranging from 7.6 to 14.2 times those for nonsmokers.
2. A dose-response relationship between cigarette smoking and risk of lung cancer for both men and women has been demonstrated in numerous studies, with risks for men who are heavy smokers ranging from 5 to 24 times those for nonsmokers. Light smokers are at an intermediate risk.
3. Mortality from lung cancer directly attributable to cigarette smoking is increased in the presence of "urbanization" and such occupational hazards as uranium mining and exposure to asbestos.
4. Cessation of smoking results in lowered risk of mortality from lung cancer in comparison with continuation of smoking.
5. Results from autopsy studies show that changes in bronchial mucosa that are thought to precede development of bronchogenic carcinoma are more common in smokers than in nonsmokers, and there is a dose-response relationship for these changes.
6. Chronic inhalation of cigarette smoke or the intratracheal instillation of various fractions of tobacco smoke produces lung cancer in such experimental animals as dogs and hamsters.
7. Cell culture studies show that various constituents found in tobacco and cigarette smoke condensate produce malignant transformation of cells.
8. Numerous complete carcinogens and cocarcinogens (tumor promoters) have been isolated from cigarette smoke condensate.
9. In lung tissue samples obtained from patients undergoing thoracic surgery, cigarette smokers have higher DNA adduct levels than nonsmokers, and there is a linear relationship between adduct levels and the amount of cigarettes consumed over time.[28] People who have given up smoking for at least five years have adduct levels similar to those of nonsmokers.

In spite of the overwhelming evidence relating smoking to lung cancer, cigarette consumption continues at a very high level and is rising for women. In several states in the U.S. the mortality due to lung cancer now exceeds that due to breast cancer in women.

MECHANISMS OF CHEMICAL CARCINOGENESIS

Initiation and Promotion

The development of a clinically detectable cancer is a multistage process that for most cancers occurring in adults takes many years. This is clear from a number of inadvertent human "experiments" in which an inciting initiating event or exposure to carcinogen can be documented. Examples include the long latency period for: (1) the development of lung cancer in cigarette smokers (e.g., the 20-pack-year phenomenon—a pack a day for 20 years produces a high incidence of lung cancer); (2) the development of cancer in radiation workers and people exposed to atomic bomb fallout or development of thyroid cancer long after exposure to radiation; and (3) the appearance of certain iatrogenically induced cancers such as cancers occurring in patients exposed to a radiocontrast solution containing radioactive thorium. In most of these instances the detection of cancer occurs many years after the initial exposure to the probable initiating cause. The reasons for this latency period have been experimentally examined in animals and can now be fairly accurately defined. As will be discussed below, the initiating event appears to induce a genetic change in cells, which becomes amplified by clonal expression of a very small percentage of the altered cells over many years, probably via continued exposure to "promoting" agents that stimulate the proliferation of the altered cells.

The first solid evidence for the multistage process of cancer development came from the work of Peyton Rous and his colleagues, who found that virus-induced skin papillomas in rabbits regressed after a period of time but could be made to reappear if the skin was stressed by punching holes in it or by the application of such irritant substances as turpentine or chloroform. These findings led Rous and his associates to conclude that tumor cells could exist in a latent or dormant state and that the tumor induction process and subsequent growth of the tumor involved different mechanisms, which they called *initiation* and *promotion*.[29]

In the early 1940s, reports appeared that creosote or croton oil, at doses that were not themselves carcinogenic, increased the number of skin tumors in mice whose skin was treated with polycyclic aromatic hydrocarbons.[30] It was also noted that when the croton oil was given after the polycyclic aromatic hydrocarbon, the augmentation in numbers of skin tumors was still observed. Experiments on the events involved in the initiation and promotion phases of carcinogenesis have been greatly aided by the identification of agents that have primarily initiating activity, such as urethane, and the purification of the components of croton oil that have only promoting activity. Diesters of the diterpene alcohol phorbol are the tumor-promoting substances in croton oil. One of these, 12-O-tetradecanoylphorbol-13-acetate (TPA) is one of the most potent promoters known and has been widely used in studies of initiation and promotion. Some carcinogens, such as certain polycyclic aromatic hydrocarbons, have both initating and promoting action and are said to be "complete" carcinogens.

An experimental protocol often used to study the initiation and promotion phases of carcinogenesis is the mouse skin model (Fig. 12-5). In this model tumor initiation is brought about by the single application of a potent initiator. Promotion is elicited by the repeated application of a promoter such as TPA. Benign papillomas begin to appear by 12 to 20 weeks, and by about 52 weeks 40 to 60 percent of the animals develop squamous cell carcinomas. If the promoting agent is given alone or if it is administered before the initiating agent, no malignant tumors occur. Once the initiating event occurs, the promoter can be given up to 1 year later and still produce carcinomas, which indicates that the initiating agent produces a stable genetic change in the cell. This is consistent with the idea that the initiating event involves a genetic mutation (see below). The promotion phase, on the other hand, is a slow, gradual process, and a prolonged exposure to the promoting agent is required. Promotion occupies the greater part of the latent period of carcinogenesis, it is at least partially reversible, and it can be arrested by certain anticarcinogenic agents (*antipromoters*).[9] The tumor promotion phase of carcinogenesis is really a continuum and probably involves several events. First, a cell proliferation phase fosters the propagation of a clone of initiated cells. Most (if not all) promoting agents are *mitogens* (stimulators of cell replication) for the target tissue in which promotion occurs. The second

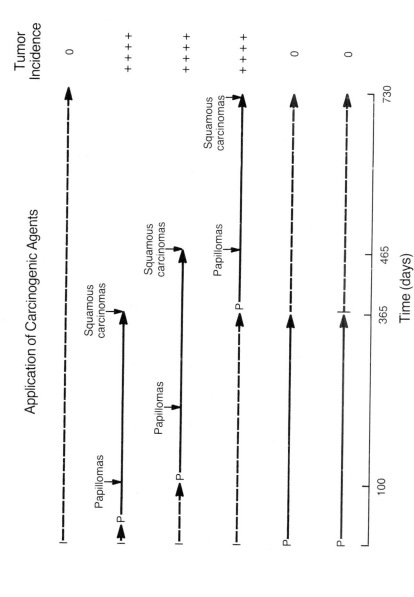

Fig. 12-5. Scheme of initiation and promotion phases of induction of carcinogenesis in mouse skin. Initiation is caused by the single application of a subcarcinogenic dose of an agent such as 7,12-dimethylbenz[a]anthracene, benzo[a]pyrene, or urethane. Promotion is carried out by repeated application (e.g., three times per week) of an agent such as the phorbol ester TPA. Papillomas develop within 12 to 20 weeks, squamous carcinomas in about 1 year. Solid lines, continual application of agent; dotted lines, duration of time without exposure to agents. Note that promoter may be added up to 1 year after a single application of the initiating agent and tumors still occur. I, initiator; P, promoter. (From Ruddon,[9] with permission.)

part of the promotion phase is one of genetic instability in the tumor cell population, during which cells with a more malignant phenotype (i.e., loss of response to growth regulatory signals, increased invasiveness, ability to metastasize) evolve. During this phase tumor growth progresses to a clinically detectable stage.

Mechanism of Action and Cellular Targets for Initiating Agents

The vast majority of tumor-initiating agents have the capability to react with cellular DNA, and most likely (as for mutagenic agents discussed in Chapter 11) nuclear DNA is the cellular target for these chemicals. Indeed, most initiating carcinogens are mutagenic in the various tests described in Chapter 11. Thus, the dictum that all (initiating) carcinogens are mutagens but not all mutagens are carcinogens has become well established. The targets in DNA for carcinogenic agents appear to be the same as those described for mutagenic agents (e.g., the N-7 and 0^6 of guanine for carcinogenic alkylating agents, the C-8 position of guanine for acetylaminofluorene, the 2-amino group of guanine for polycyclic aromatic hydrocarbons).

The evidence that tumor initiation involves a mutagenic event is strong. Agents that damage DNA are frequently carcinogenic in animals. Ultraviolet (UV) and ionizing radiation also damage DNA at doses that are carcinogenic. In one interesting experimental system this has been shown directly. Cultured cells of the fish *Poecilia formosa* can be treated in vitro with UV light to produce pyrimidine dimers, as described in Chapter 11. In this species, pyrimidine dimers can be repaired by exposure to visible light, the so-called photoreactivation repair system. If UV-irradiated cells are injected into the fish before photoreactivation occurs, thyroid carcinomas are elicited. However, no tumors appear if the irradiated cells are exposed to photoreactivating illumination prior to injection.[31]

About 90 percent of all known carcinogens are mutagenic in the Ames test (see Ch. 11).[32] Moreover, only a few noncarcinogens show significant mutagenicity in this test system. Malignant transformation can be induced in a variety of cultured mammalian cells by agents that are mutagenic for the same cells. For example, carcinogenic polycylic hydrocarbons induce mutation to purine antimetabolite resistance in Chinese hamster V79 cells if the cells are cocultured with lethally irradiated rodent cells that can metabolize the hydrocarbons to their active DNA-binding metabolite.[33] There is no mutagenic effect with noncarcinogenic hydrocarbons, and the degree of mutagenicity correlates with the in vivo carcinogenic potential of all the polycyclic aromatic hydrocarbons in the series of compounds tested.

Perhaps the most powerful evidence that mutational events are responsible in large part for initiation of malignant tumors comes from studies of patients with known DNA repair defects. One of these defects, a recessively inherited condition called xeroderma pigmentosum, is characterized by defective repair of DNA damage induced by UV light and by extreme sensitivity to sunlight. Virtually 100 percent of affected individuals will eventually develop skin cancer. Cultured cells taken from patients with xeroderma pigmentosum are also less efficient at repairing chemically induced damage to their DNA. Patients with ataxia telangiectasia, also an autosomal recessive trait, have a progressive cerebellar ataxia and immune deficiencies. Their cells are three to four times as sensitive to damage by x-irradiation and by certain carcinogenic chemicals. These patients also have a DNA repair defect and are more prone to develop leukemia and cancers of the ovary, breast, gallbladder, and lymph nodes than the general population.[34] Fanconi's anemia, another rare, autosomal recessively inherited disease, is characterized by growth retardation and hematologic insufficiency. Cells from affected individuals have more spontaneous chromosomal aberrations than normal cells and show more chromosomal damage after treatment with DNA-binding agents, such as nitrogen mustard or mitomycin C.[35] Patients with Fanconi's anemia are at increased risk to develop leukemia and various other forms of cancer.

Mechanism of Action and Cellular Targets for Promoting Agents

Tumor-promoting agents produce a wide variety of biochemical changes in cells. The tumor-promoting phorbol esters, particularly TPA, have been studied in most detail. A number of the biochemical alterations induced by these compounds may be involved in the proliferation of carcinogen-initiated tumor cells in vivo, and many of these alterations are reminiscent of the transformed phenotype depicted in Figure 12-2. The effects of phorbol esters on cultured cells include: (1) induction of enzymes such as ornithine decarboxylase, 5′-nucleotidase, ATPase, and the protease plasminogen activator; (2) stimulation of glucose uptake, DNA synthesis, and cell proliferation; and (3) alteration of cell morphology with a loss of cell surface fibronectin and the appearance of diffuse actin-containing cytoskeletal elements.[9,36] In addition, phorbol esters have been shown to stimulate anchorage-independent growth of oncogenic virus-transformed cells and to inhibit the terminal differentiation of muscle cells, chondrocytes, lipocytes, and mammary epithelial cells in culture.[9,37,38] These cell culture effects are brought about by biologically relevant concentrations (nanomolar range), and there is generally a correlation between the potencies of phorbol esters in producing the above biochemical effects and their potencies as promoters in the mouse skin carcinogenesis assay. Interestingly, TPA has been shown to stimulate DNA synthesis in cultured preneoplastic colonic epithelial cells from patients with familial polyposis but not in similar cultures of normal colonic epithelial cells,[39] which suggests that the "initiated" cells of polyposis patients are somehow "primed" to be stimulated by a tumor-promoting agent. Similarly, it has been suggested that tumor promoters increase the proliferation and colony-forming ability of mouse fibroblasts bearing an amplified gene (for dihydrofolate reductase),[40] which implies that cells with an altered DNA content may have a selective advantage in their ability to respond to the proliferative stimulus of tumor-promoting agents.

High-affinity cellular receptors for phorbol esters have been found in mammalian cells.[41–44] These receptors have high specificity for phorbol esters, are both cytosolic and membrane-associated, and have a K_D in the 10 nM range. A parallel finding, namely that tumor-promoting phorbol esters activate a calcium-requiring, phospholipid-dependent protein kinase called protein kinase C,[45] (see Ch. 2) led to the startling conclusion that, in fact, protein kinase C is itself a receptor for phorbol ester.[46,47]

Protein kinase C is widely distributed in mammalian tissues. The gene for the enzyme has been cloned, and there appear to be at least three distinct isozymes.[48] The complete enzyme is a polypeptide chain with a molecular mass of about 77,000 daltons, which is composed of two different functional domains—a 51,000-dalton fragment released after proteolysis contains the kinase catalytic domain (this fragment is catalytically active in the absence of phospholipid, calcium, and diacylglycerol), and a 32,000-dalton regulatory domain binds diacylglycerol in a phospholipid- and calcium-dependent manner.[48] Both calcium ion and phospholipid, particularly phosphatidylserine, are required for activation of the complete enzyme. Diacylglycerol, which is released from the phospholipid phosphatidylinositol in response to a number of cell-stimulatory signals, favors attachment of protein kinase C to cell membranes and activates the enzyme. It is thought that TPA and other phorbol esters can substitute for diacylglycerol as activators of protein kinase C. Various phorbol derivatives with tumor-promoting activity can activate protein kinase C, and the structural requirements of phorbol esters for tumor promotion are similar to those for protein kinase C activation.[45]

Protein kinase C has a broad substrate specificity, phosphorylating serine and threonine but not tyrosine residues in proteins. It has catalytic properties different from those of protein kinase A and is not stimulated by cyclic AMP. There is some evidence that tumor-promoting phorbol esters are intercalated into membranes, and this may explain their prolonged action in stimulating protein kinase C activity and cell proliferation, since the normal activator diacylglycerol has a very short half-life in intact cells and its stimulatory activity would be transient.[49]

It is not yet clear which substrates, if any, of protein kinase C are involved in the growth-stimulatory effects of phorbol esters. A number of substrates for protein kinase C have, however, been identified in intact cells. When platelets are activated by thrombin, a normal physiologic activator, or by phorbol esters, phosphorylation of two proteins is stimulated; one of these is a 40,000-dalton and the other a 20,000-dalton protein. This phosphorylation event is coupled to platelet aggregation and serotonin release.[49] The 20,000-dalton protein has been identified as a myosin light chain.[50] Phorbol esters have also been shown to rapidly stimulate the phosphorylation of an 80,000-dalton protein in intact nonproliferating mouse 3T3 fibroblasts.[51] Vinculin, a cytoskeletal protein involved in cellular adhesion, has also been shown to be a substrate for protein kinase C.[52]

In summary, the tumor-promoting phorbol esters have the ability to stimulate a cascade of cellular events leading to cellular proliferation. In this respect, they have certain features in common with other growth-stimulatory factors, such as epidermal growth factor. In the case of the phorbol esters there is considerable evidence indicating that the biologic effects of these agents are mediated through the action of protein kinase C, probably by modulation of the phosphorylation state and thereby the activity of a number of key cellular enzymes and structural proteins involved in cell proliferation. This mechanism appears to be a general one for tumor promoters. Mezerein, teleocidin, and aplysiatoxin are tumor promoters that are structurally different from TPA, but they also activate protein kinase C in vitro.[53]

Why tumor promoters tend to favor the proliferation of carcinogen-initiated cells is not clear, but it may relate to multiple actions of the phorbol esters. These agents, as well as other promoters in the mouse skin system, cause inflammation in the treated area, producing migration of phagocytic cells into the tissue. TPA has the ability to stimulate production by these cells of oxygen radicals,[54] which can in turn produce a number of cellular effects, including DNA strand breakage. In general, the degree of stimulation of oxygen free radical production correlates with promoting efficiency. Superoxide dismutase, an enzyme that destroys superoxide anions, and catalase, which breaks down hydrogen peroxide, prevent DNA strand breakage by TPA.[54] Thus, tumor promoters may be acting as a two-edge sword that cuts both ways: first, they damage cells in a tissue already harboring cells that are genetically altered by a mutagenic carcinogen, thereby stimulating the release of signals for cell proliferation to replace damaged cells; and, second, they foster cell proliferation by stimulating a number of the enzymes necessary for cell replication.

It is interesting that certain antipromoters have been identified, a number of which belong to the class of retinoids that are analogs of vitamin A, a vitamin essential for normal epithelial cell differentiation. The retinoids appear to block the promotion-progression phase of carcinogenesis because they are ineffective when given before or together with an initiating carcinogen, but they block the promoting effect of phorbol esters.[55] Retinoids can also prevent activated oxygen production induced in phagocytic cells by tumor promoters.

Interaction of Chemical Carcinogens with *onc* Genes

It is impossible to consider the potential mechanisms by which chemical carcinogens induce the malignant transformation of cells without considering their role in activating so-called proto-oncogenes, which are normal cellular genes that are the precursors of oncogenes that have been identified in a wide variety of animal and human cancer cells (Table 12-3).[56] During evolution, certain RNA tumor viruses (retroviruses) have apparently picked up portions of these genes, which thus have become part of the tumor virus genome. Indeed, the cellular proto-oncogenes have been identified by their sequence homology with virus *onc* genes. The first of these to be identified was the *src* gene of Rous sarcoma virus,[57] which causes sarcomas in chickens and is known to encode the structure of a tyrosine kinase termed pp60^{src}.[58,59]

It is now realized that many human tumors contain DNA sequences that, after isolation and transfection into normal mouse fibroblasts, can induce transformation of the cell to a malignant phenotype. Among the human tumors known to carry such genes are carcinomas of the colon, lung, urinary bladder, pancreas, skin, and breast; fibro- and rhabdomyosarcomas; glioblastomas; neuroblastomas; and a variety of leukemias and lymphomas.[56] The oncogenes associated with these cancers are presumed to be important in giving the cells their malignant character, but definitive proof of this remains to be obtained.

Cellular proto-oncogenes can be activated in three general ways: (1) they may become associated with retroviruses and be introduced into cells via the virus; (2) they may be turned on by regulatory elements carried by certain viruses; or (3) they may become altered via mutational events such as those produced by chemical carcinogens. Five different molecular events have been associated with proto-oncogene activation (reviewed by Land et al.[56]).

1. Overexpression of proto-oncogene following acquisition of a novel transcriptional promoter. A number of retroviruses may activate cellular proto-oncogenes by forcing overexpression after integration of a viral promoter sequence.
2. Overexpression due to amplification of the proto-oncogene or viral oncogene. For example, the *myc* proto-oncogene is amplified 30- to 50-fold in human myelocytic leukemia (HL-60) cells and in a neuroendocrine colon tumor. The Ki-*ras* gene is amplified 3- to 5-fold in a human colon carcinoma and 60-fold in an adrenocortical tumor of mice.
3. Overexpression due to increased oncogene transcription via action of "enhancer" sequences inserted into DNA in a way that increases the activity of transcriptional promoter sequences. An example of this is the presence of retrovirus enhancer region (but not its promoter region) downstream from the *myc* gene in avian lymphomas.
4. Overexpression following a chromosomal translocation event that allows transcription of a formerly silent oncogene. An example of this is the juxtaposition of the

Table 12-3. Examples of Cellular Oncogenes

Acronym	Origin	Species of Isolation	Subcellular Localization of Virally Encoded Protein	Activity of Virally Encoded Protein
src	Rous sarcoma virus	Chicken	Plasma membrane	Tyrosine kinase
yes	Y73 sarcoma virus	Chicken		Tyrosine kinase
fps(=fes)	Fujinami (ST feline) sarcoma virus	Chicken (cat)	Cytoplasm	Tyrosine kinase
abl	Abelson murine leukemia virus	Mouse	Plasma membrane	Tyrosine kinase
ros	UR II avian sarcoma virus	Chicken	Cytoplasmic membrane	Tyrosine kinase
fgr	Gardner-Rasheed feline sarcoma virus	Cat		Tyrosine kinase
erbB	Avian erythroblastosis virus	Chicken		EGF receptor
fms	McDonough feline sarcoma virus	Cat	Cytoplasm	
mos	Moloney murine sarcoma virus	Mouse	Cytoplasm	
raf	3611 murine sarcoma virus	Mouse		
Ha-ras1	Harvey murine sarcoma virus	Rat	Plasma membrane	Guanosine diphosphate or guanosine triphosphate binding
Ki-ras2	Kirsten murine sarcoma virus	Rat	Plasma membrane	
myc	Avian MC29 myelocytomastosis virus	Chicken	Nuclear matrix	
myb	Avian myeloblastosis virus	Chicken	Nuclear matrix	
fos	FBJ osteosarcoma virus	Mouse	Nucleus	Transcription activating factor
ski	Avian SKV770 virus	Chicken		
rel	Retriculoendotheliosis virus	Turkey		
sis	Simian sarcoma virus	Woolly monkey	Cytoplasm	PDGF-like growth factor
jun	Avian sarcoma virus (ASV 17)	Chicken	Nucleus	Transcription activating factor
Related Oncogenes Known from Sequence Hybridization or Transfection				
N-myc	Neuroblastoma	Human		
N-ras	Neuroblastoma, leukemia, sarcoma	Human		
Unrelated Oncogenes Known Only from Transfection				
Blym	Bursal lymphoma	Chicken		
mam	Mammary carcinoma	Mouse, human		
HER-2/neu	Neuroglioblastoma	Rat		

The retrovirus-associated oncogenes are grouped into three gene families (*src* to *raf*; Ha- and Ki-*ras*; *myc* and *myb*) and a group of genes having no known homology to one another or to any other oncogene. Each gene is presumably found in one or more copies in the genomes of all vertebrates, although this is not yet documented for many genes in this table.

(Modified from Land et al.,[56] with permission.)

myc and immunoglobulin genes in Burkitt's lymphoma cells due to chromosomal translocation. This appears to result in deregulation of the *myc* gene due to loss of its regulatory sequences and juxtaposition of the *myc* gene next to regulatory sequences involved in immunoglobulin production.[60]

5. Expression of an altered proto-oncogene product due to somatic mutation. This has been demonstrated for the *ras* genes in a human bladder carcinoma cell line, which

contains a proto-oncogene with a single point mutation that converts the Ha-*ras* proto-oncogene into a potent oncogene. This mutation results from a G to T base transversion that causes a valine to be substituted for a glycine in residue 12 of the 21,000-dalton protein coded by the gene.[56] Other known mutations of the *ras* gene family include substitution of an aspartate for glycine in position 12 and amino acid substitutions at residue 61 of the 21,000-dalton protein. These mutations alter the structure and function of the *ras* gene product.

One can visualize how chemical carcinogens could induce expression of oncogenes resident in cells by a number of the mechanisms listed above. For example, overexpression of an oncogene due to mutation in a promoter or enhancer sequence could stimulate transcription of these genes. Chromosomal strand breaks introduced by certain chemicals could produce translocations and alter the regulatory sequences adjacent to an oncogene, as in the case of the *myc* gene in Burkitt's lymphoma. Point mutations in an oncogene sequence itself could produce an altered gene product that could enhance its transforming properties. A clear example of the latter is activation of an Ha-*ras* locus in rats during induction of mammary carcinoma after injection of *N*-nitroso-*N*-methylurea (NMU), a potent alkylating carcinogen.[61] Induction of mammary carcinoma by NMU involves the specific activation of the Ha-*ras*-1 locus by a single point mutation at position 12 in the 21,000-dalton protein, similar to that noted in the human bladder carcinoma cell line, but in this case a glutamic acid is substituted for glycine. This can be explained by alkylation of guanosine at the N-7 or O^6 position, leading to a G $\rightarrow$ A base transition, as described in Chapter 11. This is exactly what would be predicted, since conversion of a GGA to a GAA in the triplet code would change the encoded amino acid from glycine to glutamic acid. In fact, precisely this change in the coding for residue 12 was shown by sequence analysis of the NMU-induced *ras* gene.[61]

Investigations in several laboratories have now shown that DNA samples prepared from chemically transformed cell lines are able to induce transformation of cultured normal mouse fibroblasts, suggesting that chemical carcinogens can induce alterations that give rise to dominant transforming genes. Examples of this include dimethylbenzanthracene-induced mouse mammary tumors, mineral oil–induced B- and T-lymphocytic leukemias, 3-methylcholanthrene-transformed mouse fibroblasts, a benzpyrene-induced rabbit bladder carcinoma, and nitrosoethylurea-induced glioblastoma and neuroblastoma in mice.[62]

The expression of *onc* genes has been linked in a number of instances to the production or action of growth factors, and this may explain how turning these genes on can lead to unregulated cellular proliferation. For example, it has been discovered that the *sis* oncogene encodes a protein very similar to platelet-derived growth factor (PDGF),[63,64] and the *erb*B transforming protein of avian erythroblastosis virus has very close sequence homology to part of the receptor for epidermal growth factor.[65] Moreover, PDGF and other mitogens have been shown to stimulate expression of the *myc* gene.[66] These data point to a relationship between growth factor production, *onc* gene transcription, and potential autostimulation of tumor cell proliferation by the induced growth factors or receptors for their activity.

The Concept of Antioncogenes

A number of human tumor samples obtained at the time of surgery have been shown to contain mutations similar to those originally detected in cell culture systems. For example, about 20 percent of human tumors appear to have activated *ras* genes.[67] Several studies have shown the presence of point mutations in Ha-*ras*, Ki-*ras*, and N-*ras* proto-oncogenes in human colon and lung carcinomas and in both acute nonlymphocytic leukemia and myelodysplasia.[68] Interestingly, an N-*ras* mutation in codon 13 was observed in an acute nonlymphocytic leukemia following extensive treatment with anticancer alkylating drugs.[68] However, deletions of parts of chromosome 5 and 7 were even more common in such cases, suggesting that loss of heterozygosity for specific alleles on the two chromosomes may play a more important role in human leukemogenesis than *onc* gene activation. As more human tumors have been examined, such a loss of chromosomal material has been observed with increasing frequency. This has led to the concept of *antioncogenes*, genes whose expression appears to regulate cell proliferation in a way that is opposite to the *onc* genes, many of which stimulate cell proliferation.

The classic example of such an oncogene is the RB gene originally described in hereditary retinoblastoma.[69] Patients with hereditary retinoblastoma are born with one germ line mutation in the RB gene, and they usually develop tumors in early childhood when the remaining normal allele of the RB gene of a retinal cell is deleted or acquires a mutation. Patients with this type of retinoblastoma are predisposed to develop tumors in both eyes and to develop malignancies in other tissues as well. It now appears that RB gene inactivation also occurs in other cancers, including breast and small cell lung carcinomas. It has been demonstrated that introduction of a cloned RB gene into cultured retinoblastoma and osteosarcoma cells suppresses the neoplastic phenotype of these cells.[70]

The RB gene codes for a 105,000-dalton protein that is thought to regulate transcription of cellular genes involved in growth control. This notion is derived from the observation that the RB gene product is a nuclear phosphoprotein that binds transcription activating factors, such as the E1A protein of adenovirus and the large T antigen of the monkey tumor virus SV40.[71] This suggests that a balance between positive and negative activators of gene transcription is lost when the normal RB alleles are lost.

It is now clear that loss of chromosomal material is a common phenomenon in human solid tumors, and this may reflect the loss during carcinogenesis of suppressor genes or antioncogenes similar to the RB genes.[68] For example, deletions of portions of human chromosome 13 have been noted in osteogenic sarcoma and breast cancer as well as in retinoblastoma. Loss of part of chromosome 11 has been seen in bladder cancer and in certain pediatric tumors (e.g., Wilms' tumor and some other embryonal cell carcinomas). Portions of chromosome 3 are lost in small cell lung cancer, renal cell carcinoma, and malignant mesothelioma. In most of these cases the loss of chromosomal material appears to represent heterozygous deletion of specific alleles, suggesting that loss of genes that negatively regulate cell proliferation may not have to be complete in order to tip the balance in favor of uncontrolled cell proliferation.

This latter point brings up an important question: Is cancer a dominant or a recessive disease? The answer seems to be that it is both. Although activation of a single oncogene can transform cells in culture to a neoplasticlike phenotype, complete malignant transformation of cells requires the action of two or more activated *onc* genes in many experimental systems.[72] In many human cancers both the presence of activated oncogenes and heterozygous deletion of certain alleles have been detected. Thus, although activation of *onc* genes appears to act like a dominant genetic cause of cancer, carcinogenesis is clearly a multistep process that most likely involves both activation of oncogenes (by chemicals and other carcinogenic factors) and loss of suppressor genes (antioncogenes) that control cell proliferation.

THE PRINCIPAL GROUPS OF CHEMICAL CARCINOGENS

Historical Perspectives

The evidence that chemicals can induce cancer in animals and humans has been accumulating for over two centuries (reviewed by Miller[73]). Percival Pott is generally given credit for making the first observation of chemical carcinogenesis in humans when in 1775 he reported a high incidence of scrotal skin cancer among men who had spent their childhood as chimney sweeps. However, it was John Hill who made the first report of chemical carcinogenesis in humans when he noted in 1761 the occurrence of nasal cancer in people who used snuff excessively. These observations slumbered for about 100 years, until Volkman in Germany and Bell in Scotland observed skin cancer in workers whose skin was in prolonged contact with tar and paraffin oils, which we now know contain polycyclic aromatic hydrocarbons. In 1895 Rehn in Germany reported the development of urinary bladder cancer in aniline dye workers. Similar observations were later made in several countries and established a relationship between bladder cancer and heavy exposure to 2-naphthylamine, benzidine, or 4-aminobiphenyl. Thus, the observation of chemical carcinogenesis in humans was well established before it was demonstrated in animal models.

One of the first successful attempts to induce cancer in animal models was reported in 1915 by Yamagiwa and Ichikawa, who elicited skin cancers on the ears of rabbits by repeated application of coal tar to the skin. The nature of the carcinogenic components in coal tar was established in the 1930s with the demonstration that synthetic 1,2,5,6-dibenzanthracene is a carcinogen, and with the identification of the carcinogen 3,4-benzpyrene in coal tar. Soon to follow were observations that other chemicals and hormones could induce cancers in animals, for example, the induction of liver tumors in rats and mice with 2'-3-dimethyl-4-aminoazobenzene, of urinary bladder cancer in dogs with 2-naphthylamine, and of mammary cancer in male mice with estrone. The list of known carcinogenic chemicals has expanded continually on the basis of both animal experimentation and human epidemiologic studies (Table 12-2) and keeps growing as new data are accumulated. The difficult questions now are (1) What is the relative risk of these agents based on actual human exposure? (2) How can dangerous carcinogens be accurately identified before they come on the market? (3) What can be done to limit exposure to known carcinogens, particularly exposure of people most susceptible by reason of their genetic make-up?

Polycyclic Aromatic Hydrocarbons

The structures of noncarcinogenic and carcinogenic polycyclic aromatic hydrocarbons are shown in Figure 12-6. As noted above, studies in the 1930s led to the identification of polycyclic aromatic hydrocarbons as the carcinogenic compounds in coal tar. A major coal tar carcinogen and one of the first identified was 3,4-benzpyrene. This led to the synthesis and biologic testing of many related compounds. Consequently, a rather detailed picture of structure-activity relationships in this group has emerged. Figure 12-6 shows that all the carcinogenic hydrocarbons may be regarded as derivatives of phenanthrene. Phenanthrene itself, like the simpler anthracene and napththacene molecules, is devoid of carcinogenicity, and 1,2,3,4-tetramethylphenanthrene (not shown) is weakly carcinogenic. Addition of a fourth benzene ring yields benz[a]anthracene, which is highly carcinogenic. Methyl substituents increase the carcinogenic potency of phenanthrene in a regular way—5,6-dimethylphenanthrene is nearly as potent as 1,2,5,6-dibenzanthracene

Typical Polycyclic Aromatic Hydrocarbons

Noncarcinogenic

Carcinogenic

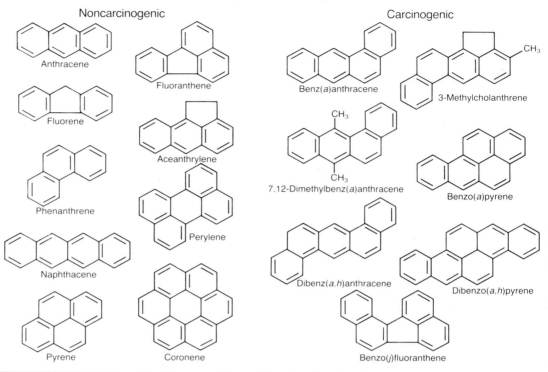

Carcinogenic Natural Products

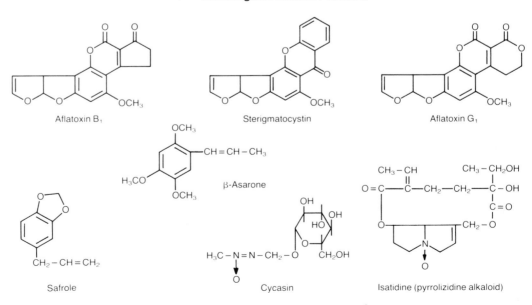

Fig. 12-6. Structures of some known carcinogens. (From Ruddon,[9] with permission.) (*Figure continues*).

Carcinogenic Aminoazo Dyes

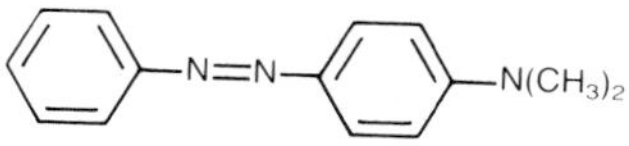

4-Dimethylaminoazobenzene

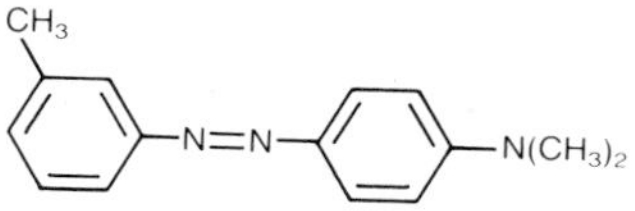

3-Methyl-4-dimethylaminoazobenzene

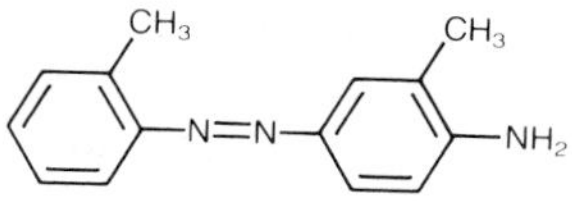

4-(*o*-Tolylazo)-*o*-toluidine

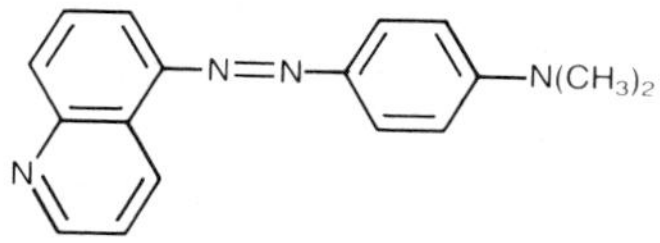

5[*p*-(Dimethylamino)phenylazo]quinoline

Carcinogenic Nitroso Compounds

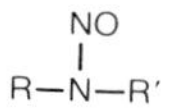

$$\begin{array}{c} NO \\ | \\ R-N-R' \end{array}$$

$R',R=CH_3,C_2H_5,C_3H_7-$
Dialkylnitrosamine

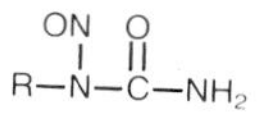

$$\begin{array}{cc} ON & O \\ | & \| \\ R-N-C-NH_2 \end{array}$$

$R=CH_3,C_2H_5,C_3H_7-$
Alkylnitrosourea

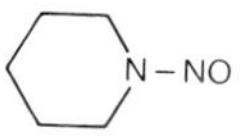

N—NO

N-Nitrosopiperidine

$$\begin{array}{c} NO \\ | \\ N-CH_3 \end{array}$$

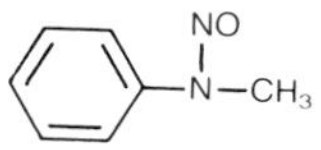

N-Methylnitrosoaniline

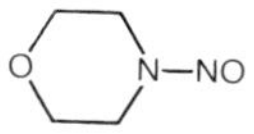

N—NO

Nitrosomorpholine

$$\begin{array}{c} NO \\ | \\ H_3C-N-COOC_2H_5 \end{array}$$

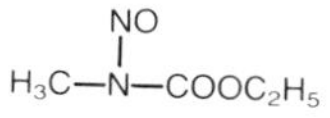

Nitrosomethylurethane

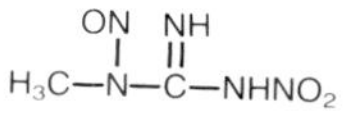

$$\begin{array}{cc} ON & NH \\ | & \| \\ H_3C-N-C-NHNO_2 \end{array}$$

N-Methyl-N'-nitro-N-nitrosoguanidine

Carcinogenic Alkylating Agents

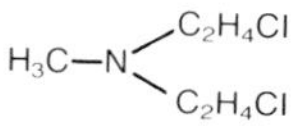

$$H_3C-N\begin{array}{c} C_2H_4Cl \\ C_2H_4Cl \end{array}$$

Nitrogen mustard

$$S\begin{array}{c} C_2H_4Cl \\ C_2H_4Cl \end{array}$$

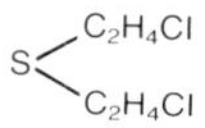

Sulfur mustard (mustard gas)

$ClH_2C-O-CH_2Cl$

Bis(chloromethyl)ether

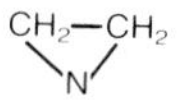

$$\begin{array}{c} CH_2-CH_2 \\ N \end{array}$$

Ethylene imine

$$\begin{array}{c} O-CH=O \\ | \\ CH_2-CH_2 \end{array}$$

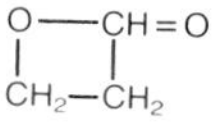

β-Propiolactone

$CH_3-SO_2-OCH_3$

Methylmethanesulfonate

Carcinogenic Aromatic Amines

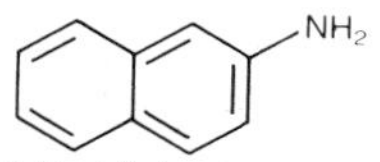

2-Naphthylamine

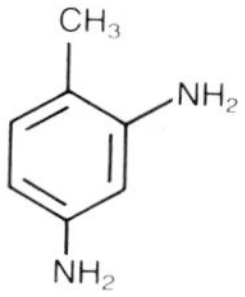

2,4-Toluenediamine

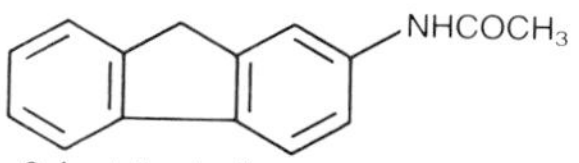

2-Acetylaminofluorene

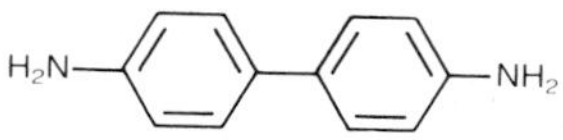

Benzidine

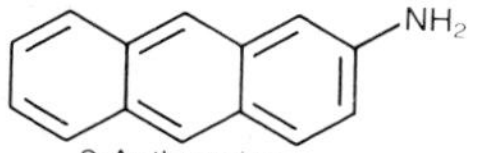

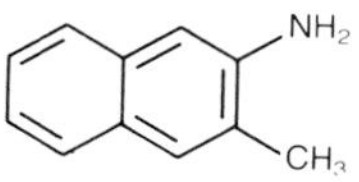

3-Methyl-2-naphthylamine

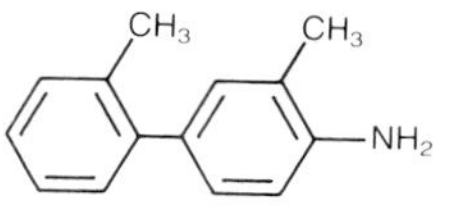

3,2-Dimethyl-4-biphenylamine

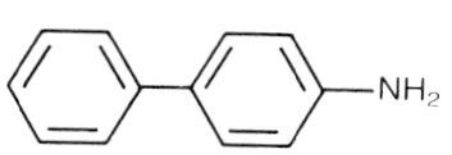

2-Anthramine

4-Biphenylamine

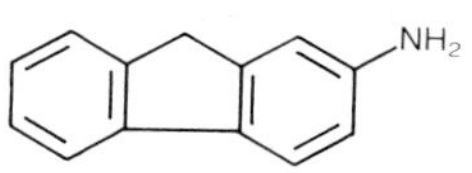

2-Fluorenamine

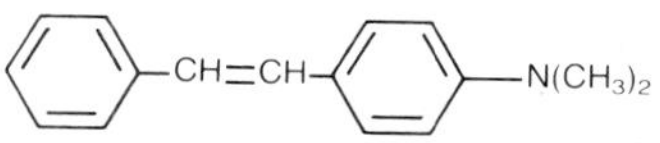

4-Dimethylaminostilbene

Fig. 12-6. (*Continued*).

(dibenz[a,h]anthracene in the newer terminology). The related 3-methylcholanthrene is a very potent carcinogen, yet the homologous anthracene derivative aceanthrylene, lacking the benzene ring at the 1,2 position, is completely inactive.

The principal requirements for carcinogenicity may be summarized as follows: The entire polycyclic hydrocarbon must be coplanar. A phenanthrene nucleus must be present together with some substituents, preferably at least one additional benzene ring. The convex edge of the phenanthrene moiety must be free of substituents. In the series of tetracyclic hydrocarbons (Fig. 12-6), most of the noncarcinogenic compounds fail to conform to the necessary specification; for example, many of them lack the phenanthrene nucleus. The potency of the carcinogenic hydrocarbons is usually enhanced by methyl substitution at appropriate positions, and the cyclization of adjacent methyl groups (as in 3-methylcholanthrene) further increases potency.

In 1950 Boyland[74] suggested that the carcinogeneity of polycyclic aromatic hydrocarbons was mediated through metabolically formed epoxides. It was hypothesized that the key epoxide formation involved the so-called K region of the hydrocarbon ring structure (Fig. 12-7). However, subsequent studies demonstrated that K region epoxides had little direct carcinogenic action. An extensive amount of work has been conducted since the 1950s to define the metabolism of polycyclic aromatic hydrocarbons and to determine the proximate and ultimate carcinogenic intermediates generated from these compounds (reviewed by Conney[75]). It is now generally accepted that carcinogenic polycyclic aromatic hydrocarbons are metabolized via the P-450 monooxygenase system to form an arene oxide on the terminal angular benzene ring, followed by hydration of the arene oxide to form a trans dihydrodiol (the "proximate" carcinogen), and subsequent epoxidation of the so-called bay-region double bond of the dihydrodiol to form the "ultimate" carcinogen that reacts with cellular targets (Fig. 12-7). Studies from a number of laboratories, for instance, have indicated that 7β,8α-dihydroxy-9α,10α-epoxy-7,8,9,10-tetrahydrobenzo-[a]pyrene is the ultimate mutagenic and carcinogenic metabolite of benzo[a]pyrene.[76,77] The analogous metabolites of benz[a]anthracene, dibenzo[a,h]pyrene, and dibenzo-[a,i]pyrene and certain other methylbenz[a]anthracenes appear to be the carcinogenic intermediates of these compounds.[75]

When the various metabolites of benzo[a]pyrene (BP) were tested for mutagenicity in the Ames test by using tester strains of *Salmonella typhimurium* and Chinese hamster V-79 cells (see Ch. 11) and tested for carcinogenicity by injection into newborn mice, it became clear that the most potent mutagen/carcinogen was the (+) enantiomer of BP 7,8-diol-9,10-epoxide-1.[75] When the (+) and (−) enantiomers were allowed to react with double-stranded DNA, it was determined that the (+) enantiomer was covalently bound preferentially to the 2-amino group of guanine and that the (+) form was bound to a 20-fold greater extent than the (−) form, in agreement with the greater mutagenic and carcinogenic effect of this isomer. Surprisingly, both BP 7,8-diol-9,10-epoxide-1 and epoxide-2 are weak carcinogens in the mouse skin painting assay compared with BP itself, most likely because they are not well absorbed or (since they are unstable in aqueous solution) undergo rapid solvolysis to biologically inactive tetraols. However, when they are injected into newborn mice, they are more potent than the parent compound. The predominant tumors formed were lung adenomas or adenocarcinomas, malignant lymphomas, and liver tumors, with the target tissue depending on the dose of carcinogen and duration of treatment. By using synthetically prepared compounds, it was shown that BP 7,8-dihydrodiol and BP 7,8-diol-9,10-epoxide were, respectively, 15 and 40 times as active at equimolar doses as the parent compound BP in producing pulmonary tumors in newborn mice. The

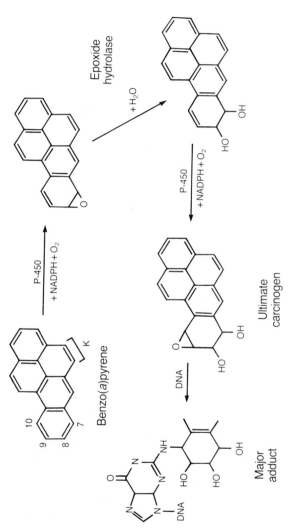

Fig. 12-7. The major route for the metabolic activation of benzo[a]pyrene and the major adduct formed with nucleic acids by interaction of the diol epoxide metabolite with the 2-amino group of guanine. (From Miller,[73] with permission.)

diol epoxide was about 2.5 times as active as the diol, which supports the view that the diol is a proximate carcinogen and the diol-epoxide the ultimate carcinogen of BP. The other potential metabolites of BP were either much less active or inactive in this system. It is somewhat disconcerting to note that liver P-450 systems acting in vivo predominantly form the more active carcinogenic (+) enantiomers of BP-7,8-diol-9,10-epoxides from BP.[75]

Amines

Aromatic Amines

Studies on the induction of bladder cancers by aromatic amines in experimental animals have shed light of how differences in metabolic pathways may affect carcinogenicity. It is clear now that the aromatic amines themselves are not carcinogenic but give rise to

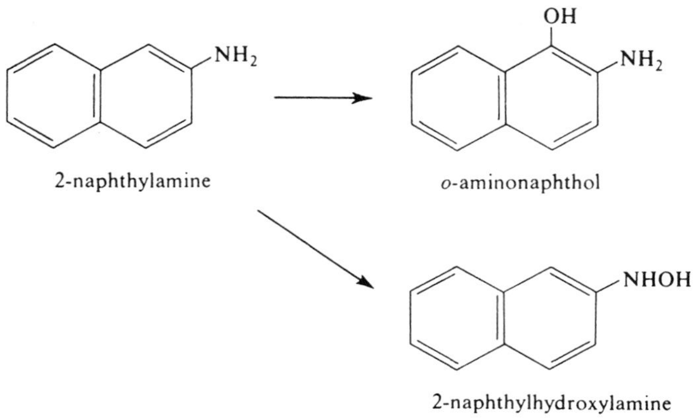

2-naphthylamine

o-aminonaphthol

2-naphthylhydroxylamine

carcinogenic metabolites in vivo. Thus, 2-naphthylamine is transformed in the liver to two principal metabolites, the o-aminonaphthol and the hydroxylamine (N-hydroxy) derivative. When 2-naphthylamine itself was tested for carcinogenicity by direct implantation into the mouse bladder after incorporation into a wax pellet, no tumors were elicited. On the other hand, both the phenolic derivative and the hydroxylamine were potent carcinogens in this system.[78] It is doubtful, however, that o-aminonaphthol is a proximate carcinogen. Hydrolysis of the N-glucuronide conjugate of hydroxylamine is favored by the low pH of the urine, resulting in the formation of a protonated hydroxylamine, which rearranges to form a nitrenium ion by loss of water (Fig. 12-8). The electrophilic nitrenium ion can then react with nucleophilic targets in the urinary bladder epithelium.

Because the carcinogenic metabolites formed in the liver are rapidly conjugated there with glucuronic acid, most tissues are protected from exposure to the carcinogens, for the glucuronides are inert. The glucuronides are excreted in the urine. In humans and dogs, the urine is known to contain a soluble β-glucuronidase, which under acid conditions releases free carcinogen in the ureters and bladder. This mechanism has been established in several ways.[78] It was shown that the carcinogenic activity responsible for producing bladder cancer is present in the urine rather than in the bladder circulation. Dogs were subjected to a surgical procedure whereby blind pouches of bladder were constructed; these pouches received their normal blood supply but were no longer in contact with urine. Naphthylamine administration produced no cancers in the pouches. If the ureters

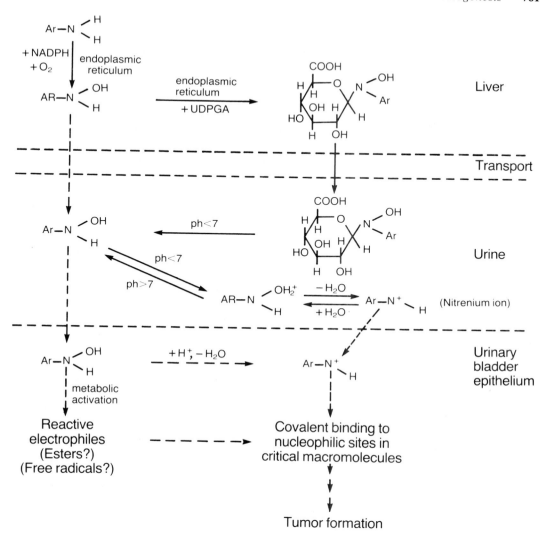

Fig. 12-8. Formation and transport of possible proximate and ultimate carcinogenic metabolites of arylamines involved in the induction of urinary bladder cancer. Ar, aryl substituent; UDPGA, uridine diphosphoglucuronic acid. (From Miller,[73] with permission.)

were transplanted to the sigmoid colon, tumors developed in them but not in the bladder. Finally, an inhibitor of β-glucuronidase (glucosaccharo-1,4-lactone) greatly reduced the incidence of bladder tumors in dogs when it was fed simultaneously with 2-naphthylamine.

It must be evident from the foregoing account that both the potency of an administered carcinogenic amine and the sites at which it will produce cancer depend upon the activity of drug-metabolizing enzymes. Conversion to *N*-hydroxy or other active products, formation of glucuronides (or sulfate esters), and enzymic hydrolysis at sites of excretion all influence the end result. It is found, for example, that in contrast to humans and dogs, mice and rats are refractory to bladder carcinogenesis by aromatic amines. Since *N*-hydroxynaphthylamine is carcinogenic by implantation in the mouse bladder and since 2-naphthylamine produces cancers at other tissue sites after it is fed to rats, it is likely that some deficiency of β-glucuronidase action in rodent urine accounts for the absence of bladder tumors in these species.

Patients with bladder tumors induced by long exposure to naphthylamine have unusually high levels of β-glucuronidase in their urine. It is not known whether these high enzyme levels predated the development of the bladder tumors; if so, this would be a good example of how genetically determined biochemical individuality might predispose to a particular kind of cancer. Administration of a β-glucuronidase inhibitor (glucosaccharo-1,4-lactone) has been proposed as a prophylactic measure for people accidentally exposed to carcinogens of the naphthylamine type.

Another aromatic amine carcinogen is 2-acetylaminofluorene (AAF). This compound, when fed in small amounts in the diet of the rat, causes cancers at many sites in the body. Most unusual has been a predilection for inducing papillomas and squamous cell carcinomas of the sebaceous gland in the external ear duct. Originally it was supposed that deacetylation occurred in the liver and that 2-aminofluorene was the active carcinogen. It became evident, however, that neither AAF nor 2-aminofluorene is directly carcinogenic. As already recounted for 2-naphthylamine, the analogous *N*-hydroxy derivative of AAF has been found to be a carcinogen.[73] The guinea pig provides a good further test of the hypothesis that metabolism to *N*-hydroxy-AAF is required for carcinogenesis, for this species does not carry out the *N*-hydroxylation reaction. Accordingly, AAF is not a carcinogen in this species. The guinea pig is not, however, intrinsically refractory; when *N*-hydroxy-AAF was fed or injected, intestinal, peritoneal, and subcutaneous cancers readily developed.

The metabolic interconversions of AAF to its carcinogenic intermediates have been worked out in detail. Although both AAF and *N*-hydroxy-AAF are carcinogenic in vivo, the early studies indicated that neither compound reacted in vitro with nucleic acids or proteins, suggesting that the ultimate carcinogen was another, as yet unidentified, metabolite. Subsequent studies showed that *N*-hydroxy-AAF is converted in rat liver to a sulfate, *N*-sulfonoxy-AAF, by the action of a cytosol sulfotransferase (Fig. 12-9). This compound reacts with nucleic acids and proteins, is highly mutagenic, and appears to be the ultimate carcinogen produced in vivo.

Other enzymatic conversions of AAF occur in rat liver; for example, *N*-hydroxy-AAF is converted to *N*-acetoxy-AAF, *N*-acetoxy-2-aminofluorene, and the glucuronide of *N*-hydroxy-AAF. The former two compounds may be important carcinogenic metabolites in nonhepatic tissues, which often have low sulfotransferase activity toward *N*-hydroxy-AAF. For instance, *N*-acetoxy-2-aminofluorene, generated by the action of acetyltransferase on *N*-hydroxy-AAF, is a strong electrophile and would be expected to react with cellular targets.

Another group of aromatic amines, important because of their widespread use in industry, includes 4-aminodiphenyl and 4-aminostilbene and their *N*-methyl derivatives. In their carcinogenicity and metabolic conversion to *N*-hydroxy derivatives in vivo, these compounds closely resemble AAF and naphthylamine. They cause tumors in various tissues in the rat after feeding, especially in the acoustic sebaceous gland, intestine, liver, and kidneys.

Finally, bladder cancers have been induced in mice by pellet implantation of saccharin,

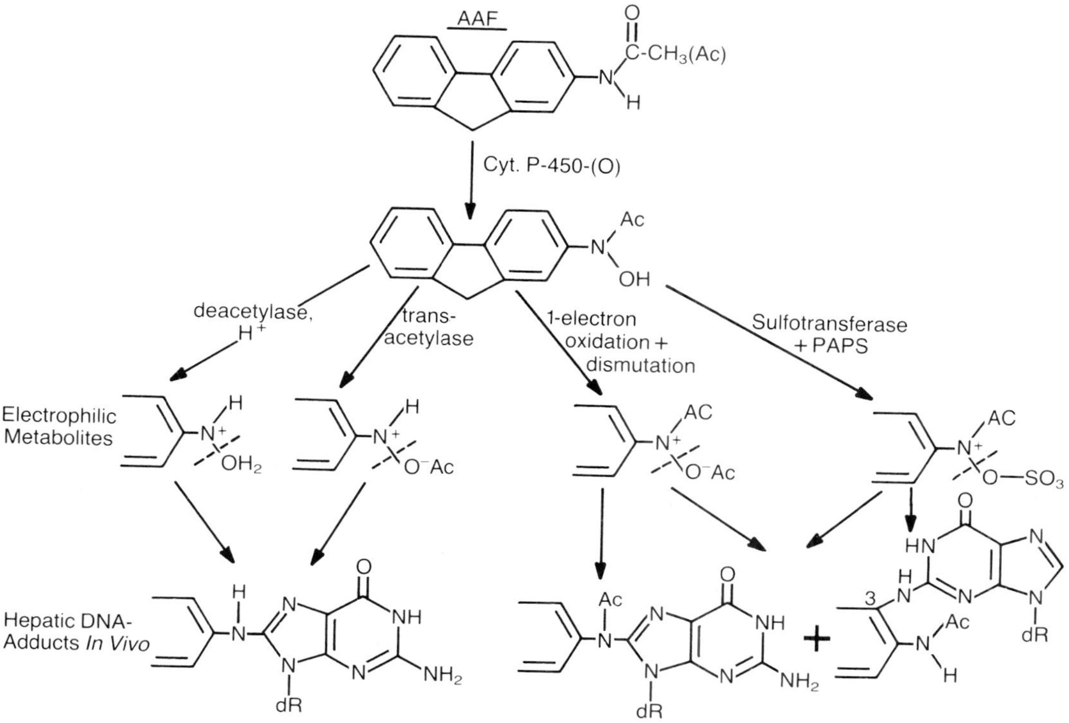

Fig. 12-9. The major metabolic pathway in rat liver for activation of AAF to the strong electrophile *N*-sulfonoxy-AAF. 3'-Phosphoadenosine-5'-phosphosulfate (PAPS) is the active sulfate donor for the sulfotransferase activity. (From Miller,[73] with permission.)

an aromatic amine that has been widely used as a noncaloric sweetening agent for human consumption.[79] Saccharin is believed to act as a tumor promoter rather than an initiating agent.

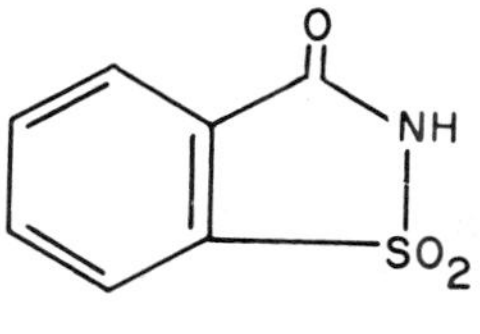

saccharin

Azo Dyes

The azo dyes first commanded attention as carcinogens when they were found to produce liver cancers after incorporation into the diet of rats. The best known member of the group is dimethylaminoazobenzene, also called "butter yellow" because of its former use as a food coloring. Numerous studies of the structure-activity relationships in this group have provided a body of empirical data about the requirements for carcinogenicity. As with the polycyclic hydrocarbons, modifications that alter the coplanar configuration abolish carcinogenicity. Methylation of the nitrogen atom at position 4 is essential for

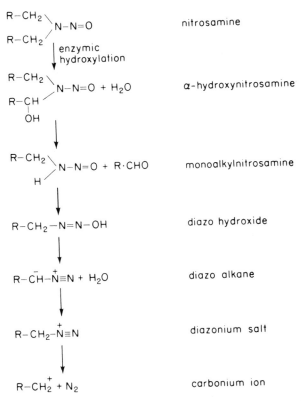

$$R-CH_2 \diagdown$$
$$\qquad\qquad N-N=O \qquad\qquad\text{nitrosamine}$$
$$R-CH_2 \diagup$$

enzymic hydroxylation

$$R-CH_2 \diagdown$$
$$\qquad\qquad N-N=O + H_2O \qquad\qquad\text{α-hydroxynitrosamine}$$
$$R-CH \diagup$$
$$\ \ |$$
$$\ \ OH$$

$$R-CH_2 \diagdown$$
$$\qquad\qquad N-N=O + R\cdot CHO \qquad\qquad\text{monoalkylnitrosamine}$$
$$H \diagup$$

$$R-CH_2-N=N-OH \qquad\qquad\text{diazo hydroxide}$$

$$R-\overset{-}{C}H-\overset{+}{N}\equiv N + H_2O \qquad\qquad\text{diazo alkane}$$

$$R-CH_2-\overset{+}{N}\equiv N \qquad\qquad\text{diazonium salt}$$

$$R-\overset{+}{C}H_2 + N_2 \qquad\qquad\text{carbonium ion}$$

Fig. 12-10. Transformation of nitrosamine to an active carcinogen. A general scheme for the probable in vivo metabolic transformation is shown. The active alkylating agent may be the diazoalkane, the diazonium compound, or the carbonium ion. The R groups represent alkyl groups, usually methyl or ethyl. Dimethylnitrosamine is a potent carcinogen in vivo; the ultimate metabolic products would be methylating agents. (From Brookes,[84] with permission.)

activity, but the monomethyl and dimethyl derivatives are equally effective; in any case, metabolic demethylation occurs in vivo. Substituents are tolerated (and sometimes increase potency) in position 3 (ortho to the amine nitrogen), as in the potent carcinogen 4-(*o*-tolylazo)-*o*-toluidine (see Fig. 12-6), but substitution of any kind in position 2 (meta to the amino group) abolishes activity. Alkyl groups larger than methyl on the amine nitrogen decrease potency.

It now appears that the azo dyes, like other aromatic amines, are metabolized to *N*-hydroxy derivatives, which in turn are further metabolized to *N*-hydroxy esters. Sulfate esters appear to be especially potent proximate carcinogens. For instance, *N*-methyl-4-aminoazobenzene, like 2-acetylaminofluorene, is activated by *N*-hydroxylation and sulfonation of the *N*-hydroxy derivatives, and the major nucleic acid adducts, like those formed by metabolites of AAF, involve substitution of C-8 of guanine residues.[73] However, the *N*-oxidation of the aminoazo dyes is catalyzed by a flavoprotein that does not require P-450, and it appears that different hepatic sulfotransferases act on the two classes of substrates.[73]

Nitrosamines

Nitrosamines constitute an interesting group of very potent carcinogens, of special significance because they may be formed in the stomach after ingestion of nitrites,[80–82] and are present in tobacco smoke.[83] These agents are converted by hydroxylation reactions to alkylating agents. Figure 12-10 shows the probable scheme of metabolic transformation, but it is not certain if the actual alkylating intermediate is the diazoalkane (e.g., diazomethane from dimethylnitrosamine), the diazonium salt, or carbonium ion.[84] When dimethylnitrosamine was fed to rats, tumors of the liver, kidney, and lung were produced. The degree of methylation of tissue DNA and protein paralleled the carcinogenic potency for various tissues. Cycasin, a naturally occurring carcinogen, found in certain nuts (Cycad nuts), alkylates by a similar mechanism.[85] The compound is a glucoside of methylazoxymethanol. In vivo it breaks down to diazomethane, and its methyl group is transferred to the 7-position of nucleic acid guanine.[86] It has also been shown to be mutagenic in bacteria.

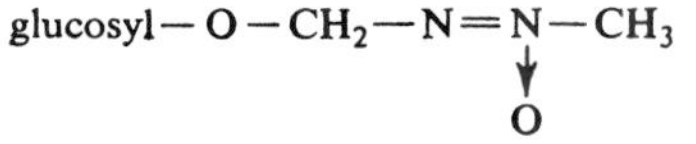

$$glucosyl - O - CH_2 - N = N - CH_3$$
$$\downarrow$$
$$O$$

cycasin

Urethane

Urethane is another chemically inert compound known to be carcinogenic. Urethane is converted to an alkylating agent by *N*-hydroxylation in rats, rabbits, and humans.[87] Al-

$$CH_3 - CH_2 - O - \overset{\overset{\displaystyle O}{\|}}{C} - NH_2 \longrightarrow CH_3 - CH_2 - O - \overset{\overset{\displaystyle O}{\|}}{C} - NHOH$$

urethane   N-hydroxyurethane

ternative modes of alkylation are indicated by isolation of two types of product from tissues. The urethane ethyl group may be transferred to form ethylmercapturic acid or *S*-ethylglutathione, both of which have been isolated after urethane administration. On the other hand, the entire *N*-hydroxyurethane moiety may be transferred; in this way, for example, *N*-acetyl-*S*-carbethoxycysteine is formed.

Alkylating Agents

The chemical reactivity of the alkylating agents and their mode of action as mutagens was discussed in Chapter 11. The bifunctional alkylating agents can cross-link the strands of the DNA duplex. That alkylating agents as a group are carcinogenic strengthens the analogy between carcinogenesis and mutagenesis. The most widely studied carcinogenic alkylating agents have been mechlorethamine (nitrogen mustard), sulfonyl esters such as 1,4-dimethanesulfonoxybutane (busulfan), and epoxy compounds such as the cyclohexane derivative shown below:

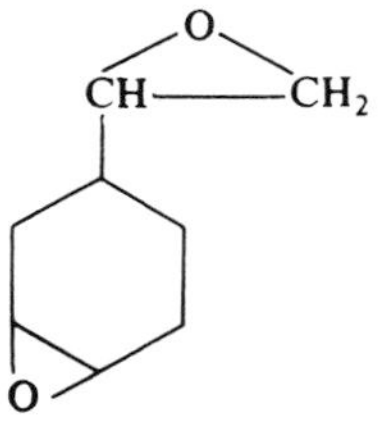

1-ethyleneoxy-3,4-epoxycyclohexane

Certain plant alkaloids (from *Senecio* species) are of great interest because they are alkylating agents with a pyrrolizidine structure.[88,89] If added to the diet, they produce liver cancer in rats. Since plants containing them are used in folk medicine or to prepare bush teas in Africa and India, they might contribute to the high incidence of hepatoma in certain geographic areas. The general structure is given below:

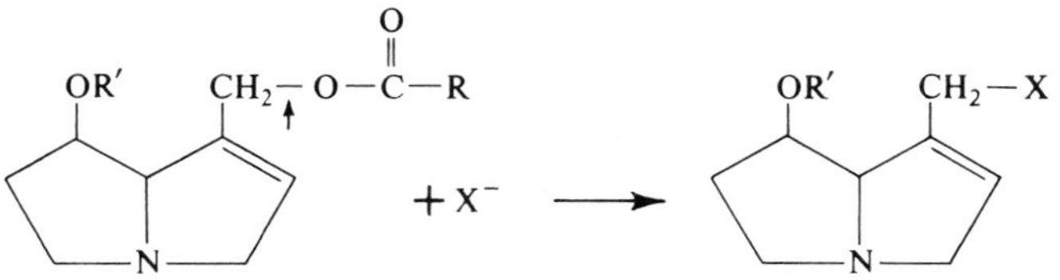

pyrrolizidine alkaloid   alkylation product

Both R and R' are usually branched alkyl chains. The ester bond is an absolute requirement for carcinogenicity; the alcohols are inert. A double bond in the 1,2-position of the pyrrolizidine ring is also required; its function is evidently to labilize the bond between oxygen and the methylene group, indicated by the small arrow. The reaction shown represents the alkylation of any nucleophilic receptor anion, such as a sulfhydryl group.

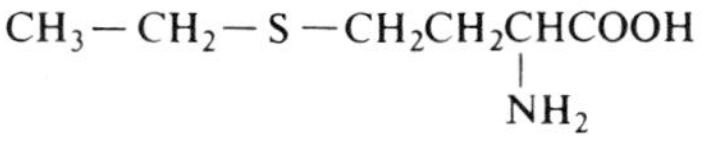

$$CH_3-CH_2-S-CH_2CH_2\underset{\underset{\displaystyle NH_2}{|}}{CH}COOH$$

ethionine

Ethionine, the ethyl analog of the amino acid methionine, is a liver carcinogen when it is fed to the rat.[90] The body's normal mechanism for methylation, in which methionine acts as a methyl donor, becomes a means of ethylation in the presence of ethionine. Normally, *S*-adenosylmethionine participates in the methylation of purines in transfer-RNA. When *S*-adenosylethionine is formed, the ethyl group (shown below in bold type) is transferred to purines and other acceptors:

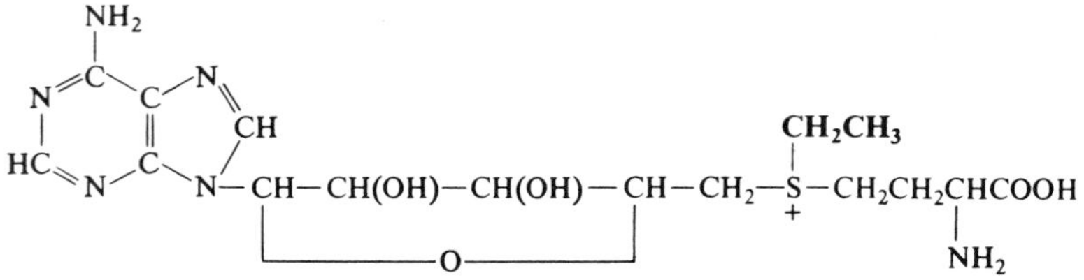

S-adenosylethionine

A number of lactones have been found to have carcinogenic activity, and some of these occur in fungi and higher plants.[91] The prototype of the group is β-propiolactone. The

β-propiolactone   ethyleneimine   epoxide

basis of the alkylating action of this compound is its strained ring structure, a feature common to such typical alkylating compounds as ethyleneimines and epoxides. β-Propiolactone is subject to two kinds of nucleophilic attack: nonionized nucleophiles form addition products at the ester bond and ionized nucleophiles at the -CH_2-O-bond, yielding carboxyethyl derivatives. For example, *S*-(2-carboxyethyl)-cysteine and 7-(2'-carboxyethyl)guanine have been isolated from organisms treated with β-propiolactone. In the same way, after exposure to the simple epoxide ethylene oxide, 7-(2'-hydroxyethyl)guanine could be isolated. That the intact lactone ring is essential to carcinogenesis was indicated by the finding that sarcomas were produced by subcutaneous injection of β-propiolactone in rats, whereas its hydrolysis product β-hydroxypropionic acid was inert.

Another interesting carcinogen found in plants is safrole, present in oils of sassafras, nutmeg, and cinnamon. It is ingested in sassafras tea, and it was used as a flavoring agent in root beer until 1960, when it was banned in the United States following the demonstration of its hepatocarcinogenic properties in the rat. It is converted in vivo to a highly reactive electrophilic product, 1'-hydroxysafrole.[92,93]

safrole   1'-hydroxysafrole

Alkylation and Arylation in the Carcinogenic Process

Advances in our understanding of drug metabolism are leading to a unitary view of the biochemistry of carcinogenesis. Some years ago, when such compounds as the polycyclic hydrocarbons, the aromatic amines, and the azo dyes were thought of as rather nonreactive molecules, it was difficult to discern any common pathway that could account for the carcinogenic effects of such diverse chemical structures. The position has changed completely as a result of these developments, discussed earlier in detail: (1) the discovery of the carcinogenic properties of alkylating agents and the relationship between their carcinogenic and mutagenic properties; (2) the elaboration of a theory that stressed the chemical reactivity of a particular region in the polycyclic hydrocarbon molecule and the proof of that reactivity by isolation of complexes with tissue proteins and nucleic acids; (3) the demonstration that all the seemingly unreactive carcinogens undergo extensive metabolic transformation in vivo, that some of the metabolites are more carcinogenic than the parent compounds, that metabolites are often active locally whereas the parent compounds are not, and that electrophilic metabolites are mutagenic although the parent compounds are not; and (4) the fact that metallic carcinogens—beryllium, cadmium, cobalt, nickel, and lead—are also, in their ionic forms, electrophilic reactants.[94,95] These results have led to the conclusion that ultimate chemical carcinogens are strong electrophilic reactants, bringing considerable order to the confusing variety of chemical carcinogens.[96] It remains to be proved that the important nucleophilic reactant in vivo is a component (e.g., guanine) of DNA, and that the somatic mutations thus induced lead to cancer.

ROLE OF DRUG-METABOLIZING ENZYMES IN CHEMICAL CARCINOGENESIS

As discussed in Chapters 5 and 6, there are multiple P-450s with characteristic but overlapping substrate specificities. These P-450s are involved in metabolism of polycyclic aromatic hydrocarbons and other precarcinogens to their proximate and ultimate carcinogenic metabolites. Paradoxically, the same enzymes are involved in the detoxification of these compounds. Thus, changes in the activity or amount of specific forms of cytochrome P-450 can alter both the extent of metabolism and the relative amounts of individual metabolites that appear. As also indicated in Chapter 7, there is marked individual genetic variation in drug-metabolizing systems that handle carcinogens. Moreover, the taking of drugs, the smoking of cigarettes, the exposure to environmental pollutants such as halogenated hydrocarbons, and the nature of the diet can all influence the metabolism of potential carcinogens in humans.

It might be supposed that since metabolic activation of many carcinogens is important for their ultimate carcinogenic action, inducers of the microsomal drug-metabolizing system (e.g., phenobarbital, aromatic hydrocarbons, chlorinated hydrocarbons) would enhance carcinogenic potency, yet this has frequently proved not to be the case. The data on this point are variable, probably because the metabolic detoxification pathways are also often induced by the same agents. Furthermore, the route of administration may have a considerable effect on the results obtained. For example, if a carcinogen is given orally and is detoxified by induced enzymes in the liver before it reaches the target tissue, the carcinogenic effect may be reduced. On the other hand, if the liver is the target tissue, carcinogenic potency for that organ may be increased. In some situations the induction of the P-450 monooxygenase system represents a "two-edged sword."[97] Animals or patients who, for genetic reasons or because they are exposed to exogenous inducing agents, have elevated xenobiotic metabolizing enzyme activities may have increased risk of developing cancer in tissue sites that are in direct contact with the carcinogen activated as a result of the induced enzymes. However, in animals or patients with lower metabolizing activities, tissues in distant sites of the body may be more susceptible to developing cancer because more carcinogen reaches that tissue owing to decreased metabolism in the liver (or other site of primary metabolism). These data have been explained by a "first-pass elimination effect" or "presystemic drug elimination"[97,98] (cf. Ch. 3).

THE PROBLEM OF ELIMINATING AND EXCLUDING CARCINOGENS FROM THE ENVIRONMENT

Guidelines for the protection of the population against the hazards of environmental carcinogenesis are very difficult to formulate. The course of the controversy over smoking is very revealing of the economic, political, and psychologic barriers that impede action even after the scientific determination has been made. Certainly the evidence implicating cigarette smoking as a prime cause of cancer in humans is as thorough and convincing as one can expect to obtain. Nevertheless, cigarette consumption has continued at a high level among young people, in whom the risk is greatest because their total exposure will be longest. And although in the United States some minor modifications of cigarette advertising techniques have been enforced, no major regulatory action by government has been forthcoming. Many argue, indeed, that the principle of personal liberty includes liberty to indulge in a pleasure such as smoking at the expense of future illness and premature death.

What, then, of drugs, food additives, insecticides, industrial wastes, and air pollutants, about which there may be only indecisive evidence of carcinogenicity? Suppose such a substance proved to be carcinogenic at some particular dosage and route of administration in laboratory animals. How is one to extrapolate the result to humans? We do not even know if there is a threshold dosage below which no cancers would occur regardless of the size of the exposed population.[99-101] And suppose a food additive or air pollutant were tested in 100 animals, or even 1,000, and yielded no cancers. It might then be asserted that the substance was not a strong carcinogen. But might it be capable, nevertheless, of causing an unacceptable cancer rate in a large exposed population? If only 1 person in 1,000 were affected, there would be about 200,000 new cases of cancer in the United States. This result would be the more appalling because, unlike cigarette smokers, these victims would be exposed to the carcinogen through no choice of their own. This problem has been dealt with legislatively in the United States in the most conservative way possible. The so-called Delaney Amendment to the Food and Drug Act prohibits the use, in processed foodstuffs, of any substance that has been shown (at any dose) to produce cancer in any experimental animal.

Unlike most drug toxicities, which are manifested fairly soon after exposure so that timely action is demanded by the public and can be taken by Federal agencies, the long-delayed effects of carcinogens rob the issue of urgency. Air pollution in our cities illustrates the contrast. Epidemics of smog-induced respiratory disease occur periodically. These episodes may be characterized by a high mortality rate and therefore may have a high "visibility" in the arena of public affairs. As a rule, urgent measures are then called for to institute more rigid control measures. Yet this ever-present hazard appears too remote to engender demands for immediate action, especially when drastic controls might be expensive or disrupt an accustomed way of life. The position adopted by regulatory agencies is necessarily a compromise between the desire to eliminate all carcinogenic hazards and the necessity of weighing the magnitude of each hazard against the benefits derived from the hazardous substance or environment.

REFERENCES

1. Greenwald P, Barlow JJ, Nasca PC, Burnett WS: Vaginal cancer after maternal treatment with synthetic estrogens. N Engl J Med 285:390, 1971
2. Adamson RH, Sieber SM: Antineoplastic agents as potential carcinogens. p. 429. In Hiatt

HH, Watson JD, Winsten JA (eds): Origins of Cancer. Cold Spring Harbor Laboratory, Cold Spring Harbor, NY, 1977

3. Weber WW, Hein DW: Acetylation pharmacogenetics. Pharmacol Rev 37:25, 1985
4. Pincus G, Vollmer EP (eds): Biological Activities of Steroids in Relation to Cancer. Academic Press, Orlando, FL, 1960
5. Bielschowski F, Horning ES: Aspects of endocrine carcinogenesis. Br Med Bull 14:106, 1958
6. Mühlbock O, Boot LM: The mechanism of hormonal carcinogenesis. p. 83. In Wolstenholme GEW, O'Conner M (eds): Ciba Foundation Symposium on Carcinogenesis. Little, Brown, Boston, 1958
7. Coombs MM, Bhatt TS, Croft CJ: Correlation between carcinogenicity and chemical structure in cyclopenta[a]phenanthrenes. Cancer Res 33:832, 1973
8. Bryan WR, Shimkin MB: Quantitative analysis of dose-response data obtained with three carcinogenic hydrocarbons in strain C3H male mice. JNCI 3:503, 1943
9. Ruddon RW: Cancer Biology. 2nd Ed. Oxford University Press, New York, 1987
10. Nicolson GL: Trans-membrane control of the receptors on normal and tumor cells. II. Surface changes associated with transformation and malignancy. Biochim Biophys Acta 458:1, 1976
11. Weber G: Enzymology of cancer cells. N Engl J Med 296:541, 1977
12. Dippold WG, Lloyd KO, Li LTC, et al.: Cell surface antigens of human malignant melanoma: Definition of six antigenic systems with mouse monoclonal antibodies. Proc Natl Acad Sci USA 77:6114, 1980
13. Collett MS, Erikson RL: Protein kinase activity associated with the avian sarcoma virus *src* gene product. Proc Natl Acad Sci USA 75:2021, 1978
14. Levinson AD, Oppermann H, Levintow L, et al: Evidence that the transforming gene of avian sarcoma virus encodes a protein kinase associated with a phosphoprotein. Cell 15:561, 1978
15. Marquardt H, Hunkapiller MW, Hood LE, et al: Transforming growth factors produced by retrovirus-transformed rodent fibroblasts and human melanoma cells: Amino acid sequence homology with epidermal growth factor. Proc Natl Acad Sci USA 80:4684, 1983
16. Doll R: Introduction. p. 1. In Hiatt HH, Watson JD, Winsten JA (eds): Origins of Human Cancer. Cold Spring Harbor Laboratory, Cold Spring Harbor, NY, 1977
17. Doll R, Peto R: The Causes of Cancer. Oxford University Press, New York, 1981
18. Blot WJ, Mason TJ, Hoover R, Fraumeni JF: Cancer by county: Etiological implications. p. 21. In Hiatt HH, Watson JD, Winsten JA (eds): Origins of Human Cancer. Cold Spring Harbor Laboratory, Cold Spring Harbor, NY, 1977
19. US Department of Health and Human Services: The Health Consequences of Smoking. Publication No. (CDC) 74-8704, Washington, 1974, pp. 35–37
20. International Agency for Research on Cancer. Report on an IARC working group: An evaluation of chemicals and industrial processes associated with cancer in humans based on human and animal data: IARC Monogr Vols. 1–20. Cancer Res 40:1, 1980
21. Jolley RL: Chlorination effects on organic constituents in effluents from domestic sanitary sewage treatment plants. Publication No. 565, Environmental Science Division, Oak Ridge National Laboratory, Oak Ridge, TN, 1973
22. Junk GA, Stanley SE: Organics in drinking water. Part I: Listing of identified chemicals. National Technical Information Services, Springfield, VA, 1975
23. Weisburger JH, Cohen LA, Wynder EL: On the etiology and metabolic epidemiology of the main human cancers. p. 567. In Hiatt HH, Watson JD, Winsten JA (eds): Origins of Human Cancer. Cold Spring Harbor Laboratory, Cold Spring Harbor, NY, 1977
24. Carroll KK: Experimental evidence of dietary factors and hormone-dependent cancers. Cancer Res 35:3374, 1975
25. Reddy BS, Wynder EL: Metabolic epidemiology of colon cancer: Fecal bile acids and neutral sterols in colon cancer patients and patients with adenomatous polyps. Cancer 39:2533, 1977
26. Ames BN: Dietary carcinogens and anticarcinogens. Science 221:1256, 1983
27. Lacassagne A: Apparition d'adénocarcinomes mammaires chez des souris mâles, traitées par une substance oestrogène synthétique. Compt Rend Soc Biol 129:641, 1938

28. Phillips DH, Hewer A, Martin CN, et al: Correlation of DNA adduct levels in human lung with cigarette smoking. Nature 336:790, 1988
29. Friedewald WF, Rous P: The initiating and promoting elements in tumor production: An analysis of the effects of tar, benzpyrene, and methylcholanthrene on rabbit skin. J Exp Med 80:101, 1944
30. Sall RD, Shear MJ: Studies in carcinogenesis. XII. Effect of the basic fraction of creosote oil on the production of tumors in mice by chemical carcinogens. JNCI 1:45, 1940
31. Hart RW, Setlow RB: Direct evidence that pyrimidine dimers in DNA result in neoplastic transformation. p. 719. In Hanawalt PC, Setlow RB (eds): Molecular Mechanisms for Repair of DNA. Plenum Press, New York, 1975
32. Mc Cann J, Choi E, Yamasaki E, Ames BN: Detection of carcinogens as mutagens in the Salmonella/microsome test: Assay of 300 chemicals. Proc Natl Acad Sci USA 72:5135, 1975
33. Huberman E, Sachs L: Mutability of different genetic loci in mammalian cells by metabolically activated carcinogenic polycyclic hydrocarbons. Proc Natl Acad Sci USA 73:188, 1976
34. Swift M, Sholman L, Perry M, Chase C: Malignant neoplasms in the families of patients with ataxia-telangiectasia. Cancer Res 36:209, 1976
35. Setlow RB: Repair deficient human disorders and cancer. Nature 271:713, 1978
36. Rifkin DB, Crowe RM, Pollack R: Tumor promoters induce changes in the chick embryo fibroblast cytoskeleton. Cell 18:361, 1979
37. Dlugosz AA, Tapscott SJ, Holtzer H: Effects of phorbol 12-myristate 13-acetate on the differentiation program of embryonic chick skeletal myoblasts. Cancer Res 43:2780, 1983
38. Taketani Y, Oka T: Tumor promoter 12-*O*-tetradecanoylphorbol 13-acetate, like epidermal growth factor, stimulates cell proliferation and inhibits differentiation of mouse mammary epithelial cells in culture. Proc Natl Acad Sci USA 80:1646, 1983
39. Friedman E, Gillin S, Lipkin M: 12-*O*-Tetradecanoylphorbol-13-acetate stimulation of DNA synthesis in cultured preoplastic familial polyposis colonic epithelial cells but not in normal colonic epithelial cells. Cancer Res 44:4078, 1984
40. Barsoum J, Varshavsky A: Mitogenic hormones and tumor promoters greatly increase the incidence of colony-forming cells bearing amplified dihydrofolate reductase genes. Proc Natl Acad Sci USA 80:5330, 1983
41. Shoyab M, Todaro GJ: Specific high affinity cell membrane receptors for biologically active phorbol and ingenol esters. Nature 288:451, 1980
42. Horowitz AD, Greenebaum E, Weinstein IB: Identification of receptors for phorbol ester tumor promoters in intact mammalian cells and of an inhibitor of receptor binding in biologic fluids. Proc Natl Acad Sci USA 78:2315, 1981
43. Solanki V, Slaga TJ: Specific binding of phorbol ester tumor promoters to intact primary epidermal cells from Sencar mice. Proc Natl Acad Sci USA 78:2549, 1981
44. Sando JJ, Young MC: Identification of high-affinity phorbol ester receptor in cytosol of EL4 thymoma cells: Requirement for calcium, magnesium, and phospholipids. Proc Natl Acad Sci USA 80:2642, 1983
45. Castagna M, Takai Y, Kaibuchi K, et al: Direct activation of calcium-activated, phospholipid-dependent protein kinase by tumor-promoting phorbol esters. J Biol Chem 257:7847, 1982
46. Niedel JE, Kuhn LJ, Vandenbark GR: Phorbol diester receptor copurifies with protein kinase C. Proc Natl Acad Sci USA 80:36, 1983
47. Kikkawa U, Takai Y, Tanaka Y, et al: Protein kinase C as a possible receptor protein of tumor-promoting phorbol esters. J Biol Chem 258:11442, 1983
48. Knopf J, Lee MH, Sultzman LA, et al: Cloning and expression of multiple protein kinase C cDNAs. Cell 46:491, 1986
49. Nishizuka Y: Phospholipid degradation and signal translation for protein phosphorylation. Trends Biochem Sci 8:13, 1983
50. Naka M, Nishikawa M, Adelstein RS, Hidaka H: Phorbol ester-induced activation of human platelets is associated with protein kinase C phosphorylation of myosin light chains. Nature 306:490, 1983

51. Rozengurt E, Rodriguez-Pena M, Smith KA: Phorbol esters, phospholipase C, and growth factors rapidly stimulate the phosphorylation of a M_r 80,000 protein in intact quiescent 3T3 cells. Proc Natl Acad Sci USA 80:7244, 1983

52. Werth DK, Niedel JE, Pastan I: Vinculin, a cytoskeletal substrate of protein kinase C. J Biol Chem 258:11423, 1983

53. Nishizuka Y: Protein kinase C in signal transduction and tumor promotion. Nature 308:693, 1984

54. Birnboim HC: DNA strand breakage in human leukocytes exposed to a tumor promoter, phorbol myristate acetate. Science 215:1247, 1982

55. Sporn MB: Chemoprevention of cancer. Nature 272:402, 1978

56. Land H, Parada LF, Weinberg RA: Cellular oncogenes and multistep carcinogenesis. Science 222:771, 1983

57. Stehelin D, Guntaka RV, Varmus HE, Bishop JM: Purification of DNA complementary to nucleotide sequences required for neoplastic transformation of fibroblasts by avian sarcoma viruses. J Mol Biol 101:349, 1976

58. Collett MS, Erikson RL: Protein kinase activity associated with the avian sarcoma virus *src* gene product. Proc Natl Acad Sci USA 75:2021, 1978

59. Hunter T, Sefton BM: Transforming gene product of Rous sarcoma virus phosphorylates tyrosine. Proc Natl Acad Sci USA 77:1311, 1980

60. Leder P, Batley J, Lenoir G, et al: Translocations among antibody genes in human cancer. Science 222:765, 1983

61. Sukumar S, Notario V, Martin-Zanca D, Barbacid M: Induction of mammary carcinomas in rats by nitroso-methylurea involves malignant activation of H-*ras*-1 locus by single point mutations. Nature 306:658, 1983

62. Cooper CS, Blair DG, Oskarsson MK, et al: Characterization of human transforming genes from chemically transformed, teratocarcinoma, and pancreatic carcinoma cell lines. Cancer Res 44:1, 1984

63. Waterfield MD, Scrace GT, Whittle N, et al: Platelet-derived growth factor is structurally related to the putative transforming protein p28^{sis} of simian sarcoma virus. Nature 304:35, 1983

64. Doolittle RF, Hunkapiller MW, Hood LE, et al: Simian sarcoma virus *onc* gene, v-*sis,* is derived from the gene (or genes) encoding a platelet-derived growth factor. Science 221:275, 1983

65. Downward J, Yarden Y, Mayes E, et al: Close similarity of epidermal growth factor receptor and v-*erb-B* oncogene protein sequences. Nature 307:521, 1984

66. Kelly K, Cochran BH, Stiles CD, Leder P: Cell-specific regulation of the c-*myc* gene by lymphocyte mitogens and platelet-derived growth factor. Cell 35:603, 1983

67. Ananthaswamy HN, Price JE, Goldberg LH, et al: Detection and identification of activated oncogenes in human skin cancers occurring on sun-exposed body sites. Cancer Res 48:3341, 1988

68. Pedersen-Bjergaard J, Janssen JWG, Lyons J, et al: Point mutation of the *ras* protooncogenes and chromosome alterations in acute nonlymphocytic leukemia and preleukemia related to therapy with alkylating agents. Cancer Res 48:1812, 1988

69. Knudson AG: Hereditary cancer, oncogenes, and antioncogenes. Cancer Res 45:1437, 1985

70. Huang HJS, Yee JK, Shew JY, et al: Suppression of the neoplastic phenotype by replacement of the RB gene in human cancer cells. Science 242:1563, 1988

71. Green MR: When the products of oncogenes and anti-oncogenes meet. Cell 56:1, 1989

72. Compere SJ, Baldacci P, Sharpe AH, et al: The *ras* and *myc* oncogenes cooperate in tumor induction in many tissues when introduced into midgestation mouse embryos by retroviral vectors. Proc Natl Acad Sci USA 86:2224, 1989

73. Miller EC: Some current perspectives on chemical carcinogenesis in humans and experimental animals: Presidential address. Cancer Res 38:1479, 1978

74. Boyland E: The biological significance of metabolism of polycyclic compounds. Biochem Soc Symp 5:40, 1950
75. Conney AH: Induction of microsomal enzymes by foreign chemicals and carcinogenesis by polycyclic aromatic hydrocarbons: GHA Clowes Memorial Lecture. Cancer Res 42:4875, 1982
76. Huberman E, Sachs L, Yang SK, Gelboin HV: Identification of mutagenic metabolites of benzo(a)pyrene in mammalian cells. Proc Natl Acad Sci USA 73:607, 1976
77. Chang RL, Levin W, Wood AW, et al: Tumorigenicity of bay-region diol-epoxides and other benzo-ring derivatives of dibenzo(a,h)pyrene and dibenzo(a,i)pyrene on mouse skin and in newborn mice. Cancer Res 42:25, 1982
78. Clayson DB: The aromatic amines. Br Med Bull 20:115, 1964
79. Bryan GT, Erturk E, Yoshida O: Production of urinary bladder carcinomas in mice by sodium saccharin. Science 168:1238, 1970
80. Magee PN, Schoental R: Carcinogenesis by nitroso compounds. Br Med Bull 20:102, 1964
81. Wolff IA, Wasserman AE: Nitrates, nitrites and nitrosamines. Science 177:15, 1972
82. Archer MC, Clark SD, Thilly JE, Tannenbaum SR: Environmental nitroso compounds: Reaction of nitrite with creatine and creatinine. Science 174:1341, 1971
83. Johnson DE, Rhoades JW: N-Nitrosamines in smoke condensate from several varieties of tobacco. JNCI 48:1845, 1972
84. Brookes P: Quantitative aspects of the reaction of some carcinogens with nucleic acids and the possible significance of such reactions in the process of carcinogenesis. Cancer Res 26:1994, 1966
85. Smith DWE: Mutagenicity of cycasin aglycone (methylazoxymethanol), a naturally occurring carcinogen. Science 152:1273, 1966
86. Druckrey H, Lange A: Carcinogenicity of azoxymethane dependent on age in BD rats. Fed Proc 31:1482, 1972
87. Boyland E, Nery R: The metabolism of urethane and related compounds. Biochem J 94:198, 1965
88. Miller JA, Miller EC: Natural and synthetic chemical carcinogens in the etiology of cancer. Cancer Res 25:1292, 1965
89. Culvenor CCJ, Dann AT, Dick AT: Alkylation as the mechanism by which the hepatotoxic pyrrolizidine alkaloids act on cell nuclei. Nature 195:570, 1962
90. Farber E: Ethionine carcinogenesis. Adv Cancer Res 7:383, 1963
91. Dickens F: Carcinogenic lactones and related substances. Br Med Bull 20:96, 1964
92. Borchert P, Wislocki PG, Miller JA, Miller EC: The metabolism of the naturally occurring hepatocarcinogen safrole to 1'-hydroxysafrole and the electrophilic reactivity of 1'-acetoxysafrole. Cancer Res 33:575, 1973
93. Borchert P, Miller JA, Miller EC, Shires TK. 1'-Hydroxysafrole, a proximate carcinogenic metabolite of safrole in the rat and mouse. Cancer Res 33:590, 1973
94. Clayson DB: Chemical Carcinogenesis. William & Wilkins, Baltimore, 1962
95. Sunderman FW, Jr: Nickel carcinogenesis. Dis Chest 54:527, 1968
96. Miller JA: Carcinogenesis by chemicals: An overview. GHA Clowes Memorial Lecture. Cancer Res 30:559, 1970
97. Nebert DW: Pharmacogenetics: An approach to understanding chemical and biologic aspects of cancer. JNCI 64:1279, 1980
98. Routledge PA, Shand DG: Presystemic drug elimination. Annu Rev Pharmacol Toxicol 19:447, 1979
99. Boyland E: The biological examination of carcinogenic substances. Br Med Bull 14:93, 1958
100. Mantel N: The concept of threshold in carcinogenesis. Clin Pharmacol Ther 4:104, 1963
101. Hatch TF: Thresholds: Do they exist? Arch Environ Health 22:687, 1971

13

Chemical Teratogenesis

Raymond W. Ruddon

Teratology (from the Greek *teras*, "monster") is the study of developmental malformations. A *teratogen* is an agent that causes such malformations. The births of "monsters" have been recorded since ancient times, when the birth of an abnormal fetus was taken as a sign from the gods (for review of historical aspects, see Warkany[1]). These events were often incorporated into folklore, and the stories of fantastic creatures were passed down through generations. Tales of creatures with three heads or the torso of a man and the head of an animal were commonplace. Unusual births, since they were both rare and frightening, were looked upon as portentous and religiously significant events. The Babylonians kept records of congenital malformations and these were used for foretelling the future. Similar observations and divinations were used by other ancient cultures as well. During the Middle Ages the interpretation of "monster births" as portents continued, and they were thought to predict catastrophes or punishments to come.

Abnormally formed fetuses were often thought to result from animal-human fertilization or from association of human beings with demons or witches. In later, more "sophisticated" cultures, unfortunate or inappropriate maternal mental impressions were thought to cause abnormal fetuses. For example, Montaigne, one of the better educated men of the sixteenth century, stated: "We know by experience that women impart the marks of their fancy to the bodies of the children they carry in their womb." Even in 1899 Keatings' *Cyclopedia of the Diseases of Children* listed 90 examples of defective children caused by maternal impression. As late as the 1950s it was believed by some that a mother's stressful fright could release enough cortisone to produce teratogenic effects.[2]

The scientific phase of teratology developed from experimentation with the artificial incubation of fowl eggs. It was observed that abnormal chicks would be produced under certain conditions such as shaking of eggs or shifts in incubation temperature. In 1891 Camille Dareste showed clearly that malformations could result from incubating fowl eggs at abnormal temperatures. Subsequently (between 1893 and 1901), Charles Féré found that alcohol, nicotine, and other chemicals, when injected into the egg, were teratogenic. Other investigators began to study the effects of various treatments on the developmental embryology of reptiles, amphibia, and fish.

In 1929 a report by Goldstein and Murphy[3] noted a higher incidence of fetal abnormalities in women and animals exposed to ionizing radiation. This was one of the first reports that external environmental factors could induce fetal malformations, but it was not immediately appreciated. In the 1940s Warkany and his associates[4,5] definitively showed that environmental factors such as maternal dietary deficiency and x-irradiation could act as teratogens in rats. Although it was known in 1941 that maternal infection with rubella virus could induce fetal abnormalities[6] and in 1951 that cortisone injections into pregnant mice could produce cleft palates,[7] it took the thalidomide disaster of 1960 and 1961 to make people keenly aware of the possibility that extrinsic chemical agents could cause fetal abnormalities in humans.

GENERAL PRINCIPLES OF TERATOGENESIS

A more remarkable process than embryogenesis is hard to imagine. The finely balanced interplay of cell proliferation, differentiation, migration, and finally organogenesis represents a precisely programmed sequence of events, repeating itself in each detail for every zygote of a species.[8-10] Underlying the morphologic development of the embryo is a progressive unfolding of biochemical potentialities, a temporally regulated transcription and translation of genetic messages, the details of which we do not fully understand. Embryogenesis involves complex interactions in both time and space. In the earliest stages, rapid cell multiplication is the rule. The numerous products of these early cell divisions have different potentialities, depending upon their relative positions in the embryonic mass and upon exposure to various chemical signals. Differentiation begins very early, in some species as early as the two- or four-cell stage. Subsequent development of primordial tissue components and organ precursors depends strongly upon mutual interactions of adjacent cell groups, apparently through chemical mediators or modifiers.[11] Migration, infolding, interpenetration, and encompassing of one cell group by another characterize a later stage of organogenesis. These spatial rearrangements account for the ectodermal origin of many internal viscera, the encapsulation of the nervous elements of the adrenal medulla by the mesodermally derived cortex, the segregation of germ cells in the gonads, and so on. Still later, midline closures of bilaterally symmetric tissues occur, such as the facial structures (lip and palate), the cranium, vertebrae, and anterior body wall. Final morphologic and functional development occurs at various times in different organs and is sometimes completed only after birth.

Two predictions could be made, a priori, on the basis of our knowledge of embryonic development: first, that so complicated a series of events could be interfered with in very specific ways; and second, that the result of such interference could depend strongly upon the timing. Because each step in embryogenesis may depend upon a previous one and because numerous tissues and organs are developing in parallel, even a temporary delay in the development of one group of cells may throw it out of phase with the rest of the embryo and thus lead to an eventual malformation. This has been shown quite clearly to be the case for renoureteral defects induced by folic acid deficiency in rats. Here the vitamin deficiency disturbed the migration of primordial cell groups so that later, after the brief vitamin deficiency was terminated, they could no longer attain their correct anatomic position.[12]

Certain general principles of teratology can be applied to the study of chemical teratogens.[13-15] The sections that follow will review these principles.

Developmental Stage Specificity of the Teratogenic Effects of Chemical Agents

Susceptibility to teratogenic agents varies during gestation and hence depends on the stage of development of the fetus. Very early in embryonic development, during the early cleavage stages in which cells are still undifferentiated and totipotent (i.e., can form any one of the organism's differentiated cell types), exposure to harmful agents may cause death of the embryo. If the exposure is less severe, those cells that survive can recover and normal embryogenesis may ensue. Thus, the effect of teratogenic agents at this stage is probably all or none in that either the embryo is destroyed or so few cells are damaged that the embryo can recover.[13,14]

The period of organogenesis, characterized by segregation of cells into tissue primordia and the beginnings of morphologic and biochemical differentiation, is the stage most sensitive to teratogenic agents. In rodents, this sensitive period extends from about the fifth to the fourteenth day of a 23-day gestation period. In the human there is only meager experimental evidence, but the timetable of embryologic development[15] suggests a period extending roughly from the third week through the third month of pregnancy. At the twentieth day after fertilization the cephalocaudal segmentation of the embryo into somites is just beginning. These segments are the precursors of the axial skeleton and musculature. At about 30 days the limb buds make their appearance, and by 60 days organ differentiation in the fetus (now 30 mm long) is well under way. Accordingly, rubella-induced malformations of the eye, ear, and heart occur principally between the fourth and eight weeks. Data from thalidomide cases indicate that interference with limb formation is chiefly a hazard of the same period, the second month of pregnancy. After organogenesis has occurred, the likelihood of major structural malformations diminishes, but exposure to exogenous chemical agents may still lead to retardation of fetal growth or mental development (or to fetal death if the dose of a toxic agent is high enough).

Depending on when exposure to a teratogen occurs, a variety of organs may be affected, and hence a typical pattern of malformation may occur. Figure 13-1 illustrates a relationship between the timing of organogenesis in the rat and the incidence of specific organ malformation.[16] Thus, for example, an exposure to a teratogen on day 8 to 9 would be expected to affect primarily the brain, eyes, heart, and skeletal system; exposure on day 12 to 13 would significantly affect the palate; and exposure on day 15 to 16 would affect the urogenital system.

Although gross morphologic or structural defects in development are the most obvious teratogenic effects of chemicals, functional abnormalities without obvious structural changes may also occur. That functional changes result from external teratogens is often difficult to document. Furthermore, it is difficult to dissociate functional effects from underlying genetically caused defects. In juvenile diabetes, for example, a deficiency of insulin production could result from a developmental defect in the number of functional islet cells or from reduced secretion by a normal number of cells. There are a number of examples of mental retardation that occur in infants without gross structural defects of the brain or spinal cord. For example, the effects of heavy maternal alcohol consumption on the mental development of the offspring represent a continuum of disorders ranging from the severe fetal alcohol syndrome (consisting of microcephaly, small midface, cardiac and renal anomalies, and severe mental retardation) to attention deficit syndromes in children with relatively normal intelligence.[17]

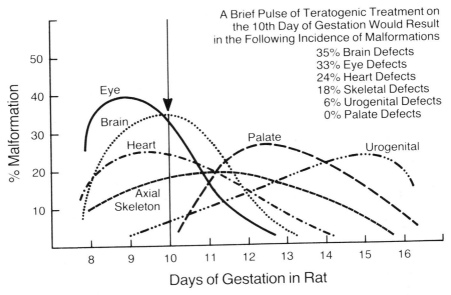

Fig. 13-1. Group of curves representing the susceptibility of particular organs and organ systems in rat embryos to a hypothetical teratogenic agent given on different days of gestation. If the agent were applied on day 10, the resulting syndrome would involve the organs indicated by the curves that are intersected by the vertical line, with percentages of incidence corresponding to the points at which the curves were crossed. Shifting the time of treatment from day 10 to another day would alter the composition of the syndrome both qualitatively and quantitatively. (From Wilson,[16] with permission.)

Dose-Response Effects with Teratogenic Agents

Although this principle may appear obvious, the concept of a safe threshold dose below which no teratogenic effects will occur has been debated for a number of years. In experimental animal studies in which intrauterine death and fetal malformation are used as the criteria of an adverse effect, a no-effect dose level of known teratogens has usually been found.[13] Different threshold doses have been found for different embryotoxicities of a given agent. Not unexpectedly, as exposure time or dosage of a teratogen increases, the frequency and severity of teratogenic effects also increases.[14]

The concept of the placenta as a "barrier" protecting the fetus from drugs taken by the mother has proved to be false as more and more drug effects on the fetus have been observed. Virtually all unbound chemicals in the maternal plasma gain access to the fetal circulation, and the amount of fetal absorption of a given chemical depends on factors similar to those noted for transport across other biologic membranes (i.e., lipophilicity, ionic charge, molecular size, etc. [see Ch. 3]).

Dose-response curves for embryotoxic effects of cytotoxic agents (e.g., alkylating agents, actinomycin D) are typically steep, with a doubling of the dose often causing a shift from a minimal to a maximal response.[13] Many such agents are also toxic to the mother if the dose is high, and the cause of fetal death in these instances may be related to maternal toxicity. One of the surprising things about thalidomide (see below) was that it proved to be teratogenic in humans and higher primates at relatively small doses, but it did not induce fetal death until several multiples of the teratogenic dose were used.

Furthermore, the drug had minimal or no maternal toxicity at teratogenic doses.[13] Potent embryotoxic drugs, such as actinomycin D, begin to be embryolethal at the same doses that induce malformations.

Species Dependence of Susceptibility to Teratogenic Agents

Some species are more susceptible than others to the teratogenic effects of drugs and other chemicals. The variations probably relate to pharmacologic differences (e.g., differences in absorption, distribution, metabolism, and excretion) and to differences in gestational duration, in mechanisms of organogenesis, and possibly also in the structure of the genetic material itself (e.g., chromatin packaging, regulatory processes for gene transcription). Mouse embryos, for example, are susceptible to induction of cleft palate by glucocorticoids, whereas most other mammalian embryos are resistant.[13,18] The interspecies variability in thalidomide susceptibility is another case in point. Other than humans and higher primates, few species are susceptible. Unfortunately, the usual species used in teratogenicity testing (mice, rats, and rabbits) are relatively insensitive to the teratogenic effects of thalidomide, and therefore such tests did not predict the disastrous effects later found in humans. It was subsequently found that certain species of macaque monkeys, baboons, and marmosets were the only animal species that show teratogenic sensitivity similar to that of humans.[19]

Selectivity of Teratogenesis and Interaction with Genetic Influences

Of principal interest are teratogens that interfere directly with fetal development at doses that do not disturb placental function or cause serious maternal toxicity. A great many teratogenic agents meet this criterion of selective toxicity for the fetus. As noted above, with some drugs such as thalidomide there is a considerable range between the dose that induces fetal malformation and the dose that causes maternal death. Indeed in some ways the most dangerous teratogens are those that are well tolerated by the mother in a dose range that is selectively damaging to fetal organogenesis but is not seriously toxic to the fetus as a whole. An agent that is selectively toxic to the mother or one that is so toxic to the fetus that fetal death and resorption (or abortion) occur would not present much hazard as a teratogen.[20] It has been shown that even such maternal disorders as severe hemorrhagic anemia and liver damage do not have teratogenic consequences.[21] Most teratogens do not impair placental function, and the most convincing experiments on teratogenesis include a morphologic demonstration of placental integrity. That experimental fetal malformatons are so easy to produce without significant harm to the mother is consistent with the effects of rubella and of thalidomide in humans and points up the risk that drugs and other environmental agents, innocuous otherwise, might be responsible for unexplained human malformations.

All teratogens, when administered at high dosage or very early in embryonic development, can cause fetal death followed by abortion or resorption of the fetus. For example, actinomycin D (which inhibits DNA-dependent RNA synthesis) was administered once intraperitoneally to pregnant rats at various times in gestation.[22] On the twentieth day of gestation the rats were sacrificed, and all fetuses and implantation sites were examined. The peak effects occurred when the drug was given between the seventh and tenth day. Fetal death and the incidence of malformations among survivors ran a parallel course. Both effects were dose-related, and the sensitivity to both was maximum at the same time in gestation.

Many substances can kill fetuses selectively but are not necessarily teratogenic for survivors, and these effects may vary between species. The mitotic poisons colchicine and podophyllotoxin are examples of agents that have selective fetal effects at certain doses. Lipopolysaccharides from *Brucella abortus* kill all rat fetuses when administered on the eleventh day of gestation and display the same sharp dependence on time of administration as do compounds with teratogenic action. Lipopolysaccharides from several enteric bacteria are teratogenic in rats, and they are known to cause abortion in humans. Aminopterin, at a dose that kills most rat fetuses, is not teratogenic for survivors; yet aminopterin in the human, if it fails to produce abortion, results in fetal malformations.

Embryogenesis is a programmed sequence of gene expression leading to a progressive selectivity of gene transcription in various tissues. Although we do not yet understand what controls the timing of gene expression or repression during embryogenesis nor exactly how the products of gene expression intervene in embryonic differentiation, it is nevertheless obvious that genetic defects could derange the process in very selective ways. It is therefore not surprising to find many examples of a genetic role in congenital malformations. Down's syndrome and chondrodystrophy (a defect in the formation of bone from cartilage) are malformations whose causes appear to be primarily genetic, one associated with trisomy for chromosome 21, the other caused by a gene mutation. Such malformations do not fall under the heading of teratogenesis since the basic defect was presumably present in the zygote and will affect the germ cells as well as all the somatic cells of the affected individual.

The distinction between heritable and nonheritable abnormalities is not completely sharp, however. If a mutagenic agent acted at an early enough stage in fetal development to affect germ cells and somatic cells alike and if the alteration were compatible with survival, the phenotypic manifestations could occur in the affected individual as well as in the offspring of that individual. Experimentally it has been shown, for example, that when the vitamin antagonist 6-aminonicotinamide was injected into pregnant mice on the thirteenth day of gestation, cleft palate was produced in the offspring. Chromosome abnormalities were also produced (polyploidy and fragmentation), not only in the region of the deformed palates but also in other cells throughout the body of the fetus. Furthermore, similar chromosome changes were observed in the maternal bone marrow after treatment, but never in untreated controls.[23]

In the experiment with 6-aminonicotinamide, the teratogen was administered fairly late in fetal development; therefore, the induced chromosome abnormalities must all have arisen during faulty mitoses. However, if such an agent were administered to a female at about the time of fertilization, the result could be a similar disturbance of meiosis in the ovum about to be fertilized. The consequent changes in chromosome number or morphology might be indistinguishable from those regarded as having been inherited from earlier generations. This may happen in human populations.[24] A "run" of sex chromosome aberrations was noted among infants born in one city during a particular 5-month period. The study began as a routine systematic examination of the sex chromatin in human newborns. The sex chromatin is material with distinctive staining properties that is associated with one of the X chromosomes.[25] It is easy to establish, therefore, by staining and microscopic examination of cells from the amniotic membrane or the infant's buccal mucosa, whether the genetic constitution is normal XX or XY or whether abnormalities such as XXY, XXX, or XO are present. During the first 18 months of the study no abnormalities were found among 1,541 infants; in the next 5 months there were 6 out of 1,009; and finally in the next 4 months there were none out of 817. Although the actual number of abnormalities was very small, the clustering of these few in a particular short period of time was most unlikely to have occurred by chance. Most interesting, during the same 5-month period there was an increase in the number (also small) of cases of Down's syndrome in this same community. The implication of the findings is that some mutagenic or teratogenic factor, perhaps a drug or virus, may have been at work in this community during the relevant period.

That certain agents have mutagenic and carcinogenic as well as teratogenic activity is hardly surprising.[26,27] At the crucial time in embryonic development, induced mutation or chromosomal abnormality, if it did not cause fetal death, might well cause abnormal fetal development. Alkylating agents, for example, are well known to be mutagens and carcinogens, and some (but not all) are potent teratogens. However, such associations are by no means the rule, and numerous teratogens are neither mutagenic nor carcinogenic. This is entirely reasonable, since all that is required for teratogenesis is a significant transient disturbance of cell function during a short critical period of organogenesis, whereas a *heritable* alteration in a cell line is required in mutagenesis and carcinogenesis.

Most congenital malformations are not associated with any obvious abnormality of the chromosomes and are not heritable. The nonheritable nature of the abnormalities has been demonstrated by brother-sister matings of malformed animals and also on a large scale in human populations. Genetic factors, however, may play an important part in determining sensitivity to teratogens as well as the probability of spontaneous malformation.[28] One indication of the role of genetic factors is the considerable difference in sensitivity between species and between strains of the same species. In three rat strains the azo dye trypan blue produced exencephalic offspring at wholly different frequencies—17, 50, and 97 percent, respectively. Cortisone produced cleft palate in all mouse fetuses of one strain but in only 20 percent of another; this difference was traced to earlier midline fusion of the palate in the more resistant strain. Cortisone also produced cleft palate in rabbits but no malformations whatsoever in rats, yet cortisone strongly potentiated the actions of another teratogen, vitamin A, in rats. Such genetically determined differences are not necessarily due to differences in metabolism or transplacental passage of teratogens.

Findings such as those described above have led some investigators to the view that chemical teratogens act by bringing out "concealed weaknesses" of the developmental processes, which have a genetic basis. It has been suggested that many induced defects are really phenocopies (i.e., phenotypic changes of exactly the same kinds as are produced by faulty genes), brought about through the same biochemical disturbances. Supporting evidence was obtained in experiments with 6-aminonicotinamide in chicks.[29] This vitamin antagonist produces skeletal anomalies, principally micromelia and parrot beak, which also occur as mutations. Specially bred stocks heterozygous for these defects had increased sensitivity to the teratogen. Conversely, in a stock possessing modifying alleles that reduce the frequency of mutant defects of the skeleton (chondrodystrophy), the teratogen had reduced efficacy.

METHODS OF EXPERIMENTAL TERATOGENESIS

Animal experiments have chiefly employed mice, rabbits, and rats, although primates have also been used.[30] Like humans, these mammals have a placenta, so that drugs are exposed to maternal tissues and subjected to maternal metabolism before entering the fetus. Moreover, the gestation period is conveniently short (only 3 weeks in a rat or mouse), multiple births are the rule (so that each treated female yields a large amount of experimental data), and housing and maintenance of large numbers of animals is simple because of their small size and low cost. The most serious limitation in the use of rodents is the different structure (and possibly function) of their placentae as compared with that of the human. Rhesus monkeys and other primates have therefore also been used,[31] since their placental structure and function, as well as the pattern of embryologic development, are like those in the human. Also although primates are very expensive, so that large-scale studies are impractical, they respond to the known teratogens that affect humans, such as thalidomide, rubella virus, and androgenic steroids.

Chick embryos are useful when the purpose of an experiment is to study the action of a proximate teratogen, which acts directly, without the necessity of prior metabolic transformation. The teratogen can be placed in direct contact with the developing embryo. A good correlation was found for the teratogenic effects of diverse compounds in chick embryos and in rodents.[32] The presence of a yolk sac in both species may explain why some agents that are teratogenic in chicks and rodents are less active in primates.

Experiments on teratogenesis in rodents begin with isolation of virgin females and determination of the estrous cycle by vaginal smears. Matings can then be arranged at the time of ovulation. Since the timing of teratogenic treatments is extremely critical, it is essential to know precisely when conception occurs. After mating, the females are isolated again, treated as desired with a teratogen, and sacrificed just before term. Since cannibalism is frequent among rodents, the offspring must be obtained by caesarean section in order to obtain reliable data. This procedure permits all implantation sites to be examined and every product of conception to be accounted for as a resorbed, dead, malformed live, or fully developed normal fetus. Gross examination will reveal the most obvious malformations; microscopic examination will reveal others. To be certain all anomalies are detected, an exhaustive gross and microscopic analysis of each fetus is required. Investigations of teratogenesis have usually focused upon morphologic abnormalities; now increasing attention is paid to effects of teratogens on biochemical processes in the developing and mature fetus.[33–35] Agents that block DNA synthesis,[36] RNA synthesis, or protein synthesis may be teratogenic, if delivered at a crucial time and the fetus as a whole survives.

INCIDENCE AND ETIOLOGY OF HUMAN TERATOGENESIS

An estimated 3 to 7 percent of human babies are born with some sort of malformation.[18] The etiology of these abnormalities is most often unknown (in about 65 percent of cases). About 20 percent are due to transmission of a known genetic defect, and 5 percent are associated with chromosomal abnormalities, 2 to 3 percent with maternal infections (e.g., rubella, toxoplasmosis, syphilis, herpes, cytomegalovirus), 4 percent with maternal metabolic disorders (diabetes, other endocrine disorders, nutritional deficiencies, or drug addictions), 1 to 2 percent with mechanical problems such as uterine structural problems and umbilical cord constrictions, and 1 to 5 percent with exposure to drugs and environmental chemicals.[14,19]

Teratogenic Agents in Animals and Humans

Table 13-1 lists some of the drugs and environmental chemicals that have been shown to be teratogenic in at least one mammalian species. Some of these are cytotoxic agents (e.g., alkylating agents, antimetabolites) and some are teratogenic in animals only at doses not usually used in humans (e.g., aspirin, penicillin). Thus, one view[19] is that drugs should be categorized according to the weight of the evidence as: (1) established as embryotoxic in humans (e.g., thalidomide, androgenic hormones, folic acid antagonists); (2) suspected

Table 13-1. Some Types of Drugs and Environmental Chemicals That Have Been Shown to be Teratogenic in One or More Species of Mammals[a]

Salicylates (e.g., aspirin, oil of wintergreen)
Certain alkaloids (e.g., caffeine, nicotine, colchicine)
Tranquilizers (e.g., meprobamate, chlorpromazine, reserpine, diazepam)
Antihistamines (e.g., buclizine, meclizine, cyclizine)
Antibiotics (e.g., chloramphenicol, streptonigrin, penicillin)
Hypoglycemics (e.g., carbutamide, tolbutamide, hypoglycins)
Corticoids (e.g., triamcinolone, cortisone)
Alkylating agents (e.g., busulfan, chlorambucil, cyclophosphamide, TEM)
Antimalarials (e.g., chloroquine, quinacrine, pyrimethamine)
Anesthetics (e.g., halothane, urethane nitrous oxide, pentobarbital)
Antimetabolites (e.g., folic acid, purine and pyrimidine analogs)
Solvents (e.g., benzene, dimethyl sulfoxide, propylene glycol)
Pesticides (e.g., aldrin, malathion, carbaryl, 2,4,5-T, captan, folpet)
Industrial effluents (e.g., some compounds of Hg, Pb, As, Li, Cd)
Plants (e.g., locoweed, lupins, jimsonweed, sweet peas, tobacco stalks)
Miscellaneous (e.g., trypan blue, triparanol, diamox)

[a] Teratogenic effects were usually seen only at doses well above therapeutic levels for the drugs, or above likely exposure levels for the environmental chemicals.

(From Wilson,[19] with permission.)

to be embryotoxic in humans (e.g., anticonvulsants, amphetamines, warfarin, oral hypoglycemics); and (3) possibly embryotoxic in humans (e.g., female sex hormones, meprobamate, chlordiazepoxides, and gaseous anesthetics such as halothane).

Agents reported to be teratogenic in humans are listed in Table 13-2. A few brief comments about some of these will serve as examples.

Alcohol

It was suspected for a long time that chronic alcohol intake by pregnant women can induce mental retardation and other physical abnormalities in their offspring. As noted above, these abnormalities can vary from severe to mild. Several studies have shown that heavy, chronic maternal alcohol intake can produce the fetal alcohol syndrome (FAS), including intrauterine growth retardation, microcephaly, maxillary hypoplasia, cardiac abnormalities, and severe mental retardation.[37–39] Although the dose-response relationships have not been clearly established, consumption of 6 ounces of alcohol per day constitutes a high risk.[39] There is some evidence to suggest that the FAS involves the actions of both alcohol and its metabolite acetaldehyde.[40] Complicating factors are poor nutrition and cigarette smoking, which often go hand in hand with heavy alcohol consumption.

Folic Acid Analogs

At one time the folic acid antagonist aminopterin was used to induce therapeutic abortions. In some of the failed abortions or those that occurred later, hydrocephalus, cleft palate, and meningomyelocele were noted.[41] The fetuses from some women who became or were pregnant during a time of treatment with the anticancer folate antagonist methotrexate showed the absence of frontal bones and digits, craniosynostosis, and rib defects. Exposure to methotrexate during the first 2 months of pregnancy or for several days between the eighth and tenth weeks of gestation produced these effects.[42,43] Most often, treatment with folate antagonists during the early months of pregnancy results in intra-

Table 13-2. Teratogenic Agents of Humans

Agents	Reported Effects and/or Associations	Comments
Alcohol	Fetal alcohol syndrome: intrauterine growth retardation, microcephaly; maxillary hypoplasia, reduction in width of palpebral fissure, mental retardation.	Direct cytotoxic effects of alcohol and acetaldehyde and indirect effects of alcoholism (poor nutrition, smoking, use of other drugs). Consumption of 6 ounces of alcohol or more per day constitutes a high risk.
Aminopterin, methotrexate	Hydrocephalus, cleft palate, meningomyelocele, intrauterine growth retardation, abnormal cranial ossification, reduction in derivatives of first branchial arch.	Folic acid antagonists that inhibit dihydrofolate reductase, resulting in cell death.
Androgens	Masculinization of female embryo: clitoromegaly with or without fusion of labia minora.	Effects are dose-dependent; stimulation of growth and differentiation of receptor-containing tissue.
Coumarin derivatives	Nasal hypoplasia, stippling of secondary epiphysis; intrauterine growth retardation, anomalies of eyes, hands, neck, variable CNS effects in gestation.	Metabolic inhibitor; bleeding is an unlikely explanation for effects. 10–25% risk from exposure during 8th–14th week of pregnancy.
Diethylstilbesterol	Masculinization of female, vaginal adenocarcinoma, anomalies of cervix and uterus. Affected males show hypotrophic testes, epidymal cysts, abnormal spermatozoa. Effects are dose-dependent.	Stimulates estrogen receptor-containing tissue, may cause misplaced tissue; 75% risk for vaginal adenosis for exposures before 9th week of pregnancy; risk of vaginal adenocarcinoma is low (1 in 10,000). Risk for anomalies in males (including minor variations) is 25%.
Diphenylhydantoin	Hydantoin syndrome: hypoplastic nails and distal phalanges, cleft lip/palate, microcephaly, mental retardation.	Direct effect on cell membranes, folate and vitamin K metabolism. Wide variation in reported risk. Associations documented only with chronic exposure.
Methylmercury	Minamata disease: cerebral palsy, microcephaly, mental retardation, blindness.	Cell death due to inhibition of enzymes, especially sulfhydryl enzymes.
Oxazolidine-2,4-diones	Fetal trimethadione syndrome: V-shaped eyebrows, low-set ears with anteriorly folded helix, high-arched palate, irregular teeth, CNS anomalies, developmental delay.	Affects cell membrane permeability. Wide variation in reported risk. Associations documented only with chronic exposure.
Polychlorinated biphenyls	Cola-colored children: pigmentation of gums, nails, and groin, hypoplastic deformed nails, intrauterine growth retardation.	Polychlorinated biphenyls and commonly occurring contaminants are cytotoxic.
Progestins	Masculinization of female embryo exposed to high doses.	Stimulates growth and differentiation of receptor-containing tissue.
Radiation	Microcephaly, mental retardation, eye anomalies, intrauterine growth retardation, visceral malformations depending on dose and stage of exposure.	Cell death and mitotic delay. Little or no risk with exposures of 5 rads or less of x-radiation.
Tetracycline	Hypoplastic tooth enamel, tooth and bone staining.	Effects seen only if exposure is during second or third trimester.

(Continued)

Table 13-2. (*continued*)

Agents	Reported Effects and/or Associations	Comments
Thalidomide	Bilateral limb reduction defects (preaxial preferential effects, phocomelia), facial hemangioma, esophageal or duodenal atresia, anomalies of external ears, kidneys, and heart.	Increased programmed cell death in the early limb bud causing retarded growth in the apical ectodermal ridge, especially in the preaxial border. Primary mechanism unknown. Very high risk of major malformations during critical periods.
Thyroid: Iodides, radioiodine, antithyroid drugs (propylthiouracil)	Hypothyroidism, goiter.	Fetopathic effect specific for the thyroid. Metabolic block resulting in decreased thyroid hormone synthesis and gland development. Maternal intake of 12 mg of iodide per day or more increases the risk of fetal goiter.

(From Beckman et al.,[14] with permission.)

uterine fetal death, but 20 to 30 percent of fetuses that survive to term have a variety of malformations.[19]

Androgens

Masculinization, characterized by clitoromegaly and sometimes by fusion of the labia, has been reported in infant girls born after maternal exposure to large doses of testosterone or methyltestosterone.[44,45] Since differentiation of external genitalia is usually complete by the twelfth week of gestation, hormone treatment after that time would have little effect on these organs.[19]

Diethylstilbestrol

In the 1950s and early 1960s diethylstilbestrol (DES) was an accepted treatment for threatened abortions in women at risk for or with a history of spontaneous abortion. In 1970 it was first reported that young women whose mothers had been given DES during the first trimester of pregnancy had an increased incidence of vaginal adenocarcinoma.[46] Subsequent studies showed that most of the vaginal adenocarcinomas in the daughters occurred after age 14 and only in those exposed before week 18 of gestation.[47,48] Although the risk of developing adenocarcinoma is very low in DES-exposed female offspring, there is a high rate of vaginal dysplasia (75 to about 90 percent depending on the study).[14,19] About 25 percent of males exposed to DES in utero exhibit genital lesions and low sperm counts, but an increased incidence of malignant neoplasia has not been reported.[49]

Methylmercury

Environmental exposure to methylmercury has occurred in some areas of the world owing to contamination of seed grains resulting from the use of this agent as a fungicide. In Iraq, for example, several pregnant women who consumed badly contaminated bread gave birth to children with cerebral palsy and other mental defects.[50] In Minamata, Japan, there were a series of well publicized cases of methylmercury poisoning due to the consumption of fish from the heavily contaminated bay. Infants born to exposed women had an increased incidence of microcephaly and cerebral palsy.[51]

Polyhalogenated Biphenyls

Polyhalogenated biphenyls, sold as fire retardants, were accidentally mixed with livestock feed in Michigan in 1975. Cattle that were inadvertently fed this material developed a variety of toxic symptoms, and some deformities in their newborn calves were claimed (for review see Wilson[52]). A variety of human illnesses were believed to have been caused by exposure to the meat and milk from these cattle. Pregnant mice fed polybrominated biphenyls at 50 to 1,000 ppm gave birth to growth-retarded young with some malformations[53]; thus these agents, at high doses at least, have teratogenic potential, but such effects have not been well documented in humans.

Our environment is rife with polychlorinated biphenyls, which have been used as lubricants, as insulators, and in paints, varnishes, and resins. Although manufacturing has been halted, the long environmental half-life of these compounds means that they will be with us for a long time. These agents have been shown to be carcinogenic in animals at high doses and to produce growth retardation, but no major malformations, in newborn rats exposed in utero. "Cola-colored" infants with low birth weight, hypoplastic nails, and enlarged eyelid sebaceous glands have been born to mothers who had consumed cooking oil contaminated with polychlorinated biphenyls,[54] but other major birth defects have not been documented.

Other Environmental Chemicals

A variety of natural substances including plants (e.g., locoweed, lupins, jimsonweed, creeping indigo, podophyllin), mycotoxins (e.g., aflatoxins, ochratoxin A, rubratoxin B), plant alkaloids and extracts (e.g., nicotine, colchicine, cycasin), and toxins (e.g., certain snake venoms, tetanus toxin, and endotoxin) have been shown to be embryotoxic in animals, usually under laboratory or controlled conditions.[52] A number of the plant products may be eaten by domestic animals, and some have been administered to pregnant mice or rats to confirm their teratogenic potential. The teratogenic effect of these substances in humans, if any, has not been confirmed.

Insecticides have not been associated with human embryotoxicity in any definitive way. Among herbicides, the defoliant 2,4,5-T is teratogenic in several rodent species when relatively large doses are used, and this effect is most likely due to the presence of the dioxin TCDD present as an impurity in 2,4,5-T. The use of 2,4,5-T in Viet Nam and in certain other countries, including the United States, has initiated several claims that its use is associated with abortions and fetal abnormalities. This is still an area of heated controversy and awaits further study.

The possible teratogenic effect in humans of numerous other pollutants such as polycyclic aromatic hydrocarbons, nitrogen oxides, and chlorinated hydrocarbons, many of which are mutagenic and carcinogenic under experimental conditions, can only be surmised at the present time. It seems likely, however, that these agents, if present in high amounts in the environment at crucial times during gestation, would have damaging effects on the fetus.

Salicylates

Occasional reports have appeared in the literature about the embryotoxic effects of aspirin (for review see Wilson[19]). Some studies have indicated an increased incidence of low birth weight and fetal abnormalities when salicylates were taken during the first trimester, while others show no increased number of congenital anomalies. The conclusion seems to be that salicylates have low teratogenic potential in humans, particularly when taken in usual occasional doses.

Antibiotics

In general, the teratogenic potential of antibiotics is quite low under usual dosage conditions.[19] Some reports, however, indicate an increase in oral clefts with the use of penicillin, tetracyclines, or chloramphenicol during the first trimester.[55] In utero exposure to tetracyclines during the second or third trimester has been shown to discolor teeth and, in very high doses, to depress skeletal bone growth and produce hypoplastic tooth enamel.[56] In utero streptomycin induction of hearing loss and vestibular defects has been reported in several studies (for review see Gal and Sharpless[17]).

General Anesthetics

Reports that anesthetists and operating room nurses who are repeatedly exposed to inhalation anesthetics have higher than expected rates of miscarriages has raised concern about the embryotoxicity of such agents (for review see Wilson[19]). Exposure of pregnant mice or rats to halothane in some studies produced an increased incidence of cleft palate[57] and some subtle ultrastructural changes in brain, kidney, and liver[58]; however, other studies showed no or very low levels of developmental abnormalities in rats.[59] The teratogenic potential of halothane, methoxyflurane, and nitrous oxide appears to be very low on the basis of the experimental animal studies.[19]

Radiation

Growth retardation, eye malformations, microcephaly, and other central nervous system defects have been reported for infants born to mothers receiving radiation therapy and for infants born to mothers surviving atomic bomb fallout in Hiroshima.[14]

Thalidomide

Thalidomide was introduced in the late 1950s in West Germany, England, and other countries as a tranquilizing agent and hypnotic. It was effective and seemed remarkably nontoxic. Although a typical therapeutic dose was about 100 mg, patients recovered from ingestion of as much as 14 g taken with suicidal intent. About 1960 some scattered reports indicated that patients receiving this drug for a long time sometimes developed neurologic disturbances.

thalidomide

Shortly after the introduction of thalidomide into therapy, there was an increase in the number of infants born with phocomelia, a shortening or complete absence of the limbs.[60] At the University Pediatric Clinic in Hamburg, for example, not a single case of phocomelia was seen in the decade 1949 to 1959. In 1959 there was a single case and; in 1960, 30 cases; and in 1961, 154 cases. Comparable increases in the frequency of this anomaly, previously almost unknown, occurred simultaneously in many parts of the world where thalidomide was in use. Finally, in November 1961, an astute pediatrician[61] suspected an association between phocomelia and the ingestion of thalidomide by the pregnant mother. Subsequent investigations in several countries[62,63] indicated that in virtually every case of phocomelia the mother had taken thalidomide between the third and eighth weeks of pregnancy. Sometimes only a few doses during the critical period sufficed.

The critical period for each kind of malformation produced in the human fetus has been established by careful retrospective analysis.[64] When thalidomide was taken 35 to 36 days after the last menstrual period (approximately 21 to 22 days of gestation), absence of the external ears and paralysis of the cranial nerves resulted. If the drug was taken 3 to 5 days later (about 24 to 27 days of gestation), the phocomelia effect was at its maximum, affecting principally the arms. A day or two later, similar defects of the legs occurred. The sensitive period terminated 48 to 50 days after the last period (34 to 36 days of gestation) with the production of hypoplastic thumbs and anorectal stenosis.

That thalidomide was responsible for the outbreak of phocomelia is beyond reasonable doubt, but it is still uncertain what exact degree of risk is attached to the ingestion of this drug by a pregnant woman. If a large number of pregnant women were given thalidomide during the critical period, what fraction of the infants would be malformed? Some investigators believe that practically all would be affected, since it was difficult to find well authenticated instances of thalidomide ingestion followed by the birth of normal infants. Others place the risk very much lower, believing that the retrospective method of investigation exaggerates such an association to an extreme degree.[65] Thus, a woman who has given birth to a malformed child will readily recall (or even imagine) taking thalidomide, especially when the effects of the drug have been publicized, but a woman with a normal child, who may also have taken thalidomide during pregnancy, has no particular interest in recalling that fact.

Thalidomide was withdrawn from the market at the end of 1961, and the outbreak of phocomelia subsided promptly. In the United States the drug had not been approved by the Food and Drug Administration and was therefore never in general use. The total number of infants throughout the world that were deformed by thalidomide must be around 10,000. Although phocomelia is the most obvious and directly disabling abnormality, congenital malformations of the internal organs are also common in the affected children.

Several key lessons were learned from the thalidomide catastrophe. A major consequence was the institution of improved procedures for screening new drugs. Teratogenic effects had not been examined routinely in the past, partly because the potential seriousness of the problem had been underestimated, but also because effective methods had not been developed. As had been shown for numerous other teratogenic agents, thalidomide displays a strong species specificity. In rats, for example, congenital abnormalities could not at first be produced by this drug. In certain strains of white rabbits, it was found that carefully timed administration of thalidomide between the eighth and sixteenth days of pregnancy led to typical limb malformations.[66] Subsequent work with rats showed that this species was sensitive after all, but only on the twelfth day of gestation.[67] Eventually, a syndrome of thalidomide-induced malformations was produced in monkeys, which is very much like that seen in humans.[68]

A possible cause of species differences in the teratogenicity of thalidomide and of differences in sensitivity among humans may be variations in metabolic pathways. Thalidomide is extensively metabolized; evidently, a metabolite rather than thalidomide itself is the proximate teratogenic agent.[69] Hydrolysis of amide bonds and ring hydroxylation alone could account for more than 100 metabolites, of which a dozen or so have been identified in vivo.[62] When the piperidine ring is opened, a glutamine or glutamic acid derivative is formed, as shown:

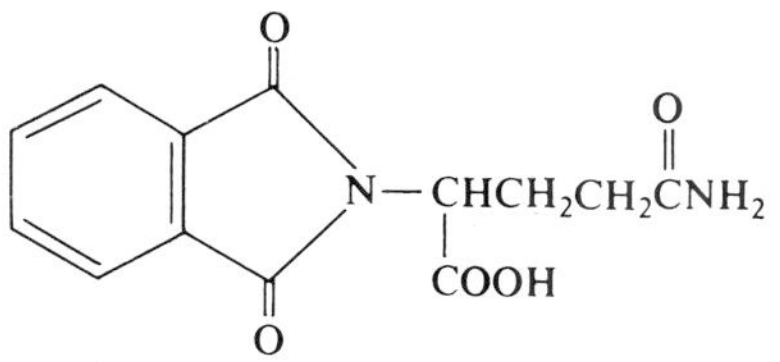

$$N\!-\!CHCH_2CH_2CNH_2$$

glutamine derivative
of thalidomide

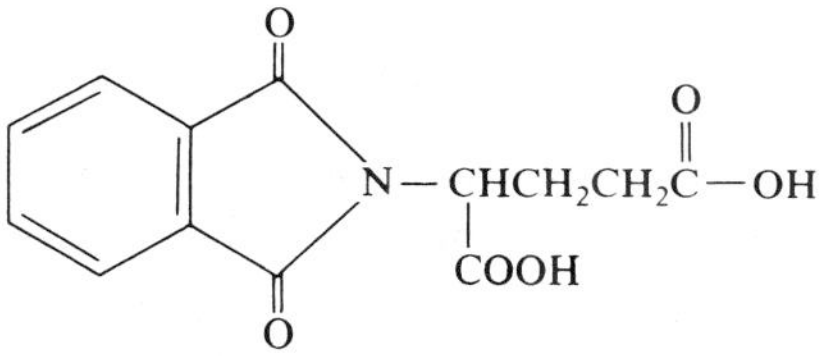

$$N\!-\!CHCH_2CH_2C\!-\!OH$$

deaminated derivative
(phthalylglutamic acid)

Decarboxylation of phthalylglutamic acid yields a monocarboxylic acid, which is the most abundant metabolite.

Early studies showed that none of the metabolites were teratogenic when injected into pregnant rabbits under the same conditions in which thalidomide showed its characteristic actions. It was discovered, however, that this was due to the inability of the metabolites to pass from maternal plasma into the fetus in appreciable quantity. Figure 13-2 shows that when thalidomide was administered, it was all converted to the monocarboxylic acid in the fetus.[69] Radioactive thalidomide was used, and samples of the plasma and of allantoic fluid were subjected to paper electrophoresis. Localization of the radioactivity peaks shows that after 4 hours thalidomide itself, the monocarboxylic acid, and a dicarboxylic acid were all present in plasma, but only the monocarboxylic acid could be found in the allantoic fluid. This experiment, together with the previously demonstrated inability of the carboxylic acid metabolites to pass the placental barrier in the rabbit, shows that thalidomide is metabolized in the fetus, or at least on the fetal side of the placenta. Without knowledge of the teratogenic potency of the monocarboxylic and dicarboxylic acid metabolites, however, it was impossible to conclude which (if either) was the proximate teratogen.

Subsequent experiments showed[70,71] that in mice, the dicarboxylic acid (phthalyl-L-glutamic acid) was teratogenic when administered to the pregnant female on days 7 to 9 of gestation. The D isomer was completely inactive, as were various products of further metabolism. It is likely, therefore, that phthalyl-L-glutamic acid is a proximate teratogen in thalidomide teratogenesis. An analog of thalidomide in which one of the CO groups in the phthalyl moiety has been reduced to CH_2 is also a potent teratogen.[72]

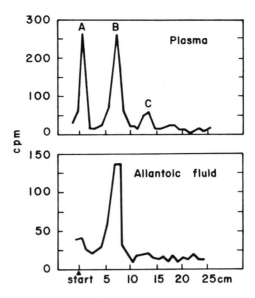

Fig. 13-2. Conversion of thalidomide to a monocarboxylic acid derivative in the rabbit fetus. Samples of plasma (above) and allantoic fluid (below) were subjected to paper electrophoresis 4 hours after administration of radioactive thalidomide to a pregnant rabbit. Anodal migration is toward the right; distance is shown on the x axis. Radioactivity in the paper is shown on the y axis. Peak A, thalidomide; peak B, monocarboxylic acid derivative; peak C, dicarboxylic acid derivative. Neither carboxylic acid passed from plasma into allantoic fluid if injected into the rabbit. (From Keberle et al.,[69] with permission.)

In the aftermath of the thalidomide episode there was intensified investigation of various drugs, both established ones and new ones, with respect to teratogenicity. An antihistaminic, meclizine hydrochloride, and a related compound, cyclizine, were found to cause skeletal abnormalities in rats.[73] Both compounds yield the same metabolite, norchlorcyclizine:

which is found in the rat fetus and may be the proximate teratogen.[74] The finding of teratogenicity by an antihistamine was alarming because drugs of this kind were widely available without prescription, and since they relieve nausea, they were likely to be used precisely at the critical period of pregnancy for relief of "morning sickness." This, indeed, was a major reason why thalidomide had such devastating effects.[65] However, extensive prospective studies in populations of pregnant women have not revealed any abnormal frequency of malformations or abortions in women taking these drugs.[75,76] Anti-inflammatory steroids have been shown to cause cleft palate in the mouse,[77–79] but their possible teratogenicity in humans remains an open question. Even caffeine, probably the most widely used of all drugs, has been reported to produce fetal abnormalities in mice,[80] although at doses (per kilogram) at least 50 times higher than those taken by people.

CONCERNS IN HUMAN TERATOGENESIS

Drugs with known teratogenic effects should obviously not be used by pregnant women, but these same drugs might well be effective and harmless in men, in women beyond the menopause, and in children. A practical question is whether pregnancy can be recognized soon enough to avoid inadvertent administration of teratogens during the time of fetal sensitivity. The problem is presented schematically in Figure 13-3. We know that the sensitive period for teratogenesis coincides with the phase of organ differentiation. In the human embryo the period of organogenesis begins at about the twentieth day of gestation (the first somite stage) and continues most vigorously through the third month.[8] A continuing process of finer morphologic and biochemical differentiation goes on throughout the second trimester; and even premature infants born in the seventh or eighth month are incompletely developed in some respects. In women with regular menses, ovulation occurs approximately 14 days (12 to 16 days) prior to the onset of the next menstrual period, and fertilization takes place within a day or two after ovulation.[81,82] Thus, at fetal age 20 days the missed period is more than a week overdue, and most pregnancy tests are already positive.[83] This hypothetical woman with perfectly regular menstrual cycles will know

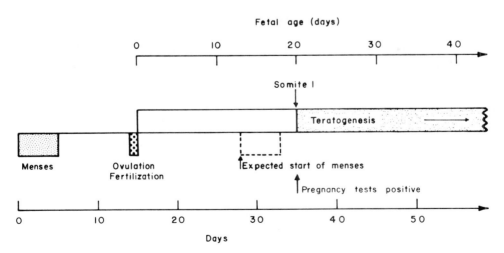

Fig. 13-3. Relationship of teratogenic susceptibility to diagnosis of pregnancy. The diagram applies to a hypothetical, perfectly regular 28-day menstrual cycle. Pregnancy will be recognized before the earliest time the fetus is susceptible to teratogenic action; before fetal age 20 days, abortion will be the likely result of damage to the fetus. Variability in the time of ovulation will delay recognition of pregnancy until beyond fetal age 20 days.

she is pregnant just in time to discontinue potentially teratogenic medications. Unfortunately, however, the length of the menstrual period varies widely, not only between women but also in the individual woman.[84] Fully one-third of all women have a range of 13 days or more between their shortest and longest cycles, whereas only 1 women in 10 varies by less than 5 days. The greater the irregularity of past periods, the longer will be the time needed for the missed period to be noted and for the woman to consider herself pregnant. It follows that for the population as a whole, if women of childbearing age are permitted access to medications that are potentially teratogenic, an unacceptably large proportion of them will have exposed their embryos to the risk of malformation before pregnancy is recognized. Clearly, then, the only safe course is to set up special safeguards for the administration of drugs to all women of childbearing age.

It is clear that the risks of chemical teratogenesis, like those of chemical mutagenesis (cf. Ch. 11), are accentuated during the first trimester, although the risk of the fetus being damaged remains throughout the gestation period. Until much more information becomes available, the very diversity of known teratogens and mutagens should dictate caution.[85,86] Whenever a drug is being administered to a woman of childbearing age, the possibility of pregnancy should be kept in mind. A woman who is known to be pregnant should not be exposed to drugs at all during pregnancy (especially during the first trimester), unless the need is pressing. Moreover, since self-medication has been found to be very common among pregnant women,[87] positive warnings should be given by the physician.

The thalidomide experience served to bring drug-induced teratogenesis out of the realm of laboratory curiosities and into the social arena. It focused attention throughout the world upon the need for more thorough testing of all possible adverse drug effects in many animal species before drugs are approved for human use. Because exhaustive animal testing is time-consuming and expensive and because new techniques often have to be devised, one consequence is a slowing of the rate at which new drugs are introduced into therapeutics.[88]

The problem of congenital malformation in the human is similar in some respects to the problems of mutation and cancer. All three occur spontaneously and can also be produced by external physical or chemical treatments. In none of the three have the causes of the spontaneous events been ascertained. Deliberate experiments are for the most part confined to laboratory animals, while human data must be largely of a statistical nature. More prospective statistical investigations in humans might bring to light associations, as yet unsuspected, between environmental influences during pregnancy (including exposure to drugs) and the subsequent birth of a malformed child.

Chemical teratogenesis, like chemical mutagenesis and chemical carcinogenesis, is a challenging area of pharmacologic investigation. Our present understanding of the teratogenic mechanisms of chemicals is primitive. With increasing knowledge about the biochemical events in normal embryogenesis should come better understanding of teratogenesis.

REFERENCES

1. Warkany J: History of teratology. p.3. In Wilson JG, Fraser FC (eds): Handbook of Teratology. Vol. 1. Plenum, New York, 1977
2. Strean LP: The Birth of Normal Babies. Twayne Publishers, New York, 1958
3. Goldstein L, Murphy DP: Etiology of ill-health in children born after maternal pelvic irradiation. II. Defective children born after postconception pelvic irradiation. AJR 22:322, 1929

4. Warkany J, Nelson RC: Appearance of skeletal abnormalities in the offspring of rats reared on a deficient diet. Science 92:383, 1940

5. Warkany J, Shraffenberger E: Congenital malformations induced in rats by roentgen rays. AJR 57:455, 1947

6. Gregg NM: Congenital cataract following German measles in the mother. Trans Ophthalmol Soc Aust 3:35, 1941

7. Fraser FC, Fainstat TD: The production of congenital defects in the offspring of pregnant mice treated with cortisone. A progress report. Pediatrics 8:527, 1951

8. Hamilton WJ, Boyd JD, Mossman HW: Human Embryology. 3rd Ed. Williams & Wilkins, Baltimore, 1962

9. Fuhrmann W: Genetics of growth and development of the fetus. Pediat Clin North Am 12:457, 1965

10. Kalter H: Teratology of the Central Nervous System. University of Chicago Press, Chicago, 1968

11. Symposium on Specificity of Cell Differentiation and Interaction. J Cell Comp Physiol 60:suppl 1:1, 1962

12. Nelson MM: Teratogenic effects of pteroylglutamic acid deficiency in the rat. p.134. Wolstenholme GWE, O'Connor CM (eds): Congenital Malformations. Ciba Foundation Symposium, Little Brown, Boston, 1960

13. Wilson JG: Current status of teratology: General principles and mechanisms derived from animal studies. p.47. In Wilson JG, Fraser FC (eds): Handbook of Teratology. Vol. 1. Plenum, New York, 1977

14. Beckman DA, Brent RL: Mechanisms of teratogenesis. Annu Rev Pharmacol Toxicol 24:483, 1984

15. Johnson EM, Kochlar DM (eds): Teratogenesis and Reproductive Toxicology. Vol. 65. Handbook of Experimental Pharmacology. Springer-Verlag, Berlin, 1983

16. Wilson JG: Embryological considerations in teratology. In Wilson JG, Warkany J (eds.): Teratology: Principles and Techniques. University of Chicago Press, Chicago, 1965.

17. Gal P, Sharpless MK: Fetal drug exposure—behavioral teratogenesis. Drug Intell Clin Pharm 18:186, 1984

18. Fraser FC: Relation of animal studies to the problem in man. p.75. In Wilson JG, Fraser FC (eds): Handbook of Teratology. Vol. 1. Plenum, New York, 1977

19. Wilson JG: Embryotoxicity of drugs in man. p.309. In Wilson JG, Fraser FC (eds): Handbook of Teratology. Vol. 1. Plenum, New York, 1977

20. West GB: Teratogenic activity of drugs. J Pharm Pharmacol 16:63, 1964

21. Wilson JG: Influence on the offspring of altered physiologic states during pregnancy in the rat. Ann NY Acad Sci 57:517, 1954

22. Wilson JG: Embryological considerations in teratology. Ann NY Acad Sci 123:219, 1965

23. Ingalls TH, Ingenito EF, Curley FJ: Acquired chromosomal anomalies induced in mice by injection of a teratogen in pregnancy. Science 141:810, 1963

24. Robinson A, Puck TT: Sex chromatin in newborns: Presumptive evidence for external factors in human nondisjunction. Science 148:83, 1965

25. Ferguson-Smith MA: The techniques of human cytogenetics. Am J Obstet Gynecol 90:1035, 1964

26. DiPaolo JA, Kotin P: Teratogenesis oncogenesis: A study of possible relationships. Arch Pathol 81:3, 1966

27. Kalter H: Correlation between teratogenic and mutagenic effects of chemicals in mammals. In Hollaender A (ed): Chemical Mutagens: Principles and Methods for Their Detection. Vol. 1. Plenum, New York, 1971

28. Wilson JG: Experimental studies on congenital malformations. J Chronic Dis 10:111, 1959

29. Landauer W: Gene and phenocopy: Selection experiments and tests with 6-aminonicotinamide. J Exp Zool 160:345, 1965

30. Axelrod LR: Drugs and nonhuman primate teratogenesis. Adv Teratol 4:217, 1970

31. Wilson JG: Use of rhesus monkeys in teratological studies. Fed Proc 30:104, 1971
32. Gebhardt DOE: The use of the chick embryo in applied teratology. Adv Teratol 5:97, 1972
33. Lietman PS: Pharmacologic effects on developing enzyme systems. Fed Proc 31:62, 1972
34. Mirkin BL: Ontogenesis of the adrenergic nervous system: Functional and pharmacologic implications. Fed Proc 31:65, 1972
35. Sparber SB: Effects of drugs on the biochemical and behavioral responses of developing organisms. Fed Proc 31:74, 1972
36. Short RD, Rao KS, Gibson JE: The in vivo biosynthesis of DNA, RNA and proteins by mouse embryos after a teratogenic dose of cyclophosphamide. Teratology 6:129, 1972
37. Jones KL, Smith DW: The fetal alcohol syndrome. Teratology 12:1, 1975
38. Mulvihill JJ, Yeager AM: Fetal alcohol syndrome. Teratology 13:345, 1976
39. Streissguth AP, Landesman-Dwyer S, Martin JC, Smith DW: Teratogenic effects of alcohol in humans and laboratory animals. Science 209:353, 1980
40. Veghelyi PV: Fetal abnormality and maternal ethanol metabolism. Lancet 2:53, 1983
41. Goetsch C: An evaluation of aminopterin as an abortifacient. Am J Obstet Gynecol 83:1474, 1962
42. Powell HR, Ekert H: Methotrexate-induced congenital malformations. Med J Aust 2:1076, 1971
43. Milunsky A, Graef JW, Gaynor MF: Methotrexate-induced congenital malformations with a review of the literature. J Pediatr 72:790, 1968
44. Grumbach MM, Conte FA: Disorders of sex differentiation. In Williams RH (ed): Textbook of Endocrinology. WB Saunders, Philadelphia, 1981
45. Moncrieff A: Non-adrenal female pseudohermaphroditism associated with hormone administration in pregnancy. Lancet 2:267, 1958
46. Herbst AL, Scully RE: Adenocarcinoma of the vagina in adolescents—a report of 7 cases including 6 clear-cell carcinomas (so-called mesonephromas). Cancer 25:745, 1970
47. Herbst AL, Scully RE, Robboy SJ: Effects of maternal DES ingestion on the female genital tract. Hosp Pract 10:51, 1975
48. Herbst AL, Poskanzer DC, Robboy SJ, et al: Prenatal exposure to stilbestrol: A prospective comparison of exposed female offspring with unexposed controls. N Engl J Med 292:334, 1975
49. Gill WB, Schumacher GFB, Bibbo M: Structural and functional abnormalities in the sex organs of male offspring of mothers treated with diethylstilbestrol (DES). J Reprod Med 16:147, 1976
50. Amin-Zake L, Majeed MA, Elhassani SB, et al: Prenatal mercury poisoning: Clinical observations over five years. Am J Dis Child 133:172, 1979
51. Murakami U: Organic mercury problem affecting intrauterine life. Adv Exp Med Biol 27:301, 1972
52. Wilson JG: Environmental chemicals. p.357. In Wilson JG, Fraser FC (eds): Handbook of Teratology. Vol. 1. Plenum, New York, 1977
53. Corbett TH, Beaudoin AR, Cornell RG: Teratogenicity of polybrominated biphenyls. Teratology 11:15A, 1975
54. Rogan WJ: PCBs and cola-colored babies: Japan, 1976, and Taiwan, 1979. Teratology 26:259, 1982
55. Saxen I: Associations between oral clefts and drugs taken during pregnancy. Int J Epidemiol 4:37, 1975
56. Cohlan SQ, Bevelander G, Tiamsic T: Growth inhibition of prematures receiving tetracycline: Clinical and laboratory investigation. Am J Dis Child 105:453, 1963
57. Smith BE, Usubiaga LE, Lehrer SB: Cleft palate induced by halothane anesthesia in C-57 black mice. Teratology 4:242, 1971
58. Chang LW, Dudley AW, Katz J, Martin AH: Nervous system development following in utero exposure to trace amounts of halothane. Teratology 9:A-15, 1974
59. Basford AB, Fink BR: The teratogenicity of halothane in the rat. Anesthesiology 29:1167, 1968
60. Taussing HB: A study of the German outbreak of phocomelia. The thalidomide syndrome. JAMA 180:1106, 1962

61. Lenz W: Kindliche Missbildungen nach Medikament-Einnahme während der Gravidität? Dtsch Med Wochenschr 86:2555, 1961
62. Williams RT: Teratogenic effects of thalidomide and related substances. Lancet 1:723, 1963
63. McBride WG: The teratogenic action of drugs. Med J Aust 2:689, 1963
64. Lenz W: Epidemiology of congenital malformations. Ann NY Acad Sci 123:228, 1965
65. Woollam DHM: Principles of teratogenesis: Mode of action of thalidomide. Proc R Soc Med 58:497, 1965
66. Larsen V: The teratogenic effects of thalidomide, imipramine HCl and imipramine-N-oxide HCl on white Danish rabbits. Acta Pharmacol Toxicol (Copenh) 20:186, 1963
67. Bignami G, Bovet D, Bovet-Nitti F, Rosnati V: Drugs and congenital abnormalities. Lancet 2:1333, 1962
68. Delahunt CS, Lassen LJ: Thalidomide syndrome in monkeys. Science 146:1300, 1964
69. Keberle H, Loustalot P, Maller RK, et al: Biochemical effects of drugs on the mammalian conceptus. Ann NY Acad Sci 123:252, 1965
70. Ockenfels H, Kohler F: Das L-Isomere als teratogenes Prinzip der N-Phthalyl-DL-glutamin-saure. Experientia 26:1236, 1970
71. Kohler F, Meise W, Ockenfels H: Teratologische Prufung einiger Thalidomidmetabolite. Experientia 27:1149, 1971
72. Schumacher HJ, Terapane J, Jordan RL, Wilson JG: The teratogenic activity of a thalidomide analogue, EM12, in rabbits, rats, and monkeys. Teratology 5:233, 1972
73. King CTG: Teratogenic effects of meclizine hydrochloride on the rat. Science 141:353, 1963
74. Narrod SA, Wilk AL, King CTG: Metabolism of meclizine in the rat. J Pharmacol Exp Ther 147:380, 1965
75. Yerushalmy J, Milkovich L: Evaluation of teratogenic effect of meclizine in man. Am J Obstet Gynecol 93:553, 1965
76. Mellin GW: Drugs in the first trimester of pregnancy and the fetal life of Homo sapiens. Am J Obstet Gynecol 90:1169, 1964
77. Walker BE: Cleft palate produced in mice by human-equivalent dosage with triamcinolone. Science 149:862, 1965
78. Pinsky L, Di George AM: Cleft palate in the mouse: A teratogenic index of glucocorticoid potency. Science 147:402, 1965
79. Andrew FD, Bowen D, Zimmerman EF: Glucocorticoid inhibition of RNA synthesis and the critical period for cleft palate induction in inbred mice. Teratology 7:167, 1973
80. Nishimura H, Nakai K: Congenital malformations in offspring of mice treated with caffeine. Proc Soc Exp Biol Med 104:140, 1960
81. Fluhmann CF: The Management of Menstrual Disorders. WB Saunders, Philadelphia, 1956
82. Gunn DL, Jenkin PM, Gunn AL: Menstrual periodicity; statistical observations on a large sample of normal cases. J Obstet Gynecol 44:839, 1937
83. Paschkis KE, Rakoff AE, Cantarow A: Clinical Endocrinology. 2nd Ed. Hoeber-Harper, New York, 1958
84. Arey LB: The degree of normal menstrual irregularity. Am J Obstet Gynecol 37:12, 1939
85. Apgar V: Drugs in pregnancy. JAMA 190:840, 1964
86. Marx JL: Drugs during pregnancy: Do they affect the unborn child? Science 180:174, 1973
87. Bleyer WA, Au WYW, Lange WA, Raisz LG: Studies on the detection of adverse drug reactions in the newborn, I. Fetal exposure to maternal medication. JAMA 213:2046, 1970
88. Fraser FC: Experimental teratogenesis in relation to congenital malformations in man. p.277. In Fishbein M (ed): Second International Conference on Congenital Malformations. The International Medical Congress, Ltd., New York, 1964

Index